Tenth Edition

Pearson Nursing Diagnosis Handbook With NIC Interventions and NOC Outcomes

Judith M. Wilkinson, PhD, ARNP, RN

Nurse Educator, Consultant

Shawnee, Kansas

PEARSON

Boston Columbus Indianapolis New York San Francisco Upper Saddle River
Amsterdam Cape Town Dubai London Madrid Milan Munich Paris Montreal Toronto
Delhi Mexico City São Paulo Sydney Hong Kong Seoul Singapore Taipei Tokyo

Publisher: Julie Levin Alexander
Executive Assistant: Regina Bruno
Executive Editor: Kelly Trakalo
Assistant Editor: Rosalie Hawley
Managing Editor, Production: Patrick Walsh
Production Liaison: Yagnesh Jani
Full-Service Project Management: Sneha Pant/PreMediaGlobal
Manufacturing Buyer: Lisa McDowell
Senior Art Director: Maria Guglielmo Walsh
Cover Designer: Wanda Espana
Director of Marketing: David Gesell
Senior Marketing Manager: Phoenix Harvey
Marketing Coordinator: Michael Sirinides
Composition: PreMediaGlobal
Printer/Binder: R. R. Donnelley
Cover Printer: Lehigh-Phoenix Color

Library of Congress Control Number: 2012954283

1 2 3 4 5 6 7 8 9 10—CRW—17 16 15 14 13

PEARSON

ISBN-13: 978-0-13-313904-4
ISBN-10: 0-13-313904-2

CONTENTS

PREFACE

Nursing Diagnosis Handbook with NIC Interventions and NOC Outcomes, 10th edition, is designed to help nurses and students develop individualized patient care plans. The new edition has been expanded to include all nursing diagnoses approved by the North American Nursing Diagnosis Association (NANDA International) for 2012–2014, as well as linkages to current Nursing Outcomes Classification (NOC) and Nursing Interventions Classification (NIC) research-based outcomes and interventions. NANDA International, NOC, and NIC standardized terminology is generally used under those designated headings; exceptions are enclosed in brackets [ ].

New to This Edition

- 16 new NANDA-I diagnoses
- 7 deleted NANDA-I diagnoses (retired)
- Thoroughly updated for revised NANDA-I diagnoses
- Thoroughly updated bibliography for each diagnosis
- Thoroughly updated NIC intervention
- Thoroughly updated NOC intervention

Features

NOC Suggested Outcomes

To facilitate use of a unified nursing language and computerized patient records, each nursing diagnosis lists the outcomes found in *NANDA, NOC*, and *NIC Linkages: Nursing Diagnoses, Outcomes, & Interventions* (3rd ed.) (Johnson, Moorhead, Bulechek, Butcher, Maas, & Swanson, 2012). Other "Suggested Outcomes" for the diagnosis can be found in *NOC Outcomes Classification (NOC)* (2008). NOC outcomes are nurse-sensitive; that is, they may be influenced by the nursing care given for a particular NANDA International diagnosis. This text also demonstrates ways to use NOC outcomes, outcome indicators, and measuring scales to state patient goals.

Updated NIC Interventions

NIC interventions have been updated to reflect the continuing work of the Iowa Interventions Project. The interventions given and defined for each nursing diagnosis are the "major interventions" associated with the outcomes listed for that nursing diagnosis in *NANDA, NOC*, and *NIC Linkages: Nursing Diagnoses, Outcomes, & Interventions* (3rd ed.) (Johnson, Moorhead, Bulechek, Butcher, Maas, & Swanson, 2012). In this text, we have highlighted the NIC interventions that are "suggested" rather than "major" interventions. We do not list all "suggested interventions." NIC interventions were developed and linked to the NANDA International categories by a research team using a multimethod process that included the judgments of experts in nursing practice and research.

Inclusion of NIC Nursing Activities

In an effort to further promote use of standardized language, some of the Nursing Activities for each nursing diagnosis are written in NIC language. This helps to illustrate how the NIC activities, as well as the broader NIC interventions, can be used in care planning.

Inclusion of Family, Community, and Collaborative Content

More family- and community-oriented goals have also been included in the Goals/Evaluation Criteria Examples section. More collaborative, family, and community nursing interventions and activities have also been included.

Enhanced Gerontology and Home Care Content

Recognizing that the majority of patients are older adults, we have included a section to each care plan for nursing activities that focus on older adults.

Because a great deal of nursing care is now given in the patient's home, and because self-care has become increasingly important, we also include in each care plan a section on Home Care.

Collaborative Problems

In the Clinical Conditions Guide to Nursing Diagnoses and Collaborative Problems section, each disease or medical condition includes the associated multidisciplinary (collaborative) problems. Appendices D, E, and F contain the most comprehensive listing of multidisciplinary problems available, organized for (a) diseases/pathophysiology, (b) tests and treatments, and (c) surgical treatments.

Other Features

Organized for Easy Use

The book is divided into three main parts: (a) An introduction to the use of nursing diagnoses; (b) complete plans of care for each NANDA International nursing diagnosis; and (c) a list of medical, surgical, psychiatric, perinatal, and pediatric conditions, each accompanied by nursing diagnoses and collaborative problems commonly associated with those conditions. This organization allows the nurse to begin the care planning process with either a medical condition or a nursing diagnosis.

Suggestions for Using NANDA International Diagnoses

Author suggestions help to clarify the nursing diagnosis labels and to advise how they can best be used.

Organization of Defining Characteristics

These cues have been alphabetized and categorized as subjective or objective. NANDA International no longer designates major, minor, and critical defining characteristics.

Easy to Individualize

Each plan of care is comprehensive and allows nurses to select specific content according to the patient's condition and situation. Each nursing diagnosis includes related factors or risk factors that make it easy to individualize the care plan to the specific patient situation. Creative nurses will tailor standardized outcomes, interventions, and related and risk factors to meet the needs of each individual patient.

Assessment, Teaching, and Collaborative Nursing Activities

Nursing activities are grouped under the headings: Assessments, Patient/Family Teaching, Collaborative Activities, and Other. This makes it easier to locate a particular activity and helps assure that the nurse considers each type of activity.

Critical Paths

An up-to-date discussion of nursing diagnosis and critical paths is featured, along with an example of a format for a multidisciplinary care plan (critical path).

Care Planning Checklist

A checklist (see perforated flap on back cover) is provided to assist the practitioner in evaluating the finished care plan for completeness and suitability for the client.

Audience

This pocket guide is intended to facilitate care planning for nursing students, staff nurses in a variety of settings, clinical nurse specialists, and staff development instructors.

REVIEWERS

Becky Bunn, MSN, RNC
University of Mary Hardin-Baylor
Belton, TX

Jayne Hansche Lobert, MS, RN, ACNS-BC, NP
Oakland Community College
Waterford, MI

Nancy J. Cooley, MSN, APRN
University of Maine at Augusta
Augusta, ME

Laurie D. Fishel, RN, MSN
Kent State University
New Philadelphia, OH

Section I
INTRODUCTION

Introduction

Background

In 1973 the American Nurses Association (ANA) mandated the use of nursing diagnosis. That same year, clinicians, educators, researchers, and theorists from every area of nursing practice came together to offer labels for conditions they had observed in practice. From that beginning, the North American Nursing Diagnosis Association (now NANDA International) was established as the formal body for the promotion, review, and endorsement of the current list of nursing diagnoses used by practicing nurses. The NANDA International membership convenes every 2 years. The current list of more than 200 diagnoses (see inside back cover and Appendix A) will undoubtedly expand as nurses explore the breadth and depth of nursing practice.

As the list of nursing diagnoses expanded, NANDA International developed a classification system to organize them. The current taxonomy (Taxonomy II) is found in Appendix B. Work continues to address a number of issues (e.g., there is some overlapping among the diagnostic labels). NANDA International has been working with the ANA and other organizations to include the NANDA International labels in other classification systems, for example the World Health Organization International Classification of Diseases (ICD). NANDA International diagnosis-related articles are presently indexed in the Cumulative Index of Nursing and Allied Health (CINAHL) and in the National Library of Medicine Medical Metathesaurus for a Unified Medical Language.

The growing use of computerized patient records demands a standardized language for describing patient problems. Nursing diagnosis fulfills that need and helps define the scope of nursing practice by describing conditions the nurse can independently treat. Nursing diagnosis highlights critical thinking and decision making and provides a consistent and universally understood terminology among nurses working in various settings, including hospitals, ambulatory care clinics, extended care facilities, occupational health facilities, and private practice.

Nursing Process in Relation to Nursing Diagnosis

The nursing process provides a structure for nursing practice—a framework in which nurses use knowledge and skills to express human caring. The nursing process is used continuously when planning and giving nursing care. The nurse considers the patient as the central figure in the plan of care and confirms the appropriateness of all aspects of nursing care by observing the patient's responses.

Assessment (also called data collection) is the initial step in the critical thinking and decision making that leads to a nursing diagnosis. The nurse uses the definition and defining characteristics of the nursing diagnosis to validate the diagnosis. Once the nursing diagnosis and the related factors or risk factors are determined, the plan of care is created. The nurse selects the relevant patient outcomes, including the patient's perceptions and suggestions for the outcomes, if possible. The nurse next works with the patient to determine which activities will help achieve the stated outcomes. Finally, after implementing the nursing activities, the nurse evaluates the care plan and the patient's progress. Is the nursing diagnosis still appropriate? Has the patient achieved the desired goals? Are the documentation interval and the target date still appropriate and realistic? Are certain interventions no longer needed? The individualized plan of care is revised as needed.

Standards of Care in Relation to Nursing Diagnosis

Nursing diagnosis care planning and standards of care are interrelated. Standards of care are developed for groups of patients about whom generalized predictions can be made. These standards direct a set of common nursing interventions for specific patient groups (e.g., for all patients having a total hip replacement). Where there are written standards of care, nursing diagnosis care planning is not used to communicate routine nursing actions. Instead, it is used for those exceptional patient problems that are not addressed in the standards of care.

Case Management and Critical Paths

Escalating health care costs and the demand for health care reform have brought about a restructuring of traditional practice patterns. Two multidisciplinary clinical systems that have emerged are case management and managed care.

Case Management

Case management is a system in which health care professionals coordinate care for high-risk, complex patient populations. These are the unusual, uncommon cases seen in an agency—patients whose condition changes frequently and unpredictably, and whose needs cannot be completely addressed by a standardized plan or critical path. The case manager, often an advanced practice nurse, focuses on roles and relationships and provides a well-coordinated care experience for patients and families in all settings in which the patient receives care.

Critical Paths and Managed Care

Managed Care is used to standardize practice for the common, most prevalent case types in an agency. For example, case types in a cardiac care unit might be myocardial infarction or cardiac catheterization. Managed care uses a tool called a critical path as a guide for achieving predictable client outcomes within a specified time frame. The critical path is a multidisciplinary plan of care that outlines crucial activities to be performed by nurses, physicians, and other health team members at designated times in order to achieve the desired patient outcomes (see the table at the end of this section, "Critical Pathways for Client Following Laparoscopic Cholecystectomy").

In managed care systems, the standardized critical path replaces the traditional nursing care plan for many clients. Some agencies have incorporated nursing diagnoses directly into the critical paths. Others use nursing diagnoses to name variances and develop an individualized plan for achieving revised outcomes. A variance occurs when desired outcomes are not achieved at the specified times.

Nursing Diagnosis Incorporated Into Critical Path As an example, when incorporating a nursing diagnosis into a critical path for a client newly diagnosed with insulin-dependent diabetes, the following nursing diagnosis would be a part of the preprinted multidisciplinary care plan:

Ineffective self-health management related to limited information and limited practice of skill, as evidenced by verbalization of limited knowledge and difficulty with prescribed regimens.

Client goals might be that by day 3, the client will recognize signs and symptoms of hypo/hyperglycemia, and by day 5, be able to self-inject the required dose of insulin.

Nursing Diagnosis Used to Name Variance In this system, the critical path for a newly diagnosed insulin-dependent diabetic would not include a nursing diagnosis, but rather would list teaching needs for each day. On day 5, if the patient is unable to meet the outcome of self-injection, this variance would be identified and analyzed. At that point the nursing diagnosis of *Ineffective self-health management* related to difficulty mastering psychomotor skill for injections would be used to individualize the nursing care for this patient's variance from the critical path.

Even in organizations using managed care, the nursing process is used to plan and deliver patient care via a multidisciplinary care plan, and nursing diagnoses are valuable in individualizing critical paths to meet unique, individual patient needs. It is vital that today's nurse be well versed in using nursing diagnoses in order to effectively identify and address nursing care issues within the multidisciplinary team.

Components of Nursing Diagnosis Care Plans

This book is organized into two parts: "Plans of Care" and "Clinical Conditions Guide to Nursing Diagnoses and Collaborative Problems." Information regarding these two parts, with some examples of how to use them, follows.

Plans of Care

Each plan of care includes a nursing diagnosis label, the label definition, defining characteristics, related factors or risk factors, suggestions for use, suggested alternative diagnoses, NOC outcomes, client goals, NIC interventions, and nursing activities. See the figure on p. xx.

The nursing diagnosis care plans are organized alphabetically to make the labels easy to locate. The diagnoses are worded in order to set forth the key concept in the first word of the label. For example, *Ineffective denial* is easier to find in an index when it is written as *Denial, ineffective.*

Nursing Diagnosis

The nursing diagnosis is a concise label that describes patient conditions observed in practice. These conditions may be actual or potential problems or wellness diagnoses. Using NANDA International terminology, potential problems are labeled *Risk for*. Appendix C contains a list of axis descriptors (previously called diagnosis qualifiers) that are used in many of the diagnostic labels (e.g., *acute*, *altered*, *impaired*). Add other qualifying words as needed to make diagnoses precise and descriptive.

Definition

The definition for each nursing diagnosis helps the nurse verify a particular nursing diagnosis. Unless otherwise specified, the definitions in this text were taken from the NANDA International taxonomy.

Defining Characteristics

Defining characteristics are cues that describe patient behavior, either observed by the nurse (objective) or verbalized by the patient and family (subjective). After assessing the patient, nurses organize the defining characteristics into meaningful patterns that alert them to the possibility of a patient problem. Usually, the presence of two or three defining characteristics verifies a nursing diagnosis.

In this text, all NANDA International defining characteristics have been included. NANDA International no longer designates defining characteristics as major, minor, and critical. This simplification was made in order to support: (a) the development of electronic nursing diagnosis databases, (b) diagnosis development, and (c) classification work.

Related Factors

The related factors imply a connection with the nursing diagnosis. Such factors may be described as related to, antecedent to, associated with, or contributing to the diagnosis. Related factors indicate what should change for the patient to return to optimal health, and therefore help the nurse to select effective nursing interventions. As an example, for the diagnosis *Activity intolerance*, the nursing activities for a patient whose related factor is arrhythmias would be quite different from those needed for a patient whose related factor is chronic pain.

Risk Factors

Risk factors will be found only in the "risk for" (potential) nursing diagnoses. The risk factors are similar to related factors and defining characteristics in the development of the care plan. They describe events and behaviors that put the patient at risk and suggest interventions to protect the patient. As an example, an elderly patient might be diagnosed with *Risk for trauma* and exhibit the following risk factors: weakness, poor vision, balancing difficulties, slippery floors, and unanchored rugs. As an etiology, this cluster of risk factors suggests the need for interventions to prevent falls.

Suggestions for Use

For certain labels, clarifying comments are included, along with suggestions for using the diagnosis appropriately or differentiating it from similar diagnoses.

Suggested Alternative Diagnoses

Suggested alternative diagnoses are other nursing diagnoses that may be considered when identifying the patient's problem. If a review of the definition and defining characteristics indicates that they only partially match the patient data, the nurse may consider the suggested alternative diagnoses as options. This is particularly helpful for the nurse unfamiliar with the nuances of each nursing diagnosis.

NOC Outcomes

For each NANDA International diagnosis, this text lists NOC outcomes links that have been recognized by the ANA (Johnson et al., 2006). These were taken from *NOC and NIC Linkages to NANDA-I and Clinical Conditions* (3rd ed.) (2012). A few additional NOC outcomes for some diagnoses were taken from *Nursing Outcomes Classification (NOC)* (4th ed.) (2008). NOC outcomes are neutral concepts reflecting patient states or behaviors (e.g., memory, coping, rest). These nurse-sensitive patient outcomes are not goals, but the nurse can use them along with their indicators to set goals for a specific patient. Indicators are more specific behaviors that are used to measure or rate the patient outcome.

Goals/Evaluation Criteria

Each nursing diagnosis also includes examples of patient goals/evaluation criteria that were developed by using NOC outcomes, outcome indicators, and measuring scales. Goals are statements of patient and family behaviors that are measurable or observable. For example, to evaluate a client outcome of Cognitive Orientation, the nurse might use these indicators:

Identifies self (mildly compromised)

Identifies significant other (moderately compromised)

Identifies current place (not compromised)

Use as few or as many patient outcomes and sample goals as necessary. If more are needed, refer to the *Nursing Outcomes Classification (NOC)* manual (Moorhead, Johnson, Maas, & Swanson, 2008).

Patient goals, like all components of the care planning process, are dynamic. Therefore, they change frequently. Specific, individualized patient goal statements are critical because they are used to evaluate patient responses to care and the success of the nursing care plan.

The nurse should be realistic when constructing patient goal statements, because partial behavior change may be the only attainable goal. With shortened length of hospital stay, nurses in the community setting may help patients to achieve goals and outcomes after they are discharged from the hospital. At the time of discharge, the nurse may initiate discussion with the patient to determine patient and family goals still requiring completion, with referral to appropriate community resources.

Always specify a target date and documentation interval for patient goals. The target date is the estimated date by which the outcome will be accomplished. The date is flexible and individualized to the patient. The documentation interval designates how often documentation should occur for each outcome. This interval should be determined during initial assessment and may be changed as patient nears completion of a goal. For example, in the care plan for *Fatigue*, the documentation interval for the goal "Maintains adequate nutrition" could be specified as t.i.d. This would mean that documentation must occur at least three times daily, after meals, until the outcome is accomplished.

NIC Interventions

This text lists two kinds of NIC interventions:

1. *NIC Major Interventions*—These are the interventions found in *NOC and NIC Linkages to NANDA-I and Clinical Conditions* (2012). In that book, NOC outcomes were linked to nursing diagnoses, and then NIC interventions were linked to the NOC outcomes. The major interventions are the most obvious interventions for achieving *a particular outcome* and should be considered first.

2. *NIC-Suggested Interventions*—These are also taken from the "linkages" book. Suggested interventions are the research-based interventions

developed by the Iowa Intervention Project team as the treatments of choice for a particular nursing diagnosis (NIC, 2004). They are the most logically obvious interventions to effect resolution of *a particular diagnosis*, but this does not mean that they are the only interventions to be used.

In this book, any Suggested Interventions listed that do *not* appear as "Major Interventions" in the linkages book are highlighted. Note that many of the same interventions for a diagnosis appear in both the NIC (Bulechek, Butcher, & Dochterman, 2008) and the linkages book.

A variety of interventions should always be considered. In NIC terminology, *interventions* are broad, general category labels. These category labels were linked to the NANDA International diagnosis labels through a systematic process drawing upon the judgments of experts in nursing practice and research. They were linked to NOC outcomes using expert opinion and in some instances nursing literature. Testing in the clinical setting is needed to support or modify the links.

Nursing Activities

In NIC terminology, the specific, detailed actions taken by the nurse (e.g., taking vital signs, monitoring intake and output) are called *activities*. The NIC "priority" and "major" interventions direct the nurse to review first the nursing activities related to those interventions. Other specific nursing activities can be found in the *NIC* handbook (Bulechek, Butcher, & Dochterman, 2008). Following is an example of how the NIC priority interventions can guide care planning for the nursing diagnosis *Fatigue*:

1. In the care plan for *Fatigue*, note that an NIC priority intervention is Energy Management. The definition of this intervention is shown as: "regulating energy use to treat or prevent fatigue and optimize function."

2. Look in the Nursing Activities section of the care plan for the specific activities that would accomplish Energy Management—that is, those that specifically focus on regulating energy and treating or preventing fatigue, such as the following examples:

- Monitor nutritional intake to ensure adequate energy resources.
- Instruct patient/significant other to recognize signs and symptoms of *Fatigue* that require reduction in activity.
- Discuss with patient and family ways to modify home environment to maintain usual activities and to minimize *Fatigue*.
- Teach activity organization and time management techniques to reduce fatigue (NIC).

3. Finally, review the rest of the nursing activities for *Fatigue*. There may be activities in addition to those for Energy Management that would be helpful, depending on the client's problem etiologies and individual needs.

You will be able to find effective nursing activities to deal with your patient's fatigue by using Steps. 1, 2, and 3. However, you may wish to compare your chosen nursing actions to the research-based interventions and activities listed in the 2008 *NIC* handbook (Bulechek, Butcher, & Dochterman, 2008). In the *NIC* handbook under the intervention label *Energy Management*, there are other specific nursing activities that accomplish Energy Management. Following are three examples:

- Plan activities for periods when the patient has the most energy
- Encourage an afternoon nap, if appropriate
- Assist patient to schedule rest periods

In addition to the priority interventions, the *NIC* handbook lists other nursing interventions to address *Fatigue*, for example, Exercise Promotion and Sleep Enhancement. The nursing activities for those interventions might also be used.

Nursing orders and activities should address the etiology of the patient's nursing diagnosis. From the activities listed for each care plan, choose those that apply to the patient's condition. Alter standardized nursing activities to make them specific to the patient. In certain instances, "q _____" or "specify plan" is included in the nursing activity as a reminder to individualize the nursing orders. As the patient's condition changes, other activities may be added, changed, or deleted. Frequent updating of this portion of the care plan is essential.

Clinical Conditions Guide to Nursing Diagnoses and Collaborative Problems

The second part of this handbook is organized to help nurses focus their assessments when the patient's medical condition is known, but the appropriate nursing diagnoses have not yet been established. In this section, medical, surgical, psychiatric, perinatal, and pediatric conditions are listed with associated collaborative problems and nursing diagnoses.

Nursing Diagnoses

The nursing diagnoses listed are those that most logically occur when the particular medical condition is present. Of course, a patient with one of the medical conditions will not have all of the nursing diagnoses listed. Select only those nursing diagnoses that are confirmed by assessment data. Furthermore, these lists should not be considered exhaustive. It is quite possible that a client with a particular medical condition will have nursing diagnoses that are not on the list. Because they represent unique human responses, nursing diagnoses cannot be predicted on the basis of medical condition alone. They must be based on data obtained by assessing the patient.

Multidisciplinary (Collaborative) Problems

Multidisciplinary problems, on the other hand, are associated with specific medical conditions. According to Carpenito (1997) , collaborative problems are the physiological complications associated with a particular medical condition, and nurses cannot treat them independently. The nurse's responsibility is to monitor the patient in order to detect the onset of collaborative problems, and to use both physician- and nursing-prescribed interventions to prevent or minimize the complication. Because there are a limited number of physiological complications possible for a particular disease, the same collaborative problems tend to be present any time a particular disease or treatment is present; that is, each disease or treatment has particular complications that are always associated with it.

Before making an individualized nursing diagnosis care plan, the nurse should identify the patient's collaborative problems. These will guide the common assessments and preventive care that all patients with that medical diagnosis should receive, much like a critical pathway. Collaborative problems are included for each condition listed in the Clinical Conditions Guide to Nursing Diagnoses and Collaborative Problems near the back of this book. Also refer to Appendix D, Multidisciplinary (Collaborative) Problems Associated with Diseases and Other Physiologic Disorders; Appendix E, Multidisciplinary (Collaborative) Problems Associated with Tests and Treatments; and Appendix F, Multidisciplinary (Collaborative) Problems Associated with Surgical Treatments.

The list of clinical conditions does not include rare disease conditions, so for unusual diseases it may be necessary to refer to a more general title. For example, the patient's medical diagnosis may be scleroderma. Since this condition occurs infrequently, the nurse should look under the general title Autoimmune Disorders and review the nursing diagnoses listed there.

How to Create a Nursing Diagnosis Care Plan

The following example shows how to use this book to create an individualized care plan for a patient.

Situation: Mrs. B, a 75-year-old female, has been admitted to a surgical unit from the recovery room following a hip pinning. Her history indicates that Mrs. B lives alone in an apartment. Her husband died 10 years ago. She has many friends and is involved in community affairs at the local senior center. She loves to walk and to ride a bicycle. Her current hospital admission is a result of falling off her bicycle. Mrs. B's postoperative medical orders include the following:

Foley catheter to gravity drainage
$D_5$2% NaCl with KCl 20 mEq to be infused over 8 hr
Morphine sulfate 1–2 mg, IV push, q15 min until comfortable to a maximum of 10 mg in 1 hr
Phenergan 25 mg IM q4–6h, prn nausea
CBC and electrolytes tomorrow in a.m.
Overhead trapeze to bed
Turn patient from back to unaffected side q1–2h
Pressure-reducing mattress overlay to bed to relieve pressure to bony prominences
Ambulate with assistance in a.m. and then q.i.d.

Assessment

4:00 p.m.—The nurse's initial assessment following return from the recovery room indicates that the patient is sleeping comfortably, vital signs are within normal limits, and the operative dressing is dry and intact. Foley catheter is draining clear, amber urine. The IV is infusing at the prescribed rate; skin is warm and dry.

5:30 p.m.—The nurse enters Mrs. B's room to check her vital signs and finds Mrs. B attempting to climb out of bed "because I have to go to the bathroom." The nurse reminds Mrs. B that she is in the hospital and has a Foley catheter in place. Mrs. B's responses indicate that she is disoriented to place and time.

Diagnosis

From her assessment of Mrs. B, the nurse identifies the cues of altered mobility, disorientation, pain medication, and change in environment. These seem to match the defining characteristics for a nursing diagnosis of *Risk for falls*. In this book the definition of *Risk for falls* is "increased susceptibility to falling that may cause physical harm." The nurse considers suggested alternative diagnoses to see if a better diagnosis can be found. She looks at the definition and defining characteristics for *Risk for injury*, *Risk for trauma*, and *Risk for impaired skin integrity*. After reviewing the alternatives, the nurse decides to use the nursing diagnosis, *Risk for falls* related to altered mobility, disorientation, pain medication, and change in environment.

NOC Outcomes

In order to focus her goal statements, the nurse begins with some of the NOC Suggested Outcomes for *Risk for falls*. Falls Occurrence and Physical Injury Severity allow the nurse to assess for actual occurrence of the diagnosis (falls). Others allow her to assess for falls risk factors; for example,

Balance, Coordinated Movement, Fall Prevention Behavior, and Knowledge: Fall Prevention. After reading the outcome definitions and referring to the *NOC* handbook, the nurse determines that Falls Occurrence and Physical Injury Severity are the only outcomes needed for Mrs. B's care plan.

Goals/Evaluation Criteria

Goals: The nurse chooses and modifies the following goals from the listed sample goals and NOC indicators:

Number of falls from bed (none)

Number of falls while transferring (none)

Number of falls while walking (none)

Patient will identify risks that increase her susceptibility to falls.

The goals are observable and appropriate for Mrs. B's situation. The documentation interval for the goals could be q4h, and the target date should be "at all times," except for the last goal, which should probably be 1 or 2 days after surgery. The target dates should be stated as an actual date (e.g., 1/30). The documentation interval and target dates should be reviewed at least daily to evaluate appropriateness.

Evaluation: The nurse would collect data about the goals to determine whether interventions were successful in preventing the potential problem, *Risk for falls*.

Nursing Interventions and Activities

Next, the nurse selects nursing interventions. The NIC interventions listed are: Body Mechanics Promotion, Bowel Incontinence Care, Cognitive Stimulation, Delirium Management, Environmental Management: Safety, Exercise Promotion: Strength Training, Exercise Promotion: Stretching, Exercise Therapy: Ambulation, Exercise Therapy: Balance, Exercise Therapy: Joint Mobility, Exercise Therapy: Muscle Control, Fall Prevention, Medication Management, Peripheral Sensation Management, Risk Identification, Seizure Precautions, Self-Care Assistance, Surveillance, Teaching: Infant Safety, and Teaching: Toddler Safety.

There are many possible NIC interventions because there are many risk factors for falls. The nurse determines that only Environmental Management: Safety, Fall Prevention, and Risk Identification apply to the goals chosen for Mrs. B.

The NIC interventions provide direction for choosing nursing activities, but they are general. In order to write individualized nursing orders for Mrs. B, the nurse selects the following from the list of nursing activities:

Identify characteristics of the environment that may increase potential for falls (e.g., slippery floors and open stairways) (NIC).

Reorient patient to reality and immediate environment when necessary.

Place articles within easy reach of patient (NIC).

Provide the dependent patient with a means of summoning help (e.g., bell or call light) when caregiver is not present (NIC).

All of the aforementioned nursing orders could be part of Mrs. B's care plan. Once an intervention or activity is no longer applicable, the nurse deletes it from the care plan. New activities should be added as needed. This example demonstrates the process used to develop a care plan for one nursing diagnosis. Other nursing diagnoses might also be appropriate for Mrs. B.

Creating a Critical Path

Explained very simply, creating a critical path is a matter of combining the care plans from nursing, medical, and other services and imposing a timeline upon the combined plan. All care and treatments are shown on the plan, and care is organized by days, weeks, or even hours and minutes, for example:

Day 1	Day 2	Day 3
Outcomes	Outcomes	Outcomes
Nursing orders	Nursing orders	Nursing orders
Medical orders	Medical orders	Medical orders

The timeline of a critical path is different for each institution, depending on the patient population. In some hospitals, a hernia repair might mean an overnight stay (and therefore a 2-day critical path); in others it might be an outpatient procedure, with the critical path broken up into hourly segments. Therefore, standardized times cannot be given for the interventions on the nursing diagnosis care plans in this book. However, the care plans can be used when creating critical paths, the same as they are used in creating nursing diagnosis care plans.

1. Determine the nursing diagnoses your patient population (e.g., herniorrhaphy patients) typically has pre- and postoperatively—or on day 1, day 2, and so forth. Refer to the Clinical Conditions Guide to Nursing Diagnoses and Collaborative Problems for ideas as needed.

2. Choose patient goals and nursing activities for each day (or hour), just as you would for a traditional nursing care plan. The difference is that instead of a single care plan for a nursing diagnosis, you will have, essentially, a care plan for each day of the patient's stay in the institution. The following table is an example.

Critical Pathways for Client Following Laparoscopic Cholecystectomy

	Date ___________ PREOPERATIVE	Date ___________ 1st 24 hr following surgery
Daily outcomes	Client will verbalize understanding of preoperative teaching, including turning . . .	Client will • Be afebrile • Have a dry, clean wound with well-approximated . . .
Tests and treatments	CBC Urinalysis Baseline physical assessment	Vital signs and O_2 saturation, neurovascular assessment, dressing, and . . .
Knowledge deficit	Orient to room and surroundings. Include family in teaching	Reorient to room and postoperative routine, include family in teaching
Psychosocial	Assess anxiety related to pending surgery	Assess level of anxiety Encourage verbalization . . .
Diet	NPO Baseline nutritional assessment	Advance to clear liquids . . .
Activity	OOB ad lib until premedicated for surgery	Provide safety precautions Bathroom privileges . . .
Medications	NPO except ordered medications	IM or PO analgesics Antibiotics if ordered
Transfer/ discharge plans	Assess discharge plans and support system	Probable discharge within 24 hr of surgery

Section II

NURSING DIAGNOSES WITH OUTCOMES AND INTERVENTIONS

Nursing Diagnoses—With Outcomes and Interventions

Diagnosis labels, definitions, and defining characteristics are based primarily on the NANDA International taxonomy. The number following the label indicates the year the diagnosis was accepted or revised. The Domain and Class numbers are also provided, to aid you in locating the diagnosis label in the NANDA-I Taxonomy II (see Appendix B). Suggested alternative diagnoses are provided for most labels. Consider those if a label does not fit the patient data satisfactorily. The authors' discussion and recommendations for using certain diagnoses are identified by the heading Suggestions for Use.

Individualizing Client Goals/Evaluation Criteria

NOC Outcomes and indicators presented under Goals/Evaluation Criteria are quoted verbatim from the *Nursing Outcomes Classification (NOC)* (4th ed.). To help you create goals using standardized language, examples of such goals are given. To individualize these and the Other Examples provided in the text, add patient-specific target dates and evaluation and documentation intervals. If you do not find goals appropriate to your patient, refer to the *NOC* manual for outcome indicators and scales to develop other goals, as needed. To save space in this book, some indicators have been combined into one goal; however, NOC lists them separately, and they must be evaluated separately.

Individualizing Nursing Activities

NIC Interventions are quoted verbatim from the *Nursing Interventions Classification (NIC)*. The shaded interventions are NIC Priority Interventions for the diagnoses that do not also appear in the *NNN Linkages* book. Selected nursing activities are also written in NIC terminology. Choose only those activities that address patient problems and etiologies. Individualize nursing activities to meet the unique needs of each patient (e.g., by adding times of and frequencies for nursing activities, including more specific details). If you do not find the exact activities you need, refer to the *NIC* manual for other interventions and activities.

A

ACTIVITY INTOLERANCE [SPECIFY LEVEL]

(1982) **Domain 4, Activity/Rest; Class 4, Cardiovascular/Pulmonary Responses**

Definition: Insufficient physiological or psychological energy to endure or complete required or desired daily activities

Defining Characteristics

Subjective

Exertional discomfort or dyspnea
Verbal report of fatigue or weakness

Objective

Abnormal heart rate or blood pressure in response to activity
ECG changes reflecting arrhythmia or ischemia

Related Factors

Bed rest and immobility
Generalized weakness
Imbalance between oxygen supply and demand
Sedentary lifestyle

NOTE: The preceding factors are from NANDA International. They are secondary to a wide variety of pathophysiologies and psychopathologies, including depression, cardiac disease (e.g., congestive heart failure), respiratory disease (e.g., emphysema), renal disease, cancer, anemia, obesity, infections (e.g., mononucleosis), and prolonged bed rest.

Suggestions for Use

Do not use this label unless it is possible to increase the patient's endurance. Use *Activity intolerance* only if the patient reports fatigue or weakness in response to activity. Medical conditions (e.g., heart disease or peripheral arterial disease) often cause *Activity intolerance*. The nurse cannot independently treat medical conditions, so a diagnostic statement such as "*Activity intolerance* related to coronary artery disease" is not useful.

Activity intolerance often creates other problems, such as *Self-care deficit*, *Social isolation*, or *Ineffective breastfeeding*, and you can use it most effectively as the etiology of these other problems.

Specify *Activity intolerance* by levels of endurance, as follows (Gordon, 1994, p. 110):

Level I: Walks regular pace on level ground but becomes more short of breath than normal when climbing one or more flights of stairs

Level II: Walks one city block 500 feet on level or climbs one flight of stairs slowly without stopping

Level III: Walks no more than 50 feet on level without stopping and is unable to climb one flight of stairs without stopping

Level IV: Dyspnea and fatigue at rest

The following is an example of such a diagnostic statement: *Self-care deficit (total)* related to Activity intolerance (Level IV).

Suggested Alternative Diagnoses

Fatigue (Activity intolerance is relieved by rest. Fatigue is not.)

Self-care deficit

NOC Outcomes

Activity Tolerance: Physiologic response to energy-consuming movements with daily activities

Endurance: Capacity to sustain activity

Energy Conservation: Personal actions to manage energy for initiating and sustaining activity

Fatigue Level: Severity of observed or reported prolonged generalized fatigue

Psychomotor Energy: Personal drive and energy to maintain activities of daily living, nutrition, and personal safety

Rest: Quantity and pattern of diminished activity for mental and physical rejuvenation

Self-Care: Activities of Daily Living (ADLs): Ability to perform the most basic physical tasks and personal care activities independently with or without assistive device

Self-Care: Instrumental Activities of Daily Living (IADLs): Ability to perform activities needed to function in the home or community independently with or without assistive device

Goals/Evaluation Criteria

Examples Using NOC Language

- Tolerates usual activity, as demonstrated by Activity Tolerance, Endurance, Energy Conservation, Fatigue Level, Psychomotor Energy, Rest, and Self-Care: ADLs (and IADLs)
- Demonstrates **Activity Tolerance**, as evidenced by the following indicators (specify 1–5: severely, substantially, moderately, mildly, or not compromised):

  Oxygen saturation with activity

  Respiratory rate with activity

  Ability to speak with physical activity

- Demonstrates **Energy Conservation**, as evidenced by the following indicators (specify 1–5: never, rarely, sometimes, often, or consistently demonstrated):
  - Recognizes energy limitations
  - Balances activity and rest
  - Organizes activities to conserve energy

Other Examples

Patient will:

- Identify activities or anxiety-producing situations that may contribute to activity intolerance
- Participate in necessary physical activity with appropriate increases in heart rate, respiratory rate, and blood pressure and monitor patterns within normal limits
- By (target date) will achieve an activity level of (specify desired level from the list in Suggestions for Use)
- Verbalize understanding of need for oxygen, medications, and/or equipment that may increase tolerance for activities
- Perform ADLs with some assistance (e.g., toilets with help ambulating to bathroom)
- Perform home maintenance management with some help (e.g., needs weekly cleaning help)

NIC Interventions

Activity Therapy: Prescription of and assistance with specific physical, cognitive, social, and spiritual activities to increase the range, frequency, or duration of an individual's (or group's) activity

Cardiac Care: Rehabilitative: Promotion of maximum functional activity level for a patient who has experienced an episode of impaired cardiac function that resulted from an imbalance between myocardial oxygen supply and demand

Energy Management: Regulating energy use to treat or prevent fatigue and optimize function

Environmental Management: Manipulation of the patient's surroundings for therapeutic benefit, sensory appeal, and psychological well-being

Exercise Therapy: Joint Mobility: Use of active or passive body movement to maintain or restore joint flexibility

Exercise Therapy: Muscle Control: Use of specific activity or exercise protocols to enhance or restore controlled body movement

Exercise Promotion: Strength Training: Facilitating regular resistive muscle training to maintain or increase muscle strength

Home Maintenance Assistance: Helping the patient and family to maintain the home as a clean, safe, and pleasant place to live

Mood Management: Providing for safety, stabilization, recovery, and maintenance of a patient who is experiencing dysfunctionally depressed or elevated mood

Self-Care Assistance: Assisting another to perform ADLs

Self-Care Assistance: IADL: Assisting and instructing a person to perform IADLs needed to function in the home or community

Sleep Enhancement: Facilitation of regular sleep/wake cycles

Nursing Activities

Assessments

- Assess the extent to which patient is able to move about in bed, stand, ambulate, and perform ADLs and IADLs
- Assess emotional, social, and spiritual response to activity
- Evaluate patient's motivation and desire to increase activity
- *(NIC) Energy Management:*
  - Determine causes of fatigue (e.g., treatments, pain, and medications)
  - Monitor cardiorespiratory response to activity (e.g., tachycardia, other dysrhythmias, dyspnea, diaphoresis, pallor, hemodynamic pressures, and respiratory rate)
  - Monitor patient's oxygen response (e.g., pulse rate, cardiac rhythm, and respiratory rate) to self-care or nursing activities
  - Monitor nutritional intake to ensure adequate energy resources
  - Monitor and record patient's sleep pattern and number of sleep hours

Patient/Family Teaching

Instruct patient and family in:

- Use of controlled breathing during activity, as appropriate
- Recognizing the signs and symptoms of *Activity intolerance*, including those that necessitate a call to the physician.
- The importance of good nutrition
- Use of equipment, such as oxygen, during activities
- Use of relaxation techniques (e.g., distraction, visualization) during activities
- Effect of *Activity intolerance* on family and work role responsibilities
- Measures to conserve energy, for example: Keep frequently used objects within easy reach
- *(NIC) Energy Management:*
  - Teach patient and significant other techniques of self-care that will minimize oxygen consumption (e.g., self-monitoring and pacing techniques for performance of ADLs)
  - Teach activity organization and time management techniques to prevent fatigue

A

Collaborative Activities

- Administer pain medications prior to activity, if pain is a factor
- Collaborate with occupational, physical (e.g., for resistance training), or recreational therapists to plan and monitor an activity program, as appropriate
- For patients who have psychiatric illness, refer for psychiatric home health services
- Refer to home health to obtain services of a home care aide, as needed
- Refer to dietitian for meal planning to increase intake of high-energy foods
- Refer for cardiac rehabilitation if condition is related to cardiac disease

Other

- Avoid scheduling care activities during rest periods
- Help patient to change position gradually, dangle, sit, stand, and ambulate, as tolerated
- Monitor vital signs before, during, and after activity; stop the activity if VS are not within normal limits for the patient or if there are signs that activity is not being tolerated (e.g., chest pain, pallor, vertigo, dyspnea)
- Plan activities with patient and family that promote independence and endurance, for example:
  - Encourage alternate periods of rest and activity
  - Set small, realistic, attainable goals for patient that increase independence and self-esteem
- *(NIC) Energy Management:*
  - Assist patient to identify preferences for activity
  - Plan activities for periods when the patient has the most energy
  - Assist with regular physical activities (e.g., ambulation, transfers, turning, and personal care), as needed
  - Limit environmental stimuli (e.g., light and noise) to facilitate relaxation
  - Assist patient to self-monitor by developing and using a written record of calorie intake and energy expenditure, as appropriate

Home Care

- Evaluate the home for conditions that contribute to Activity intolerance (e.g., stairs, furniture placement, location of bathrooms)
- Assess the need for assistive devices (e.g., lifts, electrical beds), oxygen, and so on, in the home

For Infants and Children

- Plan care for the infant or child to minimize the oxygen needs of the body:
  Anticipate needs for food, water, comfort, holding, and stimulation, to prevent unnecessary crying
  Avoid environments low in oxygen concentration (e.g., high altitudes, unpressurized airplanes)
  Minimize anxiety and stress
  Prevent hyperthermia and hypothermia
  Prevent infection
  Provide adequate rest

For Older Adults

- Allow extra time for treatments and ADLs
- Monitor for orthostatic hypotension, dizziness, and fainting during activity (Tinetti, McAvay, & Claus, 2003)

ACTIVITY INTOLERANCE, RISK FOR

(1982) **Domain 4, Activity/Rest; Class 4; Cardiovascular/Pulmonary Responses**

Definition: At risk for experiencing insufficient physiological or psychological energy to endure or complete required or desired daily activities

Risk Factors

Subjective

History of previous intolerance
Inexperience with the activity

Objective

Deconditioned status
Presence of circulatory and/or respiratory problems

Suggestions for Use

Discriminate among *Activity intolerance*, *Fatigue*, and *Self-care deficit*. See Activity Intolerance, Suggestions for Use.

Suggested Alternative Diagnoses

Fatigue, risk for
Self-care deficit, risk for

A

NOC Outcomes

Activity Tolerance: Physiologic response to energy-consuming movements with daily activities

Asthma Self-Management: Personal actions to prevent or reverse inflammatory condition resulting in bronchial constriction of the airways

Cardiopulmonary Status: Adequacy of blood volume ejected from the ventricles and exchange of carbon dioxide and oxygen at the alveolar level

Circulation Status: Unobstructed, unidirectional blood flow at an appropriate pressure through large vessels of the systemic and pulmonary circuits

Endurance: Capacity to sustain activity

Energy Conservation: Personal actions to manage energy for initiating and sustaining activity

Fatigue Level: Severity of observed or reported prolonged generalized fatigue

Nutritional Status: Energy: Extent to which nutrients and oxygen provide cellular energy

Physical Fitness: Performance of physical activities with vigor

Psychomotor Energy: Personal drive and energy to maintain ADLs, nutrition, and personal safety

Vital Signs: Extent to which temperature, pulse, respiration, and blood pressure are within normal range

Goals/Evaluation Criteria

Examples Using NOC Language

- Tolerates usual activity, as demonstrated by: Activity Tolerance, Endurance, and Energy Conservation
- Demonstrates **Energy Conservation**, as evidenced by the following indicators (specify 1–5: never, rarely, sometimes, often, or consistently demonstrated):
- Recognizes energy limitations
- Balances activity and rest
- Reports adequate endurance for activity

Other Examples

Patient will:

- Identify activities or anxiety-producing situations that may contribute to *Activity intolerance*
- Participate in necessary physical activity with appropriate increases in heart rate, respiratory rate, and blood pressure, and monitor such patterns within normal limits

- Report freedom from dyspnea, difficulty breathing, and fatigue with daily activities
- Make lifestyle changes necessary to conserve energy

Also see outcomes for Activity Intolerance.

NIC Interventions

Asthma Management: Identification, treatment, and prevention of reactions to inflammation/constriction in the airway passages

Energy Management: Regulating energy use to treat or prevent fatigue and optimize function

Exercise Promotion: Facilitation of regular physical activity to maintain or advance to a higher level of fitness and health

Exercise Promotion: Strength Training: Facilitating regular resistive muscle training to maintain or increase muscle strength

Nursing Activities

Assessments

- Determine the knowledge and recognition of energy limitations by client and significant other
- Monitor energy level and tolerance for activity
- Identify the obstacles to activity
- Refer to the Activity Intolerance diagnosis, p. xx, for other assessments

Patient/Family Teaching

- Develop a realistic plan for adapting to patient's limitations
- Explore with patient the specific consequences of inactivity
- Instruct patient and family to notify primary care provider if fatigue is persistent
- *(NIC) Energy Management*:

  Teach patient and significant other techniques of self-care that will minimize oxygen consumption (e.g., self-monitoring and pacing techniques for performance of ADLs)

  Teach activity organization and time management techniques to prevent fatigue

Other

- Enlist family in efforts to support and encourage the patient's completion of activities
- Provide decision-making (and other) support during periods of illness or high stress

For other activities and interventions, see Activity Intolerance.

A

ACTIVITY PLANNING, INEFFECTIVE

(2008) **Domain 5, Perception/Cognition; Class 5, Communication**

Definition: Inability to prepare for a set of actions fixed in time and under certain conditions.

Defining Characteristics

Subjective

Excessive anxieties toward a task to be undertaken
Verbalization of fear or worries toward a task to be undertaken

Objective

Failure pattern of behavior
Lack of plan
Lack of resources
Lack of sequential organization
Procrastination
Unmet goals for chosen activity

Related Factors

Compromised ability to process information
Defensive flight behavior when faced with proposed solution
Hedonism
Lack of support from family or friends
Unrealistic perception of events
Unrealistic perception of personal competence

Suggestions for Use

If the task to be undertaken is one that relates to managing the person's illness, or maintaining or improving health, you might consider a diagnosis of Ineffective Health Maintenance. Ineffective Activity Planning is broad, in the sense that it encompasses all types of tasks and is not limited to tasks related to health and illness.

NOC Outcomes

Anxiety Level: Severity of manifested apprehension, tension, or uneasiness arising from an unidentifiable source

Cognition: Ability to execute complex mental processes

Communication: Reception, interpretation, and expression of spoken, written, and nonverbal messages

Decision Making: Ability to make judgments and choose between two or more alternatives

Fear Level: Severity of manifested apprehension, tension, or uneasiness arising from an identifiable source

Health Beliefs: Perceived Ability to Perform: Personal conviction that one can carry out a given health behavior

Information Processing: Ability to acquire, organize, and use information

Motivation: Inner urge that moves or prompts an individual to positive action(s)

Goals/Evaluation Criteria

Examples Using NOC Language

- Demonstrates **Motivation**, as evidenced by the following indicators (specify 1–5: never, rarely, sometimes, often, or consistently demonstrated):
  - Develops an action plan
  - Obtains support as needed
  - Expresses belief in ability to perform action

Other Examples

Patient will:

- Express that he intends to take action to achieve the task
- Complete the task (by a specified date)
- Demonstrate and express positive self-esteem
- Express messages coherently
- Comprehend messages from others

NIC Interventions

Anxiety Reduction: Minimizing apprehension, dread, foreboding, or uneasiness related to an unidentified source of anticipated danger

Calming Technique: Reducing anxiety in patient experiencing acute distress

Decision-Making Support: Providing information and support for a patient who is making a decision regarding health care

Family Support: Promotion of family values, interests, and goals

Mutual Goal Setting: Collaborating with patient to identify and prioritize care goals, then developing a plan for achieving those goals

Self-Efficacy Enhancement: Strengthening an individual's confidence in his/her ability to perform a health behavior

Self-Modification Assistance: Reinforcement of self-directed change initiated by the patient to achieve personally important goals

Self-Responsibility Facilitation: Encouraging a patient to assume more responsibility for own behavior

Teaching: Individual: Planning, implementation, and evaluation of a teaching program designed to address a patient's particular needs

Nursing Activities

Assessments

- Assess the patient's verbal and nonverbal signs of anxiety
- Assess the patient's knowledge and level of skill in relation to the identified task
- Monitor the patient's progress in achieving the task
- Assess the amount and quality of family support

Patient/Family Teaching

- Teach relaxation techniques

Collaborative Activities

- Refer for family therapy or peer group support, as needed
- Administer medications to reduce anxiety, if needed

Other

- Encourage the patient to talk about his feelings and fears with regard to the task
- Encourage independence, but assist with the task if the patient cannot succeed alone
- Help the patient identify areas in which he could easily assume more responsibility
- Assist the patient in setting goals for change
- Assist the patient to identify the steps to take to achieve a task, and to create a timetable
- Assist the patient to identify rewards for task or step achievement
- Provide positive feedback for even small successes
- Encourage the family to express concerns, feelings, and questions

ACTIVITY PLANNING: INEFFECTIVE, RISK FOR

(2010)

Domain 9, Coping/Stress Tolerance; Class 2, Coping Responses

Definition: At risk for an inability to prepare for a set of actions fixed in time and under certain conditions.

Risk Factors

Objective

Compromised ability to process information
Defensive flight behavior when faced with proposed solution
Hedonism
History of procrastination
Ineffective or insufficient support systems
Unrealistic perception of events or of personal competence

Suggestions for Use

Ineffective Activity Planning may occur as a response to (or a symptom of) other conditions or nursing diagnoses such as Anxiety, Chronic Confusion, Ineffective Coping, Fatigue, Hopelessness, Ineffective Impulse Control, Ineffective Self-Health Management, Powerlessness, and Self-Care Deficit. If other defining characteristics are present (e.g., of Anxiety or Fatigue), that broader diagnosis is likely to be more effective for planning the patient's care.

NOC Outcomes

NOC outcomes have not yet been linked to this diagnosis. For suggestions, refer to *Ineffective Activity Planning.*

Goals/Evaluation Criteria

Refer to *Ineffective Activity Planning*, preceding.

NIC Interventions

NIC interventions have not yet been linked to this diagnosis. Some of the interventions and activities for *Ineffective Activity Planning* may be useful for the potential problem, as well.

Nursing Activities

Nursing activities for this diagnosis should focus on identifying risk factors and assessing for symptoms of actual *Ineffective Activity Planning.*

Assessments

- Assess availability and effectiveness of the patient's support systems
- Assess ability to process information (e.g., follow directions)
- Observe for procrastination
- Determine whether perceptions of events is realistic
- Assess the person's perception of her own competence

A

ADAPTIVE CAPACITY: INTRACRANIAL, DECREASED

(1994) **Domain 9, Coping/Stress Tolerance; Class 3, Neurobehavioral Stress**

Definition: Intracranial fluid dynamic mechanisms that normally compensate for increases in intracranial volumes are compromised, resulting in repeated disproportionate increases in intracranial pressure (ICP) in response to a variety of noxious and nonnoxious stimuli.

Defining Characteristics

Objective

Baseline ICP $\geq$ 10 mmHg

Disproportionate increase in ICP following single environmental or nursing maneuver stimulus

Elevated P_2 ICP waveform

Repeated increases in ICP of > 10 mmHg for more than 5 min following any of a variety of external stimuli

Volume-pressure response test variation (volume-pressure ratio > 2, note that pressure-volume index < 10)

Wide-amplitude ICP waveform

Related Factors

Brain injuries

Decreased cerebral perfusion pressure $\leq$ 50–60 mmHg

Sustained increase in ICP $\geq$ 10–15 mmHg

Systemic hypotension with intracranial hypertension

Suggestions for Use

This diagnosis requires both medical and nursing interventions. Most of the nursing care will be dictated by agency protocols. Therefore, this diagnosis may be better stated as a collaborative problem (e.g., Potential Complication of head injury: Increased ICP).

Suggested Alternative Diagnoses

Tissue perfusion, ineffective (cerebral)

NOC Outcomes

Neurological Status: Ability of the peripheral and central nervous system to receive, process, and respond to internal and external stimuli

Neurological Status: Consciousness: Arousal, orientation, and attention to the environment

Seizure Control: Personal actions to reduce or minimize the occurrence of seizure episodes

Tissue Perfusion: Cerebral: Adequacy of blood flow through the cerebral vasculature to maintain brain function

Goals/Evaluation Criteria

NOTE: The following outcomes cannot be produced by independent nursing activities alone.

Examples Using NOC Language

- Demonstrates increased *Intracranial adaptive capacity*, as demonstrated by Neurological Status, Neurological Status: Consciousness, Seizure Control
- Demonstrates **Neurological Status**, as evidenced by the following indicators (specify 1–5: extremely, substantially, moderately, mildly, or not compromised):

    Pupil size and reactivity
    Communication appropriate to situation
    Breathing pattern
    Blood pressure
    Intracranial pressure
    Spinal sensory/motor function
    Central sensory/motor function

Other Examples

- Cerebral perfusion pressure will be ≥ 70 mmHg (in adults), with fewer than five abnormal episodes in 24 hr
- ICP will stabilize at four or less episodes of abnormal waveforms in 24 hr

NIC Interventions

Cerebral Edema Management: Limitation of secondary cerebral injury resulting from swelling of brain tissue

Cerebral Perfusion Promotion: Promotion of adequate perfusion and limitation of complications for a patient experiencing or at risk for inadequate cerebral perfusion

Intracranial Pressure (ICP) Monitoring: Measurement and interpretation of patient data to regulate intracranial pressure

Neurologic Monitoring: Collection and analysis of patient data to prevent or minimize neurologic complications

A

Seizure Management: Care of a patient during a seizure and the postictal state

Seizure Precautions: Prevention or minimization of potential injuries sustained by a patient with a known seizure disorder

Surveillance: Purposeful and ongoing acquisition, interpretation, and synthesis of patient data for clinical decision making

Nursing Activities

Assessments

- Monitor ICP and cerebral perfusion pressure (CPP) continuously with alarm settings on
- Monitor neurologic status at regular intervals (e.g., vital signs; pupil size, shape, reaction to light, equality; consciousness/mental status; response to painful stimuli; ability to follow commands; symmetry of motor response; reflexes such as Babinski, blink, cough, gag)
- Note events that trigger changes in the ICP waveform (e.g., position change, suctioning)
- Determine baseline for vital signs and cardiac rhythm, and monitor for changes during and after activity
- *(NIC) Intracranial Pressure (ICP) Monitoring:*

  Monitor pressure tubing for bubbles

  Monitor amount and rate of cerebrospinal fluid drainage

  Monitor intake and output

  Monitor insertion site for infection

  Monitor temperature and WBC count

  Check patient for nuchal rigidity

Patient/Family Teaching

- Teach caregiver about signs that will indicate increased ICP (e.g., changes in eye coordination, increased seizure activity, restlessness, changes in speech). **NOTE:** Changes are specific to the patient, depending on the disability (e.g., trauma, hydrocephalus) underlying the increased ICP.
- Teach caregiver the specific situations that trigger ICP in the client (e.g., pain, anxiety); discuss appropriate interventions

Collaborative Activities

- Initiate agency protocols for lowering ICP (e.g., plan may include ventriculostomy to drain cerebrospinal fluid)
- Follow protocols to maintain systemic blood pressure adequate to keep CPP at ≥ 70 mmHg
- *(NIC) Intracranial Pressure (ICP) Monitoring:*

  Notify physician for elevated ICP that does not respond to treatment protocols

  Administer pharmacologic agents to maintain ICP within specified range

Administer antibiotics
Maintain controlled hyperventilation, as ordered

Other

- Do not use the knee gatch and avoid 90-degree hip flexion
- Stop any activity (e.g., suctioning) that triggers *Decreased intracranial adaptive capacity*
- Limit the duration of procedures and care activities; allow time for baseline ICP to recover between noxious activities such as suctioning
- For patients who are performing Valsalva maneuver, if they can follow directions, instruct them to exhale through their mouths
- Use gentle touching and talking
- Suction only if necessary—not prophylactically
- If suctioning is needed, preoxygenate, do not hyperventilate, and use only one or two catheter passes; administer intratracheal lidocaine, per protocol, to minimize coughing
- Allow family to visit
- *(NIC) Intracranial Pressure (ICP) Monitoring:*
  Calibrate and level the transducer
  Restrain patient, as needed
  Change transducer and flush system
  Change and/or reinforce insertion site dressing, as necessary
  Position the patient with head elevated 30–45 degrees and with neck in a neutral position [support with sand bags, small pillows, and/or rolled towels]
  Minimize environmental stimuli [e.g., noise, painful procedures]
  Space nursing care to minimize ICP elevation
  Maintain systemic arterial pressure within specified range

AIRWAY CLEARANCE, INEFFECTIVE

(1980, 1996, 1998) **Domain 11, Safety/Protection; Class 2, Physical Injury**

Definition: Inability to clear secretions or obstructions from the respiratory tract to maintain a clear airway

Defining Characteristics

Subjective

Dyspnea

Objective

Adventitious breath sounds (e.g., rales, crackles, rhonchi, wheezes)
Changes in respiratory rate and rhythm

Cyanosis
Difficulty vocalizing
Diminished breath sounds
Excessive sputum
Ineffective or absent cough
Orthopnea
Restlessness
Wide-eyed [look]

Related Factors

Environmental: Smoking, smoke inhalation, secondhand smoke

Obstructed Airway: Airway spasm, retained secretions, excessive mucus, presence of artificial airway, foreign body in airway, secretions in the bronchi, exudate in the alveoli

Physiological: Neuromuscular dysfunction, hyperplasia of the bronchial walls, chronic obstructive pulmonary disease, infection, asthma, allergic airways, [trauma]

Suggestions for Use

Use the key defining characteristics in Table 1 to discriminate among this label and the two alternative respiratory diagnoses. If cough and gag reflexes are ineffective or absent secondary to anesthesia, use *Risk for aspiration* instead of *Ineffective airway clearance* in order to focus on preventing aspiration rather than teaching effective coughing.

Table 1

Nursing Diagnosis	Present	Not Present
Impaired gas exchange	Abnormal blood gases Hypoxia Changes in mental status	Ineffective cough Cough
Ineffective breathing pattern	"Appearance" of the patient's breathing: nasal flaring, use of accessory muscles, pursed-lip breathing Abnormal blood gases	Tachycardia, restlessness Ineffective cough Obstruction or aspiration
Ineffective airway clearance	Cough, ineffective cough Changes in rate or depth of respirations Usual cause is increased or tenacious secretions or obstruction (e.g., aspiration)	Abnormal blood gases

Suggested Alternative Diagnoses

Aspiration, risk for
Breathing pattern, ineffective
Gas exchange, impaired

NOC Outcomes

Aspiration Prevention: Personal actions to prevent the passage of fluid and solid particles into the lung

Mechanical Ventilation Response: Adult: Alveolar exchange and tissue perfusion are effectively supported by mechanical ventilation

Respiratory Status: Airway Patency: Open, clear tracheobronchial passages for air exchange

Respiratory Status Ventilation: Movement of air in and out of the lungs

Goals/Evaluation Criteria

Examples Using NOC Language

- Demonstrates effective airway clearance, as evidenced by Aspiration Prevention; Respiratory Status: Airway Patency; and Respiratory Status: Ventilation, not compromised
- Demonstrates **Respiratory Status: Airway Patency**, as evidenced by the following indicators (specify 1–5: severe, substantial, moderate, mild, or no deviation from normal range):
  - Respiratory rate and rhythm
  - Depth of inspiration
  - Ability to clear secretions

Other Examples

Patient will:

- Cough effectively
- Expectorate secretions effectively
- Have a patent airway
- Have clear breath sounds on auscultation
- Have respiratory rate and rhythm within normal range
- Have pulmonary function within normal limits
- Be able to describe plan for care at home

NIC Interventions

Airway Management: Facilitation of patency of air passages

Airway Suctioning: Removal of airway secretions by inserting a suction catheter into the patient's oral airway and/or trachea

Aspiration Precautions: Prevention or minimization of risk factors in the patient at risk for aspiration

Asthma Management: Identification, treatment, and prevention of reactions to inflammation/constriction in the airway passages

Cough Enhancement: Promotion of deep inhalation by the patient with subsequent generation of high intrathoracic pressures and compression of underlying lung parenchyma for the forceful expulsion of air

Positioning: Deliberative placement of the patient or a body part to promote physiological and psychological well-being

Respiratory Monitoring: Collection and analysis of patient data to ensure airway patency and adequate gas exchange

Ventilation Assistance: Promotion of an optimal spontaneous breathing pattern that maximizes oxygen and carbon dioxide exchange in the lungs

Nursing Activities

Assessments

- Assess and document the following:
  - Effectiveness of oxygen administration and other treatments
  - Effectiveness of prescribed medications
  - Pulse oximetery readings
  - Trends in arterial blood gases, if available
  - Rate, depth, and effort of respirations
  - Related factors, such as pain, ineffective cough, viscous mucous, and fatigue
- Auscultate anterior and posterior chest for decreased or absent ventilation and presence of adventitious sounds
- *(NIC) Airway Suctioning:*
  - Determine the need for oral or tracheal suctioning
  - Monitor patient's oxygen status (SaO_2 and SvO_2 levels) and hemodynamic status (MAP [mean arterial pressure] level and cardiac rhythms) immediately before, during, and after suctioning
  - Note type and amount of secretions obtained

Patient/Family Teaching

- Explain proper use of supportive equipment (e.g., oxygen, suction, spirometer, inhalers, intermittent positive pressure breathing)
- Inform patient and family that smoking is prohibited in room; teach importance of smoking cessation
- Instruct patient in coughing and deep-breathing techniques to facilitate removal of secretions
- Teach patient to splint incision when coughing
- Teach patient and family the significance of changes in sputum, such as color, character, amount, and odor

- *(NIC) Airway Suctioning:* Instruct the patient and/or family how to suction the airway, as appropriate

Collaborative Activities

- Confer with respiratory therapist, as needed
- Consult with physician concerning need for percussion or supportive equipment
- Administer humidified air and oxygen according to agency policies
- Perform or assist with aerosol, ultrasonic nebulizer, and other pulmonary treatments according to agency policies and protocols
- Notify physician of abnormal blood gases

Other

- Encourage physical activity to promote movement of secretions
- Encourage use of an incentive spirometer (Smith-Sims, 2001)
- If patient is unable to ambulate, turn patient from side to side at least q2h
- Inform patient before initiating procedures, to lower anxiety and increase sense of control
- Provide emotional support (e.g., reassure the patient that coughing will not cause sutures to "break")
- Position patient to allow for maximum expansion of the chest cavity (e.g., head of bed elevated 45° unless contraindicated [Collard et al., 2003; Drakulovic et al., 1999])
- Suction the naso- and oropharynx to remove secretions (specify frequency)
- Perform endotracheal or nasotracheal suctioning, as appropriate. (Hyperoxygenate with Ambu bag before and after suctioning endotracheal tube or tracheostomy.)
- Maintain adequate hydration to decrease viscosity of secretions
- Remove or treat causative factors, such as pain, fatigue, and thick secretions

Home Care

- Instruct patient and family in plan for care at home (e.g., medications, hydration, nebulization, equipment, postural drainage, signs and symptoms of complications, community resources)
- Assess the home for presence of factors, such as allergens, that may precipitate Ineffective Airway Clearance
- Help patient and family to identify ways to avoid allergens, including exposure to secondhand smoke

A

For Infants and Children

- Stress to parents that it is important for the child to cough, and that coughs should not always be suppressed with medication
- Balance the need for airway clearance with the need to avoid fatigue produced by coughing when the cough is persistent or a symptom of dyspnea
- Let the child hold the stethoscope and listen to his breath sounds.

ALLERGY RESPONSE, RISK FOR

(2010) **Domain 11, Safety/Protection; Class 5, Defensive Processes**

Definition: Risk of an exaggerated immune response or reaction to substances

Risk Factors

Chemical products (e.g., bleach, cosmetics)
Dander
Environmental substances (e.g., mold, dust, pollen)
Foods (e.g., peanuts, shellfish, mushrooms)
Insect stings
Pharmaceutical agents (e.g., penicillin)
Repeated exposure to environmental substances

Non-NANDA-I Risk Factors

History of allergies
History of asthma
History of food sensitivities
History of medication sensitivities

Suggestions for Use

Note that all the listed risk factors are environmental, and that their presence does not produce an allergic reaction for most people. Therefore, you cannot diagnose a *Risk for allergic response* for a particular patient simply because he is exposed, for example, to cosmetics or shellfish. In that sense, everyone is at risk for allergic response. The only risk factor identified by NANDA-I that is specific to *a person* is repeated exposure to environmental substances. You should diagnose *Risk for allergic response* only if you have some reason to suspect that a patient has a greater-than-average risk to certain allergens. If you use this diagnosis, specify the allergen if that is practical (e.g., *Risk for allergic response r/t exposure to peanuts or penicillin*).

NOC Outcomes

NOC outcomes have not yet been formally linked to this diagnosis, but the following may be useful:

Allergic Response: Localized: Severity of localized hypersensitive immune response to a specific environmental (exogenous) antigen

Allergic Response: Systemic: Severity of systemic hypersensitive immune response to a specific environmental (exogenous) antigen

Goals/Evaluation Criteria

Examples Using NOC Language

- Will experience no allergy response, as evidenced by exhibiting no Allergic Response: Localized or Systemic
- Demonstrates no **Allergic Response: Localized**, as evidenced by the following indicators (specify 1–5: severe, substantial, moderate, mild, or none):
  - Sinus pain
  - Headache
  - Localized itching, rash, or erythema
- Demonstrates no **Allergic Response: Systemic**, as evidenced by the following indicators (specify 1–5: severe, substantial, moderate, mild, or none):
- Wheezing, stridor, or dyspnea at rest
- Tachycardia, decreased blood pressure, or dysrhythmias
- Hives
- Petechiae
- Nausea, vomiting, or diarrhea
- Anaphylactic shock

Other Examples

- Identify and avoid environmental allergens that apply to him
- Not exhibit localized or systemic allergic responses (e.g., skin, respiratory, cardiac, gastrointestinal, musculoskeletal)

NIC Interventions

NIC interventions have not yet been formally linked to this diagnosis, but the following may be useful:

Allergy Management: Identification, treatment, and prevention of allergic responses to food, medications, insect bites, contrast material, blood, and other substances

Environmental Management: Manipulation of the patient's surroundings for therapeutic benefit, sensory appeal, and psychological well-being

Medication Administration: Preparing, giving, and evaluating the effectiveness of prescription and nonprescription drugs

Respiratory Monitoring: Collection and analysis of patient data to ensure airway patency and adequate gas exchange

Risk Identification: Analysis of potential risk factors, determination of health risks, and prioritization of risk reduction strategies for an individual or group

Surveillance: Purposeful and ongoing acquisition, interpretation, and synthesis of patient data for clinical decision making

Tissue Integrity: Skin and Mucous Membranes: Structural intactness and normal physiological function of skin and mucous membranes

Nursing Activities

Nursing activities for *Risk for allergic response* focus on assisting the patient to identify allergens and sources of allergens to which she is, or may be, sensitive; assessing for signs/symptoms of known allergies; and assisting the patient to avoid known allergens, as needed.

Assessments

- Identify source(s) allergens to which the patient is (or may be) exposed both at work and at home
- Assess patient and family knowledge of sources of allergens to which the patient is sensitive
- Assess knowledge of sensitization and allergic reactions
- Observe for development of asthmatic response (e.g., wheezing, dyspnea)

Patient/Family Teaching

- Teach information about sensitization and allergic reactions, as needed
- Advise against self-treating if allergic reaction is suspected
- Teach to carry an epinephrine injector, if allergies are, or may be, severe

ANXIETY [SPECIFY LEVEL: MILD, MODERATE, SEVERE, PANIC]

(1973, 1982, 1998) **Domain 9, Coping/Stress Tolerance; Class 2, Coping Responses**

Definition: Vague, uneasy feeling of discomfort or dread accompanied by an autonomic response (the source often nonspecific or unknown to the individual); a feeling of apprehension caused by anticipation of danger. It is an alerting signal that warns of impending danger and enables the individual to take measures to deal with the threat.

Defining Characteristics

Behavioral

Diminished productivity
Expressed concerns due to change in life events
Extraneous movement (e.g., foot shuffling, hand/arm movements)
Fidgeting, restlessness
Glancing about
Insomnia
Poor eye contact
Scanning and vigilance

Affective

Anguish
Apprehension
Distressed
Fearful
Feelings of inadequacy
Focus on self
Increased wariness
Irritability
Jittery
Overexcited
Painful or persistent increased helplessness
Rattled
Regretful
Scared
Uncertainty
Worried

Physiological

Facial tension
Insomnia (non-NANDA)
Increased perspiration
Increased tension
Shakiness
Trembling or hand tremors
Voice quivering

A

Parasympathetic

Abdominal pain
Decreased blood pressure
Decreased pulse
Diarrhea
Faintness
Fatigue
Nausea
Sleep disturbance
Tingling in extremities
Urinary frequency
Urinary hesitancy
Urinary urgency

Sympathetic

Anorexia
Cardiovascular excitation
Diarrhea
Dry mouth
Facial flushing
Heart pounding
Increased blood pressure
Increased pulse
Increased reflexes
Increased respiration
Pupil dilation
Respiratory difficulties
Superficial vasoconstriction
Twitching
Weakness

Cognitive

Awareness of physiologic symptoms
Blocking of thought
Confusion
Decreased perceptual field
Difficulty concentrating
Diminished ability to problem solve
Diminished learning ability
Expressed concerns due to changes in life events (non-NANDA)
Fear of unspecific consequences
Focus on self (non-NANDA)

Forgetfulness
Impaired attention
Preoccupation
Rumination
Tendency to blame others

Related Factors

Exposure to toxins
Familial association/heredity
Interpersonal transmission and contagion
Situational and maturational crises
Stress
Substance abuse
Threat of death
Threat to or change in role status, role function, environment, health status, economic status, or interaction patterns
Threat to self-concept
Unconscious conflict about essential values and goals of life
Unmet needs

Suggestions for Use

When anxiety is a result of worry or fear related to death or dying, use the more specific diagnosis of *Death Anxiety*.

Anxiety should be differentiated from *Fear* because some of the nursing actions may be different. When a patient is fearful, the nurse tries to remove the source of the fear or help the patient deal with the specific fear. When a patient is anxious, the nurse helps identify the cause of anxiety; however, when the source of anxiety cannot be identified, the nurse helps the patient explore and express anxious feelings and find ways to cope with anxiety.

Fear and *Anxiety* present diagnostic difficulty because they are not mutually exclusive. A person who is afraid is usually anxious as well. Impending surgery may be the etiology for *Fear*, but most of the feelings about surgery relate to *Anxiety*. Because the etiology (surgery) cannot be changed, nursing interventions should focus on supporting patient-coping mechanisms for managing *Anxiety* (Carpenito-Moyet, 2006, p. 99).

Many of the same signs and symptoms are present in both *Fear* and *Anxiety*: increased heart and respiratory rate, dilated pupils, diaphoresis,

A

muscle tension, and fatigue. The following comparisons in Table 2 may be helpful:

Table 2

	Anxiety	**Fear**
Physiologic manifestations	Stimulation of the parasympathetic nervous system with increased gastrointestinal activity	Sympathetic response only; decreased gastrointestinal activity
Type of threat	Usually psychologic (e.g., to self-image); vague, nonspecific	Often physical (e.g., to safety); specific, identifiable
Feeling	Vague, uneasy feeling	Feeling of dread, apprehension
Source of feeling	Unknown by the person; unconscious	Known by the person

Because the level of anxiety influences the nursing activities, indicate in the diagnostic statement whether anxiety is moderate, severe, or panic level. Panic may require collaborative interventions, such as medications. Mild anxiety is not a problem, because it is a normal condition present in all human beings. Diagnose *Anxiety* only for patients who require special nursing interventions. Mild anxiety before surgery is a normal, healthy response and should be managed by routine teaching and emotional support.

Mild anxiety: Present in day-to-day living; increases alertness and perceptual fields; motivates learning and growth

Moderate anxiety: Narrows perceptual fields; focus is on immediate concerns, with inattention to other communications and details

Severe anxiety: Very narrow focus on specific detail; all behavior is geared toward getting relief

Panic: The person loses control and feels dread and terror. A state of disorganization causes increased physical activity, distorted perceptions and relationships, and loss of rational thought. Panic can lead to exhaustion and death (Fleet, Lesperance, Arsenault, Gregoire, Lavole, et al., 2005; Stuart and Sundeen, 1995).

Suggested Alternative Diagnoses

Decisional conflict
Death anxiety
Fear
Coping, ineffective

NOC Outcomes

Anxiety Level: Severity of manifested apprehension, tension, or uneasiness arising from an unidentifiable source

Anxiety Self-Control: Personal actions to eliminate or reduce feelings of apprehension, tension, or uneasiness from an unidentifiable source

Concentration: Ability to focus on a specific stimulus

Coping: Personal actions to manage stressors that tax an individual's resources

Hyperactivity Level: Severity of patterns of inattention or impulsivity in a child from 1 year through 17 years of age

Goals/Evaluation Criteria

Examples Using NOC Language

- *Anxiety* relieved, as evidenced by exhibiting only mild to moderate Anxiety Level, and consistently demonstrating Anxiety Self-Control, Concentration, Coping, and Hyperactivity Level.
- Demonstrates **Anxiety Self-Control**, as evidenced by the following indicators (specify 1–5: never, rarely, sometimes, often, or consistently demonstrated):
  - Plans coping strategies for stressful situations
  - Maintains role performance
  - Monitors sensory perceptual distortions
  - Monitors behavioral manifestations of anxiety
  - Uses relaxation techniques to reduce anxiety

Other Examples

Patient will:

- Continue necessary activities even though anxiety persists
- Demonstrate ability to focus on new knowledge and skills
- Identify symptoms that are indicators of own anxiety
- Communicate needs and negative feelings appropriately
- Have vital signs within normal limits

NIC Interventions

Anticipatory Guidance: Preparation of patient for an anticipated developmental and/or situational crisis

Anxiety Reduction: Minimizing apprehension, dread, foreboding, or uneasiness related to an unidentified source of anticipated danger

Calming Technique: Reducing anxiety in patient experiencing acute distress

Coping Enhancement: Assisting a patient to adapt to perceived stressors, changes, or threats that interfere with meeting life demands and roles

A

Emotional Support: Provision of reassurance, acceptance, and encouragement during times of stress

Relaxation Therapy: Use of techniques to encourage and elicit relaxation for the purpose of decreasing undesirable signs and symptoms such as pain, muscle tension, or anxiety

Nursing Activities

Assessments

- Assess and document patient's level of anxiety, including physical reactions, q __________
- Assess for cultural factors (e.g., value conflicts) that may contribute to anxiety
- Explore with patient techniques that have, and have not, reduced anxiety in the past
- *(NIC) Anxiety Reduction*: Determine patient's decision-making ability

Patient/Family Teaching

- Develop a teaching plan with realistic goals, including need for repetition, encouragement, and praise of the tasks learned
- Provide information about available community resources, such as friends, neighbors, self-help groups, churches, volunteer agencies, and recreation centers
- Teach symptoms of anxiety
- Teach family members how to distinguish between a panic attack and symptoms of a physical illness
- *(NIC) Anxiety Reduction:*

  Provide factual information concerning diagnosis, treatment, and prognosis

  Instruct patient on the use of relaxation techniques

  Explain all procedures, including sensations likely to be experienced during the procedure

Collaborative Activities

- *(NIC) Anxiety Reduction:* Administer medications to reduce anxiety, as appropriate

Other

- While anxiety is severe, stay with the patient, speak calmly, and provide reassurance and comfort
- Encourage patient to verbalize thoughts and feelings to externalize anxiety
- Help patient to focus on the present situation as a means of identifying coping mechanisms needed to reduce anxiety

- Provide diversion through television, radio, games, and occupational therapies to reduce anxiety and expand focus
- Try techniques such as guided imagery (Antall & Kresevic, 2004) and progressive relaxation
- Provide positive reinforcement when patient is able to continue ADLs and other activities despite anxiety
- Reassure patient by touch and empathetic verbal and nonverbal exchanges
- Encourage patient to express anger and irritation, and allow patient to cry
- Reduce excessive stimulation by providing a quiet environment, limited contact with others if necessary, and limited use of caffeine and other stimulants
- Suggest alternative therapies for reducing anxiety that are acceptable to patient
- Remove sources of anxiety when possible.
- *(NIC) Anxiety Reduction:*
  Use a calm, reassuring approach
  Clearly state expectations for patient's behavior
  Stay with patient [e.g., during procedures] to promote safety and reduce fear
  Administer back rub/neck rub, as appropriate
  Keep treatment equipment out of sight
  Help patient identify situations that precipitate anxiety

For Infants and Children

- Help parents to not exhibit their own anxiety in the child's presence
- Have the parents bring toys, underwear, and other objects from home
- Play with the child or take him to the play room on the unit and involve him in play
- Encourage the child to express his feelings
- Expect and allow for regression in an ill child
- Provide parents with information about the child's illness and behavioral changes they might expect to see in their child (to reduce parental anxiety) (Melnyk & Feinstein, 2001)
- Hold and comfort an infant or child
- *(NIC) Anxiety Reduction*:
  Rock an infant, as appropriate
  Speak softly or sing to an infant or child
  Offer pacifier to infant, as appropriate

A

For Older Adults

- Assess for depression, which is often masked by anxiety in older adults (Bartels, 2002)
- Use a calm, unhurried approach
- Strive for consistency among caregivers and in the environment (Halm & Alpen, 1993)

ANXIETY, DEATH

(1998, 2006) **Domain 9, Coping/Stress Tolerance; Class 2, Coping Responses**

Definition: Vague, uneasy feeling of discomfort or dread generated by perceptions of a real or imagined threat to one's existence

Defining Characteristics

Subjective

Reports concerns of overworking the caregiver
Reports deep sadness
Reports fear of developing terminal illness
Reports fear of loss of mental abilities when dying
Reports fear of pain related to dying
Reports fear of premature death
Reports fear of the process of dying
Reports fear of prolonged dying
Reports fear of suffering related to dying
Reports feeling powerless over dying
Reports negative thoughts related to death and dying
Reports worry about the impact of one's own death on significant others

Related Factors

Anticipating adverse consequences of general anesthesia
Anticipating impact of death on others
Anticipating pain
Anticipating suffering
Confronting reality of terminal disease
Discussions on topic of death
Experiencing dying process
Near death experience
Nonacceptance of own mortality
Observations related to death

Perceived proximity of death
Uncertainty about an encounter with a higher power
Uncertainty about the existence of a higher power
Uncertainty about life after death
Uncertainty of prognosis

Suggestions for Use

See *Anxiety*, Suggestions for Use. Always use the most specific label. If a dying patient's anxiety is related to death or dying, use *Death anxiety*; if not, use the broader label, *Anxiety*.

Suggested Alternative Diagnoses

Anxiety
Grieving
Sorrow, chronic
Spiritual distress

NOC Outcomes

Acceptance: Health Status: Reconciliation to significant change in health circumstances

Comfortable Death: Physical and psychological ease with the impending end of life

Depression Level: Severity of melancholic mood and loss of interest in life events

Dignified Life Closure: Personal actions to maintain control during approaching end of life

Fear Level: Severity of manifested apprehension, tension, or uneasiness arising from an identifiable source

Fear Level: Child: Severity of manifested apprehension, tension, or uneasiness arising from an identifiable source in a child from 1 year through 17 years of age

Hope: Optimism that is personally satisfying and life-supporting

Spiritual Health: Connectedness with self, others, higher power, all life, nature, and the universe that transcends and empowers the self

Goals/Evaluation Criteria

Examples Using NOC Language

- *Death Anxiety* relieved, as evidenced by consistently demonstrating Anxiety Level controlled, Dignified Life Closure, Fear Level controlled, and Hope; Comfortable Death and Spiritual Health not compromised; and no more than mild Depression Level

- Demonstrates **Anxiety Level**, as evidenced by the following indicators (specify 1–5: never, rarely, sometimes, often, or consistently demonstrated):
  - Restlessness
  - Muscle tension
  - Irritability
  - Difficulty concentrating
  - Verbalized anxiety
  - Increased blood pressure; increased respiratory rate
  - Dilated pupils; sweating; dizziness
- Demonstrates **Dignified Life Closure**, as evidenced by the following indicators (specify 1–5: never, rarely, sometimes, often, consistently demonstrated):
  - Expresses readiness for death
  - Resolves important issues and concerns
  - Reconciles relationships
  - Exchanges affection with others
  - Disengages gradually from significant others
  - Discusses spiritual experiences and concerns
  - Expresses hopefulness
  - Maintains sense of control of remaining time

Other Examples

Patient will:

- Maintain psychologic comfort during the process of dying
- Verbalize feelings (e.g., anger, sorrow, or loss) and thoughts with staff and/or significant others
- Report feeling less anxious
- Express concerns about how death will affect significant others
- Identify areas of personal control
- Express positive feelings about relationships with significant others
- Accept limitations and seek help as needed

NIC Interventions

Anxiety Reduction: Minimizing apprehension, dread, foreboding, or uneasiness related to an unidentified source of anticipated danger

Calming Technique: Reducing anxiety in patient experiencing acute distress

Coping Enhancement: Assisting a patient to adapt to perceived stressors, changes, or threats, which interfere with meeting life demands and roles

Decision-Making Support: Providing information and support for a patient who is making a decision regarding health care

Dying Care: Promotion of physical comfort and psychological peace in the final phase of life

Emotional Support: Provision of reassurance, acceptance, and encouragement during times of stress

Hope Inspiration: Facilitation of the development of a positive outlook in a given situation

Mood Management: Providing for safety, stabilization, recovery, and maintenance of a patient who is experiencing dysfunctionally depressed or elevated mood

Pain Management: Alleviation of pain or a reduction in pain to a level of comfort that is acceptable to the patient

Presence: Being with another, both physically and psychologically, during times of need

Religious Ritual Enhancement: Facilitating participation in religious practices

Spiritual Growth Facilitation: Facilitation of growth in patients' capacity to identify, connect with, and call upon the source of meaning, purpose, comfort, strength, and hope in their lives

Spiritual Support: Assisting the patient to feel balance and connection with a greater power

Nursing Activities

Assessments

- Monitor for signs and symptoms of anxiety (e.g., vital signs, appetite, sleep patterns, concentration level)
- Assess support provided by significant others
- Ask the patient's preferences for end-of-life care (e.g., who he wishes to have at the bedside, whether he wishes to die at home or in the hospital)
- Monitor for expressions of hopelessness or powerlessness (e.g., "I can't")
- Determine sources of anxiety (e.g., fear of pain, body malfunction, humiliation, abandonment, nonbeing, negative impact on survivors)

Patient/Family Teaching

- Provide information about the patient's illness and prognosis
- Provide honest and direct answers to the patient's questions about the dying process

Collaborative Activities

- Refer to home care or hospice care, as appropriate
- Arrange access to clergy or spiritual advisors as patient wishes
- Connect patient and family with appropriate support groups
- Refer to psychiatric home health care services as needed

A

Other

- Support spiritual needs without imposing own beliefs on patient (e.g., encourage patient to pray)
- Use therapeutic communication skills to build trusting relationship and facilitate expression of patient needs
- Listen attentively
- Offer support for difficult feelings without offering false reassurance or too much advice
- Encourage patient to express feelings with significant others
- Help patient to identify areas of personal control; offer choices and options to the extent of the patient's ability
- Spend time with patient to deter fear of being alone
- Assist patient to reminisce and review personal life positively
- Identify and support the patient's usual coping strategies
- Provide for physical comfort and security (e.g., provide measures to relieve pain and nausea, administer back massage)
- Answer questions about advance directives and assist with this process as needed
- Encourage family members to be present as much as the patient wishes; keep them informed; encourage them to touch and be physically close to the patient (Pierce, 1999; Tarzian, 2000)

ASPIRATION, RISK FOR

(1988) **Domain 11, Safety/Protection; Class 2, Physical Injury**

Definition: At risk for entry of gastrointestinal secretions, oropharyngeal secretions, solids, or fluids into tracheobronchial passages

Risk Factors

Objective

Age under 3 years (non-NANDA)
Decreased gastrointestinal motility
Delayed gastric emptying [e.g., secondary to ileus or intestinal obstruction]
Depressed cough and gag reflexes
Facial, oral, and neck surgery or trauma
Gastrointestinal tubes
Hindered elevation of upper body
Impaired swallowing

Incompetent lower esophageal sphincter
Increased gastric residual
Increased intragastric pressure
Medication administration
Presence of tracheostomy or endotracheal tube
Reduced level of consciousness [e.g., secondary to anesthesia, head injury, cerebrovascular accident, seizures]
Situations hindering elevation of upper body
Tube feedings
Wired jaws

Suggestions for Use

Always use the most specific label for which the patient has the necessary defining characteristics. Do not use *Risk for injury* if the patient has the defining characteristics or risk factors for *Risk for aspiration*. If the etiology of *Risk for Aspiration* is *Impaired Swallowing*, either diagnosis might be appropriate.

Suggested Alternative Diagnoses

Injury, risk for
Self-care deficit: feeding
Swallowing, impaired

NOC Outcomes

NOTE: For outcomes for specific etiologies (risk factors), refer to the diagnoses: Acute Confusion, Chronic Confusion, Ineffective Infant Feeding pattern, Impaired Physical Mobility, Feeding Self-Care Deficit, and Impaired Swallowing.

Aspiration Prevention: Personal actions to prevent the passage of fluid and solid particles into the lung

Respiratory Status: Airway Patency: Open, clear tracheobronchial passages for air exchange

Respiratory Status: Ventilation: Movement of air in and out of the lungs

Swallowing Status: Safe passage of fluids and/or solids from the mouth to the stomach

Goals/Evaluation Criteria

Examples Using NOC Language

- Will not aspirate, as evidenced by Aspiration Prevention; uncompromised Swallowing Status, and Respiratory Status: Ventilation

- Demonstrates **Aspiration Prevention**, as evidenced by the following indicators (specify 1–5: never, rarely, sometimes, often or consistently demonstrated):
  - Avoids risk factors
  - Positions self upright for eating and drinking
  - Chooses liquids and foods of proper consistency
  - Selects foods according to swallowing ability

Other Examples

Patient will:

- Demonstrate improved swallowing
- Tolerate oral intake and secretions without aspiration
- Tolerate enteral feedings without aspiration
- Have clear lung sounds and patent airway
- Maintain adequate muscle strength and tone

NIC Interventions

Airway Management: Facilitation of patency of air passages

Aspiration Precautions: Prevention or minimization of risk factors in the patient at risk for aspiration

Positioning: Deliberative placement of the patient or a body part to promote physiological and/or psychological well-being

Respiratory Monitoring: Collection and analysis of patient data to ensure airway patency and adequate gas exchange

Swallowing Therapy: Facilitating swallowing and preventing complications of impaired swallowing

Teaching: Infant Safety: Instruction on safety during first year of life

Vomiting Management: Prevention and alleviation of vomiting

Nursing Activities

Assessments

- Check gastric residual prior to feeding and giving medications
- Auscultate lung sounds before and after feedings
- Monitor for signs of aspiration during feedings: coughing, choking, drooling, cyanosis, wheezing, or fever
- Verify placement of enteral tube prior to feeding and giving medications
- Evaluate family's comfort level with feeding, suctioning, positioning, and so forth
- *(NIC) Aspiration Precautions:*
  - Monitor level of consciousness, cough reflex, gag reflex, and swallowing ability

Monitor pulmonary status [e.g., before and after feeding and before and after giving medication]

Patient/Family Teaching

- Instruct family in feeding and swallowing techniques
- Instruct family in use of suction for removal of secretions
- Review with patient and family signs and symptoms of aspiration and preventive measures
- Help family to create an emergency plan in case patient aspirates at home

Collaborative Activities

- Report any change in color of lung secretions that resembles food or feeding intake
- Request occupational therapy consultation
- Refer to a home care agency for nursing assistance at home
- *(NIC) Aspiration Precautions* : Suggest speech pathology consult as appropriate

Other

- Allow patient time to swallow
- Have a suction catheter available at the bedside and suction during meals, as needed
- Involve the family during patient's ingestion of food and meals
- Provide support and reassurance
- Place the patient in semi- or high-Fowler position when eating and for 1 hr afterward, if possible; use side-lying position if this is contraindicated
- Place patients who are unable to sit upright on their sides and elevate the head of the bed as much as possible during and after feedings
- Provide positive reinforcement for attempts to swallow independently
- Use a syringe, if necessary, when feeding the patient
- Vary consistency of foods to identify those foods more easily tolerated
- For patients with tracheostomy or endotracheal tubes, inflate the cuff during and after eating, and during and 1 hr after tube feedings
- *(NIC) Aspiration Precautions* :

    Keep head of bed elevated 30 to 45 min after feeding
    Cut food into small pieces
    Feed in small amounts
    Avoid liquids or use thickening agent
    Break or crush pills before administration
    Request medication in elixir form

A

Home Care

- Teach family caregivers how to use suction equipment

For Infants and Children

- Choose age-appropriate toys with no small, removable parts; do not give balloons to small children
- Avoid foods such as nuts, gum, grapes, and small candy
- Teach parents not to prop bottle
- For newborns with cleft lip and/or palate, refer to a pediatric nursing text for feeding techniques
- For normal newborns, keep in mind that they regurgitate easily when being fed; position upright and burp often during feedings; position infant on his side

For Older Adults

- The frail elderly person may require case management to maintain independent living; refer as needed and available
- May need modified swallow studies to be certain of ability to safely swallow, especially post-CVA

ATTACHMENT, RISK FOR IMPAIRED

(1994, 2008) **Domain 7, Role/Relationships; Class 2, Family Relationships**

NOTE: This label was formerly Risk for Impaired Parent/Child Attachment.

Definition: At risk for disruption of the interactive process between parent or significant other and child that fosters the development of a protective and nurturing reciprocal relationship.

Risk Factors

Anxiety associated with the parent role
Disorganized infant behavior
Ill child who is unable to effectively initiate parental contact due to altered behavioral organization
Inability of parents to meet personal needs
Lack of privacy
Parental conflict resulting from disorganized infant behavior
Physical barriers
Premature infant

Parent–child separation
Substance abuse

Suggestions for Use

Use this diagnosis when parent(s) are at risk for attachment problems. If actual signs of delayed attachment are observed, use *Risk for impaired parenting related to Impaired parent/infant/child attachment.*

Suggested Alternative Diagnoses

Parenting, impaired
Parenting, risk for impaired

NOC Outcomes

Knowledge: Parenting: Extent of understanding conveyed about provision of a nurturing and constructive environment for a child from 1 year through 17 years of age

Parent–Infant Attachment: Parent and infant behaviors that demonstrate an enduring affectionate bond

Parenting Performance: Parental actions to provide a child a nurturing and constructive physical, emotional, and social environment

Role Performance: Congruence of an individual's role behavior with role expectations

Goals/Evaluation Criteria

NOTE: Parental behaviors may vary according to cultural norms.

Examples Using NOC Language

- Demonstrate Parent–Infant Attachment, as evidenced by the following indicators (specify 1–5: never, rarely, sometimes, often, or consistently demonstrated):
  Parent will:
    Practice healthy behaviors during pregnancy
    Assign specific attributes to fetus
    Prepare for infant prior to birth
    Hold, touch, stroke, pat, kiss, and smile at infant
    Talk to infant
    Use en face position and eye contact
    Play with infant
    Respond to infant cues
    Console and soothe infant
    Keep infant dry, clean, and warm

Infant will:

Look at parent(s)

Respond to parent(s)' cues

- Demonstrate **Parenting Performance**, as evidenced by the following indicators (specify 1–5: never, rarely, sometimes, often, or consistently demonstrated):

  Stimulates [child's] cognitive and social development

  Stimulates [the child's] emotional and spiritual growth

  Exhibits a loving relationship [with child]

  Verbalizes positive attributes of child

NIC Interventions

Attachment Promotion: Facilitation of the development of the parent relationship

Developmental Care: Structuring the environment and providing care in response to the behavioral cues and states of the preterm infant

Environmental Management: Attachment Process: Manipulation of the patient's surroundings to facilitate the development of the parent–infant relationship

Parent Education: Infant: Instruction on nurturing and physical care needed during the first year of life

Parenting Promotion: Providing parenting information, support, and coordination of comprehensive services to high-risk families

Role Enhancement: Assisting a patient, significant other, and family to improve relationships by clarifying and supplementing specific role behaviors

Nursing Activities

In general, nursing actions for this diagnosis focus on assessing for risk factors and attachment behaviors, teaching, providing opportunities for parent–infant interaction after birth, and manipulating the environment (e.g., by providing privacy) to facilitate attachment.

NOTE that cultural sensitivity is needed when choosing nursing activities, as cultural norms around childbearing vary.

Assessments

- Assess parent's learning needs
- Assess for factors that may cause attachment problems (e.g., pain, substance abuse, premature infant)
- Observe for indicators of parent–infant attachment (see Goals/Evaluation Criteria)
- Identify parent's readiness to learn about infant care

- Assess parent's ability to recognize infant's physiologic needs (e.g., hunger cues)
- *(NIC) Attachment Promotion*:
  - Ascertain before birth whether parent(s) has names picked out for both sexes
  - Discuss parent's reaction to pregnancy

Patient/Family Teaching

- Teach/demonstrate care of newborn (e.g., feeding, bathing)
- Teach parent(s) about child development
- Assist parents in interpreting infant/child's cues and changing needs (e.g., nonverbal cues, crying, and vocalizations)
- Teach quieting techniques and support parent's ability to relieve child's distress
- *(NIC) Attachment Promotion*:
  - Inform parent(s) of care being given to newborn
  - Explain equipment used to monitor infant in nursery
  - Demonstrate ways to touch infant confined to Isolette
  - Share information gained from initial physical assessment of newborn with parent(s)
  - Discuss infant behavioral characteristics with parent(s)

Other

Prenatal Period

- *(NIC) Attachment Promotion*:
  - Provide parent(s) the opportunity to hear fetal heart tones as soon as possible
  - Provide parent(s) the opportunity to see the ultrasound image of the fetus
  - Encourage parent(s) to attend prenatal [or parenting] classes

Intrapartum Period

- *(NIC) Attachment Promotion*:
  - Encourage father–significant other to participate in labor and delivery [as desired]
  - Place infant on mother's body immediately after birth
  - Provide opportunity for parent(s) to see, hold, and examine newborn immediately after birth
  - Provide family privacy during initial interaction with newborn
- *(NIC) Environmental Management: Attachment Process*:
  - Limit number of people in delivery room
  - Provide comfortable chair for father or significant other
  - Maintain low level of stimuli in patient and family environment

Neonatal Period

B

- *(NIC) Attachment Promotion*:
  Assist parent(s) to participate in infant care
  Reinforce caregiver role behaviors
  Reinforce normal aspects of infant with defect
  Encourage parent(s) to bring personal items, such as toy or picture, to be put in Isolette or at bedside of infant
  Inform parent(s) of care being given to infant in another hospital
  Discuss infant behavioral characteristics with parent(s)
  Point out infant cues that show responsiveness to parent(s)
  Keep infant with parent(s) after birth, when possible
  Encourage parents to massage infant
  Encourage parent(s) to touch and speak to newborn
- *(NIC) Environmental Management: Attachment Process*:
  Permit father or significant other to sleep in room with mother [as desired]
  Reduce interruptions by hospital personnel

Home Care

Much postpartum care is provided through follow-up home visits. Continue with interventions described above. In addition, assess for postpartum depression and other complications that may not occur until after the woman returns home.

BLEEDING, RISK FOR

(2008) **Domain 11, Safety/Protection; Class 2, Physical Injury**

Definition: At risk for a decrease in blood volume that may compromise health

Risk Factors

Aneurysm
Circumcision
Deficient knowledge
Disseminated intravascular coagulopathy
History of falls
Gastrointestinal disorders (e.g., gastric ulcer disease, polyps, varices)
Impaired liver function (e.g., cirrhosis, hepatitis)

Inherent coagulopathies (e.g., thrombocytopenia)
Postpartum complications (e.g., uterine atony, retained placenta)
Pregnancy-related complications (e.g., placenta previa, molar pregnancy, placental abruption)
Trauma
Treatment-related side effects (e.g., surgery, medications, administration of platelet-deficient blood products, chemotherapy)

Suggestions for Use

If there are no independent actions you can take to help prevent bleeding for a particular patient, you might consider using a collaborative problem statement (e.g., Complication of surgery: Bleeding or hemorrhage).

NOC Outcomes

Blood Loss Severity: Severity of internal or external bleeding/hemorrhage
Circulation Status: Unobstructed, unidirectional blood flow at an appropriate pressure through large vessels of the systemic and pulmonary circuits

Goals/Evaluation Criteria

Examples Using NOC Language

- Abnormal bleeding will not occur, as evidenced by normal Circulation Status and no symptoms of Blood Loss Severity.
- Demonstrates no, or only mild, **Blood Loss Severity**, as evidenced by the following indicators (specify 1–5: severe, substantial, moderate, mild, or none):
  - Visible blood loss
  - Hematuria
  - Postsurgical bleeding
  - Decreased systolic or diastolic blood pressure
  - Increased apical heart rate
  - Skin and mucous membrane pallor
  - Decreased hemoglobin (Hgb)
  - Decreased hematocrit (Hct)

Other Examples

Patient will:

- Have minimal or no visible blood loss (e.g., saturate no more than one dressing every 4 hr)
- Have blood pressure, pulse, and respirations within normal limits
- (Postpartum) Have firm uterus on palpation.
- Have no hematemesis
- Have no abdominal distention

NIC Interventions

B

Bleeding Precautions: Reduction of stimuli that may induce bleeding or hemorrhage in at-risk patients

Circumcision Care: Preprocedural and postprocedural support to males undergoing circumcision

Incision Site Care: Cleansing, monitoring, and promotion of healing in a wound that is closed with sutures, clips, or staples

Postpartal Care: Monitoring and management of the patient who has recently given birth

Surveillance: Purposeful and ongoing acquisition, interpretation, and synthesis of patient data for clinical decision making

Nursing Activities

Assessments

- Monitor incisions and wounds for visible bleeding
- Monitor the healing process in the wound
- Monitor dressings for visible bleeding
- Monitor vital signs, especially blood pressure and pulse, as indicated by risk level
- Check hemoglobin and hematocrit levels.
- Monitor coagulation studies

For postpartum patients:

- Monitor fundal height and firmness regularly
- Observe lochia for bright red bleeding and clots

Patient/Family Teaching

- Teach signs of bleeding and advise to notify the nurse should bleeding occur
- *(NIC) Incision Site Care*: Teach the patient how to minimize stress on the incision site

  For patients with coagulation disorders:

  - Teach to avoid anticoagulants (e.g., aspirin, ibuprofen)
  - Teach to increase intake of foods rich in vitamin K

Collaborative Activities

- Administer blood products as prescribed

Other

- If patient is bleeding actively, maintain bed rest

For patients with coagulation disorders:

- Do not take rectal temperatures if patient is at risk for bleeding
- Use electric razor for shaving the patient

- Use a soft toothbrush for oral hygiene
- Avoid injections (for those with coagulation disorders)

BLOOD GLUCOSE LEVEL: UNSTABLE, RISK FOR

(2006) **Domain 2, Nutrition; Class 4, Metabolism**

Definition: Risk for variation of blood glucose/sugar levels from the normal range that may compromise health

Risk Factors

Developmental level
Dietary intake
Inadequate blood glucose monitoring
Lack of acceptance of diagnosis
Lack of adherence to diabetes management plan/action plan
Lack of diabetes management plan/action plan
Lack of knowledge of diabetes management plan/action plan
Medication management
Mental health status
Physical activity level
Physical health status
Pregnancy
Rapid growth periods
Stress
Weight gain
Weight loss

Suggestions for Use

Use this label for situations in which independent nursing actions can have an important impact on prevention. When the nursing actions are primarily to monitor the blood glucose and intervene collaboratively, it may be better to use the collaborative problem, Potential Complication of (insert physiological status): Hypoglycemia/hyperglycemia. Should glucose levels actually become abnormal, use either *Hyperglycemia* or *Hypoglycemia*

Suggested Alternative Diagnoses

Hyperglycemia
Hypoglycemia

NOC Outcomes

B

Adherence Behavior: Healthy Diet: Personal actions to monitor and optimize a healthy and nutritional dietary regimen

Blood Glucose Level: Extent to which glucose levels in plasma and urine are maintained in normal range

Diabetes Self-Management: Personal actions to manage diabetes mellitus, its treatment, and prevent disease progression

Knowledge: Diabetes Management: Extent of understanding conveyed about diabetes mellitus, its treatment, and the prevention of complications

Weight Maintenance Behavior: Personal actions to maintain optimum body weight

Goals/Evaluation Criteria

Examples Using NOC Language

- *Blood Glucose Level* stable as demonstrated by blood glucose, glycosolated hemoglobin, urine glucose, and urine ketones (specify 1–5: severe, substantial, moderate, mild, or no deviation from normal range)
- Risk factors controlled, as demonstrated by consistently demonstrated Adherence Behavior: Healthy Diet, Diabetes Self-Management, substantial Knowledge: Diabetes Management, Weight Maintenance Behavior, and no deviation in Blood Glucose Level

Other Examples

Patient will:

- Demonstrate correct procedure for testing blood glucose
- Follow prescribed regimen for monitoring blood glucose
- Adhere to recommendations for diet and exercise
- Demonstrate correct procedures for self-administering medications
- Describe symptoms of hypo- and hyperglycemia

NOTE: Goals for this diagnosis should focus on preventing unstable blood glucose, rather than on long-term diabetes management. Therefore, goals describing foot care, eye exams, and so forth are not given here.

NIC Interventions

Hyperglycemia Management: Preventing and treating above-normal blood glucose levels

Hypoglycemia Management: Preventing and treating low blood glucose levels

Surveillance: Purposeful and ongoing acquisition, interpretation, and synthesis of patient data for clinical decision making

Teaching: Disease Process: Assisting the patient to understand information related to a specific disease process

Teaching: Individual: Planning, implementation, and evaluation of a teaching program designed to address a patient's particular needs

Teaching: Prescribed Diet: Preparing a patient to correctly follow a prescribed diet

Teaching: Prescribed Medication: Preparing a patient to safely take prescribed medications and monitor for their effects

Nursing Activities

Nursing actions for this diagnosis focus on monitoring for signs and symptoms of hypo- or hyperglycemia, reducing risk factors, and teaching for self-regulation of glucose levels. They do not involve long-term diabetes management, so teaching foot care, for example, is not included here. For managing elevated or decreased glucose levels, see the diagnoses *Hypoglycemia* and *Hyperglycemia*.

Assessments

- Assess for factors that increase the risk of glucose imbalance
- Monitor serum glucose level (below 60 mg/dl indicates hypoglycemia; above 300 mg/dl indicates hyperglycemia) according to orders or protocol
- Monitor urine ketones
- Monitor intake and output
- Monitor for signs and symptoms of hypoglycemia (e.g., serum glucose $<$ 60 mg/dl, pallor, tachycardia, diaphoresis, jitteriness, blurred vision, irritability, chills, clamminess, confusion)
- Monitor for signs and symptoms of hyperglycemia (e.g., serum glucose $>$ 300 mg/dl, acetone breath, positive plasma ketones, headache, blurred vision, nausea, vomiting, polyuria, polydipsia, polyphagia, weakness, lethargy, hypotension, tachycardia, Kussmaul respirations)
- Determine causes of hypo- or hyperglycemia if they occur

Patient/Family Teaching

- Provide information about diabetes
- Provide information about using diet and exercise to achieve glucose balance
- Provide information about medications used to control diabetes
- Provide information about managing diabetes during illness
- Provide information about self-monitoring of glucose levels and ketones, as appropriate

Collaborative Activities

B

- Collaborate with patient and diabetes team to make changes in medication, as needed
- Notify physician if signs and symptoms of hypo- or hyperglycemia occur and cannot be reversed with independent activities

Other

- *(NIC) Hypoglycemia Management*:

  Provide simple carbohydrate, as indicated

  Provide complex carbohydrate and protein, as indicated

  Maintain IV access, as appropriate

BODY IMAGE, DISTURBED

(1973, 1998) **Domain 6, Perception/Cognition; Class 3, Body Image**

Definition: Confusion in mental picture of one's physical self

Defining Characteristics

Subjective

Depersonalization of [body] part or loss by impersonal pronouns

Emphasis on remaining strengths

Focus on past strength, function, or appearance

Heightened achievement

Negative feelings about body (e.g., feelings of helplessness, hopelessness, or powerlessness)

Personalization of body part or loss by name

Preoccupation with change or loss

Refusal to verify actual change

Verbalization of change in lifestyle

Objective

Actual change in [body] structure or function

Behaviors of monitoring or acknowledgment of one's body

Change in ability to estimate spatial relationship of body to environment

Change in social involvement

Extension of body boundary to incorporate environmental objects

Intentional hiding or overexposing body part (intentional or unintentional)

Missing body part

Nonverbal response to actual or perceived change in body (e.g., appearance, structure, function)

Not looking at body part

Not touching body part
Reports feelings that reflect an altered view of one's body (e.g., appearance, structure, function)
Reports perceptions that reflect an altered view of one's body in appearance
Trauma to nonfunctioning body part
Unintentional hiding or overexposing of body part

Related Factors

Biophysical [e.g., chronic illness, congenital defects, pregnancy]
Cognitive/perceptual [e.g., chronic pain]
Cultural or spiritual
Developmental changes
Illness
Perceptual
Psychosocial [e.g., eating disorders]
[Situational crisis (specify)]
Trauma or injury
Treatments [e.g., surgery, chemotherapy, radiation]

Suggestions for Use

Either (A) or (B), following, must be present to justify the diagnosis of *Disturbed Body Image*. The remaining defining characteristics may be used to validate the presence of (A) or (B).

(A) Verbalization of feelings or perceptions that reflect actual or perceived change in body appearance, structure, or function
(B) Nonverbal responses to actual or perceived change in body appearance, structure, or function

This label is related to *Chronic low self-esteem*, but is specific to negative feelings about one's body or body parts. Although *Disturbed body image* is often caused by loss of a body part or actual body changes, the changes in body structure or function can be perceived rather than actual. Patients on prolonged bed rest or who are dependent on machines (e.g., dialysis equipment, respirators) may experience distortion of body image. Eating disorders are often related to *Disturbed body image* and may require one of the Nutrition diagnoses.

Suggested Alternative Diagnoses

Nutrition: less than body requirements, imbalanced
Nutrition: more than body requirements, imbalanced
Self-esteem, chronic, or situational low

NOC Outcomes

B

Adaptation to Physical Disability: Adaptive response to a significant functional challenge due to a physical disability

Body Image: Perception of own appearance and body functions

Child Development: Middle Childhood: Milestones of physical, cognitive, and psychosocial progression from 6 years through 11 years of age.

Child Development: Adolescence: Milestones of physical, cognitive, and psychosocial progression from 12 years through 17 years of age.

Heedfulness of Affected Side: Personal actions to acknowledge, protect, and cognitively integrate body part(s) into self

Self-Esteem: Personal judgment of self-worth

Goals/Evaluation Criteria

Examples Using NOC Language

- *Disturbed body image* alleviated as evidenced by consistently demonstrated Adaptation to Physical Disability, positive Body Image, no delay in Child Development, and positive Self-Esteem
- Demonstrates **Body Image**, as evidenced by the following indicators (specify 1–5: never, rarely, sometimes, often, or consistently positive):
  - Congruence between body reality, body ideal, and body presentation
  - Satisfaction with body appearance and function
  - Willingness to touch affected body part

Other Examples

Patient will:

- Identify personal strengths
- Acknowledge impact of situation on existing personal relationships and lifestyle
- Acknowledge the actual change in body appearance
- Demonstrate acceptance of appearance
- Describe actual change in body function
- Realistically approximate relationship of body to environment
- Express willingness to use suggested resources after discharge
- Resume self-care responsibilities
- Maintain close social interaction and personal relationships

NIC Interventions

Anticipatory Guidance: Preparation of patient for an anticipated developmental or situational crisis

Body Image Enhancement: Improving a patient's conscious and unconscious perceptions and attitudes toward his or her body

Developmental Enhancement: Adolescent: Facilitating optimal physical, cognitive, social, and emotional growth of individuals during the transition from childhood to adulthood

Developmental Enhancement: Child: Facilitating or teaching parents–caregivers to facilitate the optimal gross motor, fine motor, language, cognitive, social and emotional growth of preschool and school-aged children

Parent Education: Adolescent: Assisting parents to understand and help their adolescent children

Parent Education: Childrearing Family: Assisting parents to understand and promote the physical, psychological, and social growth and development of their toddler, preschool, or school-aged child or children

Self-Esteem Enhancement: Assisting a patient to increase his personal judgment of self-worth

Unilateral Neglect Management: Protecting and safely reintegrating the affected part of the body while helping the patient adapt to disturbed perceptual abilities

Nursing Activities

In general, nursing actions for this diagnosis focus on establishing a trusting relationship with the client; exploring facts, feelings, and behaviors relevant to the loss; encouraging social interaction; and assisting parents to enhance body image in the child.

Assessments

- Assess and document patient's verbal and nonverbal responses to his body
- Identify the patient's usual coping mechanisms
- *(NIC) Body Image Enhancement*:

  Determine patient's body image expectations based on developmental stage

  Determine whether perceived dislike for certain physical characteristics creates a dysfunctional social paralysis for teenagers and other high-risk groups

  Determine whether a recent physical change has been incorporated into patient's body image

  Identify the effects of the patient's culture, religion, race, gender, and age on body image

  Monitor frequency of statements of self-criticism

Patient/Family Teaching

- Teach care and self-care, including complications of medical condition

Collaborative Activities

- Refer to social services department for planning care with patient and family
- Refer to physical therapy for strength and flexibility training, help with transfers and ambulation, or use of prosthesis
- Offer to make initial phone call to appropriate community resources for patient and family
- Refer to interdisciplinary teams for clients with complex needs (e.g., surgical complications)

Other

- Actively listen to patient and family and acknowledge reality of concerns about treatments, progress, and prognosis
- Encourage patient and family to air feelings and to grieve, as appropriate
- Support the patient's usual coping mechanisms; for example, don't ask the patient to explore feelings if he seems reluctant to do so
- Assist patient and family to identify and use coping mechanisms
- Assist patient and family to identify their personal strengths and acknowledge limitations
- Provide care in a nonjudgmental manner, maintaining the patient's privacy and dignity
- Be aware of your facial expression when caring for patients with disfiguring body changes; maintain a neutral expression
- Help the patient and family to gradually become accustomed to the body change, perhaps touching the area before looking at it
- Encourage patient to:
  - Maintain usual daily grooming routine
  - Participate in decision making
  - Verbalize concerns about close personal relationships and others' responses to the body change
  - Verbalize consequences of physical and emotional changes that have influenced self-concept
- *(NIC) Body Image Enhancement*:
  - Identify means of reducing the impact of any disfigurement through clothing, wigs, or cosmetics, as appropriate
  - Facilitate contact with individuals with similar changes in body image
  - Use self-disclosure exercises with groups of teenagers or others distraught over normal physical attributes

B

For Infants and Children

- *(NIC) Body Image Enhancement* :
  Determine how child responds to parents' reactions, as appropriate
  Determine patient's body image expectations based on developmental stage
  Use self-picture drawing as a mechanism for evaluating a child's body image perceptions
  Instruct children about the functions of the various body parts, as appropriate
  Teach parents the importance of their responses to the child's body changes and future adjustment, as appropriate

Home Care

- In addition to the preceding interventions:
  - Assess caregiver(s) acceptance of the client's body changes
  - Assess financial impact of changes, if any, and report to social services as needed
  - Assess home environment for safety and the need for adaptive equipment
  - Evaluate the need for psychiatric home health services to address the client's distorted body image

BODY TEMPERATURE: IMBALANCED, RISK FOR

(1986, 2000) **Domain 11, Safety/Protection; Class 6, Thermoregulation**

Definition: At risk for failure to maintain body temperature within normal range

Risk Factors

Objective
Altered metabolic rate
Dehydration
Exposure to extremes of environmental temperature
Extremes of age

Extremes of weight
Illness or trauma affecting temperature regulation

[Immaturity of newborn's temperature-regulating system]
[Inability to perspire]
Inactivity
Inappropriate clothing for environmental temperature
[Low birth weight (neonate)]
Medications causing vasoconstriction or vasodilation
Sedation
Vigorous activity

Suggestions for Use

If the risk factors are a pathophysiologic complication requiring medical intervention, use a collaborative problem instead of *Risk for imbalanced body temperature*. If the patient is at risk for both *Hypothermia* and *Hyperthermia*, then *Risk for imbalanced body temperature* is the appropriate diagnosis. If the patient is at risk for only an elevation in temperature, use *Risk for hyperthermia*; if at risk for only decreased body temperature, use *Risk for hypothermia*. If an actual temperature fluctuation exists, use *Ineffective thermoregulation*.

Suggested Alternative Diagnoses

Hyperthermia
Hypothermia
Thermoregulation, ineffective

NOC Outcomes

Thermoregulation: Balance among heat production, heat gain, and heat loss

Thermoregulation: Newborn: Balance among heat production, heat gain, and heat loss during the first 28 days of life

Goals/Evaluation Criteria

Examples Using NOC Language

- Exhibits **Thermoregulation**, as evidenced by the following indicators (specify 1–5: severely, substantially, moderately, mildly, or not compromised)
  - Increased skin temperature
  - Decreased skin temperature
  - Hyperthermia
  - Hypothermia

Other Examples

Patient will:

- Not exhibit goose bumps, sweating, shivering
- Maintain vital signs within normal ranges
- Report thermal comfort
- Describe adaptive measures to minimize fluctuations in body temperature
- Report early signs and symptoms of hypo- or hyperthermia

NIC Interventions

Newborn Care: Management of neonate during the transition to extrauterine life and subsequent period of stabilization

Malignant Hyperthermia Precautions: Prevention or reduction of hypermetabolic response to pharmacological agents used during surgery

Surveillance: Purposeful and ongoing acquisition, interpretation, and synthesis of patient data for clinical decision making

Temperature Regulation: Attaining or maintaining body temperature within a normal range

Temperature Regulation: Intraoperative: Attaining or maintaining desired intraoperative body temperature

Vital Signs Monitoring: Collection and analysis of cardiovascular, respiratory, and body temperature data to determine and prevent complications

Nursing Activities

In general, nursing actions for this diagnosis focus on preventing *Imbalanced body temperature* by identifying risk factors and intervening appropriately.

Assessments

- Assess for early signs and symptoms of hypothermia (e.g., shivering, pallor, cyanotic nailbeds, slow capillary refill, piloerection, dysrhythmias) and hyperthermia (e.g., absence of sweating, weakness, nausea and vomiting, headache, delirium)
- For adults, take oral (rather than tympanic or axillary) temperatures; oral temperatures are more accurate
- *(NIC) Temperature Regulation*: Monitor for and report signs and symptoms of hypo- and hyperthermia

Patient/Family Teaching

- Instruct patient and family in measures to minimize temperature fluctuations:

  For Hyperthermia

  Drink adequate fluids on hot days

  Limit activity on hot days

B

Lose weight, if obese
Maintain stable environmental temperature
Remove excess clothing

For Hypothermia
Bathe in warm room, away from drafts
Increase activity
Limit alcohol intake
Maintain adequate nourishment
Maintain stable environmental temperature
Wear adequate clothing

- Instruct patient and family to recognize and report early signs and symptoms of hypo- and hyperthermia:
  For Hyperthermia: Dry skin, headache, increased pulse, increased temperature, irritability, temperature above 37.8°C or 100°F, weakness
  For Hypothermia: Apathy; cold, hard abdomen that feels like marble; disorientation and confusion, drowsiness, hypertension, hypoglycemia, impaired ability to think; reduced pulse and respirations, skin hard and cold to touch, temperature of less than 95°F (35°C)

Collaborative Activities

- Report to physician if adequate hydration cannot be maintained
- Refer to social services for services (e.g., fans, heaters) needed in the home
- *(NIC) Temperature Regulation*: Administer antipyretic medication, as appropriate

Other

- *(NIC) Temperature Regulation:* Adjust environmental temperature to patient needs

Home Care

- Evaluate home environment for factors that may alter body temperature
- Teach caregivers how to take the temperature
- Help the client obtain a fan or an air-conditioner if needed
- Help the client identify a warm place they can go to in an emergency (e.g., a power outage)
- See suggestions in "For Infants and Children" and "For Older Adults," following

For Infants and Children

- Children tend to experience higher fevers than adults; a fever of 100 to 104°F (37.8 to 40°C) usually is not harmful. It is not necessary to treat all fevers in children unless the child has a history of febrile convulsions, or a serious illness is present, or if the fever is a result of heat stroke
- Do not administer aspirin for fever in children under age 18 because of the risk of developing Reye's syndrome (which can be fatal)
- Tepid sponging may serve as an alternative when aspirin is contraindicated, but it may cause more discomfort
- Children develop heat stroke more readily than do adults; protect from hot environments, and ensure intake of adequate amount of fluids
- Dry and swaddle infant (or place on skin-to-skin contact with mother) immediately after birth to prevent heat loss by evaporation
- Newborns lose a large amount of heat through their scalp; keep the head covered
- Maintain a room temperature of at least 72°F (22.2°C)
- (NIC) Temperature Regulation:
  Monitor newborn's temperature until stabilized
  Wrap infant immediately after birth to prevent heat loss

For Older Adults

- Older adults have decreased ability to adapt to cold temperature. In addition, they are less able to perceive temperature changes, and thus may not initiate protective measures. Therefore, they can become hyperthermic or hypothermic more easily than young adults.
- Prevent chilling when administering care (e.g., keep well draped when bathing)
- Maintain a room temperature of 68 to 72°F (20 to 22.2°C)
- Older adults are more likely to experience heat-related dehydration as a result of age-related changes in the kidneys and the thirst mechanism
- Encourage older adults to remove extra items of clothing (e.g., sweaters that may be worn habitually) in hot weather

BOWEL INCONTINENCE

B

(1975, 1998) **Domain 3, Elimination and Exchange; Class 2, Gastrointestinal Function**

Definition: Change in normal bowel habits characterized by involuntary passage of stool.

Defining Characteristics

Subjective

Inability to recognize urge to defecate
Recognizes rectal fullness but reports inability to expel formed stool
Self-report of inability to feel rectal fullness

Objective

Constant dribbling of soft stool
Fecal odor
Fecal staining of clothing and/or bedding
Inability to delay defecation
Inattention to urge to defecate
Red perianal skin
Urgency

Related Factors

Abnormally high abdominal or intestinal pressure
Chronic diarrhea
Colorectal lesions
Dietary habits
Environmental factors (e.g., inaccessible bathroom)
General decline in muscle tone
Immobility
Impaction
Impaired cognition
Impaired reservoir capacity
Incomplete emptying of bowel
Laxative abuse
Loss of rectal sphincter control
Lower motor nerve damage
Medications
Pelvic floor descent (non-NANDA-I)
Rectal sphincter abnormality
Self-care deficit—toileting

Stress
Upper motor nerve damage

Suggestions for Use

(a) Differentiate between this label and *Diarrhea*. (b) *Self-care deficit: toileting* may be the cause of *Bowel incontinence*. However, there seems to be no advantage to writing a diagnosis of *Bowel incontinence related to Toileting self-care deficit*. A diagnosis such as *Toileting self-care deficit related to inability to ambulate to toilet or commode* provides more specific information about the self-care deficit and thus more guidance for nursing interventions to alleviate the problem.

Suggested Alternative Diagnoses

Diarrhea
Self-care deficit: toileting

NOC Outcomes

Bowel Continence: Control of passage of stool from the bowel
Tissue Integrity: Skin and Mucous Membranes: Structural intactness and normal physiological function of skin and mucous membranes

Goals/Evaluation Criteria

Examples Using NOC Language

- Patient will exhibit **Bowel Continence**, as evidenced by the following indicators (specify 1–5: never, rarely, sometimes, often, or consistently demonstrated):
  - Maintains control of stool passage
  - Recognizes urge to defecate
  - Responds to urge in timely manner
  - Soils underclothing during day
  - Gets to toilet between urge and evacuation of stool

Other Examples

Patient will:

- Have soft, formed stools every 1 to 5 days
- Establish a regular routine of fecal elimination
- Have progressively fewer incontinent episodes
- Be free of skin irritation to perianal area

NIC Interventions

Bowel Incontinence Care: Promotion of bowel continence and maintenance of perianal skin integrity

B

Bowel Management: Establishment and maintenance of a regular pattern of bowel elimination

Bowel Training: Assisting the patient to train the bowel to evacuate at specific intervals

Perineal Care: Maintenance of perineal skin integrity and relief of perineal discomfort

Skin Surveillance: Collection and analysis of patient data to maintain skin and mucous membrane integrity

Nursing Activities

In general, nursing actions for this diagnosis focus on identifying factors contributing to incontinence, supporting normal elimination habits, providing bowel training, teaching about dietary requirements, and maintaining perineal skin integrity.

Assessments

- Assess the patient's ability for toileting self-care
- Assess ability [e.g., mobility, cognitive function] and motivation to participate in bowel training and use bowel elimination techniques
- Assess condition of perianal skin after each episode of incontinence
- Document frequency of incontinent episodes
- Record patterns of bowel elimination and incontinent episodes; include frequency and consistency of bowel movements and food and fluid intake
- *(NIC) Bowel Incontinence Care*:

  Determine physical or psychologic cause of fecal incontinence

  Monitor diet and fluid requirements

  Monitor for adequate bowel evacuation

  Determine goals of bowel management program with patient and family

Patient/Family Teaching

- Instruct patient and family about physiology of normal defecation
- *(NIC) Bowel Incontinence Care*:

  Instruct patient and family to record fecal output, as appropriate

  Discuss procedures and expected outcomes with patient

  Explain etiology of problem and rationale for actions

Collaborative Activities

- Obtain order from physician to institute bowel-training program (program may include bulk-forming laxative; rectal suppository q day; digital stimulation; and scheduled use of bedpan, commode, or bathroom)
- Refer for family therapy (e.g., for incontinence with emotional etiology)
- Refer to physician to evaluate the need of an anal continence plug

B

Other

- Provide care in an accepting, nonjudgmental manner
- Provide bedpan or assist to commode q ______________
- Provide privacy for defecation
- Establish a regular time for defecation
- Provide foods high in bulk and ample fluids
- Use a moisture barrier containing zinc oxide or dimethicone if incontinence is severe
- *(NIC) Bowel Incontinence Care*:

  Wash perianal area with soap and water and dry it thoroughly after each stool

  Use powder and creams on perianal area with caution

  Keep bed and clothing clean

  Place on incontinent pads, as needed

  Provide protective pants, as needed

Home Care

- Evaluate the accessibility of toileting facilities in the home
- Arrange for a bedside commode if the patient cannot reach the toilet soon enough
- Teach caregivers to monitor the perineal skin for redness and excoriation
- Teach caregivers to provide nonrestrictive clothing that can be easily changed
- Refer for home health aide services to help with hygiene and skin care as needed

For Infants and Children

- Obtain toilet training history of child, including duration of encopresis and treatment efforts
- For encopresis: Caution parents not to create feelings of anxiety, guilt, or inadequacy about toileting; teach parents ways to reward desired toileting behaviors
- Reinforce that the goal of therapy is to help the child with encopresis learn new bowel habits while avoiding excessive involvement of the parent with daily aspects of bowel function and diet

For Older Adults

- Evaluate all older adults for fecal incontinence on admittance to an inpatient facility

BREAST MILK, INSUFFICIENT

(2010) **Domain 2, Nutrition; Class 1, Ingestion**

Definition: Low production of maternal breast milk

Defining Characteristics

Infant

Constipation
Does not seem satisfied after sucking time
Frequent crying
Long breastfeeding time
Refuses to suck
Voids small amounts of concentrated urine (less than four to six times a day)
Wants to suck very frequently
Weight gain is lower than 500 g in a month (comparing two measures)

Mother

Milk production does not progress
No milk appears when mother's nipple is pressed
Volume of expressed breast milk is less than prescribed volume.

Related Factors

Infant

Ineffective latching on
Ineffective sucking
Insufficient opportunity to suckle
Rejection of breast
Short sucking time

Mother

Alcohol intake
Fluid volume depletion (e.g., dehydration, hemorrhage)
Malnutrition
Medication side effects (e.g., contraceptives, diuretics)
Pregnancy
Tobacco smoking

Suggestions for Use

Insufficient breast milk is a related factor for the diagnosis, *Ineffective breastfeeding*. If other of its related factors are present, it might be more useful to use Ineffective breastfeeding or *Risk for ineffective breastfeeding* as the diagnosis. Use *Insufficient breast milk* only if one or more of the defining characteristics for the mother is present (e.g., no milk appears when mother's nipple is pressed). Those listed under "Infant" might be present, but they could indicate *Ineffective breastfeeding* as well as *Insufficient breast milk.*

Suggestions for Use

Breastfeeding, ineffective
Breastfeeding, risk for ineffective (non-NANDA-I)

NOC Outcomes

NOC outcomes have not yet been linked to this new diagnosis; however, the following may be useful:

Breastfeeding Establishment: Maternal: Maternal establishment of proper attachment of an infant to and sucking from the breast for nourishment during the first 3 weeks of breastfeeding

Breastfeeding Maintenance: Continuation of breastfeeding from establishment to weaning for nourishment of an infant/toddler

Goals/Evaluation Criteria

Examples Using NOC Language

- Will have adequate supply of breast milk, as evidenced by Breastfeeding Establishment: Maternal, and Breastfeeding Maintenance.
- Demonstrates **Breastfeeding Establishment:** Maternal, as demonstrated by the following indicators (specify 1–5: not, slightly, moderately, substantially, or totally adequate):
    - Breast fullness prior to feeding
    - Fluid intake of mother
    - Pumping of breast
    - Use of family support
- Demonstrates **Breastfeeding Maintenance**, as demonstrated by the following indicators (specify 1–5: not, slightly, moderately, substantially, or totally adequate):
    - Infant's growth and/or development in normal range
    - Recognition of signs of decreased milk supply
    - Avoidance of self-medication without checking with health professional
    - Knowledge of resources for support

Other Examples

- Mother will verbalize satisfaction with breastfeeding process
- Infant will nurse 5 to 10 min at each breast

- Infant will have urination volume and frequency appropriate for age
- Infant will be content after feeding

NIC Interventions

NIC interventions have not yet been linked to this new diagnosis; however, the following may be useful:

Breastfeeding Assistance: Preparing a new mother to breastfeed her infant

Lactation Counseling: Use of an interactive helping process to assist in maintenance of successful breastfeeding

Nursing Activities

In general, nursing actions for this diagnosis focus on identifying factors contributing to insufficient milk production and teaching measures to promote increased milk production.

Assessments

- Assess the patient's knowledge of lactation and breastfeeding.
- Assess prior experience with breastfeeding
- Assess the infant for difficulties with sucking or swallowing

Patient/Family Teaching

- Explain the importance of having the infant nurse frequently, 5 to 10 min at each breast.
- Explain the importance of sucking to milk production, as well as the need to completely empty each breast.
- Demonstrate ways to wake the infant if he is falling asleep at the breast.
- If the baby does not suck for at least 5 min, teach to pump the breasts to provide stimulation and emptying
- Teach how to assist the baby to grasp the nipple, if that is a contributing factor.
- Explain that adequate rest is needed to support milk production

Collaborative Activities

- Refer to a lactation specialist (e.g., if there are problems with infant sucking and latching on or if the mother seems to lack confidence)
- Refer to La Leche League, as needed

Other

- Give positive feedback and reassurance
- Be available to answer the mother's questions
- Encourage questions and expression of feelings

BREASTFEEDING, INEFFECTIVE

(1988, 2010) **Domain 7, Role Relationships; Class 1, Caregiving Roles**

Definition: Dissatisfaction or difficulty a mother, infant, or child experiences with the breastfeeding process.

Defining Characteristics

Subjective

Perceived inadequate milk supply
Unsatisfactory breastfeeding process [as stated by mother]

Objective

Inadequate milk supply
Infant arching and crying at the breast
Infant crying or exhibiting fussiness within the first hour after breastfeeding
Infant inability to latch on to maternal breast correctly
Infant resisting latching on
Infant unresponsiveness to other comfort measures
Insufficient emptying of each breast per feeding
Insufficient opportunity for suckling at the breast
Lack of infant weight gain
No observable signs of oxytocin release
Persistence of sore nipples beyond the first week of breastfeeding
Unsustained suckling at the breast

Related Factors

Deficient knowledge
Infant anomaly
Infant receiving supplemental feedings with artificial nipple
Interrupted breastfeeding
Maternal anxiety or ambivalence
Maternal breast anomaly
Nonsupportive partner or family
Poor infant sucking reflex
Prematurity
Previous breast surgery
Previous history of breastfeeding failure
[Maternal fatigue or illness]
[Insufficient intake of fluids]

Suggestions for Use

This diagnosis focuses on the mother's satisfaction with the breastfeeding process and includes an actual or perceived inadequate milk supply. The comparisons in Table 3 may be helpful in determining the best diagnosis.

Table 3

Diagnosis	**Cues (Defining Characteristics)**
Ineffective breastfeeding	Dissatisfaction with feeding process
Ineffective infant feeding pattern	Inability of infant to suck or poorly coordinated suck and swallow response
Interrupted breastfeeding	Mother wishes to maintain lactation but is unable to put baby to breast for some feedings (e.g., illness or working)

If there are risk factors, such as maternal ambivalence, inverted nipples, or young maternal age, use Risk for ineffective breastfeeding (this is not a NANDA-I diagnosis).

Suggested Alternative Diagnoses

Breastfeeding, interrupted
[Breastfeeding, Risk for Ineffective]
Infant feeding pattern, ineffective

NOC Outcomes

Breastfeeding Establishment: Infant: Infant attachment to and sucking from the mother's breast for nourishment during the first 3 weeks of life

Breastfeeding Establishment: Maternal: Maternal establishment of proper attachment of an infant to and sucking from the breast for nourishment during the first 3 weeks of breastfeeding

Breastfeeding Maintenance: Continuation of breastfeeding for nourishment of an infant or toddler

Breastfeeding Weaning: Progressive discontinuation of breastfeeding

Knowledge: Breastfeeding: Extent of understanding conveyed about lactation and nourishment of an infant through breastfeeding

Goals/Evaluation Criteria

Examples Using NOC Language

- Mother and infant will experience *Effective breastfeeding* as demonstrated by Knowledge: Breastfeeding; Breastfeeding Establishment: Infant/Maternal; Breastfeeding Maintenance; and Breastfeeding Weaning

- Infant will demonstrate **Breastfeeding Establishment: Infant**, as evidenced by the following indicators (specify 1–5: not, slightly, moderately, substantially, or totally adequate):
  Proper alignment and latch on
  Proper areolar grasp and compression
  Correct suck and tongue placement
  Audible swallow
  Minimum eight feedings per day [on demand]
  Infant contentment after feeding
  Weight gain appropriate for age

Other Examples

Mother will:

- Maintain effective breastfeeding for as long as desired
- Describe increasing confidence with breastfeeding
- Recognize early hunger cues
- Indicate satisfaction with breastfeeding
- Not experience nipple tenderness
- Recognize signs of decreased milk supply

NIC Interventions

Breastfeeding Assistance: Preparing a new mother to breast-feed her infant

Lactation Counseling: Use of an interactive helping process to assist in maintenance of successful breastfeeding

Lactation Suppression: Facilitating the cessation of milk production and minimizing breast engorgement after giving birth

Nursing Activities

In general, nursing actions for this diagnosis focus on teaching to reduce or eliminate factors that contribute to *Ineffective breastfeeding*. Except for assessing and teaching, interventions are primarily self-care performed by the mother.

Assessments

- Assess maternal knowledge of and experience with breastfeeding
- Assess infant's ability to latch on and suck effectively
- Assess in the early prenatal period for risk factors for Ineffective Breastfeeding (e.g., under 20 years of age, low socioeconomic status, inverted nipples)
- Monitor infant weight and elimination patterns
- Assess for discomfort (e.g., sore nipples, engorgement)

- *(NIC) Lactation Counseling*:
  - Evaluate newborn suck and swallow pattern
  - Determine mother's desire and motivation to breastfeed
  - Evaluate mother's understanding of infant's feeding cues (e.g., rooting, sucking, and alertness)
  - Monitor maternal skill with latching infant onto the nipple
  - Monitor skin integrity of nipples
  - Evaluate understanding of plugged milk ducts and mastitis
  - Monitor ability to correctly relieve breast congestion

Patient/Family Teaching

- Instruct mother in breastfeeding techniques that increase her skill in feeding infant; consider relaxation techniques, comfortable positioning, stimulation of rooting reflex, establishment of infant alert state before attempting to feed, burping, stimulation of infant to continue to feed, and alternation of breasts
- Instruct mother to offer both breasts at each feeding, beginning with an alternate breast each time
- Instruct mother in breast-pumping equipment and techniques to maintain milk supply during interruptions or delays in infant sucking reflex
- Instruct mother in need for adequate rest and intake of fluids
- *(NIC) Lactation Counseling*:
  - Provide information about advantages and disadvantages of breastfeeding
  - Discuss alternative methods of feeding
  - Correct misconceptions, misinformation, and inaccuracies about breastfeeding
  - Demonstrate suck training, as appropriate
  - Instruct about infant stool and urination patterns, as appropriate
  - Recommend nipple care, as needed
  - Instruct on signs of problems to report to health care practitioner
  - Discuss signs of readiness to wean

Collaborative Activities

- Refer to appropriate community resources, such as La Leche League, lactation consultants, and the public health department

Other

- Encourage rooming-in
- Encourage feeding on demand; discourage supplemental feedings
- Have mother express enough milk to relieve engorgement, allowing nipples to evert
- Increase number of nursings on demand for a crying, wakeful infant

- Increase number of scheduled nursings for the sleepy infant of low birth weight
- Offer food and fluids to mother during day and evening prior to breastfeeding times
- Provide privacy for mother and infant
- Recognize *time-out* behaviors in premature infant
- Schedule rest periods, as needed
- Reinforce successful behaviors
- *(NIC) Lactation Counseling*:
  Provide support of mother's decisions
  Encourage continued lactation on return to work or school

Home Care

See Effective Breastfeeding.

- Observe a full breastfeeding session at postpartum home visits
- Teach signs, symptoms, and care of common problems (i.e., engorgement, sore nipples, candidiasis); instruct to contact primary care provider if stasis lasts more than 48 hr or if mastitis symptoms occur (i.e., chills, fever $> 104°F$ [40°C])

BREASTFEEDING, INTERRUPTED

(1992) **Domain 7, Role Relationships; Class 1, Caregiving Roles**

Definition: Break in the continuity of the breastfeeding process as a result of inability or inadvisability to put baby to breast for feeding.

Defining Characteristics

Subjective

Maternal desire to maintain lactation and provide (or eventually provide) her breast milk for her infant's nutritional needs

Objective

Deficient knowledge about expression or storage of breast milk
Infant receives no nourishment at the breast for some or all of feedings
Separation of mother and child

Related Factors

Abrupt weaning of infant
Contraindications to breastfeeding
[Engorgement]

Maternal employment [obligations outside the home]

[Maternal medications that are contraindicated for the infant]
Maternal or infant illness
[Prematurity]
[Sore or cracked nipples]

Suggestions for Use

Because this diagnosis represents a situation rather than a response, there is little the nurse can do to correct the interruption (e.g., the need for the mother to work). Therefore, this label might function best as an etiology (e.g., *Risk for ineffective breastfeeding related to Interrupted breastfeeding secondary to mother's employment*). Also see Suggestions for Use for Ineffective Breastfeeding.

Suggested Alternative Diagnoses

Breastfeeding, ineffective
[Breastfeeding, risk for ineffective]
Infant feeding pattern, ineffective

NOC Outcomes

Breastfeeding Maintenance: Continuation of breastfeeding from establishment to weaning for nourishment of an infant or toddler
Breastfeeding Weaning: Progressive discontinuation of breastfeeding
Knowledge: Breastfeeding: Extent of understanding conveyed about lactation and nourishment of infant through breastfeeding
Parent–Infant Attachment: Parent and infant behaviors that demonstrate an enduring affectionate bond

Goals/Evaluation Criteria

Examples Using NOC Language

- Mother and baby will not experience Interrupted breastfeeding, as evidenced by substantial Breastfeeding Knowledge, Breastfeeding Maintenance, and consistently demonstrated Parent–Infant Attachment.
- Mother and baby will demonstrate **Breastfeeding Maintenance**, as evidenced by the following indicators (specify 1–5: not, slightly, moderately, substantially, or totally adequate):
    - Infant's growth and development in normal range
    - Recognition of signs of decreased milk supply
    - Perceived support for continuation of lactation on return to work or school

Mother's ability to safely collect and store breast milk, if desired
Child care provider's ability to safely thaw, warm, and feed stored breast milk

Other Examples

- Mother and infant will maintain effective breastfeeding for as long as desired

Mother will:

- Choose and demonstrate preferred technique for expression of milk
- Describe safe storage techniques for expressed milk
- Maintain lactation

Baby will:

- Receive mother's milk unless contraindicated (e.g., by certain maternal drugs)
- Gain ________________ g/day or ________________ g/week

NIC Interventions

Anticipatory Guidance: Preparation of patient for an anticipated developmental and/or situational crisis

Attachment Promotion: Facilitation of the development of the parent–infant relationship

Bottle Feeding: Preparation and administration of fluids to an infant via a bottle

Environmental Management: Attachment Process: Manipulation of the patient's surroundings to facilitate the development of the parent–infant relationship

Lactation Counseling: Use of an interactive helping process to assist in maintenance of successful breastfeeding

Nursing Activities

In general, nursing actions for this diagnosis focus on providing motivation and support for continued breastfeeding, or teaching to facilitate the transition to bottle feeding.

Assessments

- Assess family's ability to support lactation and breastfeeding plan and cope with lifestyle changes
- Assess mother's desire and motivation to continue breastfeeding
- Confirm readiness for transition to breast after interruption (e.g., infant's stability when outside the Isolette; infant's coordination of sucking, swallowing, and breathing; mother's willingness to try)

B

- When the etiology is infant illness or prematurity, consider a feeding flow sheet to facilitate assessment: Document infant's state, oxygen needs, positioning, time at breast, total nursing time, daily weight, stool pattern
- *(NIC) Bottle Feeding*:
  - Determine water source used to dilute concentrated or powdered formula
  - Determine fluoride content of water used to dilute concentrated or powdered formula and refer for fluoride supplementation, if indicated
  - Monitor infant weight, as appropriate

Patient/Family Teaching

- Assist working mother to maintain lactation by including the following teaching:
  - Provide information about lactation and breast milk expression (with manual and electric pump), collection, and storage
  - Display and demonstrate variety of breast pumps, providing information about costs, effectiveness, and availability of each
  - Educate infant caretaker on topics such as storage and thawing of breast milk and avoidance of bottle feedings in the 2 hr prior to mother's return home
  - Provide information to enhance milk volume on topics such as adequate rest, regular expression of milk, and increase in mother's intake of fluid, especially toward the end of the work week
- If bottle feeding becomes necessary, teach parents how to prepare, store, warm, and feed formula
- *(NIC) Bottle Feeding*: Caution parent or caregiver about using microwave oven to warm formula
- If weaning is necessary, inform mother about return of ovulation and about appropriate contraceptive measures

Other

- Assist mother in setting realistic goals for herself
- Encourage continued feeding of breast milk on return to work or school
- Assist mother and premature infant with transition to breast:
  - Encourage skin-to-skin contact for mother and infant, using cover blanket over infant to maintain body temperature
  - Help infant open mouth wider
  - Position baby with one hand supporting head, leaving the other hand free to manipulate breast; ear, shoulder, and hips of infant should be aligned so that mother's nipples do not become sore

Provide privacy

- Assist working mother to maintain lactation and effective breastfeeding:
  - A few days before mother's return to work, introduce baby to bottle in different situations: someone other than mother presents bottle, mother is not present, baby is hungry, in a different place than usual for breastfeeding
  - Develop schedule for expression and storage of milk at work
  - Establish support network to ensure that mother has help with day-to-day lactation and breastfeeding problems as they occur
  - Provide anticipatory guidance for potential problems (e.g., engorgement, pain, leaking, diminished milk production, feelings of disappointment and anger, depression, guilt, inadequacy)
  - Allow infant, once latched on, to nurse until sucking and swallowing stop; switch baby to other breast and repeat until suck or swallow stops, then switch back. Time at breast will be longer than at bottle, but not to the point of infant's exhaustion.
- If abrupt weaning is necessary, assist mother to:
  - Introduce bottle feeding
  - Manage breast discomfort (e.g., ice packs to axillary area; breast binder; supportive, well-fitting bra; avoiding breast stimulation)
  - Verbalize feelings about sudden change in plans

Home Care

See Effective Breastfeeding.

BREASTFEEDING, READINESS FOR ENHANCED

(1990, 2010) **Domain 7, Role Relationships; Class 1, Caregiving Roles**

Definition: A pattern of proficiency and satisfaction of the mother–infant dyad that is sufficient to support the breastfeeding process and can be strengthened

Defining Characteristics

Subjective

Maternal verbalization of satisfaction with the breastfeeding process

Objective

Mother able to position infant at breast to promote a successful latch-on response

Adequate infant elimination patterns for age

Appropriate infant weight pattern for age
Eagerness of infant to nurse
Effective mother–infant communication patterns [e.g., infant cues, maternal interpretation or response]
Infant content after feeding
Regular and sustained suckling and swallowing at breast
Signs and symptoms of oxytocin release [letdown or milk ejection reflex]

Related Factors

Basic breastfeeding knowledge
Infant gestational age greater than 34 weeks
Maternal confidence
Normal breast structure
Normal infant oral structure
Support source

Suggestions for Use

This is a wellness diagnosis; therefore, it is not necessary to write it with an etiology (related factors). It represents a clinical judgment that breastfeeding is progressing satisfactorily and that there are no risk factors for *Ineffective breastfeeding*. During the first few days after childbirth, the nursing focus is to prevent or eliminate risk factors that might cause *Ineffective breastfeeding*. It is probably too soon, during that time, to conclude that there are no problems or risk factors, so a better choice might be *Risk for ineffective breastfeeding*. For mothers who are satisfied and proficient at breastfeeding, but who wish to be even more so, Carpenito-Moyet (2010) recommends using a non-NANDA diagnosis of *Readiness for enhanced breastfeeding* instead of *Effective breastfeeding*.

Suggested Alternative Diagnoses

Ineffective breastfeeding, risk for
[Potential for Enhanced Breastfeeding]

NOC Outcomes

Breastfeeding Establishment: Infant: Infant attachment to and sucking from the mother's breast for nourishment during the first 3 weeks of breastfeeding

Breastfeeding Establishment: Maternal: Maternal establishment of proper attachment of an infant to and sucking from the breast for nourishment during the first 3 weeks of breastfeeding

Breastfeeding Maintenance: Continuation of breastfeeding from establishment to weaning for nourishment of an infant/toddler

Breastfeeding Weaning: Progressive discontinuation of breastfeeding of an infant/toddler

Goals/Evaluation Criteria

Examples Using NOC Language

See Ineffective Breastfeeding.

Other Examples

- Mother and infant will establish and maintain breastfeeding for as long as desired
- Infant will demonstrate correct:
  - Alignment and areolar grasp
  - Latching-on technique and tongue placement
  - Suck and audible swallow
- Mother will:
  - Recognize early hunger cues
  - State satisfaction with breastfeeding
  - Experience no nipple tenderness
  - Verbalize knowledge of signs of decreased milk supply
  - Explain how to safely collect and store breast milk

NIC Interventions

Breastfeeding Assistance: Preparing a new mother to breastfeed her infant

Lactation Counseling: Use of an interactive helping process to assist in maintenance of successful breastfeeding

Lactation Suppression: Facilitating the cessation of milk production and minimizing breast engorgement after giving birth

Nursing Activities

Assessments

- Observe for correct breastfeeding technique
- *(NIC) Breastfeeding Assistance*:
  - Monitor infant's ability to suck
  - Monitor infant's ability to grasp the nipple correctly (i.e., latch-on skills)
  - Monitor skin integrity of nipples
  - Monitor letdown reflex

Patient/Family Teaching

B

- Discuss breastfeeding schedule, usually a "demand" time every $1^1/_2$–3 hr
- Instruct mother in usual breastfeeding norms (e.g., increased frequency of nursing in first weeks of life, baby's elimination patterns, uterine contractions during nursing)
- Provide anticipatory guidance for potential problems such as maternal fatigue; breast engorgement; sore, cracked nipples; multiple births
- Discuss ways to enhance milk supply:
  Drink plenty of fluids
  Get enough rest (e.g., between feedings)
  Nurse frequently
  Use alternate breast at start of each feeding
  Offer both breasts at each feeding
- *(NIC) Breastfeeding Assistance*:
  Assist parents in identifying infant arousal cues as opportunities to practice breastfeeding
  Encourage mother to allow infant to breastfeed as long as interested
  Inform mother of pump options available if needed to maintain lactation
  Encourage use of comfortable, cotton, supportive nursing bra
  Provide written materials to reinforce instructions at home

Collaborative Activities

- Make referrals to appropriate community resources, such as La Leche League, other nursing mothers, lactation consultant

Other

- Promote maternal confidence by providing positive feedback
- Provide opportunity to breast-feed within 1–2 hr after birth

Home Care

Assessments

- Assess breastfeeding technique within first 5–7 days after birth
- Confirm infant's elimination pattern
- Explore mother's breastfeeding plans, for example, duration, return to work, introduction of solid foods, weaning; provide anticipatory guidance

Patient/Family Teaching

- Discuss mother's need to check with physician prior to taking any medication while breastfeeding

B

- Provide instruction regarding breast engorgement, cracked/sore nipples, manual expression, infant appetite spurts, supplemental feedings

Collaborative Activities

- Encourage mother to enlist or request available resources for assistance (e.g., family, public health nurse, pediatrician, La Leche League, Nursing Mothers' Council)

Other

- Discuss impact of breastfeeding on family dynamics
- Discuss setting priorities that delegate meal preparation, increase mother's rest, and minimize care of the house
- Promote maternal confidence by providing encouragement, praise, and reassurance

BREATHING PATTERN, INEFFECTIVE

(1980, 1996, 1998, 2010) **Domain 4, Activity/Rest; Class 4, Cardiovascular/Pulmonary Responses**

Definition: Inspiration and/or expiration that does not provide adequate ventilation.

Defining Characteristics

Subjective

Dyspnea

Objective

Altered chest excursion
Assumption of three-point position
Bradypnea
Decreased inspiratory–expiratory pressure
Decreased minute ventilation
Decreased vital capacity
Alterations in depth of breathing (adults V_T 500 mL at rest, infants 6–8 mL/kg)
Increased anterior–posterior diameter
Nasal flaring
Orthopnea
Prolonged expiration phases
Pursed-lip breathing

Tachypnea
Use of accessory muscles to breathe
(Non-NANDA-I) Respiratory rate:
- Adults ages 14 or older: ≤11 or > 24 [breaths per minute]
- Ages 5–14: <15 or >25
- Ages 1–4: <20 or >30
- Infants: <25 or >60

Related Factors

Anxiety
Body position
Bony deformity
Chest wall deformity
Fatigue
Hyperventilation
Hypoventilation syndrome
Musculoskeletal impairment
Neurological damage
Neurological immaturity
Neuromuscular dysfunction
Obesity
Pain
Respiratory muscle fatigue
Spinal cord injury

Suggestions for Use

This label can be used for conditions such as hyperventilation, shallow breathing secondary to pain, or physiological dyspnea such as that which occurs as a side effect of some medications or diseases (e.g., asthma, allergic reaction). Do not use this label if the condition cannot be treated by independent nursing actions. Consider, too, that Ineffective breathing pattern may be a symptom of another more useful diagnosis, such as Anxiety; or it may be the etiology of another diagnosis, such as Activity intolerance. Differentiate carefully among this and the suggested alternative diagnoses. Also see Suggestions for Use for the diagnosis, Airway Clearance, Ineffective.

Suggested Alternative Diagnoses

Activity intolerance
Airway clearance, ineffective
Disuse Syndrome, risk for
Gas exchange, impaired

NOC Outcomes

Allergic Response: Systemic: Severity of systemic hypersensitive immune response to a specific environmental (exogenous) antigen

Mechanical Ventilation Response: Adult: Alveolar exchange and tissue perfusion are supported by mechanical ventilation

Mechanical Ventilation Weaning Response: Adult: Respiratory and psychological adjustment to progressive removal of mechanical ventilation

Respiratory Status: Airway Patency: Open, clear tracheobronchial passages for air exchange

Respiratory Status: Ventilation: Movement of air in and out of the lungs

Vital Signs: Extent to which temperature, pulse, respiration, and blood pressure are within normal range

Goals/Evaluation Criteria

Examples Using NOC Language

- Demonstrates effective breathing patterns, as evidenced by uncompromised Respiratory Status: Ventilation and Respiratory Status: Airway Patency; and no deviation from normal range in Vital Signs
- Demonstrates uncompromised **Respiratory Status: Ventilation**, as evidenced by the following indicators (specify 1–5: severely, substantially, moderately, mildly, or not compromised):
  Depth of inspiration and ease of breathing
  Symmetrical chest expansion
- Demonstrates uncompromised **Respiratory Status: Ventilation**, as evidenced by the following indicators (specify 1–5: severe, substantial, moderate, mild, or none)
  Accessory muscle use
  Adventitious breath sounds
  Orthopnea

Other Examples

Patient will:

- Demonstrate optimal breathing while on mechanical ventilator
- Have respiratory rate and rhythm within normal limits
- Have pulmonary function tests within normal limits for patient
- Request breathing assistance when needed
- Be able to describe plan for care at home
- Identify factors (e.g., allergens) that trigger ineffective breathing patterns and take measures to avoid them

NIC Interventions

Airway Management: Facilitation of patency of air passages

Airway Suctioning: Removal of airway secretions by inserting a suction catheter into the patient's oral airway or trachea

Allergy Management: Identification, treatment, and prevention of allergic responses to food, medications, insect bites, contrast material, blood, and other substances

Anaphylaxis Management: Promotion of adequate ventilation and tissue perfusion for an individual with a severe allergic (antigen–antibody) reaction

Artificial Airway Management: Maintenance of endotracheal and tracheostomy tubes and prevention of complications associated with their use

Asthma Management: Identification, treatment, and prevention of reactions to inflammation/constriction in the airway passages

Mechanical Ventilation Management: Invasive: Assisting the patient receiving artificial breathing support through a device inserted into the trachea

Mechanical Ventilatory Weaning: Assisting the patient to breathe without the aid of a mechanical ventilator

Respiratory Monitoring: Collection and analysis of patient data to ensure airway patency and adequate gas exchange

Ventilation Assistance: Promotion of an optimal spontaneous breathing pattern that maximizes oxygen and carbon dioxide exchange in the lungs

Vital Signs Monitoring: Collection and analysis of cardiovascular, respiratory, and body temperature data to determine and prevent complications

Nursing Activities

In general, nursing actions for this diagnosis focus on assessing for causes of Ineffective Breathing, monitoring respiratory status, teaching about self-management for allergies, coaching the patient to slow the breathing and to control his or her responses, assisting patients with respiratory treatments, and reassuring the patient during periods of dyspnea and shortness of breath.

Assessments

- Monitor for pallor and cyanosis
- Monitor effect of medications on respiratory status
- Determine location and extent of crepitus over rib cage
- Assess need for airway insertion
- Observe and document bilateral chest expansion of patient on ventilator
- *(NIC) Respiratory Monitoring*:
  Monitor rate, rhythm, depth, and effort of respirations

Note chest movement, watching for symmetry, use of accessory muscles, and supraclavicular and intercostal muscle retractions

Monitor for noisy respirations, such as crowing or snoring

Monitor breathing patterns: bradypnea, tachypnea, hyperventilation, Kussmaul respirations, Cheyne-Stokes respirations, apneustic breathing, Biot's respiration, and ataxic patterns

Note location of trachea

Auscultate breath sounds, noting areas of decreased/absent ventilation and presence of adventitious sounds

Monitor for increased restlessness, anxiety, and air hunger

Note changes in SaO_2, SvO_2, end-tidal CO_2, and arterial blood gas (ABG) values, as appropriate

Patient/Family Teaching

- Inform patient and family about relaxation techniques to improve breathing pattern; specify techniques
- Discuss the plan for care at home, including medications, supportive equipment, signs and symptoms of reportable complications, community resources
- Discuss ways of avoiding allergens, for example:
  - Check the home for mold in the walls
  - Do not use carpet on the floors
  - Use electrostatic filters on furnaces and air conditioners
- Teach how to cough effectively
- Inform patient and family that smoking is prohibited in room
- Instruct patient and family that they should notify the nurse at onset of ineffective breathing pattern

Collaborative Activities

- Confer with respiratory therapist to ensure adequate functioning of mechanical ventilator
- Report changes in sensorium, breath sounds, respiratory pattern, ABGs, sputum, and so forth, as needed or per protocols
- Administer medications (e.g., bronchodilators) per order or protocols
- Administer ultrasonic nebulizer treatments and humidified air or oxygen per order or agency protocols
- Give pain medications to allow optimal respiratory pattern, specify schedule

Other

- Correlate and document all assessment data (e.g., patient sensorium, breath sounds, respiratory pattern, ABGs, sputum, effect of medications)

- Help patient to use incentive spirometer, as needed
- Reassure patient during periods of respiratory distress
- Encourage slow abdominal breathing during periods of respiratory distress
- To help slow respiratory rate, coach to use pursed-lip and controlled breathing techniques
- Suction as needed to remove secretions
- Have patient turn, cough, and deep breathe q ______________
- Inform patient before beginning intended procedures, to lower anxiety and increase sense of control
- Maintain low-flow oxygen by nasal cannula, mask, hood, or tent; specify flow rate
- Position patient for optimal breathing; specify position
- Synchronize patient's breathing pattern with ventilator rate

Home Care

- If ventilator or other electrical equipment is being used, assess the home for electrical safety and notify the utility company so they can provide prompt service in case of power failure

For Infants and Children

- Remember that newborns are obligate nose-breathers; that their normal respirations are abdominal; and that because of their irregular respirations (also normal), you must count respirations for one full minute. A normal rate for newborns is 30–50 breaths per minute, and periods of apnea lasting up to 15 sec are normal
- To minimize the risk of sudden infant death syndrome (SIDS), infants should be placed on their back or side to sleep, rather than on their stomach
- Children continue to breathe abdominally until about age 5 years; and their smaller-diameter airways increase the risk of airway obstruction

For Older Adults

- Encourage to be as active as possible to increase ventilation

CARDIAC OUTPUT, DECREASED

(1975, 1996, 2000) Domain 4, Activity/Rest; Class 4, Cardiovascular/Pulmonary Responses

Definition: Inadequate blood pumped by the heart to meet metabolic demands of the body.

Defining Characteristics

Altered Heart Rate and Rhythm

Arrhythmias (tachycardia, bradycardia)
EKG changes
Palpitations

Altered Preload

Edema
Fatigue
Increased or decreased central venous pressure (CVP)
Increased or decreased pulmonary artery wedge pressure (PAWP)
Jugular vein distention
Murmurs
Weight gain

Altered Afterload

Cold and clammy skin
Decreased peripheral pulses
Dyspnea
Increased or decreased pulmonary vascular resistance (PVR)
Increased or decreased systemic vascular resistance (SVR)
Oliguria
Prolonged capillary refill
Skin color changes
Variations in blood pressure readings

Altered Contractility

Crackles
Cough
Orthopnea or paroxysmal nocturnal dyspnea
Decreased cardiac output
Decreased cardiac index
Decreased ejection fraction, stroke volume index (SVI), left ventricular stroke work index (LVSWI)
S_3 or S_4 sounds

Behavioral/Emotional

Anxiety
Restlessness

Related Factors

Altered heart rate or rhythm
Altered stroke volume
Altered preload
Altered afterload
Altered contractility

Non-NANDA International related factors:

Cardiac anomaly (specify)
Drug toxicity
Dysfunctional electrical conduction
Hypovolemia
Increased ventricular workload
Ventricular damage
Ventricular ischemia
Ventricular restriction

Suggestions for Use

This label does not suggest independent nursing actions. We include it because it is in the NANDA-I taxonomy, and many nurses do use it. However, the nurse can neither conclusively diagnose nor definitively treat this problem. For patients with physiologic decreased cardiac output, you may find it more useful to use a label that represents a human response to this pathophysiology (e.g., *Activity intolerance related to Decreased cardiac output*). If the patient is at risk for developing complications, we prefer to write them as collaborative problems (e.g., Potential complication of myocardial infarction: Cardiogenic shock).

Suggested Alternative Diagnoses

Activity intolerance
Self-care deficit

NOC Outcomes

Blood Loss Severity: Severity of internal or external bleeding/hemorrhage

Cardiac Pump Effectiveness: Adequacy of blood volume ejected from the left ventricle to support systemic perfusion pressure

Circulation Status: Unobstructed, unidirectional blood flow at an appropriate pressure through large vessels of the systemic and pulmonary circuits

Tissue Perfusion: Abdominal Organs: Adequacy of blood flow through the small vessels of the abdominal viscera to maintain organ function

Tissue Perfusion: Cardiac: Adequacy of blood flow through the coronary vasculature to maintain heart function

Tissue Perfusion: Cerebral: Adequacy of blood flow through the cerebral vasculature to maintain brain function

Tissue Perfusion: Cellular: Adequacy of blood flow through the vasculature to maintain function at the cellular level

Tissue Perfusion: Peripheral: Adequacy of blood flow through the small vessels of the extremities to maintain tissue function

Tissue Perfusion: Pulmonary: Adequacy of blood flow through pulmonary vasculature to perfuse alveoli/capillary unit

Vital Signs: Extent to which temperature, pulse, respiration, and blood pressure are within normal range

Goals/Evaluation Criteria

NOTE: The goals for *Decreased cardiac output* are not nurse sensitive. That is, nurses do not act independently to achieve them; collaborative efforts are necessary.

Examples Using NOC Language

- Demonstrates satisfactory cardiac output, as evidenced by Cardiac Pump Effectiveness; Circulation Status; Tissue Perfusion (Abdominal Organs, Cardiac, Cerebral, Cellular, Peripheral, and Pulmonary); and Vital Signs Status
- Demonstrates **Circulation Status**, as evidenced by the following indicators (specify 1–5: severe, substantial, moderate, mild, or no deviation from normal range):
  - Systolic, diastolic, and mean blood pressure (BP)
  - Right and left carotid pulse strength
  - Right and left [peripheral] pulse strengths [e.g., brachial, radial, femoral, pedal]
  - Central venous pressure and pulmonary wedge pressure
  - PaO_2 and $PaCO_2$
- Demonstrates **Circulation Status**, as evidenced by the following indicators (specify 1–5: severe, substantial, moderate, mild, or none):
  - Intermittent claudication
  - Neck vein distention
  - Peripheral edema
  - Ascites
  - Large-vessel bruits
  - Angina

Impaired cognition
Lower extremity ulcers

C

Other Examples

Patient will:

- Have cardiac index and ejection fraction within normal limits
- Have urine output, urine specific gravity, blood urea nitrogen (BUN), and plasma creatinine within normal limits
- Have normal skin color
- Demonstrate increasing tolerance for physical activity (e.g., without dyspnea, chest pain, or syncope)
- Describe the required diet, medications, activity, and limitations (e.g., for cardiac disease)
- Identify reportable signs and symptoms of worsening condition

NIC Interventions

Bleeding Reduction: Limitation of the loss of blood volume during an episode of bleeding

Cardiac Care: Limitation of complications resulting from an imbalance between myocardial oxygen supply and demand for a patient with symptoms of impaired cardiac function

Cardiac Care, Acute: Limitation of complications for a patient recently experiencing an episode of an imbalance between myocardial oxygen supply and demand resulting in impaired cardiac function

Cerebral Perfusion Promotion: Promotion of adequate perfusion and limitation of complications for a patient experiencing or at risk for inadequate cerebral perfusion

Circulatory Care: Arterial Insufficiency: Promotion of arterial circulation

Circulatory Care: Mechanical Assist Device: Temporary support of the circulation through the use of mechanical devices or pumps

Circulatory Care: Venous Insufficiency: Promotion of venous circulation

Embolus Care: Peripheral: Limitation of complications for a patient experiencing, or at risk for, occlusion of peripheral circulation

Embolus Care: Pulmonary: Limitation of complications for a patient experiencing, or at risk for, occlusion of pulmonary circulation

Hemodynamic Regulation: Optimization of heart rate, preload, afterload, and contractility

Hemorrhage Control: Reduction or elimination of rapid and excessive blood loss

Intravenous (IV) Therapy: Administration and monitoring of IV fluids and medications

Lower Extremity Monitoring: Collection, analysis, and use of patient data to categorize risk and prevent injury to the lower extremities

Neurologic Monitoring: Collection and analysis of patient data to prevent or minimize neurologic complications

Shock Management: Cardiac: Promotion of adequate tissue perfusion for a patient with severely compromised pumping function of the heart

Shock Management: Volume: Promotion of adequate tissue perfusion for a patient with severely compromised intravascular volume

Vital Signs Monitoring: Collection and analysis of cardiovascular, respiratory, and body temperature data to determine and prevent complications

Nursing Activities

In general, nursing actions for this diagnosis focus on monitoring for signs and symptoms of decreased cardiac output, assessing for underlying causes (e.g., hypovolemia, dysrhythmias), instituting protocols or medical orders to treat decreased cardiac output, and providing supportive measures such as positioning and hydration.

Assessments

- Assess and document BP, presence of cyanosis, respiratory status, and mental status
- Monitor for signs of fluid overload (e.g., dependent edema, weight gain)
- Assess patient's activity tolerance by noting onset of shortness of breath, pain, palpitations, or dizziness
- Evaluate patient's responses to oxygen therapy
- Assess for cognitive impairment
- *(NIC) Hemodynamic Regulation*:

  Monitor pacemaker functioning, if appropriate

  Monitor peripheral pulses, capillary refill, and temperature and color of extremities

  Monitor intake and output, urine output, and patient weight, as appropriate

  Monitor systemic and pulmonary vascular resistance, as appropriate

  Auscultate lung sounds for crackles or other adventitious sounds

  Monitor and document heart rate, rhythm, and pulses

Patient/Family Teaching

- Explain purpose of administering oxygen per nasal cannula or mask
- Instruct regarding maintenance of accurate intake and output

- Teach use, dose, frequency, and side effects of medications
- Teach to report and describe palpitations and pain onset, duration, precipitating factors, site, quality, and intensity
- Instruct patient and family in plan for care at home, including activity limitations, diet restrictions, and use of therapeutic equipment
- Provide information on stress-reduction techniques such as biofeedback, progressive muscle relaxation, meditation, and exercise
- Teach the need to weigh daily

Collaborative Activities

- Confer with physician regarding parameters for administering or withholding BP medications
- Administer and titrate antiarrhythmic, inotropic, nitroglycerin, and vasodilator medications to maintain contractility, preload, and afterload per medical order or protocols
- Administer anticoagulants to prevent peripheral thrombus formation, per order or protocol
- Promote afterload reduction (e.g., with intraaortic balloon pumping) per medical order or protocol
- Make referrals to advanced practice nurse for follow-up, as needed
- Consider referrals to case manager, social worker, or community and home health services
- Refer to social worker to evaluate ability to pay for prescription medications
- Refer for cardiac rehabilitation as appropriate

Other

- Change patient's position to flat or Trendelenburg when BP is in a range lower than normal for patient
- For sudden, severe, or prolonged hypotension, establish IV access for administration of IV fluids or medications to raise BP
- Correlate effects of laboratory values, oxygen, medications, activity, anxiety, and pain on the dysrhythmia
- Do not take rectal temperatures
- Turn patient every 2 hr or maintain other appropriate or required activity to decrease peripheral circulation stasis
- *(NIC) Hemodynamic Regulation*:
  Minimize or eliminate environmental stressors
  Insert urinary catheter, if appropriate

C

Home Care

- Assist in obtaining home services for activities of daily living, meal preparation, housekeeping, transportation for physician visits, and so forth
- Assess for barriers to compliance with treatment regimens (e.g., side effects of medications)
- Help client and family to plan for emergencies, such as power failure (if using respiratory support devices) or the need for cardiopulmonary resuscitation
- Be sure the client has a scale at home to check daily weights

For Older Adults

- Be aware that older adults often have jaw pain—or even no pain at all—with a myocardial infarction
- Be aware that older adults may have decreased liver and kidney function; be sure to assess for side effects from cardiac medications
- Observe for signs and symptoms of arrhythmias (e.g., dizziness, weakness, syncope, palpitations)
- Assess for signs of depression and social isolation; refer for mental health care if needed
- Assess for understanding of and compliance with medications and other treatments (e.g., activity, diet). Older adults may need frequent repetition and reinforcement of teaching
- Frail elderly may need case management to continue independent living

CAREGIVER ROLE STRAIN

(1992, 1998, 2000) **Domain 7, Role Relationships; Class 1, Caregiving Roles**

Definition: Difficulty in performing family/significant other caregiver role.

Defining Characteristics

Caregiving Activities

Apprehension about care receiver's care if caregiver unable to provide care
Apprehension about possible institutionalization of care receiver

Apprehension about the future regarding care receiver's health
Apprehension about the future regarding caregiver's ability to provide care
Difficulty performing or completing required tasks
C Dysfunctional change in caregiving activities
Preoccupation with care routine

Caregiver Health Status

Physical

Cardiovascular disease
Diabetes
Fatigue
Gastrointestinal upset (e.g., mild stomach cramps, vomiting, diarrhea, recurrent gastric ulcer episodes)
Headaches
Hypertension
Rash
Weight change

Emotional

Anger
Disturbed sleep
Feeling depressed
Frustration
Impaired individual coping
Impatience
Increased emotional lability
Increased nervousness
Lack of time to meet personal needs
Somatization
Stress

Socioeconomic

Alienation from others
Changes in leisure activities
Low work productivity
Refuses career advancement
Withdraws from social life

Caregiver–Care Receiver Relationship

Difficulty watching care receiver go through the illness
Grief or uncertainty regarding changed relationship with care receiver

Family Processes

Concerns about family members
Family conflict

Related Factors/Risk Factors

Care Receiver Health Status

Addiction or codependency
Illness chronicity
Illness severity
Increasing care needs and dependency
Instability of care receiver's health
Problem behaviors
Psychological or cognitive problems
Unpredictability of illness course

Caregiving Activities

24-hr care responsibilities
Amount of activities
Complexity of activities
Discharge of family members to home with significant care needs
Ongoing changes in activities
Unpredictability of care situation
Years of caregiving

Caregiver Health Status

Addiction or codependency
Inability to fulfill one's own or other's expectations
Marginal coping patterns
Physical problems
Psychological or cognitive problems
Unrealistic expectations of self

Socioeconomic

Alienation from family, friends, and coworkers
Competing role commitments
Insufficient recreation
Isolation from others

Caregiver–Care Receiver Relationship

History of poor relationship
Mental status of elder inhibiting conversation
Presence of abuse or violence
Unrealistic expectations of caregiver by care receiver

Family Processes

History of family dysfunction
History of marginal family coping

Resources

Assistance and support (formal and informal)
Caregiver is not developmentally ready for caregiver role
C Emotional strength
Inadequate community resources (e.g., respite services, recreational resources)
Inadequate equipment for providing care
Inadequate physical environment for providing care (e.g., housing, temperature, safety)
Inadequate transportation
Inexperience with caregiving
Insufficient finances
Insufficient time
Lack of caregiver privacy
Lack of knowledge about or difficulty accessing community resources
Lack of support
Physical energy

Suggestions for Use

Caregiver role strain focuses on the burden of the individual caregiver who has had to assume the care of a family member. It may affect the physical and/or mental health of the caregiver and the family. The family diagnoses (*Family coping* and *Interrupted family processes*) focus on the family system and the manner in which family functioning has been altered by a stressor. The stressor in those diagnoses is not necessarily the need to care for a family member. Differentiate between *Caregiver role strain* and *Chronic sorrow*, which caregivers may experience when a loved one has a serious chronic disability. If no defining characteristics exist, but risk factors are present, use *Risk for caregiver role strain.*

Suggested Alternative Diagnoses

Caregiver role strain, risk for
Coping: family, compromised
Coping: family, disabled
Coping, ineffective
Family processes, interrupted
Therapeutic regimen management: family, ineffective
Sorrow, chronic

NOC Outcomes

Caregiver Emotional Health: Emotional well-being of a family care provider while caring for a family member

Caregiver Lifestyle Disruption: Severity of disturbances in the lifestyle of a family member due to caregiving

Caregiver–Patient Relationship: Positive interactions and connections between the caregiver and care recipient

Caregiver Performance: Direct Care: Provision by family care provider of appropriate personal and health care for a family member

Caregiver Performance: Indirect Care: Arrangement and oversight by family care provider of appropriate care for a family member

Caregiver Physical Health: Physical well-being of a family care provider while caring for a family member

Caregiver Role Endurance: Factors that promote family care provider's capacity to sustain caregiving over an extended period of time

Caregiver Well-Being: Extent of positive perception of primary care provider's health status and life circumstances

Parenting Performance: Parental actions to provide a child a nurturing and constructive physical, emotional, and social environment

Role Performance: Congruence of an individual's role behavior with role expectations

Goals/Evaluation Criteria

Examples Using NOC Language

- Experiences relief from *Caregiver role strain*, as demonstrated by adequacy of Caregiver Emotional Health, Caregiver–Patient Relationship, Caregiver Performance: Direct and Indirect Care, Caregiver Physical Health, Caregiver Role Endurance, Caregiver Well-Being, Parenting Performance, and Role Performance
- Demonstrates **Caregiver Emotional Health**, as evidenced by the following indicators (specify 1–5: severely, substantially, moderately, mildly, or not compromised):

  Satisfaction with life

  Sense of control and self-esteem

  Perceived spiritual well-being
- Demonstrates **Caregiver Emotional Health**, as evidenced by the following indicators (specify 1–5: severe, substantial, moderate, mild, none):
- Anger, resentfulness, guilt, depression, frustration, perceived burden, and ambivalence concerning situation

Other Examples

Caregiver will:

- Verbalize knowledge of treatment regimen and procedures, follow-up care, and emergency care

- Verbalize knowledge of how to obtain and operate needed equipment and assistance
- Verbalize feeling supported

- Express willingness to assume caregiving role
- Ensure provision of appropriate level of care
- Balance competing family and personal needs
- Identify changes that could be made to relieve some of his or her burden and decrease stressors
- Identify and use personal strengths, social supports, and community resources

NIC Interventions

Anticipatory Guidance: Preparation of patient for an anticipated developmental and/or situational crisis

Attachment Promotion: Facilitation of the development of the parent–infant relationship

Caregiver Support: Provision of the necessary information, advocacy, and support to facilitate primary patient care by someone other than a health care professional

Consultation: Using expert knowledge to work with those who seek help in problem solving to enable individuals, families, groups, or agencies to achieve identified goals

Coping Enhancement: Assisting a patient to adapt to perceived stressors, changes, or threats that interfere with meeting life demands and roles

Decision-Making Support: Providing information and support for a patient who is making a decision regarding health care

Energy Management: Regulating energy use to treat or prevent fatigue and optimize function

Health System Guidance: Facilitating a patient's location and use of appropriate health services

Nutrition Management: Assisting with or providing a balanced dietary intake of foods and fluids

Parenting Promotion: Providing parenting information, support, and coordination of comprehensive services to high-risk families

Respite Care: Provision of short-term care to provide relief for family caregiver

Role Enhancement: Assisting a patient, significant other, and family to improve relationships by clarifying and supplementing specific role behaviors

Teaching: Disease Process: Assisting the patient to understand information related to a specific disease process

Teaching: Individual: Planning, implementation, and evaluation of a teaching program designed to address a patient's particular needs

Teaching: Prescribed Diet: Preparing a patient to correctly follow a prescribed diet

Teaching: Prescribed Medication: Preparing a patient to safely take prescribed medications and monitor for their effects

Nursing Activities

In general, nursing actions for this diagnosis focus on assessing for contributing factors, providing emotional support and encouragement, helping the family to evaluate the situation realistically, and providing teaching and referrals as needed.

Assessments

- Assess care receiver for signs of emotional or physical neglect or abuse
- Assess caregiver for signs of increasing role strain (e.g., depression, anxiety, increased use or abuse of alcohol or drugs, frustration, helplessness, sleeplessness, lowered morale, physical or emotional exhaustion, and personal health problems)
- Assess effects of caregiving responsibilities on personal and family life
- *(NIC) Caregiver Support*:

  Determine caregiver's level of knowledge

  Determine caregiver's acceptance of role

  Monitor family interaction problems related to care of patient

Patient/Family Teaching

- Acknowledge and teach that the work of the caregiver is both physical and mental and includes (Bowers, 1987):

  Anticipatory caregiving (making decisions based on possible future needs of care receiver, e.g., place of residence)

  Instrumental caregiving (direct, hands-on care)

  Preventive caregiving (taking action to prevent illness, injury, or complications, e.g., altering the physical environment, preparing meals)

  Protective caregiving (protecting care receiver from threats to self-image, identity, and change in relationship with caregiver)

  Supervisory caregiving (arranging for and monitoring care, e.g., making appointments, arranging transportation)

- Facilitate coping and adjustment by teaching caregiver and care receiver how to (Chilman, Nunnally, & Cox, 1988):

  Deal with pain, incapacitation, and illness-related symptoms

  Deal with hospital environment and disease-related treatments and procedures

  Establish and maintain workable relationships with the health care team

- *(NIC) Caregiver Support*:
    Teach caregiver stress management techniques
    Educate caregiver about the grieving process

C

Collaborative Activities

- Refer as needed for counseling and support during times of stress or crisis
- Refer for necessary assistance with preventive, supervisory, and instrumental caregiving (e.g., Visiting Nurse Association, respite care, hospice care, day treatment, secondary caregivers)
- Report to authorities signs of care receiver physical or emotional neglect or abuse

Other

- Assist caregiver to identify problems or concerns with caregiving (e.g., lack of knowledge, skill, and emotional readiness for caregiving; lack of social support; financial burden; disruptive behavior; increasing need for physical care)
- Develop a plan of care with caregiver that identifies coping mechanisms, personal strengths, social supports, and acknowledged limitations. Consider including the following:
    Assistance with household tasks
    Family therapy
    Self-help and mutual support groups for information, advocacy, and emotional support
- Explore with caregiver the possibility of institutional care (now or in the future) and feelings associated with institutionalization
- Explore with caregiver–care receiver past and current closeness, shared activities, and confiding in one another as indications of emotional investment and commitment to the caregiver role
- Facilitate family's adjustment to illness of family member by assisting them to (Chilman, Nunnally, & Cox, 1988):
    Develop flexibility regarding future goals
    Grieve for the loss of preillness family identity
    Maintain a sense of mastery over their lives
    Move toward acceptance of changes
    Pull together during short-term crisis
- Validate the caregiver's feelings
- *(NIC) Caregiver Support:*
    Accept expressions of negative emotion
    Act for caregiver if overburdening becomes apparent

C

Home Care

- At every visit, evaluate the quality of care being given and the quality of the caregiver–patient relationship. This includes an assessment of the caregiver's skills and abilities to provide care
- Refer to home health agency for home health aide services for activities of daily living and housekeeping
- Explore the need for adult day care as appropriate
- Monitor for worsening of the client's condition that might require institutionalization
- Assess for safety of the client in the home setting

For Infants and Children

- Assess parent's understanding of the child's illness and needs for care
- Arrange for parent(s) of chronically ill child to receive training in areas of child development and education and compliance-related behavior problems
- Encourage parents to meet the needs of well siblings (e.g., they may be angry, embarrassed, jealous of attention to the ill sibling)
- Suggest ways to help siblings adapt (e.g., include them in family decisions when possible, adhere to usual family routines, spend time alone with them, and encourage activities with their friends)

For Older Adults

- Monitor caregiver for signs of depression
- Maintain consistency of caregivers as much as possible, but divide workload among family members to prevent overburdening the primary caregiver
- Assess for safety needs

CAREGIVER ROLE STRAIN, RISK FOR

(1992, 2010) **Domain 7, Role Relationships; Class 1, Caregiving Roles**

Definition: At risk for caregiver vulnerability for felt difficulty in performing the family caregiver role.

Risk Factors

Objective

Amount of caregiving tasks

Care receiver exhibits deviant or bizarre behavior

Caregiver health impairment
Caregiver is female
Caregiver is not developmentally ready for caregiver role (e.g., a young adult needing to provide care for middle-aged care receiver)
Caregiver is spouse
Caregiver's competing role commitments
Codependency
Complexity and amount of caregiving tasks
Developmental delay of the care receiver or caregiver
Discharge of family member with significant home care needs
Duration of caregiving required
Family isolation
Illness severity of the care receiver
Inadequate physical environment for providing care (e.g., housing, transportation, community services, equipment)
Inexperience with caregiving
Lack of respite and recreation for caregiver
Marginal caregiver's coping patterns
Marginal family adaptation or dysfunction prior to the caregiving situation
Past history of poor relationship between caregiver and care receiver
Premature birth
Presence of abuse or violence
Presence of situational stressors that normally affect families (e.g., significant loss, disaster, or crisis; economic vulnerability; major life events)
Psychological problems in caregiver
Psychological or cognitive problems in care receiver
Substance abuse
Unpredictable illness course or instability in the care receiver's health

Suggestions for Use

See Caregiver Role Strain.

Suggested Alternative Diagnoses

Coping: family, compromised
Coping: family, disabled
Family processes, interrupted
Therapeutic regimen management: family, ineffective

NOC Outcomes

Also see Caregiver Role Strain.

Caregiver Home Care Readiness: Preparedness of a caregiver to assume responsibility for the health care of a family member in the home

Caregiver Performance: Direct Care: Provision by family care provider of appropriate personal and health care for a family member

Caregiver Performance: Indirect Care: Arrangement and oversight by family care provider of appropriate care for a family member

Caregiver Role Endurance: Factors that promote family care provider's capacity to sustain caregiving over an extended period of time

Caregiver Stressors: Severity of biopsychosocial pressure on a family care provider caring for another over an extended period of time

Parenting Performance: Parental actions to provide a child a nurturing and constructive physical, emotional, and social environment

Goals/Evaluation Criteria

Examples Using NOC Language

- Does not experience Caregiver role strain, as demonstrated by adequacy of Caregiver Emotional Health, Caregiver Home Care Readiness, Caregiver Physical Health, Caregiver Stressors, Caregiving Endurance Potential, and Parenting Performance
- Also see Caregiver Role Strain.

Other Examples

See Caregiver Role Strain.

NIC Interventions

Caregiver Support: Provision of the necessary information, advocacy, and support to facilitate primary patient care by someone other than a health care professional

Coping Enhancement: Assisting a patient to adapt to perceived stressors, changes, or threats that interfere with meeting life demands and roles

Energy Management: Regulating energy use to treat or prevent fatigue and optimize function

Family Involvement Promotion: Facilitating family participation in the emotional and physical care of the patient

Parent Education: Adolescent: Assisting parents to understand and help their adolescent children

Parent Education: Childrearing Family: Assisting parents to understand and promote the physical, psychological, and social growth and development of their toddler, preschool, or school-aged child or children

Parent Education: Infant: Instruction on nurturing and physical care needed during the first year of life

Parenting Promotion: Providing parenting information, support, and coordination of comprehensive services to high-risk families

Respite Care: Provision of short-term care to provide relief for family caregiver

Nursing Activities

In general, nursing actions for this diagnosis focus on assessing for risk factors associated with *Caregiver role strain*, teaching about the needs of the ill family member, identifying the needs of the caregiver, and providing assistance and referrals for support to prevent *Caregiver role strain*.

Assessments

- Assess caregiver's level of knowledge of medical and care regimen
- Determine caregiver's desire for and acceptance of role
- See Assessments for Caregiver Role Strain.

Patient/Family Teaching

- See Patient and Family Teaching for Caregiver Role Strain.

Collaborative Activities

- See Collaborative Activities for Caregiver Role Strain.

Other

- See Other activities for Caregiver Role Strain.

CHILDBEARING PROCESS, INEFFECTIVE

(2010)

Domain 8, Sexuality; Class 3, Reproduction

Definition: Pregnancy and childbirth process and care of the newborn* that does not match the environmental context, norms, and expectations

Defining Characteristics

During Pregnancy

Subjective

Does not report appropriate physical preparations

Does not report appropriate prenatal lifestyle (e.g., nutrition, elimination, sleep, bodily movement, exercise, personal hygiene)

Does not report availability of support systems

Does not report managing unpleasant symptoms in pregnancy

Does not report realistic birth plan

*The original Japanese term for *childbearing* . . . encompasses both childbirth and rearing of the neonate. It is one of the main concepts of Japanese midwifery.

Objective

Does not access support systems appropriately

Does not seek necessary knowledge (e.g., of labor and delivery, newborn care)

Failure to prepare necessary newborn care items

Inconsistent prenatal health visits

Lack of prenatal visits

Lack of respect for unborn baby

During Labor and Delivery

Subjective

Does not report availability of support systems

Does not report lifestyle (e.g., diet, elimination, sleep, bodily movement, personal hygiene) that is appropriate for the stage of labor

Objective

Does not access support systems appropriately

Does not demonstrate attachment behavior to the newborn baby

Does not report appropriate postpartum lifestyle (e.g., nutrition, elimination, sleep, bodily movement, exercise, personal hygiene)

Does not report availability of support systems

Does not respond appropriately to onset of labor

Lacks proactivity during labor and delivery

After Birth

Objective

Does not access support systems appropriately

Does not demonstrate appropriate baby feeding techniques

Does not demonstrate appropriate breast care

Does not demonstrate attachment behavior to the baby

Does not demonstrate basic baby care techniques

Does not provide safe environment for the baby

Related Factors

Deficient knowledge (e.g., of labor and delivery, newborn care)

Domestic violence

Inconsistent prenatal health visits

Lack of appropriate role models for parenthood

Lack of cognitive readiness for parenthood

Lack of maternal confidence

Lack of prenatal health visits

Lack of a realistic birth plan

Lack of a sufficient support system

Maternal powerlessness
Maternal psychological distress
Suboptimal maternal nutrition

Substance abuse
Unplanned pregnancy
Unsafe environment
Unwanted pregnancy

Suggestions for Use

Some of the defining characteristics for this diagnosis may also function as risk factors for *Risk for impaired attachment* or be symptoms of impaired attachment. *Ineffective Childbearing Process* is a broader diagnosis that relates to the overall pregnancy (knowledge, nutrition, prenatal visits), not just to the parent–infant relationship.

Suggested Alternative Diagnoses

Childbearing process: Ineffective, risk for
Impaired attachment, risk for

NOC Outcomes

NOC outcomes have not yet been linked to this diagnosis; however, the following may be useful:

Knowledge: Infant Care: Extent of understanding conveyed about caring for a baby from birth to first birthday

Knowledge: Labor and Delivery: Extent of understanding conveyed about labor and vaginal delivery

Knowledge: Postpartum Maternal Health: Extent of understanding conveyed about maternal health in the period following birth of an infant

Knowledge: Preconception Maternal Health: Extent of understanding conveyed about maternal health prior to conception to ensure a healthy pregnancy

Knowledge: Pregnancy: Extent of understanding conveyed about promotion of a healthy pregnancy and prevention of complications

Maternal Status: Antepartum: Extent to which maternal well-being is within normal limits from conception to the onset of labor

Maternal Status: Intrapartum: Extent to which maternal well-being is within normal limits from onset of labor to delivery

Maternal Status: Postpartum: Extent to which maternal well-being is within normal limits from delivery of placenta to completion of involution

Parent–Infant Attachment: Parent and infant behaviors that demonstrate an enduring affectionate bond

Postpartum Maternal Health Behavior: Personal actions to promote health of a mother in the period following birth of infant

Prenatal Health Behavior: Personal actions to promote a healthy pregnancy and a healthy newborn

Goals/Evaluation Criteria

Examples Using NOC Language

- Demonstrates effective childbearing process, as evidenced by moderate to extensive Knowledge: Infant care, Labor and Delivery, Postpartum Maternal Health, Preconception Maternal Health, Pregnancy, and Pregnancy and Postpartum Sexual Functioning
- Demonstrates effective childbearing process, as evidenced by no deviation from normal range for Maternal Status: Antepartum, Maternal Status: Intrapartum, Maternal Status: Postpartum, Parent–Infant Attachment, Postpartum Maternal Health Behavior, and Prenatal health behavior
- Demonstrates **Knowledge: Infant Care**, as evidenced by the following indicators (specify 1–5: no, limited, moderate, substantial, or extensive knowledge):

  Normal infant characteristics
  Proper holding of infant
  Pros and cons of infant feeding choices
- Demonstrates **Knowledge: Labor and Delivery**, as evidenced by the following indicators (specify 1–5: no, limited, moderate, substantial, or extensive knowledge):

  Birthing options
  Signs and symptoms of labor
  Effective breathing techniques
  Effective positioning techniques

Other Examples

See *Childbearing process, readiness for enhanced.*

NIC Interventions

NIC interventions have not yet been linked to this diagnosis; however, the following may be useful:

Attachment Promotion: Facilitation of the development of the parent relationship

Birthing: Delivery of a baby

Childbirth Preparation: Providing information and support to facilitate childbirth and to enhance the ability of an individual to develop and perform the parental role

Environmental Management: Attachment Process: Manipulation of the patient's surroundings to facilitate the development of the parent–infant relationship

C

Intrapartal Care: Monitoring and management of stages 1 and 2 of the birth process

Parent Education: Infant: Instruction on nurturing and physical care needed during the first year of life

Postpartal Care: Monitoring and management of the patient who has recently given birth

Preconception Counseling: Screening and providing information and support to individuals of childbearing age before pregnancy to promote health and reduce risks

Prenatal Care: Monitoring and management of patient during pregnancy to prevent complications of pregnancy and promote a healthy outcome for both mother and infant

Nursing Activities

Refer to the Nursing Activities for *Readiness for enhanced childbearing process*. Many, perhaps most, of the nursing activities involve teaching, counseling, and monitoring. In general, nursing actions for this diagnosis focus on the related factors present for the particular patient. For example, if the problem is caused by lack of knowledge, patient education is important; if it is due to lack of cognitive readiness, then support systems must be put in place. Assessments include identifying the related factors, as well as assessing for signs and symptoms of the diagnosis so that patient progress can be evaluated.

Comprehensive activities are beyond the scope of this book; you should consult a comprehensive maternal-newborn book. You might also consult the *Nursing Interventions Classification (NIC)* book for activities for each of the NIC interventions listed earlier.

CHILDBEARING PROCESS: INEFFECTIVE, RISK FOR

(2010)

Domain 8, Sexuality; Class 3, Reproduction

Definition: Risk for a pregnancy and childbirth process and care of the newborn* that does not match the environmental context, norms, and expectations

*The original Japanese term for *childbearing* . . . encompasses both childbirth and rearing of the neonate. It is one of the main concepts of Japanese midwifery.

Risk Factors

Deficient knowledge (e.g., of labor and delivery, newborn care)
Domestic violence
Inconsistent prenatal health visits
Lack of appropriate role models for parenthood
Lack of cognitive readiness for parenthood
Lack of maternal confidence
Lack of prenatal health visits
Lack of a realistic birth plan
Lack of a sufficient support system
Maternal powerlessness
Maternal psychological distress
Suboptimal maternal nutrition
Substance abuse
Unplanned pregnancy
Unwanted pregnancy

Suggestions for Use

For NOC outcomes, NIC interventions, and suggested nursing activities, see Readiness for Enhanced Childbearing Process.

CHILDBEARING PROCESS, READINESS FOR ENHANCED

(2008)

Domain 8, Sexuality; Class 3, Reproduction

Definition: A pattern of preparing for, maintaining, and strengthening a healthy pregnancy and childbirth process and care of newborn.

Defining Characteristics

During Pregnancy

Subjective

Reports appropriate prenatal lifestyle (e.g., diet, elimination, sleep, bodily movement, exercise, personal hygiene)
Reports appropriate physical preparations
Reports managing unpleasant symptoms in pregnancy
Reports a realistic birth plan
Reports availability of support systems

Objective

Demonstrates respect for unborn baby
Prepares necessary newborn care items

Seeks necessary knowledge (e.g., of labor and delivery, newborn care)
Has regular prenatal visits

During Labor and Delivery

Subjective

Reports lifestyle (e.g., diet, elimination, sleep, bodily movement, personal hygiene) appropriate for the stage of labor

Objective

Responds appropriately to onset of labor
Is proactive in labor and delivery
Uses relaxation techniques appropriate for the stage of labor
Demonstrates attachment behavior to the newborn baby
Utilizes support systems appropriately

After Birth

Subjective

Reports appropriate postpartum lifestyle (e.g., diet, elimination, sleep, bodily movement, personal hygiene)

Objective

Demonstrates appropriate baby feeding techniques
Demonstrates appropriate breast care
Demonstrates attachment behavior to the baby
Demonstrates basic baby care techniques
Provides safe environment for the baby
Utilizes support system appropriately

Suggestions for Use

This is a wellness diagnosis. To learn about the specialized care to support a healthy pregnancy, labor, and birth, refer to a maternal-child text.

NOC Outcomes

Knowledge: Infant Care: Extent of understanding conveyed about caring for a baby from birth to first birthday

Knowledge: Extent of understanding conveyed about labor and vaginal delivery

Knowledge: Postpartum Maternal Health: Extent of understanding conveyed about maternal health in the period following birth of an infant

Knowledge: Preconception Maternal Health: Extent of understanding conveyed about maternal health prior to conception to ensure a healthy pregnancy

Knowledge: Pregnancy: Extent of understanding conveyed about promotion of a healthy pregnancy and prevention of complications

Knowledge: Pregnancy and Postpartum Sexual Functioning: Extent of understanding conveyed about sexual function during pregnancy and postpartum

Maternal Status: Antepartum: Extent to which maternal well-being is within normal limits from conception to the onset of labor

Maternal Status: Intrapartum: Extent to which maternal well-being is within normal limits from onset of labor to delivery

Maternal Status: Postpartum: Extent to which maternal well-being is within normal limits from delivery of placenta to completion of involution

Parent–Infant Attachment: Parent and infant behaviors that demonstrate an enduring affectionate bond

Postpartum Maternal Health Behavior: Personal actions to promote health of a mother in the period following birth of infant

Prenatal Health Behavior: Personal actions to promote a healthy pregnancy and a healthy newborn

Goals/Evaluation Criteria

Examples Using NOC Language

- Demonstrates *Readiness for enhanced childbearing process*, as evidenced by moderate to extensive Knowledge: Infant care, Labor and Delivery, Postpartum Maternal Health, Preconception: Maternal Health, Pregnancy, Pregnancy and Postpartum Sexual Functioning.
- Demonstrates *Readiness for enhanced childbearing process*, as evidenced by no deviation from normal range for Maternal Status: Antepartum, Maternal Status: Postpartum, Parent–Infant Attachment, Postpartum Maternal Health Behavior, and Prenatal health behavior.
- Demonstrates **Knowledge: Infant Care**, as evidenced by the following indicators (specify 1–5: no, limited, moderate, substantial, or extensive knowledge):
  - Normal infant characteristics
  - Proper holding of infant
  - Pros and cons of infant feeding choices
- Demonstrates **Knowledge: Labor and Delivery**, as evidenced by the following indicators (specify 1–5: no, limited, moderate, substantial, or extensive knowledge):
  - Birthing options
  - Signs and symptoms of labor
  - Effective breathing techniques
  - Effective positioning techniques

Other Examples

Preconception

C

Patient will verbalize or demonstrate knowledge of:
Healthy diet for women before conception
Environmental hazards to avoid at work or home
Importance of avoiding alcohol, tobacco, and other drug use

Prenatal Period

Seeks early prenatal care; keeps appointments
Maintains a healthy weight gain
Obtains dental care
Attends childbirth preparation classes
Avoids use of alcohol, tobacco, and recreational drugs
Exercises regularly
Ingests a nutritious diet

Intrapartum Period

Copes well with discomforts of labor
Participates in techniques to relieve discomfort and facilitate labor
Vital signs do not deviate from expected ranges
Cervical dilation progresses normally

Postpartum Period

Holds and cuddles infant
Makes eye contact; assumes en face position
Verbalizes positive feelings about infant
Comments on family resemblances (e.g., "He has his father's nose.")
Assumes care of the infant (e.g., changes diapers)

NIC Interventions

Attachment Promotion: Facilitation of the development of the parent relationship

Birthing: Delivery of a baby

Childbirth Preparation: Providing information and support to facilitate childbirth and to enhance the ability of an individual to develop and perform the parental role

Environmental Management: Attachment Process: Manipulation of the patient's surroundings to facilitate the development of the parent–infant relationship

Intrapartal Care: Monitoring and management of stages 1 and 2 of the birth process

Parent Education: Infant: Instruction on nurturing and physical care needed during the first year of life

Postpartal Care: Monitoring and management of the patient who has recently given birth

Preconception Counseling: Screening and providing information and support to individuals of childbearing age before pregnancy to promote health and reduce risks

Prenatal Care: Monitoring and management of patient during pregnancy to prevent complications of pregnancy and promote a healthy outcome for both mother and infant

Nursing Activities

In general, nursing actions for this diagnosis focus in supporting parents in preparing for, maintaining, and strengthening a healthy pregnancy and childbirth process and care of newborn. Many, perhaps most, of the nursing activities involve teaching, counseling, and monitoring. Comprehensive activities are beyond the scope of this book; you should consult a comprehensive maternal-newborn book. You might also consult the *Nursing Interventions Classification (NIC)* book for activities for each of the NIC interventions listed above. We can provide only a few examples here.

Assessments

Antepartum Period

- Determine whether the parents have chosen names for both sexes
- Explore with the parents their reaction to the pregnancy
- Establish a trusting relationship
- Screen for physical abuse
- Obtain a thorough sexual history

Patient/Family Teaching

- *(NIC) Preconception Counseling*

  Educate about ways to avoid teratogens (e.g., handling cat litter, smoking cessation, and alcohol substitutes)

  Discuss specific ways to prepare for pregnancy, including the social, financial, and psychological demands of childbearing and childrearing

  Instruct about the relationships among early fetal development and personal habits, medication use, teratogens, and self-care requisites (e.g., prenatal vitamins and folic acid)

  Recommend self-care needed during the preconception period

Collaborative Activities

- Refer for follow-up care, if needed
- Refer for genetic counseling if there are genetic risk factors

Intrapartal Period

- *(NIC) Birthing:* Consult with attending physician about indicators of actual or potential complications

Other

Antepartum Period

- Allow parents to listen to the fetal heart tones as soon as possible
- Show parents the ultrasound image and discuss it with them
- *(NIC) Preconception Counseling*

  Develop a preconception, pregnancy-oriented health risk profile, based on history, prescription drug use, ethnic background, occupational and household exposures, diet, specific genetic disorders, and habits (e.g., smoking and alcohol and drug intake)

Intrapartal Period

- Limit the number of people in the delivery room
- Encourage the father/significant other to participate in labor and delivery
- *(NIC) Birthing*

  Maintain patient modesty and privacy in a quiet environment during delivery

  Assist patient with position for delivery

  Instruct patient on shallow breathing (e.g., "panting") with delivery of the head

  Praise maternal and support person efforts

Postpartal Period

- *(NIC) Environmental Management: Attachment Process*

  Create environment that fosters privacy

  Maintain low level of stimuli in patient and family environment

  Permit father/significant other to sleep in room with mother

  Reduce interruptions by phone calls and hospital personnel

  Allow for family visitation, as desired [but] protect family from interruption by visitors

COMFORT, IMPAIRED

(2008, 2010) **Domain 12, Comfort; Class 1, Physical Comfort; Class 2, Environmental Comfort; Class 3, Social Comfort**

Definition: Perceived lack of ease, relief, and transcendence in physical, psychospiritual, environmental, cultural, and social dimensions

Defining Characteristics

Subjective

Anxiety
Disturbed sleep pattern
Fear
Inability to relax
Reports being cold (or hot)
Reports being uncomfortable
Reports distressing symptoms
Reports hunger
Reports itching
Reports lack of contentment in situation
Reports lack of ease in situation

Objective

Crying
Irritability
Moaning
Restlessness
Sighing

Related Factors

Illness-related symptoms
Insufficient resources (e.g., financial, social support)
Lack of environmental or situational control
Lack of privacy
Noxious environmental stimuli
Treatment-related side effects (e.g., medication, radiation)
Non-NANDA-I: Examples of causes of discomfort include bright lights, NPO status, noxious smells, noisy environment, room too hot or too cold, linen damp or wrinkled, and allergic reactions.

Suggestions for Use

This is a rather broad diagnosis. If the patient has the defining characteristics to support a more specific NANDA-I diagnosis, such as Nausea or Pain, use that. When using Impaired Comfort, add qualifying terms to describe the discomfort more fully when possible (e.g., Impaired Comfort: Itching). You may also be able to use the etiology to make the diagnosis more descriptive (e.g., Impaired Comfort r/t noxious smells).

Suggested Alternative Diagnoses

Consider whether defining characteristics are present to support one of the following more specific diagnoses:

C

Family processes, interrupted
Nausea
Pain
Powerlessness
Self-esteem, chronic or situational low
Social isolation
Spiritual distress

NOC Outcomes

Agitation Level: Severity of disruptive physiological and behavioral manifestations of stress or biochemical triggers

Client Satisfaction: Physical Environment: Extent of positive perception of living environment, treatment environment, equipment, and supplies in acute or long-term care settings

Comfort Status: Overall physical, psychospiritual, sociocultural, and environmental ease and safety of an individual

Comfort Status: Environment: Environmental ease, comfort, and safety of surroundings

Comfort Status: Physical: Physical ease related to bodily sensations and homeostatic mechanisms

Comfort Status: Psychospiritual: Psychospiritual ease related to self-concept, emotional well-being, source of inspiration, and meaning and purpose in life

Comfort Status: Sociocultural: Social ease related to interpersonal, family, and societal relationships within a cultural context

Symptom Control: Personal actions to minimize perceived adverse changes in physical and emotional functioning

Examples Using NOC Language

- Exhibits/demonstrates **Comfort Status**, **Comfort Status: Environment**, **Comfort Status: Physical**, **Comfort Status: Psychospiritual**, and **Comfort Status: Sociocultural**
- Demonstrates mild or no **Agitation Level**, as evidenced by the following indicators (specify 1–5: severe, substantial, moderate, mild, none):
  - Restlessness
  - Irritability
  - Pulling at tubes or restraints
  - Emotional lability

Pacing
Interrupted sleep

Other Examples

- Verbalizes satisfaction with room temperature
- Verbalizes satisfaction with physical surroundings
- Indicates that care is consistent with his cultural and other needs
- Receives adequate social support from friends and family
- Indicates satisfaction with social relationships
- Communicates needs to caregivers
- Monitors own symptoms
- Follows suggestions for symptom relief measure

NIC Interventions

Anxiety Reduction: Minimizing apprehension, dread, foreboding, or uneasiness related to an unidentified source of anticipated danger

Calming Technique: Reducing anxiety in patient experiencing acute distress

Culture Brokerage: The deliberate use of culturally competent strategies to bridge or mediate between the patient's culture and the biomedical health care system

Dementia Management: Provision of a modified environment for the patient who is experiencing a chronic confusional state

Dementia Management: Bathing: Reduction of aggressive behavior during cleaning of the body

Environmental Management: Comfort: Manipulation of the patient's surroundings for promotion of optimal comfort

Environmental Management: Safety: Monitoring and manipulation of the physical environment to promote safety

Medication Administration: Preparing, giving, and evaluating the effectiveness of prescription and nonprescription drugs

Pain Management: Alleviation of pain or a reduction in pain to a level of comfort that is acceptable to the patient

Positioning: Deliberative placement of the patient or a body part to promote physiological and psychological well-being

Relaxation Therapy: Use of techniques to encourage and elicit relaxation for the purpose of decreasing undesirable signs and symptoms such as pain, muscle tension, or anxiety

Self-Efficacy Enhancement: Strengthening an individual's confidence in his or her ability to perform a health behavior

Self-Modification Assistance: Reinforcement of self-directed change initiated by the patient to achieve personally important goals

Spiritual Support: Assisting the patient to feel balance and connection with a greater power

Support System Enhancement: Facilitation of support to patient by family, friends, and community

Nursing Activities

In general, nursing actions for this diagnosis focus on assessing for symptoms and sources of discomfort and promoting comfort. Specific activities will depend on the particular source(s) of discomfort.

Assessments

- Assess for the sources of discomfort (e.g., damp dressings, tubing, wrinkled linens, itching, fever, thirst, room temperature, noise, lighting)
- Monitor the environment for safety hazards
- Assess the availability and adequacy of the patient's support system
- Explore the patient's self-efficacy ability:

  What is his perception of his ability to perform desired behaviors?

  What does he perceive to be the benefits of these behaviors?

  What are the barriers to changing his behaviors?

Patient/Family Teaching

- Support the patient's confidence in his ability to perform a health behavior: provide information, assist with a plan of action, and reinforce actions.

For itching

- Advise patient not to scratch
- Advise to wash clothing in mild detergent and put through two rinse cycles; do not use fabric softeners

Collaborative Activities

- Administer antianxiety medications as needed
- Refer to a self-help group as needed

For itching

- Apply antifungal/antiyeast powder or cream
- Obtain prescription for corticosteroid creams for local inflammation
- Obtain prescription for antihistamine if necessary
- Explain causes of itching and ways to help prevent it
- Refer for allergy testing, as needed

Other

- For patients on bed rest, change position at least every 2 hr
- Offer back rub, unless contraindicated

- Warm or cool room temperature, as required
- Reduce environmental noise as much as possible
- Dim the lights to suit the patient's preference; avoid direct light in the eyes
- Provide pillows and blankets to position immobile patients comfortably
- Answer call bells/lights promptly
- Keep the room clean; empty bedpans and other containers promptly.
- Provide relaxation therapy if the patient is willing and able to participate.
- *(NIC) Environmental Management: Comfort:* Give consideration to the placement of patients in multiple-bedded rooms (roommates with similar environmental concerns when possible)

For itching

- Encourage the patient to shower or bathe in cool water, as often as needed to relieve itching. Blot skin dry rather than rubbing dry
- Tub soaks may contain oatmeal, baking soda, cornstarch, or Aveeno
- Massage scar tissue with cocoa butter
- Prevent dry skin: Use moisturizer unless contraindicated. Do not use scented lotions
- Apply wet dressings to relieve itching
- Keep environmental temperature cool
- Do not use rough fabrics next to the skin. Use cotton sheets, if possible
- Use a bed cradle to keep linens away from the skin
- Provide distraction
- For children or confused adults, apply mitts to prevent scratching
- Trim and file the patient's nails
- Encourage patient to drink 3,000 mL fluid per day, unless contraindicated

COMFORT, READINESS FOR ENHANCED

(2006) Domain 12, Comfort; Class 1, Physical Comfort; Class 2, Environmental Comfort; Class 3, Social Comfort

Definition: A pattern of ease, relief, and transcendence in physical, psychospiritual, environmental, and social dimensions that is sufficient for well-being and can be strengthened

Defining Characteristics

Subjective/Objective

Expresses desire to enhance comfort
Expresses desire to enhance feeling of contentment
Expresses desire to enhance relaxation
Expresses desire to enhance resolution of complaints

Suggestions for Use

Because this is a wellness diagnosis, an etiology (i.e., related factors) is not needed. If none of the defining characteristics is present, consider whether an actual problem (e.g., *Pain*, *Nausea*) is present, or whether a different wellness diagnosis (e.g., *Readiness for enhanced spiritual well-being*) should be used.

Suggested Alternative Diagnoses

Coping, readiness for enhanced
Spiritual well-being: readiness for enhanced

NOC Outcomes

Comfort Status: Overall physical, psychospiritual, sociocultural, and environmental ease and safety of an individual

Personal Autonomy: Personal actions of a competent individual to exercise governance in life decisions.

Goals/Evaluation Criteria

Examples Using NOC Language

- Demonstrates **Comfort Status**, as evidenced by the following indicators (specify 1–5: severely, substantially, moderately, mildly, or not compromised):
- Care consistent with cultural beliefs
- Physical well-being

- Psychological well-being
- Physical surroundings
- Symptom control
- Social relationships

Other Examples

Patient will:

- Report improved physical and/or psychosocial-emotional comfort
- Report increased ability to relax
- Report or demonstrate improved coping abilities
- Report feeling more content and happy

NIC Interventions

Assertiveness Training: Assistance with the effective expression of feelings, needs, and ideas while respecting the rights of others

Decision-Making Support: Providing information and support for a patient who is making a decision regarding health care

Health Education: Developing and providing instruction and learning experiences to facilitate voluntary adaptation of behavior conducive to health in individuals, families, groups, or communities

Self-Awareness Enhancement: Assisting a patient to explore and understand his thoughts, feelings, motivations, and behaviors

Self-Efficacy Enhancement: Strengthening an individual's confidence in his ability to perform a health behavior

Self-Modification Assistance: Reinforcement of self-directed change initiated by the patient to achieve personally important goals

Nursing Activities

Because this nursing diagnosis is not developed to a high level, it is difficult to determine the specific focus of the nursing interventions. In general, the nurse would provide a holistic approach to comfort and self-care and teach or facilitate environmental management. Many nursing actions focus on empowering the patient to improve his own comfort. Refer to the nursing diagnosis, Impaired Comfort, for interventions to address specific problems that decrease comfort.

Assessments

- Explore with patient what "comfort" means to him
- Assess for barriers to increased comfort level
- Determine areas in which patient wishes to improve his comfort (e.g., physical, emotional, social, spiritual)
- Assess for barriers to assertiveness (e.g., socialization, emotional or cognitive condition)

- *(NIC) Self-Efficacy Enhancement*
  Explore individual's perception of his capability to perform the desired behavior
  Explore individual's perception of benefits of executing the desired behavior
  Explore individual's perception of risks of not executing the desired behavior

C

Patient/Family Teaching

- Explain differences between assertiveness, aggressiveness, and passive aggressiveness
- Teach strategies for using assertive behaviors (e.g., how to say no to unreasonable requests)
- Teach techniques such as simple massage and simple relaxation therapy
- Teach new coping strategies, as needed
- Provide information about the behaviors needed to achieve enhanced comfort

Other

- Provide opportunities to practice assertiveness (e.g., role playing)
- Work with the patient to develop a plan of self-care and to identify ways in which the nurse can enhance comfort
- Demonstrate interest in the patient
- Encourage patient to express both positive and negative ideas and feelings
- Provide therapeutic touch
- Give positive feedback for the person's efforts
- Assist to develop an appropriate exercise program
- *(NIC) Decision-Making Support:*
  Serve as a liaison between patient and family (or between patient and other health care providers)
  Facilitate collaborative decision making
  Help patient identify the advantages and disadvantages of each alternative

COMMUNICATION, READINESS FOR ENHANCED

(2002) **Domain 5, Perception/Cognition; Class 5, Communication**

Definition: A pattern of exchanging information and ideas with others that is sufficient for meeting one's needs and life goals and can be strengthened

Defining Characteristics

Subjective

Expresses satisfaction with ability to share information and ideas with others

Objective

Able to speak or write a language
Expresses thoughts and feelings
Expresses willingness to enhance communication
Forms words, phrases, and sentences
Uses and interprets nonverbal cues appropriately

Suggestions for Use

Because this is a wellness diagnosis, an etiology (i.e., related factors) is not needed. If situations exist that pose a risk to effective communication, use *Risk for impaired verbal communication.*

Suggested Alternative Diagnoses

Risk for impaired verbal communication

NOC Outcomes

Communication: Reception, interpretation, and expression of spoken, written, and nonverbal messages

Communication: Expressive: Expression of meaningful verbal and nonverbal messages

Communication: Receptive: Reception and interpretation of verbal and nonverbal messages

Goals/Evaluation Criteria

Examples Using NOC Language

- Demonstrates **Communication**, as evidenced by the following indicators (specify 1–5: severely, substantially, moderately, mildly, or not compromised):
- Use of written, spoken, or nonverbal language
- Use of sign language
- Use of pictures and drawings
- Acknowledgment of messages received
- Exchanges messages accurately with others

Other Examples

Patient will:

- Report improved ability to communicate verbally
- Report improved nonverbal communication

NIC Interventions

Anxiety Reduction: Minimizing apprehension, dread, foreboding, or uneasiness related to an unidentified source of anticipated danger

Assertiveness Training: Assistance with the effective expression of feelings, needs, and ideas while respecting the rights of others

Communication Enhancement: Hearing Deficit: Assistance in accepting and learning alternate methods for living with diminished hearing

Communication Enhancement: Speech Deficit: Assistance in accepting and learning alternate methods for living with impaired speech

Complex Relationship Building: Establishing a therapeutic relationship with a patient who has difficulty interacting with others

Socialization Enhancement: Facilitation of another person's ability to interact with others

Nursing Activities

In general, nursing actions for this diagnosis focus on assessing present communication and areas in which the client wishes to improve; establishing a good nurse–client relationship; modeling good communication; promoting sharing and relationship building; and providing feedback.

Assessments

- Assess clarity and effectiveness of verbal messages
- Assess for barriers to assertiveness (e.g., literacy level)
- Determine areas in which patient wishes to improve his communication (e.g., verbal, nonverbal, written)

Patient/Family Teaching

- Teach the difference between assertiveness and aggressiveness
- Role-model assertive behaviors
- Teach strategies for assertiveness (e.g., saying no appropriately, beginning and ending conversations, making requests)

Other

- Demonstrate interest in the patient
- Encourage to express both positive and negative ideas and feelings
- Use questions and feedback to improve the clarity of verbal and nonverbal messages
- Give praise for improved communication
- Assist with planning opportunities to practice communication techniques

Home Care

See Impaired Verbal Communication.

For Older Adults

- Be aware of the possibility of hearing and vision deficits that may prevent enhanced communication. Refer for correction as needed.
- Use techniques to promote self-esteem and self-care
- Be aware of the incidence of depression in older adults; assess mood
- Use touch when communicating, as appropriate and acceptable to the client

COMMUNICATION: VERBAL, IMPAIRED

(1983, 1996, 1998) **Domain 5, Perception/Cognition; Class 5, Communication**

Definition: Decreased, delayed, or absent ability to receive, process, transmit, and use a system of symbols [anything that has or transmits meaning]

Defining Characteristics

Objective

Absence of eye contact or difficulty in selective attending
Difficulty expressing thoughts verbally (e.g., aphasia, dysphasia, apraxia, dyslexia)
Difficulty forming words or sentences (e.g., aphonia, dyslalia, dysarthria)
Difficulty in comprehending and maintaining usual communication pattern
Disorientation in one or more of the three spheres of time, space, person
Does not or cannot speak
Dyspnea
Inability or difficulty in use of facial or body expressions
Inappropriate verbalization
Partial or total visual deficit
Slurring
Speaks or verbalizes with difficulty
Stuttering
Inability to speak language of caregiver
Willful refusal to speak

Related Factors

C

Absence of significant others
Alteration of central nervous system
Alteration of self-esteem or self-concept
Altered perceptions
Anatomical defect (e.g., cleft palate, alteration of the neuromuscular visual system, auditory system, or phonatory apparatus)
Brain tumor
Cultural difference
Decrease in circulation to brain
Differences related to developmental age
Emotional conditions
Environmental barriers
Lack of information
Physical barrier (e.g., tracheostomy, intubation)
Physiological conditions
Psychological barriers (e.g., psychosis, lack of stimuli)
Side effects of medications or treatments
[Stress]
Weakening of the musculoskeletal system

Suggestions for Use

Use this label for those who want to communicate but who have difficulty doing so. If communication problems are caused by psychiatric illness or coping difficulties, a diagnosis of *Fear* or *Anxiety* may be more appropriate. Note that communication problems may be receptive (i.e., difficulty hearing) as well as expressive (i.e., difficulty speaking).

Suggested Alternative Diagnoses

Anxiety
Coping, defensive
Fear
Self-esteem, chronic or situational low
Sensory perception, disturbed: visual, auditory

NOC Outcomes

Cognition: Ability to execute complex mental processes
Communication: Reception, interpretation, and expression of spoken, written, and nonverbal messages
Communication: Expressive: Expression of meaningful verbal and/or nonverbal messages

Communication: Receptive: Reception and interpretation of verbal and/or nonverbal messages

Information Processing: Ability to acquire, organize, and use information

Goals/Evaluation Criteria

Examples Using NOC Language

- Demonstrates **Communication**, as evidenced by the following indicators (specify 1–5: severely, substantially, moderately, mildly, or not compromised):
- Use of written, spoken, or nonverbal language
- Use of sign language
- Use of pictures and drawings
- Acknowledgment of messages received
- Exchanges messages accurately with others

Other Examples

Patient will:

- Communicate needs to staff and family with minimal frustration
- Communicate satisfaction with alternative means of communication

NIC Interventions

Active Listening: Attending closely to and attaching significance to a patient's verbal and nonverbal messages

Anxiety Reduction: Minimizing apprehension, dread, foreboding, or uneasiness related to an unidentified source of anticipated danger

Communication Enhancement, Hearing Deficit: Assistance in accepting and learning alternate methods for living with diminished hearing

Communication Enhancement: Speech Deficit: Assistance in accepting and learning alternate methods for living with impaired speech

Communication Enhancement: Visual Deficit: Assistance in accepting and learning alternate methods for living with diminished vision

Decision-Making Support: Providing information and support for a patient who is making a decision regarding health care

Memory Training: Facilitation of memory

Nursing Activities

In general, nursing actions for this diagnosis focus on assessing present communication and areas in which the client wishes to improve; establishing a good nurse–client relationship; modeling good communication; providing feedback; and memory training.

C

Assessments

- Assess and document patient's
- Primary language
- Ability to speak, hear, write, read, and understand
- Ability to establish communication with staff and family
- Response to touch, spatial distance, culture, and male and female roles that may influence communication

Patient/Family Teaching

- Explain to patient why he cannot speak or understand, as appropriate
- Explain to hearing-impaired patient that sounds will be heard differently with use of a hearing aid
- *(NIC) Communication Enhancement: Speech Deficit:*
  Instruct patient and family on use of speech aids (e.g., tracheal-esophageal prosthesis and artificial larynx)
  Teach esophageal speech, as appropriate

Collaborative Activities

- Consult with physician regarding need for speech therapy
- Help patient and family to locate resources for hearing aids
- Consult with a speech pathologist or other professional as needed
- *(NIC) Communication Enhancement: Speech Deficit:*
  Use interpreter, as necessary
  Reinforce need for follow-up with speech pathologist after discharge

Other

- Help patient to locate a telephone for the hearing impaired
- Encourage attendance at group meetings for interpersonal contact, specify group
- Encourage frequent family visits to provide stimulation for communication
- Encourage patient to communicate slowly and to repeat requests
- Give frequent positive reinforcement to patient efforts to communicate
- Encourage self-expression in any manner that provides information to staff and family
- Establish regular one-to-one contact with patient
- Use flash cards, pad, pencil, gestures, pictures, foreign language vocabulary lists, computer, and so forth, to facilitate optimal two-way communication
- Speak slowly, distinctly, and quietly, facing the patient
- When speaking to a patient with hearing impairment, be sure your mouth is visible; do not smoke, talk with a full mouth, or chew gum

- Obtain hearing-impaired patient's attention by touching
- Give clear and simple directions; avoid overwhelming choices that may add to the patient's confusion. For example, take patient by the arm, saying, "Walk with me now."
- Involve patient and family in developing a communication plan
- Provide care in a relaxed, unhurried, nonjudgmental manner
- Provide continuity in nursing assignment to establish trust and reduce frustration
- Reassure patient that frustration and anger are acceptable and expected
- Use family and significant person or hospital translator, as appropriate; specify name, phone number, and relationship in care plan
- *(NIC) Communication Enhancement: Speech Deficit:*

  Refrain from shouting at patient with communication disorders

  Carry on one-way conversations, as appropriate

  Listen attentively

Home Care

- Assess the impact of the communication deficit on family roles and functioning
- Encourage the family to include the patient in family activities to the extent possible

For Infants and Children

- Base your communication on the child's developmental stage
- Observe ways in which the child communicates (e.g., his writing, play, facial expressions)
- Teach the child alternate ways to communicate (e.g., by pointing)
- Refer children for speech therapy, as appropriate
- Teach parents the importance of using visual and tactile communication with deaf infants

For Older Adults

- Do not use "baby talk" or "talk down" to older adults
- For clients with hearing deficits:
- Determine whether the client has had his hearing evaluated
- Encourage the person to wear hearing aids if he has them
- Use touch, if acceptable to the person

COMMUNITY HEALTH, DEFICIENT

(2010) **Domain 1, Health Promotion; Class 2, Health Management**

Definition: Presence of one or more health problems or factors that deter wellness or increase the risk of health problems experienced by an aggregate

Defining Characteristics

Incidence of risks relating to hospitalization experienced by aggregates or populations
Incidence of risks relating to physiological states experienced by aggregates or populations
Incidence of risks relating to psychological states experienced by aggregates or populations
Incidence of health problems experienced by aggregates or populations
No program available to enhance wellness for an aggregate or population
No program available to prevent one or more health problems for an aggregate or population
No program available to reduce one or more health problems for an aggregate or population
No program available to eliminate one or more health problems for an aggregate or population

Related Factors

Lack of access to public health care providers
Lack of community experts
Limited resources
Program has inadequate budget
Program has inadequate community support
Program has inadequate consumer satisfaction
Program has inadequate evaluation plan
Program has inadequate outcome data
Program partly addresses health problem

Suggestions for Use

Comparing this problem to *Ineffective community coping* is somewhat difficult. It seems that this diagnosis could be made simply when demographic data show that there are aggregate health problems or a risk for such problems, or when there are no available programs to deal with the problems. *Deficient community health* appears to be more about the community's responses to existing health problems. In a sense, may constitute a risk factor for *Ineffective community coping*. *Deficient community health* is diagnosed on the basis of observed behaviors, rather than on demographics. Nevertheless, some the related factors (causes) for both diagnoses are similar (e.g., lack of services or resources).

Suggested Alternative Diagnoses

Community coping, ineffective
Community coping: ineffective, risk for (non-NANDA-I)

NOC Outcomes

NOC outcomes have not yet been linked to this diagnosis. However, the following may be useful:

Community Health Status: General state of well-being of a community or population

Goals/Evaluation Criteria

Examples Using NOC Language

- Demonstrates **Community Health Status**, as evidenced by the following indicators (specify 1–5: poor, fair, good, very good, or excellent):
  - Chronic disease rates
  - Substance abuse rates
  - Smoking rates
  - Sexually transmitted disease rates
  - Crime statistics

Other Examples

The community:

- Has health promotion and preventive health care services in place
- Has programs to promote healthy pregnancy
- Complies with environmental health standards
- Has health surveillance data systems in place

NIC Interventions

NIC interventions have not yet been linked to this diagnosis. However, the following may be useful:

Environmental Management: Community: Monitoring and influencing of the physical, social, cultural, economic, and political conditions that affect the health of groups and communities

Environmental Risk Protection: Preventing and detecting disease and injury in populations at risk from environmental hazards

Health Policy Monitoring: Surveillance and influence of government and organization regulations, rules, and standards that affect nursing systems and practices to ensure quality care of patients

Program Development: Planning, implementing, and evaluating a coordinated set of activities designed to enhance wellness, or to prevent, reduce, or eliminate one or more health problems for a group or community

Surveillance: Community: Purposeful and ongoing acquisition, interpretation, and synthesis of data for decision making in the community

Nursing Activities

See Nursing Activities for *Coping: community, ineffective*.

CONFUSION, ACUTE

(1994, 2006) **Domain 5, Perception/Cognition; Class 4, Cognition**

Definition: Abrupt onset of reversible disturbances of consciousness, attention, cognition, and perception that develop over a short period of time

Defining Characteristics

Subjective

Lack of motivation to initiate or follow through with goal-directed or purposeful behavior

Misperceptions

Objective

Fluctuation in cognition

Fluctuation in level of consciousness

Fluctuation in psychomotor activity

Increased agitation or restlessness

Hallucinations

Related Factors

Delirium

Dementia

Fluctuation in sleep–wake cycle

Substance abuse

Over 60 years of age

[NOTE: This is a NANDA International related factor. It does not imply that only people older than 60 can be confused; nor does it imply that one can assume confusion in older adults. What it means is that conditions causing confusion (e.g., organic brain syndrome, Alzheimer disease) are statistically more common in older than in younger adults.]

Other Possible Defining Characteristics (Non-NANDA International)

Prescribed medications
Self-medication and/or polypharmacy
Sleep deprivation

Suggestions for Use

Confusion may be used to describe a variety of cognitive impairments. It may be difficult to determine whether *Confusion* is acute or chronic. Therefore, until careful assessment and analysis have been done, it may be necessary to use the more general non-NANDA International term *Confusion*. *Acute confusion* develops suddenly and is short term. *Chronic confusion* develops over time and is caused by progressive degenerative changes in the brain.

Suggested Alternative Diagnoses

Confusion (non-NANDA International)
Confusion, chronic
Environmental interpretation syndrome, impaired
Tissue perfusion, ineffective (cerebral)

NOC Outcomes

Acute Confusion Level: Severity of disturbance in consciousness and cognition that develops over a short period of time
Cognitive Orientation: Ability to identify person, place, and time accurately
Distorted Thought Self-Control: Self-restraint of disruptions in perception, thought processes, and thought content
Information Processing: Ability to acquire, organize, and use information
Substance Withdrawal Severity: Severity of physical and psychological signs or symptoms caused by withdrawal from addictive drugs, toxic chemicals, tobacco, or alcohol

Goals/Evaluation Criteria

Examples Using NOC Language

- Demonstrates **Cognitive Orientation**, as evidenced by the following indicators (specify 1–5: severely, substantially, moderately, mildly, or not compromised):
  - Identifies self
  - Identifies significant other
  - Identifies current place

Identifies correct month/year/season
Identifies significant current events

C

Other Examples

Patient will:

- Have decreasing episodes of confusion
- Make lifestyle and behavior changes to alleviate or prevent further episodes of confusion
- Demonstrate decreased restlessness and agitation
- Not respond to hallucinations or delusions
- Demonstrate accurate interpretation of environment
- Organize and process information logically
- Correctly identify common objects and familiar persons
- Read and understand short written statements
- Add and subtract numbers accurately
- Obey verbal instructions and commands
- Retain motor responses to noxious stimuli
- Open eyes to external stimuli
- Be awake at appropriate times
- Have a normal electroencephalogram and electromyogram

NIC Interventions

Cognitive Stimulation: Promotion of awareness and comprehension of surroundings by utilization of planned stimuli

Delirium Management: Provision of a safe and therapeutic environment for the patient who is experiencing an acute confusional state

Delusion Management: Promoting the comfort, safety, and reality orientation of a patient experiencing false, fixed beliefs that have little or no basis in reality

Hallucination Management: Promoting the safety, comfort, and reality orientation of a patient experiencing hallucinations

Memory Training: Facilitation of memory

Reality Orientation: Promotion of patient's awareness of personal identity, time, and environment

Substance Use Treatment: Alcohol Withdrawal: Care of the patient experiencing sudden cessation of alcohol consumption

Substance Use Treatment: Drug Withdrawal: Care of the patient experiencing drug detoxification

Nursing Activities

In general, nursing actions for this diagnosis focus on assessing for causal factors, providing for safety, providing stimuli to promote orientation, communicating in simple terms, and promoting self-esteem.

Assessments

- Identify possible causes of delirium (e.g., pain, hypoglycemia, infection, medications)
- Monitor neurologic status
- Monitor emotional status
- Obtain baseline history of mental status and any changes
- Perform complete mental status exam
- *(NIC) Delusion Management:* Monitor delusions for presence of content that is self-harmful or violent

Patient/Family Teaching

- *(NIC) Delusion Management:*
  - Provide illness teaching to patient and significant others, if delusions are illness based (e.g., delirium, schizophrenia, or depression)
  - Provide medication teaching to patient and significant others

Collaborative Activities

- *(NIC) Delusion Management:* Administer antipsychotic and antianxiety medications on a routine and as-needed basis

Other

- Reassure patient with frequent therapeutic communication
- Use touch, as appropriate
- Avoid use of restraints, if possible
- Encourage family and significant others to stay with patient
- Use nursing measures (e.g., mouth care, positioning) to promote comfort and sleep
- Continue patient's usual rituals, to limit anxiety
- Give choices but limit options if patient becomes frustrated or confused
- Keep explanations and directions short and simple; repeat as necessary.
- Be sure patient wears an identification bracelet
- Orient patient (e.g., to staff, surroundings, and care activities), as needed
- Support the client's usual sleep–wake cycle (e.g., open curtains in the morning, keep the room dark or dimly lit at night)
- Call the patient by name when beginning an interaction
- Answer call lights in person rather than using an intercom
- Explain routines and procedures slowly, briefly, and in simple terms
- Give patient time to respond when presenting options or new information
- *(NIC) Delusion Management:*
  - Focus discussion on the underlying feelings, rather than the content of the delusion ("It appears as though you may be feeling frightened")
  - Avoid arguing about false beliefs; state doubt matter-of-factly

Encourage patient to verbalize delusions to caregivers before acting on them
Assist with self-care, as needed

Maintain a safe environment
Provide for the safety and comfort of patient and others when patient is unable to control behavior (e.g., limit setting, area restriction, physical restraint, or seclusion)
Decrease excessive environmental stimuli, as needed
Maintain a consistent daily routine
Assign consistent caregivers on a daily basis

Home Care

- *(NIC) Delusion Management:*
  Monitor self-care ability
  Educate family and significant others about ways to deal with patient who is experiencing delusions
- Assess the home for safety hazards (e.g., open stairways)

For Older Adults

- Interventions are similar, regardless of developmental stage, even though the incidence of confusion may be higher in older adults
- Be aware that older adults may underreport symptoms (e.g., of pain). Be sure to treat pain adequately

CONFUSION, ACUTE: RISK FOR

(2006) **Domain 5, Perception/Cognition; Class 4, Cognition**

Definition: At risk for reversible disturbances of consciousness, attention, cognition, and perception that develop over a short period of time

Risk Factors

Subjective

Pain

Objective

Alcohol use
Decreased mobility
Dementia
Fluctuation in sleep–wake cycle

History of stroke
Impaired cognition
Infection
Male gender
Medication/drugs
- Anesthesia
- Anticholinergics
- Diphenhydramine
- Multiple medications
- Opioids
- Psychoactive drugs

Metabolic abnormalities
- Azotemia
- Decreased hemoglobin
- Dehydration
- Electrolyte imbalances
- Increased blood urea nitrogen (BUN)/creatinine
- Malnutrition

Over 60 years of age
Restraints
Sensory deprivation
Substance abuse
Urinary retention

Suggestions for Use

Confusion may be used to describe a variety of cognitive impairments. It may be difficult to determine whether *Confusion* is acute or chronic. Therefore, until careful assessment and analysis have been done, it may be necessary to use the more general non-NANDA International term *Risk for confusion. Acute confusion* develops suddenly and short term. *Chronic confusion* develops over time and is caused by progressive degenerative changes in the brain.

Suggested Alternative Diagnoses

Risk for confusion (non-NANDA International)
Confusion, acute

NOC Outcomes

NOTE: The following outcomes are to assess and measure whether *Acute confusion* is occurring:

Acute Confusion Level: Severity of disturbance in consciousness and cognition that develops over a short period of time

Cognitive Orientation: Ability to identify person, place, and time accurately

NOTE: The following are examples of outcomes associated with risk factors for *Acute confusion*:

Cognition: Ability to execute complex mental processes

Concentration: Ability to focus on a specific stimulus

Medication Response: Therapeutic and adverse effects of prescribed medication

Risk Detection: Personal actions to identify personal health threats

Sensory Function: Extent to which an individual correctly senses skin stimulation, sounds, proprioception, taste and smell, and visual images

Goals/Evaluation Criteria

Examples Using NOC Language

- Does not develop *Acute confusion*, as evidenced by acceptable indicators of **Acute Confusion Level and Cognitive Orientation**
- Demonstrates **Cognitive Orientation**, as evidenced by the following indicators (specify 1–5: severely, substantially, moderately, mildly, or not compromised):
  - Identifies significant other
  - Identifies current place
  - Identifies current day
  - Identifies correct month (day and year)
  - Identifies significant current events

Other Examples

Patient/family will:

- Identify lifestyle changes that can be made to reduce the effect of those risk factors that are possible to change
- Recognize and report signs and symptoms of Acute confusion
- Also see goals for Acute confusion.

NIC Interventions

Medication Management: Facilitation of safe and effective use of prescription and over-the-counter drugs

Reality Orientation: Promotion of patient's awareness of personal identity, time, and environment

Sleep Enhancement: Facilitation of regular sleep–wake cycles

Surveillance: Purposeful and ongoing acquisition, interpretation, and synthesis of patient data for clinical decision making

Nursing Activities

In general, nursing actions for this diagnosis focus on identifying risk factors and instituting preventive measures specific to those risk factors. These might include medication management, orienting the patient to reality, and promoting sleep.

Assessments

- Assess for symptoms of *Acute confusion*, such as agitation; restlessness; fluctuation in cognition, level of conscious, psychomotor activity, or sleep–wake cycle; hallucinations; misperceptions; disorientation; or lack of motivation to initiate or follow through with goal-directed or purposeful behavior
- Monitor neurologic status
- Monitor emotional status
- Monitor fluid, electrolyte, and acid–base status
- Obtain baseline history of mental status and any changes

Patient/Family Teaching

- Point out the presence of lifestyle factors that increase the risk for *Acute confusion*; explain how they relate

Collaborative Activities

- Be alert for drug interactions in patients taking multiple medications; discuss with primary care providers

Other

- Avoid use of restraints, if possible
- Support the client's usual sleep–wake cycle (e.g., open curtains in the morning, keep the room dark or dimly lit at night)
- Call the patient by name when beginning an interaction
- Answer call lights in person rather than using an intercom
- Decrease excessive environmental stimuli, as needed
- Increase environmental stimuli as needed to prevent sensory deprivation

For Older Adults

- Interventions are similar, regardless of developmental stage, even though the incidence of confusion may be higher in older adults
- Be aware that older adults may underreport symptoms (e.g., of pain). Be sure to treat pain adequately

CONFUSION, CHRONIC

(1994) **Domain 5, Perception/Cognition; Class 4, Cognition**

Definition: Irreversible, long-standing, or progressive deterioration of intellect and personality characterized by decreased ability to interpret environmental stimuli [and] decreased capacity for intellectual thought processes; and manifested by disturbances of memory, orientation, and behavior

Defining Characteristics

Subjective

Impaired memory (short-term, long-term)

Objective

Altered interpretation and response to stimuli
Altered personality
Clinical evidence of organic impairment
Impaired socialization
No change in level of consciousness
Progressive or long-standing cognitive impairment

Related Factors

Alzheimer disease
Cerebrovascular accident
Head injury
Korsakoff's psychosis
Multi-infarct dementia

Suggestions for Use

See Suggestions for Use for Confusion, Acute. For clients with self-care deficits, be sure to include that diagnostic label in the care plan (e.g., *Total self-care deficit related to Chronic confusion*). It is difficult to distinguish between *Chronic confusion* and *Impaired environmental interpretation syndrome*.

Suggested Alternative Diagnoses

Confusion, acute
Environmental interpretation syndrome, impaired
Memory, impaired
Self-care deficit (specify)

NOC Outcomes

Cognition: Ability to execute complex mental processes
Cognitive Orientation: Ability to identify person, place, and time accurately
Concentration: Ability to focus on a specific stimulus
Decision Making: Ability to make judgments and choose between two or more alternatives
Distorted Thought Self-Control: Self-restraint of disruptions in perception, thought processes, and thought content
Identity: Distinguishes between self and nonself and characterize one's essence
Memory: Ability to cognitively retrieve and report previously stored information

Goals/Evaluation Criteria

Examples Using NOC Language

- Maintains or improves **Cognition, Cognitive Orientation, Concentration, Decision Making, Distorted Thought Self-Control, Identity, and Memory**
- Experiences no loss of **Identity,** as evidenced by the following indicators (specify 1–5: never, rarely, sometimes, often, and consistently demonstrated):
  Exhibits congruent verbal and nonverbal behavior about self
  Perceives environment accurately
  Verbalizes clear sense of personal identity
  Recognizes interpersonal versus intrapersonal conflict
- **Memory** intact, as evidenced by the following indicators (specify 1–5: severely, substantially, moderately, mildly, or not compromised):
  Recalls immediate information accurately
  Recalls recent information accurately
  Recalls remote information accurately
- Also see Goals/Evaluation Criteria for *Acute confusion.*

Other Examples

Patient will:

- Respond to visual and auditory cues, draw a circle, maintain attention
- Identify relevant information and choose among alternatives
- Interact appropriately with others
- Formulate coherent messages
- Obey simple directions and commands
- Not attend to hallucinations or delusions
- Attend to, perceive, and interpret the environmental stimuli correctly

- Correctly identify objects and people
- Balance activity with rest
- Exhibit a decrease in restlessness and agitation
- Participate to maximum ability in therapeutic milieu or ADLs
- Not be combative
- Be content and less frustrated by environmental stressors

NIC Interventions

Anxiety Reduction: Minimizing apprehension, dread, foreboding, or uneasiness related to an unidentified source of anticipated danger

Cognitive Stimulation: Promotion of awareness and comprehension of surroundings by utilization of planned stimuli

Decision-Making Support: Providing information and support for a patient who is making a decision regarding health care

Delusion Management: Promoting the comfort, safety, and reality orientation of a patient experiencing false, fixed beliefs that have little or no basis in reality

Dementia Management: Provision of a modified environment for the patient who is experiencing a chronic confusional state

Family Involvement Promotion: Facilitating family participation in the emotional and physical care of the patient

Hallucination Management: Promoting the safety, comfort, and reality orientation of a patient experiencing hallucination

Memory Training: Facilitation of memory

Reality Orientation: Promotion of patient's awareness of personal identity, time, and environment

Reminiscence Therapy: Using the recall of past events, feelings, and thoughts to facilitate pleasure, quality of life, or adaptation to present circumstances

Nursing Activities

In general, nursing actions for this diagnosis focus on identifying baseline behaviors, using low-stress approaches and procedures, controlling environmental stimuli, providing comfort, providing for safety, and encouraging but not pushing the client beyond his functional abilities.

Assessments

- Obtain information about past and present patterns of behavior and functional abilities (e.g., sleep, medication use, elimination, food intake, communication, hygiene, social interaction)
- Assess for signs of depression (e.g., insomnia, flat affect, withdrawal, loss of appetite)

- *(NIC) Dementia Management:*
  - Monitor cognitive functioning, using a standardized assessment tool [e.g., the Mini-Mental State Examination]
  - Determine physical, social, and psychologic history of patient, usual habits, and routines
  - Determine behavioral expectations appropriate for patient's cognitive status
  - Monitor nutrition and weight
  - Monitor carefully for physiologic causes of increased confusion that may be acute and reversible

Patient/Family Teaching

- Teach patient and significant others about patient's medications
- Explain the effect of the patient's illness on his mood (e.g., depression, premenstrual syndrome)
- As needed, explain to family members that a shower or tub bath are not the only ways to get clean, and that forcing a patient to bathe when he is resisting can be harmful and provoke aggressive behaviors.

Collaborative Activities

- Administer mood-stabilizing medications
- Refer to social services department for referral to day care programs, Meals On Wheels, respite care, and so forth.

Other

- If client experiences delusions or hallucinations, refer to Nursing Activities in the diagnosis of Confusion, Acute.
- In early dementia, when the main symptoms are those of Impaired memory, refer to Nursing Activities for the nursing diagnosis, Memory, Impaired
- Provide opportunity for physical activity
- Alternate activity with scheduled quiet times and activities (e.g., an hour in a recliner or chair, quiet music) at least twice a day to allow for resolution of anxiety and tension
- Provide appropriate outlets for patient's feelings (e.g., art therapy and physical exercise)
- Assist with reality orientation (e.g., provide clocks, calendars, personal items, seasonal decorations)
- Keep environment as quiet as possible (e.g., avoid buzzers, alarms, and overhead paging systems)
- Consider giving a towel bath instead of a tub or shower; do not force a patient to bathe if he is resisting
- Avoid change as much as possible (e.g., in routines, environment, caregivers)

- *(NIC) Dementia Management:*

  Include family members in planning, providing, and evaluating care, to the extent desired

  Provide a low-stimulation environment (e.g., quiet, soothing music; nonvivid and simple, familiar patterns in decor; performance expectations that do not exceed cognitive-processing ability; and dining in small groups)

  Identify and remove potential dangers in environment for patient

  Place identification bracelet on patient

  Prepare for interaction with eye contact and touch, as appropriate

  Address the patient distinctly by name when initiating interaction and speak slowly

  Introduce self when initiating contact

  Give one simple direction at a time [and repeat as necessary (e.g., "follow me," or "sit on the chair," or "put on your slippers")]

  Use distraction, rather than confrontation, to manage behavior

  Provide patient a general orientation to the season of the year by using appropriate cues (e.g., holiday decorations, seasonal decorations and activities, and access to contained, out-of-doors area)

  Label familiar photos with names of the individuals in photos

  Limit number of choices patient has to make, so not to cause anxiety
- Avoid use of physical restraints
- Assist with self-care, as needed [specify methods]
- Provide boundaries, such as red or yellow tape, on the floor when low-stimulus units are not available

Home Care

- The preceding activities are appropriate for home care; teach family and other caregivers as needed
- Assess the client's functional and self-care abilities and evaluate their impact on his safety
- Assess the need for assistive devices; refer to an occupational therapist, if necessary
- Assess family caregivers for *Caregiver role strain*; provide information and emotional support
- Refer for homemaker services as needed.
- Teach the family how to communicate with the patient more effectively (e.g., give one simple direction at a time)
- Evaluate the client for day care programs

For Older Adults

- Promote reminiscence and life review (e.g., ask questions about client's work and family, such as "Looking back, what was really important to you?")
- Cognitive impairment is not a normal part of aging. Most older adults do not exhibit cognitive impairment except as a result of pathology
- Institute case management when need for a variety of services exists
- Older adults are more likely to experience side effects of medications that can contribute to confusion
- Be aware that older adults often underreport pain; treat pain to prevent agitation

CONSTIPATION

(1975, 1998) **Domain 3, Elimination and Exchange; Class 2, Gastrointestinal Function**

Definition: Decrease in normal frequency of defecation accompanied by difficult or incomplete passage of stool or passage of excessively hard, dry stool

Defining Characteristics

Subjective

Abdominal pain
Abdominal tenderness with or without palpable muscle resistance
Anorexia
Feeling of rectal fullness or pressure
Generalized fatigue
Headache
Increased abdominal pressure
Indigestion
Nausea
Pain with defecation

Objective

Atypical presentations in older adults (e.g., change in mental status, urinary incontinence, unexplained falls, elevated body temperature)
Bright red blood with stool
Change in abdominal growling (borborygmi)

Change in bowel pattern
Decreased frequency
Decreased volume of stool

Distended abdomen
Dry, hard, formed stools
Hypo- or hyperactive bowel sounds
Oozing liquid stool
Palpable abdominal mass
Palpable rectal mass
Percussed abdominal dullness
Presence of soft pastelike stool in rectum
Severe flatus
Straining with defecation
Unable to pass stool
Vomiting

Related Factors

Functional

Abdominal muscle weakness
Habitual denial and ignoring of urge to defecate
Inadequate toileting (e.g., timeliness, positioning for defecation, privacy)
Insufficient physical activity
Irregular defecation habits
Recent environmental changes

Psychological

Depression
Emotional stress
Mental confusion

Pharmacological

Aluminum-containing antacids
Anticholinergics
Anticonvulsants
Antidepressants
Antilipemic agents
Bismuth salts
Calcium carbonate
Calcium channel blockers
Diuretics
Iron salts

Laxative overdose
Nonsteroidal anti-inflammatory agents
Opiates
Phenothiazides
Sedatives
Sympathomimetics

Mechanical

Electrolyte imbalance
Hemorrhoids
Megacolon (Hirschsprung disease)
Neurological impairment
Obesity
Postsurgical obstruction
Pregnancy
Prostate enlargement
Rectal abscess or ulcer
Rectal anal fissures
Rectal anal stricture
Rectal prolapse
Rectocele
Tumors

Physiological

Change in usual foods and eating patterns
Decreased motility of gastrointestinal tract
Dehydration
Inadequate dentition or oral hygiene
Insufficient fiber intake
Insufficient fluid intake
Poor eating habits

Suggestions for Use

Use *Constipation* when defining characteristics are present. Some clients incorrectly believe they are constipated, and they self-medicate with laxatives, enemas, and/or suppositories to ensure a daily bowel movement. For such clients, use *Perceived constipation*. When risk factors are present, but there are no symptoms, use *Risk for constipation*.

Suggested Alternative Diagnoses

Constipation, perceived
Constipation, risk for

NOC Outcomes

Bowel Elimination: Formation and evacuation of stool

C

Hydration: Adequate water in the intracellular and extracellular compartments of the body

Ostomy Self-Care: Personal actions to maintain ostomy for elimination

Symptom Control: Personal actions to minimize perceived adverse changes in physical and emotional functioning

Goals/Evaluation Criteria

Examples Using NOC Language

- *Constipation* alleviated, as indicated by **Bowel Elimination** (specify 1–5: severely, substantially, moderately, mildly, or not compromised):
  - Elimination pattern
  - Stool soft and formed
  - Passage of stool without aids
- *Constipation* alleviated, as indicated by **Bowel Elimination** (specify 1–5: severe, substantial, moderate, mild, none):
  - Blood in stool
  - Pain with passage of stool

Other Examples

Patient will:

- Demonstrate knowledge of bowel regimen necessary to overcome the side effects of medications
- Report the passage of stool with a reduction of pain and straining
- Demonstrate adequate hydration (e.g., good skin turgor, intake of fluids approximately equal to output)

NIC Interventions

Bowel Management: Establishment and maintenance of a regular pattern of bowel elimination

Bowel Training: Assisting the patient to train the bowel to evacuate at specific intervals

Constipation/Impaction Management: Prevention and alleviation of constipation/impaction

Fluid Management: Promotion of fluid balance and prevention of complications resulting from abnormal or undesired fluid levels

Fluid/Electrolyte Management: Regulation and prevention of complications from altered fluid and/or electrolyte levels

Ostomy Care: Maintenance of elimination through a stoma and care of surrounding tissue

Nursing Activities

In general, nursing actions for this diagnosis focus on assessing for and treating the causes of *Constipation*. Often this includes promoting regular elimination habits, hydration, exercise or mobility, and a high-fiber diet.

Assessments

- Gather baseline data on bowel regimen, activity, medications, and patient's usual pattern
- Assess and document:
  - Color and consistency of first stool postoperatively
  - Frequency, color, and consistency of stool
  - Passage of flatus
  - Presence of impaction
  - Presence or absence of bowel sounds and abdominal distention in all four quadrants
- *(NIC) Constipation/Impaction Management:*
  - Monitor for signs and symptoms of bowel rupture or peritonitis
  - Identify factors (e.g., medications, bed rest, and diet) that may cause or contribute to constipation

Patient/Family Teaching

- Inform patient of possibility of medication-induced constipation
- Instruct patient in bowel elimination aids that will promote optimal bowel pattern at home
- Teach patient the effects of diet (e.g., fluids and fiber) on elimination
- Instruct patient in consequences of long-term laxative use
- Stress the avoidance of straining during defecation to prevent change in vital signs, dizziness, or bleeding
- *(NIC) Constipation/Impaction Management:* Explain etiology of problem and rationale for actions to patient

Collaborative Activities

- Consult with dietitian for increase in fiber and fluids in diet
- Request a physician's order for elimination aids, such as dietary bran, stool softeners, enemas, and laxatives
- *(NIC) Constipation/Impaction Management:*
  - Consult with physician about a decrease or increase in frequency of bowel sounds
  - Advise patient to consult with physician if constipation or impaction persists

Other

- Encourage patient to request pain medication prior to defecation to facilitate painless passage of stool

- Encourage optimal activity to stimulate patient's bowel elimination
- Provide privacy and safety for patient during bowel elimination
- Provide care in an accepting, nonjudgmental manner
- Provide fluids of patient's choice, specify

Home Care

- Teach patient and family how to keep a food diary
- Teach patient and/or caregivers not to remove impacted stool on their own, but to notify their professional caregiver
- Assess the home for accessibility and privacy of the bathroom

For Infants and Children

- Constipation in children is defined by passage of hard stool, difficulty passing stool, blood-streaked stool, and abdominal discomfort
- For infants, add fruit (not applesauce or apple juice) to the diet, or add corn syrup to the formula
- For children, mix bran cereal in with other cereals if they do not like eating it. Offer prune juice; mix with other juices or water if they do not like the taste
- Teach parents, when they begin toilet training, to watch for voluntary withholding of stool, which is a common cause of constipation in children
- If constipation is persistent, refer to a primary care provider

For Older Adults

- Constipation is more common in older adults than in other age groups. With aging, the rectal wall becomes less elastic and less mucus is secreted in the intestines. Older adults may also have decreased activity and insufficient intake of fluids and fiber. In addition, laxative abuse and side effects of medications may contribute to constipation
- At the first symptom of constipation, institute a bowel management program

CONSTIPATION, PERCEIVED

(1988) **Domain 3, Elimination and Exchange; Class 2, Gastrointestinal Function**

Definition: Self-diagnosis of constipation and abuse of laxatives, enemas, and /or suppositories to ensure a daily bowel movement

Defining Characteristics

Subjective

Expectation of a daily bowel movement

Expectation of passage of stool at same time every day

Objective

Overuse of laxatives, enemas, and suppositories [to induce a daily bowel movement]

Related Factors

Cultural and family health beliefs

Faulty appraisal [of normal bowel function]

Impaired thought processes

Suggestions for Use

See Suggestions for Use for the diagnosis Constipation.

Suggested Alternative Diagnoses

Constipation

Constipation, risk for

NOC Outcomes

Bowel Elimination: Formation and evacuation of stool

Health Beliefs: Personal convictions that influence health behaviors

Knowledge: Health Behavior: Extent of understanding conveyed about the promotion and protection of health

Goals/Evaluation Criteria

Examples Using NOC Language

- *Perceived constipation* alleviated, as indicated by Bowel Elimination, Health Beliefs, and Knowledge: Health Behavior

- Demonstrates **Bowel Elimination**, as evidenced by the following indicators (specify 1–5: severely, substantially, moderately, mildly, or not compromised):
  Elimination pattern
  Ease of stool passage
  Passage of stool without aids

Other Examples

Patient will:

- Verbalize understanding of need to decrease use of laxatives, enemas, and suppositories
- Describe dietary regimen that will more naturally regulate bowel function
- Verbalize understanding that it is not always necessary to have a bowel movement every day

NIC Interventions

Active Listening: Attending closely to and attaching significance to a patient's verbal and nonverbal messages

Bowel Management: Establishment and maintenance of a regular pattern of bowel elimination

Health Education: Developing and providing instruction and learning experiences to facilitate voluntary adaptation of behavior conducive to health in individuals, families, groups, or communities

Teaching: Individual: Planning, implementation, and evaluation of a teaching program designed to address a patient's particular needs

Nursing Activities

In general, nursing actions for this diagnosis focus on communication and teaching to change the patient's perception of normal elimination versus constipation, and instituting measures to support normal elimination.

Assessments

- Assess patient's expectation of normal bowel function
- Assess for factors contributing to the problem (e.g., cultural beliefs)
- Observe, document, and report requests for laxatives, enemas, or suppositories
- *(NIC) Bowel Management:*
  Monitor bowel movements, including frequency, consistency, shape, volume, and color, as appropriate
  Note preexistent bowel problems, bowel routine, and use of laxatives

Patient/Family Teaching

- Instruct patient and family in diet, fluid intake, activity, exercise, and the consequence of overuse of laxatives, enemas, and suppositories
- Teach patient/family that it may be normal to have a bowel movement only every 2 or 3 days rather than every day
- Teach the characteristics of normal elimination and compare with the symptoms of constipation

Collaborative Activities

- Initiate a multidisciplinary care conference involving the patient and family to encourage positive behaviors (e.g., change in diet)

Other

- Assist patient to identify realistic use of laxatives, enemas, and suppositories
- Provide positive feedback to patient when behavior change occurs
- *(NIC) Active Listening*: Focus completely on the interaction by suppressing prejudice, bias, assumptions, preoccupying personal concerns, and other distractions.

Home Care

- The preceding activities apply to home care

For Older Adults

- The preceding activities are appropriate for older adults, taking into account the normal developmental changes of aging

CONSTIPATION, RISK FOR

(1998) **Domain 3, Elimination and Exchange; Class 2, Gastrointestinal Function**

Definition: At risk for a decrease in normal frequency of defecation accompanied by difficult or incomplete passage of stool, or passage of excessively hard, dry stool

Risk Factors

Functional

Abdominal muscle weakness
Habitual denial and ignoring of urge to defecate
Inadequate toileting (e.g., timeliness, positioning for defecation, privacy)

Insufficient physical activity
Irregular defecation habits
Recent environmental changes

Psychological

Depression
Emotional stress
Mental confusion

Physiological

Change in usual foods and eating patterns
Decreased motility of gastrointestinal tract
Dehydration
Inadequate dentition or oral hygiene
Insufficient fiber intake
Insufficient fluid intake
Poor eating habits

Pharmacological

Aluminum-containing antacids
Anticholinergics
Anticonvulsants
Antidepressants
Antilipemic agents
Bismuth salts
Calcium carbonate
Calcium channel blockers
Diuretics
Iron salts
Laxative overuse
Nonsteroidal anti-inflammatory agents
Opiates
Phenothiazines
Sedatives
Sympathomimetics

Mechanical

Electrolyte imbalance
Hemorrhoids
Megacolon (Hirschsprung disease)
Neurological impairment
Obesity
Postsurgical obstruction
Pregnancy

Prostate enlargement
Rectal abscess or ulcer
Rectal anal fissures
Rectal anal stricture
Rectal prolapse
Rectocele
Tumors

Suggestions for Use

See Suggestions for Use for the diagnosis Constipation.

Suggested Alternative Diagnoses

Constipation
Constipation, perceived

NOC Outcomes

Bowel Elimination: Formation and evacuation of stool
Self-Care: Toileting: Ability to toilet self independently with or without assistive device

Goals/Evaluation Criteria

Examples Using NOC Language

- *Risk for constipation* alleviated, as indicated by status of Bowel Elimination and Toileting Self-Care
- Demonstrates **Bowel Elimination**, as evidenced by the following indicators (specify 1–5: severely, substantially, moderately, mildly, or not compromised):
  - Elimination pattern
  - Stool soft and formed
  - Passage of stool without aids
- Demonstrates **Bowel Elimination** (specify 1–5: severe, substantial, moderate, mild, none):
  - Blood in stool
  - Pain with passage of stool

Other Examples

The patient will:

- Demonstrate knowledge of bowel regimen necessary to overcome the side effects of medications
- Describe dietary requirements (e.g., fluids and fiber) necessary to maintain usual bowel pattern
- Pass stool of usual consistency and frequency for patient
- Report the passage of stool with no pain or straining

NIC Interventions

Constipation/Impaction Management: Prevention and alleviation of constipation/impaction

Exercise Promotion: Facilitation of regular physical activity to maintain or advance to a higher level of fitness and health

Fluid Management: Promotion of fluid balance and prevention of complications resulting from abnormal or undesired fluid levels

Nutrition Management: Assisting with or providing a balanced dietary intake of foods and fluids

Risk Identification: Analysis of potential risk factors, determination of health risks, and prioritization of risk reduction strategies for an individual or group

Self-Care Assistance: Toileting: Assisting another with elimination

Nursing Activities

In general, nursing actions for this diagnosis focus on recognizing the presence of risk factors for *Constipation*, monitoring for symptoms, promoting normal elimination, and activities to minimize or remove risk factors.

Assessments

- Gather baseline data on bowel regimen, activity, and medications
- Assess and document postoperatively:
  Color and consistency of first stool
  Passage of flatus
  Presence or absence of bowel sounds and abdominal distention

Patient/Family Teaching

- Inform patient of possibility of medication-induced constipation
- Explain the effects of fluids and fiber in preventing constipation
- Instruct patient in consequences of long-term laxative use

Collaborative Activities

- Refer to dietitian, as needed, to increase fiber and fluids in diet

Other

- Encourage optimal activity to stimulate bowel elimination
- Provide privacy and safety for patient during bowel elimination
- Provide fluids of patient's choice; specify fluids

(For other interventions, refer to the care plan for Constipation.)

CONTAMINATION

(2006) **Domain 11, Safety/Protection; Class 4, Environmental Hazards**

Definition: Exposure to environmental contaminants in doses sufficient to cause adverse health effects

Defining Characteristics

Defining characteristics are dependent on the causative agent. Agents cause a variety of individual organ responses as well as systemic responses.

Biologics

Dermatological, gastrointestinal, neurological, pulmonary, or renal effects of exposure to biologics

(Biologics include toxins from living organisms [bacteria, viruses, fungi])

Chemicals

Dermatological, gastrointestinal, immunological, neurological, pulmonary, and renal effects of chemical exposure

Major chemical agents: petroleum-based agents, anticholinesterases:

- Type I agents act on proximal tracheobronchial portion of the respiratory tract
- Type II agents act on alveoli
- Type III agents produce systemic effects

Pesticides

Dermatological, gastrointestinal, neurological, pulmonary, or renal effects of pesticide exposure

Major categories of pesticides: Insecticides, herbicides, fungicides, antimicrobials, rodenticides

Major pesticides: organophosphates, carbamates, organochlorines, pyrethrum, arsenic, glycophosphates, bipyridyls, chlorophenoxy

Pollution

Neurological or pulmonary effects of pollution exposure

Major locations: air, water, soil

Major pollution agents: asbestos, radon, tobacco, heavy metal, lead, noise, exhaust

Radiation

Genetic, immunologic, neurological, or oncologic effects of radiation exposure

Categories:
Internal—exposure through ingestion of radioactive material [e.g., food/water contamination]

External—exposure through direct contact with radioactive material)

Waste

Dermatological, gastrointestinal, hepatic, or pulmonary effects of waste exposure
Categories of waste: trash, raw sewage, industrial waste

Related Factors

External

Chemical contamination of food and water
Exposure to bioterrorism
Exposure to disaster (natural or man-made)
Exposure to radiation (occupation in radiography, employment in nuclear industries and electrical generating plants, living near nuclear industries and electrical generating plants)
Flaking, peeling paint or plaster in presence of young children
Flooring surface (carpeted surfaces hold contaminant residue more than hard floor surfaces)
Geographic area (living in area where high levels of contaminants exist)
Inadequate municipal services (trash removal, sewage treatment facilities)
Inappropriate or no use of protective clothing
Lack of breakdown of contaminants once indoors (breakdown is inhibited without sun and rain exposure)
Living in poverty (increases potential for multiple exposure, lack of access to health care, and poor diet)
Paint, lacquer, etc., in poorly ventilated areas or without effective protection
Personal and household hygiene practices
Playing in outdoor areas where environmental contaminants are used
Presence of atmospheric pollutants
Use of environmental contaminants in the home (e.g., pesticides, chemicals, environmental tobacco smoke)
Unprotected contact with heavy metals or chemicals (e.g., arsenic, chromium, lead)

Internal

Age (children less than 5 years breathe more air, drink more water, and consume more food per pound than adults, increasing exposure to toxicants present in air, water, soil, and food)

Age (older adults: normal decline in function of immune, integumentary, cardiac, renal, hepatic, and pulmonary systems; increase in adipose tissue mass and decline in lean body mass)
Concomitant or previous exposures
Developmental characteristics of children
Gestational age during exposure
Gender (females have greater proportion of body fat, increasing likelihood of accumulating more lipid-soluble toxins than men)
Nutritional factors (e.g., obesity, vitamin and mineral deficiencies)
Preexisting disease states
Pregnancy
Smoking

Suggestions for Use

As written, this diagnosis appears to be intended for use with individual patients rather than communities, although some of the outcomes and interventions might be at the community level. Do not use this diagnosis for every client who has been exposed to any small amount of environmental contaminant. We are all exposed, daily, to at least some dose of environmental contamination. Use this diagnosis only if the person is experiencing adverse health effects or if the dose was high enough that adverse health effects would be expected (even though symptoms have not yet appeared). If the contaminant is latex, use the more specific *Latex allergy response*.

Suggested Alternative Diagnoses

Latex allergy response

NOC Outcomes

Goals for this diagnosis should focus on the reasons for exposure and on the specific symptoms produced by the organs affected. These will vary greatly among situations.

Community Disaster Readiness: Community preparedness to respond to a natural or man-made calamitous event

Community Disaster Response: Community response following a natural or man-made calamitous event

Gastrointestinal Function: Extent to which foods (ingested or tube-fed) are moved from ingestion to excretion

Immune Hypersensitivity Response: Severity of inappropriate immune response

Immune Status: Natural and acquired appropriately targeted resistance to internal and external antigens

Kidney Function: Filtration of blood and elimination of metabolic waste products through the formation of urine

Neurological Status: Ability of the peripheral and central nervous system to receive, process, and respond to internal and external stimuli

Personal Health Status: Overall physical, psychological, social, and spiritual functioning of an adult 18 years or older

Respiratory Status: Movement of air in and out of the lungs and exchange of carbon dioxide and oxygen at the alveolar level

Tissue Integrity: Skin and Mucous Membranes: Structural intactness and normal physiological function of skin and mucous membranes

Goals/Evaluation Criteria

Examples Using NOC Language

- Demonstrates **Kidney Function**, as evidenced by the following indicators (specify 1–5: severely, substantially, moderately, mildly, or not compromised):
  - 24-hr intake and output balance
  - Blood urea nitrogen
  - Serum electrolytes
  - Urine proteins
- Demonstrates **Respiratory Status**, as evidenced by the following indicators (specify 1–5: severe, substantial, moderate, mild, or no deviation from normal range):
  - Oxygen saturation
  - Respiratory rate and rhythm
  - Auscultated breath sounds
- Demonstrates satisfactory defense against, or recovery from, *Contamination*, as evidenced by satisfactory **Gastrointestinal Function**, **Immune Hypersensitivity Response**, **Immune Status, Kidney Function**, **Neurological Status**, **Personal Health Status**, **Respiratory Status**, and **Tissue Integrity: Skin and Mucous Membranes**.

Other Examples

Patient will:

- Identify how contamination occurred (e.g., at work, in the community, in the home)
- Identify ways to avoid future contamination
- Stabilize physiologically to precontamination status
- Remove or alter factors in his or her personal environment that contribute to contamination

NIC Interventions

Community Disaster Preparedness: Preparing for an effective response to a large-scale disaster

Emergency Care: Providing life-saving measures in life-threatening situations

Energy Management: Regulating energy use to treat or prevent fatigue and optimize function

Environmental Risk Protection: Preventing and detecting disease and injury in populations at risk from environmental hazards

Fluid Management: Promotion of fluid balance and prevention of complications resulting from abnormal or undesired fluid levels

Infection Protection: Prevention and early detection of infection in a patient at risk

Neurologic Monitoring: Collection and analysis of patient data to prevent or minimize neurologic complications

Nutrition Therapy: Administration of food and fluids to support metabolic processes of a patient who is malnourished or at high risk for becoming malnourished

Respiratory Monitoring: Collection and analysis of patient data to ensure airway patency and adequate gas exchange

Skin Care: Topical Treatments: Application of topical substances or manipulation of devices to promote skin integrity and minimize skin breakdown

Skin Surveillance: Collection and analysis of patient data to maintain skin and mucous membrane integrity

Specimen Management: Obtaining, preparing, and preserving a specimen for a laboratory test

Surveillance: Purposeful and ongoing acquisition, interpretation, and synthesis of patient data for clinical decision making

Triage: Disaster: Establishing priorities of patient care for urgent treatment while allocating scarce resources

Ventilation Assistance: Promotion of an optimal spontaneous breathing pattern that maximizes oxygen and carbon dioxide exchange in the lungs

Vital Signs Monitoring: Collection and analysis of cardiovascular, respiratory, and body temperature data to determine and prevent complications

Nursing Activities

In general, nursing actions for this diagnosis should focus on altering the related factors, or etiologies, of the *Contamination*. These will vary widely; the following are examples:

Assessments

- Monitor systemic (e.g., dermatological, gastrointestinal, neurological, pulmonary, renal) effects of exposure to the contaminant

- Determine where and how exposure to the contaminant occurred
- *(NIC) Triage: Disaster*

  Acquire about the nature of the problem, emergency, accident, or disaster

  Identify the patient's chief complaint

  Check for medical alert tags as appropriate

  Conduct a primary survey of all body systems as appropriate

  Monitor for life-threatening injuries or acute needs

Patient/Family Teaching

- Be sure the family is aware of any high levels of contaminants in their geographical area
- Provide information about use of protective clothing, for example when using pesticides
- Teach the dangers of secondhand smoke

Collaborative Activities

- Notify agencies responsible for protecting the environment about the patient's situation

Other

- Know where to find decontamination policies, procedures, and protocols quickly
- *(NIC) Triage: Disaster*

  Evaluate critical patients from the field first

  Evacuate injured as appropriate

  Participate in prioritization of patients for treatment

  Attach appropriate identification as indicated by patient's status

Home Care

- Assess the home, especially older homes, for flaking, peeling paint
- Assess the home for other contaminants, such as mold, pesticides, smoke
- Teach clients safe food preparation and storage methods
- Teach clients about control of animal vectors and hosts (e.g., mosquitoes, rats)
- Assist the patient to identify ways to avoid bringing contaminants into the home from the workplace (e.g., by removing work clothing at work, if possible; or, if not, removing work clothing and showering outside the house when returning home)

CONTAMINATION, RISK FOR

(2006) **Domain 11, Safety/Protection; Class 4, Environmental Hazards**

Definition: At risk for exposure to environmental contaminants in doses sufficient to cause adverse health effects

Risk Factors

External

Chemical contamination of food and water
Exposure to bioterrorism
Exposure to disaster (natural or man-made)
Exposure to radiation (occupation in radiography, employment in nuclear industries and electrical generating plants, living near nuclear industries and electrical generating plants)
Flaking, peeling paint or plaster in presence of young children
Flooring surface (carpeted surfaces hold contaminant residue more than hard floor surfaces)
Geographic area (living in area where high level of contaminants exist)
Inadequate municipal services (e.g., trash removal, sewage treatment facilities)
Inappropriate or no use of protective clothing
Lack of breakdown of contaminants once indoors (breakdown is inhibited without sun and rain exposure)
Living in poverty (increases potential for multiple exposure, lack of access to health care, and poor diet)
Paint, lacquer, etc., in poorly ventilated areas or without effective protection
Personal and household hygiene practices
Playing in outdoor areas where environmental contaminants are used
Presence of atmospheric pollutants
Use of environmental contaminants in the home (e.g., pesticides, chemicals, environmental tobacco smoke)
Unprotected contact with heavy metals or chemicals (e.g., arsenic, chromium, lead)

Internal

Age (children less than 5 years) [Young children breathe more air, drink more water, and consume more food per pound than adults, increasing exposure to toxicants present in air, water, soil, and food.]

Age (older adults) [Older adults experience normal decline in function of immune, integumentary, cardiac, renal, hepatic, and pulmonary systems; increase in adipose tissue mass and decline in lean body mass.]

Concomitant or previous exposures
Developmental characteristics of children
Gender [females have greater proportion of body fat, increasing likelihood of accumulating more lipid-soluble toxins than men]
Gestational age during exposure
Nutritional factors (e.g., obesity, vitamin and mineral deficiencies)
Preexisting disease states
Pregnancy
Previous exposures
Smoking

Suggestions for Use

This diagnosis is more specific than *Risk for injury* and is, therefore, preferred when the risk injury is known to be from an environmental contaminant. If the contaminant is latex, use *Latex allergy response*. If the risk factor is exposure to microorganisms, use *Risk for infection*.

Suggested Alternative Diagnoses

Infection, risk for
Injury, risk for
Latex allergy response, risk for

NOC Outcomes

Community Disaster Response: Community response following a natural or man-made calamitous event

Immune Status: Natural and acquired appropriately targeted resistance to internal and external antigens

Knowledge: Health Behavior: Extent of understanding conveyed about the promotion and protection of health

Personal Safety Behavior: Personal actions of an adult to control behaviors that can cause physical injury

Risk Control: Personal actions to prevent, eliminate, or reduce modifiable health threats

Safe Home Environment: Physical arrangements to minimize environmental factors that might cause physical harm or injury in the home

Goals/Evaluation Criteria

Examples Using NOC Language

- Demonstrate **Safe Home Environment**, as evidenced by the following indicators (specify 1–5: not, slightly, moderately, substantially, or totally adequate):
  - Safe storage and disposal of hazardous materials
  - Correction of lead hazard risks
  - Elimination of rodents and insects
  - Carbon monoxide detector maintenance
  - Placement of appropriate hazard warning labels

Other Examples

Community will:

- Show evidence of health protection measures such as fluoridation and sanitation
- Comply with environmental health standards

Patient will:

- Be aware of environmental risk factors
- Avoid exposure to environmental contaminants
- Modify lifestyle as needed to avoid exposure to environmental contaminants
- Use protective clothing and devices when exposure to contaminants is likely (e.g., wears sunscreen)

NIC Interventions

Bioterrorism Preparedness: Preparing for an effective response to bioterrorism events or disaster

Community Disaster Preparedness: Preparing for an effective response to a large-scale disaster

Environmental Risk Protection: Preventing and detecting disease and injury in populations at risk from environmental hazards

Health Education: Developing and providing instruction and learning experiences to facilitate voluntary adaptation of behavior conducive to health in individuals, families, groups, or communities

Surveillance: Purposeful and ongoing acquisition, interpretation, and synthesis of patient data for clinical decision making

Surveillance: Community: Purposeful and ongoing acquisition, interpretation, and synthesis of data for decision making in the community

Nursing Activities

In general, nursing actions for this diagnosis should focus on identifying and removing risk factors in the home and community.

C

Assessments

- Be familiar with local, state, and national procedures and mechanisms for reporting communicable diseases, as well as other data.
- Identify environmental contaminants existing in the community
- Work with community members and agencies to raise awareness of environmental contaminants that are present
- Bring individuals and groups together to discuss common and competing interests

Patient/Family Teaching

- Be sure the family is aware of any high levels of contaminants in their geographical area
- Provide information about use of protective clothing, for example when using pesticides
- Teach the dangers of secondhand smoke

Collaborative Activities

- Notify the appropriate environmental protection agencies about known environmental contaminants
- Consult with epidemiologists and infection control professionals as necessary

Other

- Know where to find decontamination policies, procedures, and protocols quickly
- Become familiar with specific environmental standards (e.g., Occupational Safety and Health Administration [OSHA] Regulations; Environmental Protection Agency [EPA])

Home Care

- Refer to Home Care activities for the diagnosis Contamination.

COPING: COMMUNITY, INEFFECTIVE

(1994, 1998) **Domain 9, Coping/Stress Tolerance; Class 2, Coping Responses**

Definition: Pattern of community activities for adaptation and problem solving that is unsatisfactory for meeting the demands or needs of the community

Defining Characteristics

Subjective

Community does not meet its own expectations

Expressed community powerlessness

Expressed community vulnerability

Stressors perceived as excessive

Objective

Deficits in community participation

Excessive community conflicts

High illness rates

Increased social problems (e.g., homicides, vandalism, arson, terrorism, robbery, infanticide, abuse, divorce, unemployment, poverty, militancy, mental illness)

Related Factors

Deficits in community social support services or resources

Inadequate resources for problem solving

Ineffective or nonexistent community systems (e.g., lack of emergency medical system, transportation system, or disaster planning systems)

Natural or man-made disasters

Suggestions for Use

This diagnosis is most useful for community health nurses who focus on the health of groups (e.g., unwed mothers, all the people in a county, patients with diabetes). It may be useful as a risk diagnosis to describe a community that needs preventive interventions.

Suggested Alternative Diagnoses

Coping: Community, readiness for enhanced

NOC Outcomes

Community Competence: Capacity of a community to collectively problem solve to achieve community goals

Community Disaster Readiness: Community preparedness to respond to a natural or man-made calamitous event

Community Health Status: General state of well-being of a community or population

Community Health Status: Immunity: Resistance of community members to the invasion and spread of an infectious agent that could threaten public health

Community Risk Control: Chronic Disease: Community actions to reduce the risk of chronic diseases and related complications

Community Risk Control: Communicable Disease: Community actions to eliminate or reduce the spread of infectious agents that threaten public health

Community Risk Control: Lead Exposure: Community actions to reduce lead exposure and poisoning

Community Risk Control: Violence: Community actions to eliminate or reduce intentional violent acts resulting in serious physical or psychological harm

Community Violence Level: Incidence of violent acts compared with local, state, or national values

(Also refer to NOC Outcomes for Readiness for Enhanced Community Coping.)

Goals/Evaluation Criteria

Examples Using NOC Language

- *Ineffective community coping* alleviated, as indicated by status of Community Competence, Community Disaster Readiness, Community Disaster Response, Community Health Status, Community Health Status: Immunity, Community Risk Control: Chronic and Communicable Diseases, Community Risk Control: Lead Exposure, Community Risk Control: Violence, and Community Violence Level
- Demonstrates **Community Health Status**, as evidenced by the following indicators (specify 1–5: poor, fair, good, very good, or excellent):
  - Prevalence of health promotion programs
  - Prevalence of health protection programs
  - Health status of infants, children, adolescents, adults, and elders
  - Compliance with environmental health standards
  - Morbidity rates
  - Mortality rates
  - Crime statistics
  - Health surveillance data systems in place

Other Examples

The community:

- Develops improved communication among its members
- Implements effective problem-solving strategies
- Develops group cohesiveness
- Expresses the power to manage change and improve community functioning

NIC Interventions

Bioterrorism Preparedness: Preparing for an effective response to bioterrorism events or disaster

Case Management: Coordinating care and advocating for specified individuals and patient populations across settings to reduce cost, reduce resource use, improve quality of health care, and achieve desired outcomes

Communicable Disease Management: Working with a community to decrease and manage the incidence and prevalence of contagious diseases in a specific population

Community Disaster Preparedness: Preparing for an effective response to a large-scale disaster

Community Health Development: Assisting members of a community to identify a community's health concerns, mobilize resources, and implement solutions

Environmental Management: Community: Monitoring and influencing of the physical, social, cultural, economic, and political conditions that affect the health of groups and communities

Environmental Management: Violence Prevention: Monitoring and manipulation of the physical environment to decrease the potential for violent behavior directed toward self, others, or environment

Environmental Risk Protection: Preventing and detecting disease and injury in populations at risk from environmental hazards

Health Education: Developing and providing instruction and learning experiences to facilitate voluntary adaptation of behavior conducive to health in individuals, families, groups, or communities

Immunization/Vaccination Management: Monitoring immunization status, facilitating access to immunization, and providing immunizations to prevent communicable disease

Program Development: Planning, implementing, and evaluating a coordinated set of activities designed to enhance wellness, or to prevent, reduce, or eliminate one or more health problems for a group or community

Surveillance: Community: Purposeful and ongoing acquisition, interpretation, and synthesis of data for decision making in the community

(Also refer to NIC Interventions for Readiness for Enhanced Community Coping.)

Nursing Activities

In general, nursing actions for this diagnosis focus on assessing for causative factors, promoting communication among community members and groups, assisting with problem solving, and providing information about resources.

C

Assessments

- Assess and identify causative or risk factors affecting the community's ability to adapt and cope effectively (e.g., lack of information about available resources)
- Assess the effects of health policies and standards on nursing practice, patient outcomes, and health care costs
- Determine the availability of resources and the extent to which they are being used
- *(NIC) Environmental Management: Community:*
  Initiate screening for health risks from the environment
  Monitor status of known health risks

Teaching

- Help to identify and mobilize available resources and supports (e.g., emergency aid from the Red Cross)
- Inform policy makers of projected effects of policies on patient welfare
- Inform health care consumers of current and proposed changes in health policies and standards and potential effects on health
- *(NIC) Environmental Management: Community:* Conduct educational programs for targeted risk groups [e.g., teenage pregnancy]

Collaborative Activities

- *(NIC) Environmental Management: Community:*
  Participate in multidisciplinary teams to identify threats to safety in the community
  Coordinate services to at-risk groups and communities
  Work with environmental groups to secure appropriate governmental regulations
  Collaborate in the development of community action programs

Other

- Participate in lobbying for changes in health policies and standards to improve health care
- Arrange opportunities for community members to meet and discuss the situation (e.g., civic organizations, church groups, town meetings)
- Assist community members to become aware of conflicts that prevent them from working together (e.g., anger, mistrust)
- Determine ways of disseminating information to the community (e.g., radio and television reports, flyers, meetings)
- Help write grant proposals to obtain funding for programs needed to improve community coping

- Advocate for the community (e.g., write letters to government agencies and newspapers)
- *(NIC) Environmental Management: Community:* Encourage neighborhoods to become active participants in community safety

COPING: COMMUNITY, READINESS FOR ENHANCED

(1994) **Domain 9, Coping/Stress Tolerance; Class 2, Coping Responses**

Definition: Pattern of community activities for adaptation and problem solving that is satisfactory for meeting the demands or needs of the community for management of current and future problems and/or stressors and can be strengthened

Defining Characteristics

Objective

One or more of the following characteristics that indicate effective coping:
Active planning by community for predicted stressors
Active problem solving by community when faced with issues
Agreement that community is responsible for stress management
Positive communication among community members
Positive communication among community, aggregates, and the larger community
Programs available for recreation and relaxation
Resources sufficient for managing stressors

Related Factors (Non-NANDA-I)

Community has a sense of power to manage stressors
Resources available for problem solving
Social supports available

Suggestions for Use

This diagnosis can be used for a community that is meeting its basic needs for a clean environment, food, shelter, and safety, and wishes to focus on higher levels of functioning, such as wellness promotion. When external threats (e.g., floods, epidemics) occur in such a community, they pose risk factors; as long as the community continues to adapt, *Risk for ineffective community coping*, a non-NANDA-I diagnosis, should be used. If the threat produces defining characteristics (symptoms) in the community, use *Ineffective community coping*.

Suggested Alternative Diagnoses

Coping: community, ineffective
Coping: community, risk for ineffective

C

NOC Outcomes

Community Competence: Capacity of a community to collectively problem solve to achieve community goals

Community Disaster Readiness: Community preparedness to respond to a natural or man-made calamitous event

Community Health Status: Immunity: Resistance of community members to the invasion and spread of an infectious agent that could threaten public health

Community Risk Control: Communicable Disease: Community actions to eliminate or reduce the spread of infectious agents that threaten public health

Community Risk Control: Lead Exposure: Community actions to reduce lead exposure and poisoning

Community Violence Level: Incidence of violent acts compared with local, state, or national values

Goals/Evaluation Criteria

Examples Using NOC Language

- Demonstrates **Community Competence**, as evidenced by the following indicators (specify 1–5: poor, fair, good, very good, or excellent):
  - Representation of all segments of the community in problem solving
  - Communication among members and groups
  - Use of external resources to meet goals
  - Effective use of conflict management strategies

Other Examples:

The community:

- Has a plan in place to deal with problems and stressors
- Accesses or develops programs designed to improve the well-being of specific groups within the population (e.g., weight-control programs, retirement-planning programs)
- Continues to enhance present methods of communication and problem solving
- Expresses the power to manage change and improve community functioning
- Builds upon existing group cohesiveness
- Expresses the power to manage change and improve community functioning

NIC Interventions

Bioterrorism Preparedness: Preparing for an effective response to bioterrorism events or disaster

Communicable Disease Management: Working with a community to decrease and manage the incidence and prevalence of contagious diseases in a specific population

Community Disaster Preparedness: Preparing for an effective response to a large-scale disaster

Environmental Management: Community: Monitoring and influencing of the physical, social, cultural, economic, and political conditions that affect the health of groups and communities

Environmental Risk Protection: Preventing and detecting disease and injury in populations at risk from environmental hazards

Environmental Management: Violence Prevention: Monitoring and manipulation of the physical environment to decrease the potential for violent behavior directed toward self, others, or environment

Health Policy Monitoring: Surveillance and influence of government and organization regulations, rules, and standards that affect nursing systems and practices to ensure quality care of patients

Immunization/Vaccination Management: Monitoring immunization status, facilitating access to immunizations, and providing immunizations to prevent communicable disease

Program Development: Planning, implementing, and evaluating a coordinated set of activities designed to enhance wellness, or to prevent, reduce, or eliminate one or more health problems for a group or community

Surveillance: Community: Purposeful and ongoing acquisition, interpretation, and synthesis of data for decision making in the community

Nursing Activities

In general, nursing actions for this diagnosis focus on assessing community needs, assisting with adaptation and problem-solving, and instituting wellness and self-actualization programs.

Assessments

- Determine the availability of resources and the extent to which they are being used
- Identify groups that are at most risk for unhealthful behavior
- Identify factors in high-risk groups that may motivate or prevent healthful behavior
- Determine sociocultural and historic context of individual and group health behaviors

- Create and implement processes for regular evaluation of client outcomes during and after completion of program or activities
- Assess the effects of health policies and standards on nursing practice, patient outcomes, and health care costs
- *(NIC) Environmental Management: Community*: Initiate screening for health risks from the environment

Teaching

- Help to identify and mobilize available resources and supports (e.g., funding sources, supplies)
- Select learning strategies based on identified characteristics of target population
- Design processes for informing health care consumers of existing and proposed changes in health policies
- Provide educational materials written at an appropriate level for the target group
- *(NIC) Environmental Management: Community*: Conduct educational programs for targeted risk groups [e.g., teenage pregnancy]

Collaborative Activities

- Help the community obtain funding for wellness programs (e.g., education, smoking prevention)
- *(NIC) Environmental Management: Community:*

  Participate in multidisciplinary teams to identify threats to safety in the community

  Collaborate in the development of community-action programs

  Work with environmental groups to secure appropriate governmental regulations

Other

- Establish a collaborative partnership with the community and explain the role of a community health nurse in wellness promotion
- Lobby or write letters to urge policies that promote health (e.g., health education guaranteed as an employee benefit; insurance premium reductions for healthy behaviors and lifestyles)
- Help write grants to obtain funding for wellness programs
- Assist in improving educational levels within the community
- *(NIC) Environmental Management: Community:*

  Promote governmental policy to reduce specified risks

  Encourage neighborhoods to become active participants in community safety

  Coordinate services to at-risk groups and communities

COPING, DEFENSIVE

(1988, 2008) **Domain 9, Coping/Stress Tolerance; Class 2, Coping Responses**

Definition: Repeated projection of falsely positive self-evaluation based on a self-protective pattern that defends against underlying perceived threats to positive self-regard

Defining Characteristics

Subjective

Denial of obvious problems and weaknesses
Difficulty in perception of reality
Reality distortion
Projection of blame and responsibility
Rationalizes failures

Objective

Grandiosity
Difficulty in establishing or maintaining relationships
Hostile laughter or ridicule of others
Hypersensitive to slight or criticism
Lack of follow-through or participation in treatment or therapy
Superior attitude toward others

Related Factors

Conflict between self-perception and value system
Deficient support system
Fear of failure, humiliation, or repercussions
Lack of resilience
Low level of confidence in others
Low level of self-confidence
Uncertainty
Unrealistic expectations of self

Suggestions for Use

This diagnosis is less specific than *Ineffective denial*, which is actually one of many manifestations of *Defensive coping*. Use the more specific diagnosis when attempts to cope involve overuse or misuse of denial. Because *Powerlessness* may lead to *Defensive coping*, it is important to determine which should be the focus of interventions when both are present.

Suggested Alternative Diagnoses

Coping, ineffective
Denial, ineffective

Health behavior, risk prone
Powerlessness

NOC Outcomes

Acceptance: Health Status: Reconciliation to significant change in health circumstances

Adaptation to Physical Disability: Adaptive response to a significant functional challenge due to a physical disability

Coping: Personal actions to manage stressors that tax an individual's resources

Participation in Health Care Decisions: Personal involvement in selecting and evaluating health care options to achieve desired outcome

Self-Esteem: Personal judgment of self-worth

Social Interaction Skills: Personal behaviors that promote effective relationships

Goals/Evaluation Criteria

Examples Using NOC Language

- Patient will not use *Defensive coping*, as demonstrated by Acceptance: Health Status, Adaptation to Physical Disability, effective Coping, positive Self-Esteem and Social Interaction Skills, and Participation in Health Care Decisions.
- Demonstrates **Coping**, as evidenced by the following indicators (specify 1–5: never, rarely, sometimes, often, or consistently demonstrated):
  - Modifies lifestyle to reduce stress
  - Seeks reputable information concerning illness and treatment
  - Obtains assistance from health care professional
  - Verbalizes acceptance of situation
  - Uses effective coping strategies

Other Examples

Patient will:

- Acknowledge specific problems and conflicts that interfere with social interactions and relationships
- Demonstrate decrease in defensiveness
- Express feelings about changes in health
- Express feelings of self-worth
- Reformulate previous concept of health
- Maintain effective interactions with others

C

NIC Interventions

Behavior Modification: Promotion of a behavior change

Behavior Modification: Social Skills: Assisting the patient to develop or improve interpersonal social skills

Complex Relationship Building: Establishing a therapeutic relationship with a patient who has difficulty interacting with others

Coping Enhancement: Assisting a patient to adapt to perceived stressors, changes, or threats that interfere with meeting life demands and roles

Counseling: Use of an interactive helping process focusing on the needs, problems, or feelings of the patient and significant others to enhance or support coping, problem solving, and interpersonal relationships

Emotional Support: Provision of reassurance, acceptance, and encouragement during times of stress

Self-Awareness Enhancement: Assisting a patient to explore and understand his thoughts, feelings, motivations, and behaviors

Self-Esteem Enhancement: Assisting a patient to increase his personal judgment of self-worth

Self-Responsibility Facilitation: Encouraging a patient to assume more responsibility for own behavior

Nursing Activities

In general, nursing actions for this diagnosis focus on establishing a therapeutic relationship, reducing stressors, and promoting self-esteem.

Assessments

- Assess degree of defensiveness and denial that interferes with self-assessment
- Assess self-esteem level
- Assess for feelings of powerlessness
- Assess for substance abuse

Patient/Family Teaching

- Teach alternative behaviors to obtain positive regard through group therapy, individual therapy, role playing, and role modeling

Collaborative Activities

- Refer to appropriate community resources (e.g., family or marriage counseling, substance-abuse groups)
- Refer to a mental health professional if necessary, especially when the client is coping with a traumatic event

Other

- Communicate acceptance, convey respect, and validate the patient's concerns

- Assist patient in recognizing negative coping behaviors
- Identify and discuss the subjects, situations, and people that trigger negative coping behaviors

- Provide feedback in a supportive environment on how behavior is being perceived by others
- Provide reality testing during times of grandiose behavior, denial of obvious problems, and projected blame and responsibility
- Use group situations in which the client can receive feedback about others' perceptions of his use of denial
- *(NIC) Self-Awareness Enhancement:*

  Assist patient to identify the impact of illness on self-concept
  Verbalize patient's denial of reality, as appropriate
  Assist patient to identify life priorities
  Assist patient to identify positive attributes of self

Home Care

- Assess family communication patterns for support and dysfunction
- Include family in treatment, as needed
- Refer for psychiatric home health care services
- Support family use of religion as a coping method

For Older Adults

- Assess for depression and/or dementia that may be contributing to *Defensive coping*

COPING: FAMILY, COMPROMISED

(1980, 1996) **Domain 9, Coping/Stress Tolerance; Class 2, Coping Responses**

Definition: Usually supportive primary person (family member, significant other, or close friend) provides insufficient, ineffective, or compromised support, comfort, assistance, or encouragement that may be needed by the client to manage or master adaptive tasks related to his health challenge

Defining Characteristics

Subjective

Client expresses a concern or complaint about significant person's response to his health problem

Significant person expresses an inadequate knowledge base or inadequate understanding, which interferes with effective supportive behaviors

Significant person describes preoccupation with personal reaction (e.g., fear, anticipatory grief, guilt, anxiety) to client's need

Objective

Significant person attempts assistive or supportive behaviors with unsatisfactory results

Significant person displays protective behavior disproportionate (too little or too much) to the client's abilities or need for autonomy

Significant person withdraws from client

Significant person enters into limited personal communication with client

Other Defining Characteristics (Non-NANDA International)

Family displays emotional lability

Family displays rigid role boundaries

Family member interferes with necessary medical and nursing actions

Family members are divisive and form unsupportive coalitions

Family verbal interaction with patient is absent or decreased

Related Factors

Coexisting situations affecting the significant person

Developmental crisis of significant person [specify]

Exhaustion of supportive capacity of significant people

Inadequate or incorrect information or understanding of information by a primary person

Lack of reciprocal support

Little support provided by client, in turn, for primary person

Prolonged disease or disability progression that exhausts supportive capacity of significant people

Situational crisis of significant person [specify]

Temporary family disorganization or role changes

Temporary preoccupation by a significant person

Suggestions for Use

(a) *Caregiver role strain* focuses on the needs of the caregiving family member, whereas *Family coping: compromised* focuses more on the needs of the patient. (b) The distinctions between this diagnosis and *Interrupted family processes* are not clear. (c) For severe malfunction or for abusive or destructive situations, use *Disabled family coping*, which is distinguished by the following defining characteristics:

Denial of existence or severity of illness of a family member

Despair, rejection

Desertion

Abuse (child, spousal, elder)

Suggested Alternative Diagnoses

Caregiver role strain (actual or risk for)

Family coping, disabled

Family processes, interrupted

Parental role conflict

Parenting, impaired

Therapeutic regimen management: Family, ineffective

NOC Outcomes

Caregiver Emotional Health: Emotional well-being of a family care provider while caring for a family member

Caregiver Role Endurance: Factors that promote family care provider's capacity to sustain caregiving over an extended period of time

(Also see NOC Outcomes for Family Coping, Disabled.)

Goals/Evaluation Criteria

Examples Using NOC Language

- Family will not use *Compromised family coping*, as demonstrated by satisfactory status of Caregiver Emotional Health, Caregiver–Patient Relationship, Caregiver Performance: Direct and Indirect Care, Caregiver Role Endurance, Caregiver Well-Being, Family Coping, and Family Normalization
- Also see Goals/Evaluation Criteria for *Family Coping, Disabled.*

NIC Interventions

Caregiver Support: Provision of the necessary information, advocacy, and support to facilitate primary patient care by someone other than a health care professional

Coping Enhancement: Assisting a patient *to* adapt to perceived stressors, changes, or threats that interfere with meeting life demands and roles

Emotional Support: Provision of reassurance, acceptance, and encouragement during times of stress

Family Involvement Promotion: Facilitating family participation in the emotional and physical care of the patient

Family Mobilization: Utilization of family strengths to influence patient's health in a positive direction

Family Process Maintenance: Minimization of family process disruption effects

Family Support: Promotion of family values, interests, and goals
Health System Guidance: Facilitating a patient's location and use of appropriate health services
Learning Facilitation: Promoting the ability to process and comprehend information
Normalization Promotion: Assisting parents and other family members of children with chronic illness or disabilities in providing normal life experiences for their children and families
Respite Care: Provision of short-term care to provide relief for family caregiver

Nursing Activities

In general, nursing actions for this diagnosis focus on assessing for abusive behaviors, promoting positive family communication patterns, teaching family members how to care for the patient, and providing information and emotional support

Assessments

- Identify level of patient's self-care deficits and dependency on family
- Assess interaction between patient and family; be alert for potential destructive behaviors
- Assess ability and readiness of family members to learn
- Determine extent to which family members wish to be involved with the patient
- Identify the family's expectations of and for the patient
- Identify family structure and roles
- *(NIC) Family Support:*
  Appraise family's emotional reaction to patient's condition
  Identify nature of spiritual support for family

Patient/Family Teaching

- Discuss the common responses to health challenges (e.g., anxiety, dependency, depression)
- Provide information about specific health challenge and necessary coping skills
- Teach the family those skills required for care of patient; specify skills
- Teach, role-model, and reinforce communication skills, which may include active listening, reflection, "I" statements, conflict resolution
- *(NIC) Family Support:*
  Teach the medical and nursing plans of care to family
  Provide necessary knowledge of options to family that will assist them to make decisions about patient care

Collaborative Activities

C

- Explore available hospital resources and support systems with family
- Request social service consultation to help the family determine post-hospitalization needs and identify sources of community support (e.g., support groups for families of Alzheimer's clients)
- Initiate a multidisciplinary patient care conference, involving the patient and family in problem solving and facilitation of communication
- *(NIC) Family Support:*
  Provide spiritual resources for family, as appropriate
  Arrange for ongoing respite care, when indicated and desired
  Provide opportunities for peer group support

Other

- Promote an open, trusting relationship with family
- Encourage patient and family to focus on positive aspects of the patient's situation
- Assist family in identifying behaviors that may be hindering prescribed treatment
- Assist family in realistically identifying the needs of patient and family unit
- Assist family with decision making and problem solving
- Encourage family to identify needed role changes to maintain family integrity
- Encourage family to recognize changes in interpersonal relationships
- Explore impact of conflicting values or coping styles on family relationships
- Encourage family to visit or care for patient whenever possible; provide privacy to facilitate family interactions
- Provide structure to family interaction. Consider content of interaction, length of visiting time, staff support during visit, and which family member(s) will visit, based on patient's treatment plan
- *(NIC) Family Support:*
  Foster realistic hope
  Listen to family concerns, feelings, and questions
  Facilitate communication of concerns and feelings between patient and family or between family members
  Answer all questions of family members or assist them to get answers
  Give care to patient in lieu of family to relieve them or when family is unable to give care
  Provide feedback for family regarding their coping

Home Care
- All of the preceding interventions apply to home care
- Institute telephone support for caregivers of a family member with dementia

For Infants and Children
- Encourage parents to play with, talk to, and sing to even a seriously ill child

For Older Adults
- Assess the needs and abilities of the spousal caregiver
- Reassure the caregiver of his ability to handle the caregiving and to look at the positive aspects of each situation

COPING: FAMILY, DISABLED

(1980, 1996, 2008) **Domain 9, Coping/Stress Tolerance; Class 2, Coping Responses**

Definition: Behavior of primary person (family member, significant other, or close friend) that disables his capacities and the client's capacities to effectively address tasks essential to either person's adaptation to the health challenge

Defining Characteristics

Subjective

Depression

Distortion of reality regarding patient's health problem [including extreme denial about its existence or severity]

Objective

Abandonment

Aggression and hostility

Agitation

Carrying on usual routines, disregarding client's needs

Client's development of dependence

Desertion

Disregarding client's needs

Family behaviors that are detrimental to well-being

Impaired individualization
Impaired restructuring of a meaningful life for self
Intolerance

Neglectful care of client in regard to basic human needs or illness treatment
Neglectful relationships with other family members
Prolonged overconcern for client
Psychosomaticism
Rejection
Taking on illness signs of client

Related Factors

Arbitrary handling of family's resistance to treatment [which tends to solidify defensiveness as it fails to deal adequately with underlying anxiety]
Dissonant coping styles for dealing with adaptive tasks by the significant person and client or among significant people
Highly ambivalent family relationships
Significant person with chronically unexpressed feelings of (hostility, anxiety, guilt, despair, and so forth)

Other Possible Related Factors (Non-NANDA International)

Emotionally disturbed family member
Substance-abusing family member
Use of violence to manage conflict

Suggestions for Use

This label is appropriate when there is severe malfunction or for abusive or destructive situations. It represents a more dysfunctional situation than does *Interrupted family processes* or *Compromised family coping*. The diagnostic label *Caregiver role strain* focuses on the needs of the caregiving family member, whereas *Disabled family coping* focuses more on the needs of the patient or the family unit. If there is actual violence in the family, the diagnosis might be *Disabled family coping related to use of violence to manage conflict*. When the abusive behavior is potential rather than actual, the label *Risk for violence* should be used.

Suggested Alternative Diagnoses

Caregiver role strain (actual or risk for)
Coping: family, compromised
Therapeutic regimen management: family/individual, ineffective

Parenting, impaired
Violence: other-directed, risk for

NOC Outcomes

Caregiver–Patient Relationship: Positive interactions and connections between the caregiver and care recipient

Caregiver Performance: Direct Care: Provision by family care provider of appropriate personal and health care for a family member

Caregiver Performance: Indirect Care: Arrangement and oversight by family care provider of appropriate care for a family member

Caregiver Well-Being: Extent of positive perception of primary care provider's health status and life circumstances

Caregiver Role Endurance: Factors that promote family care provider's capacity to sustain caregiving over an extended period of time

Caregiver Well-Being: Extent of positive perception of primary care provider's health status and life circumstances

Family Coping: Family actions to manage stressors that tax family resources

Family Normalization: Capacity of the family system to maintain routines and develop strategies for optimal functioning when a member has a chronic illness or disability

Neglect Cessation: Evidence that the victim is no longer receiving substandard care

Goals/Evaluation Criteria

Examples Using NOC Language

- Family will not experience *Disabled family coping*, as demonstrated by satisfactory status of Caregiver–Patient Relationship, Caregiver Performance: Direct and Indirect Care, Caregiver Role Endurance, Caregiver Well-Being, Family Coping, Family Normalization, and Neglect Cessation.
- *Family Coping* indicators include the following (specify 1–5: never, rarely, sometimes, often, or consistently demonstrated):

    Establishes role flexibility
    Manages family problems
    Cares for needs of all family members
    Maintains financial stability
    Obtains family assistance

Other Examples

Family will:

- Achieve financial stability to care for needs of family members
- Acknowledge needs of family unit

- Acknowledge needs of patient
- Begin to demonstrate effective interpersonal skills
- Demonstrate ability to resolve conflict without violence
- Express increased ability to cope with changes in family structure and dynamics
- Express unresolved feelings
- Identify and maintain intrafamily sexual boundaries
- Identify conflicting coping styles
- Participate in effective problem solving
- Participate in developing and implementing treatment plan

NIC Interventions

Abuse Protection Support: Identification of high-risk dependent relationships and actions to prevent further infliction of physical or emotional harm

Caregiver Support: Provision of the necessary information, advocacy, and support to facilitate primary patient care by someone other than a health care professional

Coping Enhancement: Assisting a patient to adapt to perceived stressors, changes, or threats that interfere with meeting life demands and roles

Environmental Management: Home Preparation: Preparing the home for safe and effective delivery of care

Family Involvement Promotion: Facilitating family participation in the emotional and physical care of the patient

Family Support: Promotion of family values, interests, and goals

Family Therapy: Assisting family members to move their family toward a more productive way of living

Health System Guidance: Facilitating a patient's location and use of appropriate health services

Learning Facilitation: Promoting the ability to process and comprehend information

Normalization Promotion: Assisting parents and other family members of children with chronic illnesses or disabilities in providing normal life experiences for their children and families

Respite Care: Provision of short-term care to provide relief for family caregiver

Nursing Activities

In general, nursing actions for this diagnosis focus on assessing the danger to the victim, assessing for causal or contributing factors, providing for the immediate safety of the victim, teaching, providing support for decision making, assisting the family to deal with the present situation, and making referrals.

Also refer to Nursing Activities in Coping: Family, Compromised.

Assessments

- Obtain history of family's pattern of behaviors and interactions and changes that have occurred
- Determine physical, emotional, and educational resources of family members
- Assess family members' motivation and desire for resolving areas of dissatisfaction or conflict
- *(NIC) Family Support:* Determine the psychological burden of prognosis for family

Patient/Family Teaching

- Discuss how violence is a learned behavior and can be transmitted to offspring
- Discuss with family effective ways to demonstrate feelings

Collaborative Activities

- Refer family and individual members to support groups, psychiatric treatment, social services (e.g., chemical-dependence programs, Parents United, Incest Survivors Anonymous, child protective services, battered wives' shelters)
- Report indications of physical or sexual abuse as directed by law to appropriate authorities

Other

- In family discussions, begin with the least emotionally laden subjects
- Assist family in recognizing the problem (e.g., managing conflict with violence, sexual abuse)
- Encourage family participation in all group meetings
- Encourage family to express concerns and to help plan posthospital care
- Help motivate family to change
- Assist family in finding better ways to handle dysfunctional behavior
- Provide "homework" for family members (e.g., a no-television night or eating some meals together)
- Assist family members in clarifying what they expect and need from each other
- Provide accurate, complete documentation of injuries and what the patient and caregivers say about them (e.g., type, occurrence, frequency)

Home Care

- All of the preceding interventions apply to home care

C

For Infants and Children

- See For Infants and Children in Compromised Family Coping.

For Older Adults

- Refer to senior centers and day care programs
- See For Older Adults in Compromised Family Coping

COPING: FAMILY, READINESS FOR ENHANCED

(1980) **Domain 9, Coping/Stress Tolerance; Class 2, Coping Responses**

Definition: A pattern of management of adaptive tasks by primary person (family member, significant other, or close friend) involved with the client's health challenge that is sufficient for health and growth, in regard to self and in relation to the client, and can be strengthened

Defining Characteristics

Subjective

Individual expresses interest in making contact with others who have experienced a similar situation

Significant person attempts to describe growth impact of crisis

Objective

Chooses experiences that optimize wellness

Significant person moves in direction of enriching lifestyle, or in the direction of health promotion

Related Factors

Needs sufficiently gratified and adaptive tasks effectively addressed to enable goals of self-actualization to surface (non-NANDA International)

Suggestions for Use

Use this diagnosis for a normally functioning family that wishes to preserve and improve family integrity during changes brought about by illness or developmental and situational crises. Such a family might wish to have control over outcomes or enhance their quality of life. There is some overlap between this label and the following Suggested Alternative Diagnoses. Pending further research, use *Readiness for enhanced family processes*.

Suggested Alternative Diagnoses

Readiness for enhanced family processes

NOC Outcomes

Caregiver Well-Being: Extent of positive perception of primary care provider's health status and life circumstance

Family Coping: Family actions to manage stressors that tax family resources

Family Functioning: Capacity of the family system to meet the needs of its members during developmental transitions

Family Normalization: Capacity of the family system to maintain routines and develop strategies for optimal functioning when a member has a chronic illness or disability

Family Resiliency: Positive adaptation and function of the family system following significant adversity or crisis

Health Promoting Behavior: Personal actions to sustain or increase wellness

Health Seeking Behavior: Personal actions to promote optimal wellness, recovery, and rehabilitation

Goals/Evaluation Criteria

(Also refer to Goals/Evaluation Criteria for the diagnoses Readiness for Enhanced Family Processes.)

Examples Using NOC Language

- Family will demonstrate **Family Functioning**, as evidenced by the following indicators (specify 1–5: never, rarely, sometimes, often, or consistently demonstrated):
  - Regulates behavior of members
  - Adapts to developmental transitions
  - Obtains adequate resources to meet needs of members
  - Members perform expected roles
  - Members support one another

Other Examples

Family member(s) will:

- Develop a plan for personal growth
- Evaluate and change plan as needed

- Identify and prioritize personal goals
- Implement plan

C NIC Interventions

Caregiver Support: Provision of the necessary information, advocacy, and support to facilitate primary patient care by someone other than a health care professional

Coping Enhancement: Assisting a patient to adapt to perceived stressors, changes, or threats that interfere with meeting life demands and roles

Family Involvement Promotion: Facilitating family participation in the emotional and physical care of the patient

Family Support: Promotion of family values, interests, and goals

Health Education: Developing and providing instruction and learning experiences to facilitate voluntary adaptation of behavior conducive to health in individuals, families, groups, or communities

Health System Guidance: Facilitating a patient's location and use of appropriate health services

Normalization Promotion: Assisting parents and other family members of children with chronic illnesses or disabilities in providing normal life experiences for their children and families

Resiliency Promotion: Assisting individuals, families, and communities in development, use, and strengthening of protective factors to be used in coping with environmental and societal stressors

Respite Care: Provision of short-term care to provide relief for family caregiver

Self-Modification Assistance: Reinforcement of self-directed change initiated by the patient to achieve personally important goals

Nursing Activities

In general, nursing actions for this diagnosis focus on assessing the family system and family supports, providing any information needed to care for the patient, and working with them to plan for family development.

Assessments

- Assess physical, emotional, and educational resources of the family
- Identify family cultural influences
- Identify any self-care deficits in patient
- Identify family structure and roles
- *(NIC) Family Support:*

  Appraise family's emotional reaction to patient's condition

  Determine the psychological burden of prognosis for family

  Identify nature of spiritual support for family

Patient/Family Teaching

- *(NIC) Family Support:*
  - Teach the medical and nursing plans of care to family
  - Provide necessary knowledge of options to family that will assist them to make decisions about patient care
  - Assist family to acquire necessary knowledge, skills, and equipment to sustain their decision about patient care

Collaborative Activities

- Identify community resources that can be used to enhance the health status of the patient with family members
- *(NIC) Family Support:* Arrange for ongoing respite care, when indicated and desired

Other

- Assist family member(s) in developing a plan for personal growth. Plan may include investigation of employment opportunities, school, support groups, enrichment activities, and exercise
- Provide emotional support and availability to family member(s) during implementation, evaluation, and revision of plan
- Assist family member(s) in identifying and prioritizing personal goals
- Encourage family member(s) to compare initial response to the crisis with current situation and to recognize change
- Provide an opportunity for family member(s) to reflect on impact of patient's illness on family structure and dynamics
- Discuss how strengths and resources can be used to enhance health status of the patient with family members
- *(NIC) Family Support:*
  - Assure family that best care possible is being given to patient
  - Accept the family's values in a nonjudgmental manner
  - Listen to family concerns, feelings, and questions
  - Facilitate communication of concerns and feelings between patient and family or between family members
  - Answer all questions of family members or assist them to get answers
  - Respect and support adaptive coping mechanisms used by family
  - Provide feedback for family regarding their coping
  - Encourage family decision making in planning long-term patient care affecting family structure and finances
  - Advocate for family, as appropriate
  - Foster family assertiveness in information seeking, as appropriate

Home Care

- All of the preceding interventions apply to home care

For Infants and Children

- See For Infants and Children in Compromised Family Coping

For Older Adults

- See For Older Adults in Compromised Family Coping

COPING, INEFFECTIVE

(1978, 1998) **Domain 9, Coping/Stress Tolerance; Class 2, Coping Responses**

Definition: Inability to form a valid appraisal of the stressors, inadequate choices of practiced responses, and inability to use available resources

Defining Characteristics

Subjective

Change in usual communication patterns
Fatigue
Verbalization of inability to cope or to ask for help

Objective

Decreased use of social support
Destructive behavior toward self and others
Difficulty organizing information
High illness rate
Inability to attend to information
Inability to meet basic needs
Inability to meet role expectations
Inadequate problem solving
Lack of goal-directed behavior
Lack of resolution of problems
Poor concentration
Risk taking
Sleep disturbance
Substance abuse
Use of forms of coping that impede adaptive behavior

Other Defining Characteristics (Non-NANDA International)

Evidence of physical and psychologic abuse
Expression of unrealistic expectations
High rate of accidents
Inappropriate use of defense mechanisms
Verbal manipulation

Related Factors

Disturbance in pattern of appraisal of threat
Disturbance in pattern of tension release
Gender differences in coping strategies
High degree of threat
Inability to conserve adaptive energies
Inadequate level of confidence in ability to cope
Inadequate level of perception of control
Inadequate opportunity to prepare for stressor
Inadequate resources available
Inadequate social support created by characteristics of relationships
Situational or maturational crises
Uncertainty

Suggestions for Use

Many labels represent failure to cope (e.g., *Anxiety*, *Risk for violence*, *Hopelessness*). Always use the most specific label that fits the patient's defining characteristics. *Ineffective coping* represents a more chronic or long-term pattern than does *Risk-prone health behavior*. It is also less specific than the label *Defensive coping*.

Suggested Alternative Diagnoses

Anxiety
Denial, ineffective
Fear
Grieving, complicated
Health behavior, risk-prone
Posttrauma syndrome
Violence, risk for: self-directed or other-directed

NOC Outcomes

Adaptation to Physical Disability: Adaptive response to a significant functional challenge due to a physical disability

Caregiver Adaptation to Patient Institutionalization: Adaptive response of family caregiver when the care recipient is moved to an institution

Child Adaptation to Hospitalization: Adaptive response of a child from 3 years through 17 years of age to hospitalization

Coping: Personal actions to manage stressors that tax an individual's resources

Decision Making: Ability to make judgments and choose between two or more alternatives

Impulse Self-Control: Self-restraint of compulsive or impulsive behaviors

Knowledge: Health Resources: Extent of understanding conveyed about relevant health care resources

Psychosocial Adjustment: Life Change: Adaptive psychosocial response of an individual to a significant life change

Risk Control: Alcohol Use: Personal actions to prevent, eliminate, or reduce alcohol use that poses a threat to health

Risk Control: Drug Use: Personal actions to prevent, eliminate, or reduce drug use that poses a threat to health

Role Performance: Congruence of an individual's role behavior with role expectations

Goals/Evaluation Criteria

Examples Using NOC Language

- Demonstrates effective **Coping**, as evidenced by the following indicators (specify 1–5: never, rarely, sometimes, often, or consistently demonstrated):
  - Identifies effective [and ineffective] coping patterns
  - Seeks reputable information about diagnosis and treatment
  - Uses behaviors to reduce stress
  - Identifies multiple coping strategies
  - Uses effective coping strategies
  - Reports decrease in negative feelings
- Demonstrates **Impulse Self-Control** by consistently maintain[ing] self-control without supervision

Other Examples

Patient will:

- Demonstrate interest in diversional activities
- Identify personal strengths that may promote effective coping
- Weigh and choose among alternatives and consequences
- Initiate conversation
- Participate in ADLs
- Participate in decision-making process

- Use verbal and nonverbal expressions applicable to situation
- Verbalize plan for either accepting or changing the situation

NIC Interventions

Anxiety Reduction: Minimizing apprehension, dread, foreboding, or uneasiness related to an unidentified source of anticipated danger

Anticipatory Guidance: Preparation of patient for an anticipated developmental and/or situational crisis

Behavior Modification: Promotion of a behavior change

Coping Enhancement: Assisting a patient to adapt to perceived stressors, changes, or threats that interfere with meeting life demands and roles

Counseling: Use of an interactive helping process focusing on the needs, problems, or feelings of the patient and significant others to enhance or support coping, problem solving, and interpersonal relationships

Decision-Making Support: Providing information and support for a patient who is making a decision regarding health care

Emotional Support: Provision of reassurance, acceptance, and encouragement during times of stress

Health System Guidance: Facilitating a patient's location and use of appropriate health services

Impulse Control Training: Assisting the patient to mediate impulsive behavior through application of problem-solving strategies to social and interpersonal situations

Role Enhancement: Assisting a patient, significant other, or family to improve relationships by clarifying and supplementing specific role behaviors

Self-Esteem Enhancement: Assisting a patient to increase his personal judgment of self-worth

Substance Use Prevention: Prevention of an alcoholic or drug use lifestyle

Nursing Activities

Assessments

- Assess patient's self-concept and self-esteem
- Identify causes of ineffective coping (e.g., lack of support, life crises, ineffective problem-solving skills)
- Monitor for aggressive behaviors
- Identify the patient's view of own condition and its congruence with the view of health care providers

- *(NIC) Coping Enhancement:*
  - Appraise patient's adjustment to changes in body image, as indicated
  - Appraise the impact of the patient's life situation on roles and relationships
  - Evaluate the patient's decision-making ability
  - Explore with the patient previous methods of dealing with life problems
  - Determine the risk of the patient's inflicting self-harm

Patient/Family Teaching

- *(NIC) Coping Enhancement:*
  - Provide factual information concerning diagnosis, treatment, and prognosis
  - Instruct the patient on the use of relaxation techniques, as needed
  - Provide appropriate social skills training
- Teach problem-solving
- Provide information about community resources

Collaborative Activities

- Initiate a patient care conference to review patient's coping mechanisms and to establish a plan of care
- Involve hospital resources in provision of emotional support for patient and family
- Serve as a liaison between patient, other health care providers, and community resources (e.g., support groups)

Other

- Assist patient in developing a plan for accepting or changing situation
- Assist patient in identifying personal strengths and setting realistic goals
- Encourage patient to:
  - Be involved in planning care activities
  - Initiate conversations with others
  - Participate in activity
- Ask family to visit whenever possible
- Encourage physical exercise, as the client is able
- *(NIC) Coping Enhancement:*
  - Encourage patient to identify a realistic description of change in role
  - Use a calm, reassuring approach
  - Reduce stimuli in the environment that could be misinterpreted as threatening
  - Provide an atmosphere of acceptance
  - Discourage decision making when the patient is under severe stress

Foster constructive outlets for anger and hostility
Explore patient's reasons for self-criticism
Arrange situations that encourage patient's autonomy
Assist patient in identifying positive responses from others
Support the use of appropriate defense mechanisms
Encourage verbalization of feelings, perceptions, and fears
Assist the patient to clarify misconceptions
Assist the patient to identify available support systems
Appraise and discuss alternative responses to situation

Home Care

- Observe family-coping patterns
- Teach family members to watch for suicidal tendencies and to refer to a mental health professional immediately if suicidal tendencies are present
- Refer to social services, psychiatric home health care, and appropriate support groups
- Involve family caregivers in monitoring medication use

For Infants and Children

- Base your communication on the child's developmental stage

For Older Adults

- In older adults who have had a CVA (stroke), assess for depression, apathy, and emotional lability, which can contribute to *Ineffective coping*
- Encourage and assist with reminiscence of positive memories
- Encourage social interaction (e.g., family, friends, groups)

COPING, READINESS FOR ENHANCED

(2002) **Domain 9, Coping/Stress Tolerance; Class 2, Coping Responses**

Definition: A pattern of cognitive and behavioral efforts to manage demands that is sufficient for well-being and can be strengthened

Defining Characteristics

Subjective

Acknowledges power
Defines stressors as manageable
Aware of possible environmental changes

Objective

Seeks knowledge of new strategies
Seeks social support

Uses a broad range of problem- and emotion-oriented strategies
Uses spiritual resources

Suggestions for Use

Because this is a wellness diagnosis, an etiology (e.g., related factors) is not needed. If situations exist that pose a risk to effective coping, use *Risk for ineffective coping*. Use individual, family, or community diagnosis, as appropriate.

Suggested Alternative Diagnoses

Coping: community, readiness for enhanced
Coping: family, readiness for enhanced
Coping, ineffective, risk for

NOC Outcomes

Acceptance: Health Status: Reconciliation to significant change in health circumstance

Adaptation to Physical Disability: Adaptive response to a significant functional challenge due to a physical disability

Coping: Personal actions to manage stressors that tax an individual's resources

Personal Well-Being: Extent of positive perception of one's health status

Role Performance: Congruence of an individual's role behavior with role expectations

Stress Level: Severity of manifested physical or mental tension resulting from factors that alter an existing equilibrium

Goals/Evaluation Criteria

Examples Using NOC Language

- Demonstrates **Acceptance: Health Status**, as evidenced by the following indicators (specify 1–5: never, rarely, sometimes, often, or consistently demonstrated):
- Recognizes reality of health situation
- Performs self-care tasks
- Reports positive self-regard
- Makes decisions about health
- Clarifies life priorities

Other Examples

Patient will:

- Adapt to developmental changes
- Report improved ability to cope with stressors
- Continue to use effective coping strategies
- Identify new coping strategies that may be effective
- Report psychological comfort

NIC Interventions

Anticipatory Guidance: Preparation of patient for an anticipated developmental and/or situational crisis

Anxiety Reduction: Minimizing apprehension, dread, foreboding, or uneasiness related to an unidentified source of anticipated danger

Coping Enhancement: Assisting a patient to adapt to perceived stressors, changes, or threats that interfere with meeting life demands and roles

Resiliency Promotion: Assisting individuals, families, and communities in development, use, and strengthening of protective factors to be used in coping with environmental and societal stressors

Role Enhancement: Assisting a patient, significant other, or family to improve relationships by clarifying and supplementing specific role behaviors

Self-Awareness Enhancement: Assisting a patient to explore and understand his thoughts, feelings, motivations, and behaviors

Support System Enhancement: Facilitation of support to patient by family, friends, and community

Nursing Activities

In general, nursing actions for this diagnosis focus on providing anticipatory guidance and enhancing the patient's present coping strategies and supports.

Assessments

- Identify the patient's view of own condition and its congruence with the view of health care providers
- Assist to identify usual responses to various situations
- Identify areas in which patient wishes to enhance coping
- Identify which relaxation techniques have been effective in the past
- Evaluate effectiveness of relaxation techniques
- *(NIC) Coping Enhancement:*

  Appraise the impact of the patient's life situation on roles and relationships

  Explore with the patient previous methods of dealing with life problems

Patient/Family Teaching

- Teach details of chosen relaxation technique(s) (e.g., visualization)
- Provide information about community resources, such as ministers and self-help groups
- *(NIC) Coping Enhancement:* Instruct the patient on the use of relaxation techniques, as needed

D

Other

- Assist patient in identifying personal strengths
- Promote family communication and relationships
- Encourage to develop family traditions (e.g., observance of holidays and birthdays)
- Encourage to attend religious services
- Assist to identify situations that may create role transition
- Provide opportunity for patient to role play new coping strategies
- Assist to identify life priorities
- *(NIC) Coping Enhancement:*
  Arrange situations that encourage patient's autonomy
  Assist patient in identifying positive responses from others
  Support the use of appropriate defense mechanisms
  Encourage verbalization of feelings, perceptions, and fears
  Assist the patient to clarify misconceptions
  Assist the patient to identify available support systems

Home Care

- Observe family coping patterns; support healthy patterns

For Infants and Children

- Teach parents ways to enhance and develop the self-esteem of their children

DECISION MAKING, READINESS FOR ENHANCED

(2006) **Domain 10, Life Principles; Class 3, Value/Belief/Action Congruence**

Definition: A pattern of choosing a course of action that is sufficient for meeting short- and long-term health-related goals and can be strengthened

Defining Characteristics

Subjective

Expresses desire to enhance decision making
Expresses desire to enhance congruency of decisions with personal and sociocultural values and goals
Expresses desire to enhance risk–benefit analysis of decisions
Expresses desire to enhance understanding of choices for decision making
Expresses desire to enhance understanding of the meaning of choices
Expresses desire to enhance use of reliable evidence for decisions

Risk Factors

To be developed.

Suggestions for Use

(a) The role of the nurse is to help clients make logical, informed decisions by providing information and support. The nurse should not try to influence the client to decide in a particular way. (b) Do not assume that clients facing a serious, even life-and-death, decision are conflicted. Such decisions may actually be easy to make in some cases.

Suggested Alternative Diagnoses

Coping, readiness for enhanced
Family processes, readiness for enhanced
Power, readiness for enhanced

NOC Outcomes

Adherence Behavior: Self-initiated actions to promote optional wellness, recovery, and rehabilitation
Decision Making: Ability to make judgments and choose between two or more alternatives
Health Beliefs: Personal convictions that influence health behaviors
Personal Autonomy: Personal actions of a competent individual to exercise governance in life decisions

Goals/Evaluation Criteria

Examples Using NOC Language

- *Decision Making* will be demonstrated, as evidenced by the following indicators (specify 1–5: severely, substantially, moderately, mildly, or not compromised):
  - Identifies relevant information
  - Recognizes contradiction with others' desires

Acknowledges relevant legal implications
Weighs and selects among alternatives
Identifies resources necessary to support each alternative
Acknowledges social context of the situation

D

Other Examples

Patient will:

- Report satisfaction with decision making
- Report enhanced congruency of decisions with personal and sociocultural values and goals
- Report improved ability to make risk–benefit analyses of decisions
- Report increased understanding of choices available and of the implications of those choices
- Reports use of reliable evidence for decisions

NIC Interventions

Assertiveness Training: Assistance with the effective expression of feelings, needs, and ideas while respecting the rights of others

Decision-Making Support: Providing information and support for a patient who is making a decision regarding health care

Health Education: Developing and providing instruction and learning experiences to facilitate voluntary adaptation of behavior conducive to health in individuals, families, groups, or communities

Self-Awareness Enhancement: Assisting a patient to explore and understand his thoughts, feelings, motivations, and behaviors

Values Clarification: Assisting another to clarify his own values in order to facilitate effective decision making

Nursing Activities

Assessments

- Assess decision-making skills and usual patterns of decision making
- Evaluate patient's support system

Patient/Family Teaching

- Teach problem-solving and decision-making processes
- Teach techniques for behaving assertively
- *(NIC) Decision-Making Support:* Provide information requested by patient

Collaborative Activities

- *(NIC) Decision-Making Support:*

  Serve as a liaison between patient and other health care providers
  Facilitate collaborative decision making

Other

- Facilitate recognition and expression of thoughts and feelings
- Assist patient to identify his learning style
- Help the patient to identify his strengths and abilities
- Provide opportunities for practicing assertive behaviors
- *(NIC) Values Clarification:*
  Create an accepting, nonjudgmental atmosphere
  Pose reflective, clarifying questions that give the patient something to think about
  Encourage patient to make a list of what is important and not important in life and the time spent on each
  Help patient to evaluate how values are in agreement with or in conflict with those of family members/significant others
  Help patient define alternatives and their advantages and disadvantages
- *(NIC) Decision-Making Support:*
  Establish communication with patient early in admission
  Facilitate patient's articulation of goals for care
  Help patient identify the advantages and disadvantages of each alternative
  Help patient explain decision to others, as needed
  Serve as a liaison between patient and family
- Encourage consideration of the issues and consequences of behavior
- Help the patient to prioritize goals
- Assist patient in identifying a course of action and adapt as necessary

Home Care

- The preceding interventions are appropriate in home care

For Older Adults

- Assess the client's present ability to make decisions and problem solve
- Assess for dementia, depression, hearing loss, and communication problems that may interfere with further enhancement of decision making
- Discuss with family members how they can be supportive of the patient's decisions, even when they are not in agreement

DECISIONAL CONFLICT (SPECIFY)

(1988, 2006) **Domain 10, Life Principles; Class 3, Value/Belief/Action Congruence**

D

Definition: Uncertainty about course of action to be taken when choice among competing actions involves risk, loss, or challenge to personal life values

Defining Characteristics

Subjective

Questioning moral rules, principles, and values while attempting a decision
Questioning personal values and beliefs while attempting a decision
Self-focusing
Verbalizes feelings of distress while attempting a decision
Verbalizes uncertainty about choices
Verbalizes undesired consequences of alternative actions being considered

Objective

Delayed decision making
Physical signs of distress or tension (e.g., increased heart rate, increased muscle tension, restlessness)
Vacillation among alternative choices

Related Factors

Lack of experience or interference with decision making
Lack of relevant information
Moral obligations require performing action
Moral obligations require not performing action
Moral values, principles, or rules support mutually inconsistent courses of action
Multiple or divergent sources of information
Perceived threat to value system
Support system deficit
Unclear personal values and beliefs

Suggestions for Use

(a) The role of the nurse is to help clients make logical, informed decisions by providing information and support. The nurse should not try to influence the client to decide in a particular way. (b) Do not assume that clients facing a serious, even life-and-death, decision are conflicted. Such decisions may actually be easy to make in some cases.

Suggested Alternative Diagnoses

Hopelessness
Parental role conflict
Powerlessness
Spiritual distress
Spiritual distress, risk for

NOC Outcomes

Decision Making: Ability to make judgments and choose between two or more alternatives

Information Processing: Ability to acquire, organize, and use information

Participation in Health Care Decisions: Personal involvement in selecting and evaluating health care options to achieve desired outcome

Personal Autonomy: Personal actions of a competent individual to exercise governance in life decisions

Goals/Evaluation Criteria

Examples Using NOC Language

- *Decisional conflict* will lessen, as demonstrated by Decision Making, Information Processing, Participation in Health Care Decisions, and Personal Autonomy
- **Decision Making** will be demonstrated, as evidenced by the following indicators (specify 1–5: severely, substantially, moderately, mildly, or not compromised):

    Identifies relevant information
    Recognizes contradiction with others' desires
    Acknowledges relevant legal implications
    Weighs and selects among alternatives
    Identifies needed resources to support each alternative
    Acknowledges social context of the situation

Other Examples

Patient will:

- Evaluate available choices in relation to personal values
- Report a decrease in tension or distress
- Exhibit information processing and logical thought processes
- Use problem solving to achieve chosen outcomes

NIC Interventions

Assertiveness Training: Assistance with the effective expression of feelings, needs, and ideas while respecting the rights of others

Decision-Making Support: Providing information and support for a patient who is making a decision regarding health care

Health Literacy Enhancement: Assisting individuals with limited ability to obtain, process, and understand information related to health and illness

Health System Guidance: Facilitating a patient's location and use of appropriate health services

Learning Facilitation: Promoting the ability to process and comprehend information

Values Clarification: Assisting another to clarify his own values in order to facilitate effective decision making

Nursing Activities

Assessments

- Assess patient's understanding of available choices
- Evaluate patient's level of tension or distress
- Assess decision-making skills and usual patterns of decision making
- *(NIC) Decision-Making Support:* Determine whether there are differences between the patient's view of own condition and the view of health care providers

Patient/Family Teaching

- Provide information about advance directives
- Teach problem-solving and decision-making processes
- *(NIC) Decision-Making Support:*

  Inform patient of alternative views or solutions in a clear and supportive manner

  Provide information requested by patient

Collaborative Activities

- Use resources (e.g., ethics committee) as appropriate.
- *(NIC) Decision-Making Support:*

  Serve as a liaison between patient and other health care providers

  Refer to support groups, as appropriate

  Refer to legal aid, as appropriate

  Facilitate collaborative decision making

Other

- Assist patient in identifying a course of action and adapt as necessary
- *(NIC) Decision-Making Support:*

  Establish communication with patient early in admission

  Facilitate patient's articulation of goals for care

Help patient identify the advantages and disadvantages of each alternative
Help patient explain decision to others, as needed
Serve as a liaison between patient and family
Respect patient's right to receive or not to receive information

Home Care

- Assess client and family agreement regarding the decision being made
- Provide information to assist family members who are considering placing a family member in a long-term care facility
- Provide support for the decision maker(s)

For Infants and Children

- As a rule, a surrogate (e.g., a parent) makes major decisions for a child. Be familiar with laws and agency policies regulating age of consent, as they differ among states.

For Older Adults

- Family members and other decision makers often exclude older adults from the decision-making process, believing that they are not competent, or that they would be upset by such discussions. Work with patient and decision makers to include the patient as much as possible.
- Assess the client's ability to make decisions and problem solve
- Assess for dementia, depression, hearing loss, and communication problems that may cause the patient to withdraw from active participation in decision making
- Discuss the need for making end-of-life decisions, if they are being avoided
- Discuss with family members how they can be supportive of the patient's decisions, even when they are not in agreement

DENIAL, INEFFECTIVE

(1988, 2006) **Domain 9, Coping/Stress Tolerance; Class 2, Coping Responses**

D

Definition: Conscious or unconscious attempt to disavow the knowledge or meaning of an event to reduce anxiety and fear, but leading to the detriment of health

Defining Characteristics

Subjective

Displaces fear of impact of the condition
Does not admit fear of death or invalidism
Displays inappropriate affect
Minimizes symptoms
Unable to admit impact of disease on life pattern

Objective

Delays seeking or refuses health care attention to the detriment of health
Displaces source of symptoms to other organs
Does not perceive personal relevance of symptoms or danger
Makes dismissive gestures or comments when speaking of distressing events
Uses self-treatment

Related Factors

Anxiety
Fear of death
Fear of loss of autonomy
Fear of separation
Lack of competency in using effective coping mechanisms
Lack of control of life situation
Lack of emotional support from others
Overwhelming stress
Threat of inadequacy in dealing with strong emotions
Threat of unpleasant reality

Suggestions for Use

Some denial in response to illness or other crises may be necessary in order for the client to cope with the situation. Such normal denial is gradually replaced by acceptance or change of the situation, and it does not interfere with the treatment regimen. *Ineffective denial* should be used for clients whose denial persists or interferes with the treatment regimen.

For example, a client newly diagnosed with myocardial infarction may respond with denial and, therefore, fail to make changes in lifestyle needed to prevent further heart damage.

Suggested Alternative Diagnoses

Coping, defensive
Coping, ineffective
Grieving, complicated
Noncompliance (specify)
Rape-trauma syndrome

NOC Outcomes

Acceptance: Health Status: Reconciliation to significant change in health circumstances
Anxiety Level: Severity of manifested apprehension, tension, or uneasiness arising from an unidentifiable source
Compliance Behavior: Personal actions to promote wellness, recovery, and rehabilitation recommended by a health professional
Health Beliefs: Perceived Threat: Personal conviction that a threatening health problem is serious and has potential negative consequences for lifestyle
Symptom Control: Personal actions to minimize perceived adverse changes in physical and emotional functioning

Goals/Evaluation Criteria

Examples Using NOC Language

- Patient will not use *Ineffective denial*, as evidenced by Acceptance: Health Status, Anxiety Level, Compliance Behavior, Health Beliefs (Perceived Threat), and Symptom Control
- Patient will demonstrate **Acceptance: Health Status** as indicated by (specify 1–5: never, rarely, sometimes, often, or consistently demonstrated):
  Relinquishes previous concept of personal health
  Recognizes reality of health situation
  Pursues information about health
  Copes with health situation
  Makes decisions about health

Other Examples

Patient will:

- Acknowledge and recognize significance of symptoms
- Report significant symptoms

- Not demonstrate physical and behavioral manifestations of anxiety
- Acknowledge vulnerability to health problem

NIC Interventions

D

Anxiety Reduction: Minimizing apprehension, dread, foreboding, or uneasiness related to an unidentified source of anticipated danger

Cognitive Restructuring: Challenging a patient to alter distorted thought patterns and view self and the world more realistically

Coping Enhancement: Assisting a patient to adapt to perceived stressors, changes, or threats that interfere with meeting life demands and roles

Counseling: Use of an interactive helping process focusing on the needs, problems, or feelings of the patient and significant others to enhance or support coping, problem solving, and interpersonal relationships

Emotional Support: Provision of reassurance, acceptance, and encouragement during times of stress

Health Education: Developing and providing instruction and learning experiences to facilitate voluntary adaptation of behavior conducive to health in individuals, families, groups, or communities

Security Enhancement: Intensifying a patient's sense of physical and psychological safety

Self-Awareness Enhancement: Assisting a patient to explore and understand his thoughts, feelings, motivations, and behaviors

Self-Efficacy Enhancement: Strengthening an individual's confidence in his ability to perform a health behavior

Self-Modification Assistance: Reinforcement of self-directed change initiated by the patient to achieve personally important goals

Self-Responsibility Facilitation: Encouraging a patient to assume more responsibility for own behavior

Teaching: Disease Process: Assisting the patient to understand information related to a specific disease process

Nursing Activities

Assessments

- Assess understanding of symptoms and illness
- Assess for signs of anxiety
- Determine whether patient's perception of his health status is realistic
- *(NIC) Anxiety Reduction:*
  Determine patient's decision-making ability
  Identify when level of anxiety changes

Patient Teaching

- Teach recognition of symptoms and desired patient responses
- *(NIC) Anxiety Reduction:* Provide factual information concerning diagnosis, treatment, and prognosis

Collaborative Activities

- Refer for psychiatric care, if indicated
- Include patient and family in a multidisciplinary conference to develop a plan of action. Plan may include:
  - Arranging for follow-up support after discharge
  - Meeting with patients in similar situations to learn new ways to cope and to decrease anxiety and fear

Other

- Establish a therapeutic relationship with patient that will allow exploration of denial
- Use every opportunity to reinforce consequences of patient's actions
- Engage patient in discussion about anxiety, fears, symptoms, and impact of illness
- Identify and reinforce patient strengths
- Demonstrate empathy, warmth, and genuineness
- *(NIC) Anxiety Reduction:*
  - Seek to understand the patient's perspective of a stressful situation
  - Reinforce behavior, as appropriate
  - Encourage verbalization of feelings, perceptions, and fears
  - Support the use of appropriate defense mechanisms
  - Assist patient to articulate a realistic description of an upcoming event

Home Care

- Assess family interactions to determine whether the patient may be using denial to protect a family member
- Provide numbers for emergency services and hotlines

For Older Adults

- Assess the client's perceptions and provide feedback to validate realistic perceptions
- Assess for recent losses (e.g., of function, of significant other) that might be delaying the client's adaptation to changes in health status

DENTITION, IMPAIRED

(1998) **Domain 11, Safety/Protection; Class 2, Physical Injury**

D

Definition: Disruption in tooth development and eruption patterns or structural integrity of individual teeth

Defining Characteristics

Subjective

Toothache

Objective

Asymmetrical facial expression
Crown or root caries
Erosion of enamel
Excessive calculus
Excessive plaque
Halitosis
Incomplete eruption for age (may be primary or permanent teeth)
Loose teeth
Malocclusion or tooth misalignment
Missing teeth or complete absence
Premature loss of primary teeth
Tooth enamel discoloration
Tooth fracture(s)
Worn-down or abraded teeth

Related Factors

Lack of access or economic barriers to professional care
Barriers to self-care
Bruxism
Chronic use of tobacco, coffee, tea, or red wine
Chronic vomiting
Dietary habits
Excessive intake of fluorides
Excessive use of abrasive cleaning agents
Genetic predisposition
Ineffective oral hygiene
Lack of knowledge regarding dental health
Nutritional deficits
Selected prescription medications
Sensitivity to heat or cold

Suggestions for Use

Independent nursing interventions for this diagnosis are preventive in nature and consist mostly of teaching oral hygiene measures. For an actual problem of *Impaired dentition*, professional dental care is needed. The diagnosis, therefore, might best be used as a risk diagnosis. Other diagnoses may be more useful. For example, if the risk for *Impaired dentition* is caused by self-care deficits a diagnosis of *Self-care deficit: Bathing and hygiene* might be used; if the risk factor is poor nutrition, the nursing diagnosis would be *Imbalanced nutrition*.

Suggested Alternative Diagnosis

Imbalanced nutrition

Self-care deficit: bathing and hygiene

NOC Outcomes

Oral Hygiene: Condition of the mouth, teeth, gums, and tongue

Self-Care: Oral Hygiene: Ability to care for own mouth and teeth independently with or without assistive device

Goals/Evaluation Criteria

Examples Using NOC Language

- Patient corrects *Impaired dentition*, as evidenced by Oral Hygiene and Self-Care: Oral Hygiene.
- Patient will demonstrate **Oral Hygiene**, as indicated by (specify 1–5: severely, substantially, moderately, mildly, or not compromised)
  - Cleanliness of mouth, teeth, gums, tongue, and dentures or dental appliances
  - Moistness of lips, oral mucosa, and tongue
- Patient will demonstrate **Oral Hygiene**, as indicated by (specify 1–5: severe, substantial, moderate, mild, or none)
  - Bleeding
  - Halitosis

Other Examples

Patient will:

- Be free from debris and plaque on dental surfaces
- Have firm, well-hydrated, nonbleeding gums of uniform color
- Verbalize feeling of oral cleanliness
- Demonstrate correct brushing and flossing procedures
- Follow sound nutritional practices, such as avoiding sweets between meals

- Have a checkup by a dentist every 6 months
- Be free from caries, loose teeth, or toothaches
- Parent will take child for first dentist visit by age 2 or 3
- Child will not experience premature loss of primary teeth

NIC Interventions

Oral Health Maintenance: Maintenance and promotion of oral hygiene and dental health for the patient at risk for developing oral or dental lesions

Oral Health Restoration: Promotion of healing for a patient who has an oral mucosal or dental lesion

Nursing Activities

Assessments

- Inspect mouth for loose or missing teeth, color and condition of enamel, number of dental fillings and caries, and tartar at base of teeth
- Observe for halitosis
- Determine client's usual oral hygiene practices
- Assess client's level of knowledge of measures to prevent Impaired dentition (e.g., "How often do you see your dentist?")
- Assess client's access to and resources for dental care
- Assess client's ability to perform oral care (e.g., "Do you have any problems caring for your teeth?")
- Assess client's knowledge of oral hygiene practices and routines (e.g., brushing method)
- Identify risk factors for impaired dentition (e.g., clients who are seriously ill, confused, depressed)

Collaborative Activities

- Refer to dental hygienist, dentist, or clinic, as needed

Client/Family Teaching

- Teach brushing and flossing techniques, as needed
- Explain the causes of dental problems, such as tooth decay
- Teach to avoid heavy use of tobacco, tea, coffee, and red wine to prevent discoloration
- Teach the potential complications of tongue piercing (e.g., cracking and chipping of teeth)
- Teach measures to avoid tooth decay:
  - Brush after meals and at bedtime
  - Ensure adequate intake of calcium, phosphorus, and vitamins A, C, and D

Avoid sweets between meals; take in moderation with meals
Eat cleansing foods, such as raw fruits and vegetables
If water is not fluoridated, take a fluoride supplement daily until at least age 14
Have a dental checkup every 6 months
Floss teeth daily

Other

- Provide oral hygiene for patients with *Self-care deficit* (e.g., thorough brushing and rinsing)
- Help patient establish an oral hygiene schedule after meals and at bedtime. For example:
    Use sulcular technique and soft toothbrush
    Rinse with mouthwash or solution of warm water and salt or baking soda

Home Care

- Assess facilities and supplies available for dental hygiene
- Assess environmental influences, such as fluoride-treated water supply
- Assess availability of and ability to access professional dental care
- Assist the client and family in developing a plan of dental hygiene, including brushing and flossing

For Infants and Children

- Teach parents to begin oral hygiene in infancy
- Teach parents to never let a child fall asleep with a bottle of milk or sweet liquids. Use a bottle of water or a pacifier if necessary.
- Teach parents the importance of caring for the child's primary teeth
- Teach parents to help children brush and floss, and/or inspect their mouths after brushing
- Recommend drinking fluoridated water when possible

For Older Adults

- Consider use of an ultrasonic toothbrush for patients who have impaired mobility of the hands
- Assess for lesions of the oral cavity and lips
- Remind the patient to remove and clean dentures after every meal and before bedtime

DEVELOPMENT: DELAYED, RISK FOR

(1998) **Domain 13, Growth/Development; Class 2, Development**

D

Definition: At risk for delay of 25% or more in one or more of the areas of social or self-regulatory behavior or in cognitive, language, or gross- or fine-motor skills

Risk Factors

Prenatal

Economically disadvantaged
Genetic or endocrine disorders
Illiteracy
Inadequate nutrition
Infections
Lack of, late, or inadequate prenatal care
Maternal age < 15 or > 35 years
Poverty
Unplanned or unwanted pregnancy

Individual"

Behavior disorders
Brain damage (e.g., hemorrhage in postnatal period, shaken baby, abuse, accident)
Chronic illness
Congenital or genetic disorders
Failure to thrive, inadequate nutrition
Foster or adopted child
Hearing impairment [or frequent otitis media]
Lead poisoning
Natural disaster
Positive drug-screening test
Prematurity
Seizures
Substance abuse
Technology dependent
Treatment-related side effects (e.g., chemotherapy, radiation therapy, pharmaceutical agents)
Vision impairment

Environmental

Economically disadvantaged
Violence

Caregiver

Abuse
Mental illness
Mental illness or learning disability

Suggestions for Use

(a) Use diagnosis when one or more risk factors are present and the nursing focus is on preventing developmental delays by eliminating the risk factors. (b) Because development is routinely assessed in nursing care of children, a diagnostic statement is usually not required for that application; such assessment is usually included in pediatric standards of care. (c) This label is not appropriate for a mentally impaired child (e.g., *Risk for delayed development related to Down syndrome*). Instead, diagnose the specific functional task that the child is unable to perform (e.g., *Feeding self-care deficit*, *Bowel incontinence*). (d) Instead of using this diagnosis, it may be better to focus on the risk factor and describe the problem, for example, as *Impaired parenting* or *Disabled family coping*.

Suggested Alternative Diagnoses

Bowel incontinence
Communication: verbal, impaired
Coping: family, compromised
Coping: family, disabled
Coping, ineffective
Growth, risk for disproportionate
Growth and development, delayed
Parenting, impaired
Self-care deficit (specify)
Urinary incontinence [specify]

NOC Outcomes

Child Development: 1, 2, 4, 6, and 12 months; 2, 3, 4, and 5 years; Middle Childhood (6–11 years); Adolescence (12–17 years): Milestones of physical, cognitive, and psychosocial progression by [specify age]

Hyperactivity Level: Severity of patterns of inattention or impulsivity in a child from 1 year through 17 years of age

Preterm Infant Organization: Extrauterine integration of physiologic and behavioral function by the infant born 24 to 37 weeks' (term) gestation

Social Interaction Skills: Personal behaviors that promote effective relationships

Goals/Evaluation Criteria

NOTE: This text can only provide examples of developmental milestones. Refer to pediatrics or child development texts for complete discussion of growth and development and for goals for a specific child.

D

- The child will achieve developmental milestones, that is, not experience a delay of 25% or more in one or more of the areas of social or self-regulatory behavior or cognitive, language, or gross- or fine-motor skills. For example:
  - For a 6-month-old: Rolls over, sits with support, grasps and mouths objects
  - For a 3-year-old: Demonstrates autonomy, is toilet trained

NIC Interventions

Abuse Protection Support: Identification of high-risk dependent relationships and actions to prevent further infliction of physical or emotional harm

Behavior Management: Overactivity/Inattention: Provision of a therapeutic milieu that safely accommodates the patient's attention deficit and/or overactivity while promoting optimal function

Caregiver Support: Provision of the necessary information, advocacy, and support to facilitate primary patient care by someone other than a health care professional

Developmental Care: Structuring the environment and providing care in response to the behavioral cues and states of the preterm infant

Parent Education: Childrearing Family: Assisting parents to understand and promote the physical, psychological, and social growth and development of their toddler, preschool, or school-aged child or children

Risk Identification: Analysis of potential risk factors, determination of health risks, and prioritization of risk-reduction strategies for an individual or group

Teaching: Infant Nutrition: Instruction on nutrition and feeding practices during first year of life

Teaching: Toddler Nutrition: Instruction on nutrition and feeding practices from the 13th month through the 24th month of life

Nursing Activities

NOTE: Because this nursing diagnosis is so broad and nonspecific, and because there are so many possible etiologies, it is not possible to list every nursing activity here. Refer to age-specific sections in growth and development texts.

Assessments

- Conduct a thorough health assessment (e.g., child's history, temperament, culture, family environment, developmental screening) to determine functional level
- Determine caretakers' level of knowledge, resources, support system, and coping skills
- Identify parental future expectations for child (e.g., ability to learn, developmental achievements)
- Monitor parent and child interactions (e.g., during feedings)
- Assess prenatally for presence of risk factors (e.g., poverty, substance abuse)
- Assess for postnatal risk factors (e.g., chronic illness, seizures, violence, caregiver mental illness)

Patient/Family Teaching

- Teach parents about normal developmental milestones
- Demonstrate activities that promote development
- Teach the importance of early prenatal care
- Teach mothers the importance of abstaining from alcohol and other drugs during pregnancy
- Teach ways to provide meaningful stimulation for infants and children
- Teach about age-appropriate behaviors
- Teach about age-appropriate toys and materials
- Role-model developmental care interventions for preterm infants
- Teach the importance of smoking cessation and the dangers of secondhand smoke

Collaborative Activities

- Refer pregnant patient to substance-abuse treatment program if needed

Other

- If risk factors cannot be removed (as in a natural disaster), assist family to find resources and support coping efforts
- Assist patient to achieve next level of development through appropriate mastery of tasks specific to his level (refer to growth and development text)
- Establish a therapeutic and trusting relationship with caretakers
- Provide appropriate play activities, encourage activities with other children
- Communicate with patient at appropriate cognitive level of development
- Provide positive rewards or feedback for attempts at self-expression
- Use consistent, structured behavior modification techniques

- Involve patient in self-care and ADLs as much as possible
- Encourage parents to expect and require responsible behavior in child

D

Home Care

- The preceding activities apply to home care, as well
- Assess for environmental factors that could cause Delayed Development (e.g., lead-based paints in older buildings)

DIARRHEA

(1975, 1998) **Domain 3, Elimination and Exchange; Class 2, Gastrointestinal Function**

Definition: Passage of loose, unformed stools

Defining Characteristics

Subjective

Abdominal pain
Cramping
Urgency

Objective

At least three loose liquid stools per day
Hyperactive bowel sounds

Related Factors

Psychological

High stress levels and anxiety

Situational

Adverse effects of pharmaceutical agents
Alcohol abuse
Contaminants
Laxative abuse
Radiation
Toxins
Travel
Tube feedings

Physiological

Infectious processes
Inflammation

Irritation
Malabsorption
Parasites

D

Suggestions for Use

Differentiate the watery stool accompanying fecal impaction from true *Diarrhea*. The watery stools accompanying impaction usually occur suddenly in a patient who has chronic constipation. When impaction is present, rectal exam will reveal a hard mass of dry stool in the rectum. Also differentiate from *Bowel incontinence*, which does not necessarily manifest as loose or unformed stools.

Suggested Alternative Diagnosis

Constipation
Incontinence, bowel

NOC Outcomes

Bowel Continence: Control of passage of stool from the bowel
Bowel Elimination: Formation and evacuation of stool
Symptom Severity: Severity of perceived adverse changes in physical, emotional, and social functioning

Goals/Evaluation Criteria

Examples Using NOC Language

- *Diarrhea* will be controlled or eliminated, as demonstrated by Bowel Continence, Bowel Elimination, and Symptom Severity
- Demonstrates effective **Bowel Elimination**, as evidenced by the following indicators (specify 1–5: severely, substantially, moderately, mildly, or not compromised):
  - Elimination pattern
  - Control of bowel movements
- Demonstrates effective **Bowel Elimination**, as evidenced by the following indicators (specify 1–5: severe, substantial, moderate, mild, none):
  - Diarrhea
  - Blood and mucus in stool

Other Examples

Patient will:

- Follow dietary requirements to alleviate diarrhea
- Practice hygiene adequate to prevent skin breakdown

- Verbalize understanding of the causes of his diarrhea
- Maintain electrolyte balance within normal limits
- Maintain acid–base balance within normal limits
- Be well hydrated (mucous membranes moist; afebrile; good eyeball turgor; BP, hematocrit, and urine output within normal limits)

NIC Interventions

Bowel Management: Establishment and maintenance of a regular pattern of bowel elimination

Diarrhea Management: Management and alleviation of diarrhea

Fluid Management: Promotion of fluid balance and prevention of complications resulting from abnormal or undesired fluid levels

Medication Management: Facilitation of safe and effective use of prescription and over-the-counter drugs

Nursing Activities

Assessments

- Perform guaiac test on stools
- Have patient identify usual bowel pattern
- Monitor laboratory values (electrolytes, CBC) and report abnormalities
- Weigh patient daily
- Assess and document:
  - Frequency, color, consistency, and amount (measure) of stool
  - Skin turgor and condition of oral mucosa as indicators of dehydration
- *(NIC) Diarrhea Management:*
  - Obtain stool for culture and sensitivity, if diarrhea continues
  - Evaluate medication profile for gastrointestinal side effects
  - Evaluate recorded intake for nutritional content
  - Monitor skin in perianal area for irritation and ulceration

Patient/Family Teaching

- Inform patient of possibility of medication-induced diarrhea
- Teach to avoid milk, coffee, spices, and foods irritating to the gastrointestinal tract
- *(NIC) Diarrhea Management:*
  - Teach patient about the appropriate use of antidiarrheal medications
  - Instruct patient and family members to record color, volume, frequency, and consistency of stools

Instruct patient to notify staff of each episode of diarrhea
Teach patient stress-reduction techniques, as appropriate

Collaborative Activities

- Consult with dietitian for adjustment of diet
- *(NIC) Diarrhea Management:* Consult physician if signs and symptoms of diarrhea persist

Other

- Help patient to identify stressors that may contribute to diarrhea
- Provide care in an accepting, nonjudgmental manner
- Provide fluids of patient's choice (specify)
- Provide privacy and safety for patient during bowel elimination
- *(NIC) Diarrhea Management:*
  Perform actions to rest the bowel (e.g., NPO or liquid diet)
  Encourage frequent, small feedings, adding bulk gradually

Home Care

- The preceding interventions are appropriate for home care use
- Evaluate the client's medications, including over-the-counter medications and herbal remedies
- Assess cleanliness and sanitation methods in the home (e.g., hand washing, food preparation)
- Teach safe food handling and preparation
- Teach Universal Precautions to family caregivers when there is infectious diarrhea
- Teach signs and symptoms of dehydration

For Infants and Children

- Monitor for signs of dehydration (i.e., increased thirst, dry mucous membranes, decreased skin turgor, sunken eyeballs, sunken fontanelles [in infants]; signs of severe diarrhea also include rapid, thready pulse, tachypnea, cyanosis, lethargy, and delayed capillary refill)
- Consult with pediatrician for alternative type of feeding
- Provide oral rehydration therapy (e.g., Pedialyte, Lytren), as ordered
- Breast-fed infants should continue breastfeeding; others should avoid milk and high-carbohydrate fluids
- Carefully monitor fluid and electrolyte losses

D

For Older Adults

- Loss of anal sphincter and perineal muscle tone can cause incontinence, which must be differentiated from diarrhea
- Older adults are at increased risk of dehydration in the presence of diarrhea; monitor for signs
- Monitor fluid and electrolyte losses carefully
- Assess carefully for impaction; remove as ordered

DISUSE SYNDROME, RISK FOR

(1988) **Domain 4, Activity/Rest; Class 2, Activity/Exercise**

Definition: At risk for deterioration of body systems as a result of prescribed or unavoidable musculoskeletal inactivity

NOTE: Complications from immobility can include pressure ulcer, constipation, stasis of pulmonary secretions, thrombosis, urinary tract infection or retention, decreased strength and endurance, orthostatic hypotension, decreased range of joint motion, disorientation, body image disturbance, and powerlessness.

Risk Factors

Subjective

Severe pain

Objective

Altered level of consciousness
Mechanical immobilization
Paralysis
Prescribed immobilization

Suggestions for Use

This label describes the cluster of potential complications of immobility (e.g., *Risk for constipation*, *Risk for impaired skin integrity*). It is a syndrome diagnosis under which a number of actual and potential problems are clustered. Therefore, when the risk factor is immobility, it is not necessary to write separate risk diagnoses such as *Risk for impaired skin integrity*. Those more specific labels should be used only if an actual problem develops (e.g., actual *Impaired skin integrity related to immobility*), or if the risk factor is something other than immobility (e.g., *Risk for impaired skin integrity related to malnutrition*). Furthermore, this diagnosis should not be written with an etiology. As a syndrome diagnosis, the etiology (disuse) is contained in the label itself.

Even though the NANDA International terminology is still *Risk for disuse syndrome*, Carpenito-Moyet (2006b, p. 272) recommends that syndrome diagnoses not be written with "risk for," since they include both actual and risk diagnoses. In that case, the diagnosis *Disuse syndrome* would be used both for clients with the risk factor of immobility and for those with the defining characteristics for actual *Disuse syndrome*.

Suggested Alternative Diagnoses

If an actual problem occurs as a result of immobility or if the etiology of a potential problem is something other than immobility, consider using a more restricted physiological nursing diagnosis such as one of the following:

Actual or Risk for:

Activity intolerance
Body image, disturbed
Breathing pattern, ineffective
Constipation
Physical mobility, impaired
Powerlessness
Sensory perception, disturbed: all (specify)
Sexuality patterns, ineffective
Skin integrity, impaired
Swallowing, impaired
Tissue perfusion, ineffective (peripheral)
Urinary retention

Risk for:

Infection
Injury
Peripheral neurovascular dysfunction

NOC Outcomes

Heedfulness of Affected Side: Personal actions to acknowledge, protect, and cognitively integrate affected body part(s) into self

Immobility Consequences: Physiological: Severity of compromise in physiological functioning due to impaired physical mobility

Immobility Consequences: Psychocognitive: Severity of compromise in psychocognitive functioning due to impaired physical mobility

Goals/Evaluation Criteria

Examples Using NOC Language

- Risk factors will be controlled and patient will not experience *Disuse syndrome*, as evidenced by outcomes of Heedfullness of Affected Side, and Physiological and Psychocognitive Immobility Consequences
- Patient will demonstrate **Immobility Consequences: Physiological**, as evidenced by the following indicators (specify 1–5: severe, substantial, moderate, mild, or none):

  Constipation, stool impaction, hypoactive bowel, or paralytic ileus
  Urinary calculi, urinary retention, or urinary tract infection
  Bone fracture, contracted joints, or ankylosed joints
  Orthostatic hypotension
  Venous thrombosis
  Pneumonia
- Patient will demonstrate **Immobility Consequences: Physiological**, as evidenced by the following indicators (specify 1–5: severely, substantially, moderately, mildly, or not compromised):

  Nutritional status
  Muscle strength and tone
  Joint movement
  Cough effectiveness
  Vital capacity

Other Examples

Goals of care for this label are broad. They focus on preventing complications of immobility for all body systems. For example, patient will:

- Be oriented to time, place, and person
- Have adequate peripheral circulation
- Maintain optimal respiratory function (e.g., effective cough, no lung congestion, normal vital capacity)
- Maintain satisfactory body image
- Demonstrate concentration and interest in surroundings
- Have laboratory values within normal limits (e.g., oxygen, blood glucose, hemoglobin and hematocrit, and serum electrolyte levels)

NIC Interventions

Analgesic Administration: Use of pharmacologic agents to reduce or eliminate pain

Bed Rest Care: Promotion of comfort and safety and prevention of complications for a patient unable to get out of bed

Cast Care: Maintenance: Care of a cast after the drying period

Exercise Therapy: Joint Mobility: Use of active or passive body movement to maintain or restore joint flexibility

Exercise Therapy: Muscle Control: Use of specific activity or exercise protocols to enhance or restore controlled body movement

Positioning: Deliberative placement of the patient or a body part to promote physiological and psychological well-being

Surveillance: Purposeful and ongoing acquisition, interpretation, and synthesis of patient data for clinical decision making

Unilateral Neglect Management: Protecting and safely reintegrating the affected part of the body while helping the patient adapt to disturbed perceptual abilities

Nursing Activities

NOTE: In addition to the following generic activities, the outcomes and interventions selected for this diagnosis are determined by the affected body system and the degree of disuse. For patient goals and nursing activities specific to each body system, refer to plans for the Suggested Alternative Diagnoses listed above.

Assessments

- Make all assessments indicated by the preceding Goals/Evaluation Criteria for this diagnosis.
- Monitor for depression
- *(NIC) Bed Rest Care:*

  Monitor the skin condition
  Monitor for constipation
  Monitor for urinary function
  Monitor pulmonary status

Patient/Family Teaching

- *(NIC) Bed Rest Care:*

  Explain reasons for requiring bed rest
  Teach bed exercises, as appropriate

Collaborative Activities

- Consult with physical therapy for ways to improve mobility
- Consult with dietitian about increasing intake of high-energy foods

Other

- Plan and implement a turning schedule
- *(NIC) Bed Rest Care:*

  Place on an appropriate therapeutic mattress/bed
  Position in proper body alignment
  Avoid using rough-textured linen

Place bed-positioning switch within easy reach
Facilitate small shifts of body weight
Perform passive and/or active range-of-motion exercises
Apply antiembolism stockings

Home Care

- Most of the preceding interventions can be adapted for use in home care
- Be sure the patient has all the assistive devices needed in the home
- Teach patient and family to recognize signs and symptoms of fatigue that require reduction in activity

For Infants and Children

- Assess for signs of delayed language developmental delay in children under age 4 who must be restrained (e.g., by traction)
- Observe for signs of withdrawal and regression, which may occur as a response to illness or immobility
- Ask the family to bring special toys from home
- Keep toys within the child's reach; they should fit the child's developmental age
- Take the child out of the room (e.g., to the playroom, to the lobby) to the extent possible

For Older Adults

- Age-related changes in muscles, joints, and connective tissues make older adults more vulnerable to *Disuse syndrome*
- It is especially important to resume mobility as soon as possible to prevent rapid deterioration
- If the patient is on complete bed rest, place him in an upright position several times daily
- Consider referral to physical therapy for resistance exercises and strength training
- Institute case management as needed to facilitate the patient's ability to live at home

DIVERSIONAL ACTIVITY, DEFICIENT

(1980) **Domain 1, Health Promotion; Class 1, Health Awareness**

Definition: Decreased stimulation from (or interest or engagement in) recreational or leisure activities

Defining Characteristics

Subjective

Patient's statements regarding: boredom (e.g., wish there was something to do, to read, etc.)

Objective

Usual hobbies cannot be undertaken in hospital

Other Defining Characteristics (Non-NANDA International)

Anger, hostility
Complaints of inability to initiate or continue with usual activity
Disruptive behavior
Flat affect
Increase in daytime sleep periods
Restlessness
Withdrawn behavior

Related Factors

Environmental lack of diversional activity [as in long-term hospitalization]

Other Related Factors (Non-NANDA International)

Deficit in social skills
Forced inactivity
Impaired perception of reality
Lack of motivation
Prolonged bed rest

Suggestions for Use

Deficient diversional activity must be diagnosed from the patient's point of view because only the patient can determine whether the activities available are adequate to meet his needs.

Suggested Alternative Diagnoses

Coping, ineffective
Health behavior, risk-prone
Loneliness, risk for
Social interaction, impaired

NOC Outcomes

Leisure Participation: Use of relaxing, interesting, and enjoyable activities to promote well-being

Motivation: Inner urge that moves or prompts an individual to positive action(s)

Play Participation: Use of activities by a child from 1 year through 11 years of age to promote enjoyment, entertainment, and development

Social Involvement: Social interactions with persons, groups, or organizations

Goals/Evaluation Criteria

Examples Using NOC Language

- *Deficient diversional activity* will be relieved, as evidenced by Motivation, Leisure Participation, Play Participation, and Social Involvement
- Demonstrates **Social Involvement**, as evidenced by the following indicators (specify 1–5: never, rarely, sometimes, often, or consistently demonstrated):
  - Interacts with close friends, neighbors, family members, or members of work group(s)
  - Participates as member of church, in organized activity, as officer in organization, or as volunteer

Other Examples

Patient will:

- Demonstrate socially acceptable behaviors during activities
- Verbalize acceptance of limitations that interfere with usual leisure activities
- Identify options for recreation
- Verbalize satisfaction with leisure activities
- Participate in appropriate play
- Demonstrate or verbalize enjoyment of play

NIC Interventions

Activity Therapy: Prescription of and assistance with specific physical, cognitive, social, and spiritual activities to increase the range, frequency, or duration of an individual's (or group's) activity

Family Process Maintenance: Minimization of family process disruption effects

Family Support: Promotion of family values, interests, and goals

Recreation Therapy: Purposeful use of recreation to promote relaxation and enhancement of social skills

Self-Modification Assistance: Reinforcement of self-directed change initiated by the patient to achieve personally important goals

Self-Responsibility Facilitation: Encouraging a patient to assume more responsibility for own behavior

Socialization Enhancement: Facilitation of another person's ability to interact with others

Therapeutic Play: Purposeful and directive use of toys or other materials to assist children in communicating their perception and knowledge of their world and to help in gaining mastery of their environment

Nursing Activities

Assessments

- Identify patient's interests
- Monitor emotional, physical, and social responses to diversional activity
- *(NIC) Self-Responsibility Facilitation:* Monitor level of responsibility that patient assumes

Collaborative Activities

- Identify resources, such as volunteers and occupational therapists, which could assist patient in recreational and leisure activities

Other

- Introduce and encourage new or alternative leisure-time activities, specify activities
- Introduce patient to other patients who have successfully dealt with similar situations
- Provide appropriate stimuli, such as music, games, puzzles, visitors, and relaxation therapy, to vary monotonous routines and stimulate thought
- Provide compatible roommate, if possible
- Supervise recreational activities, as necessary
- Encourage family, friends, and significant persons to visit
- *(NIC) Self-Responsibility Facilitation:*
  - Encourage patient to take as much responsibility for own self-care as possible
  - Encourage independence, but assist patient when unable to perform
  - Provide positive feedback for accepting additional responsibility and/or behavior change

Home Care

- Help patient to choose recreational activities appropriate to capabilities (e.g., physical, psychologic, and social)
- Refer to occupational therapy, as needed
- Work with friends and family to encourage visits to the patient, or at least contact by telephone or computer messaging

D

For Infants and Children

- *(NIC) Self-Responsibility Facilitation:* Assist parents in identifying age-appropriate tasks for which child could be responsible, as appropriate
- In inpatient settings, have age-appropriate toys within the child's reach, take the child to the playroom, and arrange for interaction with other children, as appropriate
- Encourage the family to bring favorite toys and games from home

For Older Adults

- Suggest taking part in volunteer activities (e.g., delivering meals to homebound individuals) for those who are able to do so
- Help the client identify areas of interest he might pursue for diversion
- Arrange for the client to attend a senior citizen's group (e.g., an exercises group, a communal meals group)
- Determine whether the client has transportation to activities; arrange, if necessary
- Provide an environment with good lighting for crafts and reading
- For inpatients in long-term care, consider an animal-assisted therapy program
- For clients in long-term care, consider daily recreational therapy exercises and leisure educational programs for those who can benefit from them

DRY EYE, RISK FOR

(2010) **Domain 11, Safety/Protection; Class 2, Physical Injury**

Definition: At risk for eye discomfort or damage to the cornea and conjunctiva due to reduced quantity or quality of tears to moisten the eye

Risk Factors

Aging

Autoimmune diseases (rheumatoid arthritis, diabetes mellitus, thyroid disease, gout, osteoporosis, etc.)

Contact lenses

Environmental factors (air-conditioning, excessive wind, sunlight exposure, air pollution, low humidity)

Female gender
History of allergy
Hormones
Lifestyle (e.g., smoking, caffeine use, prolonged reading)
Mechanical ventilation therapy
Neurological lesions with sensory or motor reflex loss (lagophthalmos, lack of spontaneous blink reflex due to decreased consciousness and other medical conditions)
Ocular surface damage
Place of living
Treatment-related side effects (e.g., pharmaceutical agents such as angiotensin-converting enzyme inhibitors, antihistamines, diureica, steroids, antidepressants, tranquilizers, analgesics, sedatives, neuromuscular blockage agents, surgical operations)
Vitamin A deficiency

Suggestions for Use

When discomfort is caused by dry eyes, you may need to use the diagnosis *Risk for impaired comfort related to dry eyes.* The NANDA-I diagnosis is for the potential problem, *Risk for dry eye*; there is no diagnosis for the actual problem.

Suggested Alternative Diagnoses

Comfort, impaired

NOC Outcomes

NOC outcomes have not yet been linked to this diagnosis. However, the following may be useful.

Discomfort Level: Severity of observed or reported mental or physical discomfort

Neurological Status: Consciousness: Arousal, orientation, and attention to the environment

Tissue Integrity: Skin and Mucous Membranes: Structural intactness and normal physiological function of skin and mucous membranes

Goals/Evaluation Criteria

Examples Using NOC Language

- Client will not experience dry eye, as demonstrated by Discomfort Level and Tissue Integrity: Skin and Mucous Membranes within expected range for the individual

- Will demonstrate mild to no **Discomfort Level**, as evidenced by the following indicators (specify 1–5: severe, substantial, moderate, mild, or none): Pain, anxiety, moaning, or thrashing

Other Examples

- Sclera and eyelids will be moist and without lesions
- Patient will be alerted, easily aroused, and oriented to time, place, and person

NIC Interventions

NIC interventions have not yet been linked to this diagnosis. However, the following may be useful.

Contact Lens Care: Prevention of eye injury and lens damage by proper use of contact lenses

Eye Care: Prevention or minimization of threats to eye or visual integrity

Nursing Activities

In general, nursing activities for *Risk for dry eye* focus in monitoring for risk factors (e.g., level of consciousness) and symptoms of dry eye (e.g., pain), as well as measures to minimize risk factors and thus prevent dry eye.

Assessments

- Assess for risk factors such as allergies and smoking. Pay special attention to older adults, those being mechanically ventilated and those with decreased level of consciousness
- If risk factors are present, monitor those regularly
- Assess the sclera and conjunctiva for moistness, color, redness, abrasions, and drainage

Patient/Family Teaching

- Teach proper handling, removal, and storage of contact lenses

Collaborative Activities

- Instill eye ointment or drops in the lower lids, as prescribed

Other

- Provide eye care every 2 to 4 hr for unconscious patients, those who have lost the blink reflex, or who are critically ill.
- If risk factors (e.g., coma) are present:
  - Lubricate the eyes with saline or artificial tears
  - Use a protective eye shield to keep the eyes closed

DYSREFLEXIA, AUTONOMIC

(1988) **Domain 9, Coping/Stress Tolerance; Class 3, Neurobehavioral Stress**

Definition: Life-threatening, uninhibited sympathetic response of the nervous system to a noxious stimulus after a spinal cord injury at T7 or above

Defining Characteristics

Subjective

Blurred vision

Chest pain

Headache (a diffuse pain in different portions of the head and not confined to any nerve distribution area)

Metallic taste in mouth

Paresthesia

Objective

Bradycardia (pulse rate of < 60 beats per minute, bpm)

Chills

Conjunctival congestion

Diaphoresis above injury

Horner syndrome [contraction of pupil, partial ptosis of eyelid, enophthalmos, and sometimes loss of sweating over affected side of face]

Nasal congestion

Pallor below injury

Paroxysmal hypertension [sudden periodic elevation of BP, where systolic is > 140 and diastolic is > 90 bpm]

Pilomotor reflex [gooseflesh formation when skin is cooled]

Red splotches on skin (above the injury)

Tachycardia [pulse rate > 100 bpm]

Related Factors

Bladder distention

Bowel distention

Deficient patient and caregiver knowledge

Skin irritation [or skin lesion]

Suggestions for Use

Autonomic dysreflexia is a potential problem for the patient with high spinal cord injury. *Autonomic dysreflexia* cannot continue as an actual nursing diagnosis. If independent nursing actions do not resolve it, medical treatment becomes necessary. As a rule, *Risk for automatic dysreflexia* is a more useful label than actual *Autonomic dysreflexia* because the patient is in a potential state most of the time (Carpenito-Moyet, 2006b, p. 285). The suggested alternative diagnoses represent noxious stimuli that can trigger a sympathetic response in the patient with spinal cord injury. They may be used as actual problems or as the etiology of *Autonomic dysreflexia* or *Risk for autonomic dysreflexia*.

Suggested Alternative Diagnoses

Constipation [fecal impaction]
Skin integrity, impaired
Urinary retention

NOC Outcomes

Neurological Status: Ability of the peripheral and central nervous systems to receive, process, and respond to internal and external stimuli

Neurological Status: Autonomic: Ability of the autonomic nervous system to coordinate visceral and homeostatic function

Vital Signs: Extent to which temperature, pulse, respiration, and BP are within normal range

Goals/Evaluation Criteria

Examples Using NOC Language

- Patient will not experience *Autonomic dysreflexia*, as demonstrated by Neurological Status; Neurological Status: Autonomic; and Vital Signs within expected range for the individual
- Patients will demonstrate satisfactory **Neurological Status**, as evidenced by the following indicators (specify 1–5: severely, substantially, moderately, mildly, or not compromised):

  Consciousness
  Central motor control
  Cranial sensory and motor function
  Breathing pattern

Other Examples

Patient will:

- Maintain vital signs in expected range: temperature, apical and radial pulse rates, respiration rate, systolic and diastolic BP
- Demonstrate ability to maintain bowel and bladder routine
- Identify early signs and symptoms of dysreflexia (e.g., headache, blurred vision, paresthesia)

NIC Interventions

Dysreflexia Management: Prevention and elimination of stimuli that cause hyperactive reflexes and inappropriate autonomic responses in a patient with a cervical or high thoracic cord lesion

Skin Surveillance: Collection and analysis of patient data to maintain skin and mucous membrane integrity

Surveillance: Purposeful and ongoing acquisition, interpretation, and synthesis of patient data for clinical decision making

Vital Signs Monitoring: Collection and analysis of cardiovascular, respiratory, and body temperature data to determine and prevent complications

Nursing Activities

Assessments

- Assess patient's knowledge of condition, including history of previous episodes, early signs and symptoms, and bowel and bladder regimen
- Assess skin condition at least daily, noting any reddened areas above level of spinal cord injury
- Obtain baseline temperature, BP, and pulse
- *(NIC) Dysreflexia Management:* Monitor for signs and symptoms of autonomic dysreflexia: paroxysmal hypertension, bradycardia, tachycardia, diaphoresis above the level of injury, facial flushing, pallor below the level of injury, headache, nasal congestion, engorgement of temporal and neck vessels, conjunctival congestion, chills without fever, pilomotor erection, and chest pain

Patient/Family Teaching

- Ask patient to report any early signs and symptoms of condition that occur
- *(NIC) Dysreflexia Management:* Instruct patient and family about causes, symptoms, treatment, and prevention of dysreflexia

Collaborative Activities

- *(NIC) Dysreflexia Management:* Administer antihypertensive agents intravenously, as ordered

Other

- *(NIC) Dysreflexia Management:* Identify and minimize stimuli that may precipitate dysreflexia (e.g., bladder distention, renal calculi, infection, fecal impaction, rectal examination, suppository insertion, skin breakdown, and constrictive clothing or bed linen)
- If symptoms occur, stop activity and have someone notify physician

- Quickly eliminate noxious stimulus in the following order:
  Bladder: Check catheter for patency, or catheterize patient
  Bowel: If distended, apply anesthetic ointment to rectal area and disimpact.
  Body temperature: Maintain normal body temperature

- During onset of crisis, carry out management plan according to *(NIC) Dysreflexia Management:*
  Administer antihypertensive agents intravenously, as ordered
  Stay with patient and monitor status every 3 to 5 min if hyperreflexia occurs
  Place head of bed in upright position, as appropriate, if hyperreflexia occurs

DYSREFLEXIA: AUTONOMIC, RISK FOR

(1998, 2000) **Domain 9, Coping/Stress Tolerance; Class 3, Neurobehavioral Stress**

Definition: At risk for life-threatening uninhibited response of the sympathetic nervous system, postspinal shock, in an individual with a spinal cord injury or lesion at T6 or above (has been demonstrated in patients with injuries at T7 and T8)

Risk Factors

An injury or lesion at T6 or above *and* at least one of the following noxious stimuli:

Cardiac/Pulmonary Stimuli

Deep-vein thrombosis
Pulmonary emboli

Gastrointestinal Stimuli

Bowel distention
Constipation
Difficult passage of feces
Enemas
Esophageal reflux
Fecal impaction
Gallstones
Gastric ulcers
Gastrointestinal system pathology
Hemorrhoids
Stimulation (e.g., digital, instrumentation, surgery)
Suppositories

Musculoskeletal-Integumentary Stimuli

Cutaneous stimulations (e.g., pressure ulcer, ingrown toenail, dressings, burns, rash)
Fractures
Heterotrophic bone
Pressure over bony prominences or genitalia
Range-of-motion exercises
Spasm
Sunburns
Wounds

Neurological Stimuli

Painful or irritating stimuli below the level of injury

Regulatory Stimuli

Extreme environmental temperatures
Temperature fluctuations

Reproductive Stimuli

Ejaculation
Labor and delivery
Menstruation
Ovarian cyst
Pregnancy
Sexual intercourse

Situational Problems

Constrictive clothing (e.g., straps, stockings, shoes)
Narcotic withdrawal
Positioning
Reactions to pharmaceutical agents (e.g., decongestants, sympathomimetics, vasoconstrictors)
Surgical procedures

Urological Problems

Bladder distention
Bladder spasm
Calculi
Catheterization
Cystitis
Detrusor sphincter dyssynergia
Epididymitis
Instrumentation or surgery
Urethritis
Urinary tract infection

Suggestions for Use

See Suggestions for Use for Autonomic Dysreflexia, preceding diagnosis.

Suggested Alternative Diagnoses

Constipation [fecal impaction]
Skin integrity, impaired
Urinary retention

NOC Outcomes

Bowel Elimination: Formation and evacuation of stool
Gastrointestinal Function: Extent to which foods (ingested or tube-fed) are moved from ingestion to excretion
Cardiopulmonary Status: Adequacy of blood volume ejected from the ventricles and exchange of carbon dioxide and oxygen at the alveolar level
Neurological Status: Autonomic: Ability of the autonomic nervous system to coordinate visceral and homeostatic function
Risk Detection: Personal actions to identify personal health threats
Urinary Elimination: Collection and discharge of urine

Goals/Evaluation Criteria

Examples Using NOC Language

- Patient will not experience *Autonomic dysreflexia*, as demonstrated by Cardiopulmonary Status and Neurological Status: Autonomic, within expected range for the individual
- Patients will demonstrate satisfactory **Neurological Status: Autonomic**, as evidenced by the following indicators (specify 1–5: severely, substantially, moderately, mildly, or not compromised):
  Cardiac pump effectiveness
  Vasodilatation and vasoconstriction responses
  Perspiration response pattern
  Intestinal motility
  Pupil reactivity
  Peripheral tissue perfusion
- Patients will demonstrate satisfactory **Neurological Status: Autonomic**, as evidenced by the following indicators (specify 1–5: severe, substantial, moderate, mild, or none):
  Bronchospasms
  Bladder spasms

Dilated or constricted pupils
Dysreflexia

Other Examples

Patient will:

- Maintain vital signs in expected range: temperature, apical and radial pulse rates, respiration rate, systolic and diastolic BP
- Demonstrate ability to maintain bowel and bladder routine
- Identify early signs and symptoms of dysreflexia (e.g., headache, blurred vision, paresthesia)

NIC Interventions

Bowel Management: Establishment and maintenance of a regular pattern of bowel elimination

Dysreflexia Management: Prevention and elimination of stimuli that cause hyperactive reflexes and inappropriate autonomic responses in a patient with a cervical or high thoracic cord lesion

Neurologic Monitoring: Collection and analysis of patient data to prevent or minimize neurological complications

Pressure Management: Minimizing pressure to body parts

Urinary Elimination Management: Maintenance of an optimum urinary elimination pattern

Surveillance: Purposeful and ongoing acquisition, interpretation, and synthesis of patient data for clinical decision making

Vital Signs Monitoring: Collection and analysis of cardiovascular, respiratory, and body temperature data to determine and prevent complications

Nursing Activities

Assessments

See Assessments for Autonomic Dysreflexia, preceding diagnosis.

Patient/Family Teaching

See Patient/Family Teaching for Autonomic Dysreflexia.

Other

- Quickly eliminate any noxious stimulus in the following order to prevent Autonomic Dysreflexia:

  Bladder: Check catheter for patency or catheterize patient

  Bowel: If distended, apply anesthetic ointment to rectal *area and* disimpact; consider enema or flatus tube

  Body temperature: Maintain normal body temperature

ELECTROLYTE IMBALANCE, RISK FOR

(2008) **Domain 2, Nutrition: Class 5, Hydration**

Definition: At risk for change in serum electrolyte levels that may compromise health

E

Risk Factors

Objective

Deficient fluid volume
Diarrhea
Endocrine dysfunction
Excess fluid volume
Impaired regulatory mechanisms (e.g., diabetes insipidus, syndrome of inappropriate secretion of antidiuretic hormone)
Renal dysfunction
Treatment-related side effects (e.g., medications, drains)
Vomiting

Suggestions for Use

Several nursing diagnoses may be risk factors for *Risk for electrolyte imbalance* (e.g., *Diarrhea*, *Deficient fluid volume*, *Excess fluid volume*). If, for example, *Diarrhea* is the only risk factor the patient has, it is better to use *Diarrhea* as the label because treating the diarrhea will prevent electrolyte imbalance. If many risk factors exist, you might use *Risk for electrolyte imbalance*.

In many cases, the problem is better stated as a collaborative problem. For example, for a patient with renal failure, *Potential complication: Electrolyte imbalance* is more useful than *Risk for electrolyte imbalance related to renal failure* because there are no independent nursing interventions for renal failure, other than to monitor and try to prevent the problem.

Suggested Alternative Diagnoses

Deficient fluid volume
Diarrhea
Excess fluid volume
Urinary Retention

NOC Outcomes

Electrolyte & Acid/Base Balance: Balance of electrolytes and nonelectrolytes in the intracellular and extracellular compartments of the body

Burn Healing: Extent of healing of a burn site
Fluid Balance: Water balance in the intracellular and extracellular compartments of the body
Gastrointestinal Function: Extent to which foods (ingested or tube-fed) are moved from ingestion to excretion
Hydration: Adequate water in the intracellular and extracellular compartments of the body
Nausea and Vomiting Severity: Severity of nausea, retching, and vomiting symptoms

Goals/Evaluation Criteria

Examples Using NOC Language

- Will not experience *Electrolyte Imbalance*, as demonstrated by acceptable range of Burn Healing, Fluid Balance, Gastrointestinal Function, Hydration, and Nausea and Vomiting Severity.
- Will demonstrate **Electrolyte & Acid/Base Balance**, as evidenced by the following indicators (specify 1–5: severe, substantial, moderate, mild, or no deviation from normal range):
  Apical heart rate and rhythm
  Neuromuscular nonirritability
  Respiratory rate and rhythm
  Serum electrolytes (e.g., sodium, potassium, chloride, calcium)
  Serum pH
- Will demonstrate **Electrolyte & Acid/Base Balance**, as evidenced by the following indicators (specify 1–5: severe, substantial, moderate, mild, or none):
  Impaired cognition
  Muscle cramps or weakness
  Abdominal cramps

Other Examples

- Will experience no dysrhythmias, restlessness, or paresthesia
- Fluid intake and output will be balanced
- No edema
- No loss of skin turgor

NIC Interventions

Diarrhea Management: Management and alleviation of diarrhea
Fluid/Electrolyte Management: Regulation and prevention of complications from altered fluid and/or electrolyte levels
Hemodialysis Therapy: Management of extracorporeal passage of the patient's blood through a dialyzer

Medication Management: Facilitation of safe and effective use of prescription and over-the-counter drugs

Peritoneal Dialysis Therapy: Administration and monitoring of dialysis solution into and out of the peritoneal cavity

Surveillance: Purposeful and ongoing acquisition, interpretation, and synthesis of patient data for clinical decision making

Vomiting Management: Prevention and alleviation of vomiting

Wound Care: Burns: Prevention of wound complications due to burns and facilitation of wound healing

Nursing Activities

In general, nursing activities for this diagnosis focus on identifying the factors that put the patient at risk for electrolyte imbalance, monitoring for signs and symptoms, and treating the specific imbalance (usually collaboratively). Nursing care depends on the etiology of the electrolyte imbalance (e.g., burns, diarrhea, dialysis). In this text you will find, nursing activities for etiologies such as *Deficient fluid volume*, *Diarrhea*, *Excess fluid volume*, and *Vomiting*. Also consult a medical-surgical textbook for care of the various etiologies, as needed.

Assessments

- Monitor for signs and symptoms of the relevant electrolyte imbalance (e.g., hypo/hyperkalemia, hypo/hypernatremia), for example:
  - Weakness
  - Muscle irritability
  - Nausea
  - Electrocardiogram (ECG) changes

[**NOTE:** Exhaustive signs/symptoms of all the electrolyte imbalances are beyond the scope of this book. Refer to a medical-surgical nursing text, as needed.]

- Monitor serum electrolyte levels
- Accurately record intake and output
- Monitor for dehydration

Patient/Family Teaching

- Teach symptoms of the relevant electrolyte imbalance

Collaborative Activities

- Monitor for side effects and therapeutic responses to supplemental electrolytes
- Consult physician if electrolyte imbalance persists or worsens

Other

- Provide fluids, as appropriate
- Encourage oral intake: place fluids in easy reach, provide fresh water
- Irrigate nasogastric tubes with normal saline, not water

- Control excessive electrolyte loss (e.g., by resting the bowel)
- Prepare the patient for dialysis

ENERGY FIELD, DISTURBED

(1994, 2004) **Domain 4, Activity/Rest; Class 3, Energy Balance**

Definition: Disruption of the flow of energy surrounding a person's being that results in disharmony of the body, mind, and spirit

Defining Characteristics

Objective

[Nurse's] perceptions of changes in patterns of energy flow, such as:
- Movement (wave, spike, tingling, dense, flowing)
- Sounds (tone, words)
- Temperature change (warmth, coolness)
- Visual changes (image, color)

Disruption of the field (deficit, hole, spike, bulge, obstruction, congestion, diminished flow in energy field)

Related Factors

Slowing or blocking of energy flows secondary to:

Maturational factors

Age-related developmental difficulties or crisis (specify)

Pathophysiologic factors

Illness [specify]
Injury
Pregnancy

Situational factors (personal, environmental)

Anxiety
Fear
Grieving
Pain

Treatment-related factors

Chemotherapy
Immobility
Labor and delivery
Perioperative experience

Suggestions for Use

This diagnosis suggests independent but nontraditional nursing interventions, which require specialized instruction and practice. Therefore, it should be used only by nurses who possess such expertise (Krieger, 1979; Meehan, 1991).

Suggested Alternative Diagnoses

Anxiety

Pain: acute, chronic

NOC Outcomes

Personal Well-Being: Extent of positive perception of one's health status and life circumstances

Symptom Control: Personal actions to minimize perceived adverse changes in physical and emotional functioning

Goals/Evaluation Criteria

Also refer to Goals/Evaluation Criteria for Anxiety and Acute Pain.

Examples Using NOC Language

- Demonstrates **Personal Well-Being**, as evidenced by the following indicators (specify 1–5: not at all, somewhat, moderately, very, or completely satisfied):
  - Performance of activities of daily living
  - Social relationships
  - Spiritual life
  - Ability to express emotions
  - Opportunities for health care choice(s)

Other Examples

Patient will:

- Verbalize relief of symptoms (e.g., pain, anxiety) after treatment
- Demonstrate physical evidence of relaxation (e.g., decrease in BP, pulse and respiration rates, and muscle tension)
- Indicate satisfaction with psychologic, social, spiritual, physiologic, and cognitive functioning
- Demonstrate adequate coping skills

NIC Interventions

NOTE: Several NOC interventions are available to address the related factors of *Disturbed energy field.* Therapeutic touch is the primary intervention.

Acupressure: Application of firm, sustained pressure to special points on the body to decrease pain, produce relaxation, and prevent or reduce nausea

Environmental Management: Comfort: Manipulation of the patient's surroundings for promotion of optimal comfort

Massage: Stimulation of the skin and underlying tissues with varying degrees of hand pressure to decrease pain, produce relaxation, and/or improve circulation

Self-Awareness Enhancement: Assisting a patient to explore and understand his thoughts, feelings, motivations, and behaviors

Therapeutic Touch: Attuning to the universal healing field, seeking to act as an instrument for healing influence, and using the natural sensitivity of the hands to gently focus and direct the intervention process

Nursing Activities

Prior to Administering Therapeutic Touch

- Provide for privacy
- Obtain the patient's permission to use therapeutic touch
- Have the client sit or lie in a relaxed position with the body in alignment
- Instruct the client to close her eyes and breathe evenly and slowly
- *(NIC) Therapeutic Touch:*
  - Focus awareness on the inner self
  - Focus on the intention to facilitate wholeness and healing at all levels of consciousness

Assessment

- *NIC (Therapeutic Touch):*
  - Place hands 1 to 2 inches from the patient's body
  - Begin the assessment by moving the hands slowly and steadily over as much of the patient as possible, from head to toe and front to back
  - Note the overall pattern of the energy flow, especially any areas of disturbance such as congestion or unevenness, which may be perceived through very subtle cues in the hands, for example, temperature change, tingling, or other subtle feelings of movement
  - [After the treatment] note whether the patient has experienced a relaxation response and any related outcomes
- Ask the patient to give feedback during the procedure

Treatment

- Focus completely on the patient, with unconditional love and compassion and the intention of helping the patient
- When working in the head area, or for those who may be sensitive to it (e.g., the mentally ill, the elderly, premature infants), use therapeutic touch gently and only for short periods of time
- Use actual, hands-on touch and massage, as needed
- Provide a rest period for the patient after the treatment
- *(NIC) Therapeutic Touch:*

  Focus intention on facilitating symmetry and healing in disturbed areas

  Begin by moving the hands in very gentle downward movements through the patient's energy field, thinking of the patient as a unitary whole and facilitating an open and balanced energy flow

  Continue the treatment by very gently facilitating the flow of healing energy into areas of disturbance

  Finish when it is judged that the appropriate amount of change has taken place (i.e., for an infant, 1 to 2 min; for an adult, 5 to 7 min), keeping in mind the importance of gentleness

Patient/Family Teaching

- Teach therapeutic touch to family members
- Teach the patient deep-breathing exercises to aid in relaxation
- Teach the patient to use guided imagery in conjunction with the therapeutic-touch treatment

Home Care

- Work with the family to provide a space in which to administer therapeutic touch

For Infants and Children

- Therapeutic touch is safe for children and is used even for premature infants
- Use gently and for 1 to 2 min per treatment

For Older Adults

- Therapeutic touch may be effective in relieving anxiety and agitation in patients with dementia

ENVIRONMENTAL INTERPRETATION SYNDROME, IMPAIRED

(1994)* **Domain 5, Perception/Cognition; Class 2, Orientation**

Definition: Consistent lack of orientation to person, place, time, or circumstances over more than 3 to 6 months, necessitating a protective environment

*This diagnosis will be retired from the 2015–2017 NANDA-I Taxonomy unless work is completed to bring it into compliance with the definition of syndrome diagnoses.

Defining Characteristics

Subjective

Consistent disorientation [in known and unknown environments]

Objective

Chronic confusional states
Loss of occupation or social functioning [e.g., from memory decline]
Inability to follow simple directions
Inability to reason
Inability to concentrate
Slow in responding to questions

Related Factors

Alcoholism (non-NANDA)
Dementia [e.g., Alzheimer disease, multi-infarct dementia, Pick disease, AIDS-related dementia]
Depression
Huntington disease
Parkinson disease (non-NANDA)

Suggestions for Use

Because this diagnosis and those in the Suggested Alternative Diagnoses overlap, careful analysis of the patient's defining characteristics is needed. This diagnosis is especially difficult to differentiate from *Chronic confusion*. As a rule, this author prefers to use *Chronic confusion*.

Suggested Alternative Diagnoses

Confusion, acute
Confusion, chronic
Injury, risk for

Memory, impaired
Tissue perfusion, ineffective (cerebral) (non-NANDA-I)

NOC Outcomes

Cognitive Orientation: Ability to identify person, place, and time accurately

Concentration: Ability to focus on a specific stimulus

Elopement Propensity Risk: The propensity of an individual with cognitive impairment to escape a secure area

Memory: Ability to cognitively retrieve and report previously stored information

Safe Wandering: Safe, socially acceptable moving about without apparent purpose in an individual with cognitive impairment

Goals/Evaluation Criteria

Examples Using NOC Language

- Maintains or improves Cognitive Orientation, Concentration, Elopement Propensity Risk, Memory, and Safe Wandering
- Demonstrates **Memory**, as evidenced by the following indicators (specify 1–5: severely, substantially, moderately, mildly, or not compromised):
  Recalls immediate information accurately
  Recalls recent information accurately
  Recalls recent information accurately

Other Examples

- Opens eyes to external stimuli
- Correctly identifies common objects
- Correctly identifies examples of time, place, and person
- Speaks coherently
- Identifies significant other, place, and day
- Remains free from injury or harm
- Participates to maximum level of independence in ADLs
- Is content and less frustrated by environmental stressors

NIC Interventions

Anxiety Reduction: Minimizing apprehension, dread, foreboding, or uneasiness related to an unidentified source of anticipated danger

Cognitive Stimulation: Promotion of awareness and comprehension of surroundings by utilization of planned stimuli

Dementia Management: Provision of a modified environment for the patient who is experiencing a chronic confusional state

Dementia Management: Bathing: Reduction of aggressive behavior during cleaning of the body

Elopement Precautions: Minimizing the risk of a patient leaving a treatment setting without authorization when departure presents a threat to the safety of patient or others

Environmental Management: Safety: Monitoring and manipulation of the physical environment to promote safety

E

Fall Prevention: Instituting special precautions with patient at risk for injury from falling

Memory Training: Facilitation of memory

Neurologic Monitoring: Collection and analysis of patient data to prevent or minimize neurological complications

Reality Orientation: Promotion of patient's awareness of personal identity, time, and environment

Risk Identification: Analysis of potential risk factors, determination of health risks, and prioritization of risk-reduction strategies for an individual or group

Surveillance: Safety: Purposeful and ongoing collection and analysis of information about the patient and the environment for use in promoting and maintaining patient safety

Nursing Activities

Also refer to Nursing Activities for Confusion, Chronic. In early dementia, when the main symptoms are those of *Impaired memory*, refer to Nursing Activities for Impaired Memory.

Assessments

- Determine patient's self-care abilities
- Identify safety needs of patient based on level of physical and cognitive function and past history of behavior
- *(NIC) Dementia Management:*
  - Identify usual patterns of behavior for such activities as sleep, medication use, elimination, food intake, and self-care
  - Monitor cognitive functioning, using a standardized assessment tool

Patient/Family Teaching

- Explain the effect of the patient's illness on his mood (e.g., depression, premenstrual syndrome)
- As needed, explain to family members that a shower or tub bath are not the only ways to get clean, and that forcing a patient to bathe when he is resisting can be harmful and provoke aggressive behaviors

Collaborative Activities

- Refer to social services for referral to day care programs

Other

- Modify physical environment to ensure safety for patient
- Employ a flexible approach to bathing (e.g., tub or sponge bath); be gentle, do not rush the procedure, keep the patient warm
- Use distraction to manage behavior
- Accompany ambulatory patient to activities away from the unit
- Encourage family to bring objects from home
- Promote consistency in caregiver assignment
- Orient patient to person, place, and time
- Limit visitors if patient becomes more agitated or disoriented
- Use a calm, unhurried approach
- *(NIC) Dementia Management:*

  Provide a low-stimulation environment (e.g., quiet, soothing music; nonvivid, simple, familiar patterns in décor; performance expectations that do not exceed cognitive-processing ability; and dining in small groups)

  Provide cues—such as current events, seasons, location, and names—to assist orientation

  Address the patient distinctly by name when initiating interaction and speak slowly

  Give one simple direction at a time

Home Care

- Teach family and caregivers actions to minimize risk factors that might precipitate falls in the home (e.g., removing throw rugs, providing night light)

FAILURE TO THRIVE, ADULT

(1998) **Domain 9, Coping/Stress Tolerance; Class 2, Coping Responses**

Definition: Progressive functional deterioration of a physical and cognitive nature. The individual's ability to live with multisystem diseases, cope with ensuing problems, and manage his care is remarkably diminished

Defining Characteristics

Subjective

Altered mood state—expresses feelings of sadness, being low in spirit

Reports loss of interest in pleasurable outlets [such as food, sex, work, friends, family, hobbies, or entertainment]

Reports desire for death

Objective

Anorexia [does not eat meals when offered; states does not have an appetite, not hungry, or "I don't want to eat"]

Apathy [as evidenced by lack of observable feeling or emotion in terms of normal ADLs and environment]

Cognitive decline [decline in mental processing; as evidenced by problems with responding appropriately to environmental stimuli and demonstrated difficulty in reasoning, decision making, judgment, memory and concentration, decreased perception]

Decreased participation in ADLs

Decreased social skills and social withdrawal [noticeable decrease from usual past behavior in attempts to form or participate in cooperative and interdependent relationships (e.g., decreased verbal communication with staff, family, friends)]

Frequent exacerbations of chronic health problems [such as pneumonia or urinary tract infections]

Inadequate nutritional intake—eating less than body requirements; consumes minimal to no food at most meals (i.e., consumes less than 75% of normal requirements at each or most meals)

Neglect of financial responsibilities

Neglect of home environment

Physical decline [decline in bodily function; evidence of fatigue, dehydration, incontinence of bowel and bladder]

Self-care deficit [no longer looks after or takes charge of physical cleanliness or appearance; difficulty performing simple self-care tasks; neglects home environment or financial responsibilities]

Weight loss (decreased from baseline weight) [5% unintentional weight loss in 1 month, 10% unintentional weight loss in 6 months]

Related Factors

Apathy (non-NANDA-I)

Depression

Fatigue (non-NANDA-I)

Suggestions for Use

(a) The list of Related Factors shown previously appears to be incomplete for this diagnosis. Considering the multisystem and multifunctional nature of the Defining Characteristics, there are a large number of factors that would cause them. (b) This diagnosis should be used only when several of the Defining Characteristics are present and when all are caused by the same related factors. Many of the Defining Characteristics are actually other nursing diagnoses (see the following Suggested Alternative Diagnoses), and when the patient has only a few of those problems, care planning may be better guided by those more narrowly focused diagnoses.

Suggested Alternative Diagnoses

Anxiety
Bowel incontinence
Confusion, acute or chronic
Coping, ineffective
Fatigue
Fluid volume, deficient
Grieving, complicated
Home maintenance, impaired
Hopelessness
Infection, risk for
Injury, risk for
Loneliness, risk for
Memory, impaired
Nutrition: less than body requirements, imbalanced
Powerlessness
Protection, ineffective
Role performance, ineffective
Self-care deficit (specify)
Self-esteem, chronic or situational low
Sexuality patterns, ineffective
Social interaction, impaired
Spiritual distress
Urinary Incontinence (specify type)

NOC Outcomes

Appetite: Desire to eat when ill or receiving treatment
Cognition: Ability to execute complex mental processes
Development: Late Adulthood: Cognitive, psychosocial, and moral progression from 65 years of age and older

Nutritional Status: Extent to which nutrients are available to meet metabolic needs
Nutritional Status: Food and Fluid Intake: Amount of food and fluid taken into the body over a 24-hr period
Self-Care: Activities of Daily Living (ADLs): Ability to perform the most basic physical tasks and personal care activities independently with or without assistive devices
Weight Gain Behavior: Personal actions to gain weight following voluntary or involuntary significant weight loss
Will to Live: Desire, determination, and effort to survive

Goals/Evaluation Criteria

NOTE: Some examples are given, but the specific goals for this diagnosis will depend on which of the defining characteristics are present. For other goals, refer to Defining Characteristics for the preceding Suggested Alternative Diagnoses (e.g., the goals for *Anxiety* and *Confusion*).

Examples Using NOC Language

- *Failure to thrive* alleviated, as demonstrated by satisfactory Appetite, Cognition, Development: Late Adulthood, Nutritional Status, Nutritional Status: Food and Fluid Intake, Self-Care (ADLs), Weight Gain Behavior, and Will to Live.
- Demonstrates **Will to Live**, as evidenced by the following indicators (specify 1–5: severely, substantially, moderately, mildly, or not compromised)
  - Expression of determination to live
  - Expression of optimism
  - Interest in one's illness and treatment
  - Use of strategies to compensate for problems associated with disease
  - Use of strategies to lengthen life

Other Examples

The patient will:

- Regain energy needed to cope with problems resulting from multisystem diseases
- Eat diet adequate to provide for body requirements
- Regain lost weight
- Not experience depression
- Not experience suicidal thoughts
- Not experience further cognitive decline
- Participate in decision making

- Restore relationships with significant others
- Perform ADLs (e.g., bathing, toileting)

NIC Interventions

Cognitive Stimulation: Promotion of awareness and comprehension of surroundings by utilization of planned stimuli

Decision-Making Support: Providing information and support for a patient who is making a decision regarding health care

Dementia Management: Provision of a modified environment for the patient who is experiencing a chronic confusional state

Fluid Monitoring: Collection and analysis of patient data to regulate fluid balance

Home Maintenance Assistance: Helping the patient and family to maintain the home as a clean, safe, and pleasant place to live

Hope Inspiration: Facilitation of the development of a positive outlook in a given situation

Nutrition Management: Assisting with or providing a balanced dietary intake of foods and fluids

Nutrition Therapy: Administration of food and fluids to support metabolic processes of a patient who is malnourished or at high risk for becoming malnourished

Nutritional Monitoring: Collection and analysis of patient data to prevent or minimize malnourishment

Resiliency Promotion: Assisting individuals, families, and communities in development, use, and strengthening of protective factors to be used in coping with environmental and societal stressors

Self-Care Assistance: Assisting another to perform ADLs

Spiritual Support: Assisting the patient to feel balance and connection with a greater power

Weight Gain Assistance: Facilitating gain of body weight

Nursing Activities

Assessments

- Assess for expressions of helplessness or hopelessness
- Assess mental status and cognition
- Assess nutritional status
- Identify stressful life events and changes that have occurred in the past year

Collaborative Activities

- Refer to mental health professionals for evaluation of depression
- Refer to a nutritionist

Other

- Because this diagnosis is so broad, a comprehensive list of nursing activities is not practical. Refer to Nursing Activities for the appropriate Suggested Alternative Diagnoses. For example, if the patient is experiencing anorexia and weight loss, refer to *Imbalanced nutrition: less than body requirements* for nursing activities that improve the patient's nutrition. If the patient is incontinent, refer to *Bowel incontinence* or *Urinary incontinence* for the appropriate nursing activities.

Home Care

- Assess availability of social interactions and extent of client's participation
- Assess self-care abilities
- Refer for home health aide or homemaker services as needed

FALLS, RISK FOR

(2000) **Domain 11, Safety/Protection; Class 2, Physical Injury**

Definition: At increased susceptibility to falling that may cause physical harm

Risk Factors

Adults

Age 65 or over
History of falls
Lives alone
Lower limb prosthesis
Use of assistive devices (e.g., walker, cane)
Wheelchair use

Children

< 2 years of age
Bed located near window
Lack of automobile restraints (i.e., infant carseats)
Lack of parental supervision
Male gender when < 1 year of age
No gate on stairs
No window guards
Unattended infant on bed, changing table, sofa, or other elevated surface

Cognitive

Diminished mental status (e.g., confusion, delirium, dementia, impaired reality testing)

Environment

Cluttered environment
No antislip material in bath or shower
Restraints
Throw or scatter rugs
Unfamiliar or dimly lit room
Weather conditions (e.g., ice)
Wet floors

F

Medications

ACE inhibitors
Alcohol use
Antianxiety agents
Antihypertensive agents
Diuretics
Hypnotics
Narcotics/opiates
Tranquilizers
Tricyclic antidepressants

Physiological

Anemia
Arthritis
Decreased strength in lower extremities
Diarrhea
Faintness when turning or extending neck
Foot problems
Gait difficulties
Hearing difficulties
Impaired balance
Impaired physical mobility
Neoplasms (i.e., causing fatigue or limited mobility)
Neuropathy
Orthostatic hypotension
Postoperative conditions
Postprandial blood sugar changes
Presence of acute illness
Proprioception deficits (e.g., unilateral neglect)
Sleeplessness
Urgency or incontinence

Vascular disease
Visual difficulties

Suggestions for Use

When risk factors specific to falls are present, use this diagnosis instead of the more general *Risk for injury* or *Risk for trauma*. If at risk for accidents in addition to falls, the more general diagnoses may be better.

Suggested Alternative Diagnoses

Injury, risk for
Trauma, risk for

NOC Outcomes

Falls Occurrence: Number of times an individual falls
Physical Injury Severity: Severity of injuries from accidents and trauma
(**NOTE:** The following outcomes are associated with risk factors for falls. They do not measure the actual occurrence of the diagnosis.)
Balance: Ability to maintain body equilibrium
Coordinated Movement: Ability of muscles to work together voluntarily for purposeful movement
Fall Prevention Behavior: Personal or family caregiver actions to minimize risk factors that might precipitate falls in the personal environment
Knowledge: Fall Prevention: Extent of understanding conveyed about prevention of falls

Goals/Evaluation Criteria

Examples Using NOC Language

- Will decrease or limit *Risk for falls*, as demonstrated by Balance, Coordinated Movement, Fall Prevention Behavior, and Knowledge: Fall Prevention
- Demonstrates **Falls Occurrence**, as evidenced by the following indicators (specify 1–5: 10 and over, 7–9, 4–6, 1–3, and none [in defined period of time]):
  - Falls while standing still
  - Falls while walking
  - Falls while sitting
  - Falls while transferring
  - Falls from bed
  - Falls climbing steps
  - Falls descending steps

Other Examples

Patient and family will:

- Provide a safe environment (e.g., eliminate clutter and spills, place handrails, and use rubber shower mats and grab bars)
- Identify risks that increase susceptibility to falls
- Avoid physical injury from falls

NIC Interventions

(**NOTE:** The following interventions are associated with prevention of falls and aimed at specific risk factors. An exhaustive list is beyond the scope of this book, so if a patient has risk factors not addressed here (e.g., substance abuse, urinary incontinence), consult a medical-surgical (or other) textbook and the *NIC* handbook.)

Body Mechanics Promotion: Facilitating the use of posture and movement in daily activities to prevent fatigue and musculoskeletal strain or injury

Bowel Incontinence Care: Promotion of bowel continence and maintenance of perianal skin integrity

Cognitive Stimulation: Promotion of awareness and comprehension of surroundings by utilization of planned stimuli

Delirium Management: Provision of a safe and therapeutic environment for the patient who is experiencing an acute confusional state

Delirium Management: Provision of a safe and therapeutic environment for the patient who is experiencing an acute confusional state

Environmental Management: Safety: Monitoring and manipulation of the physical environment to promote safety

Exercise Promotion: Strength Training: Facilitating regular resistive muscle training to maintain or increase muscle strength

Exercise Promotion: Stretching: Facilitation of systematic slow-stretch-hold muscle exercises to induce relaxation, to prepare muscles/joints for more vigorous exercise, or to increase or maintain body flexibility

Exercise Therapy: Ambulation: Promotion and assistance with walking to maintain or restore autonomic and voluntary body functions during treatment and recovery from illness or injury

Exercise Therapy: Balance: Use of specific activities, postures, and movements to maintain, enhance, or restore balance

Exercise Therapy: Joint Mobility: Use of active or passive body movement to maintain or restore joint flexibility

Exercise Therapy: Muscle Control: Use of specific activity or exercise protocols to enhance or restore controlled body movement

Fall Prevention: Instituting special precautions with patient at risk for injury from falling

Medication Management: Facilitation of safe and effective use of prescription and over-the-counter drugs

Peripheral Sensation Management: Prevention or minimization of injury or discomfort in the patient with altered sensation

Risk Identification: Analysis of potential risk factors, determination of health risks, and prioritization of risk-reduction strategies for an individual or group

Seizure Precautions: Prevention or minimization of potential injuries sustained by a patient with a known seizure disorder

Self-Care Assistance: Assisting another to perform ADLs

Surveillance: Purposeful and ongoing acquisition, interpretation, and synthesis of patient data for clinical decision making

Teaching: Infant Safety: Instruction on safety during first year of life

Teaching: Toddler Safety: Instruction on safety during the 2nd and 3rd years of life

Nursing Activities

Assessments

- Identify factors that affect safety needs, for example, changes in mental status, degree of intoxication, fatigue, maturational age, medications, and motor or sensory deficit (e.g., with gait, balance)
- Perform a falls risk assessment on every patient admitted to the facility
- *(NIC) Fall Prevention:*
  - Identify characteristics of environment that may increase potential for falls (e.g., slippery floors and open stairways)
  - Monitor gait, balance, and fatigue level with ambulation

Patient/Family Teaching

- *(NIC) Fall Prevention:*
  - Teach patient how to fall so as to minimize injury
  - Instruct patient to wear prescription glasses, as appropriate, when out of bed

Collaborative Activities

- *(NIC) Fall Prevention:* Collaborate with other health care team members to minimize side effects of medications that contribute to falling (e.g., orthostatic hypotension and unsteady gait)
- Refer to physical therapy for gait training and exercises to improve mobility, balance, and strength

Other

- Reorient patient to reality and immediate environment when necessary
- Assist patient with ambulation, as needed; use a transfer belt and the help of another person if the patient is unsteady
- If the patient is at risk for falls, place him in a room near the nurses' desk
- Provide assistive devices for walking (e.g., cane, walker)

- Use an alarm to alert caretaker when patient is getting out of bed or leaving room
- If necessary, use physical restraints to limit risk of falling
- *(NIC) Fall Prevention:*

  Provide the dependent patient with a means of summoning help (e.g., bell or call light) when caregiver is not present

  Place articles within easy reach of patient

- Instruct patient to call for assistance with movement, as appropriate
- Remove environmental hazards (e.g., provide adequate lighting)
- Make no unnecessary changes in physical environment (e.g., furniture placement)
- Ensure that patient wears proper shoes (e.g., nonskid soles, secure fasteners)

Home Care

- Instruct patient and family in techniques to prevent injury at home, specify techniques
- Provide educational materials related to strategies and measures to prevent falls
- Provide information on environmental hazards and characteristics (e.g., stairs, windows, gates)
- Teach family members about factors that contribute to falls and ways to decrease these risks
- Refer to physical therapy to teach the family how to assist with ambulation and transfer safely
- Assess for correct use of ambulation aids (e.g., walker)

For Infants and Children

- Raise side rails when not present at bedside
- For children old enough to climb over bed rails, use a crib with a net or "bubble top"
- *(NIC) Fall Prevention:*

  Remove objects that provide young child with climbing access to elevated surfaces

  Provide close supervision or restraining device (e.g., infant seat with seat belt) when placing infants or young children on elevated surfaces (e.g., table and highchair)

For Older Adults

- Assess the client's ability to ambulate safely with or without assistive devices
- Assess vision and remind client to wear glasses when ambulating
- Assess for and treat urinary incontinence, which is associated with increased incidence of falls
- Recommend and help the client obtain a personal emergency call system
- T'ai chi classes may be beneficial for those who are able to participate

FAMILY PROCESSES, DYSFUNCTIONAL*

(1994, 2008) **Domain 7, Role/Relationships; Class 2, Family Relationships**

Definition: Psychosocial, spiritual, and physiologic functions of the family unit are chronically disorganized, which leads to conflict, denial of problems, resistance to change, ineffective problem solving, and a series of self-perpetuating crises

*This diagnosis was formerly labeled *Dysfunctional family processes: Alcoholism.*

Defining Characteristics

Behaviors

Agitation
Blaming
Broken promises
Chaos
Complicated grieving
Conflict avoidance
Contradictory communication
Controlling communication and power struggles
Criticizing
Denial of problems
Dependency
Difficulty having fun
Difficulty with intimate relationships
Diminished physical contact
Disturbances in academic performance in children
Disturbances in concentration

Enabling to maintenance of substance use pattern (e.g., alcohol)
Escalating conflict
Expression of anger inappropriately
Failure to accomplish current or past developmental tasks and difficulty with life cycle transitions
Family special occasions are substance use centered
Harsh self-judgment
Immaturity
Impaired communication
Inability to accept or receive help
Inability to adapt to change
Inability to deal with traumatic experiences constructively
Inability to express or accept a wide range of feelings
Inability to meet emotional needs of its members
Inability to meet security needs of its members
Inability to meet spiritual needs of its members
Inadequate understanding or knowledge of substance abuse
Inability to accept a wide range of feelings
Inappropriate expression of anger
Lack of reliability
Loss of control of drinking
Lying
Manipulation
Nicotine addiction
Orientation toward tension relief rather than achievement of goals
Paradoxical communication
Rationalization
Refusal to get help
Seeking approval and affirmation
Self-blaming
Social isolation
Stress-related physical illnesses
Substance abuse
Verbal abuse of children, spouse, or parent

Feelings

Abandonment
Anger
Anxiety, tension, distress
Being different from other people
Being unloved
Confuses love and pity

Confusion
Decreased self-esteem and worthlessness
Depression
Dissatisfaction
Embarrassment
Emotional control by others
Emotional isolation and loneliness
Failure
Fear
Frustration
Guilt
Hopelessness
Hostility
Hurt
Insecurity
Lack of identity
Lingering resentment
Loss
Mistrust
Moodiness
Powerlessness
Rejection
Reports feeling misunderstood
Repressed emotions
Responsibility for substance abuser's behavior
Shame
Suppressed rage
Unhappiness
Vulnerability

Roles and Relationships

Altered role function and disruption of family roles
Chronic family problems
Closed communication systems
Deterioration in family relationships and disturbed family dynamics
Disrupted family rituals
Economic problems
Family denial
Family does not demonstrate respect for individuality and autonomy of its members
Inconsistent parenting and low perception of parental support
Ineffective spouse communication or marital problems

Intimacy dysfunction
Lack of cohesiveness
Lack of skills necessary for relationships
Neglected obligations
Pattern of rejection
Reduced ability of family members to relate to each other for mutual growth and maturation

Triangulating of family relationships

Related Factors

Addictive personality
Biochemical influences
Family history of resistance to treatment
Family history of substance abuse
Genetic predisposition to substance abuse
Inadequate coping skills
Lack of problem-solving skills
Substance abuse

Suggestions for Use

(a) Since being revised, this diagnosis is no longer limited to use with alcohol abuse. It has been broadened to include abuse of any substance, as well as factors other than substance abuse (e.g., inability to cope with traumatic experiences, inappropriate expression of anger). It is also a broader diagnosis now than *Compromised/disabled family coping.* (b) *Compromised/disabled family coping* may be more useful for describing a family who fails, specifically, to cope with a family member's health challenge. (c) *Interrupted family processes* describes a family that has a history of normal functioning, but which is undergoing a change in relationships or functioning (e.g., intimacy changes, power alliance changes). It seems to describe a healthier status than the other two diagnoses.

Suggested Alternative Diagnoses

Coping: family, compromised
Coping: family, disabled
Interrupted family processes
Violence: self-directed or other-directed, risk for

NOC Outcomes

Family Coping: Family actions to manage stressors that tax family resources
Family Functioning: Capacity of the family system to meet the needs of its members during developmental transitions

Family Integrity: Family members' behaviors that collectively demonstrate cohesion, strength, and emotional bonding

Family Resiliency: Positive adaptation and function of the family system following significant adversity or crisis

Family Social Climate: Supportive milieu as characterized by family member relationships and goals

Substance Addiction Consequences: Severity of change in health status and social functioning due to substance addiction

Goals/Evaluation Criteria

Examples Using NOC Language

- Family will resolve *Dysfunctional family coping* as demonstrated by satisfactory Family Coping, Family Functioning, Family Integrity, Family Resiliency, Family Social Climate, and Substance Addiction Consequences
- Family member(s) who abuse substances (e.g., alcohol) demonstrate(s) **Substance Addiction Consequences**, as evidenced by the following indicators (specify 1–5: severe, substantial, moderate, mild, or none):
  - Sustained decrease in physical activity
  - Chronic impaired motor function
  - Chronic fatigue
  - Chronic impaired cognitive function
  - Difficulty in maintaining employment
  - Arrests within the last year
  - Absenteeism from work or school

Other Examples

Patient and family will:

- Acknowledge that alcoholism is a family illness
- Acknowledge the severity of the threat to the well-being of the family
- Identify destructive behaviors
- Begin to change dysfunctional (e.g., codependent) patterns

NIC Interventions

Coping Enhancement: Assisting a patient to adapt to perceived stressors, changes, or threats which interfere with meeting life demands and roles

Decision-Making Support: Providing information and support for a patient who is making a decision regarding health care

Family Integrity Promotion: Promotion of family cohesion and unity

Family Integrity Promotion: Childbearing Family: Facilitation of the growth of individuals or families who are adding an infant to the family unit

Family Process Maintenance: Minimization of family process disruption effects

Family Therapy: Assisting family members to move their family toward a more productive way of living

Resiliency Promotion: Assisting individuals, families, and communities in development, use, and strengthening of protective factors to be used in coping with environmental and societal stressors

F

Role Enhancement: Assisting a patient, significant other, and/or family to improve relationships by clarifying and supplementing specific role behaviors

Self-Responsibility Facilitation: Encouraging a patient to assume more responsibility for own behavior

Substance Use Treatment: Supportive care of patient and family members with physical and psychosocial problems associated with the use of alcohol or drugs

Nursing Activities

Assessments

- Determine history of drug and alcohol use
- Determine which substances are being used
- Identify nature of spiritual support for family
- Ask directly about drinking (e.g., How often do you have six or more drinks a day? In the last year, how many times have you driven after having three or more drinks?)
- *(NIC) Substance Use Treatment:*
  - Identify with patient those factors (e.g., genetic, psychological distress, and stress) that contribute to chemical dependency
  - Screen patient at frequent intervals for continued substance use, using urine screens, or breath analysis, as appropriate
  - Determine whether codependent relationships exist in the family

Patient/Family Teaching

- Provide family members with information about alcoholism or help them to find other sources of information
- *(NIC) Substance Use Treatment:* Instruct patient and family about drugs used to treat specific substance use

Collaborative Activities

- *(NIC) Substance Use Treatment:* Identify support groups in the community for long-time substance abuse treatment
- Refer for pharmacological therapies to help prevent relapse

Other

- Recognize and accept that resolution of the alcoholism may not be the goal of care
- Emphasize to family members that they must allow the person to be responsible for his own drinking and behaviors
- Explore with the family the methods they use to control the alcoholic's behaviors (e.g., hiding the alcohol)
- Help family to identify realistic goals for changing family interaction patterns
- Assist family members to focus on changing their responses to the drinking instead of trying to control it
- Suggest that the patient try acupuncture and other alternative therapies
- Facilitate communication among family members
- Give positive feedback for adaptive coping mechanisms used by patient and family
- *(NIC) Substance Use Treatment:*
  Establish a therapeutic relationship with patient [and family]
  Assist patient and family to identify use of denial as a substitute for confronting the problem
  Facilitate support by significant others
  Encourage patient to take control over own behavior
  Help members recognize that chemical dependency is a family disease
  Discuss with patient the effect of associations with other users during leisure or work time
  Discuss the effect of substance use on relationships with family, coworkers, and friends
  Encourage patient to keep a detailed chart of substance use to evaluate progress
  Assist patient to learn alternate methods of coping with stress or emotional distress

Home Care

- Because alcoholism is a family problem, care is likely to be given in the home. All of the preceding interventions should be applicable in the home.

For Infants and Children

- Assess whether inappropriate role demands are being placed on the child
- Assess for behavioral and social problems that may be caused by family dynamics
- Assess drinking in children of alcoholic parents
- Recommend cognitive-behavioral alcohol intervention programs

For Older Adults

- Include assessment for alcohol and other substance abuse in your assessments of older adults

FAMILY PROCESSES, INTERRUPTED

(1982, 1998) **Domain 7, Role Relationships; Class 2, Family Relationships**

Definition: Change in family relationships or functioning. [The NANDA International definition does not necessarily describe a problem. A clearer definition might be: the state in which a family that normally functions effectively experiences dysfunction.]

Defining Characteristics

Subjective

Changes in satisfaction with family

Objective

Changes in [the following factors]:

Assigned tasks
Availability for affective responsiveness and intimacy
Availability for emotional support
Communication patterns
Effectiveness in completing assigned tasks
Expressions of conflict with or isolation from community resources
Expressions of conflict within family
Mutual support
Participation in decision making
Participation in problem solving
Patterns and rituals
Power alliances

Somatic complaints
Stress-reduction behaviors

Related Factors

Developmental transition or crisis
Family roles shift
Informal or formal interaction with community
Modification in family finances
Modification in family social status
Power shift of family members
Shift in health status of a family member
Situational transitions or crises

Suggestions for Use

This label describes a family that normally functions effectively but is experiencing a stressor that alters its functioning. The stressors causing *Interrupted family processes* tend to be situational or developmental transitions and crises, such as death of a family member, divorce, infidelity, loss of a job, serious illness, or hospitalization of a family member. In contrast, *Dysfunctional family processes* describes a chronically disorganized family. When the interrupted family processes are specifically focused, a diagnosis such as *Complicated grieving* or *Parental role conflict* may describe the problem more specifically.

This label is different from *Compromised family coping*, in which the family coping problem is caused by a change in the relationship between the family members. The stressor in *Compromised family coping* is withdrawal of support by a significant other, not necessarily an external stressor such as death or divorce (as in *Interrupted family processes*). *Compromised family coping* may involve the patient and only one significant other, whereas *Interrupted family processes* involves the entire family. Likewise, *Caregiver role strain* focuses on the individual caregiver rather than the whole family. *Interrupted family processes* describes a family that has the resources for coping effectively with stressors, in contrast with *Disabled family coping*, which describes a family that demonstrates destructive behaviors. If stressors are not effectively resolved, *Interrupted family processes* can progress to *Disabled family coping*. To differentiate among the suggested alternative diagnoses, carefully examine the defining characteristics and related factors of each.

Suggested Alternative Diagnoses

Caregiver role strain (actual and at risk for)
Coping: family, compromised

Coping: family, disabled
Family processes, dysfunctional
Grieving, complicated
Therapeutic regimen management: families, ineffective
Parental role conflict
Parenting, impaired

NOC Outcomes

Family Coping: Family actions to manage stressors that tax family resources

Family Functioning: Capacity of the family system to meet the needs of its members during developmental transitions

Family Normalization: Capacity of the family system to maintain routines and develop strategies for optimal functioning when a member has a chronic illness or disability

Family Resiliency: Positive adaptation and function of the family system following significant adversity or crisis

Family Social Climate: Supportive milieu as characterized by family member relationships and goals

Family Support During Treatment: Family presence and emotional support for an individual undergoing treatment

Goals/Evaluation Criteria

Examples Using NOC Language

- Family does not exhibit *Interrupted family processes*, as demonstrated by satisfactory Family Coping, Family Functioning, Family Normalization, Family Resiliency, Family Social Climate, and Family Support During Treatment

Other Examples

Patient and family will:

- Acknowledge change in family roles
- Identify coping patterns
- Participate in decision-making processes regarding posthospital care
- Function to provide mutual support for each family member
- Identify ways to cope more effectively

NIC Interventions

Coping Enhancement: Assisting a patient to adapt to perceived stressors, changes, or threats that interfere with meeting life demands and roles

Family Integrity Promotion: Promotion of family cohesion and unity

Family Integrity Promotion: Childbearing Family: Facilitation of the growth of individuals or families who are adding an infant to the family unit

Family Involvement Promotion: Facilitating family participation in the emotional and physical care of the patient

Family Presence Facilitation: Facilitation of the family's presence in support of an individual undergoing resuscitation and/or invasive procedures

Family Process Maintenance: Minimization of family process disruption effects

Family Support: Promotion of family values, interests, and goals

Normalization Promotion: Assisting parents and other family members of children with chronic illnesses or disabilities in providing normal life experiences for their children and families

Parent Education: Adolescent: Assisting parents to understand and help their adolescent children

Parent Education: Childrearing Family: Assisting parents to understand and promote the physical, psychological, and social growth and development of their toddler, preschool, or school-aged child or children

Parent Education: Infant: Instruction on nurturing and physical care needed during the first year of life

Resiliency Promotion: Assisting individuals, families, and communities in development, use, and strengthening of protective factors to be used in coping with environmental and societal stressors

Nursing Activities

Some of the interventions used to achieve the desired outcomes may also treat related factors, which produce symptoms of this nursing diagnosis.

Assessments

- Assess interaction between patient and family, being alert for potential destructive behaviors
- Assess child's limitations, so that accommodations can be made to allow child to participate in usual activities
- *(NIC) Family Integrity Promotion:*
  - Determine family understanding of condition
  - Determine family feelings regarding their situation
  - Determine typical family relationships for each family
  - Monitor current family relationships
  - Identify conflicting priorities among family members

Patient/Family Teaching

- Teach the family those skills (e.g., time management, treatments) required for care of patient
- Teach family the need to work with the school system to ensure access to appropriate educational opportunities for the chronically ill or disabled child

F

Collaborative Activities

- Initiate a multidisciplinary patient care conference, involving the patient and family in problem solving and facilitation of communication
- Provide continuity of care by maintaining effective communication between staff members through nurse report and care planning
- Request social service consultation to help the family determine post-hospitalization needs and identify sources of community support (e.g., for child care)
- Refer family to a financial counselor
- Refer to a support group as needed
- *(NIC) Family Integrity Promotion:* Refer for family therapy, as indicated

Other

- Assist family in identifying behaviors that may be hindering prescribed treatment
- Assist family in identifying personal strengths
- Encourage family to verbalize feelings and concerns
- Encourage family to participate in patient's care and help plan post-hospital care
- Provide flexible visiting hours to accommodate family visits
- Preserve family routines and rituals (e.g., providing for private meals together or family decision making)
- Provide positive reinforcement for effective use of coping mechanisms
- *(NIC) Family Integrity Promotion:*
  Provide for family privacy
  Facilitate open communications among family members
  Counsel family members on additional effective coping skills for their own use
  Assist family with conflict resolution

Home Care

- Explore available hospital and community resources with family
- Most of the preceding activities and interventions can be adapted for home care use

For Infants and Children

- Help family to focus on the child rather than on the illness or disability
- Encourage the family to participate in the care of a hospitalized child
- Involve social services to assess the need for foster care placement. Also assess for the possibility of reunifying the child with biological parents when appropriate.
- Encourage opportunities for normal childhood experiences for the chronically ill or disabled child

FAMILY PROCESSES, READINESS FOR ENHANCED

(2002) **Domain 7, Role Relationships; Class 2, Family Relationships**

Definition: A pattern of family functioning that is sufficient to support the well-being of family members and can be strengthened

Defining Characteristics

Objective

Activities support the safety and growth of family members
Balance exists between autonomy and cohesiveness
Boundaries of family members are maintained
Communication is adequate
Energy level of family supports ADLs
Expresses willingness to enhance family dynamics
Family adapts to change
Family functioning meets [physical, social, and psychological] needs of family members
Family resilience is evident
Family roles are flexible and appropriate for developmental stages
Relationships are generally positive; interdependent with community; family tasks are accomplished
Respect for family members is evident

Related Factors

This is a wellness diagnosis, so an etiology is not necessary. If risk factors suggest the possibility of developing *Interrupted family processes*, use the diagnosis *Risk for interrupted family processes*.

Suggestions for Use

This label describes a family that is functioning effectively but wishes to improve its functioning and ability to deal with situational or developmental transitions and crises.

Suggested Alternative Diagnoses

Coping: family, readiness for enhanced
Family processes, [risk for interrupted]
Parenting, readiness for enhanced

NOC Outcomes

Family Functioning: Capacity of the family system to meet the needs of its members during developmental transitions

Family Health Status: Overall health and social competence of family unit

Family Integrity: Family members' behaviors that collectively demonstrate cohesion, strength, and emotional bonding

Family Resiliency: Positive adaptation and function of the family system following significant adversity or crisis

Family Social Climate: Supportive milieu as characterized by family member relationships and goals

Goals/Evaluation Criteria

Examples Using NOC Language

- Family exhibits *enhanced family processes*, as demonstrated by satisfactory Family Coping, Family Functioning, Family Health Status, Family Integrity, Family Resiliency, and Family Social Climate

Other Examples

Patient and family will:

- Acknowledge changes in family roles
- Identify usual and effective coping patterns
- Use appropriate support systems
- Recognize environmental and lifestyle factors that are risks to health and act to minimize risks
- Function to provide mutual support for each family member

NIC Interventions

Coping Enhancement: Assisting a patient to adapt to perceived stressors, changes, or threats that interfere with meeting life demands and roles

Family Integrity Promotion: Promotion of family cohesion and unity

Family Integrity Promotion: Childbearing Family: Facilitation of the growth of individuals or families who are adding an infant to the family unit

Family Process Maintenance: Minimization of family process disruption effects

Health Education: Developing and providing instruction and learning experiences to facilitate voluntary adaptation of behavior conducive to health in individuals, families, groups, or communities

Health Screening: Detecting health risks or problems by means of history, examination, and other procedures

Health System Guidance: Facilitating a patient's location and use of appropriate health services

Resiliency Promotion: Assisting individuals, families, and communities in development, use, and strengthening of protective factors to be used in coping with environmental and societal stressors

Socialization Enhancement: Facilitation of another person's ability to interact with others

Nursing Activities

Assessments

- Assist family members to identify and anticipate situations that have the potential to disrupt family processes
- Identify family's spiritual supports
- Identify family role changes and their effects of family processes
- *(NIC) Family Integrity Promotion:*
  Determine typical family relationships for each family
  Monitor current family relationships
  Identify conflicting priorities among family members

Patient/Family Teaching

- Teach the family those skills (e.g., time management, treatments) that can enhance family processes
- Provide information about existing social support mechanisms that can be used in stressful situations

Other

- Assist family in identifying personal strengths
- Assist family with conflict resolution (if needed)
- Encourage family to verbalize feelings and concerns
- Encourage family to participate in patient's care and help plan post-hospital care
- Provide flexible visiting hours to accommodate family visits
- Preserve family routines and rituals (e.g., providing for private meals together or family decision making)

- Provide positive reinforcement for effective use of coping mechanisms
- *(NIC) Family Integrity Promotion:*
  Provide for family privacy
  Facilitate open communications among family members
  Counsel family members on additional effective coping skills for their own use

Home Care

- The preceding interventions can be used in home care.

For Infants and Children

- Encourage the family to have family meals together to promote good nutrition and enhance family communication

For Older Adults

- Provide positive reinforcement for family caregivers of older adults; stress the importance of their activities
- Explore with older adult families ways in which they can maintain social ties with friends and family

FATIGUE

(1988, 1998) **Domain 4, Activity/Rest; Class 3, Energy Balance**

Definition: An overwhelming, sustained sense of exhaustion and decreased capacity for physical and mental work at usual level

Defining Characteristics

Subjective

Compromised concentration
Compromised libido
Disinterest in surroundings
Drowsy
Feelings of guilt for not keeping up with responsibilities
Increased physical complaints
Introspection
Perceived need for additional energy to accomplish routine tasks
Reports feeling tired
Reports unremitting and overwhelming lack of energy

Objective

Decreased performance
Inability to maintain usual level of physical activity
Inability to maintain usual routines
Inability to restore energy even after sleep
Increase in rest requirements
Lack of energy
Lethargic or listless

Related Factors

Psychological

Anxiety
Boring lifestyle (report of)
Depression
Stress

Environmental

Humidity
Lights
Noise
Temperature

Situational

Negative life events
Occupation

Physiological

Anemia
Disease states
Increased physical exertion
Malnutrition
Poor physical condition
Pregnancy
Sleep deprivation

Other Related Factors (Non-NANDA International)

Altered body chemistry (e.g., caused by medications, drug withdrawal, chemotherapy)
Excessive social and role demands
Overwhelming psychologic or emotional demands

Suggestions for Use

Do not use this label to describe temporary tiredness resulting from lack of sleep. *Fatigue* describes a chronic condition that is not relieved by rest. The patient's previous energy levels and capabilities cannot immediately be restored, so the nursing focus is to help the patient find ways to adapt. Discriminate carefully between *Fatigue* and *Activity intolerance*. The energy deficit in *Fatigue* is overwhelming and may exist even when the patient has not performed any activities. *Fatigue* may be the etiology of other nursing diagnoses, such as *Self-care deficit* and *Impaired home maintenance*. Conversely, other labels, such as *Decreased cardiac output*, may be the etiology of *Fatigue*.

Suggested Alternative Diagnoses

Activity intolerance
Cardiac output, decreased
Insomnia
Self-care deficit

NOC Outcomes

Endurance: Capacity to sustain activity

Energy Conservation: Personal actions to manage energy for initiating and sustaining activity

Fatigue Level: Severity of observed or reported prolonged generalized fatigue

Nutritional Status: Energy: Extent to which nutrients and oxygen provide cellular energy

Psychomotor Energy: Personal drive and energy to maintain activities of daily living, nutrition, and personal safety

Goals/Evaluation Criteria

Examples Using NOC Language

- The patient will adapt to *Fatigue*, as evidenced by Endurance, Energy Conservation, Nutritional Status: Energy, and Psychomotor Energy.
- The patient will demonstrate **Energy Conservation**, as evidenced by the following indicators (specify 1–5: never, rarely, sometimes, often, or consistently demonstrated):

  Adapts lifestyle to energy level
  Balances activity and rest
  Maintains adequate nutrition
  Reports adequate endurance for activity
  Uses energy conservation techniques

Other Examples

Patient will:

- Maintain usual social interaction
- Identify psychologic and physical factors that may cause *Fatigue*

- Maintain ability to concentrate
- Attend and respond appropriately to visual, auditory, verbal, tactile, and olfactory cues
- Report that energy is restored after rest

NIC Interventions

Energy Management: Regulating energy use to treat or prevent fatigue and optimize function

Environmental Management: Manipulation of the patient's surroundings for therapeutic benefit, sensory appeal, and psychological well-being

Mood Management: Providing for safety, stabilization, recovery, and maintenance of a patient who is experiencing dysfunctionally depressed or elevated mood

Nutrition Management: Assisting with or providing a balanced dietary intake of foods and fluids

Nursing Activities

Assessments

- Determine the effects of *Fatigue* on quality of life
- *(NIC) Energy Management:*

  Monitor patient for evidence of excess physical and emotional fatigue

  Monitor cardiorespiratory response to activity (e.g., tachycardia, other dysrhythmias, dyspnea, diaphoresis, pallor, hemodynamic pressures, and respiratory rate)

  Monitor and record patient's sleep pattern and number of sleep hours

  Monitor location and nature of discomfort or pain during movement and activity

  Determine patient's and significant other's perception of causes of *Fatigue*

  Monitor nutritional intake to ensure adequate energy resources

  Monitor administration and effect of stimulants and depressants

Patient/Family Teaching

- Instruct patient in the relationship of Fatigue to disease process and condition
- *(NIC) Energy Management:*

  Instruct patient and significant other to recognize signs and symptoms of *Fatigue* that require reduction in activity

  Teach activity organization and time-management techniques to prevent *Fatigue*

F

Collaborative Activities

- Make other practitioners aware of the effects of *Fatigue*
- Refer for family therapy if *Fatigue* has interfered with family functioning
- Refer for psychiatric care if *Fatigue* interferes with client's relationships significantly
- *(NIC) Energy Management:* Consult with dietitian about ways to increase intake of high-energy foods

Other

- Encourage patient and family to express feelings related to life changes caused by *Fatigue*
- Assist patient in identifying measures that increase concentration; consider initiating tasks after rest periods and prioritizing necessary tasks
- Encourage limited social interaction at times of higher energy
- Encourage patient to:
  - Report activities that increase *Fatigue*
  - Report onset of pain that may produce *Fatigue* (severity, location, precipitating factors)
- Plan activities with patient and family that minimize *Fatigue*. Plan may include:
  - Assist with ADLs, as needed, specify
  - Reduce low-priority activities
- *(NIC) Energy Management:*
  - Reduce physical discomforts that could interfere with cognitive function and self-monitoring or regulation of activity
  - Assist the patient and significant other to establish realistic activity goals
  - Provide calming diversional activities (e.g., reading, talking to others) to promote relaxation
  - Promote bed rest and activity limitation (e.g., increase number of rest periods) with protected rest times of choice
  - Avoid care activities during scheduled rest periods
  - Limit environmental stimuli (e.g., light and noise) to facilitate relaxation
  - Limit number of visitors and interruptions by visitors, as appropriate

Home Care

- Discuss with patient and family ways to modify home environment to maintain usual activities and to minimize *Fatigue*
- Assess the home environment for factors that may increase fatigue (e.g., stairs, distance to bathroom, cleaning activities)

- If *Chronic pain* is the etiology of *Fatigue*, refer to a pain management program in the community
- Work with client and family to set priorities for activities based on realistic expectations of the client's abilities
- Encourage the family to keep the client involved in family routines (e.g., mealtimes) as much as possible
- Help the client to be assertive in setting limits on the demands of others
- Refer for home health aide and housekeeping services

For Infants and Children

- Assess for fatigue in infants and toddlers by interviewing parents and noting changes in sleep, activity/play, and eating patterns; small children cannot verbally express fatigue.

For Older Adults

- Assess for comorbid conditions, such as arthritis, which may contribute to Fatigue
- Assess for depression as a cause of Fatigue; refer to mental health professional as needed
- Monitor for medication side effects that can cause Fatigue (e.g., beta-blockers, pain medications)

FEAR [SPECIFY FOCUS]

(1980, 1996, 2000) **Domain 9, Coping/Stress Tolerance; Class 2, Coping Responses**

Definition: Response to perceived threat that is consciously recognized as a danger

Defining Characteristics

Subjective

Report of:

Alarm
Apprehension
Being scared
Decreased self-assurance
Dread
Excitement

Increased tension
Jitteriness
Panic
Terror
Worry (non-NANDA)

Cognitive

F

Diminished productivity, learning ability, problem-solving ability
Identifies object of fear
Stimulus believed to be a threat

Behaviors

Avoidance or attack behaviors
Impulsiveness
Increased alertness
Narrowed focus on the source of the fear

Physiological

Anorexia
Diarrhea
Dry mouth
Fatigue
Increased perspiration
Increased pulse
Increased respiratory rate and shortness of breath
Increased systolic blood pressure
Muscle tightness
Nausea
Pallor
Pupil dilation
Vomiting

Related Factors

Innate origin (e.g., sudden noise, height, pain, loss of physical support)
Innate releasers (neurotransmitters)
Language barrier
Learned response (e.g., conditioning, modeling from or identification with others)
Phobic stimulus
Sensory impairment
Separation from support system in potentially stressful situation (e.g., hospitalization, hospital procedures)
Unfamiliarity with environmental experience(s)

Suggestions for Use

See Suggestions for Use for the diagnosis, Anxiety.

Suggested Alternative Diagnoses

Anxiety
Posttrauma syndrome
Rape-trauma syndrome

NOC Outcomes

Fear Level: Severity of manifested apprehension, tension, or uneasiness arising from an identifiable source

Fear Level: Child: Severity of manifested apprehension, tension, or uneasiness arising from an identifiable source in a child from 1 year through 17 years of age

Fear Self-Control: Personal actions to eliminate or reduce disabling feelings of apprehension, tension, or uneasiness from an identifiable source

Goals/Evaluation Criteria

Examples Using NOC Language

- The patient will exhibit **Fear Self-Control**, as evidenced by the following indicators (specify 1–5: never, rarely, sometimes, often, or consistently demonstrated):
  - Seeks information to reduce fear
  - Monitors length of time between episodes
  - Maintains control over life
  - Maintains role performance and social relationships
  - Controls fear response
  - Remains productive

NIC Interventions

Anxiety Reduction: Minimizing apprehension, dread, foreboding, or uneasiness related to an unidentified source of anticipated danger

Calming Technique: Reducing anxiety in patient experiencing acute distress

Coping Enhancement: Assisting a patient to adapt to perceived stressors, changes, or threats that interfere with meeting life demands and roles

Presence: Being with another, both physically and psychologically, during times of need

Security Enhancement: Intensifying a patient's sense of physical and psychologic safety

Nursing Activities

Also refer to Nursing Activities for the diagnosis, Anxiety.

Assessments

F

- Assess patient's subjective and objective fear responses
- *(NIC) Coping Enhancement:* Appraise the patient's understanding of the disease process

Patient/Family Teaching

- Explain all tests and treatments to patient and family
- Help clients differentiate between rational and irrational fears
- Teach client and family how to use guided imagery when they are fearful

Collaborative Activities

- Assess need for social service or psychiatric intervention
- Encourage a patient–physician discussion of the patient's fear
- Initiate a multidisciplinary patient care conference to develop a plan of care

Other

- Provide frequent, positive reinforcement when patient demonstrates behaviors that may reduce or eliminate fear
- Stay with patient during new situations or when fear is severe
- Remove the source of the patient's fear whenever possible
- Convey acceptance of the patient's perception of fear to encourage open communication regarding the source of the fear
- Provide continuity of patient care through patient assignment and use of care plan
- Provide frequent verbal and nonverbal reassurances that may assist in reducing the patient's fear state, avoid clichés
- *(NIC) Coping Enhancement:*

  Appraise and discuss alternative responses to situation

  Use a calm, reassuring approach

  Assist the patient in developing an objective appraisal of the event

  Encourage an attitude of realistic hope as a way of dealing with feelings of helplessness

  Discourage decision making when the patient is under severe stress

  Encourage gradual mastery of the situation

  Introduce the patient to persons (or groups) who have successfully undergone the same experience

Encourage verbalization of feelings, perceptions, and fears
Reduce stimuli in the environment that could be misinterpreted as threatening

Home Care

- The preceding interventions are applicable to home-based care
- Identify whether there are sources of fear in the home (e.g., a dangerous neighborhood, an abusive family member)
- Arrange for someone to be with the client during periods when fear is severe (e.g., a home health aide)

For Infants and Children

- Use the same caregivers as much as possible
- Offer pacifier to infant
- Hold or rock child
- Place a night-light in room
- Encourage parent(s) to spend the night at the hospital with a child
- Institute play therapy as a healthy outlet for feelings
- Don't dismiss a child's fears as "not real"
- Do not tease or make fun of the child's fear
- Offer explanations or some way to control the fear (e.g., "I don't see a ghost in your room, but I'll leave the light on for you, and I'll be nearby if you call me.")

For Older Adults

- Provide consistency in scheduling caregivers to the extent possible
- Provide a consistent, safe, environment with as few changes as possible

FLUID BALANCE, READINESS FOR ENHANCED

(2002) **Domain 2, Nutrition; Class 5, Hydration**

Definition: A pattern of equilibrium between fluid volume and chemical composition of body fluids that is sufficient for meeting physical needs and can be strengthened

Defining Characteristics

Subjective

Expresses willingness to enhance fluid balance
No excessive thirst

Objective

Intake adequate for daily needs
Good tissue turgor

Moist mucous membranes
No evidence of edema
Risk for deficient fluid volume
Stable weight
Straw-colored urine with specific gravity within normal limits
Urine output appropriate for intake

Related Factors

This is a wellness diagnosis, so an etiology is not necessary.

Suggestions for Use

If there are risk factors for fluid imbalance, use *Risk for imbalanced fluid volume* or *Risk for deficient fluid volume.*

Suggested Alternative Diagnoses

Fluid volume, risk for deficient
Fluid volume, risk for imbalanced
Urinary elimination, readiness for enhanced

NOC Outcomes

Fluid Balance: Water balance in the intracellular and extracellular compartments of the body

Hydration: Adequate water in the intracellular and extracellular compartments of the body

Kidney Function: Filtration of blood and elimination of metabolic waste products through the formation of urine

Goals/Evaluation Criteria

Also refer to Goals/Evaluation Criteria for Deficient Fluid Volume and Excess Fluid Volume.

Examples Using NOC Language

- Demonstrates *Enhanced fluid balance*, as evidenced by Fluid Balance, adequate Hydration, and adequate Kidney Function

- **Fluid Balance** will be achieved, as evidenced by the following indicators (specify 1–5: severely, substantially, moderately, mildly, or not compromised):
  - Blood pressure
  - Radial pulse rate
  - Serum electrolytes
  - Urine specific gravity

Other Examples

Patient will:

- Have hemoglobin and hematocrit in normal range
- Not experience abnormal thirst
- Have balanced intake and output over 24 hr
- Exhibit good hydration (moist mucous membranes, ability to perspire, normal skin turgor)

NIC Interventions

Fluid Management: Promotion of fluid balance and prevention of complications resulting from abnormal or undesired fluid levels

Fluid Monitoring: Collection and analysis of patient data to regulate fluid balance

Urinary Elimination Management: Maintenance of an optimum urinary elimination pattern

Nursing Activities

Also refer to Nursing Activities for Excess Fluid Volume.

Assessments

- Ask to describe color, amount, and frequency of fluid loss
- Assess for and anticipate factors that may create fluid imbalances (e.g., strenuous exercise, medications, fever, stress, medical orders)
- Weigh daily
- *(NIC) Fluid Management:*
  - Monitor hydration status (e.g., moist mucous membranes, adequacy of pulses, and orthostatic blood pressure)

Patient/Family Teaching

- Teach to monitor hydration status (e.g., color of urine, quantity of urine)
- Teach normal fluid requirements for adults and children
- Teach clients about factors that may create fluid imbalances, and the need to drink water before engaging in such activities
- Instruct regarding fluid requirements

Other

- Assist, as needed, to make a plan for ingesting adequate fluids
- *(NIC) Fluid Management:*

  Promote oral intake (e.g., provide a drinking straw, offer fluids between meals, change ice water routinely, make freezer pops using child's favorite juice, cut gelatin into fun squares, use small medicine cups), as appropriate

  Give fluids, as appropriate

Home Care

- Because this is a wellness diagnosis, most interventions will be directed to clients living at home, or to family members caring for clients at home
- Assess the availability of safe drinking water; if none is available, assist the client to acquire resources for obtaining bottled water

For Older Adults

- Encourage clients to plan a schedule for drinking water, even if they are not thirsty

FLUID VOLUME, DEFICIENT

(1978, 1996) **Domain 2, Nutrition; Class 5, Hydration**

Definition: Decreased intravascular, interstitial, or intracellular fluid; this refers to dehydration—water loss alone without change in sodium

Defining Characteristics

Subjective

Thirst

Objective

Change in mental status

Decreased blood pressure, decreased pulse volume and pressure

Decreased skin and tongue turgor

Decreased urine output

Decreased venous filling

Dry skin and mucous membrane

Elevated hematocrit

Increased body temperature

Increased pulse rate
Increased urine concentration
Sudden weight loss (except in third-spacing)
Weakness

Related Factors

Active fluid volume loss
[Excessive continuous consumption of alcohol]
Failure of regulatory mechanisms [as in diabetes insipidus, hyperaldosteronism]
[Inadequate fluid intake secondary to ________________]

Suggestions for Use

Use this label for patients experiencing vascular, cellular, or intracellular dehydration. Use the label cautiously, because many fluid balance problems require nurse–physician collaboration. Do not use this label routinely, even as a potential problem, for patients who have a medical order of NPO. Independent nursing treatments for *Deficient fluid volume* are meant to prevent fluid loss (e.g., diaphoresis) and encourage oral fluid intake. For a diagnosis such as *Risk for deficient fluid volume* related to prescribed NPO, there are no independent nursing actions to prevent or treat either side of the diagnostic statement. Treatment of *Deficient fluid volume* related to NPO status requires, for example, a medical order for IV therapy.

Do not use *Deficient fluid volume* to describe patients who are at risk for hemorrhage, or are hemorrhaging or in hypovolemic shock. These situations usually represent collaborative problems.

Incorrect: *Risk for deficient fluid volume* related to postpartum hemorrhage

Correct: Potential complication of childbirth: Postpartum hemorrhage

Correct: Risk for postpartum hemorrhage related to uterine atony

The most appropriate use of the *Deficient fluid volume* label is as a diagnosis (either actual or potential) for patients who are not drinking sufficient amounts of oral fluids, especially in the presence of increased fluid loss (e.g., *Diarrhea*, vomiting, burns). Actual *Deficient fluid volume* may also be the etiology of other nursing diagnoses, such as *Impaired oral mucous membrane*.

Suggested Alternative Diagnoses

Deficient fluid volume, risk for
Fluid volume, risk for imbalanced

Oral mucous membrane, impaired
Tissue perfusion: renal, risk for ineffective

F

NOC Outcomes

Fluid Balance: Water balance in the intracellular and extracellular compartments of the body

Hydration: Adequate water in the intracellular and extracellular compartments of the body

Nutritional Status: Food and Fluid Intake: Amount of food and fluid taken into the body over a 24-hr period

Goals/Evaluation Criteria

Examples Using NOC Language

- *Fluid volume deficit* will be eliminated, as evidenced by Fluid Balance, adequate Hydration, and adequate Nutritional Status: Food and Fluid Intake
- **Fluid Balance** will be achieved, as evidenced by the following indicators (specify 1–5: severely, substantially, moderately, mildly, or not compromised):
  - Blood pressure
  - Radial pulse rate
  - Peripheral pulses
  - Serum electrolytes
  - Stable body weight

Other Examples

Patient will:

- Have normally concentrated urine. Specify baseline specific gravity
- Have hemoglobin and hematocrit within normal range for patient
- Have central venous and pulmonary wedge pressures in expected range
- Not experience abnormal thirst
- Have balanced intake and output over 24 hr
- Exhibit good hydration (moist mucous membranes, ability to perspire)
- Have adequate oral or IV fluid intake

NIC Interventions

Fluid Management: Promotion of fluid balance and prevention of complications resulting from abnormal or undesired fluid levels

Fluid Monitoring: Collection and analysis of patient data to regulate fluid balance

Hypovolemia Management: Expansion of intravascular fluid volume in a patient who is volume depleted

Intravenous (IV) Therapy: Administration and monitoring of IV fluids and medications

Shock Prevention: Detecting and treating a patient at risk for impending shock

Nursing Activities

NOTE: (a) Some of these activities are specific for patients who are hemorrhaging. Refer to the preceding Suggestions for Use before including those activities in your plan of care. (b) The focus of nursing activities for this nursing diagnosis is on restoring fluid volume.

Assessments

- Monitor color, amount, and frequency of fluid loss
- Observe especially for loss of fluids high in electrolytes (e.g., diarrhea, wound drainage, nasogastric suction, diaphoresis, ileostomy drainage)
- Monitor for bleeding (e.g., check all secretions for frank or occult blood)
- Identify contributing factors that may aggravate dehydration (e.g., medications, fever, stress, medical orders)
- Monitor results relevant to fluid balance (e.g., hematocrit, BUN, albumin, total protein, serum osmolality, electrolytes, and urine specific gravity levels)
- Assess for vertigo or postural hypotension
- Assess orientation to person, place, and time
- Consult the patient's advance directives to determine whether it is appropriate to replace fluids for a terminally ill patient
- *(NIC) Fluid Management:*

  Monitor hydration status (e.g., moist mucous membranes, adequacy of pulses, and orthostatic blood pressure, as appropriate)

  Weigh patient daily and monitor trends

  Maintain accurate intake and output record

Patient/Family Teaching

- Instruct patient to inform nurse of thirst.

Collaborative Activities

- Report and document output less than ________________ mL
- Report and document output more than ________________ mL
- Report electrolyte abnormalities
- *(NIC) Fluid Management:*

  Arrange availability of blood products for transfusion, if necessary

Administer prescribed nasogastric replacement based on output, as appropriate

Administer IV therapy, as prescribed

Other

- Provide frequent oral hygiene
- Specify amount of fluids to be ingested in 24 hr, quantifying desired intake during the day, evening, and night shifts
- Ensure that patient is well hydrated preoperatively
- Position in Trendelenburg or elevate patient's legs when hypotensive, unless contraindicated
- *(NIC) Fluid Management:*

  Promote oral intake (e.g., provide a drinking straw, offer fluids between meals, change ice water routinely, make freezer pops using child's favorite juice, cut gelatin into fun squares, use small medicine cups), as appropriate

  Insert urinary catheter, if appropriate

  Give fluids, as appropriate

Home Care

- Teach family caregivers how to monitor intake and output (e.g., in a bedpan or urinal)
- Teach caregivers the signs of complications of *Deficient fluid volume*, and when to call the physician or 911
- Teach family caregivers how to manage intravenous therapy; assess the caregiver's ability to administer fluids

For Infants and Children

- Calculate the child's daily fluid maintenance needs on the basis of weight. Fluids lost must be replaced over and above this amount.
- Monitor hydration carefully; infants are vulnerable to fluid loss.
- To measure output for infants, count or weigh diapers. A 1-gram wet diaper equals 1 mL of urine.
- Offer fluids children like (e.g., milk, gelatin, frozen juices, snow cones)
- Make a game out of drinking (e.g., have a tea party)
- Make a chart and give the child a sticker when fluid intake is adequate
- To encourage children to drink fluids, provide a drinking straw, make freezer pops out of juice, cut colorful gelatins into different shapes

For Older Adults

- Make sure the client drinks a specified amount of water on a regular schedule, even if not thirsty
- Use checklists on the unit, if necessary, to ensure that clients drink adequate amounts of water
- Older adults are at risk for fluid loss and dehydration; monitor intake and output carefully

FLUID VOLUME, EXCESS

(1982, 1996) **Domain 2, Nutrition; Class 5, Hydration**

Definition: Increased isotonic fluid retention

Defining Characteristics

Subjective

Anxiety
Dyspnea or shortness of breath
Restlessness

Objective

Adventitious breath sounds [rales or crackles]
Anasarca
Anxiety
Azotemia
Blood pressure changes
Change in mental status
Changes in respiratory pattern
Decreased hemoglobin and hematocrit
Edema
Electrolyte imbalance
Increased central venous pressure
Intake exceeds output
Jugular vein distention
Oliguria
Orthopnea
Pleural effusion
Positive hepatojugular reflex
Pulmonary artery pressure changes
Pulmonary congestion
Restlessness

S_3 heart sound
Specific gravity changes
Weight gain over short period of time

Related Factors

Compromised regulatory mechanism
Excess fluid intake

Excess sodium intake
[Increased fluid intake secondary to hyperglycemia, medications, compulsive water drinking, and so forth]
[Insufficient protein secondary to decreased intake or increased losses]
[Renal dysfunction, heart failure, sodium retention, immobility, and so forth]

Suggestions for Use

Do not use this label for conditions that nurses cannot prevent or treat (e.g., do not use *Excess fluid volume* to describe renal failure or pulmonary edema, as these are medical diagnoses). The main type of fluid volume excess that nurses can treat independently is peripheral dependent edema, which can be symptomatically relieved by elevating the patient's affected limbs. Edema (a symptom of *Excess fluid volume*) is an important risk factor for *Impaired skin integrity*, which can be addressed by patient teaching and protective measures. If the patient requires medical intervention to resolve the fluid excess, use a collaborative problem such as Potential Complication of renal failure: Generalized edema. *Excess fluid volume* can also be the cause of complications, such as Potential Complication of *Excess fluid volume*: Pulmonary edema.

Incorrect: *Excess fluid volume* related to decreased cardiac output

Correct: Potential Complication of decreased cardiac output: *Excess fluid volume*

Correct: Potential Complication of heart failure: Pulmonary edema

Correct: *Risk for impaired skin integrity* related to *Excess fluid volume*, as manifested by generalized edema

Suggested Alternative Diagnoses

Cardiac output, decreased
Fluid volume, risk for imbalanced
Skin integrity, risk for impaired
Tissue perfusion: peripheral, ineffective

NOC Outcomes

Fluid Balance: Water balance in the intracellular and extracellular compartments of the body

Fluid Overload Severity: Severity of excess fluids in the intracellular and extracellular compartments of the body

Kidney Function: Filtration of blood and elimination of metabolic waste products through the formation of urine

Goals/Evaluation Criteria

Examples Using NOC Language

- *Excess fluid volume* will be eliminated, as evidenced by Fluid Balance, minimal Fluid Overload Severity, and indicators of adequate Kidney Function
- **Fluid Balance** will not be compromised (in excess) as evidenced by the following indicators (specify 1–5: severely, substantially, moderately, mildly, or not compromised):
  - 24-hr intake and output balance
  - Stable body weight
  - Urine specific gravity
- **Fluid Balance** will not be compromised (in excess) as evidenced by the following indicators (specify 1–5: severe, substantial, moderate, mild, or none):
  - Adventitious breath sounds
  - Ascites, neck vein distention, and peripheral edema

Other Examples

Patient will:

- Verbalize understanding of fluid and dietary restrictions
- Verbalize understanding of prescribed medications
- Maintain vital signs within normal limits for patient
- Not experience shortness of breath
- Have hematocrit within normal limits

NIC Interventions

Electrolyte Monitoring: Collection and analysis of patient data to regulate electrolyte balance

Fluid Management: Promotion of fluid balance and prevention of complications resulting from abnormal or undesired fluid levels

Fluid Monitoring: Collection and analysis of patient data to regulate fluid balance

Fluid/Electrolyte Management: Regulation and prevention of complications from altered fluid and/or electrolyte levels

Hypervolemia Management: Reduction in extracellular or intracellular fluid volume and prevention of complications in a patient who is fluid overloaded

Urinary Elimination Management: Maintenance of an optimum urinary elimination pattern

Nursing Activities

Assessments

- Specify location and degree of peripheral, sacral, and periorbital edema on scale from 1+ to 4+
- Assess for pulmonary or cardiovascular complications as indicated by increased respiratory distress, increased pulse rate, increased blood pressure, abnormal heart sounds, or abnormal lung sounds
- Assess edematous extremity or body part for impaired circulation and skin integrity
- Assess effects of medications (e.g., steroids, diuretics, lithium) on edema
- Regularly monitor abdominal or limb girth
- *(NIC) Fluid Management:*
  - Weigh daily and monitor trends
  - Maintain accurate intake and output record
  - Monitor laboratory results relevant to fluid retention (e.g., increased specific gravity, increased BUN, decreased hematocrit, and increased urine osmolality levels)
  - Monitor for indications of fluid overload or retention (e.g., crackles, elevated CVP or pulmonary capillary wedge pressure, edema, neck vein distention, and ascites), as appropriate

Patient/Family Teaching

- Instruct patient regarding causes and resolutions of edema; dietary restrictions; and use, dosage, and side effects of prescribed medications
- *(NIC) Fluid Management:* Instruct patient on NPO status, as appropriate

Collaborative Activities

- Administer dialysis, if indicated
- Consult with primary care provider about using antiembolism stockings or Ace bandages
- Consult nutritionist to provide a diet adequate in protein and limited in sodium
- *(NIC) Fluid Management:*
  - Consult physician if signs and symptoms of fluid volume excess persist or worsen
  - Administer prescribed diuretics, as appropriate

Other

- Change position q ________________
- Elevate extremities to increase venous return

- Maintain and allocate patient's fluid restrictions
- *(NIC) Fluid Management:* Distribute the fluid intake over 24 hr, as appropriate

Home Care

- Assist client and family to integrate diet and exercise restrictions into their lifestyle.
- Assess compliance with medical treatments and medication
- Assist family to recognize signs and symptoms of worsening levels of excess fluid volume, and to know when to call the primary care provider and 911
- Instruct the client to weigh daily using the same scale each time; notify physician if there is more than a 3-pound weight change in 24 hr
- Determine whether there are factors that might interfere with the client's ability or motivation to comply with fluid and diet restrictions

For Infants and Children

- Calculate the child's daily fluid maintenance needs on the basis of weight. Fluids lost must be replaced over and above this amount.
- To measure output for infants, count or weigh diapers. A 1-gram wet diaper equals 1 mL of urine.

For Older Adults

- Older adults are particularly susceptible to developing excess fluid volume; monitor carefully for risk factors

FLUID VOLUME, RISK FOR DEFICIENT

(1978, 2010) **Domain 2, Nutrition; Class 5, Hydration**

Definition: At risk for experiencing decreased intravascular, interstitial, and/or intracellular fluid. This refers to a risk for dehydration, water loss alone without change in sodium

Risk Factors

Objective

Deficient knowledge

Deviations affecting access to or intake or absorption of fluids [e.g., physical immobility]

Excessive losses through normal routes (e.g., diarrhea)
Extremes of age
Extremes of weight
Factors influencing fluid needs (e.g., hypermetabolic state)
Failure of regulatory mechanisms
Loss of fluid through abnormal routes (e.g., indwelling tubes)
Medications (e.g., diuretics)

Suggestions for Use

Do not use routinely for patients who are NPO. Refer to Suggestions for Use for Deficient Fluid Volume. *Risk for deficient fluid volume* applies to patients who are at risk for body water loss. *Risk for imbalanced fluid volume* applies to those who are at risk for body fluid loss, gain, or both.

Suggested Alternative Diagnoses

Deficient fluid volume
Fluid balance, readiness for enhanced
Fluid volume, risk for imbalanced

NOC Outcomes

NOTE: There is an extensive list of NOC outcomes associated with the risk factors for *Risk for deficient fluid volume*. We provide here, the outcomes used to assess and measure actual occurrence of the diagnosis, as well a few outcomes that address selected risk factors (e.g., inadequate fluid intake).

Burn Healing: Extent of healing of a burn site

Fluid Balance: Water balance in the intracellular and extracellular compartments of the body

Hydration: Adequate water in the intracellular and extracellular compartments of the body

Nutritional Status: Food and Fluid Intake: Amount of food and fluid taken into the body over a 24-hr period

Thermoregulation: Balance among heat production, heat gain, and heat loss

Goals/Evaluation Criteria

Also refer to Goals/Evaluation Criteria for Deficient Fluid Volume.

Example Using NOC Language

- *Deficient fluid volume* will be prevented, as evidenced by Fluid Balance, Hydration, and Nutritional Status: Food and Fluid Intake

NIC Interventions

NOTE: Because the risk factors for *Deficient fluid volume* are so numerous, we have included only a selected few interventions to treat risk factors.

Diarrhea Management: Management and alleviation of diarrhea

Electrolyte Management: Hypernatremia: Promotion of sodium balance and prevention of complications resulting from serum sodium levels higher than desired

Electrolyte Monitoring: Collection and analysis of patient data to regulate electrolyte balance

Fluid Management: Promotion of fluid balance and prevention of complications resulting from abnormal or undesired fluid levels

Fluid Monitoring: Collection and analysis of patient data to regulate fluid balance

Hypovolemia Management: Expansion of intravascular fluid volume in a patient who is volume depleted

Intravenous (IV) Therapy: Administration and monitoring of IV fluids and medications

Risk Identification: Analysis of potential risk factors, determination of health risks, and prioritization of risk-reduction strategies for an individual or group

Surveillance: Purposeful and ongoing acquisition, interpretation, and synthesis of patient data for clinical decision making

Vital Signs Monitoring: Collection and analysis of cardiovascular, respiratory, and body temperature data to determine and prevent complications

Vomiting Management: Prevention and alleviation of vomiting

Wound Care: Burns: Prevention of wound complications due to burns and facilitation of wound healing

Nursing Activities

NOTE: Nursing activities for *Risk for deficient fluid volume* focus on monitoring and prevention by alleviating risk factors. Interventions/activities are essentially the same as those for actual *Deficient fluid volume* and *Readiness for enhanced fluid balance*. Refer to Suggestions for Use for Deficient Fluid Volume before including those activities in your plan of care.

FLUID VOLUME, RISK FOR IMBALANCED

(1998, 2008) **Domain 2, Nutrition; Class 5, Hydration**

Definition: At risk for a decrease, increase, or rapid shift from one to the other of intravascular, interstitial, or intracellular fluid that may compromise health. This refers body fluid loss, gain, or both

Risk Factors

Abdominal surgery
Ascites
Burns
Intestinal obstruction
Pancreatitis
Receiving apheresis
Sepsis
Traumatic injury (e.g., fractured hip)

Suggestions for Use

This diagnosis was submitted by the Association of Operating Room Nurses and may have specific applications for that setting. *Risk for imbalanced fluid volume* should be used when a patient is at risk for *Excess fluid volume* or for both *Deficient fluid volume* and *Excess fluid volume.* When the patient is at risk only for fluid loss (and not for fluid gain), use *Risk for deficient fluid volume.*

Suggested Alternative Diagnoses

Fluid balance, readiness for enhanced
Fluid volume, risk for deficient
Fluid volume, risk for excess [non-NANDA-I]

NOC Outcomes

NOTE: The following outcomes are primarily for assessing and measuring occurrence of the diagnosis. A selected few focus on risk factors for imbalanced fluid volume.

Burn Healing: Extent of healing of a burn site

Fluid Balance: Water balance in the intracellular and extracellular compartments of the body

Fluid Overload Severity: Severity of excess fluids in the intracellular and extracellular compartments of the body

Hydration: Adequate water in the intracellular and extracellular compartments of the body

Postprocedure Recovery: Extent to which an individual returns to baseline function following a procedure(s) requiring anesthesia or sedation

Goals/Evaluation Criteria

Refer to Goals/Evaluation Criteria for Deficient Fluid Volume, Excess Fluid Volume, and Readiness for Enhanced Fluid Balance.

NIC Interventions

NOTE: Interventions, of course, depend on the specific risk factors. Included here are assessment/monitoring interventions, as well as a selected few for addressing specific risk factors.

Fluid Management: Promotion of fluid balance and prevention of complications resulting from abnormal or undesired fluid levels

Fluid Monitoring: Collection and analysis of patient data to regulate fluid balance

Fluid/Electrolyte Management: Regulation and prevention of complications from altered fluid and/or electrolyte levels

Risk Identification: Analysis of potential risk factors, determination of health risks, and prioritization of risk-reduction strategies for an individual or group

Surveillance: Purposeful and ongoing acquisition, interpretation, and synthesis of patient data for clinical decision making

Wound Care: Burns: Prevention of wound complications due to burns and facilitation of wound healing

Nursing Activities

Refer to Nursing Activities for Deficient Fluid Volume, Excess Fluid Volume, and Readiness for Enhanced Fluid Balance.

GAS EXCHANGE, IMPAIRED

(1980, 1996, 1998) Domain 3, Elimination and Exchange; Class 4, Respiratory Function

Definition: Excess or deficit in oxygenation and/or carbon dioxide elimination at the alveolar–capillary membrane

Defining Characteristics

Subjective

Dyspnea
Headache on awakening
Visual disturbance

Objective

Abnormal arterial blood gases
Abnormal arterial pH
Abnormal rate, rhythm, depth of breathing
Abnormal skin color (e.g., pale, dusky)
Confusion

Cyanosis (in neonates only)
Decreased carbon dioxide
Diaphoresis
Hypercapnia
Hypercarbia
Hypoxemia
Hypoxia
Irritability
Nasal flaring
Restlessness
Somnolence
Tachycardia

Related Factors

Alveolar–capillary membrane changes
Ventilation–perfusion imbalance

Suggestions for Use

Use this label cautiously. Decreased passage of gases between the alveoli of the lungs and the vascular system can be diagnosed only by means of a medically prescribed diagnostic test—blood gas analysis. A patient might easily have most of the defining characteristics without actually having impaired alveolar gas exchange. It is better to use a diagnostic statement that describes oxygen-related problems that can be diagnosed and treated independently by nurses (e.g., *Activity intolerance*). If the Suggested Alternative Diagnoses, following, are treated, the *Impaired gas exchange* should improve. If the patient is at risk for *Impaired gas exchange*, write the appropriate collaborative problem (e.g., Potential Complication of thrombophlebitis: Pulmonary embolus). See Suggestions for Use for the diagnoses, Ineffective Airway Clearance; Ineffective Breathing Pattern; and Dysfunctional Ventilatory Weaning Response.

Impaired gas exchange may be associated with a number of medical diagnoses. For example, decreased functional lung tissue may be secondary to chronic lung disease, pneumonia, thoracotomy, atelectasis, respiratory distress syndrome, mass, and diaphragmatic hernia. In addition, decreased pulmonary blood supply may occur secondary to pulmonary hypertension, pulmonary embolus, congestive heart failure, respiratory distress syndrome, and anemia.

Suggested Alternative Diagnoses

Activity intolerance
Airway clearance, ineffective

Breathing pattern, ineffective
Dysfunctional ventilatory weaning response (DVWR)
Spontaneous ventilation, impaired

NOC Outcomes

Mechanical Ventilation Response: Adult: Alveolar exchange and tissue perfusion are supported by mechanical ventilation

Respiratory Status: Gas Exchange: Alveolar exchange of CO_2 and O_2 to maintain arterial blood gas concentrations

Tissue Perfusion: Pulmonary: Adequacy of blood flow through pulmonary vasculature to perfuse alveoli–capillary unit

Vital Signs: Extent to which temperature, pulse, respiration, and blood pressure are within normal range

Goals/Evaluation Criteria

Examples Using NOC Language

- *Impaired gas exchange* will be alleviated, as evidenced by uncompromised Allergic Response: Systemic, Electrolyte and Acid–Base Balance, Mechanical Ventilation Response: Adult, Respiratory Status: Gas Exchange, Respiratory Status: Ventilation, Pulmonary Tissue Perfusion, and Vital Signs
- **Respiratory Status: Gas Exchange** will not be compromised as evidenced by the following indicators (specify 1–5: severe, substantial, moderate, mild, or none):
  - Cognitive status
  - PaO_2, $PaCO_2$, arterial pH, and O_2 saturation
  - End-tidal CO_2
- **Respiratory Status: Gas Exchange** will not be compromised as evidenced by the following indicators (specify 1–5: severe, substantial, moderate, mild, or none):
  - Dyspnea at rest
  - Dyspnea with exertion
  - Restlessness, cyanosis, and somnolence
- **Respiratory Status: Ventilation** will not be compromised as evidenced by the following indicators (specify 1–5: severely, substantially, moderately, mildly, or not compromised):
  - Respiratory rate
  - Respiratory rhythm
  - Depth of inspiration
  - Expulsion of air
  - Dyspnea at rest
  - Auscultated breath sounds

Other Examples

Patient will:

- Have pulmonary function within normal limits
- Have symmetrical chest expansion
- Describe plan for care at home
- Not use pursed-lip breathing
- Not experience shortness of breath or orthopnea
- Not use accessory muscles to breathe

NIC Interventions

Acid–Base Management: Promotion of acid–base balance and prevention of complications resulting from acid–base imbalance

Acid–Base Management: Respiratory Acidosis: Promotion of acid–base balance and prevention of complications resulting from serum pCO_2 levels higher than desired

Acid–Base Management: Respiratory Alkalosis: Promotion of acid–base balance and prevention of complications resulting from serum pCO_2 levels lower than desired

Airway Management: Facilitation of patency of air passages

Anaphylaxis Management: Promotion of adequate ventilation and tissue perfusion for an individual with a severe allergic (antigen–antibody) reaction

Asthma Management: Identification, treatment, and prevention of reactions to inflammation/constriction in the airway passages

Electrolyte Management: Promotion of electrolyte balance and prevention of complications resulting from abnormal or undesired serum electrolyte levels

Embolus Care: Pulmonary: Limitation of complications for a patient experiencing, or at risk for, occlusion of pulmonary circulation

Hemodynamic Regulation: Optimization of heart rate, preload, afterload, and contractility

Laboratory Data Interpretation: Critical analysis of patient laboratory data in order to assist with clinical decision making

Mechanical Ventilation: Use of an artificial device to assist a patient to breathe

Oxygen Therapy: Administration of oxygen and monitoring of its effectiveness

Respiratory Monitoring: Collection and analysis of patient data to ensure airway patency and adequate gas exchange

Ventilation Assistance: Promotion of an optimal spontaneous breathing pattern that maximizes oxygen and carbon dioxide exchange in the lungs

Vital Signs Monitoring: Collection and analysis of cardiovascular, respiratory, and body temperature data to determine and prevent complications

Nursing Activities

Nursing activities for this diagnosis focus on gas exchange at the alveolar–capillary membrane. However, efforts to facilitation ventilation may improve oxygen delivery. Other interventions focus on the related factors (e.g., relieving *Anxiety* and managing *Pain*).

Assessments

- Assess lung sounds; respiratory rate, depth, and effort; and production of sputum as indicators of effective use of supportive equipment
- Monitor O_2 saturation with pulse oximeter
- Monitor blood gas results (e.g., low PaO_2 and elevated $PaCO_2$ levels suggest respiratory deterioration)
- Monitor electrolyte levels
- Monitor mental status (e.g., level of consciousness, restlessness, and confusion)
- Increase frequency of monitoring when patient appears somnolent
- Observe for cyanosis, especially of oral mucous membranes
- *(NIC) Airway Management:*
  Identify patient requiring actual or potential airway insertion
  Auscultate breath sounds, noting areas of decreased or absent ventilation and presence of adventitious sounds
  Monitor respiratory and oxygenation status, as appropriate
- *(NIC) Hemodynamic Regulation:*
  Auscultate heart sounds
  Monitor and document heart rate, rhythm, and pulses
  Monitor for peripheral edema, jugular vein distension, and S_3 and S_4 heart sounds
  Monitor pacemaker functioning, if appropriate

Patient/Family Teaching

- Explain proper use of supportive equipment (oxygen, suction, spirometer, IPPB)
- Instruct patient in breathing and relaxation techniques
- Explain to patient and family the reasons for low-flow oxygen and other treatments
- Inform patient and family that smoking is prohibited
- *(NIC) Airway Management:*
  Instruct how to cough effectively
  Teach patient how to use prescribed inhalers, as appropriate

Collaborative Activities

- Consult with physician regarding future need for arterial blood gas (ABG) test and use of supportive equipment as indicated by a change in the patient's condition
- Report changes in correlated assessment data (e.g., patient sensorium, breath sounds, respiratory pattern, ABGs, sputum, effect of medications)
- Administer prescribed medications (e.g., sodium bicarbonate) to maintain acid–base balance
- Prepare patient for mechanical ventilation, if necessary
- *(NIC) Airway Management:*
  - Administer humidified air or oxygen, as appropriate
  - Administer bronchodilators, as appropriate
  - Administer aerosol treatments, as appropriate
  - Administer ultrasonic nebulizer treatments, as appropriate
- *(NIC) Hemodynamic Regulation:* Administer antiarrhythmic medications, as appropriate

Other

- Inform patient before beginning intended procedures, to lower anxiety and increase sense of control
- Reassure patient during periods of respiratory distress or anxiety
- Provide frequent oral hygiene
- Institute measures to reduce oxygen consumption (e.g., control fever and pain, reduce anxiety)
- If oxygen is prescribed for patients with chronic respiratory conditions, monitor oxygen flow and respirations carefully because of the risk of oxygen-induced respiratory depression
- Institute plan of care for a patient on a ventilator, which may include:
  - Ensuring adequate oxygen delivery by reporting abnormal ABGs, having Ambu bag attached to oxygen source at bedside, and hyperoxygenating prior to suctioning
  - Ensuring effective breathing pattern by assessing for synchronization and possible need for sedation
  - Maintaining patent airway by suctioning patient and keeping an endotracheal tube or replacement at bedside
  - Monitoring for complications (e.g., pneumothorax, unilateral aeration)
  - Verifying correct placement of endotracheal tube
- *(NIC) Airway Management:*
  - Position patient to maximize ventilation potential
  - Position to alleviate dyspnea

Insert oral or nasopharyngeal airway, as appropriate
Remove secretions by encouraging coughing or by suctioning
Encourage slow, deep breathing; turning; and coughing
Assist with incentive spirometer, as appropriate
Perform chest physical therapy, as appropriate

- *(NIC) Hemodynamic Regulation:*
  Elevate the head of the bed, as appropriate
  Place in Trendelenburg position, if appropriate

Home Care

- Assess for sources of allergens and secondhand smoke
- Assist the client to recognize and avoid situations that cause breathing problems (e.g., use of household cleaners and solvents, stress)
- Impress on the family that no one should smoke in the home
- Refer to smoking cessation programs if needed
- Encourage family to install an air filter in the home
- Instruct patient and family in plan for care at home, for example, medications, activity, supportive equipment, reportable signs and symptoms, and community resources
- Keep home temperature above 68°F (20°C)
- Refer to home health aide and homemaker services to conserve energy
- Evaluate electrical safety (e.g., grounding) of respiratory equipment.
- If a home respirator is in use, notify the police and fire departments and the utility company

For Older Adults

- Monitor respirations carefully when using central nervous system depressants. Drug metabolism changes with aging, and older adults are susceptible to respiratory depression.
- If oxygen is prescribed, use low flow to prevent oxygen-induced respiratory depression

GASTROINTESTINAL MOTILITY, DYSFUNCTIONAL

(2008) **Domain 3, Elimination and Exchange; Class 2, Gastrointestinal Function**

Definition: Increased, decreased, ineffective, or lack of peristaltic activity within the gastrointestinal (GI) system

Defining Characteristics

Subjective

Abdominal cramping and/or pain
Difficulty passing stool
Nausea
Regurgitation

Objective

Absence of flatus

Abdominal distention
Accelerated gastric emptying
Bile-colored gastric residual
Change in bowel sounds (e.g., absent, hypoactive, hyperactive)
Diarrhea
Dry stool
Hard stool
Increased gastric residual
Vomiting

Related Factors

Aging
Anxiety
Enteral feedings
Food intolerance (e.g., gluten, lactose)
Immobility
Ingestion of contaminates (e.g., food, water)
Malnutrition
Pharmaceutical agents (e.g., narcotics/opiates, laxatives, antibiotics, anesthesia)
Prematurity
Sedentary lifestyle
Surgery

Suggestions for Use

This broad diagnosis can be used to describe either increased or decreased motility. However, increased motility is better described by the diagnosis, *Diarrhea;* and decreased motility is often the etiology of *Constipation.* It seems better to use those diagnoses when their defining characteristics are present. *Dysfunctional gastrointestinal motility* may also represent some collaborative problems (e.g., Risk for GI complications: Paralytic ileus). If the only independent nursing activities for the patient are to monitor for GI complications and notify the primary care provider, use a collaborative problem.

Suggested Alternative Diagnoses

Bowel incontinence
Constipation
Constipation, risk for
Diarrhea

NOC Outcomes

Bowel Elimination: Formation and evacuation of stool
Gastrointestinal Function: Extent to which foods (ingested or tube-fed) are moved from ingestion to excretion

Goals/Evaluation Criteria

Examples Using NOC Language

- Gastrointestinal motility within normal limits, as demonstrated by Bowel Elimination and Gastrointestinal Function in expected range for the patient.
- Will demonstrate **Bowel Elimination,** as evidenced by the following indicators (specify 1–5: severely, substantially, moderately, mildly, or not compromised):
  Elimination pattern
  Stool soft and formed
  Ease of stool passage
  Bowel sounds
- Will demonstrate **Bowel Elimination**, as evidenced by the following indicators (specify 1–5: severe, substantial, moderate, mild, or none):
  Constipation
  Diarrhea

Other Examples

- Amount of stool appropriate for amount of food ingested
- Amount of gastric residual in expected limits
- No abdominal distention
- No regurgitation
- No visible peristalsis

NIC Interventions

Bowel Management: Establishment and maintenance of a regular pattern of bowel elimination

Constipation/Impaction Management: Prevention and alleviation of constipation/impaction

Diarrhea Management: Management and alleviation of diarrhea

Gastrointestinal Intubation: Insertion of a tube into the GI tract

Tube Care: Gastrointestinal: Management of a patient with a GI tube

Vomiting Management: Prevention and alleviation of vomiting

Nursing Activities

G

NOTE: If you must use this diagnosis, also refer to *Constipation* and *Diarrhea*, because many of the nursing activities for this diagnosis are the same. For that reason, the activities are not highly developed here.

Assessments

- Monitor bowel sounds regularly
- Observe and percuss for abdominal distention; measure abdominal girth daily.
- Monitor frequency and consistency of bowel movements.
- Monitor fluid intake and output.
- (For patient with a GI tube) Monitor placement of the tube according to agency policy

Patient/Family Teaching

- Teach the importance of adequate fluid and fiber intake for preventing constipation
- Teach clients to see their primary care provider for severe stomach pain, blood in the stool, unintended weight loss, or constipation not relieved after following medical regimen
- Teach patients to wash their hands often to help prevent spreading pathogens that may be the cause of diarrhea.
- Provide information about foods that can cause diarrhea (e.g., highly spiced foods, high-fat foods).

Collaborative Activities

- Administer medications to increase or decrease GI motility, depending on which one is present.
- Administer antibiotics, if needed for infectious diarrhea

Other

- Provide early ambulation after surgery
- Encourage regular exercise, as tolerated

GASTROINTESTINAL MOTILITY: DYSFUNCTIONAL, RISK FOR

(2008) **Domain 3, Elimination and Exchange; Class 2, Gastrointestinal Function**

Definition: At risk for increased, decreased, ineffective, or lack of peristaltic activity within the gastrointestinal (GI) system

Risk Factors

Abdominal surgery
Aging
Anxiety
Change in food or water
Decreased GI circulation
Diabetes mellitus
Food intolerance (e.g., gluten, lactose)
Gastroesophageal reflux disease (GERD)
Immobility
Infection (e.g., bacterial, parasitic, viral)
Pharmaceutical agents (e.g., antibiotics, laxatives, narcotics/opiates, proton pump inhibitors)
Prematurity
Sedentary lifestyle
Stress
Unsanitary food preparation.

Suggestions for Use

For this and other related headings and content, refer to the diagnosis, Gastrointestinal Motility: Dysfunctional

GRIEVING

(1980, 1996, 2006) **Domain 9, Coping/Stress Tolerance; Class 2, Coping Responses**

Definition: A normal complex process that includes emotional, physical, spiritual, social, and intellectual responses and behaviors by which individuals, families, and communities incorporate an actual, anticipated, or perceived loss into their daily lives

Defining Characteristics

Subjective

Anger
Blame
Despair
Detachment
Experiencing relief
Pain

Personal growth
Psychological distress
Suffering

Objective

Alterations in activity level
Alterations in dream patterns
Alterations in immune function
Alterations in neuroendocrine function
Alterations in sleep patterns
Disorganization
Maintaining the connection to the deceased
Making meaning of the loss
Panic behavior

Other Defining Characteristics (Non-NANDA International)

Alteration in eating habits
Altered communication patterns
Altered libido
Bargaining
Difficulty taking on new or different roles
Denial of potential loss
Denial of the significance of the loss
Expression of distress at potential loss
Guilt

Related Factors

Anticipatory loss of significant object (e.g., possession, job, status, home, parts and processes of body)
Anticipatory loss of a significant other
Death of a significant other
Loss of significant object (e.g., possession, job, status, home, parts and processes of body)

Suggestions for Use

Grieving may be a normal, not necessarily maladaptive, response. If it requires no intervention, do not include it in the patient care plan. Anticipatory grieving occurs before the loss; it is not a NANDA-I diagnosis. However, it shares some defining characteristics with *Complicated grieving*. The following manifestations of functional impairment and failure of the grief process to follow normative expectations would rule out a diagnosis of *Grieving:*

Exaggerated and prolonged feelings of guilt
Interference with life functioning
Prolonged anger or hostility
Suicidal thoughts

Suggested Alternative Diagnoses

Coping, ineffective
Grieving, complicated
Grieving, complicated, risk for
Sorrow, chronic

NOC Outcomes

Adaptation to Physical Disability: Adaptive response to a significant functional challenge due to a physical disability

Coping: Personal actions to manage stressors that tax an individual's resources

Family Coping: Family actions to manage stressors that tax family resources

Grief Resolution: Adjustment to actual or impending loss

Psychosocial Adjustment: Life Change: Adaptive psychosocial response of an individual to a significant life change

Goals/Evaluation Criteria

Examples Using NOC Language

- Patient successfully resolves *Grieving*, as demonstrated by successful Adaptation to Physical Disability, Coping, Family Coping, Grief Resolution, and Psychosocial Adjustment: Life Change
- Patient demonstrates **Coping**, as evidenced by the following indicators (specify 1–5: never, rarely, sometimes, often, or consistently demonstrated):

    Identifies effective coping patterns
    Uses effective coping strategies
    Seeks reputable information diagnosis and treatment

Uses personal support system
Reports decrease in physical symptoms of stress and in negative feelings

- Patient demonstrates **Grief Resolution**, as evidenced by the following indicators (specify 1–5: never, rarely, sometimes, often, or consistently demonstrated):

    Resolves feelings about loss
    Verbalizes reality of loss
    Participates in planning funeral
    Shares loss with significant others
    Progresses through stages of grief
    Maintains personal grooming and hygiene
    Reports decreased preoccupation with loss
    Reports adequate nutritional intake
    Reports normal sexual desire

G

Other Examples

Patient and family will:

- Demonstrate ability to make mutual decisions regarding anticipated loss
- Express thoughts, feelings, and spiritual beliefs about loss
- Verbalize fears and concerns about potential loss
- Participate in grief work
- Not experience somatic distress
- Express feelings of productivity, usefulness, empowerment, and optimism
- Seeks help from a health care professional as appropriate

NIC Interventions

Anticipatory Guidance: Preparation of patient for an anticipated developmental or situational crisis

Coping Enhancement: Assisting a patient to adapt to perceived stressors, changes, or threats that interfere with meeting life demands and roles

Emotional Support: Provision of reassurance, acceptance, and encouragement during times of stress

Family Integrity Promotion: Promotion of family cohesion and unity

Grief Work Facilitation: Assistance with the resolution of a significant loss

Grief Work Facilitation: Perinatal Death: Assistance with the resolution of a perinatal loss

Nursing Activities

Assessments

- Assess past experience of patient and family with loss, existing support systems, and current grief work

- Determine cause and length of time since diagnosis of fetal or infant death
- *(NIC) Grief Work Facilitation:* Identify the loss

Patient/Family Teaching

- Teach characteristics of normal and abnormal grieving
- Discuss differences in individual patterns of grieving (e.g., male vs. female)
- *(NIC) Grief Work Facilitation:* Instruct in phases of the grieving process, as appropriate
- *(NIC) Anticipatory Guidance:*
  - Provide information on realistic expectations related to the patient's behavior
  - Suggest books and literature for the patient to read, as appropriate

Collaborative Activities

- Refer to appropriate resources, such as support groups, legal assistance, financial assistance, social services, chaplain, grief counselor, genetic counselor
- *(NIC) Grief Work Facilitation:* Identify sources of community support

Other

- Assist patient and family to verbalize fears and concerns of potential loss, including impact on the family unit
- Help patient and family to share mutual fears, plans, concerns, and hopes with each other
- *(NIC) Grief Work Facilitation:*
  - Assist the patient to identify the nature of the attachment to the lost object or person
  - Encourage expression of feelings about the loss
  - Encourage identification of greatest fears concerning the loss
  - Include significant others in discussions and decisions, as appropriate
  - Use clear words, such as *dead* or *died*, rather than euphemisms
  - Encourage patient to implement cultural, religious, and social customs associated with the loss
- *(NIC) Anticipatory Guidance:*
  - Provide the patient with a phone number to call for assistance, if necessary
  - Schedule follow-up phone calls to evaluate success or reinforcement needs
  - Rehearse techniques needed to cope with upcoming developmental milestone or situational crisis with the patient, as appropriate

Home Care

- Encourage family caregivers to express concerns and feelings about the client
- Arrange for respite care for family caregivers
- Encourage family to involve client in as many family routines and activities as possible

For Infants and Children

- Provide opportunities for the child to talk about concerns and feelings
- Base your communication on the child's developmental stage
- Help child to clarify misconceptions about death, dying, or loss
- Explain clearly that the child did not cause the impending death
- Help parents understand that the child needs to grieve and that they should not try to distract them from it or "make it go away"
- Explore the use of music therapy
- Help the family to decide whether a child should attend the funeral, making sure a trusted adult is available to care for the child during the funeral
- For perinatal loss, encourage parents to hold infant while and after the baby dies, as appropriate
- *(NIC) Grief Work Facilitation:* Encourage expression of feelings in ways comfortable to the child, such as writing, drawing, or playing

For Older Adults

- Consider referral to a bereavement counselor to help dying clients and their families
- Assist with advance directives to ensure that the patient's preferences for care are known

GRIEVING, COMPLICATED

(1980, 1986, 2004, 2006)

Domain 9, Coping/Stress Tolerance; Class 2, Coping Responses

Definition: A disorder that occurs after the death of a significant other, in which the experience of distress accompanying bereavement fails to follow normative expectations and manifests in functional impairment

Defining Characteristics

Subjective

Decreased sense of well-being
Depression
Fatigue
Longing for the deceased
Persistent emotional distress
Preoccupation with thoughts of the deceased
Rumination
Verbalizes anxiety
Verbalizes distressful feelings about the deceased
Verbalizes feeling dazed
Verbalizes feeling empty
Verbalizes feeling in shock
Verbalizes feeling stunned
Verbalizes feelings of anger
Verbalizes feelings of detachment from others
Verbalizes feelings of disbelief
Verbalizes feelings of mistrust
Verbalizes lack of acceptance of the death
Verbalizes persistent painful memories
Verbalizes self-blame
Yearning

Objective

Decreased functioning in life roles
Experiencing somatic symptoms of the deceased
Grief avoidance
Low levels of intimacy
Searching for the deceased
Self-blame
Separation distress
Traumatic distress

Related Factors

Death of a significant other
Emotional instability
Lack of social support

Suggestions for Use

Most of the defining characteristics may also be present in the normal grief process. Grieving is dysfunctional only if it is prolonged (perhaps for more than a year after the loss, although no absolute time period can be specified) or if the symptoms are unusually numerous or severe. *Chronic sorrow* describes the patient's feelings, whereas grieving describes behaviors used in trying to cope with the loss. See Suggestions for Use for Grieving.

Suggested Alternative Diagnoses

Coping, ineffective
Grieving
Health behavior, risk-prone
Sorrow, chronic
Spiritual Distress

NOC Outcomes

Coping: Personal actions to manage stressors that tax an individual's resources

Grief Resolution: Adjustment to actual or impending loss

Role Performance: Congruence of an individual's role behavior with role expectations

Goals/Evaluation Criteria

Examples Using NOC Language

- Patient/family will satisfactorily resolve *Complicated grieving*, as demonstrated by successful Coping, Grief Resolution, and Role Performance
- See Goals/Evaluation Criteria for Grieving for indicators for **Coping** and **Grief Resolution**, and for Other Examples
- Demonstrates **Role Performance**, as evidenced by the following indicators (specify 1–5: not, slightly, moderately, substantially, or totally adequate):

  Performance of role expectations
  Performance of family role behaviors
  Performance of community role behaviors
  Reported comfort with role expectations

Other Examples

Patient/family will:

- Report adequate intake of food and fluids
- Report adequate social support
- Verbalize grief
- Verbalize meaning of loss
- Demonstrate ability to make mutual decisions regarding anticipated loss

- Express thoughts, feelings, and spiritual beliefs about loss
- Verbalize fears and concerns about potential loss
- Participate in grief work
- Not experience somatic distress
- Express feelings of productivity, usefulness, empowerment, and optimism

NIC Interventions

Coping Enhancement: Assisting a patient to adapt to perceived stressors, changes, or threats that interfere with meeting life demands and roles

Emotional Support: Provision of reassurance, acceptance, and encouragement during times of stress

Family Integrity Promotion: Promotion of family cohesion and unity

Grief Work Facilitation: Assistance with the resolution of a significant loss

Grief Work Facilitation: Perinatal Death: Assistance with the resolution of a perinatal loss

Resiliency Promotion: Assisting individuals, families, and communities in development, use, and strengthening of protective factors to be used in coping with environmental and societal stressors

Role Enhancement: Assisting a patient, significant other, and/or family to improve relationships by clarifying and supplementing specific role behaviors

Self-Awareness Enhancement: Assisting a patient to explore and understand his thoughts, feelings, motivations, and behaviors

Nursing Activities

Also see Nursing Activities for Grieving.

Assessments

- Assess and document the presence and source of patient's grief
- *(NIC) Family Integrity Promotion:*

  Determine typical family relationships for each family

  Monitor current family relationships

  Identify typical family coping mechanisms

  Identify conflicting priorities among family members

Patient/Family Teaching

- Provide patient and family with information about hospital and community resources, such as self-help groups

Collaborative Activities

- Initiate a patient care conference to review patient and family needs related to their stage of the grieving process and to establish a plan of care

- Seek support among peers and others to provide patient care as needed
- *(NIC) Grief Work Facilitation: Perinatal Death:* Notify laboratory or funeral home, as appropriate, for disposition of body

Other

- Acknowledge patient's and family's grief reactions while continuing necessary care activities
- Discuss with patient and family the impact of the loss on the family unit and its functioning
- Avoid confrontation of denial and, at the same time, do not reinforce denial
- Balance any misperceptions with reality
- Encourage independence in performance of self-care, assisting patient only as necessary
- Establish a schedule for contact with patient
- Establish a trusting relationship with patient and family
- Help patient and family to participate actively in decision-making process
- Provide a safe, secure, and private environment to facilitate patient and family grieving process
- Recognize and reinforce the strength of each family member

For Infants and Children

- Refer to interventions for Grieving
- *(NIC) Grief Work Facilitation: Perinatal Death:*
  Assist in keeping infant alive until parents arrive
  Baptize the infant, as appropriate
  Discuss plans that have been made (e.g., burial, funeral, and infant name)
  Describe mementos that will be obtained, including footprints, handprints, pictures, caps, gowns, blankets, diapers, and blood pressure cuffs, as appropriate
  Prepare infant for viewing by bathing and dressing, including parents in activities as appropriate
  Encourage family members to view and hold infant for as long as desired
  Focus on normal features of infant while sensitively discussing anomalies
  Transfer infant to morgue or prepare body to be transported by family to funeral home

For Older Adults

- Use reminiscence therapy or refer to a reminiscence group
- Assess the client's support system, remind family of the client's need for support

GRIEVING, COMPLICATED, RISK FOR

(2004, 2006) **Domain 9, Coping/Stress Tolerance; Class 2, Coping Responses**

Definition: At risk for a disorder that occurs after the death of a significant other, in which the experience of distress accompanying bereavement fails to follow normative expectations and manifests in functional impairment

Risk Factors

Death of a significant other
Emotional instability
Lack of social support

Suggested Alternative Diagnoses

Coping, ineffective
Health behavior, risk-prone
Loneliness, risk for
Religiosity, risk for impaired
Social isolation
Spiritual distress, risk for

NOC Outcomes

Comfort Status: Psychospiritual: Psychospiritual ease related to self-concept, emotional well-being, source of inspiration, and meaning and purpose in life

Comfort Status: Sociocultural: Social ease related to interpersonal, family, and societal relationships within a cultural context

Coping: Personal actions to manage stressors that tax an individual's resources

Grief Resolution: Adjustment to actual or impending loss

Goals/Evaluation Criteria

Examples Using NOC Language

- Patient/family will not experience *Complicated grieving*, as demonstrated by successful Coping, and Grief Resolution
- See Goals/Evaluation Criteria for Grieving for indicators for **Coping** and **Grief Resolution**, and for Other Examples

NIC Interventions

G

Active Listening: Attending closely to and attaching significance to a patient's verbal and nonverbal messages

Coping Enhancement: Assisting a patient to adapt to perceived stressors, changes, or threats that interfere with meeting life demands and roles

Family Integrity Promotion: Promotion of family cohesion and unity

Grief Work Facilitation: Assistance with the resolution of a significant loss

Grief Work Facilitation: Perinatal Death: Assistance with the resolution of a perinatal loss

Presence: Being with another, both physically and psychologically, during times of need

Surveillance: Purposeful and ongoing acquisition, interpretation, and synthesis of patient data for clinical decision making

Nursing Activities

See Nursing Activities for Grieving and for Complicated Grieving.

GROWTH, DISPROPORTIONATE, RISK FOR

(1998) **Domain 13, Growth/Development; Class 1, Growth**

Definition: At risk for growth above the 97th percentile or below the 3rd percentile for age, crossing two percentile channels

Risk Factors

Caregiver

Abuse
Mental illness
Learning difficulties (mental handicap)
Mental retardation
Severe learning disability

Environmental

Deprivation
Economically disadvantaged
Lead poisoning
Natural disasters
Teratogens
Violence

Individual

Anorexia
Caregiver or individual maladaptive feeding behaviors
Chronic illness
Infection
Insatiable appetite
Malnutrition
[Organic and inorganic factors]
Prematurity
Substance abuse

Prenatal

Congenital or genetic disorders
Maternal infection
Maternal nutrition
Multiple gestation
Substance use or abuse
Teratogen exposure

Suggestions for Use

There are many conditions, including other nursing diagnoses, that create *Risk for disproportionate growth*, for example, *Ineffective breastfeeding*. The diagnosis of *Risk for disproportionate growth* related to *Ineffective breastfeeding* suggests goals focused on weight gain or loss but gives little guidance for nursing activities to correct the breastfeeding problem; whereas a diagnosis of *Ineffective breastfeeding* related to maternal anxiety or ambivalence provides direction for nursing activities to correct the breastfeeding problem and, indirectly, to correct the *Risk for disproportionate growth*. When possible, use the more specific diagnoses rather than the more general diagnosis *Risk for disproportionate growth*.

Because growth is routinely assessed in nursing care of children, a diagnostic statement is usually not required for that application—such assessment is usually included in pediatric standards of care. Likewise, this label is not appropriate for a child with failure to thrive. That condition may be described better by one of the family functioning diagnoses or by a diagnosis of *Imbalanced nutrition: less than body requirements*.

Suggested Alternative Diagnoses

Breastfeeding, ineffective
Disabled family coping
Growth and development, delayed
Ineffective coping

Infant feeding pattern, ineffective
Nutrition, imbalanced: less than body requirements
Parenting, impaired
Self-care deficit: feeding

NOC Outcomes

Growth: Normal increase in bone size and body weight during growth years

Physical Maturation: Female: Normal physical changes in the female that occur with the transition from childhood to adulthood

Physical Maturation: Male: Normal physical changes in the male that occur with the transition from childhood to adulthood

Weight: Body Mass: Extent to which body weight, muscle, and fat are congruent to height, frame, gender, and age

Goals/Evaluation Criteria

Examples Using NOC Language

- Does not experience *Disproportionate growth*, as demonstrated by Growth, Physical Maturation (Female, Male), and Weight: Body Mass
- Exhibits satisfactory **Growth**, as evidenced by the following indicators (specify 1-5: severe, substantial, moderate, mild, or no deviation from normal range):

  Weight percentile for sex (also for age and height)
  Rate of weight gain
  Rate of height gain
  Bone mass index
  Mean body mass

Other Examples

- The child will achieve expected growth norms (e.g., weight, head circumference, bone age, mean body mass), that is, not above the 97th percentile or below the 3rd percentile for age

NIC Interventions

Health Screening: Detecting health risks or problems by means of history, examination, and other procedures

Nutrition Management: Assisting with or providing a balanced dietary intake of foods and fluids

Nutritional Monitoring: Collection and analysis of patient data to prevent or minimize malnourishment

Teaching: Infant Nutrition: Instruction on nutrition and feeding practices during the first year of life

Teaching: Toddler Nutrition: Instruction on nutrition and feeding practices during the 2nd and 3rd years of life

Weight Management: Facilitating maintenance of optimal body weight and percent of body fat

Nursing Activities

NOTE: Because this nursing diagnosis is so broad, not every possible nursing activity can be listed here. Refer to age-specific sections in growth and development texts for full lists of activities.

Many of the interventions for preventing disproportionate growth are used in the prenatal period. Consult a maternity textbook for further information about preventing premature births and small-for-gestational-age infants.

Assessments

- Assess the caretakers' knowledge, resources, support system, coping skills, and level of commitment to develop a plan of care for eliminating risk factors
- Conduct a thorough health assessment (e.g., child's history, temperament, culture, family environment, developmental screening) to determine risk factors
- Monitor parent and child interactions and communication
- Assess adequacy of nutritional intake (e.g., calories, nutrients)
- Monitor trends in weight loss or gain
- Take skinfold measurements
- Determine food preferences

Patient/Family Teaching

- Teach caregivers about normal growth patterns
- Teach patient and family about nutritional needs
- Advise pregnant women to consult their primary care provider before taking any medications

Collaborative Activities

- Act as case manager to ensure comprehensive care by coordinating medical, school, rehabilitation, and social services efforts
- Refer to nutritionist for diet teaching and planning

Other

- Assist caregivers/parents to develop a plan of care (for possible care plans and interventions, refer to Nursing Activities for the Suggested Alternative Diagnoses)
- Establish a therapeutic and trusting relationship with caregivers/parents

GROWTH AND DEVELOPMENT, DELAYED*

(1986) **Domain 13, Growth/Development; Class 1, Growth; Class 2, Development**

Definition: Deviations from age-group norms

*This diagnosis will retire from the NANDA-I Taxonomy in 2015 unless additional work is completed to divide the diagnostic foci for growth and development into separate concepts.

Defining Characteristics

Objective

Altered physical growth
Decreased response time
Delay or difficulty in performing skills (e.g., motor, social, or expressive) typical of age group
Flat affect
Inability to perform self-care or self-control activities appropriate for age
Listlessness

Related Factors

Effects of physical disability
Environmental and stimulation deficiencies
Inadequate caretaking
Inconsistent responsiveness
Indifference
Multiple caretakers
Prescribed dependence
Separation from significant others
Stimulation deficiencies

Other Related Factors (Non-NANDA International)

Abuse
Changes in family system
Congenital anomaly
Fetal distress during or after birth or delivery
Inadequate bonding
Inadequate prenatal care
Loss
Maternal acute or chronic disease
Neonatal disease
Poverty
Prematurity
Serious illness/injury
Traumatic separation
Unhealthy maternal lifestyle during pregnancy

Suggestions for Use

Use of this label is not recommended. It is too broad to suggest nursing actions. There are many nursing diagnoses that could be considered *Delayed growth and development* or that could be caused by *Delayed growth and development* (e.g., *Self-care deficit*, *Urinary incontinence*, *Impaired verbal communication*, and *Impaired parenting*). When possible, use the more specific labels. If the problem is potential rather than actual, use *Risk for disproportionate growth* or *Risk for delayed development.*

Because growth and development are routinely assessed in nursing care of children, a diagnostic statement is usually not required for that application—such an assessment is usually included in pediatric standards of care. This label is not appropriate for a mentally impaired child (e.g., *Delayed growth and development* related to Down syndrome). Instead, diagnose the specific functional task that the child is unable to perform (e.g., *Feeding self-care deficit*). Likewise, this label is probably not appropriate for a child with failure to thrive. That condition may be described better by one of the family functioning diagnoses or by a diagnosis of *Imbalanced nutrition: less than body requirements. Delayed growth and development* is most appropriately used for a child who is having difficulty achieving age-specific developmental tasks and growth norms.

Suggested Alternative Diagnoses

Bowel incontinence
Breastfeeding, ineffective

Communication: verbal, impaired
Coping: family, compromised
Coping: family, disabled
Coping, ineffective
Infant feeding pattern, ineffective
Nutrition, imbalanced: less than body requirements
Parenting, impaired
Self-care deficit (specify)

NOC Outcomes

Child Development: 1 month: Milestones of physical, cognitive, and psychosocial progression by 1 month of age

[**NOTE:** There are identical NOC outcomes for Child Development: 2 months, 4 months, 6 months, 12 months, 2 years, 3 years, 4 years, 5 years, and middle childhood.]

Child Development: Adolescence: Milestones of physical, cognitive, and psychosocial progression from 12 years through 17 years of age

Development: Late Adulthood: Cognitive, psychosocial, and moral progression from 65 years of age and older

Development: Middle Adulthood: Cognitive, psychosocial, and moral progression from 40 through 65 years of age

Development: Young Adulthood: Cognitive, psychosocial, and moral progression from 18 through 39 years of age

Also refer to NOC Outcomes for Risk for Disproportionate Growth.

Goals/Evaluation Criteria

Examples Using NOC Language

- Normal progression of **Child Development: Adolescence**, as evidenced by the following indicators (specify 1–5: never, rarely, sometimes, often, or consistently demonstrated):

  Uses effective social interaction skills
  Respects others
  Uses formal operational thinking
  Observes rules
  Shows capacity for intimacy

Other Examples

This section can only provide examples. Refer to *Nursing Outcomes Classification (NOC)* manual or growth and development text for complete list of indicators for each age group: 2, 4, 6, and 12 months; 2, 3, 4, and 5 years; middle childhood; young, middle, and late adulthood.

- The child will achieve expected growth norms (e.g., weight, head circumference, bone age, mean body mass), that is, not above the 97th percentile or below the 3rd percentile for age
- The child will achieve milestones of physical, cognitive, and psychosocial progression (specify age of achievement), with no delay from expected range
- Examples of indicators of normal child development for a 6-month-old child are as follows: rolls over, sits with support, grasps and mouths objects
- Physical maturation will progress normally (e.g., for females: growth spurt between 9.5 and 14.5 years of age, breast development, and onset of menstruation; for males: growth spurt between 10.5 and 16 years of age, voice change, penis enlargement, increased muscle mass)
- The patient will achieve the highest level of wellness, independence, and growth and development possible given patient's illness or disability status

NIC Interventions

Anticipatory Guidance: Preparation of patient for an anticipated developmental and/or situational crisis

Attachment Promotion: Facilitation of the development of the parent relationship

Body Mechanics Promotion: Facilitating the use of posture and movement in daily activities to prevent fatigue and musculoskeletal strain or injury

Coping Enhancement: Assisting a patient to adapt to perceived stressors, changes, or threats that interfere with meeting life demands and roles

Developmental Care: Structuring the environment and providing care in response to the behavioral cues and states of the preterm infant

Developmental Enhancement: Adolescent: Facilitating optimal physical, cognitive, social, and emotional growth of individuals during the transition from childhood to adulthood

Developmental Enhancement: Child: Facilitating or teaching parents/caregivers to facilitate the optimal gross motor, fine motor, language, cognitive, social and emotional growth of preschool and school-aged children

Exercise Promotion: Facilitation of regular physical activity to maintain or advance to a higher level of fitness and health

Health Screening: Detecting health risks or problems by means of history, examination, and other procedures

Infant Care: Provision of developmentally appropriate family-centered care to the child under 1 year of age

Newborn Care: Management of neonate during the transition to extrauterine life and subsequent period of stabilization

Nutrition Management: Assisting with or providing a balanced dietary intake of foods and fluids

Nutritional Monitoring: Collection and analysis of patient data to prevent or minimize malnourishment

Parent Education: Adolescent: Assisting parents to understand and help their adolescent children

Parent Education: Childrearing Family: Assisting parents to understand and promote the physical, psychological, and social growth and development of their toddler, preschool, or school-age child/children

Parent Education: Infant: Instruction on nurturing and physical care needed during the first year of life

Parenting Promotion: Providing parenting information, support, and coordination of comprehensive services to high-risk families

Resiliency Promotion: Assisting individuals, families, and communities in development, use, and strengthening of protective factors to be used in coping with environmental and societal stressors

Role Enhancement: Assisting a patient, significant other, and family to improve relationships by clarifying and supplementing specific role behaviors

Self-Responsibility Facilitation: Encouraging a patient to assume more responsibility for own behavior

Teaching: Infant Stimulation (0–4 months, 5–8 months, and 9–12 months): Teaching parents and caregivers to provide developmentally appropriate sensory activities to promote development and movement [during the first year of life]

Nursing Activities

NOTE: Because this nursing diagnosis is so broad and nonspecific, not every possible nursing activity can be listed here. Refer to the *Nursing Interventions Classification (NIC)* manual and to age-specific sections in growth and development texts for full lists of activities.

Assessments

- Assess the caretakers' knowledge, resources, support systems, coping skills, and level of commitment to develop a plan of care
- Conduct a thorough health assessment (e.g., child's history, temperament, culture, family environment, developmental screening) to determine functional level

- Identify potential related physical problems (e.g., dehydration, falls, upper respiratory infection, skin breakdown) and initiate plans to prevent them
- Monitor parent and child interactions and communication
- Assess adequacy of nutritional intake (e.g., calories, nutrients)
- Monitor trends in weight loss or gain
- Take skinfold measurements
- Determine food preferences
- *(NIC) Self-Responsibility Facilitation:* Monitor level of responsibility that patient assumes

Patient/Family Teaching

- *(NIC) Developmental Enhancement:*
  - Teach caregivers about normal developmental milestones and associated behaviors
  - Demonstrate activities that promote development to caregivers

Collaborative Activities

- Act as case manager to ensure comprehensive care by coordinating medical, nutritional, school, rehabilitation, and social services
- *(NIC) Developmental Enhancement: Child:* Refer caregivers to support group, as appropriate

Other

- Assist caretakers to develop a plan of care (for possible care plans and interventions, refer to Family Coping: Family, Compromised; and Coping: Family, Disabled)
- Assist patient in achieving next level of growth and development through appropriate mastery of tasks specific to his level
- Create an environment where ADLs can be performed with maximum independence
- Establish a therapeutic and trusting relationship with caretakers
- Help the family develop a strategy to integrate the patient as an accepted member of the family and community
- *(NIC) Developmental Enhancement: Child:*
  - Provide activities that encourage interaction among children
  - Encourage child to express self through positive rewards or feedback for attempts
  - Offer age-appropriate toys or materials
  - Be consistent and structured with behavior management or modification strategies
- *(NIC) Self-Responsibility Facilitation:* Encourage patient to take as much responsibility for own self-care as possible

Home Care

The preceding interventions are appropriate for home care.

For Infants and Children

The preceding interventions are for patients who are infants and children. However, some interventions are directed at the patient, whereas others are directed at parents and caregivers.

H

HEALTH BEHAVIOR, RISK-PRONE

(1986, 1998, 2006, 2008) **Domain 1, Health Promotion; Class 2, Health Management**

Definition: Impaired ability to modify lifestyle and/or behaviors in a manner that improves health status

Defining Characteristics

Subjective

Minimizes health status change
Failure to achieve optimal sense of control

Objective

Demonstrates nonacceptance of health status change
Failure to take action that prevents health problems

Related Factors

Excessive alcohol
Inadequate comprehension
Inadequate social support
Low self-efficacy
Low socioeconomic status
Multiple stressors
Negative attitude toward health care
Smoking

Suggestions for Use

This diagnosis is not specific enough to be clinically useful. If you use it, add clarifying phrases (e.g., *Risk-Prone health behavior: Excessive alcohol consumption*). When possible, use a different diagnostic label that identifies the specific risk-prone behavior (e.g., *Ineffective denial*, *Risk for other-directed Violence*).

Suggested Alternative Diagnoses

Coping, ineffective
Denial, ineffective
Grieving, complicated
Violence: other-directed, risk for
Violence: self-directed, risk for

NOC Outcomes

Acceptance: Health Status: Reconciliation to significant change in health circumstances

Adaptation to Physical Disability: Adaptive response to a significant functional challenge due to a physical disability

Compliance Behavior: Personal actions taken to promote wellness, recovery, and rehabilitation recommended by a health professional

Coping: Personal actions to manage stressors that tax an individual's resources

Health-Seeking Behavior: Personal actions to promote optimal wellness, recovery, and rehabilitation

Motivation: Inner urge that moves or prompts an individual to positive action(s)

Psychosocial Adjustment: Life Change: Adaptive psychosocial response of an individual to a significant life change

Risk Control: Personal actions to prevent, eliminate, or reduce modifiable health threats

Goals/Evaluation Criteria

Examples Using NOC Language

- Demonstrates adjustment to changes in health status as evidenced by Acceptance: Health Status, Adaptation to Physical Disability, Compliance Behavior, Coping, Health-Seeking Behavior, Motivation, Psychosocial Adjustment: Life Change, and Risk Control
- Demonstrates **Acceptance: Health Status**, as evidenced by the following indicators (specify 1–5: never, rarely, sometimes, often, or consistently demonstrated):

  Relinquishes previous concept of personal health
  Pursues information about health

Reports positive self-regard
Makes decisions about health

Other Examples

Patient will:

- Verbalize acceptance of changes in health status
- Verbalize feelings about the required lifestyle and behavior changes
- Begin to make lifestyle and behavior changes
- Identify priorities for own health outcomes
- Demonstrate decreased anxiety and fear in independent activities
- Comply with prescribed treatments

NIC Interventions

Anticipatory Guidance: Preparation of patient for an anticipated developmental and/or situational crisis

Behavior Modification: Promotion of a behavior change

Coping Enhancement: Assisting a patient to adapt to perceived stressors, changes, or threats that interfere with meeting life demands and roles

Counseling: Use of an interactive helping process focusing on the needs, problems, or feelings of the patient and significant others to enhance or support coping, problem solving, and interpersonal relationships

Decision-Making Support: Providing information and support for a patient who is making a decision regarding health care

Emotional Support: Provision of reassurance, acceptance, and encouragement during times of stress

Health Education: Developing and providing instruction and learning experiences to facilitate voluntary adaptation of behavior conducive to health in individuals, families, groups, or communities

Mutual Goal Setting: Collaborating with patient to identify and prioritize care goals, then developing a plan for achieving those goals

Patient Contracting: Negotiating an agreement with an individual that reinforces a specific behavior change

Risk Identification: Analysis of potential risk factors, determination of health risks, and prioritization of risk-reduction strategies for an individual or group

Self-Efficacy Enhancement: Strengthening an individual's confidence in his ability to perform a health behavior

Self-Modification Assistance: Reinforcement of self-directed change initiated by the patient to achieve personally important goals

Self-Responsibility Facilitation: Encouraging a patient to assume more responsibility for own behavior

Values Clarification: Assisting another to clarify his own values in order to facilitate effective decision making

Nursing Activities

Assessments

- Assess patient's need for social support
- Assess amount and quality of social support available
- *(NIC) Coping Enhancement:*
  - Appraise patient's adjustment to changes in body image, as indicated
  - Appraise the impact of the patient's life situation on roles and relationships
  - Evaluate the patient's decision-making ability

Collaborative Activities

- Refer patient to community agencies and/or support groups
- Include patient and family in a multidisciplinary conference to establish a plan of care, for example:
  - Identify obstacles that hinder lifestyle and behavior changes
  - Identify personal strengths that will facilitate goal achievement
  - Review necessary lifestyle and behavior changes and select one as an initial goal

Other

- Provide a nonjudgmental environment in which patient and family can share concerns, anxieties, and fears
- *(NIC) Coping Enhancement:*
  - Assist the patient to identify available support systems [to learn new ways to cope and to decrease isolation and fear]
  - Appraise and discuss alternative responses to situation

Home Care

- The preceding interventions can be used in home care
- Assess the support system available
- Assess family communication and interaction patterns

For Older Adults

- Assess for depression or agitation in response to changes

HEALTH MAINTENANCE, INEFFECTIVE

(1982) **Domain 1, Health Promotion; Class 2, Health Management**

Definition: Inability to identify, manage, or seek out help to maintain health

H

Defining Characteristics

Subjective

Lack of expressed interest in improving health behaviors

Objective

Demonstrated lack of adaptive behaviors to environmental changes
Demonstrated lack of knowledge regarding basic health practices
History of lack of health-seeking behavior
Impairment of personal support system
Inability to take responsibility for meeting basic health practices

Other Defining Characteristics (Non-NANDA International)

History of untreated, chronic symptoms of disease process
Limited use of health care agencies and personnel
Limited use of preventive health measures
Need to adhere to cultural and religious beliefs

Related Factors

Complicated grieving
Deficient communication skills (e.g., written, verbal, or gestural)
Diminished or lack of gross- or fine-motor skills
Ineffective family coping
Ineffective individual coping
Inability to make appropriate judgments
Insufficient resources (e.g., equipment, finances)
Perceptual or cognitive impairment
Spiritual distress
Unachieved developmental tasks

Other Related Factors (Non-NANDA International)

Cultural beliefs
Lack of social supports
Motor impairment
Religious beliefs

Suggestions for Use

It may be difficult to differentiate among this diagnosis, *Risk-prone health behavior*, *Ineffective self-help management*, and *Readiness for enhanced self-health management*. Use *Ineffective health maintenance* for patients who lack the ability to maintain their overall health (e.g., due to cognitive impairment or developmental delay), and who have no expressed interest in improving their health behaviors.

Risk-prone health behavior is similar to *Ineffective health maintenance* in that the person does not have the ability to maintain health. However, it is focused more on inability to make lifestyle changes, whereas *Ineffective health maintenance* may focus more on seeking help or access to health care.

Use *Ineffective self-health management* for those who have difficulty following a therapeutic regimen for a specific health problem (e.g., because the treatment regimen is complex or because of excessive competing family demands) and who have expressed a desire to manage their illness. In comparison, *Readiness for enhanced self-health management* is a wellness diagnosis to be used for clients with a generally healthy lifestyle who are seeking to attain a higher level of wellness (e.g., a client who wishes information about BP screening).

The best approach is to choose the diagnosis for which the patient has the most Defining Characteristics, even though there is overlap among these labels.

Suggested Alternative Diagnoses

Coping, ineffective
Denial, ineffective
Health behavior, risk-prone
Knowledge, deficient
Therapeutic regimen management: family, ineffective
Noncompliance (specify)
Self-health management, ineffective
Self-health management, readiness for enhanced

NOC Outcomes

Client Satisfaction: Access to Care Resources: Extent of positive perception of access to nursing staff, supplies, and equipment needed for care

Health Beliefs: Perceived Resources: Personal conviction that one has adequate means to carry out a health behavior

Health-Promoting Behavior: Personal actions to sustain or increase wellness

Health-Seeking Behavior: Personal actions to promote optimal wellness, recovery, and rehabilitation

Knowledge: Health Behavior: Extent of understanding conveyed about the promotion and protection of health

Knowledge: Health Promotion: Extent of understanding conveyed about information needed to obtain and maintain optimal health

Knowledge: Health Resources: Extent of understanding conveyed about relevant health care resources

Participation in Health Care Decisions: Personal involvement in selecting and evaluating health care options to achieve desired outcome

Risk Detection: Personal actions taken to identify personal health threats

Social Support: Reliable assistance from others

Goals/Evaluation Criteria

Examples Using NOC Language

- Will demonstrate **Participation in Health Care Decisions**, as evidenced by the following indicators (specify 1–5: never, rarely, sometimes, often, or consistently demonstrated):
  - Exhibits self-direction in decision making
  - Seeks reputable information
  - Identifies barriers to desired outcome achievement
  - Uses problem-solving techniques to achieve desired outcomes
  - Seeks health care services to meet desired outcomes

Other Examples

Patient will:

- Develop and follow strategies to maximize health
- Acknowledge adverse effects of health beliefs
- Demonstrate awareness that healthy behavior requires some effort, and confidence in ability to manage it
- Follow recommended treatment regimens
- Identify potential health risks created by lifestyle
- Verbalize and demonstrate knowledge of preventive health measures (e.g., performs self-examinations, participates in health screenings)

NIC Interventions

Case Management: Coordinating care and advocating for specified individuals and patient populations across settings to reduce cost, reduce resource use, improve quality of health care, and achieve desired outcomes

Decision-Making Support: Providing information and support for a patient who is making a decision regarding health care

Family Involvement Promotion: Facilitating family participation in the emotional and physical care of the patient

Financial Resource Assistance: Assisting an individual/family to secure and manage finances to meet health care needs

Health Education: Developing and providing instruction and learning experiences to facilitate voluntary adaptation of behavior conducive to health in individuals, families, groups, or communities

Health Screening: Detecting health risks or problems by means of history, examination, and other procedures

Health Literacy Enhancement: Assisting individuals with limited ability to obtain, process, and understand information related to health and illness

Health System Guidance: Facilitating a patient's location and use of appropriate health services

Mutual Goal Setting: Collaborating with patient to identify and prioritize care goals, then developing a plan for achieving those goals

Risk Identification: Analysis of potential risk factors, determination of health risks, and prioritization of risk-reduction strategies for an individual or group

Risk Identification: Childbearing Family: Identification of an individual or family likely to experience difficulties in parenting and prioritization of strategies to prevent parenting problems

Self-Care Assistance: Assisting another to perform activities of daily living

Self-Care Assistance: IADL: Assisting and instructing a person to perform instrumental activities of daily living (IADL) needed to function in the home or community

Self-Efficacy Enhancement: Strengthening an individual's confidence in his ability to perform a health behavior

Self-Modification Assistance: Reinforcement of self-directed change initiated by the patient to achieve personally important goals

Self-Responsibility Facilitation: Encouraging a patient to assume more responsibility for own behavior

Support Group: Use of a group environment to provide emotional support and health-related information for members

Support System Enhancement: Facilitation of support to patient by family, friends, and community

Teaching: Individual: Planning, implementation, and evaluation of a teaching program designed to address a patient's particular needs

Nursing Activities

Assessments

- Identify beliefs and knowledge deficits that interfere with health maintenance
- Assess availability and adequacy of support system

- *(NIC) Self-Modification Assistance:*
  Appraise the patient's reasons for wanting to change
  Appraise the patient's present knowledge and skill level in relationship to the desired change

Patient/Family Teaching

- *(NIC) Health System Guidance:*
  Explain the immediate health care system, how it works, and what the patient and family can expect
  Give written instructions for purpose and location of health care activities, as appropriate
  Inform the patient the meaning of signing a consent form
  Inform patient of the cost, time, alternatives, and risks involved in a specific test or procedure
  Provide patient with copy of Patient's Bill of Rights [or similar document]
- *(NIC) Self-Modification Assistance:*
  Explain to the patient the function of cues and triggers in producing behavior
  Instruct the patient on the use of "cue expansion"—increasing the number of cues that prompt a desired behavior
  Instruct the patient on the use of "cue restriction or limitation"—decreasing the frequency of cues that elicit an undesirable behavior

Collaborative Activities

- Consult with social services to plan for health maintenance needs on discharge
- *(NIC) Health System Guidance:*
  Inform patient of appropriate community resources and contact persons
  Advise use of second opinion
  Coordinate referrals to relevant health care providers, as appropriate
  Coordinate and schedule time needed by each service to deliver care, as appropriate

Other

- *Health System Guidance:* Encourage the patient and family to ask questions about services and charges
- *(NIC) Self-Modification Assistance:*
  Assist the patient in identifying a specific goal for change
  Explore with the patient potential barriers to change behavior

Encourage the patient to identify appropriate, meaningful reinforcers and rewards

Foster moving toward primary reliance on self-reinforcement versus family or nurse for rewards

Assist the patient in evaluating progress by comparing records of previous behavior with present behavior

Home Care

- Encourage discussion of preventive health measures specific to patient needs, such as dietary changes, cessation of smoking, stress reduction, and implementation of exercise program
- Provide aids to help the client follow the therapeutic regimen (e.g., obtain a medication container and demonstrate how to put a week's medication in it)
- Consider use of a written contract with the client for making changes
- Help the client find ways to incorporate health-related changes (e.g., a low-fat diet) into his usual lifestyle
- *(NIC) Health System Guidance:*

  Inform patient of appropriate community resources and contact persons

  Assist individual to complete forms for assistance, such as housing and financial aid, as needed

For Infants and Children

- Identify risk factors for adolescent smoking (e.g., parents who smoke)
- Describe to adolescents the risks of smoking, especially the risks associated with appearance and image
- Inform about the risks of smokeless tobacco
- Explore with adolescents assertive behaviors to help them cope with peer pressure to smoke
- Explain that most people who smoke would like to quit, but that it is a difficult habit to break
- Explain to pregnant women the effects of smoking on the fetus (e.g., low birthweight)
- Teach parents that secondhand smoke contributes to sudden infant death syndrome and to allergies, otitis media, asthma, and respiratory infections in children

For Older Adults

- Assess vision, hearing, and psychomotor function; be sure eyeglasses, hearing aids, walkers, and other assistive devices are available and functioning properly
- Help the client to formulate realistic goals for changes that need to be made, recognizing that change is difficult for many older adults
- Perform or encourage the client to have screening exams (e.g., for breast cancer)
- Assess for elder abuse

HOME MAINTENANCE, IMPAIRED

(1980) **Domain 4, Activity/Rest; Class 5, Self-Care**

Definition: Inability to independently maintain a safe, growth-promoting immediate environment

Defining Characteristics

Subjective

Household members describe outstanding debts or financial crises
Household members report difficulty in maintaining their home in a comfortable fashion
Household members request assistance with home maintenance

Objective

[Accumulation of dirt, food wastes, or hygienic wastes]
Disorderly or unclean surroundings
Inappropriate household temperature
Lack of necessary equipment
Offensive odors
Overtaxed (e.g., exhausted, anxious) family members
Presence of vermin
Repeated unhygienic disorders or infections
Unavailable, insufficient, or lack of cooking equipment, clothes, linen

Related Factors

Deficient knowledge
Disease or illness
Impaired functioning
Inadequate support system
Injury

Insufficient family organization or planning
Insufficient finances
Lack of role modeling
Unfamiliarity with neighborhood resources

Other Related Factors (Non-NANDA International)

Developmental disability
Home environment obstacles

Suggestions for Use

This diagnosis emphasizes inability to manage the home environment (e.g., laundry, cleaning, and cooking). If the difficulty is with managing medications or treatments, use *Ineffective family management of therapeutic regimen* or *Ineffective self-help management.* If it is primarily a difficulty in managing self-care, such as bathing and dressing, use *Self-care deficit (specify).* Differentiate also between this label and *Caregiver role strain.*

Suggested Alternative Diagnoses

Caregiver role strain
Family coping, compromised
Health maintenance, ineffective
Injury, risk for (trauma, falls)
Therapeutic regimen management: family, ineffective
Self-care deficit (specify)

NOC Outcomes

Safe Home Environment: Physical arrangements to minimize environmental factors that might cause physical harm or injury in the home

Self-Care: Instrumental Activities of Daily Living (IADLs): Ability to perform activities needed to function in the home or community independently with or without assistive device

Goals/Evaluation Criteria

Examples Using NOC Language

- *Impaired home maintenance* will be eliminated or moderated, as demonstrated by Safe Home Environment and Self-Care: Instrumental Activities of Daily Living (IADL)
- **Safe Home Environment** will be demonstrated, as evidenced by the following indicators (specify 1–5: not, slightly, moderately, substantially, or totally adequate):
  - Building maintenance
  - Availability of clean water

Cleanliness of dwelling
Safe storage of hazardous materials

- **Self-Care: Instrumental Activities of Daily Living (IADL)** will be demonstrated, as evidenced by the following indicators (specify 1–5: severely, substantially, moderately, mildly, or not compromised):
  Shops for groceries
  Performs housework
  Manages money
  Opens containers

H

Other Examples

Patient and family/household member will:

- Follow specific plan for home maintenance
- Identify options to overcome financial constraints
- Verbalize awareness of constraints on home situation due to illness of family member
- Verbalize knowledge of available resources
- Perform home maintenance tasks (e.g., shopping, meal preparation, laundry, yard work, housework)
- Drive car (e.g., for shopping)
- Remove environmental hazards from the home
- Provide for the physical needs of dependents in the home
- Provide supervision for children (e.g., of playmates, day care workers)

NIC Interventions

Environmental Management: Manipulation of the patient's surroundings for therapeutic benefit, sensory appeal, and psychological well-being

Environmental Management: Safety: Monitoring and manipulation of the physical environment to promote safety

Home Maintenance Assistance: Helping the patient and family to maintain the home as a clean, safe, and pleasant place to live

Self-Care Assistance: IADL: Assisting and instructing a person to perform IADL needed to function in the home or community

Nursing Activities

Assessments

- *(NIC) Home Maintenance Assistance:* Determine patient's home maintenance requirements

Patient/Family Teaching

- Provide written material regarding home maintenance
- *(NIC) Home Maintenance Assistance:* Provide information on how to make home environment safe and clean

Collaborative Activities

- Assess and document need for postdischarge follow-through with public health nurse
- Contact discharge planner or social worker to establish realistic plan for home maintenance
- For inpatients, make a referral for a home visit to assess the client's abilities to function independently after discharge from the institution
- *(NIC) Home Maintenance Assistance:*

  Provide information on respite care, as needed

  Order homemaker services, as appropriate

Other

- Accept and support without judgment the realities of the home situation
- Help patient and family/household member identify obstacles and hazards in home that may impede home maintenance
- Help patient and family/household member identify strengths in family unit, as well as support systems that will assist in home maintenance
- Initiate discussion with patient and family about health status of all family members, as illness of other family members may affect home maintenance management
- *(NIC) Home Maintenance Assistance:*

  Involve patient and family in deciding home maintenance requirements

  Suggest necessary structural alterations to make home accessible

  Suggest services for pest control, as needed

  Suggest services for home repair, as needed

  Discuss cost of needed maintenance and available resources

Home Care

- All of the preceding interventions are appropriate for home care, the focus of this nursing diagnosis

For Older Adults

- Assess whether the client can function independently in the home (e.g., assess vision, hearing, mobility, and other functional abilities)
- Help client to obtain assistive devices (e.g., walkers, alarms) needed to maintain independent functioning
- Refer for home health aide and homemaker services as needed
- Be sure that family members are aware of the client's need for assistance in order to continue living at home

- Assist client to locate community resources to assist with IADL (e.g., senior centers that serve meals, parish nurses, Meals on Wheels)
- Assess the home environment for safety hazards (e.g., be sure there are stair rails, safety rails in the bathroom, adequate lighting)
- Assess for elder abuse

HOPE, READINESS FOR ENHANCED

(2006) **Domain 10, Life Principles; Class 1, Values**

Definition: A pattern of expectations and desires that is sufficient for mobilizing energy on one's own behalf that is sufficient for well-being and can be strengthened

Defining Characteristics

Expresses desire to enhance:

Ability to set achievable goals
Belief in possibilities
Congruency of expectations with desires
Hope
Interconnectedness with others
Problem-solving to meet goals
Sense of spirituality and meaning to life

Related Factors

Because this is a wellness diagnosis, an etiology (related factors) is not needed.

Suggestions for Use

This diagnosis can be used for both well and ill clients. Differentiate between this label and *Readiness for enhanced power. Readiness for enhanced hope* implies that the person believes there are solutions to his problem and that he wishes to improve his problem-solving abilities and to be sure that his goals and expectations are realistic. *Readiness for enhanced power* focuses more on the ability to choose and be involved in making changes.

Readiness for enhanced spiritual well-being and *Readiness for enhanced religiosity* are not as broad as this diagnosis, which is partly defined by a desire to enhance aspects of spirituality.

Suggested Alternative Diagnoses

Power, readiness for enhanced
Religiosity, readiness for enhanced
Spiritual well-being, readiness for enhanced

NOC Outcomes

Decision Making: Ability to make judgments and choose between two or more alternatives

Health Beliefs: Perceived Ability to Perform: Personal conviction that one can carry out a given health behavior

Hope: Optimism that is personally satisfying and life supporting

Spiritual Health: Connectedness with self, others, higher power, all life, nature, and the universe that transcends and empowers the self

Goals/Evaluation Criteria

Examples Using NOC Language

- Client will experience enhanced hope, as evidenced by improved Decision Making, Health Beliefs: Perceived Ability to Perform, Hope, and Spiritual Health
- Improved **Decision Making** will be demonstrated, as evidenced by the following indicator (specify 1–5: severely, substantially, moderately, mildly, or not compromised): Weighs and chooses among alternatives
- Increased **Hope** will be exhibited, as evidenced by the following indicators (specify 1–5: never, rarely, sometimes, often, or consistently demonstrated):

  Expresses faith, will to live, reasons to live, meaning in life, optimism, and belief in self and others

  Exhibits a zest for life

Other Examples

Patient will:

- Identify personal strengths
- Report extent and pattern of sleep adequate to produce mental and physical rejuvenation
- Demonstrate appropriate mood and affect
- Maintain or improve appropriate hygiene and grooming
- Demonstrate increased interest in social and personal relationships
- Show interest in or satisfaction with achieving life goals

NIC Interventions

Decision-Making Support: Providing information and support for a patient who is making a decision regarding health care

Hope Inspiration: Facilitation of the development of a positive outlook in a given situation

Self-Modification Assistance: Reinforcement of self-directed change initiated by the patient to achieve personally important goals

Spiritual Growth Facilitation: Facilitation of growth in patients' capacity to identify, connect with, and call upon the source of meaning, purpose, comfort, strength, and hope in his life

Values Clarification: Assisting another to clarify his own values in order to facilitate effective decision making

Nursing Activities

Assessments

- Assess decision-making ability
- Assess nutrition: intake and body weight
- Assess spiritual needs
- Determine adequacy of relationships and other social supports

Patient/Family Teaching

- Provide information on community resources, such as community agencies, social agencies, self-improvement classes, stress-reduction classes, counseling
- *(NIC) Hope Inspiration:* Teach reality recognition by surveying the situation and making contingency plans

Collaborative Activities

- Refer for spiritual counseling, if this is acceptable to the patient
- *(NIC) Hope Inspiration:* Provide patient and family opportunity to be involved with support groups

Other

- Encourage active participation in group activities to provide opportunity for social supports and problem solving
- Schedule time with patient to provide opportunity to explore coping measures
- Provide positive feedback when appropriate
- Explore with the client her sources or spirituality.
- Recommend spending some time outdoors each day; for inpatients, place bed near the window.
- *(NIC) Hope Inspiration:*
  - Assist patient and family to identify areas of hope in life
  - Demonstrate hope by recognizing the patient's intrinsic worth and viewing the patient's illness as only one facet of the individual
  - Help the patient expand spiritual self

Employ guided life review or reminiscence, as appropriate
Avoid masking the truth
Involve the patient actively in own care
Encourage therapeutic relationships with significant others

Home Care

- The preceding interventions are all appropriate for home-based care
- Assess and facilitate family communication
- If the client must remain in bed, place the bed in an area central to family activities
- Suggest outdoor activities, such as gardening
- Encourage involvement in church and other community activities

For Infants and Children

- Teach parents about age-appropriate expectations for their children
- Encourage participation in school activities

For Older Adults

- Identify losses that may interfere with enhanced hope
- Assist clients to recognize and cope with emotional responses to identified losses
- Suggest activities such as dance, music, and art
- Recommend some form of daily exercise, based on client's ability and interests
- Use pet therapy if possible

HOPELESSNESS

(1986) **Domain 6, Self-Perception; Class 1, Self-Concept**

Definition: Subjective state in which an individual sees limited or no alternatives or personal choices available and is unable to mobilize energy on own behalf

Defining Characteristics

Subjective

Verbal cues (e.g., despondent content, "I can't," sighing)

Objective

Closing eyes
Decreased affect
Decreased appetite
Decreased response to stimuli
Decreased verbalization
Lack of initiative
Lack of involvement in care
Passivity
Shrugging in response to speaker
Sleep pattern disturbance
Turning away from speaker
Avoiding eye contact (non-NANDA International)

Related Factors

Abandonment
Deteriorating physical condition
Long-term stress
Lost belief in transcendent values or spiritual power
Prolonged activity restrictions
Social isolation
Lack of social supports (non-NANDA International)

Suggestions for Use

Differentiate between this label and *Powerlessness*. *Hopelessness* implies that the person believes there is no solution to his problem ("no way out"). In *Powerlessness*, the person may know of a solution to the problem but believes it is beyond his control to achieve the solution. Long-term feelings of *Powerlessness* may lead to *Hopelessness*. Although both diagnoses share some defining characteristics, the following are specific only to *Powerlessness:* irritability, resentment, anger, guilt, and fear of alienation from caregivers. For some patients, *Hopelessness* may be a risk factor for suicide.

Suggested Alternative Diagnoses

Anxiety, death
Coping, ineffective
Decisional conflict
Failure to thrive, adult
Grieving, complicated (may be an etiology of *Hopelessness*)
Powerlessness
Sorrow, chronic

Spiritual distress, actual/risk
Violence: self-directed, risk for

NOC Outcomes

Depression Level: Severity of melancholic mood and loss of interest in life events

Depression Self-Control: Personal actions to minimize melancholy and maintain interest in life events

Hope: Optimism that is personally satisfying and life supporting

Mood Equilibrium: Appropriate adjustment of prevailing emotional tone in response to circumstances

Psychomotor Energy: Personal drive and energy to maintain activities of daily living, nutrition, and personal safety

Quality of Life: Extent of positive perception of current life circumstances

Will to Live: Desire, determination, and effort to survive

Goals/Evaluation Criteria

Examples Using NOC Language

- *Hopelessness* will be eliminated, as evidenced by consistent Depression Level, Depression Self-Control, presence of Hope, Mood Equilibrium, Psychomotor Energy, expressed satisfaction with Quality of Life, and Will to Live
- **Quality of Life** will be demonstrated, as evidenced by the following indicator (specify 1–5: not at all, somewhat, moderately, very, or completely satisfied): Social circumstances, close relationships, achievement of life goals, self-concept
- **Hope** will be exhibited, as evidenced by the following indicators (specify 1–5: never, rarely, sometimes, often, or consistently demonstrated):
  - Expresses faith, will to live, reasons to live, meaning in life, optimism, and belief in self and others
  - Exhibits a zest for life

Other Examples

Also see *Other Examples* for Readiness for Enhanced Hope.

Patient will:

- Initiate behaviors that may reduce feelings of hopelessness

NIC Interventions

Also refer to NIC Interventions for Readiness for Enhanced Hope.

Coping Enhancement: Assisting a patient to adapt to perceived stressors, changes, or threats that interfere with meeting life demands and roles

Counseling: Use of an interactive helping process focusing on the needs, problems, or feelings of the patient and significant others to enhance or support coping, problem solving, and interpersonal relationships

Mood Management: Providing for safety, stabilization, recovery, and maintenance of a patient who is experiencing dysfunctionally depressed mood or elevated mood

Resiliency Promotion: Assisting individuals, families, and communities in development, use, and strengthening of protective factors to be used in coping with environmental and societal stressors

Values Clarification: Assisting another to clarify his own values in order to facilitate effective decision making

Nursing Activities

Also refer to Nursing Activities for Readiness for Enhanced Hope.

Assessments

- Assess and document potential for suicide
- Monitor affect and decision-making ability
- Monitor nutrition: intake and body weight

Patient/Family Teaching

- *(NIC) Hope Inspiration:* Teach reality recognition by surveying the situation and making contingency plans

Collaborative Activities

- Obtain psychiatric consultation

Other

- Encourage active participation in group activities to provide opportunity for social supports and problem solving
- Explore with patient factors that contribute to feelings of hopelessness
- Provide positive reinforcement for behaviors that demonstrate initiative, such as eye contact, self-disclosure, reduction in amount of sleep time, self-care, increased appetite

HUMAN DIGNITY, COMPROMISED, RISK FOR

(2006) **Domain 6, Self-Perception; Class 1, Self-Concept**

Definition: At risk for perceived loss of respect and honor

Risk Factors

Cultural incongruity
Disclosure of confidential information

Exposure of the body
Inadequate participation in decision making
Loss of control of body functions
Perceived dehumanizing treatment
Perceived humiliation
Perceived intrusion by clinicians
Perceived invasion of privacy
Stigmatizing label
Use of undefined medical terms

Suggestions for Use

The author does not recommend using this nursing diagnosis, except perhaps in very unusual circumstances, until it is developed further. Every ill person, and certainly every patient in an institution, is at risk for compromised human dignity. Therefore, I believe it would be difficult to find a patient to whom this diagnosis does *not* apply.

Furthermore, professional and moral imperatives dictate that the nurse should attend to human dignity with every nursing action taken. Therefore, I question what interventions this diagnosis suggests that are over and above "normal" nursing care. In addition, this diagnosis seems to suggest the need for a certain nursing attitude or approach, rather than specific nursing interventions.

In situations where the risk factors result from the actions of someone other than nurses, the nurse's role as a patient advocate should dictate intervention without need of a nursing diagnosis.

NOC Outcomes

Client Satisfaction: Caring: Extent of positive perception of nursing staff's concern for the client

Client Satisfaction: Protection of Rights: Extent of positive perception of protection of a client's legal and moral rights provided by the nursing staff

Comfort Status: Physical: Physical ease related to bodily sensations and homeostatic mechanisms

Comfort Status: Psychospiritual: Psychospiritual ease related to self-concept, emotional well-being, source of inspiration, and meaning and purpose in life

Comfort Status: Sociocultural: Social ease related to interpersonal, family, and societal relationships within a cultural context

Dignified Life Closure: Personal actions to maintain control during approaching end of life

Goals/Evaluation Criteria

Examples Using NOC Language

- Human dignity will be preserved, as evidenced by Client Satisfaction: Caring and Client Satisfaction: Protection of Rights
- Human dignity will be preserved, as evidenced by Comfort Status: Physical, Psychospiritual, and Sociocultural; and by Dignified Life Closure
- **Client Satisfaction: Protection of Rights** will be demonstrated, as evidenced by the following indicators (specify 1–5: not at all, somewhat, moderately, very, or completely satisfied):
  - Maintenance of privacy
  - Confidentiality of client information maintained
  - Included in decisions about care

Other Examples

Patient will state satisfaction with:

- The courtesy and respect shown by caregivers
- Staff attention to cultural practices
- Emotional support provided by staff
- Clarity and appropriateness of communication shown by staff

NIC Interventions

Admission Care: Facilitating entry of a patient into a health care facility

Anticipatory Guidance: Preparation of patient for an anticipated developmental and/or situational crisis

Bowel Incontinence Care: Promotion of bowel continence and maintenance of perianal skin integrity

Culture Brokerage: The deliberate use of culturally competent strategies to bridge or mediate between the patient's culture and the biomedical health care system

Decision-Making Support: Providing information and support for a patient who is making a decision regarding health care

Discharge Planning: Preparation for moving a patient from one level of care to another within or outside the current health care agency

Health System Guidance: Facilitating a patient's location and use of appropriate health services

Patient Rights Protection: Protection of health care rights of a patient, especially a minor, incapacitated, or incompetent patient unable to make decisions

Risk Identification: Analysis of potential risk factors, determination of health risks, and prioritization of risk-reduction strategies for an individual or group

Surveillance: Purposeful and ongoing acquisition, interpretation, and synthesis of patient data for clinical decision making

Nursing Activities

Assessments

- Assess patient's satisfaction with nursing care
- Observe the respect for human dignity shown by other caregivers
- Determine the patient's wishes about his care
- Determine who is legally responsible for providing consent for treatments
- Determine whether the patient has advance directives

Patient/Family Teaching

- *(NIC) Patient Rights Protection:* Provide patient with "Patient's Bill of Rights" [or other similar document]

Collaborative Activities

- *(NIC) Patient Rights Protection:*
  - Work with physician and hospital administration to honor patient's and family's wishes
  - Honor written "Do Not Resuscitate" (DNR) orders

Other

- Provide for privacy (e.g., pull curtains, drape the patient) during procedures
- Arrange for privacy for conversations between the patient and family and care providers
- Never force or coerce (e.g., by using scare tactics) a patient to consent to a treatment
- Protect the confidentiality of the patient's health information
- Honor the wishes expressed in the patient's living will (or other advance directive)
- *(NIC) Patient Rights Protection:* Intervene in situations involving unsafe or inadequate care

For Infants and Children

- Be familiar with state laws and agency policies regarding the age at which children are considered legally able to give consent for treatments

For Older Adults

- Assess the client's ability to provide legal consent for care and treatment

HYPERTHERMIA

(1986) **Domain 11, Safety/Protection; Class 6, Thermoregulation**

Definition: Body temperature elevated above normal range

Defining Characteristics

Objective

Flushed skin
Increase in body temperature above normal range
[Increased respiratory rate]
Seizures or convulsions
Skin warm to touch
Tachycardia
Tachypnea

Related Factors

Anesthesia or pharmaceutical agents
Decreased perspiration
Dehydration
Illness or trauma
Inappropriate clothing
Increased metabolic rate
[Prolonged] exposure to hot environment
Vigorous activity

Suggestions for Use

Nursing activities, such as removal of clothing or a cool sponge bath, are effective for mild *Hyperthermia*. However, severe *Hyperthermia* is a life-threatening condition requiring both medical and nursing intervention. Consider also that an elevated temperature may not be a problem, but merely a symptom of a disease process or infection; in that case, it is treated by a medication such as acetaminophen or aspirin. Most hyperthermias require collaborative treatment.

Suggested Alternative Diagnoses

Body temperature, imbalanced, risk for
Hyperthermia, risk for (non-NANDA)
Thermoregulation, ineffective

NOC Outcomes

Thermoregulation: Balance among heat production, heat gain, and heat loss

Thermoregulation: Newborn: Balance among heat production, heat gain, and heat loss during the first 28 days of life

Vital Signs: Extent to which temperature, pulse, respiration, and blood pressure are within normal range

Goals/Evaluation Criteria

Examples Using NOC Language

- Patient will demonstrate **Thermoregulation**, as evidenced by the following indicators (specify 1–5: severe, substantial, moderate, mild, or none):
  - Increased skin temperature
  - Hyperthermia
  - Dehydration
  - Drowsiness
- Patient will demonstrate **Thermoregulation**, as evidenced by the following indicators (specify 1–5: severely, substantially, moderately, mildly, or not compromised):
  - Sweating when hot
  - Radial pulse rate
  - Respiratory rate

Other Examples

Patient and family will:

- Demonstrate proper method of taking temperature
- Describe measures to prevent or minimize increase in body temperature
- Report early signs and symptoms of *Hyperthermia*

Infants will:

- Experience no respiratory distress, restlessness, or lethargy
- Use heat-dissipation posture

NIC Interventions

Fever Treatment: Management of a patient with hyperpyrexia caused by nonenvironmental factors

Malignant Hyperthermia Precautions: Prevention or reduction of hypermetabolic response to pharmacologic agents used during surgery.

Newborn Care: Management of neonate during the transition to extrauterine life and subsequent period of stabilization

Newborn Monitoring: Measurement and interpretation of physiologic status of the neonate the first 24 hr after delivery

Temperature Regulation: Attaining or maintaining body temperature within a normal range

Vital Signs Monitoring: Collection and analysis of cardiovascular, respiratory, and body temperature data to determine and prevent complications

Nursing Activities

Also see Nursing Activities for Body Temperature, Imbalanced, Risk for.

Assessments

- Monitor for seizure activity
- Monitor hydration (e.g., skin turgor, moist mucous membranes)
- Monitor blood pressure, pulse, and respirations
- Assess appropriateness of clothing for the environmental temperature
- *For surgery patients:*
  - Obtain personal and family history of malignant hyperthermia, deaths from anesthesia, or postoperative fever
  - Monitor for signs of malignant hyperthermia (e.g., fever, tachypnea, arrhythmias, BP changes, mottled skin, rigidity, profuse sweating)
- *(NIC) Temperature Regulation:*
  - Monitor temperature at least every 2 hr, as appropriate
  - Institute a continuous core temperature monitoring device, as appropriate
  - Monitor skin color and temperature

Patient/Family Teaching

- Instruct patient and family in measures for prevention and early recognition of hyperthermia (e.g., heatstroke and heat exhaustion)
- *(NIC) Temperature Regulation:* Teach indications of heat exhaustion and appropriate emergency treatment, as appropriate

Collaborative Activities

- *(NIC) Temperature Regulation:*
  - Administer antipyretic medication, as appropriate
  - Use cooling mattress and tepid baths to adjust altered body temperature, as appropriate

Other

- Remove excess clothing and cover patient with only a sheet
- Apply cool washcloths (or ice bag covered with a cloth) to axilla, groin, forehead, and nape of neck
- Encourage intake of oral fluids, at least 2,000 mL a day, with additional fluids during strenuous activities or moderate activities in hot weather

- Use a circulating fan in patient's room
- Use a cooling blanket
- For malignant hyperthermia:
  Perform emergency care according to protocol
  Keep emergency equipment in operative areas according to protocol

Home Care

- Many of the preceding interventions may be appropriate for home care use
- Teach patient and family how to use an oral or tympanic thermometer (nonmercury containing)
- Assess the temperature in the home; assist to obtain fans or air conditioner if necessary

For Infants and Children

- Teach parents not to give aspirin for fever to children under 18 years of age
- Teach parents that it is not necessary to treat all fevers in children. As a general rule, fevers in children with no history of convulsion do not need to be treated unless they are higher than 104°F (40°C).
- Tepid sponging can be used to treat fever, but it does increase the child's discomfort and can cause crying and agitation that may counteract the cooling effect of the sponging

For Older Adults

- Teach patients and family that older adults are at increased risk for hyperthermia and dehydration
- Teach patients and caregivers/family the early signs of hyperthermia or heatstroke
- Instruct to avoid alcohol and caffeine in hot weather
- Consider an oral temperature greater than 99°F (37.2°C), or an increase of 1.5° to 2.0°F (0.8° to 1.1°C), to be a fever in older adults
- Do not take rectal temperature in clients with dementia, as it may be upsetting
- Teach older adult clients to call their primary care physician if they have a fever

HYPOTHERMIA

(1986, 1988) **Domain 11, Safety/Protection; Class 6, Thermoregulation**

Definition: Body temperature below normal range

Defining Characteristics

Objective

Body temperature below normal range
Cool skin
Cyanotic nail beds
Hypertension
Pallor
Piloerection
Shivering
Slow capillary refill
Tachycardia

Related Factors

Aging
Consumption of alcohol
Damage to hypothalamus
Decreased metabolic rate
Evaporation from skin in cool environment
Exposure to cool environment
Illness or trauma
Decreased ability to shiver
Inactivity
Inadequate clothing
Malnutrition
Medications [causing vasodilation]

Other Related Factors (Non-NANDA International)

Hypothyroidism
Immaturity of newborn's temperature regulatory system
Loss of subcutaneous fat and malnutrition
Low birth weight

Suggestions for Use

Because severe *Hypothermia* (rectal temperature below 35°C or 95°F) may cause complications such as impaired myocardial or respiratory function, such low readings should be reported to the physician so that collaborative interventions may be instituted. Mild *Hypothermia* (95–97°F or 35–36°C) should respond to nursing interventions.

Suggested Alternative Diagnoses

Body temperature, imbalanced, risk for
Infant behavior: disorganized, risk for
Thermoregulation, ineffective

NOC Outcomes

Thermoregulation: Balance among heat production, heat gain, and heat loss

Thermoregulation: Newborn: Balance among heat production, heat gain, and heat loss during the first 28 days of life period

Vital Signs: Extent to which temperature, pulse, respiration, and blood pressure are within normal range

Goals/Evaluation Criteria

Also see Goals/Evaluation Criteria for Hyperthermia and for Risk for Imbalanced Body Temperature.

Examples Using NOC Language

- Patient will demonstrate **Thermoregulation**, as evidenced by the following indicators (specify 1–5: severe, substantial, moderate, mild, or none):
  - Decreased skin temperature
  - Skin color changes
- Patient will demonstrate **Thermoregulation**, as evidenced by the following indicators (specify 1–5: severely, substantially, moderately, mildly, or not compromised):
  - Presence of goose bumps when cold
  - Shivering when cold
  - Reported thermal comfort

Other Examples

Patient and family will:

- Describe measures to prevent/minimize decrease in body temperature
- Report early signs and symptoms of hypothermia
- Maintain patient body temperature of at least 97°F (36°C)

Infant will:

- Use heat-retaining posture
- Have blood glucose within normal limits
- Not be lethargic

NIC Interventions

Hypothermia Treatment: Rewarming and surveillance of a patient whose core body temperature is below 35°C

Newborn Care: Management of neonate during the transition to extrauterine life and subsequent period of stabilization

H

Newborn Monitoring: Measurement and interpretation of physiologic status of the neonate the first 24 hr after delivery

Temperature Regulation: Attaining or maintaining body temperature within a normal range

Temperature Regulation: Intraoperative: Attaining or maintaining desired intraoperative body temperature

Vital Signs Monitoring: Collection and analysis of cardiovascular, respiratory, and body temperature data to determine and prevent complications

Nursing Activities

Also see Nursing Activities for Risk for Imbalanced Body Temperature.

Assessments

- Record baseline vital signs
- Place patient on cardiac monitor
- Use a low-range thermometer, if necessary, to obtain accurate temperature
- Assess for symptoms of hypothermia (e.g., skin color changes, shivering, fatigue, weakness, apathy, slurred speech)
- Assess for medical conditions that contribute to hypothermia (e.g., diabetes, myxedema)
- *(NIC) Temperature Regulation:*

  Institute use of a continuous core temperature monitoring device, as appropriate

  Monitor temperature at least every 2 hr, as appropriate

Patient/Family Teaching

- *(NIC) Temperature Regulation:*

  Teach patient, particularly elderly patients, actions to prevent hypothermia from cold exposure

Teach indications of hypothermia and appropriate emergency treatment, as appropriate

Collaborative Activities

- For severe hypothermia, assist with core-warming techniques (e.g., hemodialysis, peritoneal dialysis, colonic irrigation)

Other

- Provide warmth, dry clothing, heated blankets, mechanical heating devices, adjusted room temperature, hot-water bottles, submersion in warm water, and warm oral fluids, as tolerated
- Do not give intramuscular (IM) or subcutaneous medications to hypothermic patient

For intraoperative patient:

- Regulate room temperature to maintain patient's warmth
- Cover patient's head and exposed body parts
- Warm blood before administering
- Cover patient with warm blanket for transport after surgery

Home Care

- Be sure there is a thermometer in the home, that someone can read it, and that it is accurate
- Teach the client or family to take a temperature
- *(NIC) Temperature Regulation:*

  Teach patient, particularly elderly patients, actions to prevent hypothermia from cold exposure

  Teach indications of hypothermia and appropriate emergency treatment, as appropriate

For Infants and Children

- Keep room temperature above 72°F (22.2°C)
- Keep the infant's clothing dry; replace damp clothing as soon as possible
- *(NIC) Temperature Regulation:*

  Monitor newborn's temperature until stabilized

  Wrap infant immediately after birth to prevent heat loss

  Apply stockinette cap to prevent heat loss of newborn

  Place newborn in Isolette or under warmer, as needed

For Older Adults

- Keep room temperature above 70°F (21.1°C); older adults are susceptible to heat loss, so operating room temperatures should also be raised before surgery
- Advise clients to dress warmly if it is not possible to raise room temperature enough—even wearing a jacket, hat, and gloves if necessary
- Assess carefully for confusion and decreased level of consciousness; older adults may not shiver or complain of feeling cold

IDENTITY: PERSONAL, DISTURBED

(1978, 2008) **Domain 6, Self-Perception; Class 1, Self-Concept**

Definition: Inability to maintain an integrated and complete perception of self

Defining Characteristics

Contradictory personal traits
Delusional description of self
Disturbed body image
Gender confusion
Ineffective coping
Ineffective relationships
Ineffective role performance
Reports feelings of emptiness or strangeness
Reports fluctuating feelings about self
Unable to distinguish between inner and outer stimuli
Uncertainty about cultural values (e.g., beliefs, religion, moral questions)
Uncertainty about ideological values (e.g., beliefs, religion, moral questions)

Related Factors

Chronic or situational low self-esteem
Cult indoctrination
Cultural discontinuity
Discrimination
Dysfunctional family processes

Ingestion or inhalation of toxic chemicals
Manic states
Multiple personality disorder
Organic brain syndromes
Perceived prejudice
Psychiatric disorders (e.g., psychoses, depression, dissociative disorder)
Situational crises
Social role change
Stages of growth and/or development
Use of psychoactive pharmaceutical agents

Suggested Alternative Diagnoses

Confusion, acute
Confusion, chronic
Self-esteem, chronic low
Self-esteem, situational low

NOC Outcomes

Distorted Thought Control: Self-restraint of disruptions in perception, thought processes, and thought content
Identity: Distinguishes between self and nonself and characterizes one's essence
Sexual Identity: Acknowledgement and acceptance of own sexual identity

Goals/Evaluation Criteria

Examples Using NOC Language

- Demonstrates **Identity**, as evidenced by the following indicators (specify 1–5: never, rarely, sometimes, often, or consistently demonstrated):
  - Verbalizes clear sense of personal identity
  - Verbalizes affirmations of personal identity
  - Exhibits congruent verbal and nonverbal behavior about self
  - Differentiates self from environment
  - Differentiates self from other human beings
  - Establishes personal boundaries

Other Examples

Patient will:

- Express willingness to use suggested resources on discharge
- Identify personal strengths
- Maintain close personal relationships

NIC Interventions

Delusion Management: Promoting the comfort, safety, and reality orientation of a patient experiencing false, fixed beliefs that have little or no basis in reality

Environmental Management: Manipulation of the patient's surroundings for therapeutic benefit, sensory appeal, and psychological well-being

Hallucination Management: Promoting the safety, comfort, and reality orientation of a patient experiencing hallucinations

Self-Awareness Enhancement: Assisting a patient to explore and understand his thoughts, feelings, motivations, and behaviors

Self-Esteem Enhancement: Assisting a patient to increase his personal judgment of self-worth

Teaching: Sexuality: Assisting individuals to understand physical and psychosocial dimensions of sexual growth and development

Nursing Activities

Also refer to Nursing Activities for Self-Esteem, Chronic Low and Self-Esteem, Situational Low.

Assessments

- Assess need for assistance from social services department for planning care with patient and family
- *(NIC) Self-Esteem Enhancement:*
  Monitor patient's statements of self-worth
  Determine patient's confidence in own judgment
  Monitor frequency of self-negating verbalizations

Patient/Family Teaching

- *(NIC) Delusion Management:* Educate family and significant others about ways to deal with patient who is experiencing delusions

Collaborative Activities

- Offer to make initial phone call to appropriate community resources for patient and family
- Request psychiatric consultation
- *(NIC) Delusion Management:* Administer antipsychotic and antianxiety medications on a routine and as-needed basis

Other

- Encourage patient to verbalize concerns about close personal relationships
- Encourage patient to verbalize consequences of physical and emotional changes that have influenced self-concept

- Encourage patient and family to air feelings and to grieve
- Provide care in a nonjudgmental manner, maintaining the patient's privacy and dignity
- Always address the patient by name
- Involve the patient in decisions about care
- Refrain from talking to others about the patient in his presence; include the patient in the discussion
- *(NIC) Delusion Management:*
  Avoid arguing about false beliefs; state doubt matter-of-factly
  Maintain a consistent daily routine
  Maintain a safe environment
- *(NIC) Self-Esteem Enhancement:*
  Encourage patient to identify strengths
  Provide experiences that increase patient's autonomy, as appropriate
  Refrain from negatively criticizing
  Convey confidence in patient's ability to handle situation
  Encourage the patient to evaluate own behavior

Home Care

- The preceding interventions can be adapted for home care
- Explain to the family ways in which they can provide feedback to the client about ego boundaries
- Refer to counseling and self-help groups as needed; involve the family in checking to see that the client actually attends the group
- Monitor medications
- Obtain psychiatric home health services if client is homebound

For Infants and Children

- *(NIC) Self-Esteem Enhancement:* Instruct parents on the importance of their interest and support in their children's development of a positive self-concept

For Older Adults

- Assess for depression, common in older adults, which may be masked by *Disturbed personal identity*
- Do not use "pet" names (e.g., "dear," or "sweetie")
- Orient the patient to time, place, and person frequently

IDENTITY: PERSONAL, RISK FOR DISTURBED

(2010) **Domain 6, Self-Perception; Class 1, Self-Concept**

Definition: Risk for the inability to maintain an integrated and complete perception of self

Risk Factors

Chronic or situational low self-esteem
Cult indoctrination
Cultural discontinuity
Discrimination
Dysfunctional family processes
Ingestion or inhalation of toxic chemicals
Manic states
Multiple personality disorder
Organic brain syndromes
Perceived prejudice
Psychiatric disorders (e.g., psychoses, depression, dissociative disorder)
Situational crises
Social role change
Stages of growth and/or development
Use of psychoactive pharmaceutical agents

Suggested Alternative Diagnoses

Confusion, acute: risk for
Confusion, chronic
Identity: personal, disturbed
Self-esteem, risk for chronic low
Self-esteem, risk for situational low

NOC Outcomes

NOTE: NOC outcomes have not been linked to this diagnosis. The following may be helpful.

Distorted Thought Self-Control: Self-restraint of disruptions in perception, thought processes, and thought content

Identity: Distinguishes between self and non-self and characterizes ones essence

Self-Esteem: Personal judgment of self-worth

Sexual Identity: Acknowledgement and acceptance of own sexual identity

Goals/Evaluation Criteria

Examples Using NOC Language

See Examples Using NOC Language for the diagnosis *Disturbed personal identity*, preceding.

- Does not develop *Disturbed personal identity*, as demonstrated by Distorted Thought Self-Control, Identity, Self-Esteem, and Sexual Identity.

Other Examples

See Other Examples for the diagnosis *Disturbed personal identity*, preceding.

NIC Interventions

NIC interventions have not been developed for this diagnosis. Select from the NIC Interventions for the diagnosis *Disturbed personal identity*, preceding.

Nursing Activities

Nursing activities should focus on preventing and monitoring for symptoms of *Disturbed personal identity.* Prevention measures must be specific to the patient's risk factors. Select appropriate interventions from the Nursing Activities section for the diagnosis *Disturbed personal identity,* preceding.

IMMUNIZATION STATUS, READINESS FOR ENHANCED

(2006)

Domain 1, Health Promotion; Class 2, Health Management

Definition: A pattern of conforming to local, national, and/or international standards of immunization to prevent infectious disease(s) that is sufficient to protect a person, family, or community and can be strengthened

Defining Characteristics

Expresses desire to enhance:

Behavior to prevent infectious disease

Identification of possible problems associated with immunizations

Identification of providers of immunizations

Immunization status

Knowledge of immunization standards
Record-keeping of immunizations

Related Factors

This is a wellness diagnosis, so an etiology is not necessary.

Suggested Alternative Diagnoses

None

NOC Outcomes

Immunization Behavior: Personal actions to obtain immunization to prevent a communicable disease

Risk Control: Personal actions to prevent, eliminate, or reduce modifiable health threats

Goals/Evaluation Criteria

Examples Using NOC Language

- Demonstrates **Immunization Behavior** as evidenced by the following indicators (specify 1–5: never, rarely, sometimes, often, or consistently demonstrated):
  - Describes risks associated with specific immunization
  - Obtains immunizations recommended for age, chronic illness, and/or occupational risk by the American Academy of Pediatrics or United States Public Health Service
  - Identifies community resources for immunization
  - Describes relief measures for vaccine side effects

NIC Interventions

Immunization/Vaccination Management: Monitoring immunization status, facilitating access to immunizations, and providing of immunizations to prevent communicable disease

Nursing Activities

Assessments

- Obtain medical history, including history of allergies
- Assess immunization status at each health visit
- Assess patient's knowledge about recommended immunization schedules
- Assess for contraindications to specific vaccines

Patient/Family Teaching

- *(NIC) Immunization/Vaccination Management:*
  Inform individuals of immunization protective against illness but not presently required by law (e.g., influenza, pneumococcal, and hepatitis B vaccinations)
  Teach individual/families about vaccinations available in the event of special incidence and/or exposure (e.g., cholera, influenza, plague, rabies, Rocky Mountain spotted fever, smallpox, typhoid fever, typhus, yellow fever, and tuberculosis)
  Inform travelers of vaccinations appropriate for travel to foreign countries
  Provide and update diary for recording date and type of immunizations

Collaborative Activities

- Follow appropriate guidelines for immunizations (e.g., American Academy of Pediatrics, U.S. Public Health Service, and American Academy of Family Physicians)

Other

- Notify the patient when immunizations are not up to date
- Obtain informed consent before administering a vaccine
- Observe the client for the specified period after giving a vaccine

Home Care

- This is a wellness diagnosis, so all of the interventions apply to home care

For Infants and Children

- *(NIC) Immunization/Vaccination Management:*
  Teach parents recommended immunizations necessary for children, their routes of medication administration, reasons and benefits of use, adverse reactions, and side effects schedule (e.g., hepatitis B, diphtheria, tetanus, pertussis, *Haemophilus influenzae*, polio, measles, mumps, rubella, and varicella)
  Inform families which immunizations are required by law for entering preschool, kindergarten, junior high, high school, and college
  Audit school immunization records for completeness on a yearly basis
  Identify providers who participate in federal "Vaccine for Children" program to provide free vaccines
  Inform parents of comfort measures helpful after medication administration to a child

For Older Adults

- Urge older adults to follow recommended schedule for obtaining influenza and pneumonia vaccines
- Help arrange for transportation to immunization clinics

IMPULSE CONTROL, INEFFECTIVE

(2010) **Domain 5, Perception/Cognition; Class 4, Cognition**

Definition: A pattern of performing rapid, unplanned reactions to internal or external stimuli without regard for the negative consequences of these reactions to the impulsive individual or to others

Defining Characteristics

Acting without thinking
Asking personal questions of others despite their discomfort
Inability to save money or regulate finances
Irritability
Pathological gambling
Sensation seeking
Sexual promiscuity
Sharing personal details inappropriately temper outbursts
Too familiar with strangers
Violence

Related Factors

Anger
Chronic low self-esteem
Codependency
Compunction
Delusion
Denial
Disorder of cognition
Disorder of development
Disorder of mood or personality
Disturbed body image
Economically disadvantaged
Environment that might cause frustration or irritation

Fatigue
Hopelessness
Ineffective coping
Insomnia
Organic brain disorders
Smoker
Social isolation
Stress vulnerability
Substance abuse
Suicidal feeling
Unpleasant physical symptoms

I

Suggestions for Use

Ineffective impulse control may be caused by conditions/diagnoses such as *Chronic low self-esteem*, cognitive disorders, developmental disorders, *Disturbed body image*, *Fatigue*, *Hopelessness*, *Ineffective coping*, *Insomnia*, and *Social isolation*, or it may be a symptom. You will need to identify the focus your outcomes and interventions, as well as choosing the diagnosis with the Defining Characteristics that best fit the patient.

NOC Outcomes

NOC outcomes have not been developed for this diagnosis. The following may be useful.

Distorted Thought Self-Control: Self-restraint of disruptions in perception, thought processes, and thought content

Impulse Self-Control: Self-restraint of compulsive or impulsive behaviors

Social Interaction Skills: Personal behaviors that promote effective relationships

Examples Using NOC Language

- Client will not experience *Ineffective impulse control*, as demonstrated by Distorted Thought Self-Control, Impulse Self-Control, and Social Interaction Skills
- Will demonstrate **Impulse Self-Control**, as evidenced by the following indicators (specify 1–5: never, rarely, sometimes, often, or consistently demonstrated):
  - Identifies harmful impulsive behaviors
  - Identifies consequences of impulsive actions
  - Avoids high-risk situations
  - Controls impulses

Other Examples

- Observes personal boundaries when interacting with others
- Exhibits sensitivity to the feelings and discomfort of others
- Refrains from inappropriate sharing of personal details
- Refrains from gambling
- Refrains from sexual promiscuity
- Controls temper outbursts

NIC Interventions

NIC interventions have not been developed for this diagnosis. The following may be useful.

I

Anger Control Assistance: Facilitation of the expression of anger in an adaptive, nonviolent manner

Behavior Management: Overactivity/Inattention: Provision of a therapeutic milieu that safely accommodates the patient's attention deficit and/or overactivity while promoting optimal function

Impulse Control Training: Assisting the patient to mediate impulsive behavior through application of problem-solving strategies to social and interpersonal situations

Limit Setting: Establishing the parameters of desirable and acceptable patient behavior

Nursing Activities

Assessments

- Assess for underlying causes of impulsive behavior (e.g., low self-esteem, anger, cognitive disorders, developmental delay)
- Determine the patient's cognitive baseline and developmental level
- Observe for inappropriate expressions of anger, inappropriate personal sharing, and other signs and symptoms of *Ineffective impulse control*

Patient/Family Teaching

- *(NIC) Behavior Management: Overactivity/Inattention:*
  Instruct in problem-solving skills
  Teach/reinforce appropriate social skills

Collaborative Activities

Administer medications as needed (e.g., for hyperactivity)

Other

Set limits with the patient
Do not argue with the patient
Assist the person to recognize when she is feeling angry or frustrated

Remind the person that a feeling is a signal to stop and think (and maybe use words), not a signal to act
Provide practice in expressing feelings with words rather than aggressive behavior
Provide opportunities for the patient to practice problem solving and encourage the patient to practice in situations outside the therapeutic environment
Provide positive reinforcement (e.g., praise efforts at self-control)
Help the patient to evaluate the outcomes of a chosen course of action

INFANT BEHAVIOR, DISORGANIZED

(1994, 1998) **Domain 9, Coping/Stress Tolerance; Class 3, Neurobehavioral Stress**

Definition: Disintegrated physiological and neurobehavioral responses of infant to the environment

Defining Characteristics

Attention-Interaction System

Abnormal response to sensory stimuli (e.g., difficult to soothe, inability to sustain alert status)

Motor System

Altered primitive reflexes
Finger splay, fisting, or hands to face
Hyperextension of arms and legs
Increased, decreased, or limp motor tone
Jittery
Tremors, startles, twitches
Uncoordinated movement

Physiological

Bradycardia, tachycardia, or arrhythmias
[Bradypnea, tachypnea, apnea]
Desaturation [oximetry reading]
Feeding intolerances [e.g., aspiration or emesis]
Skin color changes [e.g., pale, cyanotic, mottled, or flushed color]
"Time-out" signals (e.g., gaze, grasp, hiccough, cough, sneeze, sigh, slack jaw, open mouth, tongue thrust)

Regulatory Problems

Inability to inhibit startle
Irritability

State-Organization System

Active–awake (fussy, worried gaze)
Diffuse sleep, state oscillation
Irritable crying
Quiet–awake (staring, gaze aversion)

Related Factors

I

Caregiver

Cue misreading
Deficient knowledge regarding behavioral cues
Environmental stimulation contribution

Environmental

Lack of containment within the environment
Physical environment inappropriateness
Sensory deprivation or overstimulation
Sensory inappropriateness

Individual

Illness
Immature neurologic system
Low postconceptual age
Prematurity

Prenatal

Congenital or genetic disorders
Teratogenic exposure

Postnatal

Feeding intolerance
Invasive procedures
Malnutrition
Oral or motor problems
Pain

Suggestions for Use

This diagnosis is most useful for infants, especially premature infants, in neonatal intensive care units. Immature neurologic development and increased or noxious environmental stimuli create a situation in which the infant must use energy for adaptation rather than for growth and development.

Suggested Alternative Diagnoses

Development: delayed, risk for
Growth, disproportionate, risk for
Growth and development, delayed
Infant behavior: disorganized, risk for
Thermoregulation, ineffective

NOC Outcomes

Child Development: 1 month and 2 months: Milestones of physical, cognitive, and psychosocial progression by 1 month and 2 months of age. [**NOTE:** NOC lists these separately for each age group.]

Neurologic Status: Ability of the peripheral and central nervous systems to receive, process, and respond to internal and external stimuli

Preterm Infant Organization: Extrauterine integration of physiological and behavioral function by the infant born 24–37 (term) weeks' gestation

Sleep: Natural periodic suspension of consciousness during which the body is restored

Thermoregulation, Newborn: Balance among heat production, heat gain, and heat loss during the first 28 days of life

Goals/Evaluation Criteria

Examples Using NOC Language

- **Neurologic Status** is normal, as evidenced by the following indicators (specify 1–5: severely, substantially, moderately, mildly, or not compromised):
  - Consciousness, central motor control, cranial sensory or motor function, spinal sensory and motor function, and autonomic function
  - Breathing pattern
  - Sleep–rest pattern
- **Thermoregulation** is not compromised, as evidenced by the following indicators (specify 1–5: severe, substantial, moderate, mild, or none):
  - Increased skin temperature
  - Decreased skin temperature
  - Skin color changes

Hyperthermia and hypothermia
Muscle twitching

Other Examples

Infant will:

- Experience no seizure activity
- Experience no restlessness or lethargy
- Exhibit organized neurobehavioral functioning in all systems
- Utilize nonshivering thermogenesis
- Demonstrate no delay from expected range of development: 1 month (e.g., holds head erect momentarily) and 2 months (e.g., displays some head control in upright position). **NOTE:** Refer to a child development or pediatrics text for a comprehensive list of developmental milestones for each age.
- Exhibit adequate muscle function (e.g., tone and contraction of muscle; control, steadiness, and speed of muscle movement)

Parent/caregiver will:

- Recognize infant behavioral cues that communicate stress
- Modify the environment in response to infant's behaviors
- Demonstrate appropriate handling techniques to enhance normal development

NIC Interventions

Developmental Care: Structuring the environment and providing care in response to the behavioral cues and states of the preterm infant

Environmental Management: Manipulation of the patient's surroundings for therapeutic benefit, sensory appeal, and psychological well-being

Infant Care: Provision of developmentally appropriate family-centered care to the child under 1 year of age

Neurologic Monitoring: Collection and analysis of patient data to prevent or minimize neurological complications

Newborn Care: Management of neonate during the transition to extrauterine life and subsequent period of stabilization

Newborn Monitoring: Measurement and interpretation of physiologic status of the neonate the first 24 hr after delivery

Positioning: Deliberative placement of the patient or a body part to promote physiological and psychological well-being

Sleep Enhancement: Facilitation of regular sleep–wake cycles

Temperature Regulation: Attaining or maintaining body temperature within a normal range

Nursing Activities

Assessments

- Determine whether infant is achieving developmental milestones
- Monitor for signs of stress and maladaptation
- Identify infant's self-regulatory behaviors (e.g., sucking, hand-to-mouth movements)
- Observe for causative external environmental factors (e.g., lights, handling, noise)
- Assess for causative internal factors, such as pain and hunger
- Monitor sleep pattern

Patient/Family Teaching

- Teach parents about infant's needs and abilities
- Demonstrate gentle handling of the baby
- Model appropriate response to infant's behavioral cues
- Instruct parents on normal growth and development
- Prepare parents for skills needed to care for a preterm infant (e.g., feeding, skin care)

Other

- Use sheepskin, water bed, or other protective mattress or pad for infants who do not tolerate frequent position changes
- Encourage parents to hold infant and participate in care to the extent possible
- Provide a consistent caregiver
- Help parents to identify their infant's capabilities and limitations
- Observe for signs of pain and intervene aggressively to treat pain or remove painful stimuli (e.g., medicate with analgesics before painful procedures)
- Space interventions and handling to allow infant to have uninterrupted sleep for 3–4 hr at a time
- Position infant in correct body alignment
- Provide boundaries (e.g., swaddle, hold close) during all treatments and activities
- *(NIC) Environmental Management:*

  Avoid unnecessary exposure, drafts, overheating, or chilling

  Control or prevent undesirable or excessive noise, when possible

  Reduce environmental stimuli, as appropriate [e.g., speak in a soft tone at the bedside, limit conversation, open and close incubator slowly and quietly, do not tap on incubator, place rolled blankets near infant's head to absorb sound; cover incubator or warmer during sleep periods]

Home Care

- Although this nursing diagnosis is especially useful for preterm infants in NICUs, the preceding interventions can also be adapted for use in home care after the infant leaves the hospital.
- Assess the home environment for a balance of stimuli (e.g., light, sound) to prevent sensory overload and sensory deprivation
- Help parents locate parent support groups in the community

INFANT BEHAVIOR: DISORGANIZED, RISK FOR

(1994) **Domain 9, Coping/Stress Tolerance; Class 3, Neurobehavioral Stress**

Definition: At risk for alteration in integrating and modulating of the physiologic and behavioral systems of functioning (i.e., autonomic, motor, state-organization, self-regulatory, and attentional–interactional systems)

Risk Factors

Environmental overstimulation
Invasive or painful procedures
Lack of containment within environment
Motor problems
Oral problems
Painful procedures
Prematurity

Suggestions for Use

This diagnosis is most useful for infants, especially premature infants, in neonatal intensive care units. Immature neurologic development and increased or noxious environmental stimuli create the risk for a situation in which the infant must use energy for adaptation rather than for growth and development.

Suggested Alternative Diagnoses

Disorganized infant behavior
Development: delayed, risk for
Growth, disproportionate, risk for
Growth and development, delayed
Infant behavior: organized, readiness for enhanced
Thermoregulation, ineffective

NOC Outcomes

Child Development: 1 month, 2 months, 4 months, 6 months, and 12 months: Milestones of physical, cognitive, and psychosocial progression by 1, 2, 4, 6, and 12 months of age [**NOTE:** NOC lists a separate outcome for each age group.]

Coordinated Movement: Ability of muscles to work together voluntarily for purposeful movement

Knowledge: Infant Care: Extent of understanding conveyed about caring for a baby from birth to first birthday

Knowledge: Preterm Infant Care: Extent of understanding conveyed about the care of a premature infant born 24 to 37 weeks' (term) gestation

Neurological Status: Ability of the peripheral and central nervous system to receive, process, and respond to internal and external stimuli

Preterm Infant Organization: Extrauterine integration of physiologic and behavioral function by the infant born 24 to 37 (term) weeks' gestation

Goals/Evaluation Criteria

Refer to Goals/Evaluation Criteria for Disorganized Infant Behavior.

NIC Interventions

Developmental Care: Structuring the environment and providing care in response to the behavioral cues and states of the preterm infant

Environmental Management: Attachment Process: Manipulation of the patient's surroundings to facilitate the development of the parent–infant relationship

Environmental Management: Comfort: Manipulation of the patient's surroundings for promotion of optimal comfort

Infant Care: Provision of developmentally appropriate family-centered care to the child under 1 year of age

Kangaroo Care: Promoting closeness between parent and physiologically stable preterm infant by preparing the parent and providing the environment for skin-to-skin contact

Neurologic Monitoring: Collection and analysis of patient data to prevent or minimize neurologic complications

Newborn Monitoring: Measurement and interpretation of physiologic status of the neonate the first 24 hr after delivery

Positioning: Deliberative placement of the patient or a body part to promote physiological and psychological well-being

Risk Identification: Analysis of potential risk factors, determination of health risks, and prioritization of risk-reduction strategies for an individual or group

Surveillance: Purposeful and ongoing acquisition, interpretation, and synthesis of patient data for clinical decision making

Teaching: Infant Safety:0–3, 4–6, 7–9, and 10–12 months: Instruction on safety during first year of life

Teaching: Infant Stimulation (0–4 months, 5–8 months, and 9–12 months): Teaching parents and caregivers to provide developmentally appropriate sensory activities to promote development and movement [during the first year of life]

Nursing Activities

Refer to Nursing Activities for Infant Behavior, Disorganized

I

Assessment

The following assessments should be performed the first 24 hr after delivery:

- *(NIC) Newborn Monitoring:*
  - Perform Apgar evaluation at 1 and 5 min after birth
  - Monitor newborn's temperature, until stabilized
  - Monitor respiratory rate and breathing pattern
  - Monitor respiratory status, noting signs of respiratory distress: tachypnea, nasal flaring, grunting, retractions, rhonchi, or rales
  - Monitor for respiratory distress, hypoglycemia, and anomalies, if mother has diabetes
  - Monitor newborn's color
  - Monitor for signs of hyperbilirubinemia
  - Infant's ability to suck
  - Monitor newborn's first feeding
  - Newborn's weight
  - Record newborn's first voiding and bowel movement
  - Monitor umbilical cord
  - Monitor male newborn's response to circumcision

INFANT BEHAVIOR: ORGANIZED, READINESS FOR ENHANCED

(1994) **Domain 9, Coping/Stress Tolerance; Class 3, Neurobehavioral Stress**

Definition: A pattern of modulation of the physiologic and behavioral systems of functioning (i.e., autonomic, motor, state-organizational, self-regulatory, and attentional-interactional systems) in an infant that is sufficient for well-being and can be improved

Defining Characteristics

Objective

Definite sleep–wake states
Response to stimuli (e.g., visual and auditory)
Stable physiological measures
Use of some self-regulatory behaviors

Related Factors

This is a wellness diagnosis; no etiology is needed in the diagnostic statement

Suggested Alternative Diagnoses

Infant behavior, disorganized, risk for

NOC Outcomes

Child Development: 1 Month, 2 Months, 4 Months, 6 Months, and 12 Months: Milestones of physical, cognitive, and psychosocial progression by 1 month, 2 months, and 4 months of age [**NOTE:** NOC lists a separate outcome for each age group.]

Newborn Adaptation: Adaptive response to the extrauterine environment by a physiologically mature newborn during the first 28 days

Sleep: Natural periodic suspension of consciousness during which the body is restored

Goals/Evaluation Criteria

See Goals/Evaluation Criteria for Disorganized Infant Behavior.

Examples Using NOC Language

- Demonstrates no delay from expected range of **Child Development (1, 2, 4, 6, and 12 Months)** [**NOTE:** Refer to pediatrics or child development text or NOC manual for specific examples of normal growth and development in each age group.]

Other Examples

Infant will:

- Have blood glucose within normal limits
- Demonstrate no maladaptive or abnormal compensatory behaviors
- Have normal pattern, amount, and quality of sleep
- Be wakeful at appropriate times

NIC Interventions

Anticipatory Guidance: Preparation of patient for an anticipated developmental and/or situational crisis

Health Screening: Detecting health risks or problems by means of history, examination, and other procedures

Infant Care: Provision of developmentally appropriate family-centered care to the child under 1 year of age

Newborn Care: Management of neonate during the transition to extrauterine life and subsequent period of stabilization

Newborn Monitoring: Measurement and interpretation of physiologic status of the neonate the first 24 hr after delivery

Parent Education: Infant: Instruction on nurturing and physical care needed during the first year of life

Sleep Enhancement: Facilitation of regular sleep–wake cycles

Nursing Activities

Assessments

- Monitor infant's pattern and amount of sleep
- Assess ability to regulate all physical and behavioral systems (e.g., cardiac, respiratory, sleep–wake states, reciprocal interactions, self-regulatory)

Patient/Family Teaching

- Teach family measures to promote sleep (e.g., comforting behaviors, lifestyle changes, consistent schedules)
- Review the developmental needs of infants (e.g., stimulation, sleep requirements)
- Help parents identify the infant's signs of overstimulation and stress
- Role-model and teach parents to provide age-appropriate auditory, visual, tactile, vestibular, and gustatory stimulation daily; some examples are the following:

  Auditory: Classical music; high-pitched, melodic speaking

  Visual: Face-to-face positioning with eye contact; mobiles and toys in black, white, and red contrasting colors

  Tactile: Skin-to-skin contact; massage; firm, gentle touch

Vestibular: Rocking
Gustatory: Pacifier, sucking fingers (nonnutritive sucking)

- Explain that developmental stimulation should occur when infant is alert
- Teach parents to provide developmental stimulation frequently and for short periods rather than long periods
- Role-model and teach parents to use gentle touch; a soft, melodic tone of voice; and mutual gazing
- Teach parents to respond to all of the infant's vocalizations

Collaborative Activities

- Schedule medications and treatments to support infant's sleep pattern
- Advocate for policies that allow significant others to be present as much as desired

Other

- Adjust environment (e.g., light, noise, temperature, mattress, and bed) to promote sleep
- Maintain infant's usual bedtime routines (e.g., rocking, pacifier)
- Use massage, positioning, and touch to relax infant and promote sleep
- Schedule treatments to minimize interference with infant's sleep (allow cycle of at least 90 min)
- Support the infant's self-regulatory behaviors (e.g., hand-to-mouth movements, sucking on fingers, limb flexion) for coping with environmental stimuli
- *(NIC) Infant Care*
  Feed infant foods that are developmentally appropriate
  Keep side rails up when not caring for infant
  Talk to infant while giving care
  Comfort infant after painful procedures
  Encourage family visitation
  Maintain infant's daily routine during hospitalization

Home Care

- The preceding interventions are appropriate for home care

INFANT FEEDING PATTERN, INEFFECTIVE

(1992, 2006) Domain 2, Nutrition; Class 1, Ingestion

Definition: Impaired ability of an infant to suck or coordinate the suck/swallow response resulting in inadequate oral nutrition for metabolic needs

Defining Characteristics

Objective

Inability to coordinate sucking, swallowing, and breathing
Inability to initiate or sustain an effective suck

Related Factors

Anatomical abnormality
Neurologic impairment or delay
Oral hypersensitivity
Prematurity
Prolonged NPO

Suggestions for Use

This label describes a baby with sucking or swallowing difficulties. It focuses on the nutritional needs of the infant rather than the mother–baby interaction. The goal of nursing activities is to prevent weight loss or promote weight gain. Use the defining characteristics in Table 3 (under Breastfeeding, Ineffective) to discriminate among this label and the suggested alternative diagnoses. If inadequate nutrition is caused by factors other than a feeding problem, use the diagnosis *Imbalanced nutrition*.

Suggested Alternative Diagnoses

Breastfeeding, ineffective
Breastfeeding, interrupted
Growth, disproportionate, risk for
Nutrition, imbalanced: less than body requirements

NOC Outcomes

Breastfeeding Establishment: Infant: Infant attachment to and sucking from the mother's breast for nourishment during the first 3 weeks of breastfeeding

Breastfeeding Maintenance: Continuation of breastfeeding for nourishment of an infant/toddler

Swallowing Status: Oral Phase: Preparation, containment, and posterior movement of fluids and/or solids in the mouth

Goals/Evaluation Criteria

Examples Using NOC Language

- Demonstrates **Breastfeeding Establishment: Infant**, as evidenced by the following indicators (specify 1–5: not, slightly, moderately, substantially, or totally adequate):
  - Proper alignment and latch on
  - Proper areolar grasp and compression
  - Correct suck and tongue placement
  - Audible swallow
  - Urinations per day appropriate for age
- Demonstrates **Breastfeeding Maintenance**, as evidenced by the following indicators (specify 1–5: not, slightly, moderately, substantially, or totally adequate):
- Infant's growth and development in normal range
- Techniques to prevent breast tenderness

Other Examples

- Infant coordinates suck and swallow with respirations while maintaining heart rate and color
- Oral food and fluid intake are adequate

NIC Interventions

Bottle Feeding: Preparation and administration of fluids to an infant via a bottle

Breastfeeding Assistance: Preparing a new mother to breast-feed her infant

Lactation Counseling: Use of an interactive helping process to assist in maintenance of successful breastfeeding

Nonnutritive Sucking: Provision of sucking opportunities for infant

Nutritional Monitoring: Collection and analysis of patient data to prevent or minimize malnourishment

Parent Education: Infant: Instruction on nurturing and physical care needed during the first year of life

Nursing Activities

Assessments

- Assess infant's readiness for nipple feeding:
  - Coordination of sucking, swallowing, and breathing (34 weeks)
  - Presence of gag reflex (32 weeks)
  - Presence of mature sucking reflex (32–34 weeks)
  - Presence of rooting reflex (28–36 weeks)

- Assess daily whether the infant is ready to advance. Consider a feeding flow sheet to facilitate assessment; document infant's state, oxygen needs, preferred nipple, position, formula type and temperature, amount of feeding taken in first 10 min, total feeding, total feeding time, daily weight, and stool pattern
- At each feeding, assess infant's nipple feeding skills by evaluating if infant:
  - Actively initiates swallow in coordination with suck
  - Actively sucks liquid from bottle
  - Completes feeding in acceptable time
  - Coordinates sucking, swallowing, and breathing
  - Loses minimal liquid from mouth
- At each feeding, assess respiratory function and behavioral state and monitor infant for problems such as regurgitation, abdominal distention, and increased residuals
- If infant must be tube-fed:
  - Monitor for proper placement of the tube (e.g., check for gastric residual or follow appropriate protocol)
  - Monitor for presence of bowel sounds
- *(NIC) Lactation Counseling:*
  - Determine knowledge base about breastfeeding
  - Determine mother's desire and motivation to breast-feed
  - Evaluate mother's understanding of infant's feeding cues (e.g., rooting, sucking, alertness)
  - Monitor maternal skill with latching infant to the nipple

Patient/Family Teaching

- Teach the following to increase success with nipple feeding:
  - Avoid techniques that interrupt infant's learning by allowing passive flow of liquid without infant's active participation (e.g., jiggling bottle, moving nipple up and down, moving nipple in and out of infant's mouth, moving infant's jaw up and down)
  - Burp the infant frequently
  - Choose the most appropriate nipple (consider size, shape, firmness, size of hole)
  - Consider varying formula (e.g., by thickness, taste, temperature)
  - Calm the infant prior to feeding; during feeding, remove nipple at first sign of respiratory or state changes
  - Feed the premature infant when fully alert and eager
  - Overfill bottle above amount of scheduled feeding to make sucking easier and to minimize sucking of air
  - Position the infant in a semiupright position with head slightly forward and chin tilting down

Provide consistent caregivers to better read infant's cues and facilitate infant learning; involve mother at earliest opportunity
Remain relaxed and patient during feeding, allow brief rest periods, pace the infant to complete feeding in appropriate time (too quickly may compromise safety, too slowly may increase fatigue and calorie expenditure)
Use facilitation techniques (e.g., prior to feeding, increase oral sensitivity by stroking the infant's lips, cheeks, and tongue; during feeding, place your fingers on each cheek and under the jaw midway between the chin and throat to provide inward and forward support of the cheeks and tongue)

- If infant must be tube-fed, inform parents on importance of meeting infant sucking needs
- *(NIC) Lactation Counseling:*
  Demonstrate suck training, as appropriate
  Instruct about infant's stool and urination patterns, as appropriate
  Instruct on signs of problems to report to health care practitioner

Collaborative Activities

- Establish support network to ensure that mother has help with day-to-day lactation or breastfeeding problems as they occur
- Refer to a lactation specialist or breastfeeding support group, as needed
- Refer to a physical or occupational therapist any infant who is not progressing with feeding or has structural or oral motor defects
- If infant cannot maintain oral nutrition, provide enteral tube feedings, according to protocol
- Consult with physician or nutritionist regarding type and strength of enteral feeding

Other

- Arrange for home visit within 72 hr of discharge
- Determine most appropriate feeding method (e.g., nipple feeding; intermittent gavage; continuous feeding with nasogastric [NG] tube, jejunal tube, or gastrostomy)
- If infant must be tube-fed:
  Elevate head of the bed or hold infant during feedings
  Offer pacifier to infant during feeding
  Talk to infant during feeding
  Perform daily skin care around feeding device, keep feeding site dry
  Change feeding containers and tubing every 24 hr

Home Care

- The preceding interventions can be used in home-based care
- If feeding problems are present or suspected before discharge from hospital, refer the family to community resources for early interventions
- Teach parents how to monitor intake, output, and hydration status

INFECTION, RISK FOR

(1986, 2010) **Domain 11, Safety/Protection; Class 1, Infection**

Definition: At increased risk for being invaded by pathogenic organisms

Risk Factors

Chronic disease (e.g., diabetes mellitus, obesity)
Deficient knowledge to avoid exposure to pathogens
Inadequate primary defenses
Altered peristalsis
Broken skin (e.g., intravenous catheter placement, invasive procedures)
Change in pH of secretions
Decrease in ciliary action
Premature rupture of amniotic membranes
Prolonged rupture of amniotic membranes
Smoking
Stasis of body fluids
Traumatized tissue (e.g., trauma, tissue destruction)
Inadequate secondary defenses
Decreased hemoglobin
Immunosuppression (e.g., inadequate acquired immunity; pharmaceutical agents including immunosuppressants, steroids, monoclonal antibodies, immunomodulators)
Leukopenia
Suppressed inflammatory response
Inadequate vaccination
Increased environmental exposure to pathogens (e.g., outbreaks)
Invasive procedures
Malnutrition

Suggestions for Use

Do not use this label routinely for patients with surgical incisions. For the common surgical population, maintaining routine standards of care will prevent incision infection. Likewise, do not use *Risk for infection* routinely for patients who have an indwelling catheter. Aseptic technique is expected. Everyone is, in a sense, at risk for infection. Therefore, use this nursing diagnosis only for those patients who are at higher than "usual" risk, for example, those with nutritional deficits or compromised immune systems. For patients with actual infection, use a collaborative problem (e.g., Potential Complication: sepsis).

Suggested Alternative Diagnoses

Injury, risk for
Nutrition, imbalanced: less than body requirements
Protection, ineffective
Skin integrity, impaired
Tissue integrity, impaired

NOC Outcomes

Community Risk Control: Communicable Disease: Community actions to eliminate or reduce the spread of infectious agents that threaten public health

Immune Status: Natural and acquired appropriately targeted resistance to internal and external antigens

Infection Severity: Severity of infection and associated symptoms

Infection Severity: Newborn: Severity of infection and associated symptoms during the first 28 days of life

Risk Control: Infectious Process: Personal actions to prevent, eliminate, or reduce the threat of infection

Risk Control: Sexually Transmitted Diseases (STD): Personal actions to prevent, eliminate, or reduce behaviors associated with sexually transmitted diseases

Wound Healing: Primary Intention: Extent of regeneration of cells and tissue following intentional closure

Wound Healing: Secondary Intention: Extent of regeneration of cells and tissue in an open wound

Goals/Evaluation Criteria

Examples Using NOC Language

- Risk factors for infection will be eliminated as evidenced by Community Risk Control: Communicable Disease; Immune Status; Risk Control: Infectious Process; Risk Control: Sexually Transmitted Diseases; and Wound Healing: Primary and Secondary Intention

- Patient will demonstrate **Risk Control: Sexually Transmitted Diseases (STD)**, as evidenced by the following indicators (specify 1–5: never, rarely, sometimes, often, or consistently demonstrated):
  Monitors personal behaviors for STD exposure risk
  Follows selected exposure control strategies
  Uses methods to control STD transmission

Other Examples

Patient/family will:

- Be free of signs and symptoms of infection
- Demonstrate adequate personal hygiene
- Indicate gastrointestinal, respiratory, genitourinary, and immune status within normal limits
- Describe factors contributing to infection transmission
- Report signs and symptoms of infection and follow screening and monitoring procedures

NIC Interventions

Communicable Disease Management: Working with a community to decrease and manage the incidence and prevalence of contagious diseases in a specific population

Immunization/Vaccination Management: Monitoring immunization status, facilitating access to immunizations, and providing immunizations to prevent communicable disease

Incision Site Care: Cleansing, monitoring, and promotion of healing in a wound that is closed with sutures, clips, or staples

Infection Control: Minimizing the acquisition and transmission of infectious agents

Infection Protection: Prevention and early detection of infection in a patient at risk

Surveillance: Purposeful and ongoing acquisition, interpretation, and synthesis of patient data for clinical decision making

Teaching: Safe Sex: Providing instruction concerning sexual protection during sexual activity

Tube Care: Urinary: Management of a patient with urinary drainage equipment

Wound Care: Prevention of wound complications and promotion of wound healing

Nursing Activities

Assessments

- Monitor for signs and symptoms of infection (e.g., temperature, pulse rate, drainage, appearance of wound, secretions, appearance of urine, skin temperature, skin lesions, fatigue, malaise)

- Assess for factors that increase vulnerability to infection (e.g., advanced age, age younger than 1 year, immunocompromise, malnutrition)
- Monitor laboratory values (e.g., CBC, absolute granulocyte count, differential results, cultures, serum protein, and albumin)
- Observe performance of personal hygiene practices to protect against infection

Patient/Family Teaching

- Explain to patient and family why illness or therapy increases the risk for infection
- Instruct on performance of personal hygiene practices (e.g., handwashing) to protect against infection
- Explain rationale and benefits for and side effects of immunizations
- Provide patient and family a method for keeping a record of immunizations (e.g., form, diary)
- *(NIC) Infection Control:*
  Instruct patient on appropriate handwashing techniques
  Instruct visitors to wash hands on entering and leaving the patient's room

Collaborative Activities

- Follow agency protocol for reporting suspected infections or positive cultures
- *(NIC) Infection Control:* Administer antibiotic therapy, as appropriate

Other

- Protect patient from cross-contamination by not assigning same nurse to another patient with an infection and not rooming patient with an infected patient
- *(NIC) Infection Control:*
  Clean the environment appropriately after each patient use
  Maintain isolation techniques, as appropriate
  Institute universal precautions
  Limit the number of visitors, as appropriate

Home Care

- Teach basic hygiene measures such as handwashing, not sharing towels and cups.
- Teach safe methods of food handling, preparation, or storage
- Help patient and family identify factors in their environment, lifestyle, or health practices that increase risk of infection
- Teach family how to dispose of soiled dressings and other biological wastes
- Do not make a home visit if you are ill

- Refer patient and family to social services or community resources to assist in managing home hygiene and nutrition
- *(NIC) Infection Control:* Teach patient and family about signs and symptoms of infection and when to report them to the health care provider

For Infants and Children

- Teach parents recommended immunization schedule for diphtheria, tetanus, pertussis, polio, measles, mumps, and rubella
- Refer to social services for help in paying for immunizations (e.g., insurance coverage and health department clinics)
- Monitor for frequent antibiotic use in infants and children; reassure parents that the common cold should not be treated with antibiotics

For Older Adults

- Recognize that as the immune system declines, older adults may not show typical symptoms, even in the presence of serious infections. Observe for a low-grade temperature or confusion
- Refer to a podiatrist for foot care (e.g., ingrown toenails, removal of calluses) beyond trimming toenails
- Recommend influenza and pneumonia immunizations; recommend limiting exposure to other people during peak of the influenza season
- Assess for factors that increase the client's risk for infection (e.g., chronic illness, depression)

INJURY, RISK FOR

(1978) **Domain 11, Safety/Protection; Class 2, Physical Injury**

Definition: At risk of injury as a result of environmental conditions interacting with the individual's adaptive and defensive resources

Risk Factors

Internal

Abnormal blood profile (e.g., leukocytosis or leucopenia, altered clotting factors, thrombocytopenia, sickle cells, thalassemia, decreased hemoglobin)
Biochemical dysfunction (e.g., sensory dysfunction)
Developmental age (physiological, psychosocial)
Effector dysfunction
Immune or autoimmune disorder
Integrative dysfunction

Malnutrition
Physical (e.g., broken skin, altered mobility)
Psychological (affective orientation)
Sensory dysfunction
Tissue hypoxia

External

Biological (e.g., immunization level of community, microorganisms)
Chemical (e.g., poisons, pollutants, drugs, pharmaceutical agents, alcohol, caffeine, nicotine, preservatives, cosmetics, and dyes)
Human (e.g., nosocomial agents; staffing patterns; cognitive, affective, or psychomotor factors)
Mode of transport or transportation
Nutritional (e.g., vitamins, food types)
Physical (e.g., design, structure, and arrangement of community, building, or equipment)

Suggestions for Use

This is a broad label that includes internal risk factors such as altered clotting factors and decreased hemoglobin. It is important to identify only those patients who are at unusually high risk for this problem. Everyone has at least some risk for accidents and injury, but the label should be used only for those who require nursing intervention to prevent injury.

NOTE: It may be useful to use the label *Disturbed sensory perception* as an etiology for *Risk for injury*.

Several diagnoses describe injury more specifically: *Risk for falls; Latex allergy response; Risk for latex allergy response*; and *Risk for: suffocation, poisoning, trauma, vascular aspiration, reaction to iodinated contrast media, impaired skin integrity, neonatal jaundice,* and *disuse syndrome*. When possible, use these more specific labels instead of *Risk for injury* because they provide clearer direction for nursing care. They need no further specification except for *Risk for trauma*, which includes wounds, burns, and fractures, as well as many other risk factors.

Some nurses use the label *Risk for injury* to describe the potential for such conditions as malignant hyperthermia. It is also sometimes used as a general description for the potential for fetal distress that exists during labor. Those conditions are more usefully described as collaborative problems; however, for nurses who do not use collaborative problems, this text includes goals and nursing interventions for those situations.

Suggested Alternative Diagnoses

Aspiration, risk for
Bleeding, risk for
Falls, risk for
Home maintenance, impaired
Infection, risk for
Latex allergy response
Latex allergy response, risk for
Poisoning, risk for
Protection, ineffective
Suffocation, risk for
Trauma, risk for
Violence: self-directed, risk for

NOC Outcomes

Abuse Protection: Protection of self and/or dependent others from abuse

Falls Occurrence: Number of times an individual falls

Personal Safety Behavior: Personal actions of an adult to control behaviors that can cause physical injury

Physical Injury Severity: Severity of injuries from accidents and trauma

Risk Control: Personal actions to prevent, eliminate, or reduce modifiable health threats

Risk Detection: Personal actions to identify personal health threats

Safe Home Environment: Physical arrangements to minimize environmental factors that might cause physical harm or injury in the home

Sensory Function: Extent to which an individual correctly senses skin stimulation, sounds, proprioception, taste and smell, and visual images

Tissue Integrity: Skin and Mucous Membranes: Structural intactness and normal physiological function of skin and mucous membranes

Goals/Evaluation Criteria

Examples Using NOC Language

- *Risk for injury* will be decreased, as evidenced by Personal Safety Behavior, Risk Control, and Safe Home Environment
- **Risk Control** will be demonstrated, as evidenced by the following indicators (specify 1–5: never, rarely, sometimes, often, or consistently demonstrated):

  Monitors environmental and personal behavior risk factors
  Develops effective risk control strategies
  Follows selected risk control strategies
  Modifies lifestyle to reduce risk

Other Examples

Patient and family will:

- Provide a safe environment (e.g., eliminate clutter and spills, place handrails, and use rubber shower mats and grab bars)
- Identify risks that increase susceptibility to injury
- Avoid physical injury

Parents will:

- Recognize risk of and monitor for abuse
- Screen playmates, caregivers, and other social contacts
- Recognize signs of gang membership and other high-risk social behaviors

I

NIC Interventions

Abuse Protection Support: Identification of high-risk dependent relationships and actions to prevent further infliction of physical or emotional harm

Allergy Management: Identification, treatment, and prevention of allergic responses to food, medications, insect bites, contrast material, blood, and other substances

Environmental Management: Safety: Monitoring and manipulation of the physical environment to promote safety

Fall Prevention: Instituting special precautions with patient at risk for injury from falling [**NOTE:** If a patient requires Falls Prevention, the author recommends using the nursing diagnosis *Risk for falls*.]

Latex Precautions: Reducing the risk of a systemic reaction to latex [**NOTE:** If the patient requires Latex Precautions, use a diagnosis of *Risk for* or actual *Latex allergy response* instead of *Risk for injury*.]

Malignant Hyperthermia Precautions: Prevention or reduction of a hypermetabolic response to pharmacologic agents used during surgery. [**NOTE:** If the patient requires Malignant Hyperthermia Precautions, use a nursing diagnosis of *Risk for hyperthermia* instead of *Risk for injury*.]

Physical Restraint: Application, monitoring, and removal of mechanical restraining devices or manual restraints to limit physical mobility of patient

Pressure Management: Minimizing pressure to body parts

Risk Identification: Analysis of potential risk factors, determination of health risks, and prioritization of risk-reduction strategies for an individual or group

Sports-Injury Prevention: Youth: Reducing the risk of sports-related injury in young athletes

Surveillance: Safety: Purposeful and ongoing collection and analysis of information about the patient and the environment for use in promoting and maintaining patient safety

Nursing Activities

Because this diagnostic label is so broad, nursing activities vary greatly depending on the problem etiology. It is not possible to anticipate every possible nursing activity that might be used for this diagnosis.

Assessments

I

- Identify factors that affect safety needs, for example, changes in mental status, degree of intoxication, fatigue, maturational age, medications, and motor or sensory deficit (e.g., with gait, balance)
- Identify environmental factors that create risk for falls (e.g., slippery floors, throw rugs, open stairways, windows, swimming pools)
- Check patient for presence of constrictive clothing, cuts, burns, or bruises
- Review obstetrical history for pertinent information that may influence induction, such as gestational age and length of prior labor and such contraindications as complete placenta previa, classical uterine incision, and pelvic structural deformities

Patient/Family Teaching

- Instruct patient to use caution in use of heat-therapy devices
- Provide educational materials related to strategies and measures to prevent injury

Collaborative Activities

- Refer to educational classes in the community

Other

- Reorient patient to reality and immediate environment when necessary
- Assist patient with ambulation, as needed
- Provide assistive devices for walking (e.g., cane, walker)
- Use heating devices with caution to prevent burns in patients with sensory deficit
- Use an alarm to alert caretaker when patient is getting out of bed or leaving room
- If necessary, use physical restraints to limit risk of falling
- Place bell or call light within reach of dependent patient at all times
- Instruct patient to call for assistance with movement, as appropriate
- Remove environmental hazards (e.g., provide adequate lighting)

- Make no unnecessary changes in physical environment (e.g., furniture placement)
- Ensure that patient wears proper shoes (e.g., nonskid soles, secure fasteners)

Home Care

- Identify factors that affect safety needs, for example, changes in mental status, degree of intoxication, fatigue, maturational age, medications, and motor or sensory deficit (e.g., with gait, balance)
- Identify environmental factors that create risk for falls (e.g., slippery floors, throw rugs, open stairways, windows, swimming pools)
- Provide information on environmental hazards and characteristics (e.g., stairs, windows, cupboard locks, swimming pools, streets, gates)
- Instruct patient and family in techniques to prevent injury at home, specify techniques
- Make no unnecessary changes in physical environment (e.g., furniture placement)

For Infants and Children

- Institute electronic fetal monitoring during intrapartal care, according to agency protocols
- Raise crib rails when not present at bedside
- For children old enough to climb over bed rails, use a crib with a net or bubble top
- Caution parents about the need to supervise young children when they are around water (e.g., bathtub)
- Teach parents fire and burn safety (e.g., always supervise young children in the kitchen; keep handles of cooking pans turned toward the back of the stove)
- Teach parents the necessity of play safety (e.g., wearing a helmet when riding a bike)
- Teach gun safety to parents and children

For Older Adults

- Teach client to wear glasses and hearing aids and to use assistive devices when walking; be sure these aids are in working order, properly fitted, and so on
- Assess for orthostatic hypotension
- Assess whether client can drive safely and whether his night vision is adequate for driving at night
- Monitor and teach client to monitor blood glucose
- Provide a medical identification bracelet, if needed

INSOMNIA

(2006) Domain 4, Activity/Rest; Class 1, Sleep/Rest

Definition: A disruption in amount and quality of sleep that impairs functioning

Defining Characteristics

Observed changes in affect
Observed lack of energy
Increased work/school absenteeism
Patient reports:
Changes in mood
Decreased health status
Decreased quality of life
Difficulty concentrating
Difficulty falling asleep or staying asleep
Dissatisfaction with sleep (current)
Increased accidents
Lack of energy
Nonrestorative sleep
Sleep disturbances that produce next-day consequences
Waking up too early

Related Factors

Activity pattern (e.g., timing, amount)
Anxiety
Depression
Environmental factors (e.g., ambient noise, daylight/darkness exposure, ambient temperature/humidity, unfamiliar setting)
Fear
Gender-related hormonal shifts
Grief
Impairment of normal sleep pattern (e.g., travel, shift work, parental responsibilities, interruptions for interventions)
Inadequate sleep hygiene (current)
Intake of alcohol
Intake of stimulants
Medications/pharmaceutical agents
Physical discomfort (e.g., body temperature, pain, shortness of breath, cough, gastroesophageal reflux, nausea, incontinence/urgency)
Stress (e.g., ruminative presleep pattern)

Suggestions for Use

Insomnia is used when disruption of sleep causes discomfort or interferes with the patient's desired lifestyle. *Insomnia* is a general diagnosis. The etiologic factors can sometimes make it specific enough to direct nursing intervention, as in *Insomnia related to frequent awakening of infant during the night.* When possible, the specific type of *Insomnia* should be identified (on the problem side of the diagnosis) in order to better direct nursing care. Following are examples of appropriate diagnoses:

Insomnia (early awakening) related to depression

Insomnia (delayed onset of sleep) related to overstimulation prior to bedtime

Suggested Alternative Diagnoses

Activity intolerance

Fatigue

Sleep deprivation

Sleep pattern, disturbed

NOC Outcomes

Fatigue Level: Severity of observed or reported prolonged generalized fatigue

Personal Well-Being: Extent of positive perception of one's health status

Sleep: Natural periodic suspension of consciousness during which the body is restored

Goals/Evaluation Criteria

Examples Using NOC Language

- Patient demonstrates **Sleep**, as evidenced by the following indicators (specify 1–5: severely, substantially, moderately, mildly, or not compromised):
  - Hours of sleep (at least 5 hr/24 hr for adults)
  - Sleep pattern, quality, and routine
  - Feelings of rejuvenation after sleep
  - Wakeful at appropriate times

Other Examples

- Identifies measures that will increase rest or sleep
- Demonstrates physical and psychologic well-being

NIC Interventions

Anxiety Reduction: Minimizing apprehension, dread, foreboding, or uneasiness related to an unidentified source of anticipated danger

Coping Enhancement: Assisting a patient to adapt to perceived stressors, changes, or threats that interfere with meeting life demands and roles

Environmental Management: Manipulation of the patient's surroundings for therapeutic benefit, sensory appeal, and psychological well-being

Energy Management: Regulating energy use to treat or prevent fatigue and optimize function

Mood Management: Providing for safety, stabilization, recovery, and maintenance of a patient who is experiencing dysfunctionally depressed or elevated mood

Pain Management: Alleviation of pain or a reduction in pain to a level of comfort that is acceptable to the patient

I

Sleep Enhancement: Facilitation of regular sleep–wake cycles

Nursing Activities

Assessments

- *(NIC) Sleep Enhancement:*
  - Determine the effects of the patient's medications on sleep pattern
  - Monitor patient's sleep pattern and note physical (e.g., sleep apnea, obstructed airway, pain or discomfort, and urinary frequency) or psychologic (e.g., fear or anxiety) circumstances that interrupt sleep

Patient/Family Teaching

- Explain that alcohol may help the person fall asleep, but that it also decreases sleep quality by causing frequent awakenings and nightmares; advise to avoid alcohol within 4 to 6 hr of bedtime
- Discourage the use of over-the-counter sleeping pills; explain that they interfere with the quality of sleep, cause daytime drowsiness, and lose their effectiveness after a few weeks; advise patient to consult his primary care provider
- *(NIC) Sleep Enhancement:*
  - Explain the importance of adequate sleep during pregnancy, illness, psychosocial stresses, and so on.
  - Instruct patient to avoid bedtime foods and beverages that interfere with sleep
  - Instruct the patient and significant others about factors (e.g., physiologic, psychologic, lifestyle, frequent work-shift changes, rapid time-zone changes, excessively long work hours, and other environmental factors) that contribute to sleep pattern disturbances

Collaborative Activities

- Confer with physician regarding need to revise medication regimen when it interferes with sleep pattern
- Refer to a sleep clinic, if necessary

- *(NIC) Sleep Enhancement:* Encourage use of sleep medications that do not contain REM-sleep suppressor(s)

Other

- Avoid loud noises and use of overhead lights during nighttime sleep, providing a quiet, peaceful environment, and minimizing interruptions
- Find a compatible roommate for the patient, if possible
- Help patient identify possible underlying causes of sleeplessness, such as fear, unresolved problems, and conflicts
- Reassure patient that irritability and mood alterations are common consequences of sleep deprivation
- Assist the client to take a warm bath in the evening
- *(NIC) Sleep Enhancement:*

  Facilitate maintenance of patient's usual bedtime routine, presleep cues or props, and familiar objects (e.g., for children, a favorite blanket or toy, rocking, pacifier, or story; for adults, a book to read), as appropriate

  Assist patient to limit daytime sleep by providing activity that promotes wakefulness, as appropriate

  Initiate or implement comfort measures of massage, positioning, and affective touch

  Provide for naps during the day, if indicated, to meet sleep requirements

  Group care activities to minimize number of awakenings; allow for sleep cycles of at least 90 min

Home Care

- All of the preceding interventions can be adapted for use in home care
- Interview the sleep partner to assess sleep behaviors and possible contributing causes (e.g., ask whether the patient snores)
- Have the client keep a sleep diary
- Teach relaxation techniques

For Infants and Children

- Maintain the child's usual bedtime routine. Provide familiar objects such as a favorite blanket or toy, rocking, or pacifier; read a story; sing to the child; and so on
- Help the child feel comfortable and safe at night: use a nightlight, assure him that you will be close by
- Help the child transition to bedtime by switching him to quieter, less lively activities in the hour before bedtime (e.g., snuggling, reading a story)

For Older Adults

- Because of changes in sleep quality that occur with aging, older adults need more time in bed to achieve a restorative effect. However, actual sleep time decreases with age.
- Be aware that older adults find it more difficult to fall asleep and are more easily awakened than younger adults
- Suggest that the client limit fluid intake in the evening to decrease the possibility of being awakened by the need to void
- Advise the client to take diuretics early in the morning if possible
- Evaluate for depression or anxiety, which are common among older adults
- Assist the client in choosing daytime physical and social activities appropriate to his functional abilities (e.g., walking)
- Advise client to reduce daytime napping, or if naps are needed to take them as early in the day as possible and limit their duration
- Teach clients the changes in sleep that occur with normal aging
- Use a nightlight for safety
- For clients with dementia, help families obtain a hospital-type bed that has side rails and that can be put in a low position
- Consider keeping a commode by the bedside for nighttime use, even if not needed during the daytime

IODINATED CONTRAST MEDIA, RISK FOR ADVERSE REACTION TO

(2010) **Domain 11, Safety/Protection; Class 5, Defensive Processes**

Definition: At risk for any noxious or unintended reaction associated with the use of iodinated contrast media that can occur within 7 days after contrast agent injection

Risk Factors

Anxiety
Concurrent use of medications (e.g., beta-blockers, interleukin-2, metformin, nephrotoxic medications)
Dehydration
Extremes of age
Fragile veins (e.g., prior or actual chemotherapy treatment or radiation in the limb to be injected, multiple attempts to obtain intravenous access, indwelling IV lines in place for more than 24 hr, previous axillary

lymph node dissection in the limb to be injected, distal IV access sites: hand, wrist, foot, ankle)
Generalized debilitation
History of allergies
History of previous adverse effect from iodinated contrast media
Physical and chemical properties of the contrast media (e.g., iodine concentration, viscosity, high osmolality, ion toxicity)
Unconsciousness
Underlying disease (e.g., heart disease, pulmonary disease, blood dyscrasias, endocrine disease, renal disease, pheochromocytoma, autoimmune disease)

Suggestions for Use

Because the independent nursing actions for this diagnosis are primarily for monitoring for risk factors, it may be better stated as a collaborative problem. Many of the risk factors would respond only to collaborative treatment. This diagnosis is very specifically focused on a single allergen and should be used instead of *Risk for allergy response* if risk factors reaction to iodinated contrast media are present.

Suggested Alternative Diagnoses

Allergy response, risk for
Injury, risk for

NOC Outcomes

NOC outcomes have not yet been formally linked to this diagnosis, but the following may be useful:

Allergic Response: Localized: Severity of localized hypersensitive immune response to a specific environmental (exogenous) antigen
Allergic Response: Systemic: Severity of systemic hypersensitive immune response to a specific environmental (exogenous) antigen

Goals/Evaluation Criteria

Examples Using NOC Language

- Will experience no allergy response, as evidenced by exhibiting no Allergic Response: Localized or Systemic.
- Demonstrates no **Allergic Response: Systemic,** as evidenced by the following indicators (specify 1–5: severe, substantial, moderate, mild, or none):
    - Anaphylactic shock
    - Decreased blood pressure
    - Facial edema

Hives
Laryngeal edema
Nausea, vomiting
Tachycardia or dysrhythmias
Wheezing, stridor, or dyspnea at rest

Other Examples

- Will exhibit no hoarseness (sign of laryngeal edema)
- Will not experience seizure activity
- Will not exhibit localized or systemic allergic responses (e.g., skin, respiratory, cardiac, gastrointestinal, musculoskeletal)

I

NIC Interventions

NIC interventions have not yet been formally linked to this diagnosis, but the following may be useful:

Allergy Management: Identification, treatment, and prevention of allergic responses to food, medications, insect bites, contrast material, blood, and other substances

Environmental Management: Manipulation of the patient's surroundings for therapeutic benefit, sensory appeal, and psychological well-being

Medication Administration: Preparing, giving, and evaluating the effectiveness of prescription and nonprescription drugs

Respiratory Monitoring: Collection and analysis of patient data to ensure airway patency and adequate gas exchange

Risk Identification: Analysis of potential risk factors, determination of health risks, and prioritization of risk-reduction strategies for an individual or group

Surveillance: Purposeful and ongoing acquisition, interpretation, and synthesis of patient data for clinical decision making

Tissue Integrity: Skin and Mucous Membranes: Structural intactness and normal physiological function of skin and mucous membranes

Nursing Activities

Nursing activities for this diagnosis focus on assessing for risk factors for reaction to iodinated contrast media, assessing for signs/symptoms of allergic reaction, and notifying the appropriate medical care provider of such findings.

Assessments

- Determine whether there is a history of prior reaction to iodinated contrast agents

- Assess for history of asthma or multiple, severe allergies
  - Assess for risk factors such as underlying disease (e.g., renal insufficiency)
  - Check lab results for serum creatinine and/or estimated glomerular filtration rate
  - Obtain a list of the patient's recent and present medications (e.g., metformin)
  - Observe for symptoms of a reaction to the contrast medium (e.g., hypotension, wheezing, facial edema, hoarseness/laryngeal edema, change in mental status)
  - Observe for extravasation of the medium

Collaborative Activities

- Apply and manage pulse oximetry
- Be certain that oxygen is available. Administer as needed
- Check to be sure that proper equipment is available in the room(s) where a reaction might occur (e.g., mouth-to-mask breather, Code Cart, IV fluids, pulse oximetry)
- Be familiar with the medications in the contrast reaction medication boxes and be ready to assist with administration as needed (e.g., epinephrine, atropine, corticosteroids)

Other

After the procedure:

- Monitor pulse and blood pressure according to protocol
- Auscultate lungs according to protocol
- Monitor pulse oximetry
- Monitor for facial edema and skin color
- Notify the medical care provider immediately if symptoms of reaction are present
- If a reaction occurs, maintain a calm, reassuring demeanor

JAUNDICE, NEONATAL

(2008, 2010) Domain 2, Nutrition; Class 4, Metabolism

Definition: The yellow-orange tint of the neonate's skin and mucous membranes that occurs after 24 hr of life as a result of unconjugated bilirubin in the circulation.

Defining Characteristics

Abnormal blood profile (e.g., hemolysis; total serum bilirubin <2mg/dL; total serum bilirubin in the high-risk range on age in hour-specific nomogram)

Abnormal skin bruising
Yellow mucous membranes
Yellow-orange skin
Yellow sclera

Related factors

Abnormal weight loss (>7%–8% in breastfeeding newborn, 15% in term infant)
Feeding pattern not well established
Infant experiences difficulty making the transition to extrauterine life
Neonate age 1–7 days
Stool (meconium) passage delayed

NOC Outcomes

NOC outcomes have not yet been linked to this nursing diagnosis. The following examples may be useful.

Newborn Adaptation: Adaptive response to the extrauterine environment by a physiologically mature newborn during the first 28 days

Knowledge: Treatment Procedure: Extent of understanding conveyed about a procedure required as part of a treatment regimen

Goals/Evaluation Criteria

Examples Using NOC Language

- Infant will not experience *Neonatal jaundice*, as demonstrated by Newborn Adaptation and parental Knowledge: Treatment Procedure.
- Will demonstrate **Newborn Adaptation** as evidenced by the following indicators (specify 1–5: severe, substantial, moderate, mild, or no deviation from normal range):
    - Bilirubin level
    - Bowel elimination
    - Skin color
    - Suck reflex
    - Weight

Other Examples

- Parents/caregivers will verbalize understanding of the cause, possible outcomes, and treatment for hyperbilirubinemia
- Jaundice resolves and bilirubin levels decrease with phototherapy

NIC Interventions

NIC interventions have not yet been linked to this nursing diagnosis. The following examples may be useful.

Breastfeeding Assistance: Preparing a new mother to breast-feed her infant

Phototherapy: Neonate: Use of light therapy to reduce bilirubin levels in newborn infants

Nursing Activities

Nursing activities focus on identifying and monitoring for improvement in causal/contributing factors; monitoring the neonate's symptoms of neonatal jaundice; providing collaborative and independent interventions for correcting hyperbilirubinemia; and assessing for and preventing side effects of phototherapy.

Assessments

- Review the intrapartal record for risk factors (e.g., prematurity, sepsis, low birth weight, birth trauma, need for resuscitation at birth)
- Assess maternal prenatal nutritional levels, especially with regard to protein intake
- Observe for signs of hypoglycemia (e.g., irritability, jitteriness, lethargy); obtain heelstick glucose levels as indicated
- Assess success of breastfeeding
- Observe for pallor, edema
- Observe the skin for jaundice in natural light. Also observe sclera and oral mucosa
- Note neonate's age at onset of jaundice
- Review lab results (total serum bilirubin and albumin, hemoglobin/hematocrit, and reticulocyte count)
- Observe for behavior changes that may indicate bilirubin toxicity (e.g., lethargy, poor feeding, diminished or absent reflexes, high-pitched cry, twitching, fever, convulsions)
- Evaluate intake and output; and observe for physical signs of dehydration
- Monitor core temperature
- Monitor weight loss

Patient/Family Teaching

- Encourage feeding within 4 to 6 hr after birth
- Encourage mother to breast-feed infant 8 to 12 times a day
- Teach parents/caregivers to not apply lotion or oils to the skin of the neonate receiving phototherapy

Collaborative Activities

- Initiate and manage phototherapy per protocol or primary care provider's prescription

- Apply eye patches during phototherapy to prevent retinal injury. Remove for feedings and other activities
- Administer breast milk substitute for 24 to 48 hr, if indicated/prescribed
- Prepare for and assist with exchange transfusion, if necessary
- Arrange for home phototherapy if necessary
- Make arrangements for follow-up serum bilirubin testing, if necessary

Other

- Keep neonate warm and dry
- Give the parents/caregivers the name and number of a person to contact if jaundice increases or other symptoms are noted

JAUNDICE: NEONATAL, RISK FOR

(2010)

Domain 2, Nutrition; Class 4, Metabolism

Definition: At risk for the yellow-orange tint of the neonate's skin and mucous membranes that occurs after 24 hr of life as a result of unconjugated bilirubin in the circulation

Risk Factors

Abnormal weight loss (>7%–8% in breastfeeding newborn, 15% in term infant)
Feeding pattern not well established
Infant experiences difficulty making the transition to extrauterine life
Neonate age 1–7 days
Prematurity
Stool (meconium) passage delayed

Suggestions for Use

Monitoring skin color, including observing for jaundice, is a routine assessment made for all newborns. Therefore, this diagnosis should be used only for those infants who have one or more of the preceding Risk Factors. Do not use it routinely for all newborns.

NOC Outcomes

NOC outcomes have not yet been linked to this nursing diagnosis. The following examples may be useful.

Newborn Adaptation: Adaptive response to the extrauterine environment by a physiologically mature newborn during the first 28 days

Goals/Evaluation Criteria

Examples Using NOC Language

- Infant will not experience *Neonatal jaundice*, as demonstrated by Newborn Adaptation
- Also see Examples Using NOC Language for the diagnosis *Neonatal Jaundice*

Other Examples

- Parents/caregivers will verbalize understanding of the cause, possible outcomes, and signs and symptoms for hyperbilirubinemia

J

NIC Interventions

NIC interventions have not yet been linked to this nursing diagnosis. The following examples may be useful.

Breastfeeding Assistance: Preparing a new mother to breast-feed her infant

Newborn Care: Management of neonate during the transition to extrauterine life and subsequent period of stabilization

Newborn Monitoring: Measurement and interpretation of physiologic status of the neonate the first 24 hr after delivery

Nursing Activities

Nursing activities focus on identifying and modifying risk factors for *Neonatal jaundice* and monitoring for symptoms of neonatal jaundice (e.g., skin color).

Abnormal weight loss (>7%–8% in breastfeeding newborn, 15% in term infant)

Assessments

- Review the intrapartal record for risk factors (e.g., prematurity, sepsis, low birth weight, birth trauma, need for resuscitation at birth)
- Assess maternal prenatal nutritional levels, especially with regard to protein intake.
- Observe for signs of hypoglycemia (e.g., irritability, jitteriness, lethargy); obtain heelstick glucose levels as indicated
- Assess success of breastfeeding
- Observe the skin for jaundice in natural light. Also observe sclera and oral mucosa.

- Determine neonate's gestational age
- Review lab results (total serum bilirubin and albumin, hemoglobin/hematocrit, and reticulocyte count)
- Evaluate intake and output; and observe for physical signs of dehydration.
- Monitor core temperature
- Monitor weight loss

Patient/Family Teaching

- Encourage feeding within 4 to 6 hr after birth
- Encourage mother to breast-feed infant 8 to 12 times a day

Collaborative Activities

- Administer breast milk substitute for 24 to 48 hr, if indicated/prescribed
- Notify primary care provider of risk factors or of jaundice.

Other

- Keep neonate warm and dry
- Give the parents/caregivers the name and number of a person to contact if jaundice increases of other symptoms are noted

KNOWLEDGE, DEFICIENT (SPECIFY)

(1980) **Domain 5, Perception/Cognition; Class 4, Cognition**

Definition: Absence or deficiency of cognitive information related to specific topic

Defining Characteristics

Subjective

Reports the problem

Objective

Inaccurate follow-through of instruction

Inaccurate performance on tests

Inappropriate or exaggerated behaviors (e.g., hysteria, hostility, agitation, or apathy)

Related Factors

Cognitive limitation

Information misinterpretation

Lack of exposure

Lack of interest in learning
Lack of recall
Unfamiliarity with information resources

Suggestions for Use

The author does not recommend *Deficient knowledge* as a problem label for the following reasons:

- *Deficient knowledge* is not truly a human response. "Response" suggests a behavior or action; *Deficient knowledge* is simply a state of being.
- *Deficient knowledge* does not necessarily describe a health state.
- *Deficient knowledge* does not necessarily describe a problem. Nursing diagnoses should reflect altered functioning, but *Deficient knowledge* simply means the person lacks some knowledge, not that his functioning is changed as a result of that lack of knowledge.

Deficient knowledge can contribute to a number of problem responses, including *Anxiety*, *Impaired parenting*, *Self-care deficit*, or *Ineffective coping*. Therefore, it may be used effectively as the etiology of a nursing diagnosis (e.g., *Risk for injury* [*trauma*] related to lack of knowledge of proper application of seat belts when pregnant or *Anxiety related to lack of knowledge of procedures involved in bone marrow aspiration*).

If *Deficient knowledge* is used as the problem part of a nursing diagnosis, one goal must be "Patient will acquire knowledge about...." This causes the nurse to focus on giving information rather than focusing on the behaviors caused by the patient's lack of knowledge, reinforcing the belief that giving information will change behavior and solve problems. On the other hand, when *Deficient knowledge* is used as an etiology, it focuses attention on behaviors that indicate self-doubt, decisional conflict, anxiety, and so forth. Note the difference in nursing care suggested by the following diagnostic statements:

Deficient knowledge (bone marrow aspiration) related to lack of prior experience

Anxiety related to Deficient knowledge (bone marrow aspiration)

Patient teaching is an important intervention for most patients and for all nursing diagnoses (e.g., *Constipation, Ineffective breastfeeding*). Therefore, it is not necessary, or even desirable, to have a *Deficient knowledge* diagnosis on every patient's care plan. Nurses should include teaching as one of the nursing interventions for all the other diagnoses that they make.

Some patients, such as a newly diagnosed diabetic, require a great deal of teaching in order to acquire necessary self-care skills. Such special teaching plans should be a part of the routine care on standardized care plans for these patients and should not require an individualized nursing diagnosis. However, if the agency does not have a standardized plan or protocol, it will be necessary to write an individualized teaching plan. Even then, *Deficient knowledge* should be used as the etiology of a response, for example, *Risk for ineffective health maintenance (diabetes management) related to Deficient knowledge (medication, diet, exercise, and skin care) secondary to new diagnosis.*

If used at all, *Deficient knowledge* should describe conditions in which the patient needs new or additional knowledge. It should not be used for problems involving the patient's ability to learn (e.g., *Deficient knowledge related to severe anxiety about outcome of surgery*). Rakel and Bulechek (1990) propose a diagnosis of *Situational learning disability: Impaired ability to learn* or *Situational learning disability: Lack of motivation to learn* for such conditions. However, these are not NANDA International labels.

At least two studies have shown that *Deficient knowledge* is one of the diagnoses most frequently used (misused) by nurses (Gordon, 1985; Lambert & Jones, 1989). This may be due in part to premature diagnosing: It is easy to recognize a knowledge deficit, label it as a problem, and not look beyond that to the human response to the lack of knowledge. Misuse of this diagnosis also occurs because of the mistaken belief that information giving effectively changes human behavior.

Suggested Alternative Diagnoses

Coping [individual], ineffective
Denial, ineffective
Health behavior, risk prone
Health maintenance, ineffective
Home maintenance, impaired
Therapeutic regimen management: family, ineffective
Noncompliance (specify)

NOC Outcomes

Knowledge:[specify]: Extent of understanding conveyed about, [e.g.,] Breastfeeding.

[**NOTE:** NOC has 42 Knowledge outcomes: Arthritis Management, Asthma Management, Body Mechanics, Breastfeeding, Cancer Management, Cancer Threat Reduction, Cardiac Disease Management, Child Physical Safety, Conception Prevention, Congestive Heart Failure Management, Depression Management, Diabetes Management, Diet, Disease Process, Energy Conservation, Fall Prevention, Fertility Promotion, Health Behavior, Health Promotion, Health Resources, Hypertension Management, Illness Care, Infant Care, Infection Management, Labor and Delivery, Medication,

Multiple Sclerosis Management, Ostomy Care, Pain Management, Parenting, Personal Safety, Postpartum Maternal Health, Preconception Maternal Health, Pregnancy, Pregnancy and Postpartum Sexual Functioning, Prescribed Activity, Preterm Infant Care, Sexual Functioning, Substance Use Control, Treatment Procedure, Treatment Regimen, and Weight Management. Conceivably, any subject or outcome could be placed after the NOC Knowledge label to create yet another outcome.]

Goals/Evaluation Criteria

Examples Using NOC Language

NOTE: Because this diagnosis is so broad and nonspecific, useful goals will of course reflect the patient's specific knowledge deficit, as in these examples given for *Deficient knowledge* of diet.

- Demonstrates **Knowledge: Diet**, as evidenced by the following indicators (specify 1–5: no, limited, moderate, substantial, or extensive):
  [Description of]:
  Recommended diet
  Rationale for diet
  Food allowed in diet
  Strategies to change dietary habits
  Self-monitoring activities

Other Examples

Patient and family will:

- Identify need for additional information regarding prescribed treatment (e.g., diet information)
- Demonstrate ability to ________________ (specify skill or behavior)

NIC Interventions

NOTE: The following have been linked to the diagnosis *Deficient knowledge*. Other interventions can be found in the NIC domain "Patient Education"—for example, Chemotherapy Management, Learning Facilitation, and Learning Readiness Enhancement.

Asthma Management: Identification, treatment, and prevention of reactions to inflammation/constriction in the airway passages

Body Mechanics Promotion: Facilitating the use of posture and movement in daily activities to prevent fatigue and musculoskeletal strain or injury

Breastfeeding Assistance: Preparing a new mother to breast-feed her infant

Cardiac Precautions: Prevention of an acute episode of impaired cardiac function by minimizing myocardial oxygen consumption or increasing myocardial oxygen supply

Childbirth Preparation: Providing information and support to facilitate childbirth and to enhance the ability of an individual to develop and perform the role of parent

Circulatory Care: Venous Insufficiency: Promotion of venous circulation

Client Satisfaction: Teaching: Extent of positive perception of instruction provided by nursing staff to improve knowledge, understanding, and participation in care

Developmental Care: Structuring the environment and providing care in response to the behavioral cues and states of the preterm infant

Energy Management: Regulating energy use to treat or prevent fatigue and optimize function

Environmental Management: Safety: Monitoring and manipulation of the physical environment to promote safety

Fall Prevention: Instituting special precautions with patient at risk for injury from falling

Family Planning: Contraception: Facilitation of pregnancy prevention by providing information about the physiology of reproduction and methods to control conception

Family Planning: Infertility: Management, education, and support of the patient and significant other undergoing evaluation and treatment for infertility

Fertility Preservation: Providing information, counseling, and treatment that facilitate reproductive health and the ability to conceive

Health Education: Developing and providing instruction and learning experiences to facilitate voluntary adaptation of behavior conducive to health in individuals, families, groups, or communities

Health Screening: Detecting health risks or problems by means of history, examination, and other procedures

Health System Guidance: Facilitating a patient's location and use of appropriate health services

Hypervolemia Management: Reduction in extracellular or intracellular fluid volume and prevention of complications in a patient who is fluid overloaded

Infection Control: Minimizing the acquisition and transmission of infectious agents

Lactation Counseling: Use of an interactive helping process to assist in maintenance of successful breastfeeding

Nutritional Counseling: Use of an interactive helping process focusing on the need for diet modification

Ostomy Care: Maintenance of elimination through a stoma and care of surrounding tissue

Pain Management: Alleviation of pain or a reduction in pain to a level of comfort that is acceptable to the patient

Parent Education: Adolescent: Assisting parents to understand and help their adolescent children

Parent Education: Childrearing Family: Assisting parents to understand and promote the physical, psychological, and social growth and development of their toddler, preschool, or school-aged child or children

Parent Education: Infant: Instruction on nurturing and physical care needed during the first year of life

Postpartal Care: Monitoring and management of the patient who has recently given birth

Preconception Counseling: Screening and providing information and support to individuals of childbearing age before pregnancy to promote health and reduce risks

Prenatal Care: Monitoring and management of patient during pregnancy to prevent complications of pregnancy and promote a healthy outcome for both mother and infant

Preparatory Sensory Information: Describing in concrete and objective terms the typical sensory experiences and events associated with an upcoming stressful health care procedure or treatment

Reproductive Technology Management: Assisting a patient through the steps of complex infertility treatment

Risk Identification: Analysis of potential risk factors, determination of health risks, and prioritization of risk-reduction strategies for an individual or group

Sexual Counseling: Use of an interactive helping process focusing on the need to make adjustments in sexual practice or to enhance coping with a sexual event/disorder

Substance Use Prevention: Prevention of an alcoholic or drug use lifestyle

Substance Use Treatment: Supportive care of patient and family members with physical and psychosocial problems associated with the use of alcohol or drugs

Teaching, Disease Process: Assisting the patient to understand information related to a specific disease process

Teaching, Individual: Planning, implementation, and evaluation of a teaching program designed to address a patient's particular needs

Teaching: Infant Safety: Instruction on safety during first year of life

Teaching: Prescribed Activity/Exercise: Preparing a patient to achieve or maintain a prescribed level of activity

Teaching: Prescribed Diet: Preparing a patient to correctly follow a prescribed diet

Teaching: Prescribed Medication: Preparing a patient to safely take prescribed medications and monitor for their effects

Teaching: Procedure/Treatment: Preparing a patient to understand and mentally prepare for a prescribed procedure or treatment

Teaching: Psychomotor Skill: Preparing a patient to perform a psychomotor skill

Teaching: Safe Sex: Providing instruction concerning sexual protection during sexual activity

Teaching: Sexuality: Assisting individuals to understand physical and psychosocial dimensions of sexual growth and development

Teaching: Toddler Safety: Instruction on safety during the second and third years of life

Weight Management: Facilitating maintenance of optimal body weight and percentage of body fat

Nursing Activities

NOTE: Because *Deficient knowledge* is such a broad label, this text provides only general activities. Refer to the NIC manual for nursing activities associated with a specific intervention, such as Teaching: Safe Sex or Teaching: Psychomotor Skill.

Assessments

- Check for accurate feedback to ensure that patient understands prescribed treatment and other relevant information
- *(NIC) Teaching: Individual:*
  - Determine the patient's learning needs
  - Appraise the patient's current level of knowledge and understanding of content [e.g., knowledge of prescribed procedure or treatment]
  - Determine the patient's ability to learn specific information (e.g., developmental level, physiologic status, orientation, pain, fatigue, unfulfilled basic needs, emotional state, and adaptation to illness)
  - Determine the patient's motivation to learn specific information (i.e., health beliefs, past noncompliance, bad experiences with health care and learning, and conflicting goals)
  - Appraise the patient's learning style

Patient/Family Teaching

- Establish rapport with the patient/family
  - Provide teaching at patient's level of understanding, repeating information as necessary
- Use multiple teaching approaches, return demonstrations, and verbal and written feedback.
- *(NIC) Teaching: Individual:*
  - Establish teacher credibility, as appropriate
  - Set mutual, realistic learning goals with the patient
  - Provide an environment conducive to learning
  - Select appropriate teaching methods and strategies
  - Select appropriate educational materials

Reinforce behavior, as appropriate
Provide time for the patient to ask questions and discuss concerns
Document the content presented, the written materials provided, and the patient's understanding of the information or patient behaviors that indicate learning on the permanent medical record
Include the family and significant others, as appropriate

Collaborative Activities

- Provide information on community resources that will help the patient maintain his treatment regimen
- Develop a coordinated multidisciplinary teaching plan, specify plan
- Plan with patient and physician adjustment in treatment to facilitate patient's ability to follow prescribed treatment

Other

- Interact with patient in a nonjudgmental manner to facilitate learning

Home Care

- Teaching is equally important in home-based and acute care settings. All of the preceding interventions can be adapted for home care.
- Find a suitable space in the home for the teaching
- Assess for low literacy; adapt materials and strategies accordingly
- Consider using video- or teleconferencing and computer programs

For Infants and Children

- Base your communication and teaching strategies on the child's developmental stage (e.g., adolescents learn well in peer groups)

For Older Adults

- Assess for physical and mental constraints to learning (e.g., hearing deficits, loss of psychomotor dexterity) and adjust your teaching as needed
- Be sure that eyeglasses and hearing aids are functioning properly
- Provide printed materials the client can use later in a more leisurely setting
- Repeat and reinforce information; keep sessions brief
- Use audiovisual materials (e.g., television, DVDs)

KNOWLEDGE (SPECIFY), READINESS FOR ENHANCED

(2002) **Domain 5, Perception/Cognition; Class 4, Cognition**

Definition: A pattern of cognitive information related to a specific topic, or its acquisition, which is sufficient for meeting health-related goals and can be strengthened

Defining Characteristics

Subjective

Explains knowledge of the topic
Expresses an interest in learning

Objective

Behaviors congruent with expressed knowledge
Describes previous experiences pertaining to the topic

Related Factors

This is a wellness diagnosis, so no etiology is needed.

Suggestions for Use

See discussion of the diagnosis *Deficient knowledge*. When possible, use a more specific diagnosis, such as one of the examples in Suggested Alternative Diagnoses.

Suggested Alternative Diagnoses

Nutrition, readiness for enhanced
Parenting, readiness for enhanced
Sleep, readiness for enhanced
Urinary elimination, readiness for enhanced

NOC Outcomes

[NOTE: Only three NOC outcomes have been linked to Readiness for Enhanced Knowledge. They are listed and defined later. However, NOC has 42 Knowledge outcomes: Arthritis Management, Asthma Management, Body Mechanics, Breastfeeding, Cancer Management, Cancer Threat Reduction, Cardiac Disease Management, Child Physical Safety, Conception Prevention, Congestive Heart Failure Management, Depression Management, Diabetes Management, Diet, Disease Process, Energy Conservation, Fall Prevention, Fertility Promotion, Health Behavior, Health Promotion, Health Resources,

Hypertension Management, Illness Care, Infant Care, Infection Management, Labor and Delivery, Medication, Multiple Sclerosis Management, Ostomy Care, Pain Management, Parenting, Personal Safety, Postpartum Maternal Health, Preconception Maternal Health, Pregnancy, Pregnancy and Postpartum Sexual Functioning, Prescribed Activity, Preterm Infant Care, Sexual Functioning, Substance Use Control, Treatment Procedure, Treatment Regimen, and Weight Management. Conceivably, any subject or outcome could be placed after the NOC Knowledge outcome to create yet another outcome.]

Knowledge: Health Behavior: Extent of understanding conveyed about the promotion and protection of health

Knowledge: Health Promotion: Extent of understanding conveyed about information needed to obtain and maintain optimal health

Knowledge: Health Resources: Extent of understanding convened about relevant health care resources

Goals/Evaluation Criteria

Other Examples

Patient and family will:

- Identify need for additional information regarding health-promoting behaviors or prescribed treatment (e.g., diet information about)
- Demonstrate ability to ________________ (specify skill or behavior)

NIC Interventions

Listed next are the NIC interventions that have been linked to the preceding NOC outcomes. Also refer to NIC Interventions for Deficient Knowledge (preceding diagnosis). Conceivably, many NIC interventions would apply, depending on the patient's situation.

Health Education: Developing and providing instruction and learning experiences to facilitate voluntary adaptation of behavior conducive to health in individuals, families, groups, or communities

Health System Guidance: Facilitating a patient's location and use of appropriate health services

Learning Facilitation: Promoting the ability to process and comprehend information

Learning Readiness Enhancement: Improving the ability and willingness to receive information

Nursing Activities

NOTE: Refer to Nursing Activities for Deficient Knowledge (preceding diagnosis). Because *Deficient knowledge* is such a broad label, this text provides only general activities.

Other

- Assist the patient in setting realistic learning goals
- Use a variety of teaching strategies
- Relate new content to previous knowledge and experience
- Allow time for the patient to ask questions

LATEX ALLERGY RESPONSE

(1998, 2006) **Domain 11, Safety/Protection: Class 5, Defensive Processes**

Definition: A hypersensitive reaction to natural latex rubber products

Defining Characteristics

Life-Threatening Reactions Occurring in the First Hour After Exposure to Latex Protein

Contact urticaria progressing to generalized symptoms
Edema of the lips, tongue, uvula, and/or throat
Hypotension, syncope, cardiac arrest
Tightness in chest, wheezing, bronchospasm leading to respiratory arrest
[Shortness of breath (dyspnea)]

Orofacial Characteristics

Edema of sclera or eyelids
Erythema and/or itching of the eyes
Facial erythema
Facial itching
Oral itching
Nasal congestion, itching, and/or erythema
Rhinorrhea
Tearing of the eyes

Gastrointestinal Characteristics

Abdominal pain
Nausea

Generalized Characteristics

Flushing
Generalized discomfort
Generalized edema
Increasing complaint of total body warmth
Restlessness

Type IV Reactions—Occurring 1 Hour or More After Exposure

Discomfort reaction to additives such as thiurams and carbamates
Eczema
Irritation
Redness

Related Factors

Hypersensitivity to natural latex rubber protein

Suggestions for Use

For situations that frequently cause sensitization allergy to latex, see Risk Factors for the diagnosis Latex Allergy Response, Risk for. For both diagnoses, nursing care focuses on avoiding exposure to latex. When an actual allergic reaction occurs, the dermatitis must be treated medically and the nursing diagnoses of *Impaired skin integrity* and *Risk for infection* may be used.

Suggested Alternative Diagnoses

Infection, risk for
Latex allergy response, risk for
Skin integrity, impaired

NOC Outcomes

Allergic Response: Localized: Severity of localized hypersensitive immune response to a specific environmental (exogenous) antigen

Allergic Response: Systemic: Severity of systemic hypersensitive immune response to a specific environmental (exogenous) antigen

Tissue Integrity: Skin and Mucous Membranes: Structural intactness and normal physiological function of skin and mucous membranes

Goals/Evaluation Criteria

Examples Using NOC Language

- Demonstrates **Allergic Response: Localized** as evidenced by the following indicators (specify 1–5: severe, substantial, moderate, slight, or none)
  - Localized itching
  - Localized rash
  - Localized pain
  - Localized edema
  - Increased localized skin temperature

Other Examples

- Regains skin integrity, as evidenced by good hydration; reduced inflammation, scaling, and flaking; decreased inflammation; and verbalizations of reduced itching

- Experiences restful sleep
- Does not experience respiratory complications (e.g., asthma)
- Exhibits a positive self-concept, as evidenced by expressed feelings of self-worth and satisfaction with interpersonal interactions
- Does not experience recurrence of the allergic response to latex

NIC Interventions

Airway Management: Facilitation of patency of air passages

Allergy Management: Identification, treatment, and prevention of allergic responses to food, medications, insect bites, contrast material, blood, or other substances

Anaphylaxis Management: Promotion of adequate ventilation and tissue perfusion for an individual with a severe allergic (antigen–antibody) reaction

Emergency Care: Providing life-saving measures in life-threatening situations

Latex Precautions: Reducing the risk of a systemic reaction to latex

Respiratory Monitoring: Collection and analysis of patient data to ensure airway patency and adequate gas exchange

Skin Surveillance: Collection and analysis of patient data to maintain skin and mucous membrane integrity

Nursing Activities

Assessments

- Identify source(s) of latex to which the patient was (or might be) exposed
- Assess skin for signs of healing (e.g., decreased redness, flaking, and scaling)
- Assess comfort level
- Assess sleep–rest pattern
- Observe for signs of *Disturbed body image* or *Social isolation*
- Observe for development of asthmatic response (e.g., wheezing, dyspnea)
- *(NIC) Latex Precautions:*

  Monitor latex-free environment

  Monitor patient for signs and symptoms of a systemic reaction

Patient/Family Teaching

- Explain the relationship between skin dryness, the symptom of itching, and the prescribed therapy (i.e., hydration)

- Explain that scratching will only produce more itching
- *(NIC) Latex Precautions:* Instruct visitors about latex-free environment

Collaborative Activities

- *(NIC) Latex Precautions:* Report information to physician, pharmacist, and other care providers, as indicated

Other

- Provide alternatives for supplies and equipment containing latex (e.g., condoms, balloons, gloves, urinary, or IV catheters)
- *(NIC) Latex Precautions:*
  Place allergy band on patient
  Post sign indicating latex precautions
  Survey environment and remove latex products

Home Care

- Assess the home for presence of latex-containing products (e.g., condoms, balloons); assist the client in obtaining alternatives to such products
- Explain that the skin lesions are not contagious (unless they are infected)
- Teach to bathe daily for 15–20 min and apply emollient or prescribed medication within 4 min after the bath
- Teach to use warm, not hot, water for bathing
- Explain that keeping the home and work environments at a constant temperature (68–75° F) and humidity (about 50%) will help decrease itching
- Suggest that the client wear loose-fitting, open-weave, cotton clothing and avoid rough or tightly woven fabrics
- Advise against self-treating with leftover medication at home
- Encourage client to maintain existing social activities
- *(NIC) Latex Precautions:*
  Instruct patient and family about latex content in household products and substitution with nonlatex products, as appropriate;
  Instruct patient to wear a medical alert tag
  Instruct patient and family about signs and symptoms of a reaction
  Instruct patient and family about emergency treatment (e.g., epinephrine), as appropriate

LATEX ALLERGY RESPONSE, RISK FOR

(1998, 2006) **Domain 11, Safety/Protection; Class 5, Defensive Processes**

Definition: Risk of hypersensitivity to natural latex rubber products that may compromise health

Risk Factors

Allergies to bananas, avocados, tropical fruits, kiwis, and chestnuts
Allergies to poinsettia plants
Conditions needing continuous or intermittent catheterization (non-NANDA)
History of allergies or asthma
History of reactions to latex [e.g., balloons, condoms, gloves]
Multiple surgical procedures, especially from infancy [e.g., spina bifida]
Professions with daily exposure to latex [e.g., medicine, nursing, dentistry]

Suggestions for Use

This label may be more useful than actual *Latex allergy response*. See Suggestions for *Latex allergy response*.

Suggested Alternative Diagnoses

Protection, ineffective
Injury, risk for

NOC Outcomes

Allergic Response: Localized: Severity of localized hypersensitive immune response to a specific environmental (exogenous) antigen

Risk Control: Personal actions to prevent, eliminate, or reduce modifiable health threats

Risk Detection: Personal actions to identify personal health threats

Tissue Integrity: Skin and Mucous Membranes: Structural intactness and normal physiological function of skin and mucous membranes

Goals/Evaluation Criteria

- Does not experience allergic reaction to latex (e.g., no skin lesions or symptoms)
- Identifies and avoids environmental sources of latex

NIC Interventions

Allergy Management: Identification, treatment, and prevention of allergic responses to food, medications, insect bites, contrast material, blood, and other substances

Environmental Management: Manipulation of the patient's surroundings for therapeutic benefit, sensory appeal, and psychological well-being

Latex Precautions: Reducing the risk of a systemic reaction to latex

Surveillance: Purposeful and ongoing acquisition, interpretation, and synthesis of patient data for clinical decision making

Nursing Activities

Also see Nursing Activities for the diagnosis, Latex Allergy Response.

Assessments

- Identify source(s) of latex to which the patient is (or may be) exposed both at work and at home
- Assess patient and family knowledge of sources of latex
- Assess knowledge of sensitization and allergic reactions
- *(NIC) Latex Precautions:*

  Question patient or appropriate other about history of neural tube defect (e.g., spina bifida) or congenital urological condition (e.g., exstrophy of the bladder)

  Question patient or appropriate other about history of systemic reactions to natural rubber latex (e.g., facial or scleral edema, tearing eyes, urticaria, rhinitis, and wheezing)

Patient/Family Teaching

- Teach information about sensitization and allergic reactions, as needed
- Advise against self-treating if allergic reaction is suspected
- *(NIC) Latex Precautions:* Instruct patient and family about risk factors for developing a latex allergy

Collaborative Activities

- Help develop agency and organizational policies to decrease worker exposure to latex products
- *(NIC) Latex Precautions:* Refer patient to allergist for allergy testing, as appropriate

Other

- For clients with risk factors (e.g., allergy to bananas, history of asthma), provide alternatives (or sources for alternatives) for supplies and equipment containing latex (e.g., condoms, balloons, gloves, urinary catheters, IV catheters)

LIVER FUNCTION, RISK FOR IMPAIRED

(2006, 2008) **Domain 2, Nutrition; Class 4, Metabolism**

Definition: At risk for liver dysfunction that may compromise health

Risk Factors

Hepatotoxic medications (e.g., acetaminophen, statins)
HIV coinfection
Substance abuse (e.g., alcohol, cocaine)
Viral infection (e.g., hepatitis A, hepatitis B, hepatitis C, Epstein–Barr)

Suggested Alternative Diagnoses

Health behavior, risk-prone
Injury, risk for

NOC Outcomes

(**NOTE:** NOC does not have an outcome that directly measures liver function. We have listed two outcomes that might occur with liver failure. Others, such as Fluid Overload Severity, might be useful. The other outcomes listed here relate to prevention of impaired liver function.)

Alcohol Abuse Cessation Behavior: Personal actions to eliminate alcohol use that poses a threat to health

Blood Coagulation: Extent to which blood clots within normal period of time

Drug Abuse Cessation Behavior: Personal actions to eliminate drug use that poses a threat to health

Infection Severity: Severity of infection and associated symptoms

Medication Response: Therapeutic and adverse effects of prescribed medication

Risk Control: Personal actions to prevent, eliminate, or reduce modifiable health threats

Risk Detection: Personal actions to identify personal health threats

Goals/Evaluation Criteria

Examples Using NOC Language

- Liver function is not impaired, as evidenced by Blood Coagulation and Medication Response

- Demonstrates **Blood Coagulation**, as evidenced by the following indicators (specify 1–5: severe, substantial, moderate, mild, or no deviation from normal range):
  - Clot formation
  - Partial thromboplastin time (PTT)
  - Prothrombin time (PT)
  - Hemoglobin (Hgb)
  - Platelet Count

Other Examples

- States absence of right upper quadrant (RUQ) pain
- Normal stool (e.g., brown, no blood or mucus)
- Stable vital signs
  - No bleeding
  - No petechiae
  - No bruising or ecchymosis
  - No hematuria, hemoptysis, or hematemesis
  - No blood in the stool
  - No bleeding of the gums

NIC Interventions

Infection Control: Minimizing the acquisition and transmission of infectious agents

Infection Protection: Prevention and early detection of infection in a patient at risk

Medication Management: Facilitation of safe and effective use of prescription and over-the-counter drugs

Risk Identification: Analysis of potential risk factors, determination of health risks, and prioritization of risk-reduction strategies for an individual or group

Substance Use Treatment: Supportive care of patient and family members with physical and psychosocial problems associated with the use of alcohol or drugs

Substance Use Treatment: Alcohol Withdrawal: Care of the patient experiencing sudden cessation of alcohol consumption

Substance Use Treatment: Drug Withdrawal: Care of the patient experiencing drug detoxification

Surveillance: Purposeful and ongoing acquisition, interpretation, and synthesis of patient data for clinical decision making

Teaching: Individual: Planning, implementation, and evaluation of a teaching program designed to address a patient's particular needs

Teaching: Prescribed Medication: Preparing a patient to safely take prescribed medications and monitor for their effects

Nursing Activities

Because this is a potential diagnosis, the focus of nursing activities is to: (a) Modify the existing risk factors to the extent possible and (b) assess for signs and symptoms of impaired liver function

Assessments

- Monitor intake and output
- Monitor vital signs, pain (especially RUQ), and mental status
- Monitor for ascites, peripheral edema, and jugular vein distention
- Monitor electrolytes
- Observe for blood in the stool
- Observe skin and sclera for jaundice

Patient/Family Teaching

- Provide information about the disease process(es) that create the risk for impaired liver function

Collaborative Activities

- Administer medications and treatments for underlying disease processes, to decrease the risk for impaired liver function

LONELINESS, RISK FOR

(1994, 2006) **Domain 6, Self-Perception; Class 1, Self-Concept**

Definition: At risk for experiencing discomfort associated with a desire or need for more contact with others

Risk Factors

Affectional deprivation [e.g., death of a spouse]
Cathectic deprivation [e.g., no one to talk to]
Physical isolation [e.g., isolation because of infectious disease]
Social isolation [e.g., shunning by peer group]

Suggestions for Use

Discriminate between this diagnosis and *Social isolation*. *Social isolation* is objective (perceived by others); *Loneliness* is subjective (an inner feeling state). *Social isolation* may be the risk factor or etiology of *Loneliness*. *Loneliness* better describes the feeling response brought about by solitude that is not desired by the person. For *Loneliness* that is brought about by physical disability or disfigurement, see *Disturbed body image*.

Suggested Alternative Diagnoses

Body image, disturbed
Grieving, complicated
Relocation stress syndrome
Social interaction, impaired
Social isolation

NOC Outcomes

Caregiver Stressors: Severity of biopsychosocial pressure on a family care provider caring for another over an extended period of time
Family Functioning: Capacity of the family system to meet the needs of its members during developmental transitions
Family Social Climate: Supportive milieu as characterized by family member relationships and goals
Grief Resolution: Adjustment to actual or impending loss
Leisure Participation: Use of relaxing, interesting, and enjoyable activities to promote well-being
Loneliness Severity: Severity of emotional, social, or existential isolation response
Psychosocial Adjustment: Life Change: Adaptive psychosocial response of an individual to a significant life change
Social Interaction Skills: Personal behaviors that promote effective relationships
Social Involvement: Social interactions with persons, groups, or organizations

Goals/Evaluation Criteria

Examples Using NOC Language

- Demonstrates prevention of *Loneliness*, as evidenced by Loneliness Severity and Social Involvement
- Demonstrates **Social Involvement**, as evidenced by the following indicators (specify 1–5: never, rarely, sometimes, often, or consistently demonstrated):
  - Interacts with close friends, neighbors, family members, or members of work group(s)
  - Participates as member of church
  - Participates in leisure activities with others
  - Participates in organized activity

Other Examples

- Uses time alone in a positive way when socialization is not possible
- Identifies reasons for feelings of loneliness
- Describes a plan for increasing meaningful relationships
- Uses effective interpersonal communication skills (e.g., self-disclosure, cooperation, sensitivity, assertiveness, consideration, genuineness, trust, and compromise); specify skills most relevant to patient
- Verbalizes adequacy of social supports (e.g., assistance provided by others)
- Indicates willingness to ask others for help
- Effectively accomplishes grief work (e.g., expresses feelings, verbalize acceptance of loss)

NIC Interventions

Attachment Promotion: Facilitation of the development of the parent relationship

L

Activity Therapy: Prescription of and assistance with specific physical, cognitive, social, and spiritual activities to increase the range, frequency, or duration of an individual's (or group's) activity

Animal Assisted Therapy: Purposeful use of animals to provide affection, attention, diversion, and relaxation

Behavior Modification: Social Skills: Assisting the patient to develop or improve interpersonal social skills

Caregiver Support: Provision of the necessary information, advocacy, and support to facilitate primary patient care by someone other than a health care professional

Emotional Support: Provision of reassurance, acceptance, and encouragement during times of stress

Family Integrity Promotion: Promotion of family cohesion and unity

Family Integrity Promotion: Childbearing Family: Facilitation of the growth of individuals or families who are adding an infant to the family unit

Family Process Maintenance: Minimization of family process disruption effects

Family Support: Promotion of family values, interests, and goals

Grief Work Facilitation: Assistance with the resolution of a significant loss

Parenting Promotion: Providing parenting information, support, and coordination of comprehensive services to high-risk families

Recreation Therapy: Purposeful use of recreation to promote relaxation and enhancement of social skills

Relocation Stress Reduction: Assisting the individual to prepare for and cope with movement from one environment to another

Risk Identification: Analysis of potential risk factors, determination of health risks, and prioritization of risk-reduction strategies for an individual or group

Sibling Support: Assisting a sibling to cope with a brother's or sister's illness/chronic condition/disability

Socialization Enhancement: Facilitation of another person's ability to interact with others

Support Group: Use of a group environment to provide emotional support and health-related information for members

Support System Enhancement: Facilitation of support to patient by family, friends, and community

Surveillance: Purposeful and ongoing acquisition, interpretation, and synthesis of patient data for clinical decision making

Visitation Facilitation: Promoting beneficial visits by family and friends

Nursing Activities

Assessments

- Assess the patient's perceived and actual support systems
- Determine risk factors for loneliness (e.g., lack of energy needed for social interaction, poor communication skills)
- Compare client's desire for visitation and social interaction to actual visitation and social interaction
- Monitor patient's response to visits from family and friends
- *(NIC) Visitation Facilitation:*

  Determine patient's preferences for visitation and release of information

  Determine need for more visits from family and friends
- Assess past and present family relationships

Patient/Family Teaching

- *(NIC) Visitation Facilitation:* Discuss policy for overnight stay of family members/significant others

Collaborative Activities

- Refer patient to group or program for increased understanding and practice of communication and interaction skills
- Refer to support groups as appropriate

Other

- *(NIC) Visitation Facilitation:*

  Facilitate visitation of children, as appropriate

  Assist family members to find adequate lodging and meals

- Encourage patient to talk about feelings of loneliness
- Role-play communication skills and techniques with patient
- Help patient identify strengths and limitations in communicating
- Give positive feedback when patient uses effective social interaction skills
- Help patient to recognize available social supports
- Encourage family members to provide care to the patient, as appropriate

Home Care

- Some of the preceding interventions can be adapted for use in home care
- Teach social skills, as needed (e.g., role-model self-disclosure)
- Teach patient to monitor own behaviors that contribute to social isolation
- Assist patient to discover new interests
- Discuss with the client the possibility of referral for visiting volunteers' services
- Encourage patient to reach out to others who have similar interests
- Encourage telephone or computer contact with friends and family

For Infants and Children

- Assess for shyness and low self-esteem, especially among adolescents
- Discuss with parents the possibility of acquiring a pet

For Older Adults

- Assess for functional limitations that may interfere with social interactions (e.g., communication difficulty, hearing or vision problems)
- Assess for depression; refer to mental health professional as needed
- Assess for changes in mental status (e.g., memory loss, confusion)
- Encourage participation in physical activity groups (e.g., water aerobics)
- Discuss the possibility of moving to a retirement community
- Arrange for the client to have one meal a day at a community center for older adults

MATERNAL–FETAL DYAD, RISK FOR DISTURBED

(2008) **Domain 8, Sexuality; Class 3, Reproduction**

Definition: At risk for disruption of the symbiotic maternal–fetal dyad as a result of comorbid or pregnancy-related conditions

Risk Factors

Complications of pregnancy (e.g., premature rupture of membranes, placenta previa or abruption, late prenatal care, multiple gestation)
Compromised oxygen transport (e.g., anemia, cardiac disease, asthma, hypertension, seizures, premature labor, hemorrhage)
Impaired glucose metabolism (e.g., diabetes, steroid use)
Physical abuse
Substance abuse (e.g., tobacco, alcohol, drugs)
Treatment-related side effects (e.g., pharmaceutical agents, surgery)

Suggestions for Use

(a) This diagnosis appears to be more narrowly defined than *Risk for impaired attachment*. This diagnosis specifies that the disruption in attachment must be caused by comorbid or pregnancy-related conditions. You will need to choose the label based on the best fit with the patient's risk factors. (b) Whereas this diagnosis is limited to the prenatal period, *Risk for impaired attachment* can be used in the neonatal and subsequent periods. (c) Although it is not entirely clear, it seems that *Risk for disturbed maternal–fetal dyad* refers to the risk to the physical maternal–fetal relationship (e.g., premature birth), rather than the psychosocial relationship (as in *Risk for impaired attachment*).

Suggested Alternative Diagnoses

Attachment, risk for impaired

NOC Outcomes

Fetal Status: Intrapartum: Extent to which fetal signs are within normal limits from onset of labor to delivery
Maternal Status: Antepartum: Extent to which maternal well-being is within normal limits from conception to the onset of labor

(**NOTE:** The preceding two outcomes are used to assess and measure the actual occurrence of disturbed maternal–fetal dyad. You may need other outcomes, depending on the risk factors present. Following are a few of those.)

Abuse Protection: Protection of self and/or dependent others from abuse

Alcohol Abuse Cessation Behavior: Personal actions to eliminate alcohol use that poses a threat to health

Blood Glucose Level: Extent to which glucose levels in plasma and urine are maintained in normal range

Cardiopulmonary Status: Adequacy of blood volume ejected from the ventricles and exchange of carbon dioxide and oxygen at the alveolar level

Prenatal Health Behavior: Personal actions to promote a healthy pregnancy and a healthy newborn

Smoking Cessation Behavior: Personal actions to eliminate tobacco use

Goals/Evaluation Criteria

Examples Using NOC Language

- Will not experience *Disturbed maternal/fetal dyad*, as demonstrated by Fetal Status: Intrapartum and Maternal Status: Intrapartum
- Demonstrates satisfactory Fetal Status: Intrapartum, as evidenced by the following indicators (specify 1–5: severe, substantial, moderate, mild, or no deviation from normal range):
  - Amniotic fluid color and amount
  - Deceleration patterns in electronic fetal monitor findings
  - Fetal heart rate (120–160 bpm)
  - Variability in electronic fetal monitor findings

Other Examples

- Fetal growth within normal limits
- Pregnancy continues to term
- Mother recognizes risk factors that may impact the pregnancy
- Mother demonstrates emotional attachment to fetus
- Maternal vital signs remain normal during pregnancy.
- Mother experiences no edema, headache, vaginal bleeding, or other signs/symptoms of complications of pregnancy.

NIC Interventions

Abuse Protection Support: Domestic Partner: Identification of high-risk dependent domestic relationships and actions to prevent possible or further infliction of physical, sexual, or emotional harm, or exploitation of a domestic partner

Cardiac Care: Limitation of complications resulting from an imbalance between myocardial oxygen supply and demand for a patient with symptoms of impaired cardiac function

Cardiac Precautions: Prevention of an acute episode of impaired cardiac function by minimizing myocardial oxygen consumption or increasing myocardial oxygen supply

Electronic Fetal Monitoring: Antepartum: Electronic evaluation of fetal heart rate response to movement, external stimuli, or uterine contractions during antepartal testing

High-Risk Pregnancy Care: Identification and management of a high-risk pregnancy to promote healthy outcomes for mother and baby

Prenatal Care: Monitoring and management of patient during pregnancy to prevent complications of pregnancy and promote a healthy outcome for both mother and infant

Risk Identification: Analysis of potential risk factors, determination of health risks, and prioritization of risk-reduction strategies for an individual or group

Smoking Cessation Assistance: Helping another to stop smoking

Substance Use Treatment: Supportive care of patient and family members with physical and psychosocial problems associated with the use of alcohol or drugs

Surveillance: Late Pregnancy: Purposeful and ongoing acquisition, interpretation, and synthesis of maternal–fetal data for treatment, observation, or admission

Ultrasonography: Limited Obstetric: Performance of ultrasound exams to determine ovarian, uterine, or fetal status

Vital Signs Monitoring: Collection and analysis of cardiovascular, respiratory, and body temperature data to determine and prevent complications

Nursing Activities: Nursing activities for this diagnosis focus on identifying risk factors and monitoring for symptoms of disruption in the maternal–fetal dyad (e.g., late or variable decelerations in the fetal heart rate).

Assessments

- Review patient records for complications with previous pregnancies (e.g., preterm labor, urinary tract or vaginal infections)
- Review patient records for family history that may affect pregnancy (e.g., sickle cell, Tay–Sachs disease)

- Determine the amount and timing of prenatal care and prenatal screening done
- Assess for comorbid conditions (e.g., hypertension, anemia)
- Assess nutritional status
- Monitor for severe nausea or vomiting, especially after first trimester.
- Inquire whether the patient has been exposed to teratogens (e.g., lead, certain medications, illegal drugs, alcohol)
- Assess for exposure to infectious diseases (e.g., rubella, Chlamydia)
- Review laboratory results (e.g., hemoglobin, blood type and Rh group, serum glucose, platelet count)
- Assist with screening for genetic disorders (e.g., phenylketonuria)
- Assess home situation (e.g., for safety); screen for abuse
- Monitor weight throughout pregnancy
- Monitor fetal heart rate throughout pregnancy and labor
- Monitor for preterm uterine contractions
- Test urine for ketones

Patient/Family Teaching

- Provide information about procedures such as amniocentesis, contraction stress test, and ultrasonography
- Teach symptoms that necessitate the need for the patient to notify the obstetrician (e.g., vaginal bleeding, persistent vomiting, headache, blurred vision, and swollen ankles)
- Review medications with patient/family
- Teach self-care techniques such as avoiding heavy lifting and scheduling rest periods during the day
- Explain and demonstrate how to monitor blood glucose levels, as appropriate
- Discuss the impact the patient's preexisting conditions may have on the pregnancy

Collaborative Activities

- Assist in treating comorbid conditions (e.g., cardiac problems)
- Refer for counseling, if needed

Other

- Develop a therapeutic, trusting relationship with the patient/family
- Assist, as needed, with developing a nutritious dietary plan
- Encourage intake of at least 2 quarts of caffeine-free fluids per day
- Encourage smoking cessation

MEMORY, IMPAIRED

(1994) **Domain 5, Perception/Cognition; Class 4, Cognition**

Definition: Inability to remember or recall bits of information or behavioral skills

Defining Characteristics

Forgets to perform a behavior at a scheduled time
Inability to recall if a behavior was performed
Inability to learn or retain new skills or information
Inability to perform a previously learned skill
Inability to recall factual information
Inability to recall [recent or past] events
Reports experience of forgetting

Related Factors

[NOTE: *Impaired memory* may be attributed to pathophysiologic or situational causes that are either temporary or permanent.]
Anemia
Decreased cardiac output
[Depression]
Excessive environmental disturbances
Fluid and electrolyte imbalance
Hypoxia [acute or chronic]
Neurologic disturbances

Suggestions for Use

Use this diagnosis only if it is possible for the patient's memory to improve. If the impairment is permanent, consider using it as an etiology of another diagnosis, for example, *Self-care deficit* or *Risk for injury*. *Impaired memory* is also a defining characteristic for some other diagnoses, such as *Chronic confusion*, in which other symptoms are also present.

Suggested Alternative Diagnoses

Confusion, chronic
Environmental interpretation syndrome, impaired

NOC Outcomes

Cognitive Orientation: Ability to identify person, place, and time accurately

Memory: Ability to cognitively retrieve and report previously stored information

Neurological Status: Ability of the peripheral and central nervous system to receive, process, and respond to internal and external stimuli

Goals/Evaluation Criteria

Examples Using NOC Language

- Demonstrates unimpaired memory, as evidenced by Cognitive Orientation, Memory, and Neurological Status
- Demonstrates **Cognitive Orientation** as evidenced by the following indicators (specify 1–5: severely, substantially, moderately, mildly, or not compromised): Identifies self; significant other; current place; and correct day, month, year, and season
- Demonstrates **Neurologic Status**, as evidenced by the following indicators (specify 1–5: severely, substantially, moderately, mildly, or not compromised):

  Cognitive orientation
  Communication appropriate to situation
  Cognitive status
  Central motor control

Other Examples

Patient will:

- Use techniques to help improve memory
- Accurately recall immediate, recent, and remote information
- Verbalize being better able to remember

NIC Interventions

Anxiety Reduction: Minimizing apprehension, dread, foreboding, or uneasiness related to an unidentified source of anticipated danger

Cerebral Perfusion Promotion: Promotion of adequate perfusion and limitation of complications for a patient experiencing, or at risk for, inadequate cerebral perfusion

Cognitive Stimulation: Promotion of awareness and comprehension of surroundings by utilization of planned stimuli

Delirium Management: Provision of a safe and therapeutic environment for the patient who is experiencing an acute confusional state

Dementia Management: Provision of a modified environment for the patient who is experiencing a chronic confusional state

Memory Training: Facilitation of memory

Neurologic Monitoring: Collection and analysis of patient data to prevent or minimize neurological complications

Reality Orientation: Promotion of patient's awareness of personal identity, time, and environment

Nursing Activities

Assessments

- Assess for depression, anxiety, and increased stressors that may be contributing to memory loss
- Assess neurologic function to determine whether patient has memory loss only or also has problems, such as dementia, which need to be referred for further treatment
- Assess extent and nature of memory loss (e.g., immediate, recent, or remote events; gradual or sudden loss)
- Determine history and present pattern of alcohol use
- Determine which medications or street drugs the client is taking that might affect memory (e.g., marijuana)
- *(NIC) Memory Training:* Monitor patient's behavior during therapy

Patient/Family Teaching

- *(NIC) Memory Training:* Structure the teaching methods according to patient's organization of information

Collaborative Activities

- Refer patients with sudden memory loss to physician
- *(NIC) Memory Training:* Refer to occupational therapy, as appropriate

Other

- Do not rearrange furniture in the room
- Help the patient to relax in order to improve concentration
- Maintain consistency of caregivers to the extent possible
- *(NIC) Memory Training:*
  - Discuss with patient and family any practical memory problems experienced
  - Stimulate memory by repeating patient's last expressed thought, as appropriate
  - Reminisce about past experiences with patient, as appropriate
  - Implement appropriate memory techniques, such as visual imagery, mnemonic devices, memory games, memory cues, association

techniques, making lists, using computers or using name tags, or rehearsing information

Assist in associated-learning tasks, such as practice learning and recalling verbal and pictorial information presented, as appropriate

Provide for orientation training, such as patient rehearsing personal information and dates, as appropriate

Provide opportunity for concentration, such as a game matching pairs of cards, as appropriate

Provide opportunity to use memory for recent events, such as questioning patient about a recent outing

Provide for picture recognition memory, as appropriate

- Encourage patient to participate in group memory training programs, as appropriate

Home Care

- Label items (e.g., the bathroom door, the sink, the refrigerator) to increase recall
- Do not rearrange furniture in the home
- Assess whether the client needs family and friends to manage schedules and communicate reminders (e.g., of appointments or medications)

For Older Adults

- Explain to the older patient that short-term memory loss frequently occurs with aging
- If memory continues to deteriorate and affect affective and cognitive functioning, refer for mental health assessment (e.g., for dementia or depression)
- Assess whether memory loss may be a side effect of the patient's medications (e.g., digitalis)
- Encourage the client to work to improve his memory; explain that improvement is possible using brain stimulating strategies

MOBILITY: BED, IMPAIRED

(1998, 2006) **Domain 4, Activity/Rest; Class 2, Activity/Exercise**

Definition: Limitation of independent movement from one bed position to another (specify level of independence using a standardized functional scale)

Defining Characteristics

Impaired ability to do the following:

Move from supine to sitting
Move from sitting to supine
Move from supine to prone
Move from prone to supine
Move from supine to long sitting
Move from long sitting to supine
Reposition self in bed
Turn from side to side

Related Factors

Cognitive impairment
Deconditioning
Environmental constraints (i.e., bed size, bed type, treatment equipment, restraints)
Insufficient muscle strength
Lack of knowledge (non-NANDA-)
Musculoskeletal impairment (e.g., contractures)
Neuromuscular impairment
Obesity
Pain
Sedating medications

Suggestions for Use

1. When the patient's bed mobility cannot be improved, this label should be used as a related or risk factor for other nursing diagnoses, such as *Risk for impaired skin integrity*.
2. Specify level of mobility, the same as you would for Impaired Physical Mobility and Impaired Wheelchair Mobility:

   Level 0: Is completely independent

   Level 1: Requires use of equipment or device

Level 2: Requires help from another person for assistance, supervision, or teaching
Level 3: Requires help from another person and equipment/device
Level 4: Is dependent; does not participate in activity

See Suggestions for Use for Mobility: Impaired Physical.

Suggested Alternative Diagnoses

Disuse syndrome, risk for
Injury, risk for
Mobility: physical, impaired
Skin integrity, risk for impaired

NOC Outcomes

Body Positioning: Self-Initiated: Ability to change own body positions independently with or without assistive device

M

Coordinated Movement: Ability of muscles to work together voluntarily for purposeful movement

Mobility: Ability to move purposefully in own environment independently with or without assistive device

Goals/Evaluation Criteria

Examples Using NOC Language

- Achieves bed mobility, as evidenced by Self-Initiated Body Positioning, Coordinated Movement, and satisfactory Mobility
- Demonstrates **Mobility**, as evidenced by the following indicators (specify 1–5: severely, substantially, moderately, mildly, or not compromised):
  - Coordination
  - Body positioning performance
  - Muscle and joint movement

Other Examples

The patient will:

- Perform full range-of-motion of all joints
- Turn self in bed or state realistic level of assistance needed
- Demonstrate correct use of assistive devices (e.g., trapeze)
- Request repositioning assistance, as needed

NIC Interventions

Bed Rest Care: Promotion of comfort and safety and prevention of complications for a patient unable to get out of bed

Body Mechanics Promotion: Facilitating the use of posture and movement in daily activities to prevent fatigue and musculoskeletal strain or injury

Exercise Promotion: Strength Training: Facilitating regular resistive muscle training to maintain or increase muscle strength

Exercise Therapy: Joint Mobility: Use of active or passive body movement to maintain or restore joint flexibility

Exercise Therapy: Muscle Control: Use of specific activity or exercise protocols to enhance or restore controlled body movement

Positioning: Deliberative placement of the patient or a body part to promote physiological and psychological well-being

Self-Care Assistance: Assisting another to perform ADLs

Nursing Activities

Assessments

- Perform ongoing assessment of patient's mobility
- Assess level of consciousness
- Assess muscle strength and joint mobility (range of motion)

Patient/Family Teaching

- Instruct in active and passive range-of-motion exercises to improve muscle strength and endurance
- Instruct in turning techniques and correct body alignment

Collaborative Activities

- Use occupational and physical therapists as resources in developing plan to maintain and increase bed mobility

Other

- Position call light or button within easy reach
- Provide assistive devices (e.g., trapeze)
- Provide positive reinforcement during activities
- Implement pain control measures before beginning exercises or physical therapy
- Ensure that care plan includes number of personnel needed to turn patient

Home Care

- The preceding interventions are also appropriate for home care
- Assess the ability of caregivers to move and turn the client; obtain home health care as needed

- Assess need for assistance from home health agency or other organization
- Assess need for durable medical equipment; assist in obtaining it as necessary
- Teach caregivers good body mechanics
- Teach caregivers and patient how to use assistive devices
- Use the client's regular bed if possible. For example, you can use blocks to raise the head of the bed.
- Obtain a hospital-type bed if the client's medical condition requires it, or if the caregivers need it to allow them to care for the patient
- Suggest moving the patient's bed into an area of the home where it is accessible and where the client can interact with other family members
- Urge caregivers to allow the client to participate in self-care to the extent possible; explain the benefits of maintaining independence

MOBILITY: PHYSICAL, IMPAIRED

(1973, 1998) **Domain 4, Activity/Rest; Class 2, Activity/Exercise**

Definition: Limitation in independent, purposeful physical movement of the body or of one or more extremities (specify level, using a standardized functional scale):

Level 0: Is completely independent
Level 1: Requires use of equipment or device
Level 2: Requires help from another person for assistance, supervision, or teaching
Level 3: Requires help from another person and equipment or device
Level 4: Is dependent; does not participate in activity

Defining Characteristics

Objective

Decreased reaction time
Difficulty turning
Engages in substitutions for movement (e.g., increased attention to other's activity, controlling behavior, focuses on pre-illness or disability activity)
Exertional dyspnea
Gait changes (e.g., decreased walk, speed, difficulty initiating gait, small steps, shuffles feet, exaggerated lateral postural sway)
Jerky movement

Limited ability to perform fine-motor skills
Limited ability to perform gross-motor skills
Limited range of motion
Movement-induced tremor
Postural instability (during performance of routine ADLs)
Slowed movement
Uncoordinated or jerky movements

Related Factors

Activity intolerance
Altered cellular metabolism
Anxiety
Body mass index above 75th age-appropriate percentile
Cognitive impairment
Cultural beliefs regarding age-appropriate activity
Deconditioning
Decreased endurance
Decreased muscle strength, control, or mass
Deficient knowledge regarding value of physical activity
Depressive mood state
Developmental delay
Discomfort
Joint stiffness or contractures
Lack of physical or social environmental supports
Limited cardiovascular endurance
Loss of integrity of bone structures
Malnutrition
Medications
Musculoskeletal impairment
Neuromuscular impairment
Pain
Prescribed movement restrictions
Reluctance to initiate movement
Sedentary lifestyle, disuse, or deconditioning
Sensoriperceptual impairments

Suggestions for Use

Use *Impaired physical mobility* to describe individuals with limited ability for independent physical movement, such as decreased ability to move arms or legs or generalized muscle weakness, or when nursing interventions will focus on restoring mobility and function or preventing further deterioration. For example, an appropriate diagnosis would be *Impaired physical mobility related to ineffective management of Chronic pain secondary to rheumatoid arthritis*.

Do not use this label to describe temporary immobility that cannot be changed by the nurse (e.g., traction, prescribed bed rest) or permanent paralysis. In these and many other instances, Impaired physical mobility can be used effectively as the etiology of a problem. For example: *Impaired tissue integrity (pressure ulcer) related to Impaired physical mobility +4*. When appropriate, use more specific labels, such as *Impaired bed mobility*, *Impaired transfer ability*, *Impaired wheelchair mobility*, or *Impaired walking*.

Suggested Alternative Diagnoses

Disuse syndrome, risk for
Injury, risk for
Mobility: bed, impaired
Mobility: wheelchair, impaired
Self-care deficit
Transfer ability, impaired
Walking, impaired

NOC Outcomes

Ambulation: Ability to walk from place to place independently with or without assistive device

Balance: Ability to maintain body equilibrium

Body Mechanics Performance: Personal actions to maintain proper body alignment and to prevent muscular skeletal strain

Client Satisfaction: Functional Assistance: Extent of positive perception of nursing assistance to achieve mobility and self-care

Coordinated Movement: Ability of muscles to work together voluntarily for purposeful movement

Joint Movement (Specify Joint): Active range of motion of ____________ (specify joint) with self-initiated movement

Joint Movement: Passive: Joint movement with assistance

Mobility: Ability to move purposefully in own environment independently with or without assistive device

Neurological Status: Central Motor Control: Ability of the central nervous system to coordinate skeletal muscle activity for body movement

Skeletal Function: Ability of the bones to support the body and facilitate movement

Transfer Performance: Ability to change body location independently with or without assistive device

Goals/Evaluation Criteria

Examples Using NOC Language

- Demonstrates **Mobility**, as evidenced by the following indicators (specify 1–5: severely, substantially, moderately, mildly, or not compromised):
  - Balance
  - Coordination
  - Body positioning performance
  - Muscle and joint movement
  - Walking
  - Moves with ease

Other Examples

- Demonstrates correct use of assistive devices with supervision
- Requests assistance with mobilization activities, as needed
- Performs ADLs independently with assistive devices (specify activity and device)
- Bears weight
- Walks with effective gait for ________________ (specify distance)
- Transfers to and from chair or wheelchair
- Maneuvers wheelchair effectively

NIC Interventions

Body Mechanics Promotion: Facilitating the use of posture and movement in daily activities to prevent fatigue and musculoskeletal strain or injury

Exercise Promotion: Facilitation of regular physical activity to maintain or advance to a higher level of fitness and health

Exercise Promotion: Strength Training: Facilitating regular resistive muscle training to maintain or increase muscle strength

Exercise Therapy: Ambulation: Promotion and assistance with walking to maintain or restore autonomic and voluntary body functions during treatment and recovery from illness or injury

Exercise Therapy: Balance: Use of specific activities, postures, and movements to maintain, enhance, or restore balance

Exercise Therapy, Joint Mobility: Use of active or passive body movement to maintain or restore joint flexibility

Exercise Therapy: Muscle Control: Use of specific activity or exercise protocols to enhance or restore controlled body movement

Positioning: Deliberative placement of the patient or a body part to promote physiological or psychological well-being

Positioning: Wheelchair: Placement of a patient in a properly selected wheelchair to enhance comfort, promote skin integrity, and foster independence

Self-Care Assistance: Transfer: Assisting a person with limitation of independent movement to learn to change body location

Nursing Activities

Assessment is an ongoing process to determine the performance level of the patient's *Impaired mobility*.

Level 1 Nursing Activities

- Assess need for home health assistance and need for durable medical equipment
- Teach patient about and monitor use of mobility devices (e.g., cane, walker, crutches, or wheelchair)
- Instruct and assist him with transfer process (e.g., bed to chair)
- Refer to physical therapist for an exercise program
- Provide positive reinforcement during activities
- Assist patient to use supportive, nonskid footwear for walking
- *(NIC) Positioning:*
  - Instruct the patient how to use good posture and good body mechanics while performing any activity
  - Monitor traction devices for proper setup

M

Level 2 Nursing Activities

- Assess patient's learning needs
- Assess need for assistance from home health agency and need for durable medical equipment
- Instruct and encourage patient in active or passive range-of-motion exercises to maintain or develop muscle strength and endurance
- Instruct and encourage patient to use a trapeze or weights to enhance and maintain strength of upper extremities.
- Teach techniques for safe transfer and ambulation
- Instruct patient regarding weight-bearing status
- Instruct patient regarding correct body alignment
- Use occupational and physical therapists as a resource in developing a plan for maintaining or increasing mobility
- Provide positive reinforcement during activities
- Supervise all mobilization attempts and assist patient, as necessary
- Use a gait belt when assisting with transfer or ambulation

Levels 3 and 4 Nursing Activities

- Determine patient motivation level for maintaining or restoring mobility of joints and muscles

- Use occupational and physical therapists as resource in planning patient care activities
- Encourage patient and family to view limitations realistically
- Provide positive reinforcement during activities
- Administer analgesics before beginning exercises
- Develop a plan specifying the following:
  Type of assistive device
  Positioning of patient in bed or chair
  Ways to transfer and turn patient
  Number of personnel needed to mobilize patient
  Necessary elimination equipment (e.g., bedpan, urinal, fracture pan)
  Schedule of activities
- *(NIC) Positioning:*
  Monitor traction devices for proper setup
  Place on an appropriate therapeutic mattress or bed
  Position in proper body alignment
  Place in the designated therapeutic position [e.g., avoid placing the amputation stump in the flexion position; elevate the affected body part, as appropriate; immobilize or support the affected body part, as appropriate]
  Turn the immobilized patient at least every 2 hr, according to a specific schedule, as appropriate
  Place bed-positioning switch and call light within easy reach
  Encourage active or passive range-of-motion exercises, as appropriate

Home Care

- Assess the home environment for barriers to mobility (e.g., stairs, uneven floors)
- Refer for home health aide services for help with ADLs
- Refer to physical therapy services for strength, balance, and gait training
- Refer to occupational therapy services for assistive devices
- Suggest exercising with a family member or friend
- Teach to get out of bed slowly

For Older Adults

- Monitor for complications of immobility (e.g., pneumonia, pressure sores), which occur more quickly in older adults
- Evaluate for depression and impaired cognition
- Monitor for orthostatic hypotension; when assisting the client out of bed, have client dangle before standing

MOBILITY: WHEELCHAIR, IMPAIRED

(1998, 2006) **Domain 4, Activity/Rest; Class 2, Activity/Exercise**

Definition: Limitation of independent operation of wheelchair within environment [specify level]

Defining Characteristics

Inability to operate:

Manual wheelchair on curbs
Power wheelchair on curbs
Manual wheelchair on even surface
Power wheelchair on even surface
Manual wheelchair on uneven surface
Power wheelchair on uneven surface
Manual wheelchair on an incline
Power wheelchair on an incline
Manual wheelchair on a decline
Power wheelchair on a decline

Related Factors

Cognitive impairment
Deconditioning
Deficient knowledge
Depressed mood
Environmental constraints (e.g., stairs, inclines, uneven surfaces, unsafe obstacles, distances, lack of assistive devices or person, wheelchair type)
Impaired vision
Insufficient muscle strength
Limited endurance
Musculoskeletal impairment (e.g., contractures)
Neuromuscular impairment
Obesity
Pain

Suggestions for Use

Specify levels of independence, which are the same as the options for *Impaired physical mobility* and *Impaired bed mobility*:

Level 0: Is completely independent
Level 1: Requires use of equipment or device
Level 2: Requires help from another person for assistance, supervision, or teaching

Level 3: Requires help from another person and equipment and device
Level 4: Is dependent; does not participate in activity

See Suggestions for Use for Mobility: Physical, Impaired.

Suggested Alternative Diagnoses

Injury, risk for
Mobility: physical, impaired
Skin integrity, risk for impaired
Transfer ability, impaired

NOC Outcomes

Ambulation: Wheelchair: Ability to move from place to place in a wheelchair
Balance: Ability to maintain body equilibrium
Coordinated Movement: Ability of muscles to work together voluntarily for purposeful movement
Mobility: Ability to move purposefully in own environment independently with or without assistive device
Transfer Performance: Ability to change body location independently with or without assistive device

Goals/Evaluation Criteria

Examples Using NOC Language

- Demonstrates **Mobility**, as evidenced by the following indicators (specify 1–5: severely, substantially, moderately, mildly, or not compromised):
  - Balance, coordination, and body positioning performance
  - Transfer performance
- Demonstrates **Ambulation: Wheelchair**, as evidenced by the following indicators (specify 1–5: severely, substantially, moderately, mildly, or not compromised):
  - Propels wheelchair safely
  - Maneuvers curbs
  - Maneuvers doorways
  - Maneuvers ramps
  - Propels wheelchair short/moderate/long distance

Other Examples

- Requests assistance with mobilization activities, as needed
- Performs ADLs independently with or without assistive devices (specify activity and device)
- Demonstrates moderate active movement of all joints or specify affected joints

M

NIC Interventions

Exercise Promotion: Strength Training: Facilitating regular resistive muscle training to maintain or increase muscle strength

Exercise Therapy: Balance: Use of specific activities, postures, and movements to maintain, enhance, or restore balance

Exercise Therapy: Muscle Control: Use of specific activity or exercise protocols to enhance or restore controlled body movement

Positioning: Wheelchair: Placement of a patient in a properly selected wheelchair to enhance comfort, promote skin integrity, and foster independence

Self-Care Assistance: Transfer: Assisting a person with limitation of independent movement to learn to change body location

Nursing Activities

Assessments

M

- Assess patient's learning needs regarding use of wheelchair
- Assess joint mobility and muscle strength
- Assess cognitive abilities
- Determine patient's motivation level for using wheelchair
- *(NIC) Positioning: Wheelchair:*
    - Check patient's position in the wheelchair while patient sits on selected pad and wears proper footwear
    - Monitor for patient's inability to maintain correct posture in wheelchair

Patient/Family Teaching

- *(NIC) Positioning: Wheelchair:*
    - Instruct patient on exercises to increase upper body strength, as appropriate
    - Instruct patient on how to operate wheelchair, as appropriate

Collaborative Activities

- Collaborate with physical and occupational therapists, as needed (e.g., to be certain that wheelchair size and type is appropriate for patient)

Other

- Provide positive reinforcement during activities
- Supervise attempts to operate wheelchair on curbs and inclines
- Encourage patient and family to view limitations realistically
- *(NIC) Positioning: Wheelchair:*
    - Check that footrests have at least 2 inches of clearance from the floor
    - Ensure that wheelchair allows at least 2–3 inches of clearance from the back of knee to front of sling seat
    - Provide modifications or appliances to wheelchair to correct for patient problems or muscle weakness

Home Care

- The preceding interventions are appropriate for home care
- Also see Home Care interventions for Impaired Physical Mobility
- Assess need for assistance from home health agency and need for special modifications to wheelchair (e.g., motor)

For Older Adults

- See interventions for Older Adults with Impaired Physical Mobility
- Avoid using restraints to keep the patient in the chair

MORAL DISTRESS

(2006) **Domain 10, Life Principles; Class 3, Values/Belief/Action Congruence**

Definition: Response to the inability to carry out one's chosen ethical/moral decision/action

Defining Characteristics

Expresses anguish (e.g., powerlessness, guilt, frustration, anxiety, self-doubt, fear) over difficulty acting on one's moral choice

Related Factors

Conflict among decision makers
Conflicting information guiding moral/ethical decision making
Cultural conflicts
End-of-life decisions
Loss of autonomy
Physical distance of decision maker
Time constraints for decision making
Treatment decisions

Suggestions for Use

Differentiate between *Moral distress* and *Decisional conflict*. If the patient is torn between two equally good (or bad) choices of action and cannot decide what to do, use *Decisional conflict*. If the person believes she knows the right thing to do, but for some reason cannot do what she has decided, use *Moral distress*. The suffering accompanying *Moral distress* may lead to *Impaired religiosity* and *Spiritual distress*. *Moral distress* is more specifically, and narrowly, defined than *Risk for impaired religiosity* and *Risk for spiritual distress*. *Powerlessness* often accompanies *Moral distress*.

Suggested Alternative Diagnoses

Decisional conflict
Powerlessness
Religiosity, risk for impaired
Spirituality, risk for impaired

NOC Outcomes

Anxiety Level: Severity of manifested apprehension, tension, or uneasiness arising from an unidentifiable source

Comfort Status: Psychospiritual: Psychospiritual ease related to self-concept, emotional well-being, source of inspiration, and meaning and purpose in life

Dignified Life Closure: Personal actions to maintain control during approaching end of life

Fear Level: Severity of manifested apprehension, tension, or uneasiness arising from an identifiable source

Personal Autonomy: Personal actions of a competent individual to exercise governance in life decisions

Spiritual Health: Connectedness with self, others, higher power, all life, nature, and the universe that transcends and empowers the self

Goals/Evaluation Criteria

Examples Using NOC Language

- *Moral distress* will be relieved, as evidenced by: Anxiety Level, Comfort Status: Psychospiritual, Dignified Life Closure, Fear Level, Personal Autonomy, and Spiritual Health
- Demonstrates **Personal Autonomy**, as evidenced by the following indicators (specify 1–5: never, rarely, sometimes, often, or consistently demonstrated):
  - Expresses independence with decision-making process
  - Asserts personal preferences
  - Makes decisions free from undue pressure by [specify:] parents, spouse, children, extended family, friends, health care provider

Other Examples

- Expresses satisfaction with spiritual life
- Demonstrates the ability to cope

- Expresses an acceptable level of happiness
- Verbalizes resolution of symptoms such as guilt, frustration, and self-doubt
- Verbalizes understanding that no moral failing occurred on his part because he was powerless to carry out his moral decision

NIC Interventions

(**NOTE:** Although Johnson, Moorhead, Bulechek, Butcher, Maas, Swanson, (2012) have linked Decision-Making Support to this nursing diagnosis, the author believes it is not needed because, by the diagnosis' definition, the patient has already made a decision.)

Anxiety Reduction: Minimizing apprehension, dread, foreboding, or uneasiness related to an unidentified source of anticipated danger

Decision-Making Support: Providing information and support for a patient who is making a decision regarding health care

Emotional Support: Provision of reassurance, acceptance, and encouragement during times of stress

Patient Rights Protection: Protection of health care rights of a patient, especially a minor, incapacitated, or incompetent patient unable to make decisions

Self-Esteem Enhancement: Assisting a patient to increase his personal judgment of self-worth

Spiritual Growth Facilitation: Facilitation of growth in patients' capacity to identify, connect with, and call upon the source of meaning, purpose, comfort, strength, and hope in their lives

Spiritual Support: Assisting the patient to feel balance and connection with a greater power

Nursing Activities

Nursing interventions for this diagnosis should assume that the patient is comfortable with the moral decision he has made and that his anguish results from being unable to carry out that decision. Activities should focus on (a) helping the patient cope with the immediate feelings of distress, (b) identifying problematic feelings (e.g., anxiety, powerlessness) more specifically in order to formulate nursing diagnoses and interventions to alleviate them. Note that *Powerlessness* is commonly associated with *Moral distress*, and (c) advocating for the patient to remove barriers to acting on his decision, or to reach a satisfactory compromise. However, in many (if not most) situations you may be unable to empower the patient—that is, no matter the intervention, he may not be able (or allowed) to carry out his moral decision. In that case, interventions would aim to empower the patient for making future decisions.

Assessments

- Observe for expressions of anguish and unhappiness
- Talk with the patient to identify his feelings more specifically (e.g., powerlessness, guilt, anger, frustration, anxiety, self-doubt)
- Assess for physical and behavioral manifestations of anxiety
- Find out who is legally empowered to make decisions for the patient
- Assess the patient's confidence in own judgment

Patient/Family Teaching

- Provide factual information about the situation that has occurred; clarify any misperceptions
- Provide information about advance directives
- Teach relaxation and guided imagery
- Provide a copy of "Patient's Bill of Rights," "Patient-Care Partnership," or similar document

Collaborative Activities

- Refer to agency ethics committee
- Refer to chaplain or other spiritual adviser of the patient's choosing
- Communicate with administrators and health team members to honor patient and family wishes

Other

- Demonstrate empathy and acceptance; establish trust; make supportive statements
- Use touch as appropriate
- Provide opportunities for spiritual activities
- Use active listening; encourage to express concerns and feelings
- Consider whether values clarification would be helpful to the patient
- Encourage to identify own strengths and reevaluate negative perceptions of self
- Explore reasons for feelings of guilt
- Arrange for privacy for conversations between patient, significant others, and health care professionals
- Do not force treatment
- Assist the patient to recognize and express feelings (e.g., of guilt, sadness, powerlessness)
- Encourage the patient to talk or cry as a way to relieve tensions
- Help the patient to identify life values
- Help the patient to identify available supports

Home Care

- The preceding interventions are appropriate for home care use

NAUSEA

(1998, 2002, 2010) **Domain 12, Comfort; Class 1, Physical Comfort**

Definition: A subjective phenomenon of an unpleasant feeling in the back of the throat and stomach that may or may not result in vomiting

Defining Characteristics

Subjective

Aversion toward food
Gagging sensation
Increased salivation
Increased swallowing
Report of nausea [or "sick to stomach"]
Sour taste in mouth

Non-NANDA International Symptoms

May be accompanied by pallor, cold and clammy skin, tachycardia, and gastric stasis. Nausea usually precedes vomiting, but may be experienced after vomiting or when vomiting does not occur.

Related Factors

Treatment Related

Gastric irritation [e.g., from pharmaceutical agents (e.g., aspirin, nonsteroidal anti-inflammatory drugs [NSAIDs], steroids, antibiotics), alcohol, iron, and blood]
Gastric distention [e.g., delayed gastric emptying caused by pharmaceutical agents such as narcotics and anesthetics]
Pharmaceutical agents (e.g., analgesics, antiviral for HIV, aspirin, opioids) and chemotherapeutic agents
Toxins (e.g., radiotherapy)

Biophysical

Biochemical disorders (e.g., uremia, diabetic ketoacidosis, pregnancy)
Esophageal or pancreatic disease
Gastric distention (e.g., due to delayed gastric emptying; pyloric intestinal obstruction; genitourinary and biliary distention; upper bowel

stasis; external compression of the stomach, liver, spleen, or other organs; enlargement that slows stomach functioning; excess food intake)
Gastric irritation [e.g., due to pharyngeal and peritoneal inflammation]
Increased intracranial pressure
Intra-abdominal tumors
Liver or splenetic capsule stretch
Localized tumors such as acoustic neuroma, primary or secondary brain tumors, bone metastases at base of skull
Meningitis
Motion sickness, Meniere's disease, or labyrinthitis
Pain
Pregnancy
Toxins (e.g., tumor-produced peptides, abnormal metabolites due to cancer)

Situational

Anxiety or fear
Noxious odors or noxious taste
Psychological factors
Unpleasant visual stimulation

Suggestions for Use

This label is appropriate for short-term episodes of nausea and vomiting (e.g., postoperatively). When *Nausea* is severe or prolonged and may compromise adequate nutrition, use *Risk for imbalanced nutrition: less than body requirements related to Nausea.*

Suggested Alternative Diagnoses

Fluid volume, risk for deficient
Nutrition: less than body requirements, risk for imbalanced

NOC Outcomes

Appetite: Desire to eat when ill or receiving treatment
Nausea and Vomiting Control: Personal actions to control nausea, retching, and vomiting symptoms
Nausea and Vomiting: Disruptive Effect: Severity of observed or reported disruptive effects of nausea, retching, and vomiting on daily functioning
Nausea and Vomiting Severity: Severity of nausea, retching, and vomiting symptoms

Goals/Evaluation Criteria

Examples Using NOC Language

- *Nausea* will be relieved, as evidenced by: substantial Appetite and uncompromised Nausea and Vomiting Control.
- Demonstrates acceptable **Nausea and Vomiting: Disruptive Effects**, as evidenced by the following indicators (specify 1–5: severe, substantial, moderate, slight, or none):
  - Decreased fluid intake
  - Decreased food intake
  - Decreased urinary output
  - Altered fluid balance
  - Altered serum electrolytes
  - Altered nutritional status
  - Weight loss

Other Examples

The patient will:

- Identify and avoid causal stimuli
- Report relief from nausea, retching, and vomiting
- Identify and implement measures that decrease nausea

NIC Interventions

Environmental Management: Manipulation of the patient's surroundings for therapeutic benefit, sensory appeal, and psychological well-being

Fluid Monitoring: Collection and analysis of patient data to regulate fluid balance

Fluid/Electrolyte Management: Regulation and prevention of complications from altered fluid or electrolyte levels

Medication Management: Facilitation of safe and effective use of prescription and over-the-counter drugs

Nausea Management: Prevention and alleviation of nausea

Nutritional Monitoring: Collection and analysis of patient data to prevent or minimize malnourishment

Vomiting Management: Prevention and alleviation of vomiting

Nursing Activities

Assessment

- Monitor patient's subjective symptoms of nausea
- Monitor urine color, quantity, and specific gravity

- Assess for causes of the nausea (e.g., bowel obstruction, medication side effects)
- *(NIC) Nutritional Monitoring:*
  Monitor trends in weight loss and gain
  Monitor energy level, malaise, fatigue, and weakness
  Monitor caloric and nutrient intake
- *(NIC) Fluid Management:*
  Monitor intake and output
  Monitor BP, heart rate, and respiratory status
  Monitor mucous membranes, skin turgor, and thirst

Patient/Family Teaching

- Explain the causes of the nausea
- If possible, tell the patient how long to expect the nausea to last
- Teach patient to use voluntary swallowing or deep breathing to suppress the vomiting reflex
- Teach to eat slowly
- Teach to restrict fluids 1 hr before, 1 hr after, and during meals

Collaborative Activities

- Administer prescribed antiemetics
- Consult with physician to provide adequate pain control with medications that do not cause nausea for the patient
- *(NIC) Fluid Monitoring:* Administer fluids, as appropriate

Other

- Elevate head of bed or place in lateral position to prevent aspiration (for clients with decreased mobility)
- Keep client and bedding clean when vomiting occurs
- Remove odor-producing substances immediately (e.g., bedpans, food)
- Do not schedule painful or nausea-producing procedures near mealtimes
- Provide oral care after vomiting
- Apply cool, damp cloth to patient's wrists, neck, and forehead
- Offer cold foods and other foods with little odor

Home Care

- Instruct to avoid the smell of food preparation at home (e.g., let someone else prepare meals, stay out of the kitchen, go for a walk during meal preparation)
- All of the preceding interventions can also be used in home care

For Infants and Children

- Infants and children are at increased risk of *Deficient fluid volume* as a result of *Nausea*, because they will usually refuse to feed.

For Older Adults

- Monitor carefully for side effects of antiemetic medications (e.g., sedation)
- Assess whether the nausea might be caused by NSAIDs the patient is taking for arthritis

NEUROVASCULAR DYSFUNCTION: PERIPHERAL, RISK FOR

(1992) **Domain 11, Safety/Protection; Class 2, Physical Safety**

Definition: At risk for disruption in circulation, sensation, or motion of an extremity

Risk Factors

Burns
Fractures
Immobilization
Mechanical compression (e.g., tourniquet, cast, brace, dressing, or restraint)
Orthopedic surgery
Trauma
Vascular obstruction

Suggestions for Use

Use this label for situations nurses can prevent by reducing or eliminating causative factors (e.g., *Risk for peripheral neurovascular dysfunction related to compression from restraints*). For situations requiring medical treatment (e.g., thrombophlebitis), use a collaborative problem such as Potential Complication of thrombophlebitis in left leg: *Peripheral neurovascular dysfunction.*

Suggested Alternative Diagnosis

Perioperative positioning injury, risk for

NOC Outcomes

Neurological Status: Peripheral: Ability of the peripheral nervous system to transmit impulses to and from the central nervous system

Sensory Function: Cutaneous: Extent to which stimulation of the skin is correctly sensed

Tissue Perfusion: Peripheral: Adequacy of blood flow through the small vessels of the extremities to maintain tissue function

Goals/Evaluation Criteria

Examples Using NOC Language

- Demonstrates **Tissue Perfusion: Peripheral**, as evidenced by the following indicators (specify 1–5: severe, substantial, moderate, mild, or no deviation from normal range):
  - Capillary refill fingers/toes
  - Extremity skin temperature
  - Localized extremity pain
  - Numbness
  - Paresthesia
  - Peripheral edema
  - Skin breakdown

Other Examples

- Blood pressure within normal limits
- Recognizes signs and symptoms of peripheral neurovascular dysfunction
- Strong pulses in the extremity
- Remains free of injury from compression devices or restraints
- Uncompromised strength in the extremity
- Demonstrates optimal healing and adaptation to cast, traction, or dressing
- Good muscle tone and strong movement of extremities

NIC Interventions

Cast Care: Maintenance: Care of a cast after the drying period

Circulatory Care: Arterial Insufficiency: Promotion of arterial circulation

Circulatory Care: Venous Insufficiency: Promotion of venous circulation

Circulatory Precautions: Protection of a localized area with limited perfusion

Lower Extremity Monitoring: Collection, analysis, and use of patient data to categorize risk and prevent injury to the lower extremities

Neurologic Monitoring: Collection and analysis of patient data to prevent or minimize neurologic complications

Peripheral Sensation Management: Prevention or minimization of injury or discomfort in the patient with altered sensation

Positioning: Neurologic: Achievement of optimal, appropriate body alignment for the patient experiencing or at risk for spinal cord injury or vertebrae irritability

Pressure Management: Minimizing pressure to body parts

Pressure Management: Minimizing pressure to body parts

Nursing Activities

Assessments

- Perform neurovascular assessments every hour for the first 24 hr following casting, injury, traction, or restraints. Then, if stable, perform the following activities q4h:
  - Assess for and report increasing and progressive pain that is present on passive movement and not relieved by narcotics, which may be first sign of compartmental syndrome
- Assess motor function, movement, and strength of the involved peripheral nerve
- *(NIC) Circulatory Care (Arterial and Venous Insufficiency):* Perform a comprehensive appraisal of peripheral circulation (e.g., check peripheral pulses, edema, capillary refill, color, and temperature)
- *(NIC) Peripheral Sensation Management:*
  - Monitor for paresthesia: numbness, tingling, hyperesthesia, and hypoesthesia
  - Monitor sharp and dull and/or hot and cold discrimination
  - Monitor fit of bracing devices, prostheses, shoes, and clothing
  - Check shoes, pockets, and clothing for wrinkles or foreign objects
  - Monitor for thrombophlebitis and deep-vein thrombosis

N

Patient/Family Teaching

- Teach patient and family routine cast care and measures to prevent complications
- Teach patient and family signs and symptoms of peripheral nerve injury and importance of immediate medical attention
- Teach patient and family to perform passive, assisted, or active range-of-motion exercises
- *(NIC) Peripheral Sensation Management:*
  - Instruct patient to use timed intervals, rather than presence of discomfort, as a signal to alter position
  - Instruct patient or family to use thermometer to test water temperature

Collaborative Activities

- Collaborate with physical therapist in developing and executing an exercise program

Other

- Avoid tight dressings and appliances to prevent ischemia
- Institute immediate treatment if compartmental syndrome is suspected: keep involved extremity at heart level; notify physician; and anticipate removal of anterior cast, occlusive bandages, and surgical intervention
- Assure that patient's clothing is not restrictive
- Perform passive or assisted range-of-motion exercises
- *(NIC) Circulatory Care (Arterial and Venous Insufficiency):*

  Elevate affected limb 20 degrees or greater above the level of the heart [to improve venous return], as appropriate

  Place extremity in a dependent position [to improve arterial circulation], as appropriate

  Maintain adequate hydration to prevent increased blood viscosity

  Change the patient's position at least every 2 hr, as appropriate

N

- *(NIC) Peripheral Sensation Management:*

  Avoid or carefully monitor use of heat or cold, such as heating pads, hot-water bottles, and ice packs

  Encourage patient to use the unaffected body part to identify location and texture of objects

  Place cradle over affected body parts to keep bed clothes off affected areas

  Encourage patient to wear well-fitting, low-heeled, soft shoes

Home Care

- Most of the preceding interventions can be adapted for use in home care
- *(NIC) Circulatory Care (Arterial and Venous Insufficiency):*

  Instruct the patient on proper foot care

  Instruct the patient on factors that interfere with circulation (e.g., smoking, restrictive clothing, exposure to cold temperatures, and crossing of legs and feet)

For Infants and Children

- Recognize that restlessness, fussiness, and crying may be nonverbal cues of physical distress in infants, children, or adults with impaired verbal communication

NONCOMPLIANCE [SPECIFY]

(1973, 1996, 1998) Domain 10, Life Principles; Class 3, Value/Belief/Action Congruence

Definition: Behavior of person or caregiver that fails to coincide with a health-promoting or therapeutic plan agreed on by the person (or family, or community) and health care professional. In the presence of an agreed-on, health-promoting or therapeutic plan, the person's or caregiver's behavior is fully or partially nonadherent and may lead to clinically ineffective or partially ineffective outcomes.

Defining Characteristics

Objective

Behavior indicative of failure to adhere [by direct observation or by statements of patient or significant others]
Evidence of development of complications
Evidence of exacerbation of symptoms
Failure to keep appointments
Failure to progress
Objective tests (e.g., physiologic measures, detection of physiologic markers)

Related Factors

Healthcare Plan

Complexity
Cost
Duration
Financial flexibility of plan
Intensity

Individual Factors

Cultural influences
Deficient knowledge of the regimen behavior
Health beliefs
Individual's value system
Motivational forces
Personal and developmental abilities
Significant others
Spiritual values

Health System

Access to and convenience of care
Communication and teaching skills of the provider

Credibility of provider
Difficulty in client–provider relationships
Individual health coverage
Provider continuity and regular follow-up
Provider reimbursement [especially of teaching and follow-up]
Satisfaction with care

Network

Involvement of members in health plan
Perceived beliefs of significant others
Social value regarding plan

Suggestions for Use

Noncompliance describes failure to adhere to a therapeutic recommendation after having made an informed decision to do so and after expressing an intention to do so. If the patient is informed and *intends* to follow instructions, then nursing intervention can be directed at finding and removing the factors that keep him from doing so. For example, a patient may state, "My husband doesn't need to lose weight, and he loves fried food and pastries. He just won't eat the diet foods, and I really don't have time to cook one meal for myself and one for the rest of the family." This client would like to comply with her diet, but situational factors make it difficult. You could write a nursing diagnosis of *Noncompliance with low-calorie diet related to inconvenience of preparing special foods and lack of family support*. That diagnosis does suggest independent nursing interventions.

Noncompliance should not be used for a patient who makes an informed decision to not follow a therapeutic recommendation, for instance, when a patient decides to stop taking a medication with unpleasant side effects. Nursing intervention might then be directed at convincing the patient of the value of continuing with the therapy, but the nurse should balance this approach with respect for the patient's autonomy when he has truly made an informed decision. Remember that a decision to refuse therapy can be as rational as a decision to have therapy.

Noncompliance should not be used for patients who are unable to follow instructions (e.g., weakness, cognitive disability) or who lack necessary information. If those factors are contributing to *Noncompliance*, then it is better to use the diagnosis *Ineffective health maintenance*.

Some nurses believe that *Noncompliance* is a negative label. When using this diagnosis, be sure to express the etiology in neutral, nonjudgmental terms. Geissler (1991) has suggested the term *nonadherence*, although it is not yet a NANDA International label.

Suggested Alternative Diagnoses

Denial, ineffective
Health maintenance, ineffective
Management of therapeutic regimen: family, ineffective
Nonadherence (non-NANDA-I)
Client–provider relationships

NOC Outcomes

Caregiver Performance: Direct Care: Provision by family care provider of appropriate personal and health care for a family member

Caregiver Performance: Indirect Care: Arrangement and oversight by family care provider of appropriate care for a family member

Compliance Behavior: Personal actions to promote wellness, recovery, and rehabilitation recommended by a health professional

Compliance Behavior: Prescribed Diet: Personal actions to follow food and fluid intake recommended by a health professional for a specific health condition

Compliance: Prescribed Medication: Personal actions to administer medication safely to meet therapeutic goals as recommended by a health professional

Motivation: Inner urge that moves or prompts an individual to positive action(s)

Treatment Behavior: Illness or Injury: Personal actions to palliate or eliminate pathology

Goals/Evaluation Criteria

Examples Using NOC Language

- *Noncompliance* will decrease, as demonstrated by Caregiver Performance: Direct and Indirect Care; Compliance Behavior; Motivation; and Treatment Behavior: Illness or Injury
- Demonstrates **Compliance Behavior**, as evidenced by the following indicators (specify 1–5: never, rarely, sometimes, often, or consistently demonstrated):

  Performs treatment regimen as prescribed
  Seeks reputable information about diagnosis and treatment
  Monitors medication and therapeutic effects
  Performs self-screening when directed

Other Examples

Patient will:

- Not abuse health care providers physically or verbally
- Use pain control measures

N

- Comply with prescribed medication and treatment regimens
- Keep appointments with health care providers
- Report significant treatment effects and side effects
- Report controlling illness symptoms

NIC Interventions

Caregiver Support: Provision of the necessary information, advocacy, and support to facilitate primary patient care by someone other than a health care professional

Health Education: Developing and providing instruction and learning experiences to facilitate voluntary adaptation of behavior conducive to health in individuals, families, groups, or communities

Health System Guidance: Facilitating a patient's location and use of appropriate health services

Learning Facilitation: Promoting the ability to process and comprehend information

N

Medication Management: Facilitation of safe and effective use of prescription and over-the-counter drugs

Mutual Goal Setting: Collaborating with patient to identify and prioritize care goals, then developing a plan for achieving those goals

Nutritional Counseling: Use of an interactive helping process focusing on the need for diet modification

Self-Efficacy Enhancement: Strengthening an individual's confidence in his ability to perform a health behavior

Patient Contracting: Negotiating an agreement that reinforces a specific behavior change

Self-Modification Assistance: Reinforcement of self-directed change initiated by the patient to achieve personally important goals

Self-Responsibility Facilitation: Encouraging a patient to assume more responsibility for own behavior

Teaching: Disease Process: Assisting the patient to understand information related to a specific disease process

Teaching: Individual: Planning, implementation, and evaluation of a teaching program designed to address a patient's particular needs

Teaching: Prescribed Diet: Preparing a patient to correctly follow a prescribed diet

Teaching: Prescribed Medication: Preparing a patient to safely take prescribed medications and monitor for their effects

Teaching: Procedure/Treatment: Preparing a patient to understand and mentally prepare for a prescribed procedure or treatment

Nursing Activities

Assessments

- Identify probable cause of patient's noncompliant behavior

Patient/Family Teaching

- Help patient and family to understand the need for following the prescribed treatment and the consequences of noncompliance
- *(NIC) Health System Guidance:*
  - Inform patient of appropriate community resources and contact persons
  - Give written instructions for purpose and location of health care activities, as appropriate

Collaborative Activities

- Consult with physician about possible alteration in medical regimen to encourage patient's compliance
- *(NIC) Health System Guidance:*
  - Coordinate referrals to relevant health care providers, as appropriate
  - Identify and facilitate communication among health care providers and patient and family, as appropriate
  - Coordinate and schedule time needed by each service to deliver care, as appropriate
  - Provide follow-up contact with patient, as appropriate
  - Assist individual to complete forms for assistance, such as housing and financial aid, as needed

Other

- Encourage the patient to express feelings and concerns about hospitalization and relationship with health care providers
- Provide emotional support to family members to help them maintain a positive relationship with patient
- Give positive reinforcement for compliance to encourage ongoing positive behaviors
- Develop a written contract with the patient and evaluate compliant behaviors on a continuing basis. Specify contract
- *(NIC) Self-Modification Assistance:*
  - Encourage the patient to examine personal values and beliefs and satisfaction with them
  - Explore with the patient potential barriers to change behavior
  - Identify with the patient the most effective strategies for behavior change

Assist the patient in formulating a systematic plan for behavior change [including intrinsic and extrinsic rewards and reinforcers]

Assist the patient in identifying even small successes

Home Care

- The preceding interventions are appropriate for use in home care
- Encourage self-management of care to the extent possible
- Assist the patient to incorporate the treatment regimen into his daily schedule
- If it becomes necessary, be sure the client understands that the home health agency will not be allowed to continue providing services if the client chooses to not adhere to the medical regimen

For Infants and Children

- Base your communication on the child's developmental stage. Keep explanations short and concrete
- Point out specific, observable benefits of adhering to the treatment regimen
- Avoid punishing the child for not adhering to the treatment regimen; as a last resort perhaps try a technique such as withholding privileges, or using time-out for younger children
- Try using rewards for desired behaviors (e.g., put stars on a chart)
- Involve the child in self-care to her abilities (e.g., an older child might draw up her own insulin; a younger one brings it to mother to draw up)

For Older Adults

- Assess for cognitive deficits that may decrease compliance
- Assess for functional deficits that may decrease compliance (e.g., arthritic hands may not be able to open medication bottles; people with failing vision may have difficulty reading labels)
- Obtain assistive devices, as needed (e.g., pill dispenser)
- Simplify the treatment regimen as much as possible
- Use reminders: written instructions, lists, calls from family or friends, a medication organizer divided into days of the week and hours of the day, and so forth
- Refer for home health services if patient cannot manage treatment regimen alone (e.g., have a home health nurse come to set up a week's medications in an organizer)
- Assess whether the patient can afford the medications
- Monitor for depression as a cause of noncompliance

NUTRITION, IMBALANCED: LESS THAN BODY REQUIREMENTS

(1975, 2000) **Domain 2, Nutrition; Class 1, Ingestion**

Definition: Intake of nutrients insufficient to meet metabolic needs

Defining Characteristics

The author recommends using this label only if one of the following NANDA cues is present:

Body weight 20% or more below ideal weight range

Food intake less than metabolic needs, either total calories or specific nutrients (non-NANDA International)

Loss of weight with adequate food intake

Reported inadequate food intake less than the recommended daily allowance (RDA)

Subjective

Abdominal cramping

Abdominal pain [with or without pathology]

Aversion to eating

Indigestion (non-NANDA International)

Perceived inability to ingest food

Reported altered taste sensation

[Reported] lack of food

Satiety immediately after ingesting food

Objective

Capillary fragility

Diarrhea or steatorrhea

[Evidence of] lack of food

Excessive loss of hair

Hyperactive bowel sounds

Lack of information, misinformation

Lack of interest in food

Misconceptions

Pale mucous membranes

Poor muscle tone

Refusal to eat (non-NANDA International)

Sore [inflamed] buccal cavity

Weakness of muscles required for swallowing or mastication

Related Factors

Inability to ingest or digest food or absorb nutrients due to biologic, psychologic, or economic factors (insufficient finances), including the following non-NANDA-I examples:
Chemical dependence (specify)
Chronic illness (specify)
Difficulty in chewing or swallowing
Economic factors
Food intolerance
High metabolic needs
Inadequate sucking reflex in the infant
Lack of basic nutritional knowledge
Limited access to food
Loss of appetite
Nausea and vomiting
Parental neglect
Psychologic impairment (specify)

Suggestions for Use

Use this label for patients who are able to eat but unable to ingest, digest, or absorb nutrients to adequately meet metabolic needs. Inadequate ingestion might occur because of decreased appetite, nausea, poverty, or many other situations. Examples of patients unable to digest food or absorb particular nutrients are those with allergies, diarrhea, lactose intolerance, or poorly fitting dentures.

Do not use this label routinely for persons who are NPO or for those completely unable to ingest food for other reasons (e.g., unconscious patients). Nurses cannot prescribe independent nursing interventions for a diagnosis such as *Imbalanced nutrition: less than body requirements related to NPO*. They cannot give the missing nutrients, and they cannot change the NPO order. Additionally, the patient is often NPO for only a short time before and after surgery; thus, any lack of nutrients is temporary and resolves without nursing intervention. Long-term NPO status is a risk factor for other nursing diagnoses, such as *Risk for impaired oral mucous membrane*, and for collaborative problems such as Potential Complication: Electrolyte imbalance.

The patient might have a total nutritional deficit or perhaps be deficient in only one nutrient. When the deficit is something other than total, it should be specified like the following example: *Imbalanced nutrition: less than body requirements for protein related to lack of knowledge of nutritious foods and limited budget for food.*

Suggested Alternative Diagnoses

Breastfeeding, ineffective
Dentition, impaired
Failure to thrive, adult
Infant feeding pattern, ineffective
Nausea
Self-care deficit: feeding
Swallowing, impaired

NOC Outcomes

Appetite: Desire to eat when ill or receiving treatment

Compliance Behavior: Prescribed Diet: Personal actions to follow food and fluid intake recommended by a health professional for a specific health condition

Gastrointestinal Function: Extent to which foods (ingested or tube-fed) are moved from ingestion to excretion

Nutritional Status: Extent to which nutrients are available to meet metabolic needs

Nutritional Status: Biochemical Measures: Body fluid components and chemical indices of nutritional status

Nutritional Status: Nutrient Intake: Nutrient intake to meet metabolic needs

Weight: Body Mass: Extent to which body weight, muscle, and fat are congruent to height, frame, gender, and age

Weight Gain Behavior: Personal actions to gain weight following voluntary or involuntary significant weight loss

Goals/Evaluation Criteria

Examples Using NOC Language

- Demonstrates **Nutritional Status**, as evidenced by the following indicators (specify 1–5: severe, substantial, moderate, mild, or no deviation from normal range):
  - Nutrient intake
  - Food intake
  - Fluid intake
  - Energy

Other Examples

Patient will:

- Maintain weight at ______________ kg or gain ______________ kg by ______________ (specify date)

N

- Describe components of nutritionally adequate diet
- Verbalize willingness to follow diet
- Tolerate prescribed diet
- Maintain body mass and weight WNL
- Have laboratory values (e.g., transferrin, albumin, and electrolytes) WNL
- Report adequate energy levels

NIC Interventions

Breastfeeding Assistance: Preparing a new mother to breast-feed her infant

Diarrhea Management: Management and alleviation of diarrhea

Eating Disorders Management: Prevention and treatment of severe diet restriction and overexercising or binging and purging of food and fluids

Fluid Management: Promotion of fluid balance and prevention of complications resulting from abnormal or undesired fluid levels

Fluid/Electrolyte Management: Regulation and prevention of complications from altered fluid or electrolyte levels

Laboratory Data Interpretation: Critical analysis of patient laboratory data in order to assist with clinical decision making

N

Lactation Counseling: Use of an interactive helping process to assist in maintenance of successful breastfeeding

Nutrition Management: Assisting with or providing a balanced dietary intake of foods and fluids

Nutrition Therapy: Administration of food and fluids to support metabolic processes of a patient who is malnourished or at high risk for becoming malnourished

Nutritional Counseling: Use of an interactive helping process focusing on the need for diet modification

Nutritional Monitoring: Collection and analysis of patient data to prevent or minimize malnourishment

Teaching: Prescribed Diet: Preparing a patient to correctly follow a prescribed diet

Self-Care Assistance: Feeding: Assisting a person to eat

Weight Gain Assistance: Facilitating gain of body weight

Weight Management: Facilitating maintenance of optimal body weight and percent of body fat

Nursing Activities

General Activities for all Imbalanced Nutrition

Assessments

- Determine patient motivation for changing eating habits
- Determine patient's ability to meet nutritional needs

- Monitor laboratory values, especially transferrin, albumin, and electrolytes
- *(NIC) Nutrition Management:*
  Ascertain patient's food preferences
  Monitor recorded intake for nutritional content and calories
  Weigh patient at appropriate intervals

Patient/Family Teaching

- Teach a method for meal planning
- Teach patient and family foods that are nutritious, yet inexpensive
- *(NIC) Nutrition Management:* Provide appropriate information about nutritional needs and how to meet them

Collaborative Activities

- Confer with dietitian to establish protein requirements for patients with inadequate protein intake or protein losses (e.g., patients with anorexia nervosa, glomerular disease, or peritoneal dialysis)
- Confer with physician regarding need for appetite stimulant, supplemental feedings, nutritional tube feedings, or TPN so that adequate caloric intake is maintained
- Refer to physician to determine cause of altered nutrition
- Refer to appropriate community nutritional programs (e.g., Meals on Wheels, food banks) if patient cannot buy or prepare adequate food
- *(NIC) Nutrition Management:* Determine—in collaboration with dietitian, as appropriate—number of calories and type of nutrients needed to meet nutrition requirements [especially for patients with high-energy needs, such as postoperative patients and those with burns, trauma, fever, and wounds].

Other

- Develop meal plan with patient to include schedule of meals, eating environment, patient likes and dislikes, food temperature
- Encourage family members to bring food of patient's preference from home
- Assist patient to write realistic weekly goals for exercise and food intake
- Encourage patient to display food and exercise goals in a prominent location and review them daily
- Offer largest meal during time of day when patient's appetite is greatest
- Create a pleasant environment for meals (e.g., remove unsightly supplies and excretions)
- Avoid invasive procedures before meals
- Feed patient, as needed

- *(NIC) Nutrition Management:*
  Provide patient with high-protein, high-calorie, nutritious finger foods and drinks that can be readily consumed, as appropriate
  Teach patient how to keep a food diary, as needed

Difficulty in Chewing and Swallowing

Also refer to Nursing Activities under the preceding General Activities for all Imbalanced Nutrition and to Nursing Activities for the diagnosis Swallowing, Impaired.

Assessments

- Assess and document degree of chewing and swallowing difficulty

Collaborative Activities

- Request occupational therapy consultation

Other

- Reassure patient and provide calm atmosphere during meals
- Have suction catheters available at bedside and suction during meals, as needed
- Place patient in semi-Fowler or high-Fowler position to facilitate swallowing; have patient remain in this position for 30 min following meals to prevent aspiration
- Place food on unaffected side of mouth to facilitate swallowing
- When feeding patient, use syringe, if necessary, to facilitate swallowing
- *(NIC) Nutrition Management:* Encourage patient to wear properly fitted dentures or acquire dental care

N

Nausea/Vomiting

Also refer to Nursing Activities under General Activities for all Impaired Nutrition, and to Nursing Activities for the diagnosis Nausea.

Assessments

- Identify factors precipitating nausea and vomiting
- Document color, amount, and frequency of emesis

Patient/Family Teaching

- Instruct patient in slow, deep breathing, and voluntary swallowing to decrease nausea and vomiting

Collaborative Activities

- Administer antiemetics and/or analgesics before eating or on prescribed schedule

Other

- Minimize factors that may precipitate nausea and vomiting, specify factors
- Offer cool, wet washcloth to be placed on forehead or back of neck

- Offer oral hygiene before meals
- Limit diet to ice chips and clear liquids when symptoms are severe; progress with diet, as appropriate

Loss of Appetite

Also refer to Nursing Activities under General Activities for all Patients with Impaired Nutrition.

Assessments

- Identify factors that may contribute to patient's loss of appetite (e.g., medications, emotional concerns)

Other

- Give positive feedback to patient who shows increased appetite
- Provide foods in accordance with patient's personal, cultural, and religious preferences
- *(NIC) Nutrition Management:* Offer snacks (e.g., frequent drinks and fresh fruits or fruit juice), as appropriate
- Provide a variety of high-calorie, nutritious foods from which to select

Eating Disorders

Also refer to Nursing Activities under General Activities for all Impaired Nutrition, preceding.

Assessments

- Monitor patient for behaviors associated with weight loss

Collaborative Activities

- Consult dietitian to determine daily caloric intake necessary to attain target weight
- Notify physician if patient refuses to eat
- Work with physician, nutritionist, and patient to set weight and intake goals
- Refer for mental health care

Other

- Establish a trusting, supportive relationship with patient
- Communicate expectations for appropriate intake of food and fluid and amount of exercise
- Confine patient's eating to scheduled meals and snacks
- Accompany patient to bathroom after meals or snacks to observe for self-induced vomiting
- Develop behavior modification program specific to patient's needs
- Provide positive reinforcement for weight gain and appropriate eating behaviors, but do not focus interactions on food or eating
- Explore with patient and significant others personal issues (e.g., body image) that contribute to eating behaviors

- Communicate that the patient is responsible for choices about eating and physical activity
- Discuss the benefits of healthy eating behaviors and the consequences of noncompliance

Home Care

- The preceding interventions are appropriate, or can be adapted, for home care
- If depression is diagnosed, refer for psychiatric home health care services

For Infants and Children

- Base your communication on the child's developmental stage
- Teach parents and children the importance of choosing healthy snacks (e.g., fresh fruits and vegetables, popcorn, boiled eggs, peanut butter, cheese) instead of foods high in sugar, salt, or fat (e.g., candy, chips, ice cream)
- If possible, and if necessary, limit the child's intake of milk so there will be an appetite for other foods; some children prefer to drink milk almost exclusively
- Teach parents about nutritional needs during different developmental stages
- Do not allow food to become a battleground for parents and children
- Encourage family to make meals a pleasant social event for the family
- Provide small portions and offer a variety of foods

For Older Adults

- Assess cognitive and functional abilities that may interfere with the patient's ability to prepare and eat foods (e.g., ability to reach shelves where food is stored, to open cans, to stand at the stove; condition of dentures or teeth)
- Assess whether client can afford adequate food
- If client lives alone, assist in finding a community center that provides meals for older adults for at least one meal a day; or minimally, arrange for Meals on Wheels
- Arrange for transportation to buy food, if needed
- Assess for protein and energy malnutrition, which is common among older adults

- Arrange for high-protein supplements as needed; offer liquid supplements, as needed
- Assess for depression as a cause of loss of appetite
- Assess for medication side effects that may be causing loss of appetite

NUTRITION, IMBALANCED: MORE THAN BODY REQUIREMENTS

(1975, 2000) **Domain 2, Nutrition; Class 1, Ingestion**

Definition: Intake of nutrients that exceeds metabolic needs

Defining Characteristics

The author recommends using this diagnosis only if one or more of the following NANDA International defining characteristics are present:

Triceps skinfold greater than 15 mm in men and 25 mm in women

Weight 20% over ideal for height and frame

Objective

Concentrating food intake at end of day

Dysfunctional eating pattern (e.g., pairing food with other activities)

Eating in response to external cues, such as time of day or social situation

Eating in response to internal cues other than hunger (e.g., anxiety, [anger, depression, boredom, stress, loneliness])

Sedentary activity level

Other Defining Characteristics (Non-NANDA International)

Rapid transition across growth percentiles in infants or children

Reported or observed higher baseline weight at beginning of each pregnancy

Related Factors

Excessive intake in relation to metabolic need

Excessive intake in relation to physical activity (caloric expenditure)

Other Related Factors (Non-NANDA International)

Chemical dependence

Decreased metabolic requirements (e.g., secondary to prescribed bed rest)

Ethnic and cultural norms

Increased appetite

Lack of basic nutritional knowledge

Medications that stimulate appetite

N

Use of food as reward or comfort measure
Obesity in one or both parents
Use of solid food as major food source before 5 months of age
Selecting foods that do not meet daily requirements
Substituting sweets for addiction

Suggestions for Use

This diagnosis is most appropriate for patients who are motivated to lose weight (e.g., a woman who has gained weight after pregnancy). For patients who are overweight but not motivated to participate in a weight loss program, consider *Ineffective health maintenance* instead. Note that *Imbalanced nutrition: more than body requirements* focuses attention on nutrition instead of on lifestyle changes necessary for weight loss (e.g., exercise). Eating in response to stressors might be better described as *Ineffective coping*.

Although some of the nursing actions and one of the NIC interventions specify "eating disorders management" as an intervention for this diagnosis, the focus of nursing for a patient who is binging and purging is much more complex than excess calorie intake. This diagnosis has limited use in that situation, although the nurse provides supportive interventions.

Suggested Alternative Diagnoses

Coping, ineffective
Health maintenance, ineffective
Nutrition, imbalanced: risk for more than body requirements

NOC Outcomes

Nutritional Status: Food and Fluid Intake: Amount of food and fluid taken into the body over a 24-hr period

Weight Loss Behavior: Personal actions to lose weight through diet, exercise, and behavior modification

Goals/Evaluation Criteria

Examples Using NOC Language

- Demonstrates **Nutritional Status: Food and Fluid Intake**, as evidenced by the following indicator (specify 1–5: not, slightly, moderately, substantially, or totally adequate): oral food and fluid intake

Other Examples

- Acknowledges weight problem
- Verbalizes desire to lose weight
- Participates in a structured weight loss program

- Participates in a regular exercise program
- Approaches ideal weight (specify)
- Refrains from binge eating
- Experiences adequate, but not excessive, intake of calories, fats, carbohydrates, vitamins, minerals, iron, and calcium

NIC Interventions

Behavior Modification: Promotion of a behavior change

Exercise Promotion: Facilitation of regular physical activity to maintain or advance to a higher level of fitness and health

Nutrition Management: Assisting with or providing a balanced dietary intake of foods and fluids

Nutritional Counseling: Use of an interactive helping process focusing on the need for diet modification

Nutritional Monitoring: Collection and analysis of patient data to prevent or minimize malnourishment

Support Group: Use of a group environment to provide emotional support and health-related information for members

Weight Reduction Assistance: Facilitating loss of weight and/or body fat

Nursing Activities

Also see Nursing Activities for Risk for Imbalanced Nutrition: More Than Body Requirements.

Assessments

- *(NIC) Weight Reduction Assistance:*
  - Determine patient's desire and motivation to reduce weight or body fat
  - Determine current eating patterns by having patient keep a diary of what, when, and where he eats
  - Weigh patient weekly
- Monitor recorded intake for nutritional content and calories

Patient/Family Teaching

- Encourage patient to follow a diet of complex carbohydrates and protein and avoid simple sugars, fast food, caffeine, soft drinks
- *(NIC) Nutrition Management:*
  - Provide appropriate information about nutritional needs and how to meet them
- *(NIC) Weight Reduction Assistance:*
  - Discuss with patient and family the influence of alcohol consumption on food ingestion

Instruct on how to read labels when purchasing food, to control amount of fat and calorie density of food to be consumed

Teach food selection, in restaurants and social gatherings, that is consistent with planned calorie and nutrient intake

Instruct on how to calculate percentage of fat in food products

Collaborative Activities

- Confer with dietitian to implement weight loss program that includes dietary management and energy expenditure
- *(NIC) Nutrition Management:* Determine, in collaboration with dietitian as appropriate, number of calories and type of nutrients needed to meet nutrition requirements
- *(NIC) Weight Reduction Assistance:* Encourage attendance at support groups for weight loss (e.g., TOPS Club or Weight Watchers)

Other

- Develop a trusting, supportive relationship with patient
- Help patient to identify physical problems that may be related to obesity or eating disorder
- For patient with compulsive eating disorder, establish expectations for appropriate eating behaviors, intake of food and fluid, and amount of exercise
- Explore with patient personal issues that may contribute to overeating
- Communicate that the patient, alone, is responsible for choices about eating and physical activity
- Provide positive reinforcement for weight loss, maintenance of dietary regimen, improved eating behaviors, and exercise
- Focus on the patient's feelings about himself rather than on the obesity
- Discuss with patient emotions or high-risk situations that stimulate eating (e.g., types of foods, social situations, interpersonal stresses, unmet personal expectations, eating in secret or in private)
- *(NIC) Weight Reduction Assistance:*

  Set a weekly goal for weight loss

  Assist patient to identify motivation for eating and internal and external cues associated with eating

  Determine with the patient the amount of weight loss desired

  Assist with adjusting diet to lifestyle and activity level

  Set a realistic plan with the patient to include reduced food intake and increased energy expenditure [plan should specify frequency of meals and snacks and include self-monitoring activities]

  Encourage substitution of undesirable habits with desirable habits

  Plan an exercise program, taking into consideration the patient's limitations

  Encourage use of internal reward systems when goals are accomplished

Home Care

- The preceding interventions can be used or adapted for home care
- Also refer to Home Care interventions for Nutrition, Imbalanced: Less Than Body Requirements

For Infants and Children

- Children should not be placed on "a diet" to lose weight. Instead, emphasize healthy eating
- Teach parents to not use food as a reward for good behavior
- Involve the child in planning meals and preparing food
- Encourage parents to limit television viewing to 1 or 2 hr a day; instead, participate with their children in physical activities (e.g., swimming, bicycling)
- Also refer to For Infants and Children, in the diagnosis Nutrition, Imbalanced: Less Than Body Requirements

For Older Adults

- Assess cognitive functional abilities that may interfere with the patient's ability to prepare and eat healthy, low-calorie foods (e.g., ability to reach shelves where food is stored, to open cans, to stand at the stove)
- Assess condition of dentures or teeth. Clients who have difficulty chewing may eat soft, packaged, and snack foods (e.g., cupcakes, ice cream)
- Assess whether client can afford to buy foods such as fresh fruits and vegetables, fish, and lean meats
- Assess client's senses of smell and taste; decreased smell and taste can cause people to add sugar and salt to foods and to feel less satisfied after eating
- Teach the client to use seasonings other than sugar and salt
- Explain that because of a slower metabolism, calorie needs decrease with age; therefore, previous eating patterns must change to avoid gaining weight

NUTRITION, IMBALANCED: RISK FOR MORE THAN BODY REQUIREMENTS

(1980, 2000)

Domain 2, Nutrition; Class 1, Ingestion

Definition: At risk for an intake of nutrients that exceeds metabolic needs

Risk Factors

Subjective

Increased appetite (non-NANDA)
Eating in response to external cues (e.g., time of day or social situation)
Eating in response to internal cues other than hunger (e.g., anxiety)
Reported use of solid food as major food source before 5 months of age

Objective

Concentrating food intake at end of day
Dysfunctional eating patterns
Higher baseline weight at beginning of each pregnancy
Observed use of food as reward or comfort measure
Pairing food with other activities
Parental obesity
Rapid transition across growth percentiles in infants or children
Sedentary lifestyle

Other Risk Factors (non-NANDA International)

Chemical dependence
Decreased metabolic requirements
Ethnic and cultural norms
Lack of basic nutritional knowledge
Lack of physical exercise

Suggestions for Use

See Suggestions for Use for Nutrition, Imbalanced: More Than Body Requirements.

Suggested Alternative Diagnoses

Coping, ineffective
Health maintenance, ineffective

NOC Outcomes

Adherence Behavior: Healthy Diet: Personal actions to monitor and optimize a healthy and nutritional dietary regimen

Knowledge: Diet: Extent of understanding conveyed about recommended diet

Nutritional Status: Food and Fluid Intake: Amount of food and fluid taken into the body over a 24-hr period

Nutritional Status: Nutrient Intake: Nutrient intake to meet metabolic needs

Weight: Body Mass: Extent to which body weight, muscle, and fat are congruent to height, frame, gender, and age

Weight Maintenance Behavior: Personal actions to maintain optimum body weight

Goals/Evaluation Criteria

Examples Using NOC Language

- Demonstrates **Nutritional Status: Food and Fluid Intake**, as evidenced by the following indicator (specify 1–5: not, slightly, moderately, substantially, or totally adequate): oral food and fluid intake [not excessive]

Other Examples

- Acknowledges presence of risk factors
- Participates in a regular exercise program
- Maintains ideal weight (specify)
- Eats a balanced diet

NIC Interventions

Nutrition Management: Assisting with or providing a balanced dietary intake of foods and fluids

Nutritional Monitoring: Collection and analysis of patient data to prevent or minimize malnourishment

Self-Modification Assistance: Reinforcement of self-directed change initiated by the patient to achieve personally important goals

Weight Management: Facilitating maintenance of optimal body weight and percent body fat

Nursing Activities

Assessments

- Monitor presence of risk factors for weight gain
- *(NIC) Weight Management:*
  Determine individual's ideal body weight
  Determine individual's ideal percent body fat
- *(NIC) Nutrition Management:* Weigh patient at appropriate intervals

Patient/Family Teaching

- Provide information regarding available community resources, such as dietary counseling, exercise programs, self-help groups
- *(NIC) Weight Management:*
  Discuss with the individual the relationships among food intake, exercise, weight gain, and weight loss
  Discuss with individual the medical conditions that may affect weight
  Discuss with individual the habits and customs and cultural and heredity factors that influence weight

Discuss risks associated with being over- and underweight
Assist in developing well-balanced meal plans consistent with level of energy expenditure

Other

- Develop a weight-management plan
- Develop a plan for management of eating to include the following:
  Frequency of meals and snacks
  Diet high in complex carbohydrates and protein
  Avoidance of simple sugars, fast food, caffeine, and soft drinks
  Recognition of high-risk situations (e.g., types of foods, social situations, interpersonal stresses, unmet personal expectations, eating in secret or in private)
- Provide frequent positive reinforcement for good nutrition and exercise

Home Care

- The preceding interventions can be used or adapted for home care
- Also refer to Home Care interventions for *Nutrition, Imbalanced: Less Than Body Requirements*

For Infants and Children

- Teach parents to emphasize healthy eating and provide a healthy diet
- Teach parents to not use food as a reward for good behavior
- Involve the child in planning meals and preparing food
- Encourage parents to limit television viewing to 1 or 2 hr a day; instead, participate with their children in physical activities (e.g., swimming, bicycling)
- Also refer to For Infants and Children in the diagnosis *Nutrition, Imbalanced: Less Than Body Requirements*

For Older Adults

See For Older Adults, in Nutrition, Imbalanced: More Than Body Requirements

NUTRITION, READINESS FOR ENHANCED

(2002)

Domain 2, Nutrition; Class 1, Ingestion

Definition: A pattern of nutrient intake that is sufficient for meeting metabolic needs and can be strengthened

Defining Characteristics

Subjective

Attitude toward eating and drinking is congruent with health goals

Expresses knowledge of healthy food and fluid choices

Expresses willingness to enhance nutrition

Objective

Consumes adequate food and fluid

Eats regularly

Follows an appropriate standard for intake (e.g., [the U.S. Department of Agriculture's MyPlate], or American Diabetic Association guidelines)

Safe preparation and storage for food and fluids

Related Factors

This is a wellness diagnosis, so an etiology is not necessary.

Suggestions for Use

If risk factors are present, use *Risk for imbalanced nutrition.*

Suggested Alternative Diagnoses

Fluid balance, readiness for enhanced

Knowledge (specify), readiness for enhanced

Nutrition, risk for imbalanced (specify more or less than body requirements)

NOC Outcomes

Adherence Behavior: Self-initiated actions to promote optional wellness, recovery, and rehabilitation

Knowledge: Diet: Extent of understanding conveyed about recommended diet

Nutritional Status: Extent to which nutrients are available to meet metabolic needs

Nutritional Status: Nutrient Intake: Nutrient intake to meet metabolic needs

Weight Maintenance Behavior: Personal actions to maintain optimum body weight

Goals/Evaluation Criteria

Examples Using NOC Language

- Demonstrates **Nutritional Status:** as evidenced by the following indicators (specify 1–5 severe, substantial, moderate, mild, or no deviation from normal range): nutrient intake, food intake, fluid intake, weight/height ratio, energy

Other Examples

- Maintains ideal weight (specify)
- Eats a balanced diet
- Reports enhanced nutritional value of foods consumed (e.g., eats more nonprocessed foods, fewer saturated fats)

NIC Interventions

Health Education: Developing and providing instruction and learning experiences to facilitate voluntary adaptation of behavior conducive to health in individuals, families, groups, or communities

Nutrition Management: Assisting with or providing a balanced dietary intake of foods and fluids

Nutritional Counseling: Use of an interactive helping process focusing on the need for diet modification

Nutritional Monitoring: Collection and analysis of patient data to prevent or minimize malnourishment

Teaching: Individual: Planning, implementation, and evaluation of a teaching program designed to address a patient's particular needs

Teaching: Prescribed Diet: Preparing a patient to correctly follow a prescribed diet

Weight Management: Facilitating maintenance of optimal body weight and percent of body fat

Nursing Activities

Assessments

- Monitor presence of risk factors for weight gain or loss
- Assess plans for improving diet
- *(NIC) Nutritional Counseling:*
  Determine patient's food intake and eating habits
  Facilitate identification of eating behaviors to be changed
  Discuss patient's food likes and dislikes
- Determine patient's ideal body weight
- Determine patient's ideal percentage of body fat
- Teach patient to weigh at appropriate intervals

Patient/Family Teaching

- Provide information regarding available community resources, such as dietary counseling, exercise programs, self-help groups
- Point out habits and cultural and hereditary factors that influence weight
- Discuss the importance of maintaining a healthy weight
- Provide information about buying, preparing, and storing nutritious foods

- Assist in developing healthful meal plans
- *(NIC) Nutritional Counseling:*
  Discuss patient's knowledge of the four basic food groups, as well as perceptions of the needed diet modification
  Provide information, as necessary, about the health need for diet modification: weight loss, weight gain, sodium restriction, cholesterol reduction, fluid restriction, and so on

Other

- Provide frequent positive reinforcement for good nutrition

Home Care

- The preceding interventions can be used or adapted for home care

For Infants and Children

- Teach parents to emphasize healthy eating and provide a healthy diet
- Teach parents to not use food as a reward for good behavior
- Involve the child in planning meals and preparing food
- Encourage parents to limit television viewing to 1 or 2 hr a day; instead, participate with their children in physical activities (e.g., swimming, bicycling)
- Also refer to For Infants and Children in the diagnosis Nutrition, Imbalanced: Less Than Body Requirements

ORAL MUCOUS MEMBRANE, IMPAIRED

(1982, 1998) **Domain 11, Safety/Protection; Class 2, Physical Injury**

Definition: Disruptions of the lips and/or soft tissue of the oral cavity

Defining Characteristics

Subjective

Difficulty eating or swallowing
Diminished [or absent] taste
Oral pain and discomfort
Reports bad taste in mouth

Objective

Bleeding
Coated tongue

Desquamation
Difficult speech
Edema
Enlarged tonsils
Fissures, cheilitis
Geographic tongue
Gingival hyperplasia
Gingival or mucosal pallor
Gingival recession
Halitosis
Hyperemia
Macroplasia
Mucosal denudation
Oral lesions or ulcers
Pocketing deeper than 4 mm
Presence of pathogens
Purulent drainage or exudates
Red or bluish masses (e.g., hemangiomas)
Smooth, atrophic tongue

Stomatitis
Vesicles, nodules, or papules
White patches or plaques, spongy patches, or white curdlike exudates
Xerostomia (dry mouth)

Other Defining Characteristics (non-NANDA International)

Discomfort with hot or cold foods
Dry, cracked lips

Related Factors

Barriers to oral self-care
Barriers to professional care
Chemotherapy
Chemical irritants (e.g., alcohol, tobacco, acidic foods, drugs, regular use of inhalers or other noxious agents)
Cleft lip or palate
Decreased platelets
Decreased salivation
Dehydration
Depression
Diminished hormone levels (women)
Immunocompromised
Immunosuppression

Ineffective oral hygiene
Infection
Loss of supportive structures
Malnutrition [or vitamin deficiency]
Mechanical (e.g., ill-fitting dentures, braces, [and ET or NG] tubes)
Medication side effects
Mouth breathing
NPO for more than 24 hr
Pathologic conditions of the oral cavity (non-NANDA International)
Radiation therapy
Stress
Surgery in oral cavity
Trauma (e.g., drugs, noxious agents)

Suggested Alternative Diagnoses

Dentition, impaired
Self-Care Deficit: (Oral) Hygiene
Tissue integrity, impaired

NOC Outcomes

Oral Hygiene: Condition of the mouth, teeth, gums, and tongue
Tissue Integrity: Skin and Mucous Membranes: Structural intactness and normal physiologic function of skin and mucous membranes

Goals/Evaluation Criteria

Examples Using NOC Language

- Demonstrates **Oral Hygiene**, as evidenced by the following indicators (specify 1–5: severely, substantially, moderately, mildly, or not compromised):
  - Cleanliness of mouth, teeth, gums, tongue, dentures, or dental appliances
  - Moisture of oral mucosa and tongue
  - Color of mucosa membranes [pink]
  - Integrity of oral mucosa, tongue, gum[s], and [teeth]
- Demonstrates **Tissue Integrity: Skin and Mucous Membranes**, as evidenced by the following indicators (specify 1–5: severe, substantial, moderate, mild, or none):
  - Mucous membrane lesions
  - Erythema
  - Necrosis

Other Examples

- Ingests foods and fluids with increasing comfort
- No halitosis
- Performs essential oral hygiene as prescribed and instructed

NIC Interventions

Oral Health Maintenance: Maintenance and promotion of oral hygiene and dental health for the patient at risk for developing oral or dental lesions

Oral Health Restoration: Promotion of healing for a patient who has an oral mucosa or dental lesion

Self-Care Assistance: Assisting another to perform ADLs

Teaching: Individual: Planning, implementation, and evaluation of a teaching program designed to address a patient's particular needs

Nursing Activities

Assessments

- Identify irritating substances such as tobacco, alcohol, food, medications, extremes in food temperature, seasonings
- Assess patient's understanding of and ability to perform oral care
- *(NIC) Oral Health Restoration:*
  Determine the patient's perception of changes in taste, swallowing, quality of voice, and comfort
  Monitor patient every shift for dryness of the oral mucosa
  Monitor for signs and symptoms of glossitis and stomatitis
  Monitor for therapeutic effects of topical anesthetics, oral protective pastes, and topical or systemic analgesics, as appropriate

O

Patient/Family Teaching

- *(NIC) Oral Health Restoration:*
  Reinforce oral hygiene regimen as part of discharge teaching
  Instruct patient to avoid commercial mouthwashes
  Instruct patient to report signs of infection to physician immediately

Collaborative Activities

- Confer with physician regarding an order for antifungal mouthwash or oral topical anesthetic if fungal infection exists.
- *(NIC) Oral Health Restoration:*
  Consult physician if signs and symptoms of glossitis and stomatitis persist or worsen
  Apply topical anesthetics, oral protective pastes, and topical or systemic analgesics, as needed

Other

- Provide mouth care prior to meals and as needed
- Avoid use of sugared candies and gum
- Clean dentures after each meal
- Remove dentures in case of severe stomatitis
- *(NIC) Oral Health Restoration:*
  - Plan small, frequent meals; select soft foods; and serve chilled or room-temperature foods
  - Assist patient to select soft, bland, and nonacidic foods
  - Increase mouth care to every 2 hr and twice at night if stomatitis is not controlled
  - Use a soft toothbrush for removal of dental debris
  - Encourage frequent rinsing of the mouth with any of the following: sodium bicarbonate solution, warm saline, or hydrogen peroxide solution
  - Avoid use of lemon-glycerin swabs
  - Discourage smoking and alcohol consumption

Home Care

- The preceding interventions can be adapted for use in home care; the chief difference is that the nurse is more likely to be performing the interventions for an inpatient, whereas in the home, the nurse will more likely teach the client or caregiver to perform the interventions
- Suggest the use of cool beverages and Popsicles® to reduce discomfort
- Suggest the use of a room humidifier if the home air is dry

For Infants and Children

- Teach parents that it is normal for a child's gums to be red and swollen during teething
- Replace the child's toothbrush about every 3 months
- Teach parents to give the child something safe to chew on while teething

For Older Adults

- Assess whether the client is able to perform his own oral hygiene
- Observe lips and oral cavity for lesions (e.g., masses, ulcerations, red or white patches, granular lesions)
- Be aware that many older adults visit a dentist only rarely. Encourage regular visits; assist to obtain transportation and financial assistance, if needed

PAIN, ACUTE

(1996) **Domain 12, Comfort: Class 1, Physical Comfort**

Definition: Unpleasant sensory and emotional experience arising from actual or potential tissue damage or described in terms of such damage (International Association for the Study of Pain); sudden or slow onset of any intensity from mild to severe with an anticipated or predictable end and a duration of less than 6 months

Defining Characteristics

Subjective

Coded report (e.g., use of pain scale)

Reports pain

Objective

Autonomic responses (e.g., diaphoresis; blood pressure, respiration, or heart rate changes; pupillary dilation)

Distraction behavior (e.g., pacing, seeking out other people and/or activities, repetitive activities)

P

Expressive behavior (e.g., restlessness, moaning, crying, vigilance, irritability, sighing)

Facial mask (e.g., eyes lack luster, beaten look, fixed or scattered movement, grimaces)

Guarding behavior or protective gestures

Narrowed focus (e.g., altered time perception, impaired thought processes, reduced interaction with people and environment)

Observed evidence of pain

Positioning to avoid pain

Protective gestures

Sleep disturbance

Other Defining Characteristics (Non-NANDA International)

Communication of pain descriptors (e.g., discomfort, nausea, night sweats, muscle cramps, itching skin, numbness, tingling of extremities)

Grimacing

Limited attention span

Pallor

Withdrawal

Related Factors

Injury agents (e.g., biologic, chemical, physical, psychologic)

Suggestions for Use

Acute pain can be diagnosed on the patient's report alone because that is sometimes the only sign of *Acute pain*. None of the other defining characteristics taken alone would be sufficient to diagnose *Acute pain*. The related factors indicate that a patient can suffer both physical and psychologic *Acute pain*. Qualifier words should be added to this diagnosis to indicate the severity, location, and nature of the pain. Two examples of appropriate diagnoses are as follows: *Severe, stabbing chest pain related to fractured ribs*, and *Mild frontal headache related to sinus congestion*.

It is important to differentiate between *Acute pain* and *Chronic pain* because the nursing focus is different for each. *Acute pain* (e.g., postoperative incision pain) is usually a collaborative problem managed primarily by administering narcotic analgesics. There are a few independent nursing interventions for *Acute pain*, such as teaching the patient to splint the incision while moving, but these alone would not provide adequate pain relief. The nurse takes a more active role in teaching patients self-management of *Chronic pain*. When pain is acute or caused by a stressor not amenable to nursing intervention (e.g., surgical incision), it may be an etiology rather than a problem, for example, *Ineffective airway clearance related to weak cough secondary to Acute pain from chest incision*. In differentiating between *Acute pain* and *Chronic pain*, the comparison in Table 4 may be helpful.

P

Table 4

Defining Characteristics	Pain	Chronic Pain
Duration less than 6 months	X	
Duration longer than 6 months		X
Autonomic responses, such as pallor, increase in vital signs, and diaphoresis	X	
Personality changes		X
Weight loss		X

Pain can also be the etiology (i.e., related factor) for other nursing diagnoses, such as *Powerlessness related to inability to cope with Acute pain, and Self-care deficit: dressing/grooming, related to joint Pain with movement.*

Suggested Alternative Diagnosis

Comfort, impaired
Pain, chronic

NOC Outcomes

Client Satisfaction: Pain Management: Extent of positive perception of nursing care to relieve pain

Discomfort Level: Severity of observed or reported mental or physical discomfort

Pain Control: Personal actions to control pain

Pain Level: Severity of observed or reported pain

Goals/Evaluation Criteria

Examples Using NOC Language

- Demonstrates **Pain Control**, as evidenced by the following indicators (specify 1–5: never, rarely, sometimes, often, or consistently demonstrated):
  - Recognizes pain onset
  - Uses preventive measures
  - Reports pain controlled
- Demonstrates **Pain Level**, as evidenced by the following indicators (specify 1–5: severe, substantial, moderate, mild, or none):
  - Facial expressions of pain
  - Restlessness or muscle tension
  - Length of pain episodes
  - Moaning and crying
  - Restlessness

P

Other Examples

Patient will:

- Demonstrate individualized relaxation techniques that are effective for achieving comfort
- Maintain pain level at (specify) or less (on scale of 0–10)
- Report physical and psychologic well-being
- Recognize causal factors and use measures to modify them
- Report pain to health care provider
- Use analgesic and nonanalgesic relief measures appropriately
- Not experience a compromise in respiratory rate, heart rate, or blood pressure
- Maintain a good appetite
- Report sleeping well
- Report ability to maintain role performance and interpersonal relationships

NIC Interventions

Analgesic Administration: Use of pharmacologic agents to reduce or eliminate pain

Medication Administration: Preparing, giving, and evaluating the effectiveness of prescription and nonprescription drugs
Medication Management: Facilitation of safe and effective use of prescription and over-the-counter drugs
Pain Management: Alleviation of pain or a reduction in pain to a level of comfort that is acceptable to the patient
Patient-Controlled Analgesia (PCA) Assistance: Facilitating patient control of analgesic administration and regulation
Sedation Management: Administration of sedatives, monitoring of the patient's response, and provision of necessary physiological support during a diagnostic or therapeutic procedure
Surveillance: Purposeful and ongoing acquisition, interpretation, and synthesis of patient data for clinical decision making

Nursing Activities

Assessments

- Use self-report as first choice to obtain assessment information
- Ask patient to rate pain or discomfort on a scale of 0–10 (0 = no pain or discomfort, 10 = worst pain)
- Use pain flow sheet to monitor pain relief of analgesics and possible side effects
- Assess the impact of religion, culture, beliefs, and circumstances on patient's pain and responses
- In assessing patient's pain, use words that are consistent with patient's age and developmental level
- *(NIC) Pain Management:*
  Perform a comprehensive assessment of pain to include location, characteristics, onset and duration, frequency, quality, intensity or severity of pain, and precipitating factors
  Observe for nonverbal cues of discomfort, especially in those unable to communicate effectively

P

Patient/Family Teaching

- Include in discharge instructions the specific medication to be taken, frequency of administration, potential side effects, potential medication interactions, specific precautions when taking the medication (e.g., physical activity limitations, dietary restrictions), and name of person to notify about unrelieved pain
- Instruct patient to inform nurse if pain relief is not achieved
- Inform patient of procedures that may increase pain and offer suggestions for coping

- Correct misconceptions about narcotic or opioid analgesics (e.g., risks of addiction and overdose)
- *(NIC) Pain Management:* Provide information about the pain, such as causes of the pain, how long it will last, and anticipated discomforts from procedures
- *(NIC) Pain Management:*
  Teach the use of nonpharmacologic techniques (e.g., biofeedback, transcutaneous electrical nerve stimulation [TENS], hypnosis, relaxation, guided imagery, music therapy, distraction, play therapy, activity therapy, acupressure, hot or cold application, and massage) before, after, and if possible, during painful activities; before pain occurs or increases; and along with other pain-relief measures

Collaborative Activities

- Manage immediate postoperative pain with scheduled opiate (e.g., q4h for 36 hr) or PCA
- *(NIC) Pain Management:*
  Use pain-control measures before pain becomes severe
  Notify physician if measures are unsuccessful or if current complaint is a significant change from patient's past experience of pain

P

Other

- Adjust frequency of dosage as indicated by pain assessment and side effects
- Help patient identify comfort measures that have worked in the past, such as distraction, relaxation, or application of heat or cold
- Attend to comfort needs and other activities to assist relaxation, including the following measures:
  Offer position change, back rubs, and relaxation
  Change bed linen, as necessary
  Provide care in an unhurried, supportive manner
  Involve patient in decisions regarding care activities
- Help patient focus on activities rather than on pain and discomfort by providing diversion through television, radio, tapes, and visitors
- Use a positive approach in order to optimize patient response to analgesics (e.g., "This will help relieve your pain")
- Explore feelings about fear of addiction; to reassure patient, ask: "If you didn't have this pain, would you still want to take this drug?"
- *(NIC) Pain Management:*
  Incorporate the family in the pain relief modality, if possible
  Control environmental factors that may influence the patient's response to discomfort (e.g., room temperature, lighting, and noise)

Home Care

- The preceding interventions can be adapted for use in home care
- Teach client and family to use the technology required for administering the medications (e.g., infusion pumps, TENS units)

For Infants and Children

- Be aware that infants are as sensitive to pain as adults. Use topical anesthetics (e.g., EMLA cream) before performing venipuncture; for neonates, use oral sucrose
- To assess pain in young children, use the Faces Pain Scale or other picture-scale

For Older Adults

- Note that older adults have increased sensitivity to analgesic effects of opiates with higher peak effect and longer duration of pain relief
- Be alert to possible drug–drug and drug–disease interactions in older adults, who often have multiple illnesses and take multiple medications
- Recognize that pain is not a normal part of aging
- Expect to reduce the usual opioid dose for older adults, as they are more sensitive to opioids
- Avoid using meperidine (Demerol) and propoxyphene (Darvon), or other drugs that are primarily metabolized in the kidney
- Avoid using drugs with a long half-life because of the increased likelihood of toxicity from drug accumulation
- When discussing pain, be sure the patient can hear you and can see any written pain scales
- When teaching about medications, repeat the information as often as necessary; leave written information with the patient
- Assess for drug interactions, including over-the-counter medications

PAIN, CHRONIC

(1986, 1996)

Domain 12, Comfort; Class 1, Physical Comfort

Definition: Unpleasant sensory and emotional experience arising from actual or potential tissue damage or described in terms of such damage (International Association for the Study of Pain); sudden or slow onset of any intensity from mild to severe, constant or recurring, without an anticipated or predictable end and with a duration of greater than 6 months

Defining Characteristics

Verbal or coded report or observed evidence of the following:

Subjective

Depression

Fatigue

Fear of reinjury

Pain

Objective

Altered ability to continue previous activities

Anorexia

Atrophy of involved muscle group

Changes in sleep pattern

Facial mask (e.g., eyes lack luster, beaten look, fixed or scattered movement, and grimace)

Guarding behavior

Irritability

Observed protective behavior

Reduced interaction with people

Restlessness

Self-focusing

Sympathetic mediated responses (e.g., temperature, cold, changes of body position, hypersensitivity)

Weight changes

Related Factors

Chronic physical or psychosocial disability (e.g., metastatic cancer, neurologic injury, arthritis)

Suggestions for Use

See Suggestions for Use for Acute Pain.

Suggested Alternative Diagnosis

Pain, acute

Comfort, impaired

NOC Outcomes

Client Satisfaction: Pain Management: Extent of positive perception of nursing care to relieve pain

Pain: Adverse Psychological Response: Severity of observed or reported adverse cognitive and emotional responses to physical pain

Pain Control: Personal actions to control pain
Pain: Disruptive Effects: Severity of observed or reported disruptive effects of chronic pain on daily functioning
Pain Level: Severity of observed or reported pain

Goals/Evaluation Criteria

Examples Using NOC Language

- Demonstrates **Pain: Disruptive Effects**, as evidenced by the following indicators (specify 1–5: severe, substantial, moderate, mild, or none):
  Impaired role performance or disrupted interpersonal relationships
  Impaired concentration
  Impaired self-care
  Interrupted sleep
  Loss of appetite
- Demonstrates **Pain Level**, as evidenced by the following indicators (specify 1–5: severe, substantial, moderate, mild, or none):
  Facial expressions of pain
  Restlessness or pacing
  Muscle tension
  Loss of appetite
  Length of pain episodes

P

Other Examples

Patient will:

- Verbalize knowledge of alternative measures for pain relief
- Report that level of pain is maintained at (specify) or less (on scale of 0–10)
- Remain productive at work or school
- Report enjoying leisure activities
- Report physical and psychologic well-being
- Recognize factors that increase pain and take preventive measures
- Appropriately use analgesic and nonanalgesic relief measures

NIC Interventions

Analgesic Administration: Use of pharmacologic agents to reduce or eliminate pain
Behavior Modification: Promotion of a behavior change
Coping Enhancement: Assisting a patient to adapt to perceived stressors, changes, or threats that interfere with meeting life demands and roles
Medication Management: Facilitation of safe and effective use of prescription and over-the-counter drugs

Mood Management: Providing for safety, stabilization, recovery, and maintenance of a patient who is experiencing dysfunctionally depressed mood or elevated mood

Pain Management: Alleviation of pain or a reduction in pain to a level of comfort that is acceptable to the patient

Patient-Controlled Analgesia (PCA) Assistance: Facilitating patient control of analgesic administration and regulation

Self-Responsibility Facilitation: Encouraging a patient to assume more responsibility for own behavior

Nursing Activities

Also refer to Nursing Activities for the Acute Pain diagnosis.

Assessments

- Assess and document effects of long-term medication use
- *(NIC) Pain Management:*

  Monitor patient satisfaction with pain management at specified intervals

  Determine the impact of the pain experience on quality of life (e.g., sleep, appetite, activity, cognition, mood, relationships, performance of job, and role responsibilities)

Patient/Family Teaching

- Convey to patient that total pain relief may not be achievable

Collaborative Activities

- Initiate a multidisciplinary patient care planning conference
- *(NIC) Pain Management:* Consider referrals for patient, family, and significant others to support groups and other resources, as appropriate

Other

- Offer patient pain-relief measures to supplement pain medication (e.g., biofeedback, relaxation techniques, back rub)
- Assist patient in identifying reasonable and acceptable level of pain
- *(NIC) Pain Management:*

  Promote adequate rest and sleep to facilitate pain relief

  Medicate prior to an activity to increase participation, but evaluate the hazard of sedation

Home Care

Refer to "Home Care" for the diagnosis Acute Pain

> **For Older Adults**
>
> Refer to "For Older Adults" in the Acute Pain diagnosis

PARENTING, IMPAIRED

(1978, 1998) **Domain 7, Role Relationships; Class 1, Caregiving Roles**

Definition: Inability of the primary caretaker to create, maintain, or regain an environment that promotes the optimum growth and development of the child

Defining Characteristics

Infant or Child

Objective

Behavioral disorders
Failure to thrive
Frequent accidents
Frequent illness
Incidence of physical and psychological trauma or abuse
Lack of attachment
Lack of separation anxiety
Poor academic performance
Poor cognitive development
Poor social competence
Runaway

Parental

Subjective

Negative statements about child
Reports frustration
Reports inability to control child
Reports role inadequacy
Statements of inability to meet child's needs

Objective

Abandonment
Child abuse
Child neglect
Frequently punitive
Inadequate attachment

Inadequate child health maintenance
Inappropriate caretaking skills [e.g., involving toilet training, sleep and rest, feeding, discipline]
Inappropriate child-care arrangements
Inappropriate visual, tactile, or auditory stimulation
Inconsistent behavior management
Inconsistent care
Inflexibility in meeting needs of child
Little cuddling
Maternal–child interaction deficit
Paternal–child interaction deficit
Rejection of or hostility to child
Unsafe home environment

Other Defining Characteristics (Non-NANDA International)

Child care from multiple caretakers without consideration of needs of infant or child
Compulsive seeking of role approval from others
Growth and development lag
Noncompliance with child's health appointments

Related Factors

Infant or Child

Altered perceptual abilities
Attention-deficit hyperactivity disorder
Difficult temperament
Handicapping condition or developmental delay
Illness
Multiple births
Not gender desired
Premature birth
[Prolonged] separation from parent
Separation from parent at birth
Temperamental conflicts with parental expectations

Knowledge

Deficient knowledge about child development
Deficient knowledge about child health maintenance
Deficient knowledge about parenting skills
Inability to respond to infant cues
Lack of cognitive readiness for parenthood
Lack of education
Limited cognitive functioning

Poor communication skills
Preference for physical punishment
Unrealistic expectation [for self, infant, partner]

Physiologicical

Physical illness

Psychological

Depression
Difficult birthing process
Disability
High number or closely spaced pregnancies
History of mental illness
History of substance abuse
Lack of [or late] prenatal care
Sleep deprivation or disturbed sleep pattern
Young parental age

Other Related Factors (non-NANDA)

Multiple births
Separation from infant or child

Social

Change in family unit
Economically disadvantaged
Father of child not involved
Financial difficulties
History of being abused
History of being abusive
Inability to put child's needs before own
Inadequate child-care arrangements
Lack of family cohesiveness
Lack of resources
Lack of social support networks
Lack of transportation
Lack of valuing parenthood
Lack of, or poor, parental role model
Legal difficulties
Low self-esteem, situational or chronic
Maladaptive coping strategies
Marital conflict
Mother of child not involved
Poor home environment
Poor problem-solving skills

Poverty
Presence of stress (e.g., financial, legal, recent crisis, cultural move)
Relocations
Role strain
Single parent
Social isolation
Unemployment or job problems
Unplanned or unwanted pregnancy

Suggestions for Use

Parenting is normally a maturational process of adjustment, requiring only nursing behaviors to prevent potential problems and promote health. This label represents a less healthy level of functioning than *Parental role conflict*, in which a parent or parents have been functioning satisfactorily but face situational challenges (e.g., divorce, illness) that create role conflict and confusion. Unresolved *Parental role conflict* may progress to *Impaired parenting*.

Suggested Alternative Diagnoses

Caregiver role strain (actual or at risk for)
Coping: family, compromised or disabled
Development, risk for delayed
Growth, risk for disproportionate
Growth and development, delayed
Family processes, interrupted
Parental role conflict
Parenting, risk for impaired
Role performance, ineffective

NOC Outcomes

Child Development (2, 4, 6, and 12 Months; 2, 3, 4, and 5 Years; Middle Childhood, and Adolescence): Milestones of physical, cognitive, and psychosocial progression by (specify months or years) of age. [**NOTE:** NOC has separate outcomes and indicators for each age.]

Parent–Infant Attachment: Parent and infant behaviors that demonstrate an enduring affectionate bond

Parenting Performance: Parental actions to provide a child a nurturing and constructive physical, emotional, and social environment

Parenting: Psychosocial Safety: Parental actions to protect a child from social contacts that might cause harm or injury

Role Performance: Congruence of an individual's role behavior with role expectations

Safe Home Environment: Physical arrangements to minimize environmental factors that might cause physical harm or injury in the home

Social Support: Reliable assistance from others

Goals/Evaluation Criteria

Also see Goals/Evaluation Criteria for the diagnoses Delayed Growth and Development and Risk for Impaired Parenting.

Examples Using NOC Language

- Demonstrates **Parent–Infant Attachment**, as evidenced by the following indicators (specify 1–5: never, rarely, sometimes, often, or consistently demonstrated):
  Parent(s):
  Verbalize positive feelings toward infant
  Touch, stroke, pat, kiss, and smile at infant
  Visit nursery
  Vocalize to infant
  Use en face position and eye contact
- Demonstrates **Parenting Performance**, as evidenced by the following indicators (specify 1–5: never, rarely, sometimes, often, or consistently demonstrated):
  Provides for child's physical needs
  Stimulates cognitive and social development
  Stimulates emotional and spiritual growth
  Exhibits a loving relationship
  Provides preventive and episodic health care
- Demonstrates **Role Performance**, as evidenced by the following indicators (specify 1–5: not, slightly, moderately, substantially, or totally adequate):
  Performance of parental role behaviors
  Performance of role expectations
- Demonstrates **Safe Home Environment**, as evidenced by the following indicators (specify 1–5: not, slightly, moderately, substantially, or totally adequate):
  Smoke detector maintenance
  Proper disposal of medications
  Safe storage of firearms
  Safe storage of hazardous materials
  Provision of a safe play area
  Use of electrical outlet covers

Other Examples

The parent(s) will:

- Demonstrate constructive discipline
- Identify effective ways to express anger and frustration that are not harmful to child
- Actively participate in counseling and parenting classes
- Identify and use community resources that assist with home care
- Identify people who can provide information and emotional support when needed
- Indicate willingness to ask others for help

The child will:

- Achieve physical, cognitive, and psychosocial milestones at expected times (refer to appropriate age group for specific developmental norms)

NIC Interventions

Abuse Protection Support: Child: Identification of high-risk, dependent child relationships and actions to prevent possible or further infliction of physical, sexual, or emotional harm or neglect of basic necessities of life

Attachment Promotion: Facilitation of the development of the parent–infant relationship

Coping Enhancement: Assisting a patient to adapt to perceived stressors, changes, or threats that interfere with meeting life demands and roles

Developmental Enhancement: Adolescent: Facilitating optimal physical, cognitive, social, and emotional growth of individuals during the transition from childhood to adulthood

Developmental Enhancement: Child: Facilitating or teaching parents and caregivers to facilitate the optimal gross-motor, fine-motor, language, cognitive, social, and emotional growth of preschool and school-aged children

Environmental Management: Attachment Process: Manipulation of the patient's surroundings to facilitate the development of the parent–infant relationship

Environmental Management: Safety: Monitoring and manipulation of the physical environment to promote safety

Family Integrity Promotion: Promotion of family cohesion and unity

Family Integrity Promotion: Childbearing Family: Facilitation of the growth of individuals or families who are adding an infant to the family unit

Family Involvement Promotion: Facilitating family participation in the emotional and physical care of the patient

Family Process Maintenance: Minimization of family process disruption effects

Family Support: Promotion of family values, interests, and goals

Kangaroo Care: Promoting closeness between parent and physiologically stable preterm infant by preparing the parent and providing the environment for skin-to-skin contact

Newborn Care: Management of neonate during the transition to extrauterine life and subsequent period of stabilization

Parent Education: Adolescent: Assisting parents to understand and help their adolescent children

Parent Education: Childrearing Family: Assisting parents to understand and promote the physical, psychological, and social growth and development of their toddler or preschool or school-aged child or children

Parent Education: Infant: Instruction on nurturing and physical care needed during the first year of life

Parenting Promotion: Providing parenting information, support, and coordination of comprehensive services to high-risk families

Risk Identification: Childbearing Family: Identification of an individual or family likely to experience difficulties in parenting and prioritization of strategies to prevent parenting problems

Role Enhancement: Assisting a patient, significant other, or family to improve relationships by clarifying and supplementing specific role behaviors

Support Group: Use of a group environment to provide emotional support and health-related information for members

Support System Enhancement: Facilitation of support to patient by family, friends, and community

Surveillance: Safety: Purposeful and ongoing collection and analysis of information about the patient and the environment for use in promoting and maintaining patient safety

Nursing Activities

Refer to Nursing Activities for Parenting, Risk for Impaired.

Assessments

- Assess for postpartum, and other, depression
- Assess parents for partner abuse
- Assess for symptoms of *Impaired parenting* (see Defining Characteristics, preceding)

Collaborative Activities

- Offer to make initial telephone call to appropriate community resources
- *(NIC) Abuse Protection Support: Child:*
  Refer families to human services and counseling professionals, as needed

Provide parents with community resource information that includes addresses and phone numbers of agencies that provide respite care, emergency child care, housing assistance, substance abuse treatment, sliding-fee counseling services, food pantries, clothing distribution centers, health care, human services, hot lines, and domestic abuse shelters

Report suspected abuse or neglect to proper authorities

Refer parents to Parents Anonymous for group support, as appropriate

Other

- Encourage expression of feelings (e.g., guilt, anger, ambivalence) regarding parenting role
- Help parent identify deficits and alterations in parenting skills
- Provide frequent opportunities for parent–child interaction
- Role-model parenting skills
- Help identify realistic expectations of parenting role
- Acknowledge and reinforce parenting strengths and skills
- *(NIC) Family Integrity Promotion:*

  Establish trusting relationship with family members

  Assist family with conflict resolution

  Assist family to resolve unrealistic feelings of guilt or responsibility, as warranted

  Facilitate a tone of togetherness within or among the family

  Facilitate open communication among family members

During Pregnancy

- *(NIC) Attachment Promotion:*

  Discuss parent's reaction to pregnancy

  Provide parent(s) the opportunity to hear fetal heart tones as soon as possible

  Discuss parent's reaction to hearing fetal heart tones, viewing ultrasound image, etc.

  Assist father or significant other during participation in labor and delivery

At Delivery

- *(NIC) Attachment Promotion:*

  Place infant on mother's body immediately after birth

  Provide father opportunity to hold newborn in delivery area

  Provide pain relief for mother

  Provide family privacy during initial interaction with newborn

  Encourage parents to touch and speak to newborn

Home Care

- Many of the preceding interventions can be adapted for use in home care
- Assess parent–child interactions while in the home
- Assess the home environment for signs of ineffective caretaking skills (e.g., old food left sitting out, trash containers overflowing, no food in refrigerator or cupboards)

For Older Adults

- Teach parents and grandparents the importance of grandparents to the child's development

PARENTING, IMPAIRED, RISK FOR

(1978, 1998) **Domain 7, Role Relationships; Class 1, Caregiving Roles**

Definition: At risk for inability of the primary caretaker to create, maintain, or regain an environment that promotes the optimum growth and development of the child

Risk Factors

Infant or Child

Altered perceptual abilities
Attention-deficit hyperactivity disorder
Developmental delay
Difficult temperament
Handicapping condition
Illness
Multiple births
Not gender desired
Premature birth
Prolonged separation from parent
Temperamental conflicts with parental expectation
Non-NANDA International:
Unplanned or unwanted child

Knowledge

Deficient knowledge about child development or child health maintenance
Deficient knowledge about parenting skills

Inability to respond to infant cues
Lack of cognitive readiness for parenthood
Low cognitive functioning
Low educational level [or attainment]
Poor communication skills
Preference for physical punishment
Unrealistic expectations of child

Physiological

Physical illness

Psychological

Closely spaced pregnancies
Depression
Difficult birth process
Disability
High number of pregnancies
History of mental illness
History of substance abuse
Sleep deprivation or disruption
Young parental age

Social

Change in family unit
Chronic or situational low self-esteem
Economically disadvantaged
Father of child not involved
Financial difficulties
History of being abused
History of being abusive
Inadequate child-care arrangements
Lack of access to resources
Lack of family cohesiveness
Lack of parental role model
Lack of, or late, prenatal care
Lack of resources
Lack of social support network
Lack of transportation
Lack of valuing of parenthood
Legal difficulties
Low self-esteem (chronic or situational)
Maladaptive coping strategies
Marital conflict
Mother of child not involved

Parent–child separation
Poor home environment
Poor parental role model
Poor problem-solving skills
Poverty
Relocation
Role strain [or overload]
Single parent
Social isolation
Stress
Unemployment or job problems
Unplanned or unwanted pregnancy

Suggestions for Use

Adjustment to parenting is a normal maturational process that calls for nursing interventions to prevent potential problems and promote health.

Suggested Alternative Diagnoses

Attachment, risk for impaired
Caregiver role strain, risk for
Coping: family, compromised
Coping: family, readiness for enhanced
Family processes, interrupted
Role conflict, parental
Role performance, ineffective

NOC Outcomes

Use the following two outcomes to assess for actual occurrence of Impaired Parenting:

Parenting Performance: Parental actions to provide a child a nurturing and constructive physical, emotional, and social environment

Parenting: Psychosocial Safety: Parental actions to protect a child from social contacts that might cause harm or injury

The following outcomes are associated with the risk factors for Impaired Parenting:

Abusive Behavior Self-Restraint: Self-restraining and neglectful behaviors toward others

Aggression Self-Control: Self-restraint of assaultive, combative, or destructive behaviors toward others

Caregiver Emotional Health: Emotional well-being of a family care provider while caring for a family member

Caregiver Physical Health: Physical well-being of a family care provider while caring for a family member

Child Development: (1, 2, 4, 6, and 12) Months: Milestones of physical, cognitive, and psychosocial progression by [specify] months of age

Child Development: 2, 3, and 4 Years: Milestones of physical, cognitive, and psychosocial progression by 2 years of age

Child Development: Middle Childhood: Milestones of physical, cognitive, and psychosocial progression from 6 years through 11 years of age

Child Development: Adolescence: Milestones of physical, cognitive, and psychosocial progression from 12 years through 17 years of age

Family Coping: Family actions to manage stressors that tax family resources

Knowledge: Parenting: Extent of understanding conveyed about provision of a nurturing and constructive environment for a child from 1 year through 17 years of age

Social Support: Reliable assistance from others

Stress Level: Severity of manifested physical or mental tension resulting from factors that alter an existing equilibrium

P

Goals/Evaluation Criteria

Also see Goals/Evaluation Criteria for the preceding diagnosis, Parenting, Impaired.

Examples Using NOC Language

- Demonstrates **Parenting Performance**, as evidenced by the following indicators (specify 1–5: never, rarely, sometimes, often, or consistently demonstrated):
  - Uses age-appropriate discipline
  - Expresses satisfaction with parental role
  - Verbalizes positive attributes of child
  - Exhibits a loving relationship

Other Examples

Parent(s) will:

- Exhibit attachment behaviors during pregnancy and at birth of the infant
- Identify own risk factors that may lead to ineffective parenting
- Identify high-risk situations that may lead to ineffective parenting
- Recognize and compensate for physical, cognitive, or psychologic limitations for caregiving
- Demonstrate recovery from past emotional abuses (e.g., verbalize confidence and self-esteem)

- Seek help for emotional problems/neuroses
- Verbalize a sense of control over own behaviors and life situation
- Report having positive interpersonal relationships

NIC Interventions

Abuse Protection Support: Child: Identification of high-risk, dependent child relationships and actions to prevent possible or further infliction of physical, sexual, or emotional harm or neglect of basic necessities of life

Anger Control Assistance: Facilitation of the expression of anger in an adaptive, nonviolent manner

Attachment Promotion: Facilitation of the development of the parent–infant relationship

Caregiver Support: Provision of the necessary information, advocacy, and support to facilitate primary patient care by someone other than a health care professional

Childbirth Preparation: Providing information and support to facilitate childbirth and to enhance the ability of an individual to develop and perform the parental role

Developmental Enhancement: Adolescent: Facilitating optimal physical, cognitive, social, and emotional growth of individuals during the transition from childhood to adulthood

Developmental Enhancement: Child: Facilitating or teaching parents/caregivers to facilitate the optimal gross-motor, fine-motor, language, cognitive, social and emotional growth of preschool and school-aged children

Family Integrity Promotion: Promotion of family cohesion and unity

Family Integrity Promotion: Childbearing Family: Facilitation of the growth of individuals or families who are adding an infant to the family unit

Normalization Promotion: Assisting parents and other family members of children with chronic illnesses or disabilities in providing normal life experiences for their children and families

Parent Education: Adolescent: Assisting parents to understand and help their adolescent children

Parent Education: Childrearing Family: Assisting parents to understand and promote the physical, psychological, and social growth and development of their toddler or preschool or school-aged child or children

Parenting Promotion: Providing parenting information, support, and coordination of comprehensive services to high-risk families

Prenatal Care: Monitoring and management of patient during pregnancy to prevent complications of pregnancy and promote a healthy outcome for both mother and infant

Surveillance: Purposeful and ongoing acquisition, interpretation, and synthesis of patient data for clinical decision making

Nursing Activities

Nursing activities for this potential problem focus on supportive actions to modify risk factors and prevent Impaired Parenting. Also refer to Nursing Activities for *Readiness for Enhanced Parenting* (the following diagnosis).

Assessment

- Determine whether parents have unrealistic expectations for child's behavior or negative attributions for their child's behavior
- *(NIC) Abuse Protection Support: Child:*

  Identify parents who have had another child removed from the home or have placed previous children with relatives for extended periods

  Identify parents who have a history of substance abuse, depression, or major psychiatric illness

  Identify parents who have a history of domestic violence or a mother who has a history of numerous "accidental" injuries

  Identify crisis situations that may trigger abuse (e.g., poverty, unemployment, divorce, homelessness, and domestic violence)

  Identify infants or children with high-care needs (e.g., prematurity, low birth weight, colic, feeding intolerances, major health problems in the first year of life, developmental disabilities, hyperactivity, and attention-deficit disorders)
- During pregnancy, ask whether parent(s) has chosen names for both sexes
- Observe new parents for behaviors indicating lack of attachment (e.g., disgust when changing diaper, fear, or disappointment in gender)
- Assess parent's knowledge of infant or child basic care needs
- *(NIC) Family Integrity Promotion:*

  Determine typical family relationships for each family

  Monitor current family relationships

P

Patient/Parent Teaching

- *(NIC) Abuse Protection Support: Child:*

  Instruct parents on problem-solving, decision-making, and childrearing and parenting skills or refer parents to programs where these skills can be learned

  Provide parents with information on how to cope with protracted infant crying, emphasizing that they should not shake the baby

Provide the parents with noncorporal punishment methods for disciplining children

- *(NIC) Developmental Enhancement: Child:* Teach caregivers about normal developmental milestones and associated behaviors

Collaborative Activities

- Refer to community support and educational programs to assist with development of parenting skills and provide anticipatory guidance
- Encourage parents to attend prenatal education classes
- *(NIC) Abuse Protection Support: Child:*

  Refer at-risk pregnant women and parents of newborns to nurse home visitation services

  Provide at-risk families with a public health nurse referral to ensure that the home environment is monitored, that siblings are assessed, and that families receive continued assistance

Other

- *(NIC) Family Integrity Promotion: Childbearing Family:*

  Listen to family's concerns, feelings, and questions

  Prepare parent(s) for expected role changes involved in becoming a parent

  Encourage parent(s) to maintain individual hobbies or outside interests

Home Care

- The preceding interventions can be adapted for use in home care
- For an ill child, assess the need for respite care for care providers

PARENTING, READINESS FOR ENHANCED

(2002) **Domain 7, Role Relationship; Class 1, Caregiving Roles**

Definition: A pattern of providing an environment for children or other dependent person(s) that is sufficient to nurture growth and development and can be strengthened

Defining Characteristics

Subjective

Children or other dependent person(s) express satisfaction with home environment

Expresses willingness to enhance parenting

Objective

Emotional support of children [or dependent person(s)]
Evidence of attachment [bonding]
[Physical and emotional] needs of children [or dependent person(s)] are met
Exhibits realistic expectations of children [or dependent person(s)]

Related Factors

This is a wellness diagnosis, so an etiology is not needed. If risk factors exist, use *Risk for impaired parenting.*

Suggestions for Use

In general, adjustment to parenting is a normal maturational process that calls for nursing interventions to prevent potential problems and promote health. If interventions are not limited to parenting, consider one of the Suggested Alternative Diagnoses.

Suggested Alternative Diagnoses

Coping: family, readiness for enhanced
Family processes, readiness for enhanced

NOC Outcomes

Family Functioning: Capacity of the family system to meet the needs of its members during developmental transitions

Knowledge: Child Physical Safety: Extent of understanding conveyed about safely caring for a child from 1 year through 17 years of age

Knowledge: Infant Care: Extent of understanding conveyed about caring for a baby from birth to first birthday

Knowledge: Parenting: Extent of understanding conveyed about provision of a nurturing and constructive environment for a child from 1 year through 17 years of age

Parenting: Adolescent Physical Safety: Parental actions to prevent physical injury in an adolescent from 12 years through 17 years of age

Parenting: Early/Middle Childhood Physical Safety: Parental actions to avoid physical injury of a child from 3 years through 11 years of age

Parenting: Infant/Toddler Physical Safety: Parental actions to avoid physical injury of a child from birth through 2 years of age

Parenting Performance: Parental actions to provide a child a nurturing and constructive physical, emotional, and social environment

Parenting: Psychosocial Safety: Parental actions to protect a child from social contacts that might cause harm or injury

Goals/Evaluation Criteria

Also see Goals/Evaluation Criteria for *Parenting, Impaired.*

Examples Using NOC Language

- Demonstrates **Parenting Performance**, as evidenced by the following indicators (specify 1–5: never, rarely, sometimes, often, or consistently demonstrated):
  - Uses age-appropriate discipline
  - Expresses realistic expectations of parental role
  - Verbalizes positive attributes of child
- Demonstrates **Knowledge: Parenting**, as evidenced by the following indicators (specify 1–5: no, limited, moderate, substantial, or extensive knowledge):
  - Normal growth and development
  - Physical care needs
  - Psychological and socialization needs
  - Effective communication strategies

Other Examples

Parent(s) will:

- Identify personal risk factors that may lead to ineffective parenting
- Identify high-risk situations that may lead to ineffective parenting
- Recognize and compensate for physical, cognitive, or psychologic limitations for caregiving
- Verbalize a sense of control over own behaviors and life situation
- Report having positive interpersonal relationships
- Demonstrate constructive discipline
- Identify and use community resources that assist with home care
- Identify people who can provide information and emotional support when needed
- Indicate willingness to ask others for help

The child will:

- Achieve physical, cognitive, and psychosocial milestones at expected times (refer to appropriate age group for specific developmental norms)

NIC Interventions

Developmental Enhancement: Adolescent: Facilitating optimal physical, cognitive, social, and emotional growth of individuals during the transition from childhood to adulthood

Developmental Enhancement: Child: Facilitating or teaching parents and caregivers to facilitate the optimal gross-motor, fine-motor, language, cognitive, social, and emotional growth of preschool and school-aged children

Family Integrity Promotion: Promotion of family cohesion and unity

Family Integrity Promotion: Childbearing Family: Facilitation of the growth of individuals or families who are adding an infant to the family unit

Parent Education: Adolescent: Assisting parents to understand and help their adolescent children

Parent Education: Childrearing Family: Assisting parents to understand and promote the physical, psychological, and social growth and development of their toddler or preschool or school-aged child or children

Parent Education: Infant: Instruction on nurturing and physical care needed during the first year of life

Parenting Promotion: Providing parenting information, support, and coordination of comprehensive services to high-risk families

Teaching: Infant Nutrition: Instruction on nutrition and feeding practices during the first year of life

Teaching: Infant Safety: Instruction on safety during first year of life

Teaching: Toddler Safety: Instruction on safety during the second and third years of life

Nursing Activities

Assessment

P

- Determine whether parents have realistic expectations for child's behavior
- Assess parent's knowledge of infant or child basic care needs
- *(NIC) Family Integrity Promotion:*
  Determine typical family relationships for each family
  Monitor current family relationships

Patient/Parent Teaching

- Provide information about child care, as needed
- Teach problem-solving, decision-making, and childrearing skills, as needed
- Instruct regarding noncorporal punishment methods for disciplining children
- Teach parents ways to provide appropriate stimulation to infants, especially premature infants
- Teach about age-appropriate toys
- For infants confined to an Isolette, demonstrate ways to touch
- *(NIC) Developmental Enhancement: Child:* Teach caregivers about normal developmental milestones and associated behaviors

Collaborative Activities

- *(NIC) Developmental Enhancement: Child:* Facilitate caregivers' contact with community resources, as appropriate

Other

- Promote parent–infant attachment during pregnancy and at birth; for example:
  - Encourage father or significant other to be present during the birth process
  - Provide privacy and allow the parent(s) to see, hold, and examine newborn immediately after birth
  - While performing the initial newborn assessment, point out characteristics and abilities of the newborn to the parent(s)
  - Acknowledge and reinforce positive parenting behaviors
- *(NIC) Family Integrity Promotion:*
  - Be a listener for the family members
  - Facilitate a tone of togetherness within/among the family
  - Facilitate open communications among family members

Home Care

- The preceding interventions can be used in home care

For Older Adults

- Explain the importance of grandparents to the child's development

PERFUSION: GASTROINTESTINAL, RISK FOR INEFFECTIVE

(2008) **Domain 4, Activity/Rest; Class 4, Cardiovascular/Pulmonary Responses**

Definition: At risk for decrease in gastrointestinal circulation that may compromise health

Risk Factors

Abdominal aortic aneurysm
Abdominal compartment syndrome
Abnormal partial thromboplastin time
Abnormal prothrombin time
Acute gastrointestinal hemorrhage
Age >60 years
Anemia
Coagulopathy (e.g., sickle cell anemia)
Diabetes mellitus

Disseminated intravascular coagulation
Female gender
Gastroesophageal varices
Gastrointestinal disease (e.g., duodenal or gastric ulcer, ischemic colitis, ischemic pancreatitis)
Hemodynamic instability
Liver dysfunction
Myocardial infarction
Poor left ventricular performance
Renal failure
Smoking
Stroke
Trauma
Treatment-related side effects (e.g., cardiopulmonary bypass, pharmaceutical agents, gastric surgery)
Vascular disease (e.g., peripheral vascular disease, aortoiliac occlusive disease

Suggestions for Use

Actual ineffective gastrointestinal perfusion would represent a medical diagnoses or condition. The outcomes and interventions would be for medical/surgical treatments. The nurse's role is to monitor and detect changes in the patient's condition. Therefore, nursing care may be better directed by the use of collaborative problems (e.g., Potential Complication of renal failure: Ineffective gastrointestinal perfusion).

Suggested Alternative Diagnoses

Cardiac output, decreased

NOC Outcomes

NOTE: The following outcome is used to assess actual occurrence of ineffective gastrointestinal perfusion:

Tissue Perfusion: Abdominal Organs: Adequacy of blood flow through the small vessels of the abdominal viscera to maintain organ function

NOTE: Examples of outcomes associated with risk factors for ineffective gastrointestinal perfusion include the following:

Alcohol Abuse Cessation Behavior: Personal actions to eliminate alcohol use that poses a threat to health

Cardiac Pump Effectiveness: Adequacy of blood volume ejected from the left ventricle to support systemic perfusion pressure

Circulation Status: Unobstructed, unidirectional blood flow at an appropriate pressure through large vessels of the systemic and pulmonary circuits

Fluid Overload Severity: Severity of excess fluids in the intracellular and extracellular compartments of the body

Gastrointestinal Function: Extent to which foods (ingested or tube-fed) are moved from ingestion to excretion

Hydration: Adequate water in the intracellular and extracellular compartments of the body

Examples Using NOC Language

- Demonstrates **Circulation Status**, as evidenced by the following indicators (specify 1–5: severe, substantial, moderate, mild, or no deviation from normal range): Systolic and diastolic BP
- Demonstrates **Hydration**, as evidenced by the following indicators (specify 1–5: severely, substantially, moderately, mildly, or not compromised): urine output, serum sodium, moist mucous membranes
- Demonstrates **Hydration**, as evidenced by the following indicators (specify 1–5: severe, substantial, moderate, mild, or none):
  [Abnormal] thirst
  Increased hematocrit
  Increased blood urea nitrogen

Other Examples

- Demonstrates adequate food, fluid, and nutrient intake
- Reports sufficient energy
- Displays body mass and weight in expected range

P

NIC Interventions

Bleeding Reduction: Gastrointestinal: Limitation of the amount of blood loss from the upper and lower gastrointestinal tract and related complications

Cardiac Care: Limitation of complications resulting from an imbalance between myocardial oxygen supply and demand for a patient with symptoms of impaired cardiac function

Circulatory Care: Arterial Insufficiency: Promotion of arterial circulation

Circulatory Care: Venous Insufficiency: Promotion of venous circulation

Fluid Management: Promotion of fluid balance and prevention of complications resulting from abnormal or undesired fluid levels

Hemodynamic Regulation: Optimization of heart rate, preload, afterload, and contractility

Nursing Activities

Assessments

- Monitor vital signs
- Monitor cardiac rhythm

- Keep accurate record of fluid intake and output
- Assess for signs of altered fluid balance (e.g., dry mucous membranes, cyanosis, and jaundice)

Collaborative Activities

- *(NIC) Fluid Management:*
  Administer IV therapy, as prescribed

Patient/Family Teaching

- Explain all procedures and expected sensations to patient
- Explain the need for fluid restrictions, as needed

Collaborative Activities

- Administer diuretics, as ordered
- Notify physician if signs and symptoms of fluid volume excess develop

PERIOPERATIVE POSITIONING INJURY, RISK FOR

(1994, 2006) **Domain 11, Safety/Protection; Class 2, Physical Injury**

P

Definition: At risk for inadvertent anatomical and physical changes as a result of posture or equipment used during an invasive/surgical procedure

Risk Factors

[Advanced age]
Disorientation
Edema
Emaciation
Immobilization
Muscle weakness
Obesity
Sensory or perceptual disturbances due to anesthesia

Suggestions for Use

This diagnosis is a specific variation of *Risk for injury*. All surgery patients have at least some risk for *Perioperative positioning injury (PPI)*. For those with no preexisting risk factors, no etiology is needed because the perioperative positioning itself is the etiology. When there are preexisting risk factors (e.g., edema, advanced age, diabetes, arthritis, vascular disease), include them as the etiology (e.g., *Risk for PPI related to generalized edema*). A long surgical procedure also increases the risk for *PPI*. Actual *PPI* may be the etiology of other nursing diagnoses (e.g., *Impaired skin integrity*).

Suggested Alternative Diagnoses

Neurovascular dysfunction: peripheral, risk for
Skin integrity, risk for impaired
Tissue integrity, impaired [risk for]
Trauma, risk for

NOC Outcomes

To assess for actual occurrence of Perioperative Positioning Injury, use the following outcome:

Physical Injury Severity: Severity of injuries from accidents and trauma

The following are some outcomes associated with risk factors for Perioperative Positioning Injury:

Circulation Status: Unobstructed, unidirectional, blood flow at an appropriate pressure through large vessels of the systemic and pulmonary circuits

Post-Procedure Recovery: Extent to which an individual returns to baseline function following a procedure(s) requiring anesthesia or sedation

Tissue Perfusion: Cellular: Adequacy of blood flow through the vasculature to maintain function at the cellular level

Tissue Perfusion: Peripheral: Adequacy of blood flow through the small vessels of the extremities and maintains tissue function

Goals/Evaluation Criteria

Examples Using NOC Language

- *PPI* will not occur, as demonstrated by uncompromised Circulation Status, Tissue Perfusion: Cellular, and Tissue Perfusion: Peripheral.
- Demonstrates **Circulation Status**, as evidenced by the following indicators (specify 1–5: severe, substantial, moderate, mild, or no deviation from normal range):

  [Bilateral] brachial, radial, femoral, and pedal pulses
  Systolic and diastolic blood pressure

Other Examples

Patient will have:

- No skin, tissue, or neuromuscular injury as a result of perioperative positioning

- Brisk capillary refill
- Normal peripheral sensation
- Normal skin color and temperature
- Unimpaired muscle function
- No peripheral edema
- No localized extremity pain

NIC Interventions

Nursing interventions focus on preventing positioning injuries.

Circulatory Precautions: Protection of a localized area with limited perfusion

Peripheral Sensation Management: Prevention or minimization of injury or discomfort in the patient with altered sensation

Positioning: Intraoperative: Moving the patient or body part to promote surgical exposure while reducing the risk of discomfort and complications

Pressure Management: Minimizing pressure to body parts

Skin Surveillance: Collection and analysis of patient data to maintain skin and mucous membrane integrity

Nursing Activities

Assessments

- Determine preexisting factors (e.g., poor nutrition, diseases) that create risk for PPI
- *(NIC) Positioning: Intraoperative:*
  - Determine patient's range of motion and stability of joints
  - Check peripheral circulation and neurologic status
  - Monitor patient's position intraoperatively
- *(NIC) Skin Surveillance [postoperative period]:*
  - Observe extremities for color, warmth, swelling, pulses, texture, edema, and ulcerations
  - Monitor skin for areas of discoloration, bruising, and breakdown
  - Monitor skin color and temperature

Patient/Family Teaching

- *(NIC) Skin Surveillance:* Instruct family member or caregiver about signs of skin breakdown, as appropriate

Collaborative Activities

- Report on transfer to postanesthesia nurses any preexisting risk factors or any symptoms observed during surgery and immediate postoperative recovery

Other

- Lift patient when positioning; do not slide or pull patient
- Always reposition patient slowly and gently
- Ensure that surgical team members do not lean on the patient
- *(NIC) Positioning: Intraoperative:*

 Use assistive devices [e.g., leg restraint strap] for immobilization

 Use an adequate number of personnel to transfer patient

 Support the head and neck during transfer

 Protect IV lines, catheters, and breathing circuits

 Maintain patient's proper body alignment [refer to agency procedures or a surgical textbook for details of supine, prone, lateral, and lithotomy positions]

 Elevate extremities, as appropriate

 Apply padding [e.g., to bony prominences] or avoid pressure to superficial nerves

 Apply safety strap and arm restraint, as needed

 Protect the eyes, as appropriate

For Older Adults

- Be especially vigilant to prevent pressure on bony prominences; older adults are vulnerable to tissue damage because of loss of subcutaneous fat, muscle wasting, and nutritional deficits

POISONING, RISK FOR

(1980, 2006) **Domain 11, Safety/Protection; Class 4, Environmental Hazards**

Definition: At risk of accidental exposure to, or ingestion of, drugs or dangerous products in sufficient doses that may compromise health

Risk Factors

External (Environmental)

Availability of illicit drugs potentially contaminated by poisonous additives

Dangerous products placed or stored within the reach of children or confused persons

[Insufficient finances]

Large supplies of pharmaceutical agents in house

Pharmaceutical agents stored in unlocked cabinets accessible to children or confused persons

Internal (Individual)

Cognitive or emotional difficulties
Deficient knowledge regarding pharmaceutical agents
Deficient knowledge regarding poisoning prevention
Lack of proper precautions
Reduced vision
Reports occupational setting is without adequate safeguards

Other Risk Factors (Non-NANDA)

Chemical contamination of food and water
Flaking, peeling paint or plaster in presence of young children
Paint, lacquer, and so forth in poorly ventilated areas or without effective protection
Presence of atmospheric pollutants
Presence of poisonous vegetation
Unprotected contact with heavy metals or chemicals

Suggestions for Use

Use the most specific label for which defining characteristics are present (i.e., if required risk factors are present, use *Risk for poisoning* instead of *Risk for injury*).

Suggested Alternative Diagnoses

Home maintenance, impaired
Injury, risk for
Parenting, impaired
Violence: self-directed, risk for

NOC Outcomes

Knowledge: Child Physical Safety: Extent of understanding conveyed about safely caring for a child from 1 year through 17 years of age

Safe Home Environment: Physical arrangements to minimize environmental factors that might cause physical harm or injury in the home

Symptom Severity: Severity of perceived adverse changes in physical, emotional, and social functioning

Personal Safety Behavior: Personal actions of an adult to control behaviors that cause physical injury

Goals/Evaluation Criteria

Examples Using NOC Language

- Demonstrates **Safe Home Environment**, as evidenced by the following indicators (specify 1–5: not, slightly, moderately, substantially, or totally adequate):
  - Carbon monoxide detector maintenance
  - Safe storage of medications
  - Correction of lead hazard risks
  - Placement of appropriate hazard warning labels

Other Examples

- Develops strategies to prevent poisoning
- Demonstrates understanding of safe use of medication, as indicated by description of proper methods of administration, dosage, storage, and disposal
- Seeks information about potential risks
- Reports keeping contact numbers for poison control centers in an easily accessible location

NIC Interventions

Environmental Management, Safety: Monitoring and manipulation of the physical environment to promote safety

Health Education: Developing and providing instruction and learning experiences to facilitate voluntary adaptation of behavior conducive to health in individuals, families, groups, or communities

Risk Identification: Analysis of potential risk factors, determination of health risks, and prioritization of risk-reduction strategies for an individual or group

Surveillance, Safety: Purposeful and ongoing collection and analysis of information about the patient and the environment for use in promoting and maintaining patient safety

Teaching: Infant (and Toddler) Safety: Instruction on safety during the first [three years] of life

Nursing Activities

Assessments

- **(NIC) Environmental Management: Safety:** Monitor the environment for changes in safety status
- **(NIC) Surveillance: Safety:**
  - Monitor patient for alterations in physical or cognitive function that might lead to unsafe behavior

Determine degree of surveillance required by patient, based on level of functioning and the hazards present in environment

Patient/Family Teaching

- Provide educational materials related to safety strategies and countermeasures for poisons
- *(NIC) Environmental Management: Safety:*
  Educate high-risk individuals and groups about environmental hazards (e.g., lead and radon)
  Provide patient with emergency phone numbers (e.g., police, local health department, and poison control center)

Collaborative Activities

- Refer to community classes (e.g., cardiopulmonary resuscitation [CPR], first aid)
- *(NIC) Environmental Management: Safety:* Collaborate with other agencies (e.g., health department, police, and Environmental Protection Agency [EPA]) to improve environmental safety

Other

- *(NIC) Environmental Management: Safety:*
  Modify the environment to minimize hazards and risk
  Use protective devices (e.g., restraints, side rails, locked doors, fences, and gates) to physically limit mobility or access to harmful situations
- *(NIC) Surveillance: Safety:* Provide appropriate level of supervision and surveillance to monitor patient and to allow for therapeutic actions, as needed

Home Care

- The preceding interventions are appropriate for use in home care
- Provide a list of telephone numbers for local poison control centers and other emergency numbers
- Assist the family to identify poisonous substances in or near the home (e.g., paint, fertilizer, weed spray, gasoline, rodent poison)
- Be sure there is a carbon monoxide detector in the home
- Recommend having annual inspection of the furnace
- Recommend installing a chimney screen to prevent animals (e.g., squirrels) from nesting there and blocking the chimney

For Infants and Children

- Obtain "Mr. Yuk" labels for parents to use on poisonous substances (to obtain stickers, go to http://www.chp.edu/CHP/mryuk)
- Use child-resistant packaging, but do not assume any container is completely childproof
- Store medications and toxic substances in their original containers, never in food containers
- When administering medications to children, do not tell them it is candy
- Teach parents that syrup of ipecac is no longer recommended for use in the home
- Teach parents that some household plants are poisonous; they should be removed from the home, or at least stored out of reach of children

For Older Adults

- If the client uses two similar-appearing medications, advise client and family to not store them in the same location

POST-TRAUMA SYNDROME

(1986, 1998)

Domain 9, Coping/Stress Tolerance; Class 1, Post-Trauma Responses

Definition: Sustained maladaptive response to a traumatic, overwhelming event

Defining Characteristics

Subjective

Anger or rage
Anxiety
Fear
Flashbacks
Gastric irritability
Grieving
Guilt
Headaches
Hopelessness
Intrusive dreams or nightmares

Intrusive thoughts
Palpitations
Reports feeling numb
Shame

Objective

Aggression
Alienation
Altered mood states
Avoidance
Compulsive behavior
Denial
Depression
Detachment
Difficulty concentrating
Enuresis (in children)
Exaggerated startle response
Horror
Hypervigilance
Irritability
Neurosensory irritability
Panic attacks
Psychogenic amnesia
Repression
Substance abuse

Related Factors

Abuse (physical and psychological)
Being held prisoner of war
Criminal victimization
Disasters
Epidemics
Events outside the range of usual human experience
[Military combat]
[Rape]
Serious accidents (e.g., industrial, motor vehicle)
Serious threat or injury to self or loved ones
Sudden destruction of one's home or community
Torture
Tragic occurrence involving multiple deaths
Wars
Witnessing mutilation or violent death

Suggestions for Use

(a) If the related factor is rape, use the *Rape-trauma syndrome* diagnosis. (b) Because this is a syndrome diagnosis, the diagnostic statement does not need related factors and the second part of the statement (etiology) is omitted. (c) Other nursing diagnoses (e.g., *Risk for suicide*) may be needed in addition to *Rape-trauma syndrome* in order to focus nursing interventions more specifically.

Suggested Alternative Diagnoses

Coping: family, compromised or disabled
Coping, ineffective
Rape-trauma syndrome
Self-mutilation, risk for
Suicide, risk for
Violence: self-directed, risk for

NOC Outcomes

Abuse Recovery: Emotional: Extent of healing of psychologic injuries due to abuse

Abuse Recovery: Financial: Extent of control of monetary and legal matters following financial exploitation

Abuse Recovery: Sexual: Extent of healing of physical and psychological injuries due to sexual abuse or exploitation

Anxiety Level: Severity of manifested apprehension, tension, or uneasiness arising from an unidentifiable source

Coping: Personal actions to manage stressors that tax an individual's resources

Depression Level: Severity of melancholic mood and loss of interest in life events

Fear Level: Severity of manifested apprehension, tension, or uneasiness arising from an identifiable source

Fear Level: Child: Severity of manifested apprehension, tension, or uneasiness arising from an identifiable source in a child from 1 year through 17 years of age

Impulse Self-Control: Self-restraint of compulsive or impulsive behaviors

Self-Mutilation Restraint: Personal actions to refrain from intentional self-inflicted injury (nonlethal)

Goals/Evaluation Criteria

Examples Using NOC Language

- Demonstrates **Abuse Recovery: Sexual**, as evidenced by the following indicators (specify 1–5: none, limited, moderate, substantial, or extensive):
  - Expressions of right to have been protected from abuse
  - Healing of physical injuries
  - Relief of anger in nondestructive ways
  - Evidence of non-abusive opposite-sex (or same-sex) relationships
- Demonstrates **Abuse Recovery: Sexual**, as evidenced by the following indicators (specify 1–5: extensive, substantial, moderate, limited, or none):
  - Verbalization of feelings about the abuse
  - Sleep disturbances
  - Depression
  - Self-mutilation
  - Suicide attempts

Other Examples

- Acknowledges value of counseling
- Expresses hopefulness and empowerment
- Does not exhibit eating disorders
- Identifies feelings and situations that lead to impulsive actions
- Controls destructive and harmful impulses without supervision
- Seeks help when unable to control impulses
- Reports relief from physical symptoms (e.g., headache, gastrointestinal upset)

NIC Interventions

Anxiety Reduction: Minimizing apprehension, dread, foreboding, or uneasiness related to an unidentified source of anticipated danger

Behavior Management: Self-Harm: Assisting the patient to decrease or eliminate self-mutilating or self-abusive behaviors

Coping Enhancement: Assisting a patient to adapt to perceived stressors, changes, or threats that interfere with meeting life demands and roles

Counseling: Use of an interactive helping process focusing on the needs, problems, or feelings of the patient and significant others to enhance or support coping, problem-solving, and interpersonal relationships

Financial Resource Assistance: Assisting an individual and family to secure and manage finances to meet health care needs

Impulse Control Training: Assisting the patient to mediate impulsive behavior through application of problem-solving strategies to social and interpersonal situations

Mood Management: Providing for safety, stabilization, recovery, and maintenance of a patient who is experiencing dysfunctionally depressed mood or elevated mood

Security Enhancement: Intensifying a patient's sense of physical and psychological safety

Suicide Prevention: Reducing the risk for self-inflicted harm with intent to end life

Support System Enhancement: Facilitation of support to patient by family, friends, and community

Therapy Group: Application of psychotherapeutic techniques to a group, including the utilization of interactions between members of the group

Trauma Therapy: Child: Use of an interactive helping process to resolve a trauma experienced by a child

Nursing Activities

Also refer to Nursing Activities for the diagnosis Post-Trauma Syndrome, Risk for.

Collaborative Activities

- Follow hospital and agency policy regarding legal responsibility for reporting to authorities

Other

- Enhance patient's feeling of safety in the following ways:
  - Monitor and hold phone calls at patient's request
  - Monitor and limit visitation
  - Consider private versus semiprivate assignment and choice of roommate
  - Institute precautions to prevent physical harm to the patient or others
- *(NIC) Counseling:*
  - Establish a therapeutic relationship based on trust and respect
  - Demonstrate empathy, warmth, and genuineness
  - Use techniques of reflection and clarification to facilitate expression of concerns
  - Encourage expression of feelings
  - Reveal selected aspects of your own experiences or personality to foster genuineness and trust, as appropriate
  - Discourage decision making when the patient is under severe stress, when possible

POST-TRAUMA SYNDROME, RISK FOR

(1998) **Domain 9, Coping/Stress Tolerance; Class 1, Post-Trauma Response**

Definition: At risk for sustained maladaptive response to a traumatic or overwhelming event

Risk Factors

Diminished ego strength
Displacement from home
Duration of the event
Exaggerated sense of responsibility
Inadequate social support
Occupation (e.g., police, fire, rescue, corrections, emergency room staff, mental health)
Perception of event
Survivor's role in the event
Unsupportive environment

Suggestions for Use

(a) As a rule, syndrome diagnoses are one-part diagnostic statements, omitting the related factors. However, because this is a "risk for" (potential) diagnosis, it may be helpful to write a two-part statement with the related factors as the etiology (e.g., *Risk for post-trauma syndrome related to inadequate social support to aid in coping with aftermath of surviving a fire in which friends died*). (b) If defining characteristics are present for any of the Suggested Alternative Diagnoses, the nurse will need to decide whether it is more useful to write an actual diagnosis (e.g., *Social isolation related to unacceptable social values*) or to use the alternative diagnosis as an etiology (e.g., *Risk for post-trauma syndrome related to Social isolation*).

Suggested Alternative Diagnoses

Coping: community, ineffective
Coping: family, compromised or disabled
Coping: ineffective
Family processes, interrupted
Identity: personal, disturbed
Self-esteem, situational low
Social isolation
Spiritual distress

NOC Outcomes

Abuse Recovery: Extent of healing following physical or psychological abuse that may include sexual or financial exploitation

Anxiety Level: Severity of manifested apprehension, tension, or uneasiness arising from an unidentifiable source

Comfort Status: Psychospiritual: Psychospiritual ease related to self-concept, emotional well-being, source of inspiration, and meaning and purpose in life

Coping: Personal actions to manage stressors that tax an individual's resources

Health Beliefs: Perceived Threat: Personal conviction that a threatening health problem is serious and has potential negative consequences for lifestyle

Personal Resiliency: Positive adaptation and function of an individual following significant adversity or crisis

Risk Control: Personal actions to prevent, eliminate, or reduce modifiable health threats

Risk Detection: Personal actions to identify personal health threats

Self-Esteem: Personal judgment of self-worth

Social Support: Reliable assistance from others

Stress Level: Severity of manifested physical or mental tension resulting from factors that alter an existing equilibrium

Goals/Evaluation Criteria

Examples Using NOC Language

- Recovery from *Post-trauma syndrome* is indicated by Abuse Recovery (if appropriate); Anxiety Level; Comfort Status: Psychospiritual; Coping; Personal Resiliency; Self-Esteem; and Stress Level.

Other Examples

Risk factors will be identified and controlled or eliminated so that *Post-trauma syndrome* does not occur.

- Displays adequate ego strength
- Has adequate social support
- Demonstrates appropriate affect for the situation
- Demonstrates adequate social interaction
- Identifies and use effective coping strategies

NIC Interventions

Anxiety Reduction: Minimizing apprehension, dread, foreboding, or uneasiness related to an unidentified source of anticipated danger

Coping Enhancement: Assisting a patient to adapt to perceived stressors, changes, or threats that interfere with meeting life demands and roles

Counseling: Use of an interactive helping process focusing on the needs, problems, or feelings of the patient and significant others to enhance or support coping, problem-solving, and interpersonal relationships

Family Mobilization: Utilization of family strengths to influence patient's health in a positive direction

Guilt Work Facilitation: Helping another to cope with painful feelings of actual or perceived responsibility

Hope Inspiration: Facilitation of the development of a positive outlook in a given situation

Resiliency Promotion: Assisting individuals, families, and communities in development, use, and strengthening of protective factors to be used in coping with environmental and societal stressors

Risk Identification: Analysis of potential risk factors, determination of health risks, and prioritization of risk-reduction strategies for an individual or group

Security Enhancement: Intensifying a patient's sense of physical and pshychological safety

Self-Esteem Enhancement: Assisting a patient to increase his personal judgment of self-worth

Spiritual Support: Assisting the patient to feel balance and connection with a greater power

Support Group: Use of a group environment to provide emotional support and health-related information for members

Support System Enhancement: Facilitation of support to patient by family, friends, and community

Surveillance: Purposeful and ongoing acquisition, interpretation, and synthesis of patient data for clinical decision making

Nursing Activities

Assessments

- Assess psychologic response to the trauma
- Assess adequacy and availability of support system and community resources
- Assess family situation

Patient/Family Teaching

- Explain to significant others how they can provide support

Collaborative Activities

- Provide information on or referral to community resources (e.g., rape counselors, clergy, crisis centers, support groups, mental health professionals, social services, Victims' Assistance, Survivors of Trauma)

Other

- Provide opportunity for social supports and problem solving (e.g., participation in social and community activities)
- Encourage patient to verbalize account of the event
- Support the patient needing an invasive medical procedure, which may precipitate flashbacks:
  Explain necessity of procedure
  Premedicate if needed to minimize distress and discomfort
  Stay with patient during procedure
  Encourage patient to discuss feelings after procedure

Home Care

- The preceding interventions may be adapted for home care use
- Encourage the family to continue daily activities as they were before the trauma occurred
- If the trauma was to one family member only, be sure to assess the impact of the trauma on other family members
- Provide support to significant others, as well as to the traumatized member

For Infants and Children

- Use play therapy (e.g., drawing, playing with dolls) to help the child express feelings of fear, anger, guilt, and so forth
- Base your explanations on the child's developmental level
- Assist the parents to understand the child's needs
- Work with the schools to institute counseling and other programs to deal with post-traumatic stress after a disaster or other traumatic event
- Refer for psychological evaluation and counseling for a child who has experienced trauma, who has a disfiguring injury, or who has cancer or other serious illness

For Older Adults

- Assess for multiple losses or crises that may exhaust coping skills
- Help the client to draw on skills used to cope successfully with past crises
- Assess for depression; refer as appropriate
- For clients who live alone, encourage social interaction and assist them to develop a support system

POWER, READINESS FOR ENHANCED

(2006) **Domain 9, Coping/Stress Tolerance; Class 2, Coping Responses**

Definition: A pattern of participating knowingly in change that is sufficient for well-being and can be strengthened

Defining Characteristics

Expresses readiness to enhance:

- Awareness of possible changes to be made
- Freedom to perform actions for change
- Identification of choices that can be made for change
- Involvement in creating change
- Knowledge for participation in change
- Participation in choices for daily living and health
- Power

NOTE: Even though power (a response) and empowerment (an intervention approach) are different concepts, the literature related to both concepts supports the defining characteristics of this diagnosis.

Suggestions for Use

None

Suggested Alternative Diagnoses

Decision making, readiness for enhanced
Hope, readiness for enhanced
Powerlessness, risk for
Therapeutic regimen management, readiness for enhanced

NOC Outcomes

Health Beliefs: Perceived Control: Personal conviction that one can influence a health outcome

Health Promoting Behavior: Personal actions to sustain or increase wellness

Knowledge: Health Promotion: Extent of understanding conveyed about information needed to obtain and maintain optimal health

Participation in Health Care Decisions: Personal involvement in selecting and evaluating health care options to achieve desired outcome

Personal Autonomy: Personal actions of a competent individual to exercise governance in life decisions

Personal Resiliency: Positive adaptation and function of an individual following significant adversity or crisis

Goals/Evaluation Criteria

Examples Using NOC Language

- Demonstrates enhanced power, as evidenced by Health Beliefs: Perceived Control, Health Promoting Behavior, Knowledge: Health Promotion, Participation in Health Care Decisions, Personal Autonomy, and Personal Resiliency.
- Demonstrates **Participation in Health Care Decisions**, as evidenced by the following indicators (specify 1–5: never, rarely, sometimes, often, or consistently demonstrated):
  Identifies health outcome priorities
  Uses problem-solving techniques to achieve desired outcomes
  Negotiates for care preferences

Other Examples

- Identifies actions that are within his control

NIC Interventions

Coping Enhancement: Assisting a patient to adapt to perceived stressors, changes, or threats that interfere with meeting life demands and roles

Decision-Making Support: Providing information and support for a patient who is making a decision regarding health care

Health Education: Developing and providing instruction and learning experiences to facilitate voluntary adaptation of behavior conducive to health in individuals, families, groups, or communities

Health System Guidance: Facilitating a patient's location and use of appropriate health services

Mutual Goal Setting: Collaborating with patient to identify and prioritize care goals, then developing a plan for achieving those goals

Self-Efficacy Enhancement: Strengthening an individual's confidence in his ability to perform a health behavior

Self-Modification Assistance: Reinforcement of self-directed change initiated by the patient to achieve personally important goals

Self-Responsibility Facilitation: Encouraging a patient to assume more responsibility for own behavior

Resiliency Promotion: Assisting individuals, families, and communities in development, use, and strengthening of protective factors to be used in coping with environmental and societal stressors

Nursing Activities

Refer to the Nursing Activities for Powerlessness, following.

POWERLESSNESS

(1982, 2010) **Domain 9, Coping/Stress Tolerance; Class 2, Coping Responses**

Definition: The lived experience of lack of control over a situation, including a perception that one's actions do not significantly affect an outcome

Defining Characteristics

Subjective

Reports alienation
Reports doubt regarding role performance
Reports frustration over inability to perform previous activities
Reports lack of control
Reports shame

Objective

Dependence on others
Depression over physical deterioration
Nonparticipation in care

P

Related Factors

Illness-related regimen [e.g., long term, difficult, complex]
Institutional environment
Unsatisfying interpersonal interactions
Chronic or terminal illness (non-NANDA International)
Complications threatening pregnancy (non-NANDA International)

Suggestions for Use

Differentiate between *Powerlessness* and *Hopelessness*. *Hopelessness* implies that the person believes there is no solution to his problem (i.e., "no way out"). In *Powerlessness*, patients may know of a solution to their problem but believe it is beyond their control to achieve the solution. If *Powerlessness* is prolonged, it can lead to *Hopelessness*. Nurses should be careful to diagnose *Powerlessness* from the patient's perspective and not assume the patient perceives the situation as they would. Cultural and individual differences exist in a person's need to feel in control of a situation (e.g., to be told they have a fatal illness).

Suggested Alternative Diagnoses

Anxiety
Coping, ineffective

Death anxiety
Fear
Grieving, complicated
Hopelessness
Post-trauma syndrome
Rape-trauma syndrome
Self-esteem, chronic low
Spiritual distress

NOC Outcomes

Depression Self-Control: Personal actions to minimize melancholy and maintain interest in life events

Health Beliefs: Perceived Ability to Perform: Personal conviction that one can carry out a given health behavior

Health Beliefs: Perceived Control: Personal conviction that one can influence a health outcome

Health Beliefs: Perceived Resources: Personal conviction that one has adequate means to carry out a health behavior

Participation in Health Care Decisions: Personal involvement in selecting and evaluating health care options to achieve desired outcome

Personal Autonomy: Personal actions of a competent individual to exercise governance in life decisions

Goals/Evaluation Criteria

Examples Using NOC Language

- Demonstrates Depression Self-Control; Health Beliefs: Perceived Ability to Perform, Perceived Control, and Perceived Resources; Participation in Health Care Decisions; and Personal Autonomy (specify level, 1–5)
- Demonstrates **Participation in Health Care Decisions**, as evidenced by the following indicators (specify 1–5: never, rarely, sometimes, often, or consistently demonstrated):
  Identifies health outcome priorities
  Uses problem-solving techniques to achieve desired outcomes
  Negotiates for care preferences

Other Examples

Patient will:

- Verbalize any feelings of powerlessness
- Identify actions that are within his control
- Relate absence of barriers to action

- Verbalize ability to perform necessary actions
- Report adequate support from significant others, friends, and neighbors
- Report sufficient time, personal finances, and health insurance
- Report availability of equipment, supplies, services, and transportation

NIC Interventions

Also refer to the NIC Interventions for the diagnosis *Readiness for Enhanced Power*, preceding.

Cognitive Restructuring: Challenging a patient to alter distorted thought patterns and view self and the world more realistically

Decision-Making Support: Providing information and support for a patient who is making a decision regarding health care

Emotional Support: Provision of reassurance, acceptance, and encouragement during times of stress

Financial Resource Assistance: Assisting an individual/family to secure and manage finances to meet health care needs

Health System Guidance: Facilitating a patient's location and use of appropriate health services

P

Mood Management: Providing for safety, stabilization, recovery, and maintenance of a patient who is experiencing dysfunctionally depressed mood or elevated mood

Mutual Goal Setting: Collaborating with patient to identify and prioritize care goals, then developing a plan for achieving those goals

Patient Rights Protection: Protection of health care rights of a patient, especially a minor, incapacitated, or incompetent patient unable to make decisions

Self-Efficacy Enhancement: Strengthening an individual's confidence in his ability to perform a health behavior

Self-Esteem Enhancement: Assisting a patient to increase his personal judgment of self-worth

Self-Responsibility Facilitation: Encouraging a patient to assume more responsibility for own behavior

Support System Enhancement: Facilitation of support to patient by family, friends, and community

Nursing Activities

Assessments

- *(NIC) Self-Esteem Enhancement:*
  - Determine patient's locus of control
  - Determine patient's confidence in own judgment
  - Monitor levels of self-esteem over time, as appropriate

- *(NIC) Self-Responsibility Facilitation:*
  Monitor level of responsibility that patient assumes
  Determine whether patient has adequate knowledge about health care condition

Collaborative Activities

- Initiate a multidisciplinary patient care conference to discuss and develop patient care routine

Other

- Help patient to identify factors that may contribute to powerlessness
- Discuss with patient realistic options in care, providing explanations for these options
- Involve patient in decision making about care
- Explain to patient the rationale for any change in the plan of care
- *(NIC) Self-Esteem Enhancement:*
  Explore previous achievements of success
  Reinforce the personal strengths that patient identifies
  Convey confidence in patient's ability to handle situation
- *(NIC) Self-Responsibility Facilitation:*
  Encourage verbalizations of feelings, perceptions, and fears about assuming responsibility
  Encourage independence but assist patient when unable to perform

Home Care

- The preceding interventions are appropriate for home care
- Assess for abuse
- If abuse is suspected, make appropriate reports and help the victim take actions to ensure safety
- Assess for negative family attitudes toward the client that could contribute to a sense of powerlessness

For Older Adults

- Assess for multiple losses, common in aging, which may lead to *Powerlessness*
- Assess locus of control (internal or external)
- Assess for physical conditions (e.g., loss of mobility) that could contribute to *Powerlessness*
- Encourage and facilitate interaction with peers (e.g., senior citizens' center, groups)
- Encourage as much independence as possible in activities of daily living
- Assess for *Powerlessness* in caregivers
- Refer for homemaker services as needed

POWERLESSNESS, RISK FOR

(2000, 2010)

Definition: At risk for the lived experience or lack of control over a situation, including a perception that one's actions do not significantly affect an outcome

Risk Factors

Anxiety
Caregiving
Chronic low self-esteem
Deficient knowledge
Economically disadvantaged
Illness
Ineffective coping patterns
Lack of social support
Pain
Progressive debilitating disease
Situational low self-esteem
Social marginalization
Stigmatized condition or disease
Unpredictable course of illness

Suggested Alternative Diagnoses

Chronic low self-esteem
Grieving, complicated
Relocation stress syndrome
Situational low self-esteem
Spiritual distress, risk for

NOC Outcomes

Health Beliefs: Perceived Ability to Perform: Personal conviction that one can carry out a given health behavior

Health Beliefs: Perceived Control: Personal conviction that one can influence a health outcome

Participation in Health Care Decisions: Personal involvement in selecting and evaluating health care options to achieve desired outcome

Personal Autonomy: Personal actions of a competent individual to exercise governance in life decisions

Self-Direction of Care: Care recipient actions taken to direct others who assist with or perform physical tasks and personal health care

Goals/Evaluation Criteria

Examples Using NOC Language

Refer to examples for *Powerlessness* and *Readiness for enhanced powerlessness*

Other Examples

- Identifies actions that are within his control
- Relates absence of barriers to action
- Verbalizes ability to perform necessary actions
- Reports adequate support from significant others, friends, and neighbors
- Reports sufficient time, personal finances, and health insurance
- Reports availability of equipment, supplies, services, and transportation

NIC Interventions

Assertiveness Training: Assistance with the effective expression of feelings, needs, and ideas while respecting the rights of others

Body Image Enhancement: Improving a patient's conscious and unconscious perceptions and attitudes toward his body

Coping Enhancement: Assisting a patient to adapt to perceived stressors, changes, or threats that interfere with meeting life demands and roles

Dying Care: Promotion of physical comfort and psychological peace in the final phase of life

Financial Resource Assistance: Assisting an individual/family to secure and manage finances to meet health care needs

Health System Guidance: Facilitating a patient's location and use of appropriate health services

Self-Efficacy Enhancement: Strengthening an individual's confidence in his ability to perform a health behavior

Self-Esteem Enhancement: Assisting a patient to increase his personal judgment of self-worth

Nursing Activities

Refer to Nursing Activities for *Powerlessness*.

PROTECTION, INEFFECTIVE

(1990) **Domain 1, Health Promotion; Class 2, Health Management**

Definition: Decrease in the ability to guard self from internal or external threats such as illness or injury

Defining Characteristics

Subjective

Chilling
Dyspnea
Fatigue
Itching

Objective

Altered clotting
Anorexia
Cough
Deficient immunity
Disorientation
Immobility
Impaired healing
Insomnia
Maladaptive stress response
Neurosensory alteration
Perspiring
Pressure ulcers
Restlessness
Weakness

Related Factors

Abnormal blood profiles (e.g., leukopenia, thrombocytopenia, anemia, coagulation)
Diseases (e.g., cancer, immune disorders)
Drug therapies (e.g., antineoplastic, corticosteroid, immune, anticoagulant, thrombolytic)
Extremes of age
Inadequate nutrition
Substance abuse
Treatment-related side effects (e.g., surgery, radiation)
Abuse (non-NANDA International)

Suggestions for Use

(a) When possible, use a more specific label such as *Risk for infection*, *Impaired skin integrity*, *Impaired tissue integrity*, *Impaired oral mucous membrane*, or *Fatigue*. (b) *Ineffective protection* should not be used as a "catch-all" diagnosis for patients who are immunosuppressed or who have abnormal clotting factors. For example, the author does not recommend routine use of *Ineffective protection* during labor.

Suggested Alternative Diagnoses

Coping: family, compromised or disabled
Infection, risk for
Injury, risk for
Neurovascular dysfunction: peripheral, risk for
Parenting, impaired
Perioperative positioning injury, risk for
Skin integrity, risk for impaired

NOC Outcomes

Blood Coagulation: Extent to which blood clots within normal period of time

Cognitive Orientation: Ability to identify person, place, and time accurately

Fatigue Level: Severity of observed or reported prolonged generalized fatigue

Immune Status: Natural and acquired appropriately targeted resistance to internal and external antigens

Immunization Behavior: Personal actions to obtain immunization to prevent a communicable disease

Mobility: Ability to move purposefully in own environment independently with or without assistive device

Neurological Status: Peripheral: Ability of the peripheral nervous system to transmit impulses to and from the central nervous system

Nutritional Status: Extent to which nutrients are available to meet metabolic needs

Respiratory Status: Movement of air in and out of the lungs and exchange of carbon dioxide and oxygen at the alveolar level

Symptom Control: Personal actions to minimize perceived adverse changes in physical and emotional functioning

Tissue Integrity: Skin and Mucous Membranes: Structural intactness and normal physiological function of skin and mucous membranes

Wound Healing: Primary Intention: Extent of regeneration of cells and tissue following intentional closure

Goals/Evaluation Criteria

Examples Using NOC Language

- Demonstrates **Immune Status**, as evidenced by the following indicators (specify 1–5: severe, substantial, moderate, mild, or none):
    - Recurrent infections
    - Chronic fatigue

- Demonstrates **Immune Status**, as evidenced by the following indicators (specify 1–5: severely, substantially, moderately, mildly, or not compromised):
  - Immunizations current
  - Antibody titers
  - Differential WBC
  - T4-cell, T8-cell, and complement levels

Other Examples

- Demonstrates behaviors that decrease risk of injury, infection, or bleeding
- Reports early signs and symptoms of injury, infection, or bleeding
- Remains free of signs and symptoms of injury, infection, or bleeding
- Verbalizes a plan to provide safety for self and children (e.g., obtaining a restraining order)
- Demonstrates adequate nutritional status
- Exhibits respiratory status within normal limits

NIC Interventions

Bleeding Precautions: Reduction of stimuli that may induce bleeding or hemorrhage in at-risk patients

Eating Disorders Management: Prevention and treatment of severe diet restriction and overexercising or binging and purging of food and fluids

Energy Management: Regulating energy use to treat or prevent fatigue and optimize function

Exercise Therapy: Ambulation: Promotion and assistance with walking to maintain or restore autonomic and voluntary body functions during treatment and recovery from illness or injury

Exercise Therapy: Balance: Use of specific activities, postures, and movements to maintain, enhance, or restore balance

Health Education: Developing and providing instruction and learning experiences to facilitate voluntary adaptation of behavior conducive to health in individuals, families, groups, or communities

Immunization/Vaccination Management: Monitoring immunization status, facilitating access to immunizations, and providing immunizations to prevent communicable disease

Incision Site Care: Cleansing, monitoring, and promotion of healing in a wound that is closed with sutures, clips, or staples

Infection Control: Minimizing the acquisition and transmission of infectious agents

Infection Protection: Prevention and early detection of infection in a patient at risk

Nutrition Therapy: Administration of food and fluids to support metabolic processes of a patient who is malnourished or at high risk for becoming malnourished

Nutritional Counseling: Use of an interactive helping process focusing on the need for diet modification

Peripheral Sensation Management: Prevention or minimization of injury or discomfort in the patient with altered sensation

Pressure Management: Minimizing pressure to body parts

Reality Orientation: Promotion of patient's awareness of personal identity, time, and environment

Respiratory Monitoring: Collection and analysis of patient data to ensure airway patency and adequate gas exchange

Risk Identification: Analysis of potential risk factors, determination of health risks, and prioritization of risk-reduction strategies for an individual or group

Ventilation Assistance: Promotion of an optimal spontaneous breathing pattern that maximizes oxygen and carbon dioxide exchange in the lungs

Wound Care: Prevention of wound complications and promotion of wound healing

Nursing Activities

Because there are so many risk factors for this diagnosis, there are also many possible nursing activities. Choose activities that focus on the patient's particular risk factors.

Prevention of Infection

See Nursing Activities for the diagnosis *Risk for Infection.*

Prevention of Injury

See Nursing Activities for the diagnosis *Risk for Injury.*

Assessments

- Monitor the safety of items brought in by visitors

Other

- Remove sharp objects and other potential weapons from patient area
- Lock utility and storage rooms

Prevention of Bleeding

Assessments

- Evaluate extent of patient's bleeding risk

Patient/Family Teaching

- Advise patient to wear medical identification bracelet and to alert dentist or physician
- Instruct patient to avoid trauma (e.g., from contact sports, sharp objects, stiff toothbrush)
- Teach patient signs and symptoms of bleeding and when to report it
- Teach patient first aid for bleeding

Intraoperative and Postoperative Periods

Refer to Nursing Activities for the diagnosis *Perioperative Positioning Injury.*

Assessments

- Monitor oxygenation
- Monitor and record vital signs q15 minutes or more often, as appropriate
- Monitor urinary output
- Monitor level of consciousness
- Monitor surgical site
- Assess pain q15 minutes during first hour
- Observe patient's skin for injury after use of electrosurgery

Other

- Document and communicate allergies
- Inspect the patient's skin under the grounding pad
- Encourage deep breathing and coughing
- Be certain the equipment is functioning correctly
- Assist with counts of sponges, sharps, and instruments

Restoration and Growth

Patient/Family Teaching

- Provide information on community resources and support groups

Collaborative Activities

- Consult dietitian for suggestions to improve nutrition
- Confer with social services to identify appropriate referral for counseling

Other

- Explore with patient ways to enhance sleep and rest
- Assist patient in achieving optimum sleep, rest, nutrition, activity, and stress management
- Discuss relaxation techniques with patient/family
- Assist patient and family in identifying and planning an appropriate exercise program

Home Care

- Assess for abuse
- Only a few of the preceding nursing activities are suitable for use in home care
- Teach safe food handling and storage, especially for clients with depressed immune function

For Infants and Children

- For preterm and low-birth-weight infants, use alcohol hand rub for handwashing; wear gloves for patient care
- Do not use topical antibiotic ointment routinely for preterm infants
- Encourage breastfeeding for low-birth-weight infants

For Older Adults

- Help clients adapt an exercise program suitable for their functional abilities
- Recommend supplemental vitamins and minerals

RAPE-TRAUMA SYNDROME

(1980, 1998) **Domain 9, Coping/Stress Tolerance; Class 1, Post-Trauma Response**

Definition: Sustained maladaptive response to a forced, violent sexual penetration against the victim's will and consent

Defining Characteristics

Subjective

Anger
Anxiety
Chronic low self-esteem
Confusion
Embarrassment
Fear
Guilt
Humiliation
Mood swings
Muscle tension or spasms
Nightmares and sleep disturbances

Powerlessness
Self-blame
Shame

Objective
Aggression
Agitation
Change in relationships
Denial
Dependence
Depression
Disorganization
Dissociative disorders
Helplessness
Hyperalertness
Impaired decision making
Paranoia
Phobias
Physical trauma (e.g., bruising, tissue irritation)
Revenge
Sexual dysfunction
Shock
Substance abuse
Suicide attempts
Vulnerability

Related Factors

Rape [patient's biopsychosocial response to event]

NOC Outcomes

Abuse Protection: Protection of self or dependent others from abuse
Abuse Recovery: Emotional: Extent of healing of psychological injuries due to abuse
Abuse Recovery: Physical: Extent of healing of physical injuries due to abuse
Abuse Recovery: Sexual: Extent of healing of physical and psychological injuries due to sexual abuse or exploitation
Sexual Functioning: Integration of physical, socioemotional, and intellectual aspects of sexual expression and performance

Goals/Evaluation Criteria

Examples Using NOC Language

- Demonstrates **Abuse Recovery: Sexual**, as evidenced by the following indicators (specify 1–5: extensive, substantial, moderate, limited, or none):
  - Verbalization of details of abuse
  - Verbalization of feelings about the abuse
  - Verbalization of feelings of guilt
  - Sleep disturbances
- Demonstrates **Abuse Recovery: Sexual**, as evidenced by the following indicators (specify 1–5: none, limited, moderate, substantial, or extensive):
  - Verbalization of accurate information about sexual functioning
  - Expressions of right to have been protected from abuse
  - Expressions of hope
  - Evidence of non-abusive same-sex and opposite-sex relationships

Other Examples

Patient will:

- Identify and use effective coping strategies
- Report cessation of sexual abuse
- Engage in positive interpersonal relationships
- Resolve feelings of depression
- Have appropriate affect for situation
- Obtain treatment for, and resolve, emotional problems and behaviors resulting from the trauma
- Be able to control negative or destructive impulses

NIC Interventions

Abuse Protection Support: Identification of high-risk, dependent relationships and actions to prevent further infliction of physical or emotional harm

Abuse Protection Support: Child: Identification of high-risk, dependent child relationships and actions to prevent possible or further infliction of physical, sexual, or emotional harm or neglect of basic necessities of life

Abuse Protection Support: Domestic Partner: Identification of high-risk, dependent domestic relationships and actions to prevent possible or further infliction of physical, sexual, or emotional harm or exploitation of a domestic partner

Abuse Protection Support: Elder: Identification of high-risk, dependent elder relationships and actions to prevent possible or further infliction of physical, sexual, or emotional harm; neglect of basic necessities of life; or exploitation

Behavior Management: Sexual: Delineation and prevention of socially unacceptable sexual behaviors

Counseling: Use of an interactive helping process focusing on the needs, problems, or feelings of the patient and significant others to enhance or support coping, problem solving, and interpersonal relationships

Health Screening: Detecting health risks or problems by means of history, examination, and other procedures

Rape-Trauma Treatment: Provision of emotional and physical support immediately following a reported rape

Risk Identification: Analysis of potential risk factors, determination of health risks, and prioritization of risk-reduction strategies for an individual or group

Sexual Counseling: Use of an interactive helping process focusing on the need to make adjustments in sexual practice or to enhance coping with a sexual event/disorder

Therapy Group: Application of psychotherapeutic techniques to a group, including the utilization of interactions between members of the group

Trauma Therapy: Child: Use of an interactive helping process to resolve a trauma experienced by a child

Nursing Activities

Assessments

- Assess whether patient presents a safety risk to self or others
- *(NIC) Rape-Trauma Treatment:*

  Document whether patient has showered, douched, or bathed since incident

  Document mental state, physical state (clothing, dirt, and debris), history of incident, evidence of violence, and prior gynecological history

  Determine presence of cuts, bruises, bleeding, lacerations, or other signs of physical injury

Patient/Family Teaching

- Support and educate significant others; discuss therapeutic response to victim and changes in victim's behaviors that can be anticipated
- *(NIC) Rape-Trauma Treatment:*

  Inform patient of HIV testing, as appropriate

  Give clear, written instructions about medication use, crisis support services, and legal support

  Explain legal proceedings available to patient

Collaborative Activities

- *(NIC) Rape-Trauma Treatment:*

  Refer patient to rape advocacy program

  Offer medication to prevent pregnancy, as appropriate

  Offer prophylactic antibiotic medication against venereal disease

Other

- Approach patient in a nonjudgmental and supportive manner
- Allow adequate time for patient to respond to even simple questions
- Counsel immediate family, spouse, or partner to maintain close relationship with victim, with attention to dispelling feelings of blame (e.g., self or projected)
- Encourage patient and family to verbalize feelings
- *(NIC) Rape-Trauma Treatment:*

  Provide support person to stay with patient

  Implement rape protocol (e.g., label and save soiled clothing, vaginal secretions, and vaginal hair combings)

  Implement crisis intervention counseling

Home Care

- A few of the preceding nursing activities can be used in home care
- Facilitate the development of a long-term support system
- Explain to family that recovery may occur very slowly—over several years
- Advise the client to follow up with her primary care provider to be tested for pregnancy and sexually transmitted infections

For Infants and Children

- Be aware that a child is most likely to have been raped by an acquaintance and usually within the child's home or neighborhood
- Evaluate the potential for suicide, especially when the victim is an adolescent boy
- Adapt your communication to the child's developmental level
- Use art play to promote expression of feelings and description of the event
- Help the parents to understand the child's responses following the rape
- Correct any incorrect conclusions the child has drawn about the trauma (e.g., feeling guilty)
- Stress to parents the need to reestablish the child's sense of security in his life

For Older Adults

- Assess for depression, helplessness, and powerlessness, which are more common in older adults in response to rape
- If symptoms are present, be alert for sexual abuse of institutionalized elders (e.g., in long-term facilities); these patients are very vulnerable and also may be hesitant to report such abuse

RELATIONSHIP, INEFFECTIVE

(2010) **Domain 7, Role Relationships; Class 3, Role Performance**

Definition: A pattern of mutual partnership that is insufficient to provide for each other's needs

Defining Characteristics

Subjective

Does not identify partner as a key person
Inability to communicate in a satisfying manner between partners
Reports dissatisfaction with complementary relation between partners
Reports dissatisfaction with fulfilling emotional or physical needs between partners
Reports dissatisfaction with sharing of ideas or information between partners

Objective

Does not meet developmental goals appropriate for family life-cycle stage
No demonstration of mutual respect between partners
No demonstration of mutual support in daily activities between partners
No demonstration of understanding of partner's insufficient (physical, social, psychological) functioning

Related Factors

Cognitive changes in one partner
Developmental crises
History of domestic violence
Incarceration of one partner
Poor communication skills

Stressful life events
Substance abuse
Unrealistic expectations

NOC Outcomes

NOC outcomes have not yet been published for this problem. The following may be useful.

Development: Late Adulthood: Cognitive, psychosocial, and moral progression from 65 years of age and older

Development: Middle Adulthood: Cognitive, psychosocial, and moral progression from 40 through 65 years of age

Development: Young Adulthood: Cognitive, psychosocial, and moral progression from 18 through 39 years of age

Family Functioning: Capacity of the family system to meet the needs of its members during developmental transitions

Family Integrity: Family members' behaviors that collectively demonstrate cohesion, strength, and emotional bonding

Role Performance: Congruence of an individual's role behavior with role expectations

Goals/Evaluation Criteria

Examples Using NOC Language

- Relationship will be effective, as evidenced by normal Development: Late (Middle, or Young) Adulthood and satisfactory Role Performance by both partners.
- Demonstrates **Development: Middle Adulthood**, as evidenced by the following indicators (specify 1–5: never, rarely, sometimes, often, or consistently demonstrated):

  Maintains a healthy intimate relationship with partner
  Adjusts to sexual function changes
  Acknowledges values and opinions of others [i.e., partner]
  Respects others
  Recognizes that mutual trust is necessary in healthy relationships

Other Examples

- Identifies partner as an important person in her or his life
- Reports satisfaction with the relationship
- Reports sharing of ideas and/or information with each other
- Reports satisfactory fulfilling of physical and emotional needs
- Partners demonstrate mutual support in daily activities
- Partners openly and honestly discuss differences and tolerate differences of opinion
- Partners express anger appropriately

NIC Interventions

NIC interventions have not yet been linked to this diagnosis; however, the following may be useful.

Coping Enhancement: Assisting a patient to adapt to perceived stressors, changes, or threats that interfere with meeting life demands and roles

Family Integrity Promotion: Promotion of family cohesion and unity

Role Enhancement: Assisting a patient, significant other, and family to improve relationships by clarifying and supplementing specific role behaviors

Socialization Enhancement: Facilitation of another person's ability to interact with others

Nursing Activities

Assessments

- Assist each partner to identify the ways in which they wish to improve the relationship
- Assess partners' use of effective communication skills
- Determine how the partners deal with conflict
- Assess each partners feelings about the sexual aspects of their relationship
- Assess the overall functioning of the family

Patient/Family Teaching

- Teach communication skills (provide opportunity for role playing)
- Recommend Web sites that might be useful.
- Describe the technique of active listening and explain its importance
- Teach conflict resolution skills (e.g., win–win strategies)

Collaborative Activities

- Refer to couple support groups, to assertiveness training classes, and to other resources as indicated by the couple's needs
- Refer for medical care for psychological or physical problems of either partner

Other

- Role play ways to de-escalate an argument
- Role play active listening
- Maintain a positive attitude and approach
- Encourage open communication of concerns and questions
- Discuss the importance of not blaming the other partner
- Encourage the partners to ask for each other's opinion about problems
- Encourage partners to share feelings with each other. Monitor these exchanges at first, to assure that it will be a safe exchange with no blaming or anger.

RELATIONSHIP, INEFFECTIVE, RISK FOR

(2010) **Domain 7, Role Relationships; Class 3, Role Performance**

Definition: Risk for a pattern of mutual partnership that is insufficient to provide for each other's needs

Risk Factors

Cognitive changes in one partner
Developmental crises
History of domestic violence
Incarceration of one partner
Poor communication skills
Stressful life events
Substance abuse
Unrealistic expectations

NOC Outcomes

NOC outcomes have not yet been published for this problem. The following may be useful.

Development: Late Adulthood: Cognitive, psychosocial, and moral progression from 65 years of age and older

Development: Middle Adulthood: Cognitive, psychosocial, and moral progression from 40 through 65 years of age

Development: Young Adulthood: Cognitive, psychosocial, and moral progression from 18 through 39 years of age

Role Performance: Congruence of an individual's role behavior with role expectations

Goals/Evaluation Criteria

Examples Using NOC Language

- *Ineffective relationship* will not occur, as evidenced by normal Development: Late (Middle, or Young) Adulthood and satisfactory Role Performance by both partners.
- Demonstrates **Development: Middle Adulthood**, as evidenced by the following indicators (specify 1–5: never, rarely, sometimes, often, or consistently demonstrated):

    Maintains a healthy intimate relationship with partner
    Adjusts to sexual function changes
    Acknowledges values and opinions of others [i.e., partner]

Respects others [i.e., partner]
Recognizes that mutual trust is necessary in healthy relationships

Other Examples

- Identifies partner as an important person in her or his life
- Reports satisfaction with the relationship
- Reports sharing of ideas and/or information with each other
- Reports satisfactory fulfilling of physical and emotional needs
- Partners demonstrate mutual support in daily activities
- Partners openly and honestly discuss differences and tolerate differences of opinion
- Partners express anger appropriately

NIC Interventions

NIC interventions have not yet been linked to this diagnosis; however, the following may be useful.

Coping Enhancement: Assisting a patient to adapt to perceived stressors, changes, or threats that interfere with meeting life demands and roles

Family Integrity Promotion: Promotion of family cohesion and unity

Role Enhancement: Assisting a patient, significant other, and family to improve relationships by clarifying and supplementing specific role behaviors

Socialization Enhancement: Facilitation of another person's ability to interact with others

Nursing Activities

Because this is a potential problem, nursing activities focus on assessing for symptoms of the actual problem, identifying risk factors, and moderating or removing risk factors.

Assessments

- Assist the couple to identify stressors on the relationship (i.e., risk factors)
- Assess partners' use of effective communication skills
- Determine how the partners deal with conflict
- Assess each partner's feelings about the sexual aspects of their relationship
- Assess the overall functioning of the family
- Assess for risk factors (e.g., substance abuse)

Patient/Family Teaching

- Teach communication skills (provide opportunity for role playing), as needed
- Recommend Web sites that might be useful in dealing with existing risk factors
- Describe the technique of active listening and explain its importance

Collaborative Activities

- Refer to couple support groups, to assertiveness training classes, and to other resources (e.g., substance-abuse treatment) as indicated by the couple's needs
- Refer for medical care for psychological or physical problems of either partner

Other

- Maintain a positive attitude and approach
- Encourage open communication of concerns and questions
- Discuss the importance of not blaming the other partner
- Encourage partners to share feelings with each other. Monitor these exchanges at first, to assure that it will be a safe exchange with no blaming or anger

RELATIONSHIP, READINESS FOR ENHANCED

(2010) **Domain 7, Role Relationships; Class 3, Role Performance**

Definition: A pattern of mutual partnership that is insufficient to provide for each other's needs and can be strengthened

Defining Characteristics

Subjective

Reports desire to enhance communication between partners
Reports satisfaction with complementary relationship between partners
Reports satisfaction with fulfilling emotional needs by one's partner
Reports satisfaction with fulfilling physical needs by one's partner
Reports satisfaction with sharing of ideas between partners
Reports satisfaction with sharing of information between partners

Objective

Demonstrates mutual respect between partners
Demonstrates mutual support in daily activities between partners
Demonstrates understanding of partner's insufficient (physical, social, psychological) function
Demonstrates well-balanced autonomy between partners
Demonstrates well-balanced collaboration between partners
Identifies each other as a key person
Meets developmental goals appropriate for family life-cycle stage

NOC Outcomes

Development: Late Adulthood: Cognitive, psychosocial, and moral progression from 65 years of age and older

Development: Middle Adulthood: Cognitive, psychosocial, and moral progression from 40 through 65 years of age

Development: Young Adulthood: Cognitive, psychosocial, and moral progression from 18 through 39 years of age

Role Performance: Congruence of an individual's role behavior with role expectations

Goals/Evaluation Criteria

Examples Using NOC Language

- *Ineffective relationship* will not occur, as evidenced by normal Development: Late (Middle, or Young) Adulthood and satisfactory Role Performance by both partners
- Demonstrates **Development: Middle Adulthood**, as evidenced by the following indicators (specify 1–5: never, rarely, sometimes, often, or consistently demonstrated):
  - Maintains a healthy intimate relationship with partner
  - Adjusts to sexual function changes
  - Acknowledges values and opinions of others [i.e., partner]
  - Respects others [i.e., partner]
  - Recognizes that mutual trust is necessary in healthy relationships

R

Other Examples

- Identifies partner as an important person in her or his life
- Reports satisfaction with the relationship
- Reports sharing of ideas and/or information with each other
- Reports satisfactory fulfilling of physical and emotional needs
- Partners demonstrate mutual support in daily activities
- Partners openly and honestly discuss differences and tolerate differences of opinion

NIC Interventions

Family Integrity Promotion: Promotion of family cohesion and unity

Family Support: Promotion of family values, interests, and goals

Role Enhancement: Assisting a patient, significant other, and family to improve relationships by clarifying and supplementing specific role behaviors

Self-Awareness Enhancement: Assisting a patient to explore and understand his thoughts, feelings, motivations, and behaviors

Values Clarification: Assisting another to clarify her or his own values in order to facilitate effective decision making

Nursing Activities

Assessments

- Assist the couple to identify factors that could become stressors on the relationship
- Assess partners' use of effective communication skills
- Determine what improvements the partners want to make in their relationships
- Determine how the partners deal with conflict
- Assess the overall functioning of the family
- Assess partners' perceptions of each of their roles

Patient/Family Teaching

- Teach communication skills (provide opportunity for role playing), as needed
- Recommend Web sites dealing with healthy relationships
- Describe the technique of active listening and explain its importance
- Teach partners about nonverbal communication, as needed

Other

- Maintain a positive attitude and approach
- Encourage open communication of concerns and questions
- Encourage partners to share feelings with each other
- Encourage the use of play and humor in the relationship

RELIGIOSITY, IMPAIRED

(2004) **Domain 10, Life Principles; Class 3, Value/Belief/Action Congruence**

Definition: Impaired ability to exercise reliance on beliefs and/or participate in rituals of a particular faith tradition

Defining Characteristics

Subjective

Difficulty adhering to prescribed religious beliefs
Expresses a need to reconnect with previous belief patterns
Expresses a need to reconnect with previous customs

Expresses emotional distress because of separation from faith community
Questions religious belief patterns
Questions religious customs

Objective

Difficulty adhering to prescribed religious rituals (e.g., religious ceremonies, dietary regulations, clothing, prayer, worship or religious services, private religious behaviors, reading religious materials or media, holiday observances, meetings with religious leaders)

Related Factors

Developmental and Situational

Aging
End-stage life crises
Life transitions

Physical

Illness
Pain

Psychological

Anxiety
Fear of death
Ineffective coping
Ineffective support
R
Lack of security
Personal crisis
Use of religion to manipulate

Sociocultural

Cultural barriers to practicing religion
Environmental barriers to practicing religion
Lack of social integration
Lack of sociocultural interaction

Spiritual

Spiritual crises
Suffering

Suggestions for Use

Based on the NANDA-I definition, this diagnosis is appropriate when something blocks the patient's ability to participate in religious practices. For example, if a homebound patient can no longer attend church services, the nurse could help arrange for transportation. If the barrier cannot be removed, use the diagnosis *Spiritual distress.*

Suggested Alternative Diagnoses

Religiosity, impaired, risk for
Spiritual distress
Spiritual distress, risk for

NOC Outcomes

Comfort Status: Psychospiritual: Psychospiritual ease related to self-concept, emotional well-being, source of inspiration, and meaning and purpose in life

Hope: Optimism that is personally satisfying and life supporting

Spiritual Health: Connectedness with self, others, higher power, all life, nature, and the universe that transcends and empowers the self

Goals/Evaluation Criteria

Examples Using NOC Language

- Demonstrates **Spiritual Health**, as evidenced by the following indicators (specify 1–5: severely, substantially, moderately, mildly, or not compromised):
  - Ability to pray
  - Ability to worship
  - Participation in spiritual rites and passages
  - Interaction with spiritual leaders
  - Quality of faith

Other Examples

- Verbalizes experiencing meaning and purpose in life
- Participates in religious rituals such as singing and music
- Reports reading spiritual materials
- Expresses feelings of connectedness with inner self and with others

NIC Interventions

Anxiety Reduction: Minimizing apprehension, dread, foreboding, or uneasiness related to an unidentified source of anticipated danger

Hope Inspiration: Facilitation of the development of a positive outlook in a given situation

Religious Ritual Enhancement: Facilitating participation in religious practices

Spiritual Growth Facilitation: Facilitation of growth in patients' capacity to identify, connect with, and call upon the source of meaning, purpose, comfort, strength, and hope in their lives

Spiritual Support: Assisting the patient to feel balance and connection with a greater power

Values Clarification: Assisting another to clarify her or his own values in order to facilitate effective decision making

Assessments

- Assess for obstacles to religious practices (e.g., limitations imposed by disease process, lack of transportation)
- Determine whether the client wishes to participate in religious rituals and services
- Use established tools to assess spiritual well-being

Patient/Family Teaching

- Inform patient/family of the religious resources available in the institution
- Inform client of religious books and articles available in Braille, in large print, or on tape

Collaborative Activities

- Refer to chaplain, pastor, or other spiritual adviser
- Obtain a medical order to allow fasting, if patient wishes to do so

Other

- *(NIC) Spiritual Growth Facilitation:*
  - Offer individual and group prayer support, as appropriate
  - Assist the patient to explore beliefs as related to healing of body, mind, and spirit

- Share own spiritual perspectives and beliefs, as appropriate
- Pray with the patient, if requested to do so
- Use therapeutic communication to build trust
- Demonstrate empathy and acceptance
- Facilitate patient's use of religious rituals (e.g., provide physical support, allow to wear religious medals)
- Provide privacy and quiet for prayer and other religious practices
- Be accepting and nonjudgmental about the client's religious practices
- Turn on religious programs on radio or television if the client desires

Home Care

- Most of the preceding interventions can be adapted for home care use
- Identify organizations within the community that will provide transportation to religious services, as needed

> **For Infants and Children**
> - Base interventions on developmental level
> - Adhere to the parents' religious practices (e.g., have the child pray before meals and at bedtime if they do so at home)
> - Assess whether the child believes his illness to be punishment for doing wrong

RELIGIOSITY, IMPAIRED, RISK FOR

(2004) **Domain 10, Life Principles; Class 3, Value/Belief/Action Congruence**

Definition: At risk for an impaired ability to exercise reliance on religious beliefs and/or participate in rituals of a particular faith tradition

Related Factors

Developmental

Life transitions

Environmental

Barriers to practicing religion
Lack of transportation

Physical

Hospitalization
Illness
Pain

Psychological

Depression
Ineffective caregiving
Ineffective coping
Ineffective support
Lack of security

Sociocultural

Cultural barrier to practicing religion
Lack of social interaction
Social isolation

Spiritual

Suffering

Suggestions for Use

Based on the NANDA-I definition, this diagnosis is appropriate when a situation exists that may block the patient's ability to participate in religious practices, but the patient is not exhibiting any defining characteristics. For example, if a homebound patient can no longer attend church services, the nurse could help arrange for transportation to prevent *Impaired religiosity*. If the barrier cannot be removed, use the diagnosis *Spiritual distress*.

Suggested Alternative Diagnoses

Religiosity, impaired
Spiritual distress
Spiritual distress, risk for

NOC Outcomes

Comfort Status: Psychospiritual: Psychospiritual ease related to self-concept, emotional well-being, source of inspiration, and meaning and purpose in life

Spiritual Health: Connectedness with self, others, higher power, all life, nature, and the universe that transcends and empowers the self

Goals/Evaluation Criteria

See Goals/Evaluation Criteria for the Impaired Religiosity diagnosis, preceding.

NIC Interventions

Anxiety Reduction: Minimizing apprehension, dread, foreboding, or uneasiness related to an unidentified source of anticipated danger

Coping Enhancement: Assisting a patient to adapt to perceived stressors, changes, or threats that interfere with meeting life demands and roles

Culture Brokerage: The deliberate use of culturally competent strategies to bridge or mediate between the patient's culture and the biomedical health care system

Family Mobilization: Utilization of family strengths to influence patient's health in a positive direction

Pain Management: Alleviation of pain or a reduction in pain to a level of comfort that is acceptable to the patient

Religious Ritual Enhancement: Facilitating participation in religious practices

Relocation Stress Reduction: Assisting the individual to prepare for and cope with movement from one environment to another

Risk Identification: Analysis of potential risk factors, determination of health risks, and prioritization of risk-reduction strategies for an individual or group

Security Enhancement: Intensifying a patient's sense of physical and psychological safety

Socialization Enhancement: Facilitation of another person's ability to interact with others

Spiritual Growth Facilitation: Facilitation of growth in patients' capacity to identify, connect with, and call upon the source of meaning, purpose, comfort, strength, and hope in their lives

Support System Enhancement: Facilitation of support to patient by family, friends, and community

Surveillance: Purposeful and ongoing acquisition, interpretation, and synthesis of patient data for clinical decision making

Nursing Activities

Assessments

- Assess for obstacles to religious practices (e.g., limitations imposed by disease process, lack of transportation)
- Determine whether the client wishes to participate in religious rituals and services
- Use established tools to assess spiritual well-being

Patient/Family Teaching

- Inform patient/family of the religious resources available in the institution
- Inform client of religious books and articles available in Braille, in large print, or on tape

Collaborative Activities

- Refer to chaplain, pastor, or other spiritual adviser
- Obtain a medical order to allow fasting, if patient wishes to do so

Other

- Encourage the patient to express feelings such as anger or sadness
- Encourage the patient to talk or cry to relieve tensions
- Share own spiritual perspectives and beliefs, as appropriate
- Pray with the patient, if requested to do so
- Use therapeutic communication to build trust
- Demonstrate empathy and acceptance
- Facilitate patient's use of religious rituals (e.g., provide physical support, allow to wear religious medals)
- Provide privacy and quiet for prayer and other religious practices

- Be accepting and nonjudgmental about the client's religious practices
- Turn on religious programs on radio or television if the client desires

Home Care

- Most of the preceding interventions can be adapted for home care use
- Identify organizations within the community that will provide transportation to religious services, as needed

For Infants and Children

- Base interventions on developmental level
- Adhere to the parents' religious practices (e.g., have the child pray before meals and at bedtime if they do so at home)
- Assess whether the child believes his illness to be punishment for doing wrong

RELIGIOSITY, READINESS FOR ENHANCED

(2004)

Domain 10, Life Principles;
Class 3, Value/Belief/Action Congruence

R

Definition: A pattern of reliance on religious beliefs and/or participation in rituals of a particular faith tradition that is sufficient for well-being and can be strengthened

Defining Characteristics

Expresses desire to strengthen religious belief patterns that have provided comfort in the past

Expresses desire to strengthen religious belief patterns that have provided comfort in the past

Expresses desire to strengthen religious customs that have provided comfort in the past

Questions belief patterns that are harmful

Questions customs that are harmful

Rejects belief patterns that are harmful

Rejects customs that are harmful

Requests for assistance in expanding religious options

Requests for assistance to increase participation in prescribed religious beliefs (e.g., religious ceremonies, dietary regulations, dietary rituals, clothing, prayer, worship, religious services, private religious behaviors, reading religious materials, religious media, holiday observances)

Requests forgiveness
Requests meeting with religious leaders or facilitators
Requests reconciliation
Requests religious experiences
Requests religious materials

Suggestions for Use

This wellness diagnosis needs no etiology.

Suggested Alternative Diagnoses

Religiosity, risk for impaired
Spiritual well-being, readiness for enhanced

NOC Outcomes

Hope: Optimism that is personally satisfying and life supporting

Spiritual Health: Connectedness with self, others, higher power, all life, nature, and the universe that transcends and empowers the self

Goals/Evaluation Criteria

See Goals/Evaluation Criteria for the diagnosis, Impaired Religiosity.

Other Examples

Patient will express satisfaction with:

- Ability to perform activities of daily living (ADLs)
- Role performance
- Level of happiness
- Physical health
- Mental health

NIC Interventions

Hope Inspiration: Facilitation of the development of a positive outlook in a given situation

Religious Ritual Enhancement: Facilitating participation in religious practices

Spiritual Growth Facilitation: Facilitation of growth in patient's capacity to identify, connect with, and call upon the source of meaning, purpose, comfort, strength, and hope in her or his life

Spiritual Support: Assisting the patient to feel balance and connection with a greater power

Nursing Activities

See Nursing Activities for the diagnosis, Impaired Religiosity.

RELOCATION STRESS SYNDROME

(1992, 2000) **Domain 9, Coping/Stress Tolerance; Class 1, Post-Trauma Responses**

Definition: Physiological or psychosocial disturbance following transfer from one environment to another

Defining Characteristics

Subjective

Alienation
Aloneness
Anger
Anxiety (e.g., separation)
Depression
Fear
Frustration
Loneliness
Loss of identity or self-worth
Low self-esteem, chronic or situational
Sleep disturbance
Worry

Objective

R

Dependency
Increased physical symptoms or illness (e.g., GI disturbance, weight change)
Increased verbalization of needs
Insecurity
Pessimism
Unwillingness to move, or concern over relocation
Withdrawal

Related Factors

Decreased health status
Feelings of powerlessness
Impaired psychosocial health
Isolation [from family and friends]
Lack of adequate support system
Lack of predeparture counseling
Language barrier
Losses

Move from one environment to another
Passive coping
Past, concurrent, and recent losses (non-NANDA International)
Unpredictability of experience

Suggestions for Use

Because this is a syndrome diagnosis, no etiology is needed in the diagnostic statement. A syndrome nursing diagnosis represents a group of other nursing diagnoses that are present together. If only one or two of the defining characteristics are present (e.g., anxiety, loneliness), write separate nursing diagnoses for those responses (e.g., *Anxiety*) instead of using *Relocation stress syndrome*.

Suggested Alternative Diagnoses

Anxiety
Confusion, acute
Grieving, complicated
Hopelessness
Insomnia
Loneliness, risk for
Powerlessness
Sorrow, chronic
Spiritual distress

NOC Outcomes

Anxiety Level: Severity of manifested apprehension, tension, or uneasiness arising from an unidentifiable source
Child Adaptation to Hospitalization: Adaptive response of a child from 3 years through 17 years of age to hospitalization
Coping: Personal actions to manage stressors that tax an individual's resources
Depression Level: Severity of melancholic mood and loss of interest in life events
Loneliness Severity: Severity of emotional, social, or existential isolation response
Psychosocial Adjustment: Life Change: Adaptive psychosocial response of an individual to a significant life change
Quality of Life: Extent of positive perception of current life circumstances
Stress Level: Severity of manifested physical or mental tension resulting from factors that alter an existing equilibrium

Goals/Evaluation Criteria

Examples Using NOC Language

- Demonstrates **Coping**, as evidenced by the following indicators (specify 1–5: never, rarely, sometimes, often, or consistently demonstrated):
  - Verbalizes acceptance of situation
  - Reports decrease in negative feelings
  - Reports decrease in physical symptoms of stress
  - Modifies lifestyle to reduce stress
- Demonstrates **Psychosocial Adjustment: Life Change**, as evidenced by the following indicators (specify 1–5: never, rarely, sometimes, often, consistently demonstrated):
  - Maintains self-esteem
  - Reports feeling useful
  - Uses available social support

Other Examples

Patient will:

- Demonstrate ability to adjust to new environment
- Verbalize satisfaction with new living arrangements
- Express optimism about the present and the future
- Express satisfaction with life achievements
- Participate in diversions (e.g., hobbies)

Child will:

- Adapt to hospitalization (e.g., will not demonstrate agitation, regressive behaviors, anxiety, fear, or anger)
- Respond to play therapy and comfort measures
- Show resolution of separation anxiety

NIC Interventions

Anxiety Reduction: Minimizing apprehension, dread, foreboding, or uneasiness related to an unidentified source of anticipated danger

Coping Enhancement: Assisting a patient to adapt to perceived stressors, changes, or threats that interfere with meeting life demands and roles

Family Involvement Promotion: Facilitating family participation in the emotional and physical care of the patient

Hope Inspiration: Facilitation of the development of a positive outlook in a given situation

Mood Management: Providing for safety, stabilization, recovery, and maintenance of a patient who is experiencing dysfunctionally depressed or elevated mood

Relocation Stress Reduction: Assisting the individual to prepare for and cope with movement from one environment to another

Security Enhancement: Intensifying a patient's sense of physical and psychological safety

Socialization Enhancement: Facilitation of another person's ability to interact with others

Spiritual Support: Assisting the patient to feel balance and connection with a greater power

Trauma Therapy: Child: Use of an interactive helping process to resolve a trauma experienced by a child

Values Clarification: Assisting another to clarify his own values in order to facilitate effective decision making

Nursing Activities

Assessments

- Assess patient's orientation, mood (e.g., depressed, angry, anxious), and physiologic status on admission and q _______________
- Identify patient's previous schedules and routines
- Assess readiness for discharge
- *(NIC) Coping Enhancement*: Appraise patient's needs or desires for social support

Collaborative Activities

- Maintain consistency in caregivers and care routines as much as possible, consider a case manager
- Utilize other resources to assist in transition to new environment
- Coordinate referrals among health care providers and agencies to effect a smooth transfer or relocation

R

Other

- Orient patient to new environment as often as needed
- Establish new environment as close to previous environment as possible to maintain consistency in placement of personal belongings, furniture, pictures, and so forth
- To ease the transfer, encourage family to stay with patient, bring familiar objects from home, and provide familiar socialization
- Avoid unplanned or abrupt transfers; also avoid transfers at night or at change of shift
- *(NIC) Coping Enhancement:*
  - Assist the patient in developing an objective appraisal of the event
  - Use a calm, reassuring approach
  - Seek to understand the patient's perspective of a stressful situation
  - Discourage decision making when the patient is under severe stress
  - Foster constructive outlets for anger and hostility
  - Arrange situations that encourage patient's autonomy

Introduce patient to persons (or groups) who have successfully undergone the same experience

Encourage verbalization of feelings, perceptions, and fears [about the relocation]

- *(NIC) Security Enhancement:*

  Offer to remain with patient in a new environment during initial interactions with others

  Present change gradually
- Provide information about whether the move will be temporary or permanent
- Assist patient and family to recall and appreciate past achievements and experiences
- Provide an environment in which the patient can practice his religion
- Involve the patient actively in own care to the extent possible

Home Care

- Most of the preceding nursing activities can be adapted for home care

For Infants and Children

- Try to avoid relocation during the school year. If it is necessary to do so, assist the child or adolescent in transition to the new environment (e.g., by assigning a "big sister" or by providing counseling)
- Support parents who must relocate for a child's treatment
- Consider the child's developmental level when assessing responses to relocation
- Expect changes in sleeping and eating habits of toddlers and preschoolers
- Hold a young child, as needed
- Encourage parents to stay overnight in the hospital with a child
- Have parents bring the hospitalized child's favorite toys

For Older Adults

- Arrange for supports so that older adults can remain in their home as long as possible
- Help the family to accept that, up to a point, less than ideal conditions in the home may be preferable to institutionalization of the older family member
- Attend to the safety of the home environment to facilitate keeping the client in the home as long as possible

- Arrange for home care aides, Meals on Wheels, and similar services to assist with Instrumental Activities of Daily Living (IADLs), to allow the client to remain at home
- Offer as many choices as possible regarding the relocation (e.g., timing, mode of transportation, choice of facility)
- Assess for depression and hopelessness, as well as anger and feelings of powerlessness, especially when relocating to a nursing home
- Assess the risk for suicide
- When a client is admitted to a long-term care facility, assess the spouse's ability to cope, as well as the client's; put support systems in place for the spouse
- Plan with clients well in advance of their admission to a long-term care facility

RELOCATION STRESS SYNDROME, RISK FOR

(2000) **Domain 9, Coping/Stress Tolerance; Class1, Post-Trauma Responses**

Definition: At risk for physiological or psychosocial disturbance following transfer from one environment to another

Risk Factors

Subjective

Feelings of powerlessness

Objective

Decreased [psychosocial or physical] health status
Lack of adequate support system
Lack of predeparture counseling
Losses
Moderate mental competence (e.g., alert enough to experience changes)
Moderate-to-high degree of environmental change
Move from one environment to another
Passive coping
Unpredictability of experiences

Suggested Alternative Diagnoses

Loneliness, risk for
Powerlessness, risk for
Relocation stress syndrome

NOC Outcomes

Discharge Readiness: Supported Living: Readiness of a patient to relocate from a health care institution to a lower level of supported living

Personal Health Status: Overall physical, psychological, social, and spiritual functioning of an adult 18 years or older

Psychosocial Adjustment: Life Change: Adaptive psychosocial response of an individual to a significant life change

Goals/Evaluation Criteria

See Goals/Evaluation Criteria for Relocation Stress Syndrome, preceding.

NIC Interventions

Anticipatory Guidance: Preparation of patient for an anticipated developmental and/or situational crisis

Coping Enhancement: Assisting a patient to adapt to perceived stressors, changes, or threats that interfere with meeting life demands and roles

Discharge Planning: Preparation for moving a patient from one level of care to another within or outside the current health care agency

Relocation Stress Reduction: Assisting the individual to prepare for and cope with movement from one environment to another

Transport: Interfacility: Moving a patient from one facility to another

Nursing Activities

See Nursing Activities for the preceding diagnosis, Relocation Stress Syndrome.

RENAL PERFUSION: RISK FOR INEFFECTIVE

(2008) **Domain 4, Activity/Rest; Class 4, Cardiovascular/Pulmonary Responses**

Definition: At risk for a decrease in blood circulation to the kidney that may compromise health

Risk Factors

Abdominal compartment syndrome
Advanced age
Bilateral cortical necrosis
Burns
Cardiac surgery

Cardiopulmonary bypass
Diabetes mellitus
Exposure to nephrotoxins
Female gender
Glomerulonephritis
Hypertension
Hypovolemis
Hypoxemia
Hypoxia
Infection (e.g., sepsis, localized infection)
Interstitial nephritis
Malignancy
Malignant hypertension
Metabolic acidosis
Multitrauma
Polynephritis
Renal artery stenosis
Renal disease (polycystic kidney)
Smoking
Substance abuse
Systemic inflammatory response syndrome
Treatment-related side effects (e.g., pharmaceutical agents, surgery)
Vascular embolism
Vasculitis

Suggestions for Use

If actual ineffective renal tissue perfusion occurs, it is a medical problem. Instead of this potential (risk for) diagnosis, you may prefer to use a collaborative problem based on the existing risk factor, such as Potential Complication of substance abuse: Ineffective renal tissue perfusion; or Potential Complication of sepsis: Ineffective renal tissue perfusion.

Suggested Alternative Diagnoses

Fluid volume excess
Fluid volume imbalance, risk for
Ineffective Peripheral Tissue Perfusion

NOC Outcomes

NOTE: To assess for actual ineffective renal perfusion, use the following two outcomes:

Kidney Function: Filtration of blood and elimination of metabolic waste products through the formation of urine

Tissue Perfusion: Abdominal Organs: Adequacy of blood flow through the small vessels of the abdominal viscera to maintain organ function

NOTE: The following outcomes are associated with risk factors for ineffective renal perfusion:

Blood Loss Severity: Severity of internal or external bleeding/hemorrhage

Cardiopulmonary Status: Adequacy of blood volume ejected from the ventricles and exchange of carbon dioxide and oxygen at the alveolar level

Circulation Status: Unobstructed, unidirectional blood flow at an appropriate pressure through large vessels of the systemic and pulmonary circuits

Electrolyte and Acid/Base Balance: Balance of electrolytes and nonelectrolytes in the intracellular and extracellular compartments of the body

Fluid Balance: Water balance in the intracellular and extracellular compartments of the body

Knowledge: Diabetes Management: Extent of understanding conveyed about diabetes mellitus, its treatment, and the prevention of complications

Knowledge: Hypertension Management: Extent of understanding conveyed about high blood pressure, its treatment, and the prevention of complications

Vital Signs: Extent to which temperature, pulse, respiration, and blood pressure are within normal range

Goals/Evaluation Criteria

Examples Using NOC Language

- Patient will demonstrate adequate kidney perfusion, as evidenced by Kidney Function and Tissue Perfusion: Abdominal Organs.
- Demonstrates **Electrolyte and Acid–Base Balance**, as evidenced by the following indicators (specify 1–5: severely, substantially, moderately, mildly, or not compromised):
  - Mental alertness, cognitive orientation, and muscle strength
  - Lab tests (e.g., serum Na^+, K^+, Cl^-, Ca^{2+}, Mg^{2+}, bicarbonate, BUN, creatinine)
- **Kidney Function** will be demonstrated, as evidenced by the following indicators (specify 1–5: severely, substantially, moderately, mildly, or not compromised):
  - 24-hr intake and output balance
  - Blood urea nitrogen
  - Serum creatinine

Urine specific gravity
Urine color
Urine pH

Other Examples

- Laboratory tests within normal limits (e.g., urine specific gravity, glucose, ketone, pH, and protein levels and microscopic results)
- Arterial PCO within normal limits
- No hematuria
- Blood pressure within normal limits
- No weight gain
- No nausea, fatigue, or malaise

NIC Interventions

Nursing interventions focus on identifying early onset of and preventing ineffective renal perfusion by treating risk factors.

Bleeding Reduction: Limitation of the loss of blood volume during an episode of bleeding

Bleeding Reduction: Gastrointestinal: Limitation of the amount of blood loss from the upper and lower gastrointestinal tract and related complications

Blood Products Administration: Administration of blood or blood products and monitoring of patient's response

Circulatory Care: Arterial Insufficiency: Promotion of arterial circulation

Embolus Care: Peripheral: Limitation of complications for a patient experiencing, or at risk for, occlusion of peripheral circulation

Fluid Management: Promotion of fluid balance and prevention of complications resulting from abnormal or undesired fluid levels

Hemodynamic Regulation: Optimization of heart rate, preload, afterload, and contractility

Hypovolemia Management: Expansion of intravascular fluid volume in a patient who is volume depleted

Medication Management: Facilitation of safe and effective use of prescription and over-the-counter drugs

Teaching: Disease Process: Assisting the patient to understand information related to a specific disease process

Thrombolytic Therapy Management: Collection and analysis of patient data to expedite safe, appropriate provision of an agent that dissolves a thrombus

Vital Signs Monitoring: Collection and analysis of cardiovascular, respiratory, and body temperature data to determine and prevent complications

Nursing Activities

Assessments

- *(NIC) Fluid Management:*
  Monitor hydration status (e.g., moist mucous membranes, adequacy of pulses, and orthostatic blood pressure), as appropriate
  Monitor lab results relevant to fluid retention (e.g., increased specific gravity, increased BUN, decreased hematocrit, and increased urine osmolality levels)
  Monitor for indications of fluid overload or retention (e.g., crackles, elevated CVP or pulmonary capillary wedge pressure, edema, neck vein distention, and ascites), as appropriate
  Maintain accurate intake and output record
  Insert urinary catheter, if appropriate
  Monitor vital signs, as appropriate
  Monitor patient's response to prescribed electrolyte therapy
  Weigh patient daily and monitor trends
- **For hemodialysis patients:**
  Monitor serum electrolyte levels
  Monitor blood pressure
  Weigh patient before and after procedure
  Monitor BUN, serum creatinine, serum electrolytes, and hematocrit levels between dialysis treatments
  Assess for signs of dialysis disequilibrium syndrome (e.g., headache, nausea and vomiting, hypertension, and altered level of consciousness)
  Observe for dehydration, muscle cramps, or seizure activity
  Assess for bleeding at the dialysis access site or elsewhere
  Observe for transfusion reaction, if appropriate
  Assess patency of arteriovenous fistula (e.g., palpate for pulse, auscultate for bruit)
  Assess mental status (e.g., consciousness, orientation)
  Monitor clotting times
- **For peritoneal dialysis patients**:
  Assess temperature, orthostatic BP, apical pulse, respirations, and lung sounds before dialysis
  Weigh patient daily
  Measure and record abdominal girth
  Note BUN, serum electrolyte, creatinine, pH, and hematocrit levels prior to dialysis and periodically during the procedure
  During instillation and dwell periods, observe for respiratory distress

Record amount and type of dialysate instilled, dwell time, and amount and appearance of the drainage

Monitor for signs of infection at exit site and in peritoneum

Patient/Family Teaching

- Explain all procedures and expected sensations to patient
- Explain the need for fluid restrictions, as needed
- For dialysis patients:

  Teach patient signs and symptoms that indicate the need to contact a physician (e.g., fever, bleeding)

  Teach procedure to patients having home dialysis

Collaborative Activities

- Administer diuretics, as ordered
- Notify physician if signs and symptoms of fluid volume excess worsen
- (For hemodialysis patients) administer heparin according to protocol and adjust dosage

Other

- Distribute prescribed fluid intake appropriately over 24-hr period
- Maintain fluid and diet restrictions (e.g., low sodium, no salt), as ordered
- (For hemodialysis patients) do not perform venipunctures or take blood pressures on the arm with a fistula
- For peritoneal dialysis patients:

  Use strict aseptic technique at all times

  Warm dialysate to body temperature before dialysis

  Place in semi-Fowler position and slow instillation rate if respiratory distress occurs

RESILIENCE, IMPAIRED INDIVIDUAL

(2008) **Domain 9, Coping/Stress Tolerance; Class 2, Coping Responses**

Definition: Decreased ability to sustain a pattern of positive responses to an adverse situation or crisis

Defining Characteristics

Subjective

Decreased interest in academic or vocational activities

Depression

Guilt

Low self-esteem
Lower perceived health status
Renewed elevation of distress
Shame

Objective

Isolation
Social isolation
Using maladaptive coping skills (i.e., drug use, violence, etc.)

Related Factors

Demographics that increase chance of maladjustment
Gender
Inconsistent parenting
Large family size
Low intelligence
Low maternal education
Minority status
Neighborhood violence
Parental mental illness
Poor impulse control
Poverty
Psychological disorders
Substance abuse
Violence
Vulnerability factors that encompass indices that exacerbate the negative effects of the risk condition

Suggestions for Use

A diagnosis should be stated in terms of human responses to disease, injury, or other stressors. However, resilience is a characteristic of a person, rather than a human response. Also, a patient might have more than one of the defining characteristics, but still be resilient. If that is the case, consider using a diagnostic label that describes that condition—for example, *Ineffective coping*, or *Compromised family coping*.

Suggested Alternative Diagnoses

Coping: family, compromised or disabled
Coping, ineffective
Parenting, impaired
Social isolation
Self-esteem: low, chronic or situational

NOC Outcomes

NOTE: The author does not recommend using this diagnosis. However, because NOC outcomes have been linked to it, those are included here.

Coping: Personal actions to manage stressors that tax an individual's resources

Depression Level: Severity of melancholic mood and loss of interest in life events

Personal Resiliency: Positive adaptation and function of an individual following significant adversity or crisis

Goals/Evaluation Criteria

Examples Using NOC Language

- Patient will demonstrate resilience, as evidenced by Coping, Depression Level, and Personal Resiliency.
- **Personal Resilience** will be demonstrated, as evidenced by the following indicators (specify 1–5: never, rarely, sometimes, often, or consistently demonstrated):
  - Verbalizes positive outlook
  - Verbalizes an enhanced sense of control
  - Adapts to adversities and challenges
  - Avoids drug (or alcohol) misuse
  - Participates in employment
  - Participates in curricular (and extracurricular) school activities
  - Expresses self-efficacy

R

Other Examples

- Seeks and uses available resources to support adaptation and resilience

NIC Interventions

NOTE: Although the author does not recommend using this diagnosis, NIC interventions have been linked to it; so examples are included here.

Coping Enhancement: Assisting a patient to adapt to perceived stressors, changes, or threats that interfere with meeting life demands and roles

Crisis Intervention: Use of short-term counseling to help the patient cope with a crisis and resume a state of functioning comparable to or better than the precrisis state

Decision-Making Support: Providing information and support for a patient who is making a decision regarding health care

Mood Management: Providing for safety, stabilization, recovery, and maintenance of a patient who is experiencing dysfunctionally depressed or elevated mood

Resiliency Promotion: Assisting individuals, families, and communities in development, use, and strengthening of protective factors to be used in coping with environmental and societal stressors

Role Enhancement: Assisting a patient, significant other, or family to improve relationships by clarifying and supplementing specific role behaviors

Nursing Activities

Assessments

- Identify underlying stressors and related factors (e.g., chronic illnesses, unemployment)

  Assess family dynamics and communication patterns

  Determine patient's education level

  Assess coping behavior patterns

  Assess family resources (e.g., financial, support groups)

  Identify cultural and spiritual beliefs and practices

Patient/Family Teaching

- Provide information, as needed (e.g., nutrition, substance use)

Collaborative Activities

- Refer to support groups, as needed (e.g., for substance-abuse or domestic violence programs)

R

Other

- Encourage the client to express feelings, pointing out the difference between feelings and behavior
- Acknowledge the difficulty of making changes in the situation
- Facilitate communication among the client and family members
- Focus on and reinforce client strengths
- Reinforce self-responsibility for choices and actions

RESILIENCE, READINESS FOR ENHANCED

(2008) **Domain 9, Coping/Stress Tolerance; Class 2, Coping Responses**

Definition: A pattern of positive responses to an adverse situation or crisis that is sufficient for optimizing human potential and can be strengthened

Defining Characteristics

Subjective

Expressed desire to enhance resilience
Identifies available resources
Identifies support systems
Reports enhanced sense of control
Reports self-esteem

Objective

Access to resources
Demonstrates a positive outlook
Effective use of conflict management strategies
Enhances personal coping skills
Increases positive relationships with others
Involvement in activities
Makes progress toward goals
Presence of a crisis
Safe environment is maintained
Sets goals
Takes responsibilities for actions
Use of effective communication skills

Suggestions for Use

Because this is a wellness diagnosis, no Related Factors are needed.

Suggested Alternative Diagnoses

Coping, readiness for enhanced
Resilience, risk for compromised

NOC Outcomes

Coping: Personal actions to manage stressors that tax an individual's resources

Personal Resiliency: Positive adaptation and function of an individual following significant adversity or crisis

Goals/Evaluation Criteria

Examples Using NOC Language

- Patient will demonstrate resilience, as evidenced by Coping and Personal Resiliency.
- **Personal Resilience** will be demonstrated, as evidenced by the following indicators (specify 1–5: never, rarely, sometimes, often, or consistently demonstrated):

Verbalizes positive outlook
Verbalizes an enhanced sense of control
Adapts to adversities and challenges
Avoids drug (or alcohol) misuse
Participates in employment
Participates in curricular (and extracurricular) school activities
Expresses self-efficacy

Other Examples

- Seeks and uses available resources to support adaptation and resilience

NIC Interventions

Coping Enhancement: Assisting a patient to adapt to perceived stressors, changes, or threats that interfere with meeting life demands and roles

Resiliency Promotion: Assisting individuals, families, and communities in development, use, and strengthening of protective factors to be used in coping with environmental and societal stressors

Nursing Activities

Assessments

- Identify underlying stressors and related factors (e.g., chronic illnesses, unemployment)
- Assess family dynamics and communication patterns
- Determine patient's education level
- Assess coping behavior patterns
- Assess family resources (e.g., financial, support groups)
- Identify cultural and spiritual beliefs and practices

Patient/Family Teaching

- Provide information, as needed (e.g., nutrition, substance use)

Other

- Encourage the client to express feelings, pointing out the difference between feelings and behavior
- Acknowledge the difficulty of making changes
- Facilitate communication among the client and family members
- Focus on and reinforce client strengths
- Reinforce self-responsibility for choices and actions

RESILIENCE, RISK FOR COMPROMISED

(2008) **Domain 9, Coping/Stress Tolerance; Class 2, Coping Responses**

Definition: At risk for decreased ability to sustain a pattern of positive responses to an adverse situation or crisis

Risk Factors

Chronicity of existing crises
Multiple coexisting adverse situations
Presence of an additional new crisis (e.g., unplanned pregnancy, death of a spouse, loss of job, illness, loss of housing, death of family member)

Suggestions for Use

See the diagnosis *Resilience, Impaired Individual.*

Suggested Alternative Diagnoses

Parenting, impaired
Social isolation
Self-esteem: low, chronic, or situational

NOC Outcomes

Personal Resiliency: Positive adaptation and function of an individual following significant adversity or crisis

Goals/Evaluation Criteria

Examples Using NOC Language

- Resilience will not be compromised, as evidenced by Personal Resiliency.
- **Personal Resiliency** will be demonstrated, as evidenced by the following indicators (specify 1–5: never, rarely, sometimes, often, or consistently demonstrated):
  - Verbalizes positive outlook
  - Verbalizes an enhanced sense of control
  - Adapts to adversities and challenges
  - Avoids drug (or alcohol) misuse
  - Participates in employment
  - Participates in curricular (and extracurricular) school activities
  - Expresses self-efficacy

Goals/Evaluation Criteria

Examples Using NOC Language

- Resilience will not be compromised, as evidenced by Personal Resiliency.
- **Personal Resiliency** will be demonstrated, as evidenced by the following indicators (specify 1–5: never, rarely, sometimes, often, or consistently demonstrated):
  - Verbalizes positive outlook
  - Verbalizes an enhanced sense of control
  - Adapts to adversities and challenges
  - Avoids drug (or alcohol) misuse
  - Participates in employment
  - Participates in curricular (and extracurricular) school activities
  - Expresses self-efficacy

Other Examples

- Seeks and uses available resources to support adaptation and resilience

NIC Interventions

Anticipatory Guidance: Preparation of patient for an anticipated developmental and/or situational crisis

Behavior Modification: Promotion of a behavior change

Case Management: Coordinating care and advocating for specified individuals and patient populations across settings to reduce cost, reduce resource use, improve quality of health care, and achieve desired outcomes

Crisis Intervention: Use of short-term counseling to help the patient cope with a crisis and resume a state of functioning comparable to or better than the precrisis state

Culture Brokerage: The deliberate use of culturally competent strategies to bridge or mediate between the patient's culture and the biomedical health care system

Health System Guidance: Facilitating a patient's location and use of appropriate health services

Hope Inspiration: Facilitation of the development of a positive outlook in a given situation

Multidisciplinary Care Conference: Planning and evaluating patient care with health professionals from other disciplines

Risk Identification: Analysis of potential risk factors, determination of health risks, and prioritization of risk-reduction strategies for an individual or group

Self-Efficacy Enhancement: Strengthening an individual's confidence in his ability to perform a health behavior

Sustenance Support: Helping an individual/family in need to locate food, clothing, or shelter

Nursing Activities

Assessments

- Identify underlying stressors and related factors (e.g., chronic illnesses, unemployment)
- Assess family dynamics and communication patterns
- Determine patient's education level
- Assess coping behavior patterns
- Assess family resources (e.g., financial, support groups)
- Identify cultural and spiritual beliefs and practices

Patient/Family Teaching

- Provide information, as needed (e.g., nutrition, substance use)

Collaborative Activities

- Refer to support groups, as needed (e.g., for substance-abuse or domestic violence programs)

Other

- Encourage the client to express feelings, pointing out the difference between feelings and behavior
- Acknowledge the difficulty of making changes in the situation
- Facilitate communication among the client and family members
- Focus on and reinforce client strengths
- Reinforce self-responsibility for choices and actions

R

ROLE CONFLICT, PARENTAL

(1988) **Domain 7, Role Relationships; Class 3, Role Performance**

Definition: Parental experience of role confusion and conflict in response to crisis

Defining Characteristics

Subjective

Anxiety

Expresses concern about perceived loss of control over decisions relating to the child

Fear
Express(es) concern(s) about changes in parental role
Express(es) concern(s) about family (e.g., functioning, communication, health)
Express(es) feeling(s) of inadequacy to provide for child's needs (e.g., physical, emotional)
Verbalizes feelings of frustration
Verbalizes feelings of guilt

Objective

Demonstrates disruption in caretaking routines
Reluctant to participate in usual caretaking activities

Related Factors

Change in marital status [e.g., career, roles]
[Financial crisis]
Home care of a child with special needs [e.g., apnea monitoring, postural drainage, hyperalimentation]
Interruptions in family life due to home care regimen [e.g., treatments, caregivers, lack of respite]
Intimidation by invasive or restrictive modalities [e.g., isolation, intubation]
Separation from child due to chronic illness
Specialized care centers [policies]

Suggestions for Use

Use this label when a situation causes unsatisfactory role performance by previously effective caregivers (parents).

Suggested Alternative Diagnoses

Caregiver role strain (actual or risk for)
Coping: family, compromised
Family processes, interrupted
Parenting, impaired
Parenting, impaired, risk for

NOC Outcomes

Caregiver Home Care Readiness: Extent of preparedness of a caregiver to assume responsibility for the health care of a family member in the home

Caregiver Lifestyle Disruption: Severity of disturbances in the lifestyle of a family member due to caregiving

Knowledge: Parenting: Extent of understanding conveyed about provision of a nurturing and constructive environment for a child from 1 year through 17 years of age

Parenting Performance: Parental actions to provide a child a nurturing and constructive physical, emotional, and social environment

Role Performance: Congruence of an individual's role behavior with role expectations

Goals/Evaluation Criteria

Examples Using NOC Language

- *Parental role conflict* will be resolved or alleviated, as evidenced by Caregiver Home Care Readiness, Caregiver Lifestyle Disruption, Knowledge: Parenting, Parenting Performance, and Role Performance.
- **Parenting Performance** will be demonstrated, as evidenced by the following indicators (specify 1–5: never, rarely, sometimes, often, or consistently demonstrated):

  Provides for child's physical needs
  Provides for child's special needs
  Stimulates cognitive and social development
  Stimulates emotional and spiritual growth
  Exhibits a loving relationship
- **Role Performance** will be demonstrated, as evidenced by the following indicators (specify 1–5: not, slightly, moderately, substantially, or totally adequate): Performance of family and work role behaviors

Other Examples

The parent or caregiver will:

- Identify and use social supports available in the community
- Use effective coping strategies
- Demonstrate ability to modify parenting role in response to crisis
- Express a sense of adequacy in providing for child's needs
- Be available to support child and give consent for treatments
- Develop trust in health care providers
- Request information about the patient's illness and treatment
- Express willingness to assume caregiving role
- Demonstrate knowledge of the child's illness, treatment regimen, and emergency care

NIC Interventions

Anticipatory Guidance: Preparation of patient for an anticipated developmental and/or situational crisis

Caregiver Support: Provision of the necessary information, advocacy, and support to facilitate primary patient care by someone other than a health care professional

Coping Enhancement: Assisting a patient to adapt to perceived stressors, changes, or threats that interfere with meeting life demands and roles

Counseling: Use of an interactive helping process focusing on the needs, problems, or feelings of the patient and significant others to enhance or support coping, problem solving, and interpersonal relationships

Crisis Intervention: Use of short-term counseling to help the patient cope with a crisis and resume a state of functioning comparable to or better than the precrisis state

Decision-Making Support: Providing information and support for a patient who is making a decision regarding health care

Developmental Enhancement: Adolescent: Facilitating optimal physical, cognitive, social, and emotional growth of individuals during the transition from childhood to adulthood

Developmental Enhancement: Child: Facilitating or teaching parents and caregivers to facilitate the optimal gross motor, fine motor, language, cognitive, social, and emotional growth of preschool and school-aged children

Discharge Planning: Preparation for moving a patient from one level of care to another within or outside the current health care agency

Family Involvement Promotion: Facilitating family participation in the emotional and physical care of the patient

R

Family Process Maintenance: Minimization of family process disruption effects

Parent Education: Adolescent: Assisting parents to understand and help their adolescent children

Parent Education: Childrearing Family: Assisting parents to understand and promote the physical, psychological, and social growth and development of their toddler, preschool, or school-aged child or children

Parenting Promotion: Providing parenting information, support, and coordination of comprehensive services to high-risk families

Role Enhancement: Assisting a patient, significant other, or family to improve relationships by clarifying and supplementing specific role behaviors

Nursing Activities

Assessments

- Ask parents to describe how they want to be involved in the care of their hospitalized child

- *(NIC) Family Process Maintenance:*
  Determine typical family processes
  Identify effects of role changes on family processes

Patient/Family Teaching

- Teach new role behaviors created by the crisis situation
- Explain rationale for treatments and encourage questions to minimize misunderstandings and maximize participation
- *(NIC) Family Process Maintenance*: Teach family time management and organization skills when performing patient home care, as needed

Collaborative Activities

- *(NIC) Family Process Maintenance*: Assist family members to use existing support mechanisms

Other

- Confront parents with their ineffective parenting behaviors (during this crisis) and discuss alternatives
- Encourage parents to express feelings about the child's illness
- Involve parents in care to the extent possible, and to the extent they desire
- Make parents comfortable in the hospital setting (e.g., provide sleeping accommodations at the child's bedside)
- Help parents to identify personal strengths and coping skills that may be useful in resolving the crisis
- Discuss with parent(s) a strategy for meeting personal and family current needs
- Give positive reinforcement for constructive parental actions
- *(NIC) Family Process Maintenance:*
  Keep opportunities for visiting flexible to meet needs of family members and patient
  Provide mechanisms for family members staying at health care agency to communicate with other family members (e.g., telephones, tape recordings, open visiting, photographs, e-mail messages, and videotapes)
  Assist family members to facilitate home visits by patient, when appropriate

Home Care

- The preceding nursing activities are appropriate or can be adapted for use in home care

ROLE PERFORMANCE, INEFFECTIVE

(1978, 1996, 1998) **Domain 7, Role Relationships; Class 3, Role Performance**

Definition: Patterns of behavior and self-expression that do not match the environmental context, norms, and expectations

Defining Characteristics

Subjective

Altered role perceptions
Anxiety or depression
Change in self-perception of role
Inadequate confidence
Inadequate motivation
Powerlessness
Role ambivalence, conflict, confusion, denial, dissatisfaction, overload, or strain
Uncertainty

Objective

Change in capacity to resume role
Change in other's perception of role
Change in usual patterns of responsibility
R Deficient knowledge
Discrimination
Domestic violence
Harassment
Inadequate adaptation to change [or transition]
Inadequate external support for role enactment
Inadequate opportunities for role enactment
Inadequate role competency and skills
Inadequate self-management
Inappropriate developmental expectations
Ineffective coping
Ineffective role performances
Pessimism
System conflict

Related Factors

Knowledge

Inadequate role preparation (e.g., role transition, skill, rehearsal, validation)
Lack of education

Lack of or inadequate role model
Unrealistic role expectations

Non-NANDA International

Developmental transitions
Lack of knowledge about role
Role transition

Physiological

Body image alteration
Cognitive deficits
Depression
Fatigue
Low self-esteem
Mental illness
Neurological defects
Pain
Physical illness
Substance abuse

Social

Conflict
Developmental level, young age
Domestic violence
[Family conflict]
[Inadequate or] inappropriate linkage with health care system
Inadequate role socialization [e.g., role model, expectations, responsibilities]
Inadequate support system
Job schedule demands
Lack of resources
Lack of rewards
Low socioeconomic status
Stress
Young age

Suggestions for Use

When applicable, use more specific labels such as *Parental role conflict*, *Sexual dysfunction*, and *Interrupted family processes*. Some degree of role conflict and disruption is present for everyone. If the patient is having difficulty with role performance, consider using *Ineffective role performance* as the etiology of another diagnosis that describes the impact on functioning (e.g., *Impaired home maintenance related to Ineffective role performance*).

Suggested Alternative Diagnoses

Caregiver role strain, actual and risk for
Family processes, interrupted
Home maintenance, impaired
Role conflict, parental
Self-esteem, situational low

NOC Outcomes

Caregiver Performance: Direct Care: Provision by family care provider of appropriate personal and health care for a family member

Caregiver Performance: Indirect Care: Arrangement and oversight by family care provider of appropriate care for a family member

Coping: Personal actions to manage stressors that tax an individual's resources

Depression Level: Severity of melancholic mood and loss of interest in life events

Parenting Performance: Parental actions to provide a child a nurturing and constructive physical, emotional, and social environment

Psychosocial Adjustment: Life Change: Adaptive psychosocial response of an individual to a significant life change

Role Performance: Congruence of an individual's role behavior with role expectations

Goals/Evaluation Criteria

Examples Using NOC Language

- Demonstrates **Role Performance**, as evidenced by the following indicators (specify 1–5: not, slightly, moderately, substantially, or totally adequate):
  - Performance of role expectations
  - Knowledge of role transition periods
  - Performance of family, community, work, intimate, and friendship role behaviors
  - Reported strategies for role change(s)

Other Examples

- Acknowledges impact of situation on existing personal relationships, lifestyle, and role performance
- Describes actual change in function
- Expresses willingness to use resources upon discharge
- Verbalizes feelings of productivity and usefulness
- Demonstrates ability to manage finances

NIC Interventions

Anticipatory Guidance: Preparation of patient for an anticipated developmental or situational crisis

Coping Enhancement: Assisting a patient to adapt to perceived stressors, changes, or threats that interfere with meeting life demands and roles

Hope Inspiration: Facilitation of the development of a positive outlook in a given situation

Mood Management: Providing for safety, stabilization, recovery, and maintenance of a patient who is experiencing dysfunctionally depressed or elevated mood

Parenting Promotion: Providing parenting information, support, and coordination of comprehensive services to high-risk families

Role Enhancement: Assisting a patient, significant other, and family to improve relationships by clarifying and supplementing specific role behaviors

Self-Efficacy Enhancement: Strengthening an individual's confidence in his ability to perform a health behavior

Nursing Activities

Assessments

- Assess the anticipated duration of the role difficulties
- Assess need for assistance from social services department for planning care with patient and family

Patient/Family Teaching

- *(NIC) Role Enhancement*: Teach new behaviors needed by patient/parent to fulfill a role

Other

- Assist patient in identifying personal strengths
- Actively listen to patient and family and acknowledge reality of concerns
- Encourage patient and family to air feelings and to grieve
- *(NIC) Role Enhancement:*
  Assist patient to identify various roles in life cycle
  Assist patient to identify usual role in family
  Assist patient to identify role insufficiency

Home Care

- The preceding nursing activities are appropriate for use in home care
- Assess the impact of communication on family roles and functioning
- Facilitate discussion of role adaptations related to children leaving home (i.e., empty-nest syndrome), as appropriate

For Infants and Children

- *(NIC) Role Enhancement*: Facilitate discussion of how siblings' roles will change with newborn's arrival, as appropriate

For Older Adults

- *(NIC) Role Enhancement*: Assist adult children to accept elderly parent's dependency and the role changes involved, as appropriate
- Monitor the health status of grandparents raising grandchildren
- Refer to support groups to facilitate adjustment to role changes
- Assess for memory loss that might interfere with role performance; refer for memory rehabilitation therapy as needed

SEDENTARY LIFESTYLE

(2004)

Domain 1, Health Promotion; Class 1, Health Awareness

Definition: Reports a habit of life that is characterized by a low physical activity level

Defining Characteristics

S

Objective

Chooses a daily routine lacking physical exercise
Demonstrates physical deconditioning
Reports preference for activities low in physical activity

Related Factors

Deficient knowledge of health benefits of physical exercise
Lack of interest or motivation
Lack of resources (time, money, companionship, facilities)
Lack of training for accomplishment of physical exercise

Suggestions for Use

If other unhealthful behaviors are present (e.g., poor eating habits, insufficient sleep), and if these are related to the patient's limited abilities, consider a broader diagnosis, such as *Ineffective health maintenance*.

Suggested Alternative Diagnosis

Activity intolerance
Health maintenance, ineffective
Noncompliance

NOC Outcomes

Motivation: Inner urge that moves or prompts an individual to positive action(s)
Physical Fitness: Performance of physical activities with vigor

Goals/Evaluation Criteria

Examples Using NOC Language

- Demonstrates **Physical Fitness**, as evidenced by the following indicators (specify 1–5: severely, substantially, moderately, mildly, or not compromised):
  - Blood pressure
  - Body mass index
  - Target heart rate during exercise
  - Resting heart rate

Other Examples

- Verbalizes awareness of the risks of a sedentary lifestyle
- Describes the benefits of regular exercise
- Gradually increases the amount of physical exercise performed
- Increases his physical endurance when exercising
- Improves muscle strength
- Improves joint flexibility

NIC Interventions

Activity Therapy: Prescription of and assistance with specific physical, cognitive, social, and spiritual activities to increase the range, frequency, or duration of an individual's (or group's) activity
Exercise Promotion: Facilitation of regular physical activity to maintain or advance to a higher level of fitness and health
Exercise Promotion: Strength Training: Facilitating regular resistive muscle training to maintain or increase muscle strength
Self-Modification Assistance: Reinforcement of self-directed change initiated by the patient to achieve personally important goals

Self-Responsibility Facilitation: Encouraging a patient to assume more responsibility for own behavior

Teaching: Prescribed Activity/Exercise: Preparing a patient to achieve or maintain a prescribed level of activity

Nursing Activities

Assessments

- Assess the client's regular pattern of exercise
- Assess the client's activity tolerance (e.g., changes in vital signs with activity)
- Assess the client's motivation to incorporate exercise into her lifestyle
- Determine the reasons for the lack of physical exercise (e.g., lack of time, resources, depression, and so forth)

Patient/Family Teaching

- Explain the benefits of regular exercise
- Stress the need to begin exercising gradually

Collaborative Interventions

- Refer to a trainer or physical therapist for special conditioning exercises, as needed

Other

S

- Assist the client in developing an exercise program appropriate for his physical capabilities, personal preferences, and daily routines
- Suggest walking as an exercise that is easy to work into daily routines, is inexpensive to do, does not demand top physical conditioning, can be done with a partner for support
- For those who are not in top physical condition, suggest water aerobics and swimming (in addition to walking)
- Assist the client in developing short-term goals that will serve as motivation to continue exercise program
- Suggest exercising with a friend or family member
- Assist in setting priorities to make time for exercise
- Suggest keeping a record of activity and exercise

Home Care

- The preceding nursing activities are appropriate for home care use
- Evaluate the home for barriers to mobility

For Infants and Children

- Help the child make a plan to walk more; encourage wearing a pedometer
- For adolescents, stress the benefits of exercise for strength and physical appearance

For Older Adults

- Stress the contribution of physical activity to healthy aging (e.g., in preventing osteoporosis in women)
- Use the Get Up and Go test to screen the client's mobility and endurance (sit in a chair, rise to standing position, walk 10 feet, turn, return to the chair, and sit)
- Suggest low-impact exercise, such as tai chi
- Refer to physical therapist for resistance exercises to retard muscle atrophy
- Assess for depression
- Assist client to obtain any assistive devices for mobility (e.g., a walker)

SELF-CARE, READINESS FOR ENHANCED

(2006) **Domain 4, Activity/Rest; Class 5, Self-Care**

Definition: A pattern of performing activities for oneself that helps to meet health-related goals and can be strengthened

Defining Characteristics

Expresses desire to enhance:
- Independence in maintaining health
- Independence in maintaining life
- Independence in maintaining personal development
- Independence in maintaining well-being
- Knowledge of strategies for self-care
- Responsibility for self-care
- Self-care

Suggestions for Use

The definition and defining characteristics show this to be a very broadly stated diagnosis. If it were limited to enhancing bathing/hygiene, dressing/grooming, feeding, and toileting, the nurse could assist the client in strengthening self-care in ADLs. In that case, goals and activities for the *Self-care deficit* diagnoses could be used.

As stated, however, this diagnosis is all-inclusive and could involve almost every area of a person's life. Therefore, it is not possible to specifically state goals and interventions for it.

If the person expresses a desire to focus on knowledge of strategies of self-care, consider *Readiness for enhanced knowledge*; if it involves maintaining personal development, consider *Readiness for enhanced self-concept.*

Suggested Alternative Diagnoses

Readiness for enhanced knowledge
Readiness for enhanced self-concept

NOC Outcomes

NOTE: Although it is not possible to state specific goals for this diagnosis, NOC outcomes have been published for this diagnosis. Therefore, we list them here.

Discharge Readiness: Independent Living: Readiness of a patient to relocate from a health care institution to living independently

Self-Care: ADLs: Ability to perform the most basic physical tasks and personal care activities independently with or without assistive device

Self-Care: IADLs: Ability to perform activities needed to function in the home or community independently with or without assistive device

S

Self-Care: Non-Parenteral Medication: Ability to administer oral and topical medications to meet therapeutic goals independently with or without assistive device

Self-Care: Parenteral Medication: Ability to administer parenteral medications to meet therapeutic goals independently with or without assistive device

Self-Care Status: Ability to perform personal care activities and instrumental activities of daily living

Goals/Evaluation Criteria

See Suggestions for Use, preceding.

NIC Interventions

NOTE: Although it is not possible to state specific interventions for this diagnosis, NIC interventions have been published for this diagnosis. Therefore, we list them here.

Discharge Planning: Preparation for moving a patient from one level of care to another within or outside the current health care agency

Environmental Management: Home Preparation: Preparing the home for safe and effective delivery of care

Self-Efficacy Enhancement: Strengthening an individual's confidence in his ability to perform a health behavior

Teaching: Individual: Planning, implementation, and evaluation of a teaching program designed to address a patient's particular needs

Teaching: Prescribed Medication: Preparing a patient to safely take prescribed medications and monitor for their effects

Nursing Activities

See Suggestions for Use, preceding.

SELF-CARE DEFICIT—DISCUSSION

Self-care deficit describes a state in which a person experiences impaired ability to perform self-care activities such as bathing, dressing, eating, and toileting. If the person is unable to perform any self-care, the situation is described as *Total self-care deficit.* However, the diagnoses are classified into more specific problems, each with its own defining characteristics; these problems can exist alone or in various combinations, such as *Feeding self-care deficit* and *Feeding and bathing/hygiene self-care deficit.*

Self-care deficits are often caused by *Activity intolerance*, *Impaired physical mobility*, *Pain*, *Anxiety*, or perceptual or cognitive impairment (e.g., *Feeding self-care deficit +2 related to disorientation*). As an etiology, *Self-care deficit* can cause depression, *Fear* of becoming dependent, and *Powerlessness* (e.g., *Fear of becoming totally dependent related to total self-care deficit +2 secondary to residual weakness from CVA [stroke]*).

S

Self-care deficit should be used to label only those conditions in which the focus is to support or improve the patient's self-care abilities. Outcome and evaluation criteria for these labels must reflect improved functioning. Therefore, if the diagnosis is used for states not amenable to treatment, there is no hope of achieving the stated outcomes. The focus of nursing interventions in this case is twofold: (a) to increase the patient's ability to perform self-care and (b) to help patients with limitations and perform care the patient cannot do.

SELF-CARE DEFICIT, BATHING

(1980, 1998, 2008) **Domain 4, Activity/Rest; Class 5, Self-Care**

Definition: Impaired ability to perform or complete bathing or hygiene activities for oneself

Defining Characteristics

Objective

Inability to [perform the following tasks]:
Access bathroom
Dry body
Get bath supplies
Obtain water source
Regulate [temperature or flow of] bathwater
Wash body [or body parts]

Related Factors

Decreased motivation
Environmental barriers
Inability to perceive body part
Inability to perceive spatial relationship
Musculoskeletal impairment
Neuromuscular impairment
Pain
Perceptual or cognitive impairment
Severe anxiety
Weakness [and fatigue]

Other Related Factors (Non-NANDA International)

Depression
Developmental disability
Intolerance to activity
Medically imposed restrictions
Psychologic impairment (specify)

Suggestions for Use

See Self-Care Deficit—Discussion, preceding.

In order to promote efforts to restore functioning, the patient's functional level must be classified using a standardized scale such as the following:

0 = Completely independent
1 = Requires use of equipment or device
2 = Requires help from another person for assistance, supervision, or teaching
3 = Requires help from another person and equipment or device
4 = Dependent, does not participate in activity

The definitions and descriptors in Table 5 may be helpful in determining which number to assign to a patient's functional level:

Table 5

	Totally Dependent (+4)	**Moderately Dependent (+3)**	**Semi-dependent (+2)**
Bathing	Patient needs complete bath; cannot assist at all	Nurse supplies all equipment; positions patient; washes back, legs, perineum, and all other parts, as needed; patient can assist	Nurse provides all equipment; positions patient in bed and bathroom. Patient completes bath, except for back and feet
Oral Hygiene	Nurse completes entire procedure	Nurse prepares brush, rinses, mouth, positions patient	Nurse provides equipment; patient does task

Suggested Alternative Diagnoses

Activity intolerance
Mobility: physical, impaired
Self-care deficit, total

NOC Outcomes

Self-Care: Bathing: Ability to cleanse own body independently with or without assistive device

Self-Care: Hygiene: Ability to maintain own personal cleanliness and kempt appearance independently with or without assistive device

Goals/Evaluation Criteria

Examples Using NOC Language

- Demonstrates **Self-Care: Bathing** as evidenced by the following indicators (specify 1–5: severely, substantially, moderately, mildly, or not compromised):
  - Gets bath supplies
  - Bathes in tub (sink, shower)
  - Cleans perineal area

Other Examples

- Accepts assistance or total care by caregiver, if needed
- Verbalizes satisfactory body cleanliness and oral hygiene
- Maintains mobility needed to get to bathroom and get bath supplies
- Turns on and regulates water temperature and flow
- Washes and dries body
- Performs mouth care
- Applies deodorant

NIC Interventions

Select other NIC interventions as appropriate for the patient's particular self-care deficits (e.g., Nail Care, Hair Care, Foot Care). The following are examples.

Bathing: Cleaning of the body for the purposes of relaxation, cleanliness, and healing

Oral Health Maintenance: Maintenance and promotion of oral hygiene and dental health for the patient at risk for developing oral or dental lesions

Self-Care Assistance, Bathing/Hygiene: Assisting patient to perform personal hygiene

Nursing Activities

Assessments

- Assess ability to use assistive devices
- Assess oral mucous membranes and body cleanliness daily
- Assess skin condition during bath
- Monitor for changes in functional abilities
- *(NIC) Self-Care Assistance: Bathing/Hygiene*: Monitor cleaning of nails, according to patient's self-care ability

S

Patient/Family Teaching

- Instruct patient and family in alternative methods for bathing and oral hygiene

Collaborative Activities

- Offer pain medications prior to bathing
- Refer patient and family to social services for home care
- Use occupational and physical therapy as resources in planning patient care activities (e.g., to provide adaptive equipment)

Other

- Encourage independence in bathing and oral hygiene, assisting patient only as necessary
- Encourage patient to set own pace during self-care

- Include family in provision of care
- Accommodate patient's preferences and needs as much as possible (e.g., bath versus shower, and time of day)
- *(NIC) Self-Care Assistance: Bathing/Hygiene:*
  - Provide assistance until patient is fully able to assume self-care
  - Place towels, soap, deodorant, shaving equipment, and other needed accessories at bedside or in bathroom
  - Facilitate patient's brushing teeth, as appropriate
- Shave patient, as indicated
- Offer handwashing after toileting and before meals

Home Care

- In addition to the activities in this section, most of the preceding activities are appropriate for home care
- Recommend the installation of grab bars and nonskid surfaces in bathrooms
- Refer for home health aide services as appropriate
- Teach bathing skills to caregivers, as needed
- Do not insist on bathing a terminally ill client who does not wish it

For Infants and Children

- Allow the child to perform self-care to the extent possible, to promote self-concept

For Older Adults

- Assess ability to perform ADLs independently, using acceptable scales
- Assess for and accommodate cognitive or physical changes that may contribute to self-care deficits
- Encourage walking and strength-building exercises
- Ensure that there are grab bars and nonslip surfaces in the bathing room
- Use a no-rinse cleanser instead of soap; use lukewarm water
- Keep the bathing environment warm; and expose only the area of the body being bathed
- Provide a full bath once or twice a week, partial baths on other days, to prevent skin dryness
- Bathe and dry gently to protect fragile skin
- Promote independence to the extent of the client's abilities

SELF-CARE DEFICIT: DRESSING

(1980, 1998, 2008) **Domain 4, Activity/Rest; Class 5, Self-Care**

Definition: Impaired ability to perform or complete dressing activities for self

Defining Characteristics

Objective

Impaired ability to:

- Fasten clothing
- Obtain clothing
- Put on or take off necessary items of clothing
- Put on or take off shoes or socks

Inability to:

- Choose clothing
- Maintain appearance at a satisfactory level
- Pick up clothing
- Put on clothing on lower body
- Put on clothing on upper body
- Put on shoes or socks
- Remove shoes or socks
- Remove clothes
- Use assistive devices
- Use zippers

Related Factors

Decreased motivation
Discomfort
Environmental barriers
Fatigue
Musculoskeletal impairment
Neuromuscular impairment
Pain
Perceptual or cognitive impairment
Severe anxiety
Weakness [or tiredness]

Other Related Factors (Non-NANDA International)

Depression
Developmental disability
Intolerance to activity
Psychologic impairment (specify)

Suggestions for Use

See Self-Care Deficit—Discussion, preceding. Classify functional level using a standardized scale such as the following:

0 = Completely independent
1 = Requires use of equipment or device
2 = Requires help from another person for assistance, supervision, or teaching
3 = Requires help from another person and equipment or device
4 = Dependent; does not participate in activity

The following definitions and descriptors in Table 6 may be helpful in determining which number to assign to a patient's functional level:

Table 6

	Totally Dependent (+4)	**Moderately Dependent (+3)**	**Semi-dependent (+2)**
Dressing or grooming	Patient needs to be dressed and cannot assist the nurse; nurse combs patient's hair	Nurse combs patient's hair, assists with dressing, buttons and zips clothing, ties shoes	Nurse gathers items for patient; may button, zip, or tie clothing. Patient dresses self

Suggested Alternative Diagnoses

Activity intolerance
Fatigue
Mobility: physical, impaired
Self-care deficit, total (non-NANDA-International)

NOC Outcomes

Self-Care: Dressing: Ability to dress self independently with or without assistive device

Goals/Evaluation Criteria

Examples Using NOC Language

- Demonstrates **Self-Care: Dressing** as evidenced by the following indicators (specify 1–5: severely, substantially, moderately, mildly, or not compromised):
  - Puts clothing on upper (and/or lower) body
  - Puts on socks (and shoes)
  - Ties shoes

Other Examples

Patient will:

- Accept care by caregiver
- Express satisfaction with dressing
- Use adaptive devices to facilitate dressing
- Choose clothes and obtain them from closet or drawers
- Zip and button clothing
- Be neatly dressed
- Be able to remove clothing, socks, and shoes

NIC Interventions

Environmental Management: Manipulation of the patient's surroundings for therapeutic benefit, sensory appeal, and psychological well-being

Self-Care Assistance: Dressing/Grooming: Assisting patient with clothes and makeup

Nursing Activities

Assessments

- Assess ability to use assistive devices
- Monitor energy level and activity tolerance
- Monitor for improved or deteriorating ability to dress and perform hair care
- Monitor for sensory, cognitive, or physical deficits that may make dressing difficult for the patient

Patient/Family Teaching

- Demonstrate use of assistive devices and adaptive activities
- Instruct patient in alternative methods for dressing and hair care, specify methods

Collaborative Activities

- Offer pain medications prior to dressing and grooming
- Refer patient and family to social services for obtaining home health aide, as needed
- Use occupational and physical therapy as resource in planning patient care activities and for assistive devices
- *(NIC) Self-Care Assistance: Dressing/Grooming*: Facilitate assistance of a barber or beautician, as necessary

Other

- Encourage independence in dressing and grooming, assisting patient only as necessary
- Accommodate cognitive deficits in the following ways:
  - Use nonverbal cues (e.g., give patient one article of clothing at a time, in the order needed)

- Speak slowly and keep directions simple
- Use Velcro fasteners and closures when possible
- Create opportunities for small successes, specify
- Encourage patient to set own pace during dressing and grooming
- Help patient choose clothing that is loose fitting and easy to put on
- Provide for safety by keeping environment uncluttered and well-lighted
- *(NIC) Self-Care Assistance: Dressing/Grooming:*
  Provide patient's clothes in accessible area (e.g., at bedside) [and in the order they will be needed for dressing]
  Maintain privacy while the patient is dressing
  Help with laces, buttons, and zippers, as needed
  Use extension equipment [e.g., long-handled shoehorn, buttonhook, zipper pull] for pulling on clothing, if appropriate
  Reinforce efforts to dress self

Home Care

- The preceding activities are appropriate for home care
- Refer for home health aide services as appropriate

For Infants and Children

- Allow the child to perform self-care to the extent possible, to promote self-concept
- Allow the child to choose what he wants to wear

For Older Adults

- Assess ability to perform ADLs independently, using accepted scales
- Assess for and accommodate cognitive or physical changes that may contribute to self-care deficits
- Encourage walking and strength-building exercises
- Promote independence to the extent of the client's abilities

S

SELF-CARE DEFICIT: FEEDING

(1980, 1998) **Domain 4, Activity/Rest; Class 5, Self-Care**

Definition: Impaired ability to perform or complete feeding activities

Defining Characteristics

Objective

Inability to:

- Bring food from a receptacle to the mouth
- Chew food
- Complete a meal
- Get food onto utensil
- Handle utensils
- Ingest food in a socially acceptable manner
- Ingest food safely
- Ingest sufficient food
- Manipulate food in mouth
- Open containers
- Pick up cup or glass
- Prepare food for ingestion
- Swallow food
- Use assistive device

Related Factors

Decreased motivation
Discomfort
Environmental barriers
Fatigue

Musculoskeletal impairment
Neuromuscular impairment
Pain
Perceptual or cognitive impairment
Severe anxiety
Weakness

Other Related Factors (Non-NANDA International)

Depression
Developmental disability
Intolerance to activity
Psychologic impairment

Suggestions for Use

Feeding self-care deficit may be the etiology (i.e., related factor) for *Imbalanced nutrition: less than body requirements*. Also see Self-Care

Deficit—Discussion in a preceding section. Use a standardized scale, such as the following, to classify patient's functional level:

0 = Completely independent
1 = Requires use of equipment or device
2 = Requires help from another person for assistance, supervision, or teaching
3 = Requires help from another person and equipment or device
4 = Dependent, does not participate in activity

The following definitions and descriptors in Table 7 may be helpful in determining which number to assign to a patient's functional level:

Table 7

	Totally Dependent (+4)	Moderately Dependent (+3)	Semi-dependent (+2)
Feeding	Patient needs to be fed totally	Nurse cuts food, opens containers, positions patient, monitors, and encourages eating	Nurse positions patient, gathers supplies, and monitors eating

Suggested Alternative Diagnoses

Activity intolerance
Mobility, physical, impaired
[Self-care deficit, total]

S

NOC Outcomes

Nutritional Status: Food and Fluid Intake: Amount of food and fluid taken into the body over a 24-hr period

Self-Care: Eating: Ability to prepare and ingest food and fluid independently with or without assistive device

Swallowing Status: Safe passage of fluids or solids from the mouth to the stomach

Goals/Evaluation Criteria

Examples Using NOC Language

- Demonstrates **Self-Care: Eating**, as evidenced by the following indicator (specify 1–5: severely, substantially, moderately, mildly, or not compromised):

  Gets food onto the utensil
  Brings food to mouth with fingers (or container or utensil)
  Chews food

Swallows fluid
Completes a meal

Other Examples

- Accepts feeding by caregiver
- Feeds self independently (or specify level)
- Expresses satisfaction with eating and with ability to feed self
- Demonstrates adequate intake of food and fluids
- Uses adaptive devices to eat
- Opens containers and prepares food

NIC Interventions

Feeding: Providing nutritional intake for patient who is unable to feed self

Nutrition Management: Assisting with or providing a balanced dietary intake of foods and fluids

Nutritional Monitoring: Collection and analysis of patient data to prevent or minimize malnourishment

Referral: Arrangement for services by another care provider or agency

Self-Care Assistance: Feeding: Assisting a person to eat

Swallowing Therapy: Facilitating swallowing and preventing complications of impaired swallowing

Nursing Activities

Assessments

S

- Assess ability to use assistive devices
- Assess energy level and activity tolerance
- Assess for improved or deteriorating ability to feed self
- Assess for sensory, cognitive, or physical deficits that may make self-feeding difficult
- Assess ability to chew and swallow
- Assess intake for nutritional adequacy

Patient/Family Teaching

- Demonstrate use of assistive devices and adaptive activities
- Instruct patient in alternative methods for eating and drinking, specify method and teaching plan

Collaborative Activities

- Refer patient and family to social services for obtaining home health aide
- Use occupational and physical therapy as resources in planning patient care activities
- *(NIC) Self-Care Assistance: Feeding*: Provide for adequate pain relief before meals, as appropriate

Other

- Accommodate cognitive deficits in the following ways:
  Avoid using sharp eating utensils (e.g., steak knives)
  Check for food in cheeks
  Have meals in quiet environment to limit distraction from task
  Keep verbal communication short and simple
- Serve one food at a time in small amounts
- Acknowledge and reinforce patient's accomplishments
- Encourage independence in eating and drinking, assisting patient only as necessary
- Encourage patient to wear dentures and eyeglasses
- Provide for privacy while eating if patient is embarrassed
- When feeding, allow patient to determine order of foods
- Sit down while feeding; do not hurry
- Serve finger foods (e.g., fruit, bread) to promote independence
- Include parents and family in feeding and meals
- *(NIC) Self-Care Assistance: Feeding:*
  Create a pleasant environment during mealtime (e.g., put bedpans, urinals, and suctioning equipment out of sight)
  Provide for oral hygiene before meals
  Fix food on tray, as necessary, such as cutting meat or peeling an egg
  Avoid placing food on a person's blind side
  Provide a drinking straw, as needed or desired
  Provide adaptive devices to facilitate patient's feeding self (e.g., long handles, handle with large circumference, or small strap-on utensils), as needed
  Provide frequent cueing and close supervision, as appropriate

Home Care

- For clients who must be fed, teach caregivers to observe for and report the signs and symptoms of dysphagia (e.g., gurgling when speaking, clearing of the throat, coughing, choking)
- Do not insist that a terminally ill client eat if he does not wish to

For Infants and Children

- Base your communication on the child's developmental stage

For Older Adults

- Arrange for clients to eat with others; when possible, allow the patient to fill his plate from a serving bowl
- Assess denture fit and condition
- Do not rush the patient during feedings

SELF-CARE DEFICIT: TOILETING

(1980, 1998, 2008) **Domain 4, Activity/Rest; Class 5, Self-Care**

Definition: Impaired ability to perform or complete own toileting activities

Defining Characteristics

Objective

Inability to carry out proper toilet hygiene
Inability to flush toilet or commode
Inability to get to toilet or commode
Inability to manipulate clothing for toileting
Inability to sit on or rise from toilet or commode

Related Factors

Decreased motivation
Environmental barriers
Fatigue
Impaired mobility status
Impaired transfer ability
Musculoskeletal impairment
Neuromuscular impairment
Pain
Perceptual or cognitive impairment
Severe anxiety
Weakness

Other Defining Characteristics (Non-NANDA International)

Depression
Developmental disability
Intolerance to activity
Medically imposed restrictions
Psychologic impairment (specify)

Suggestions for Use

Self-care deficit: toileting may be an etiology (i.e., related factor) for *Impaired skin integrity* or *Social isolation*. Also see Self-Care

Deficit—Discussion, in a preceding section. Use a standardized scale, such as the following, to classify functional levels:

0 = Completely independent
1 = Requires use of equipment or device
2 = Requires help from another person for assistance, supervision, or teaching
3 = Requires help from another person and equipment or device
4 = Dependent, does not participate in activity

The following definitions and descriptors in Table 8 may be helpful in determining which number to assign to a patient's functional level:

Table 8

	Totally Dependent (+4)	Moderately Dependent (+3)	Semi-dependent (+2)
Toileting	Patient is incontinent; nurse places patient on bedpan or commode	Nurse provides bedpan, positions patient on or off bedpan, places patient on commode	Patient can walk to bathroom or commode with assistance; nurse helps with clothing

Suggested Alternative Diagnoses

Activity intolerance
Bowel incontinence
Fatigue
Mobility, physical, impaired
Total self-care deficit (non-NANDA-I)
Transfer ability, impaired
Urinary incontinence (functional, reflex, stress, urge)

NOC Outcomes

Ostomy Self-Care: Personal actions to maintain ostomy for elimination
Self-Care: Toileting: Ability to toilet self independently with or without assistive device

Goals/Evaluation Criteria

Examples Using NOC Language

- Demonstrates **Self-Care: Toileting,** as evidenced by the following indicators (specify 1–5: severely, substantially, moderately, mildly, or not compromised):
  Positions self on toilet or commode
  Empties bladder (or bowel)

Gets up from toilet or commode
Adjusts clothing after toileting

Other Examples

- Accepts help from caregiver
- Recognizes or acknowledge need for help with toileting
- Recognizes and respond to urge to urinate and/or defecate
- Able to get to and from toilet
- Wipes self after toileting

NIC Interventions

Bowel Management: Establishment and maintenance of a regular pattern of bowel elimination

Ostomy Care: Maintenance of elimination through a stoma and care of surrounding tissue

Self-Care Assistance: Toileting: Assisting another with elimination

Teaching: Individual: Planning, implementation, and evaluation of a teaching program designed to address a patient's particular needs

Nursing Activities

Also see Nursing Activities for the diagnoses, Bowel Incontinence and Urinary Incontinence: Functional, Reflex, Stress, Total, and Urge.

Assessments

- Assess ability to ambulate independently and safely
- Assess ability to manipulate clothing
- Assess ability to use assistive devices (e.g., walkers, canes)
- Monitor energy level and activity tolerance
- Assess for improved or deteriorating ability to toilet self
- Assess for sensory, cognitive, or physical deficits that may limit self-toileting

Patient/Family Teaching

- Instruct patient and family in transfer and ambulation techniques
- Demonstrate use of assistive equipment and adaptive activities
- *(NIC) Self-Care Assistance: Toileting*: Instruct patient and appropriate others in toileting routine

Collaborative Activities

- Offer pain medications prior to toileting
- Refer patient and family to social services for obtaining home health aide
- Use occupational and physical therapy as resources in planning patient care activities and obtaining necessary assistive equipment

Other

- Specify functional level and assist with toileting or provide basic care, as needed
- Avoid use of indwelling catheters and condom catheters if possible
- Encourage patient to wear clothes that are easy to manage; assist with clothing, as needed
- Keep bedpan or urinal within patient's reach
- *(NIC) Self-Care Assistance: Toileting:*
  - Assist patient to toilet, commode, bedpan, fracture pan, and urinal at specified intervals
  - Facilitate toilet hygiene after completion of elimination
  - Flush toilet; cleanse elimination utensil (commode, bedpan)
  - Replace patient's clothing after elimination
  - Provide privacy during elimination
- Remove objects that impair access to the toilet (e.g., loose rugs and small, movable furniture)
- Use room deodorizers, as needed
- Be sure the patient has a way to summon nurse or other caregivers and let the patient and family know they will be answered immediately

Home Care

- Most of the preceding activities are also appropriate for home care
- *(NIC) Environmental Management*: Provide family and significant other with information about making home environment safe for patient

For Older Adults

- Accommodate cognitive deficits (e.g., keep verbal instructions short and simple)
- Allow sufficient time for toileting to avoid fatigue and frustration
- Recommend and assist with strength-building exercises
- Assist the client to ambulate for a few minutes when up to the toilet
- Provide a footstool at the commode or toilet as needed to elevate the knees above the hips

SELF-CONCEPT, READINESS FOR ENHANCED

(2002) **Domain 6, Self-Perception; Class 1, Self-Concept**

Definition: A pattern of perceptions or ideas about the self that is sufficient for well-being and can be strengthened

Defining Characteristics

Subjective

Accepts strengths and limitations

Expresses confidence in abilities

Expresses satisfaction with, sense of worthiness, role performance, body image, personal identity, and thoughts about self

Expresses willingness to enhance self-concept

Objective

Actions are congruent with verbal expression [e.g., of feelings and thoughts]

Related Factors

This is a wellness diagnosis, so an etiology is not needed.

Suggestions for Use

S

Self-concept is a broad diagnosis that includes body image, self-esteem, personal identity, and role performance. *Readiness for enhanced self-concept* can be used when there are no risk factors for the more specific problems (e.g., *Chronic or situational low self-esteem*, *Ineffective role performance*). If risk factors are present, consider a diagnosis such as *Risk for situational low self-esteem*.

Suggested Alternative Diagnoses

Coping, readiness for enhanced

Self-esteem, risk for situational low

NOC Outcomes

Body Image: Perception of own appearance and body functions

Personal Well-Being: Extent of positive perception of one's health status

Self-Esteem: Personal judgment of self-worth

Goals/Evaluation Criteria

Examples Using NOC Language

- Demonstrates **Self-Esteem**, as evidenced by the following indicators (specify 1–5: never, rarely, sometimes, often, or consistently positive):
  Verbalizations of self-acceptance
  Acceptance of compliments from others
  Description of success in work, school, or social groups

Other Examples

- Acknowledges personal strengths
- Exhibits realistic self-appraisal
- Expresses a willingness to enhance self-concept
- Participates in making decisions regarding plan of care
- Practices behaviors that generate self-confidence
- Verbalizes positive feelings about body, self, abilities, and role performance

NIC Interventions

Body Image Enhancement: Improving a patient's conscious and unconscious perceptions and attitudes toward his body

Self-Awareness Enhancement: Assisting a patient to explore and understand his thoughts, feelings, motivations, and behaviors

Self-Esteem Enhancement: Assisting a patient to increase his personal judgment of self-worth

Nursing Activities

S

Assessments

- Assess for evidence of positive self-concept (e.g., mood, positive body image, satisfaction with role responsibilities, perception of and satisfaction with self in general)
- *(NIC) Self-Esteem Enhancement:*
  Monitor patient's statements of self-worth
  Determine patient's confidence in own judgment

Patient/Family Teaching

- Teach positive behavioral skills through role play, role modeling, discussion, and so forth

Other

- Help client to anticipate developmental and situational changes that may influence role performance and self-esteem
- *(NIC) Self-Esteem Enhancement:*
  Convey confidence in patient's ability to handle situation(s)
  Encourage patient to accept new challenges

Reinforce the personal strengths that patient identifies
Assist patient to identify positive responses from others
Assist in setting realistic goals to achieve higher self-esteem
Explore previous achievements of success
Reward or praise patient's progress toward reaching goals

Home Care

- Preceding activities are also appropriate for use in home care

For Infants and Children

- *(NIC) Self-Esteem Enhancement*: Instruct parents on the importance of their interest and support in their children's development of a positive self-concept

SELF-ESTEEM, CHRONIC LOW

(1988, 1996, 2008) **Domain 6, Self-Perception; Class 2, Self-Esteem**

Definition: Long-standing, negative self-evaluation or feelings about self or self-capabilities

Defining Characteristics

Subjective

Evaluation of self as unable to deal with events
Reports feelings of shame and guilt
Exaggerates negative feedback about self
Rejects positive feedback about self

Objective

Dependent on others' opinions
Excessively seeks reassurance
Frequent lack of success [in work or other] life events
Hesitant to try new things and situations
Indecisive behavior
Lack of eye contact
Nonassertive or passive
Overly conforming

Other Defining Characteristics (Non-NANDA International)

Projection of blame or responsibility for problems
Self-destructive behaviors (e.g., alcohol, drug abuse)
Self-negating verbalization
Self-neglect

Related Factors

Ineffective adaptation to loss
Lack of affection
Lack of approval
Lack of membership in group
Perceived discrepancy between self and cultural norms
Perceived discrepancy between self and spiritual norms
Perceived lack of belonging
Perceived lack of respect from others
Psychiatric disorder
Repeated failures
Repeated negative reinforcement
Traumatic event or situation

Related Factors (Non-NANDA International)

Chronic illness
Congenital anomaly
Repeated unmet expectations

Suggestions for Use

Chronic low self-esteem is different from *Situational low self-esteem* in that the symptoms are long-standing and seem to result from frequent, actual, or perceived lack of success in work or role performance.

Suggested Alternative Diagnoses

Coping, ineffective
Hopelessness
Powerlessness
Self-concept disturbance (non-NANDA International)
Self-esteem, situational low

NOC Outcomes

Depression Level: Severity of melancholic mood and loss of interest in life events

Self-Esteem: Personal judgment of self-worth

Goals/Evaluation Criteria

Examples Using NOC Language

- Demonstrates **Self-Esteem**, as evidenced by the following indicators (specify 1–5: never, rarely, sometimes, often, or consistently positive):
- Verbalizations of self-acceptance
- Maintenance of erect posture

- Maintenance of eye contact
- Maintenance of grooming and hygiene
- Acceptance of compliments from others
- Description of success in work, school, or social groups

Other Examples

- Acknowledges personal strengths
- Expresses a willingness to seek counseling
- Participates in making decisions regarding plan of care
- Practices behaviors that generate self-confidence

NIC Interventions

Hope Inspiration: Facilitation of the development of a positive outlook in a given situation

Mood Management: Providing for safety, stabilization, recovery, and maintenance of a patient who is experiencing dysfunctionally depressed or elevated mood

Self-Esteem Enhancement: Assisting a patient to increase his personal judgment of self-worth

Nursing Activities

Assessments

- *(NIC) Self-Esteem Enhancement:*
  Monitor patient's statements of self-worth
  Determine patient's confidence in own judgment
  Monitor frequency of self-negating verbalizations

S

Patient/Family Teaching

- Provide information about the value of counseling and available community resources
- Teach positive behavioral skills through role play, role modeling, discussion, and so forth

Collaborative Activities

- Seek assistance from hospital resources (e.g., social workers, psychiatric clinical specialist, pastoral care services), as needed

Other

- Set limits about negative verbalization (e.g., regarding frequency, content, audience)
- *(NIC) Self-Esteem Enhancement:*
  Reinforce the personal strengths that patient identifies
  Assist patient to identify positive responses from others

Refrain from teasing
Assist in setting realistic goals to achieve higher self-esteem
Assist patient to reexamine negative perceptions of self
Assist the patient to identify the impact of peer group on feelings of self-worth
Explore previous achievements of success
Reward or praise patient's progress toward reaching goals
Facilitate an environment and activities that will increase self-esteem

Home Care

- Most of the preceding activities are appropriate for home care
- Monitor attendance at self-help groups
- Assess for side-effects and knowledge of psychotropic medications, if the client is taking them

For Infants and Children

- *(NIC) Self-Esteem Enhancement*: Instruct parents on the importance of their interest and support in their children's development of a positive self-concept

For Older Adults

- Encourage client to participate in group activities (e.g., church, exercise groups)
- Suggest participation in groups that help others (e.g., delivering mid-day meals to home-bound persons)

SELF-ESTEEM, RISK FOR CHRONIC LOW

(2010) **Domain 6, Self-Perception; Class 2, Self-Esteem**

Definition: At risk for long-standing negative self-evaluating/feelings about self or self-capabilities

Risk Factors

Ineffective adaptation to loss
Lack of affection
Lack of approval

Lack of membership in group
Perceived discrepancy between self and cultural norms
Perceived discrepancy between self and spiritual norms
Perceived lack of belonging
Perceived lack of respect from others
Psychiatric disorder
Repeated failures
Repeated negative reinforcement
Traumatic event or situation

Suggested Alternative Diagnoses

Powerlessness, Risk for
Self-Esteem, Risk for Situational Low

NOC Outcomes

NOTE: NOC outcomes have not yet been linked to this diagnosis. However, the following seems logical.

Self-Esteem: Personal judgment of self-worth

Goals/Evaluation Criteria

See Goals/Evaluation Criteria for the diagnosis Chronic Low Self-Esteem, preceding.

NIC Interventions

NOTE: NIC interventions have not yet been linked to this diagnosis; however, the following may be useful.

Hope Inspiration: Facilitation of the development of a positive outlook in a given situation

Mood Management: Providing for safety, stabilization, recovery, and maintenance of a patient who is experiencing dysfunctionally depressed or elevated mood

Self-Esteem Enhancement: Assisting a patient to increase his personal judgment of self-worth

Nursing Activities

Nursing activities focus on (a) promoting self-esteem and (b) minimizing risk factors in order to prevent Chronic Low Self-Esteem. Activities will depend on the patient's particular risk factors.

Assessments

- *(NIC) Self-Esteem Enhancement:*

  Monitor patient's statements of self-worth

  Determine patient's confidence in own judgment

  Monitor frequency of self-negating verbalizations

Patient/Family Teaching

- Provide information about the value of counseling and available community resources
- Teach positive behavioral skills through role play, role modeling, discussion, and so forth

Collaborative Activities

- Seek assistance from hospital resources (e.g., social workers, psychiatric clinical specialist, pastoral care services), as needed

Other

- *(NIC) Self-Esteem Enhancement:*

  Reinforce the personal strengths that patient identifies

  Assist patient to identify positive responses from others

  Assist patient to reexamine negative perceptions of self

  Assist the patient to identify the impact of peer group on feelings of self-worth

  Reward or praise patient's progress toward reaching goals

  Facilitate an environment and activities that will increase self-esteem

Home Care

- Most of the preceding activities are appropriate for home care
- Monitor attendance at self-help groups

For Infants and Children

- *(NIC) Self-Esteem Enhancement*: Instruct parents on the importance of their interest and support in their children's development of a positive self-concept

For Older Adults

- Encourage client to participate in group activities (e.g., church, exercise groups)
- Suggest participation in groups that help others (e.g., delivering midday meals to home-bound persons)

SELF-ESTEEM, RISK FOR SITUATIONAL LOW

(2000) **Domain 6, Self-Perception; Class 2, Self-Esteem**

Definition: At risk for developing negative perception of self-worth in response to a current situation [specify]

Risk Factors

Subjective

Disturbed body image
Unrealistic self-expectations

Objective

Behavior inconsistent with values
Decreased [power or] control over environment
Developmental changes (specify)
Failures or rejections
Functional impairment (specify)
History of abuse, neglect, or abandonment
History of learned helplessness
Lack of recognition
Loss
Physical illness (specify)
Social role changes (specify)

Suggested Alternative Diagnoses

Body image, disturbed
Coping, ineffective
Identity, personal, disturbed
Self-concept, readiness for enhanced
Self-esteem, situational low

NOC Outcomes

NOTE: The primary outcome, Self-Esteem, is needed to determine whether the patient has developed actual *Situational Low Self-Esteem*. Other outcomes you choose depend on the risk factors you are attempting to remove or minimize. It is beyond the scope of this book to list outcomes for all possible risk factors. Following are a few examples:

Abuse Recovery: Extent of healing following physical or psychological abuse that may include sexual or financial exploitation

Neglect Recovery: Extent of physical, emotional, and spiritual healing following the cessation of substandard care

Self-Esteem: Personal judgment of self-worth

Goals/Evaluation Criteria

Refer to Goals/Evaluation Criteria for Self-Esteem: Situational Low, following.

NIC Interventions

NOTE: Choose interventions to treat the patient's particular risk factors. The following are a few examples.

Abuse Protection Support: Identification of high-risk, dependent relationships and actions to prevent further infliction of physical or emotional harm

Body Image Enhancement: Improving a patient's conscious and unconscious perceptions and attitudes toward his body

Resiliency Promotion: Assisting individuals, families, and communities in development, use, and strengthening of protective factors to be used in coping with environmental and societal stressors

Self-Esteem Enhancement: Assisting a patient to increase his personal judgment of self-worth

Values Clarification: Assisting another to clarify her or his own values in order to facilitate effective decision making

Nursing Activities

Nursing activities focus on preventing Situational Low Self-Esteem. Refer to Nursing Activities for Self-Esteem, Situational Low, following.

S

SELF-ESTEEM, SITUATIONAL LOW

(1988, 1996, 2000) **Domain 6, Self-Perception; Class 2, Self-Esteem**

Definition: Development of a negative perception of self-worth in response to a current situation [specify]

Defining Characteristics

Subjective

Evaluation of self as unable to deal with situations or events

Expressions of helplessness and uselessness

Self-negating verbalizations

Reports current situational challenge to self-worth

Objective

Indecisive or nonassertive behavior

Related Factors

Behavior inconsistent with values
Developmental changes (specify)
Disturbed body image
Failures and rejections
Functional impairment
Lack of recognition
Loss
Social role changes

Related Factors (Non-NANDA International)

Situational crisis

Suggestions for Use

Situational low self-esteem can be differentiated from *Chronic low self-esteem* in that the symptoms are episodic. Symptoms occur in a person with previously good self-esteem and are in response to some actual or perceived event or situation. Goals and nursing activities, therefore, may focus on problem solving the situation in addition to building the patient's self-esteem.

Suggested Alternative Diagnoses

Body image, disturbed
Coping, ineffective
Personal identity, disturbed
Risk-prone health behavior

Self-esteem, chronic low

NOC Outcomes

Adaptation to Physical Disability: Adaptive response to a significant functional challenge due to a physical disability

Grief Resolution: Adjustment to actual or impending loss

Personal Resiliency: Positive adaptation and function of an individual following significant adversity or crisis

Psychosocial Adjustment: Life Change: Adaptive psychosocial response of an individual to a significant life change

Self-Esteem: Personal judgment of self-worth

Goals/Evaluation Criteria

Examples Using NOC Language

- Demonstrates **Self-Esteem**, as evidenced by the following indicators (specify 1–5: never, rarely, sometimes, often, or consistently positive):
  - Verbalization of self-acceptance
  - Open communication

Fulfillment of personally significant roles
Acceptance of compliments from others
Willingness to confront others
Description of success in work, school, and social groups

- Demonstrates **Psychosocial Adjustment: Life Change**, as evidenced by the following indicators (specify 1–5: never, rarely, sometimes, often, or consistently demonstrated):
  Reports feeling useful
  Verbalizes optimism about future
  Uses effective coping strategies

Other Examples

- Acknowledges personal strengths
- Practices behaviors that generate self-confidence
- Verbalizes episodic change/loss

NIC Interventions

Anticipatory Guidance: Preparation of patient for an anticipated developmental or situational crisis

Body Image Enhancement: Improving a patient's conscious and unconscious perceptions and attitudes toward his body

Coping Enhancement: Assisting a patient to adapt to perceived stressors, changes, or threats that interfere with meeting life demands and roles

Grief Work Facilitation: Assistance with the resolution of a significant loss

Grief Work Facilitation: Perinatal Death: Assistance with the resolution of a perinatal loss

Resiliency Promotion: Assisting individuals, families, and communities in development, use, and strengthening of protective factors to be used in coping with environmental and societal stressors

Self-Esteem Enhancement: Assisting a patient to increase his personal judgment of self-worth

Nursing Activities

Also refer to Nursing Activities for Self-Esteem, Chronic Low, preceding.

Patient/Family Teaching

- Teach positive behavioral skills through role play, role modeling, discussion, and so forth

Collaborative Activities

- Refer to appropriate community resources
- Seek assistance from hospital resources (social worker, clinical nurse specialist, pastoral care services), as needed

Other

- Explore recent changes with patient that may have influenced low self-esteem
- *(NIC) Self-Esteem Enhancement:*
  Convey confidence in patient's ability to handle situation
  Encourage increased responsibility for self, as appropriate
  Explore reasons for self-criticism or guilt
  Encourage patient to accept new challenges

Home Care

- The preceding activities are also appropriate for home care. Also see Nursing Activities for Self-Esteem, Chronic Low, preceding

SELF-HEALTH MANAGEMENT, INEFFECTIVE

(1994, 2008) **Domain 1, Health Promotion; Class 2, Health Management**

Definition: Pattern of regulating and integrating into daily living a therapeutic regimen for the treatment of illness and its sequelae that is unsatisfactory for meeting specific health goals

Defining Characteristics

S

Objective

Failure to include treatment regimens in daily living
Failure to take action to reduce risk failures
Ineffective choices in daily living for meeting health goals

Subjective

Reports desire to manage the illness
Reports difficulty with prescribed regimens

Related Factors

Complexity of health care system or of therapeutic regimen
Decisional conflicts
Deficient knowledge
Economic difficulties
Excessive demands made (e.g., individual, family)
Family conflict
Family patterns of health care
Inadequate number of cues to action
Perceived barriers

Perceived benefits
Perceived susceptibility
Powerlessness
Regimen
Social support deficit

Suggestions for Use

Use this diagnosis for patients who wish to follow a therapeutic regimen and are motivated to do so but are having difficulty with it. For example, this diagnosis is appropriate for a patient who is trying to lose weight and has the necessary information but finds it difficult to adhere to a low-calorie diet because her business requires her to eat out frequently. It is not appropriate for an obese patient who is not interested in dieting or losing weight.

Suggested Alternative Diagnoses

Risk-prone health behavior
Denial, ineffective
Health maintenance, ineffective
Noncompliance (specify)

NOC Outcomes

Alcohol Abuse Cessation Behavior: Personal actions to eliminate alcohol use that poses a threat to health

Asthma Self-Management: Personal actions to prevent or reverse inflammatory condition resulting in bronchial constriction of the airways

Blood Glucose Level: Extent to which glucose levels in plasma and urine are maintained in normal range

Cardiac Disease Self-Management: Personal actions to manage heart disease and prevent disease progression

Compliance Behavior: Personal actions to promote wellness, recovery, and rehabilitation recommended by a health professional

Compliance Behavior: Prescribed Diet: Personal actions to follow food and fluid intake recommended by a health professional for a specific health condition

Compliance Behavior: Prescribed Medication: Personal actions to administer medication safely to meet therapeutic goals as recommended by a health professional

Diabetes Self-Management: Personal actions to manage diabetes mellitus and prevent disease progression

Drug Abuse Cessation Behavior: Personal actions to eliminate drug use that poses a threat to health

Health Beliefs: Perceived Control: Personal conviction that one can influence a health outcome

Medication Response: Therapeutic and adverse effects of prescribed medication

Multiple Sclerosis Self-Management: Personal actions to manage multiple sclerosis and prevent disease progression

Participation in Health Care Decisions: Personal involvement in selecting and evaluating health care options to achieve desired outcome

Postpartum Maternal Health Behavior: Personal actions to promote health of a mother in the period following birth of infant

Prenatal Health Behavior: Personal actions to promote a healthy pregnancy and a healthy newborn

Seizure Control: Personal actions to reduce or minimize the occurrence of seizure episodes

Self-Care: Non-Parenteral Medication: Ability to administer oral and topical medications to meet therapeutic goals independently with or without assistive device

Self-Care: Parenteral Medication: Ability to administer parenteral medications to meet therapeutic goals independently with or without assistive device

Smoking Cessation Behavior: Personal actions to eliminate tobacco use

Symptom Control: Personal actions to minimize perceived adverse changes in physical and emotional functioning

Systemic Toxin Clearance: Dialysis: Clearance of toxins from the body with peritoneal dialysis or hemodialysis

Treatment Behavior: Illness or Injury: Personal actions to palliate or eliminate pathology

Goals/Evaluation Criteria

Examples Using NOC Language

- Demonstrates **Compliance Behavior**, as evidenced by the following indicators (specify 1–5: never, rarely, sometimes, often, or consistently demonstrated)
- Performs treatment regimen as prescribed
- Monitors treatment response
- Performs self-screening when directed
- Performs activities of daily living as prescribed

Other Examples

- Changes or modifies health regimen as directed by health professional
- Reports symptom control
- Monitors personal behavior risk factors

NIC Interventions

Asthma Management: Identification, treatment, and prevention of reactions to inflammation/constriction in the airway passages

Bedside Laboratory Testing: Performance of laboratory tests at the bedside or point of care

Cognitive Restructuring: Challenging a patient to alter distorted thought patterns and view self and the world more realistically

Counseling: Use of an interactive helping process focusing on the needs, problems, or feelings of the patient and significant others to enhance or support coping, problem-solving, and interpersonal relationships

Decision-Making Support: Providing information and support for a patient who is making a decision regarding health care

Environmental Management: Safety: Monitoring and manipulation of the physical environment to promote safety

Health System Guidance: Facilitating a patient's location and use of appropriate health services

Hemodialysis Therapy: Management of extracorporeal passage of the patient's blood through a dialyzer

Laboratory Data Interpretation: Critical analysis of patient laboratory data in order to assist with clinical decision making

Medication Management: Facilitation of safe and effective use of prescription and over-the-counter drugs

Nutritional Counseling: Use of an interactive helping process focusing on the need for diet modification

Peritoneal Dialysis Therapy: Administration and monitoring of dialysis solution into and out of the peritoneal cavity

Postpartal Care: Monitoring and management of the patient who has recently given birth

Prenatal Care: Monitoring and management of patient during pregnancy to prevent complications of pregnancy and promote a healthy outcome for both mother and infant

Self-Awareness Enhancement: Assisting a patient to explore and understand his thoughts, feelings, motivations, and behaviors

Self-Care Assistance: Assisting another to perform ADLs

Self-Efficacy Enhancement: Strengthening an individual's confidence in his ability to perform a health behavior

Self-Modification Assistance: Reinforcement of self-directed change initiated by the patient to achieve personally important goals

Self-Responsibility Facilitation: Encouraging a patient to assume more responsibility for own behavior

Smoking Cessation Assistance: Helping another to stop smoking

Substance Use Treatment: Supportive care of patient and family members with physical and psychosocial problems associated with the use of alcohol or drugs

Teaching: Disease Process: Assisting the patient to understand information related to a specific disease process

Teaching: Individual: Planning, implementation, and evaluation of a teaching program designed to address a patient's particular needs

Teaching: Prescribed Activity/Exercise: Preparing a patient to achieve or maintain a prescribed level of activity

Teaching: Prescribed Diet: Preparing a patient to correctly follow a prescribed diet

Teaching: Prescribed Medication: Preparing a patient to safely take prescribed medications and monitor for their effects

Teaching: Procedure/Treatment: Preparing a patient to understand and mentally prepare for a prescribed procedure or treatment

Teaching: Psychomotor Skill: Preparing a patient to perform a psychomotor skill

Nursing Activities

Assessments

- Assess patient's level of understanding of illness, complications, and recommended treatments to determine knowledge deficit
- Interview patient and family to determine problem areas in integrating treatment regimen into lifestyle
- *(NIC) Self-Modification Assistance:*
  - Appraise the patient's reasons for wanting to change
  - Appraise the patient's present knowledge and skill level in relationship to the desired change
  - Appraise the patient's social and physical environment for extent of support of desired behaviors

Patient/Family Teaching

- Identify essential treatments
- Offer information on community resources specific to health goals of patient (e.g., support groups)
- Assist patient to identify situational obstacles that interfere with adherence to therapeutic regimen
- Provide information on illness, complications, and recommended treatments

- *(NIC) Self-Modification Assistance:* Instruct the patient on how to move from continuous reinforcement to intermittent reinforcement

Collaborative Activities

- Collaborate with other health care providers to determine how to modify therapeutic regimen without jeopardizing patient's health

Other

- Assist patient to develop realistic plan to achieve adherence to therapeutic regimen. Plan should include the following:
  - Identification of modifications or adaptations in ADLs
  - Identification of support systems to achieve therapeutic goals
  - Identification of actions patient and family are willing to take (e.g., dietary changes, exercise modification, sleep pattern changes, medication and treatment schedules, sexual activity modifications, role changes)
- Provide coaching and support to motivate patient's continued adherence to therapy
- *(NIC) Self-Modification Assistance:*
  - Assist the patient in identifying a specific goal for change
  - Assist the patient in identifying target behaviors that need to change to achieve the desired goal
  - Explore with the patient potential barriers to change behavior
  - Identify with the patient the most effective strategies for behavior changes
  - Encourage the patient to identify appropriate, meaningful reinforcers and rewards
  - Foster moving toward primary reliance on self-reinforcement versus family or nurse rewards
  - Assist the patient in identifying the circumstances or situations in which the behavior occurs (e.g., cues or triggers)
  - Explain to the patient the importance of self-monitoring in attempting behavior change

Home Care

- The preceding activities can be used or adapted for home care
- Assist the patient or family to find ways to integrate the therapeutic regimen into their activities of daily living

SELF-HEALTH MANAGEMENT, READINESS FOR ENHANCED

(2002, 2008) **Domain 1, Health Promotion; Class 2, Health Management**

Definition: Pattern of regulating and integrating into daily living a therapeutic program for the treatment of illness and its sequelae that is sufficient for meeting health-related goals and can be strengthened

Defining Characteristics

Objective

Choices of daily living are appropriate for meeting goals (e.g., treatment, prevention)

No unexpected acceleration of illness symptoms

Subjective

Describes reduction of risk factors

Expresses desire to manage the illness (e.g., treatment, prevention of sequelae)

Expresses little difficulty with prescribed regimens

Suggestions for Use

This diagnosis does not need to include related factors because it is a wellness diagnosis.

S

NOC Outcomes

Adherence Behavior: Self-initiated actions to promote optimal wellness, recovery, and rehabilitation

Compliance Behavior: Personal actions to promote wellness, recovery, and rehabilitation recommended by a health professional

Health Orientation: Personal commitment to health behaviors as lifestyle priorities

Knowledge: Treatment Regimen: Extent of understanding convened about a specific treatment regimen

Participation in Health Care Decisions: Personal involvement in selecting and evaluating health care options to achieve desired outcome

Risk Control: Personal actions to prevent, eliminate, or reduce modifiable health threats

Treatment Behavior: Illness or Injury: Personal actions to palliate or eliminate pathology

Goals/Evaluation Criteria

Examples Using NOC Language

- Demonstrates **Adherence Behavior**, as evidenced by the following indicators (specify 1–5: never, rarely, sometimes, often, or consistently demonstrated):
  - Uses reputable health information to develop health strategies
  - Provides rationale for adopting a health regimen
  - Describes rationale for deviating from a recommended health regimen
  - Performs self-monitoring of health status
- Demonstrates **Participation in Health Care Decisions**, as evidenced by the following indicator (specify 1–5: never, rarely, sometimes, often, or consistently demonstrated): Evaluates satisfaction with health care outcomes
- Demonstrates **Risk Control**, as evidenced by the following indicators (specify 1–5: never, rarely, sometimes, often, or consistently demonstrated):
  - Monitors environmental and personal behavior risk factors
  - Participates in screening for associated health problems and identified risks

Other Examples

- Describes and follows prescribed health regimens (e.g., diet, exercise)
- Changes or modifies health regimen as directed by health provider
- Reports symptom control

NIC Interventions

Anticipatory Guidance: Preparation of patient for an anticipated developmental or situational crisis

Decision-Making Support: Providing information and support for a patient who is making a decision regarding health care

Family Involvement Promotion: Facilitating family participation in the emotional and physical care of the patient

Health Education: Developing and providing instruction and learning experiences to facilitate voluntary adaptation of behavior conducive to health in individuals, families, groups, or communities

Health System Guidance: Facilitating a patient's location and use of appropriate health services

Mutual Goal Setting: Collaborating with patient to identify and prioritize care goals, then developing a plan for achieving those goals

Risk Identification: Analysis of potential risk factors, determination of health risks, and prioritization of risk-reduction strategies for an individual or group

Self-Modification Assistance: Reinforcement of self-directed change initiated by the patient to achieve personally important goals

Teaching: Individual: Planning, implementation, and evaluation of a teaching program designed to address a patient's particular needs

Teaching: Procedure/Treatment: Preparing a patient to understand and mentally prepare for a prescribed procedure or treatment

Nursing Activities

Assessments

- Assess patient's knowledge of health promotion and disease prevention
- Identify patient's usual methods of coping and problem solving

Patient/Family Teaching

- Help patient to plan for the future by providing information on the usual course of the patient's illness
- Teach stress management techniques
- *(NIC) Health System Guidance:*

  Explain the immediate health care system, how it works, and what the patient and family can expect

  Inform the patient of accreditation and state health department requirements for judging the quality of a facility

  Give written instructions for purpose and location of health care activities, as appropriate

  Inform patient how to access emergency services by telephone and vehicle, as appropriate

S

Collaborative Activities

- Offer information on community resources specific to health goals of the patient (e.g., support groups)
- *(NIC) Health System Guidance:* Identify and facilitate communication among health care providers and patient and family, as appropriate

Other

- Help patient to identify and prepare for upcoming developmental milestones, role changes, or situational crises
- Help patient to identify situational obstacles that interfere with adherence to therapeutic regimen
- Plan to visit patient at strategic developmental or situational times
- *(NIC) Health System Guidance:* Encourage the patient and family to ask questions about services and charges

SELF-MUTILATION

(2000) **Domain 11, Safety/Protection; Class 3, Violence**

Definition: Deliberate self-injurious behavior causing tissue damage with the intent of causing nonfatal injury to attain relief of tension

Defining Characteristics

Objective

Abrading
Biting
Constricting a body part
Cuts or scratches on body
Hitting
Ingestion or inhalation of harmful substances [or objects]
Insertion of object(s) into body orifice(s)
Picking at wounds
Self-inflicted burns (e.g., eraser, cigarette)
Severing

Related Factors

Subjective

Disturbed body image
Feels threatened with [actual or potential] loss of significant relationship (e.g., loss of parent or parental relationship)
Irresistible urge to cut self
Irresistible urge for self-directed violence
Low or unstable self-esteem
Mounting tension that is intolerable
Negative feelings (e.g., depression, rejection, self-hatred, separation anxiety, guilt, depersonalization)
Unstable body image

Objective

Adolescence
Autistic individual
Battered child
Borderline personality disorder
Character disorder
Childhood illness or surgery
Childhood sexual abuse
Depersonalization
Developmentally delayed individual

Dissociation
Disturbed interpersonal relationships
Eating disorders
Emotionally disturbed
Family alcoholism
Family divorce
Family history of self-destructive behaviors
History of inability to plan solutions or see long-term consequences
History of self-injurious behaviors
Impulsivity
Inability to express tension verbally
Incarceration
Ineffective coping
Isolation from peers
Labile behavior (mood swings)
Lack of family confidant
Living in nontraditional setting (e.g., foster, group, or institutional care)
Needs quick reduction of stress
Peers who self-mutilate
Perfectionism
Poor parent–adolescent communication
Psychotic state (command hallucinations)
Sexual identity crisis
Substance abuse

Use of manipulation to obtain nurturing relationship with others
Violence between parental figures

Suggestions for Use

Use *Self-mutilation* for a patient who has already inflicted injury on self. Use *Risk for self-mutilation* when risk factors are present, but the person has not actually exhibited injurious behavior.

Suggested Alternative Diagnoses

Suicide, risk for

NOC Outcomes

Identity: Distinguishes between self and nonself and characterizes one's essence

Impulse Self-Control: Self-restraint of compulsive or impulsive behaviors

Self-Mutilation Restraint: Personal actions to refrain from intentional self-inflicted injury (nonlethal)

Goals/Evaluation Criteria

See Goals/Evaluation Criteria for the diagnosis Self-Mutilation, Risk for, following.

NIC Interventions

Behavior Management: Self-Harm: Assisting the patient to decrease or eliminate self-mutilating or self-abusive behaviors

Cognitive Restructuring: Challenging a patient to alter distorted thought patterns and view self and the world more realistically

Counseling: Use of an interactive helping process focusing on the needs, problems, or feelings of the patient and significant others to enhance or support coping, problem-solving, and interpersonal relationships

Environmental Management: Safety: Monitoring and manipulation of the physical environment to promote safety

Impulse Control Training: Assisting the patient to mediate impulsive behavior through application of problem-solving strategies to social and interpersonal situations

Limit Setting: Establishing the parameters of desirable and acceptable patient behavior

Patient Contracting: Negotiating an agreement with an individual which reinforces a specific behavior change

Self-Awareness Enhancement: Assisting a patient to explore and understand his thoughts, feelings, motivations, and behaviors

Wound Care: Prevention of wound complications and promotion of wound healing

S

Nursing Activities

For All Patients

Assessments

- Assess self-injury behaviors, including methods used, known triggers, and so forth
- Assess nature and extent of the injuries
- *(NIC) Behavior Management: Self-Harm*: Determine the motive or reason for the behaviors

Collaborative Activities

- Obtain medical orders, as needed, to treat self-inflicted injuries (e.g., cuts, abrasions)

Patient/Family Teaching

- Provide support and education to family regarding patient status and methods of treatment
- *(NIC) Behavior Management: Self-Harm*: Instruct patient in coping strategies (e.g., assertiveness training, impulse control training, and progressive muscle relaxation), as appropriate

Other

- Provide patient safety, using least restrictive measures (e.g., environmental manipulation, assign roommate, assign patient room close to nursing station, family and visitor restriction, patient within eyesight at all times, patient within arm's length, other interventions specific to patient)
- Accompany patient to activities outside of the unit, as needed
- *(NIC) Behavior Management: Self-Harm:*

  Develop appropriate behavioral expectations and consequences, given the patient's level of cognitive functioning and capacity for self-control

  Remove dangerous items from the patient's environment

  Use a calm, nonpunitive approach when dealing with self-harmful behaviors
- Use physical or manual restraint and time-outs as needed to calm patient who is expressing anger inappropriately
- Identify consequences of inappropriate expression of anger
- Establish trust and rapport

S

Psychotic Patients

Assessments

- Observe for behavioral changes from baseline assessment (e.g., increased withdrawal, agitation)
- Assess patient for morbid preoccupation with suicide, self-mutilation, hopelessness, and worthlessness
- Assess patient with command hallucinations to determine content and source (e.g., ask patient: "Whose voice is it? What did the voice tell you to do? Did the voice tell you to hurt yourself and how? Does the voice have control over you?")
- Monitor intensity of hallucinations and delusions and attempt reality testing (specify frequency)
- Determine whether religious, persecutory, or somatic delusions contributed to the self-injury

Collaborative Activities

- Obtain physician order if intervention is a denial of rights
- *(NIC) Behavior Management: Self-Harm*: Administer medications, as appropriate, to decrease anxiety, stabilize mood, and decrease self-stimulation

Other

- If patient exhibits calmness abruptly following a period of agitation, provide increased safety measures to prevent self-injury
- Assist patient to differentiate internal stimuli from outside world
- Encourage patient to verbalize thoughts and impulses instead of storing up tension
- Search patient and environment for potentially harmful items
- Trim patient's fingernails and toenails to prevent scratching
- Encourage physical activity
- Contract with patient to not injure self
- If patient is unable to make contract or follow directions, stay with patient at all times until either patient reports a decrease in command hallucinations, delusions, or self-mutilation impulses, or until seclusion or restraint is used
- *(NIC) Behavior Management: Self-Harm:*

  Place patient in a more protective environment (e.g., area restriction and seclusion) if self-harmful impulses or behaviors escalate

  Apply, as appropriate, mitts, splints, helmets, or restraints to limit mobility and ability to initiate self-harm

  Assist patient to identify situations and feelings that may prompt self-harm

Personality Disorder Patients

Assessments

- Assess patient's level of impulsivity and frustration tolerance

Patient/Family Teaching

- Teach patient alternative stress-tension-relieving measures (e.g., relaxation techniques; physical exercise; journal writing; self-affirmations; and distracting techniques such as music, television, and conversation)
- Provide family and significant other with guidelines explaining how self-harmful behavior can be managed outside the care environment
- *(NIC) Behavior Management: Self-Harm*: Provide illness teaching to patient and significant others if self-harmful behavior is illness based (e.g., borderline personality disorder or autism)

Collaborative Activities

- Consider antianxiety or neuroleptic medications according to physician order
- Provide the consistent responses to patient by collaborating closely with other health care providers. Review treatment plan frequently to prevent staff splitting and conflict regarding treatment goals.

Other

- Encourage patient to seek out staff and peers instead of using alcohol or drugs
- Establish regular and frequent check-in times with assigned staff
- *(NIC) Behavior Management: Self-Harm:*
  Contract with patient, as appropriate, for "no self-harm"
  Provide the predetermined consequences if patient is engaging in self-harmful behaviors

Retarded or Autistic Patients

Assessments

- Assess patient's response to environment to determine if there were stressors that led to self-injury

Patient/Family Teaching

- *(NIC) Behavior Management: Self-Harm*: Provide illness teaching to patient and significant others if self-harmful behavior is illness based (e.g., borderline personality disorder or autism)

Other

- Alter environmental situations that produce stress that provokes self-injury behaviors
- Remove reinforcement that may induce self-injury behavior (e.g., comforting patient after headbanging, excusing patient from perceived unpleasant tasks)
- Develop behavioral plan that will decrease the incidence of self-injury
- Use protective devices to prevent self-injury (e.g., mitts, helmet, jacket restraint, protective clothing)

S

SELF-MUTILATION, RISK FOR

(1992, 2000) **Domain 11, Safety/Protection; Class 3, Violence**

Definition: At risk for deliberate self-injurious behavior causing tissue damage with the intent of causing nonfatal injury to attain relief of tension

Risk Factors

Subjective

Depersonalization
Disturbed body image

Feels threatened with [actual or potential] loss of significant relationship
Irresistible urge to cut or damage self
[Low or unstable body image]
Low or unstable self-esteem
Mounting tension that is intolerable
Needs quick reduction of stress
Negative feelings (e.g., depression, rejection, self-hatred, separation anxiety, guilt)
Perfectionism
Psychotic state (command hallucinations)

Objective

Adolescence
Autistic individuals
Battered child
Borderline personality disorder
Character disorders
Childhood illness or surgery
Childhood sexual abuse
Developmentally delayed individual
Dissociation
Disturbed interpersonal relationships
Eating disorders
Emotionally disturbed child
Family alcoholism
Family divorce
Family history of self-destructive behaviors
History of inability to plan solutions or see long-term consequences
History of self-injurious behavior
Impulsivity
Inability to express tension verbally
Inadequate coping
Incarceration
Isolation from peers
Living in nontraditional setting (e.g., foster, group, or institutional care)
Loss of control over problem-solving situations
Loss of significant relationships
Peers who self-mutilate
Sexual identity crisis
Substance abuse
Use of manipulation to obtain nurturing relationship with others
Violence between parental figures

Suggestions for Use

Risk for self-mutilation is a more specific diagnosis than *Risk for self-directed violence*, although the two diagnoses have some of the same defining characteristics (i.e., risk factors). *Risk for self-directed violence* includes actions such as drug and alcohol abuse and high-risk lifestyle (e.g., driving fast), which are not included in *Risk for self- mutilation.*

Suggested Alternative Diagnoses

Self-directed violence, risk for
Self-mutilation
Suicide, risk for

NOC Outcomes

(**NOTE:** Self-Mutilation Restraint is the essential outcome to enable you to determine whether this potential diagnosis is progressing to actual Self-Mutilation. Other outcomes should be chosen according to the patient's risk factors.)

Impulse Self-Control: Self-restraint of compulsive or impulsive behaviors

Self-Mutilation Restraint: Personal actions to refrain from intentional self-inflicted injury (nonlethal)

Goals/Evaluation Criteria

Examples Using NOC Language

S

- Demonstrates **Self-Mutilation Restraint**, as evidenced by the following indicators (specify 1–5: never, rarely, sometimes, often, or consistently demonstrated):
  - Upholds contract to not harm self
  - Refrains from gathering means for self-injury
  - Maintains self-control without supervision

Other Examples

- Refrains from injuring self
- Verbalizes reduction or absence of command hallucinations or delusions
- Identifies feelings that lead to impulsive actions
- Identifies and avoids high-risk environments and situations

NIC Interventions

Anger Control Assistance: Facilitation of the expression of anger in an adaptive nonviolent manner

Anxiety Reduction: Minimizing apprehension, dread, foreboding, or uneasiness related to an unidentified source of anticipated danger

Behavior Management: Self-Harm: Assisting the patient to decrease or eliminate self-mutilating or self-abusive behaviors

Environmental Management, Safety: Monitoring and manipulation of the physical environment to promote safety

Impulse Control Training: Assisting the patient to mediate impulsive behavior through application of problem-solving strategies to social and interpersonal situations

Nursing Activities

NOTE: Choose interventions and nursing activities directed at modifying risk factors and preventing self-mutilation.

For All Patients

Assessments

- Assess patient for history of self-injury behaviors, including methods used, known triggers, and so forth
- *(NIC) Anger Control Assistance*: Monitor potential for inappropriate aggression and intervene before its expression
- *(NIC) Behavior Management: Self-Harm*: Determine the motive or reason for the behaviors

Patient/Family Teaching

- Provide support and education to family regarding patient status and methods of treatment
- *(NIC) Behavior Management: Self-Harm*: Instruct patient in coping strategies (e.g., assertiveness training, impulse control training, and progressive muscle relaxation, as appropriate)

S

Other

- Provide patient safety, using least restrictive measures (e.g., environmental manipulation, assign roommate, assign patient room close to nursing station, family and visitor restriction, patient within eyesight at all times, patient within arm's length, other interventions specific to patient)
- Accompany patient to activities outside of the unit, as needed
- *(NIC) Behavior Management: Self-Harm:*

  Develop appropriate behavioral expectations and consequences, given the patient's level of cognitive functioning and capacity for self-control

  Remove dangerous items from the patient's environment

  Use a calm, nonpunitive approach when dealing with self-harmful behaviors

- *(NIC) Anger Control Assistance:*
  - Use external controls (e.g., physical or manual restraint, time-outs) as needed (as last resort) to calm patient who is expressing anger in a maladaptive manner
  - Identify consequences of inappropriate expression of anger
  - Establish basic trust and rapport with patient

Psychotic Patients

Assessments

- Observe for behavioral changes from baseline assessment (e.g., increased withdrawal, agitation)
- Assess patient for morbid preoccupation with suicide, self-mutilation, hopelessness, and worthlessness
- Assess patient with command hallucinations to determine content and source (e.g., ask patient: "Whose voice is it? What is the voice telling you to do? Is the voice telling you to hurt yourself and how? Does the voice have control over you?")
- Monitor intensity of hallucinations or delusions and attempt reality testing (specify frequency)
- Assess patient for religious or persecutory delusions that may lead to self-injury
- Assess patient for somatic delusions that may lead to self-injury (e.g., beliefs that part of body is diseased, rotten, or unnecessary)

Collaborative Activities

- Obtain physician order if intervention is a denial of rights
- *(NIC) Behavior Management: Self-Harm*: Administer medications, as appropriate, to decrease anxiety, stabilize mood, and decrease self-stimulation

Other

- If patient exhibits calmness abruptly following a period of agitation, provide increased safety measures to prevent self-injury
- Assist patient to differentiate internal stimuli from outside world
- Encourage patient to verbalize thoughts and impulses instead of storing up tension
- Search patient as needed for potentially harmful items
- Trim patient's fingernails and toenails to prevent scratching
- Encourage physical activity
- Contract with patient to not injure self
- If patient is unable to make contract or follow directions, stay with patient at all times until either patient reports a decrease in command hallucinations, delusions, or self-mutilation impulses or until seclusion or restraint is used

- *(NIC) Behavior Management: Self-Harm:*
  Place patient in a more protective environment (e.g., area restriction and seclusion) if self-harmful impulses or behaviors escalate
  Apply, as appropriate, mitts, splints, helmets, or restraints to limit mobility and ability to initiate self-harm
  Assist patient to identify situations and feelings that prompt self-harmful behavior

Personality Disorder Patients

Assessments

- Assess patient's level of impulsivity and frustration tolerance

Patient/Family Teaching

- Teach patient alternative stress-tension-relieving measures (e.g., relaxation techniques; physical exercise; journal writing; self-affirmations; and distracting techniques such as music, television, and conversation)
- Provide family and significant other with guidelines explaining how self-harmful behavior can be managed outside the care environment
- *(NIC) Behavior Management: Self-Harm*: Provide illness teaching to patient and significant others if self-harmful behavior is illness based (e.g., borderline personality disorder or autism)

Collaborative Activities

- Consider antianxiety or neuroleptic medications according to physician order
- Provide consistent responses to patient by collaborating closely with other health care providers. Review treatment plan frequently to prevent staff splitting and conflict regarding treatment goals.

Other

- Encourage patient to seek out staff and peers instead of using alcohol or drugs
- Establish regular and frequent check-in times with assigned staff
- *(NIC) Behavior Management: Self-Harm:*
  Contract with patient, as appropriate, for "no self-harm"
  Provide the predetermined consequences if patient is engaging in self-harmful behaviors

Retarded/Autistic Patients

Assessments

- Assess patient's response to environment to determine if there is a stressor that may lead to self-injury

Patient/Family Teaching

- *(NIC) Behavior Management: Self-Harm*: Provide illness teaching to patient and significant others if self-harmful behavior is illness based (e.g., borderline personality disorder or autism)

Other

- Alter environmental situations that may produce stress that provokes self-injury behaviors
- Remove reinforcement that may induce self-injury behavior (e.g., comforting patient after headbanging, excusing patient from perceived unpleasant tasks)
- Develop behavioral plan that will prevent or decrease incidence of self-injury
- Use protective devices to prevent self-injury (e.g., mitts, helmet, jacket restraint, protective clothing)

SELF-NEGLECT

(2008) **Domain 4, Activity/Rest; Class 5, Self-Care**

Definition: A constellation of culturally framed behaviors involving one or more self-care activities in which there is a failure to maintain a socially accepted standard of health and well-being (Gibbons, Lauder, & Ludwick, 2006).

Defining Characteristics

Objective

Inadequate environmental hygiene
Inadequate personal hygiene
Nonadherence to health activities

Related Factors

Capgras syndrome
Cognitive impairment (e.g., dementia)
Depression
Executive processing ability
Fear of institutionalization
Frontal lobe dysfunction
Functional impairment
Learning disability
Lifestyle choice
Maintaining control

Major life stressor
Malingering
Obsessive-compulsive disorder
Paranoid personality disorders
Schizotypal personality disorders
Substance abuse

Suggested Alternative Diagnosis

Home maintenance, impaired
Self-care deficit, bathing, dressing, or toileting

NOC Outcomes

Self-Care: Activities of Daily Living (ADL): Ability to perform the most basic physical tasks and personal care activities independently with or without assistive device

Self-Care: Bathing: Ability to cleanse own body independently with or without assistive device

Self-Care: Dressing: Ability to dress self independently with or without assistive device

Self-Care: Hygiene: Ability to maintain own personal cleanliness and kempt appearance independently with or without assistive device

Self-Care: IADLs: Ability to perform activities needed to function in the home or community independently with or without assistive device

Self-Care: Oral Hygiene: Ability to care for own mouth and teeth independently with or without assistive device

Self-Care: Toileting: Ability to toilet self independently with or without assistive device

Goals/Evaluation Criteria

Examples Using NOC Language

- Client will not neglect self, as demonstrated by Self-Care: Activities of Daily Living, IADLs, Bathing, Dressing, Hygiene, Oral Hygiene, and Toileting
- Will demonstrate **Self-Care: Hygiene**, as evidenced by the following indicators (specify 1–5: severely, substantially, moderately, mildly, or not compromised):

  Cleans perineal area
  Keeps nose blown and clean
  Combs or brushes hair
  Maintains body hygiene

Other Examples

- Performs activities of daily living (e.g., toileting, bathing, dressing)
- Caregiver assists patient with environmental management, as needed

NIC Interventions

Oral Health Maintenance: Maintenance and promotion of oral hygiene and dental health for the patient at risk for developing oral or dental lesions

Self-Care Assistance: Assisting another to perform ADLs

Self-Care Assistance, Bathing/Hygiene: Assisting patient to perform personal hygiene

Self-Care Assistance: Dressing/Grooming: Assisting patient with clothes and makeup

Self-Care Assistance: IADL: Assisting and instructing a person to perform instrumental activities of daily living (IADL) needed to function in the home or community

Self-Care Assistance: Toileting: Assisting another with elimination

Nursing Activities

Nursing activities focus on identifying the etiological factors for the patient's *Self-Neglect*, determining the severity of the problem, correcting the problem, or facilitating the patient's efforts to cope with it.

Assessments

- Perform a mental status examination
- Perform a complete physical assessment, paying close attention to personal hygiene
- Assess living arrangement and people available to help with activities of daily living
- Perform a home safety assessment
- Determine level of involvement and support among family members and significant others
- Inquire about recent changes in circumstances and life circumstances (e.g., loss of a partner, physical changes)
- Assess the patient's desire and ability to change the situation
- Monitor for indicators of resolution of *Self-Neglect*
- *(NIC) Self-Care Assistance:*
  - Monitor patient's ability for independent self-care
  - Monitor patient's need for adaptive devices for personal hygiene, dressing, grooming, toileting, and eating

S

Patient/Family Teaching

- *(NIC) Self-Care Assistance*: Teach parents/family to encourage independence, to intervene only when the patient is unable to perform
- Provide information specific to client needs (e.g., discuss dietary requirements)

Collaborative Activities

- Develop a multidisciplinary team, if possible (e.g., case manager, dietitian, physician, occupational therapist)
- Refer to Meals on Wheels or other meals-at-home plan, as needed
- Recommend alternative placements if satisfactory home- and self-care cannot be achieved.

Other

- Develop a therapeutic relationship with client and family
- Encourage client to express concerns
- Help client identify goals and priorities
- Encourage family members to participate in care planning and decision making
- Assist with setting up a safe medication regimen
- *(NIC) Self-Care Assistance*:
  - Consider age of patient when promoting self-care activities
  - Encourage patient to perform normal activities of daily living to level of ability
  - Establish a routine for self-care activities

SEXUAL DYSFUNCTION

(1980, 2006) **Domain 8, Sexuality; Class 2, Sexual Function**

S

Definition: The state in which an individual experiences a change in sexual function during the sexual response phases of desire, excitation, and/or orgasm, which is viewed as unsatisfying, unrewarding, or inadequate

Defining Characteristics

Subjective

Alterations in achieving sexual satisfaction
Change of interest in self or others
Inability to achieve desired satisfaction
Perceived alteration in sexual excitation
Perceived deficiency of sexual desire
Perceived limitations imposed by disease or therapy
Verbalization of problem

Objective

Actual limitations imposed by disease or therapy
Alterations in achieving perceived sex role
Seeking confirmation of desirability

Other Defining Characteristics (Non-NANDA International)

Concern over adequacy in meeting sexual desire of partner
Painful coitus
Phobic avoidance of sexual experience

Related Factors

Absent or ineffectual role models
Altered body function or structure (e.g., pregnancy, recent childbirth, drugs, surgery, anomalies, disease process, trauma, radiation)
Biopsychosocial alteration of sexuality
Lack of privacy
Lack of significant other
Misinformation or lack of knowledge
Physical abuse
Psychosocial abuse (e.g., harmful relationships)
Values conflict
Vulnerability

Other Related Factors (Non-NANDA International)

Body image disturbance
Disturbance in self-esteem
Hormonal changes
Medical treatment
Pain
Sexual trauma or exploitation
Unrealistic expectations of self and partner
Vaginal dryness

Suggestions for Use

If patient data does not fit the defining characteristics, consider the more general label *Ineffective sexuality patterns*. **Note**: *Sexual dysfunction* may be a symptom of other diagnoses, such as *Rape-trauma syndrome*. Or it may be the etiology of other diagnoses, such as *Anxiety* or *Situational low self-esteem*.

Suggested Alternative Diagnoses

Body image, disturbed
Rape-trauma syndrome
Self-esteem, chronic or situational low
Sexuality pattern, ineffective

NOC Outcomes

Abuse Recovery: Sexual: Extent of healing of physical and psychological injuries due to sexual abuse or exploitation

Knowledge: Pregnancy and Postpartum Sexual Functioning: Extent of understanding conveyed about sexual function during pregnancy and postpartum

Physical Aging: Normal physical changes that occur with the natural aging process

Risk Control: Sexually Transmitted Diseases (STDs): Personal actions to prevent, eliminate, or reduce behaviors associated with sexually transmitted disease

Sexual Functioning: Integration of physical, socioemotional, and intellectual aspects of sexual expression and performance

Sexual Identity: Acknowledgment and acceptance of own sexual identity

Goals/Evaluation Criteria

Examples Using NOC Language

- Demonstrates **Abuse Recovery: Sexual**, as evidenced by the following indicators (specify 1–5: none, limited, moderate, substantial, or extensive):
  Evidence of non-abusive same-sex relationships
  Evidence of non-abusive opposite-sex relationships
  Expressions of comfort with gender identity and sexual orientation
- Demonstrates **Sexual Functioning**, as evidenced by the following indicators (specify 1–5: never, rarely, sometimes, often, or consistently demonstrated):
  Attains sexual arousal
  Sustains arousal through orgasm
  Expresses ability to be intimate
  Expresses acceptance of partner
  Expresses willingness to be sexual

Other Examples

Patient and partner will:

- Demonstrate willingness to discuss changes in sexual function
- Request needed information about changes in sexual function
- Verbalize understanding of medically imposed restrictions
- Adapt modes of sexual expression to accommodate age- or illness-related physical changes
- Verbalize ways to avoid STDs

NIC Interventions

Abuse Protection Support: Identification of high-risk, dependent relationships and actions to prevent further infliction of physical or emotional harm

Behavior Modification: Promotion of a behavior change

Counseling: Use of an interactive helping process focusing on the needs, problems, or feelings of the patient and significant others to enhance or support coping, problem solving, and interpersonal relationships

Infection Control: Minimizing the acquisition and transmission of infectious agents

Postpartal Care: Monitoring and management of the patient who has recently given birth

Prenatal Care: Monitoring and management of patient during pregnancy to prevent complications of pregnancy and promote a healthy outcome for both mother and infant

Risk Identification: Analysis of potential risk factors, determination of health risks, and prioritization of risk-reduction strategies for an individual or group

Self-Awareness Enhancement: Assisting a patient to explore and understand his thoughts, feelings, motivations, and behaviors

Sexual Counseling: Use of an interactive helping process focusing on the need to make adjustments in sexual practice or to enhance coping with a sexual event or disorder

Teaching: Sexuality: Assisting individuals to understand physical and psychosocial dimensions of sexual growth and development

Teaching: Safe Sex: Providing instruction concerning sexual protection during sexual activity

Nursing Activities

Assessments

- Monitor for indicators of resolution of *Sexual dysfunction* (e.g., capacity for intimacy)
- *(NIC) Sexual Counseling:*
  - Preface questions about sexuality with a statement that tells the patient that many people experience sexual difficulties
  - Determine amount of sexual guilt associated with the patient's perception of the causative factors of the illness

Patient/Family Teaching

- Provide information necessary to enhance sexual function (e.g., anticipatory guidance, educational materials, stress-reduction exercises, sensation-enhancing exercises, prosthetics, implants, focused counseling)

- *(NIC) Sexual Counseling:*
  - Discuss the effect of the illness, health situation, and medication on sexuality, as appropriate [e.g., medication side effects; normal aspects of aging; postsurgical adjustments, especially after surgery on sexual organs or ostomy; postmyocardial infarction]
  - Discuss the necessary modifications in sexual activity, as appropriate
  - Inform patient early in the relationship that sexuality is an important part of life and that illness, medications, and stress (or other problems or events the patient is experiencing) often alter sexual functioning
  - Provide factual information about sexual myths and misinformation that patient may verbalize
  - Instruct the patient only on techniques compatible with [the patient's] values and beliefs

Collaborative Activities

- Encourage continuation of counseling after discharge
- *(NIC) Sexual Counseling:*
  - Provide referral or consultation with other members of the health care team, as appropriate
  - Refer the patient to a sex therapist, as appropriate

Other

- Encourage verbalization of sexual concerns by utilizing caregivers who have an established rapport with patient and are comfortable discussing patient's sexual concerns, specify caregiver
- Allow time and privacy to address patient's sexual concerns
- Alert patient and partner to possibility of disinterest in, decreased capacity for, or discomfort during sexual activity
- *(NIC) Sexual Counseling:*
  - Encourage patient to verbalize fears and to ask questions
  - Help patient to express grief and anger about alterations in body functioning and appearance, as appropriate
  - Include the spouse or sexual partner in the counseling as much as possible, as appropriate
  - Introduce patient to positive role models who have successfully conquered a similar problem, as appropriate
  - Provide reassurance and permission to experiment with alternative forms of sexual expression, as appropriate

Home Care

- The preceding activities are appropriate for home care
- Assist the client and partner to create a time and place for privacy in which to develop their sexual relationship; assist them to be assertive and communicate this need to others in the family, as needed

For Older Adults

- Assess the older client's sexual needs and functioning
- Inform clients of normal changes of aging, such as reduced vaginal lubrication in women and less firm erections in men
- Suggest methods to improve sexual functioning (e.g., use of water-soluble lubricant and Kegel exercises for women)

SEXUALITY PATTERNS, INEFFECTIVE

(1986, 2006) **Domain 8, Sexuality; Class 2, Sexual Function**

Definition: Expressions of concern regarding own sexuality

Defining Characteristics

Subjective

Alterations in achieving perceived sex role
Alteration in relationship with significant other
Values conflict

Objective

Reports changes in sexual activities or behaviors
Reports difficulties with sexual activities or behaviors
Reports limitations in sexual activities or behaviors

Related Factors

Conflicts with sexual orientation or variant preferences
Fear of pregnancy
Fear of acquiring sexually transmitted infection
Impaired relationship with significant other
Ineffective or absent role models
Knowledge or skill deficit about alternative responses to health-related transitions, altered body function or structure, illness, or medical treatment
Lack of privacy
Lack of significant other

Other Related Factors (Non-NANDA International)

Body image disturbance
Low self-esteem
Illness or medical treatments

Suggestions for Use

When possible, use a more specific label, such as *Sexual dysfunction*.

Suggested Alternative Diagnoses

Body image, disturbed
Rape-trauma syndrome
Self-esteem, situational low
Sexual dysfunction

NOC Outcomes

Abuse Recovery: Sexual: Extent of healing of physical and psychological injuries due to sexual abuse or exploitation

Physical Maturation: Female: Normal physical changes in the female that occur with the transition from childhood to adulthood

Physical Maturation: Male: Normal physical changes in the male that occur with the transition from childhood to adulthood

Sexual Identity: Acknowledgement and acceptance of own sexual identity

Goals/Evaluation Criteria

Examples Using NOC Language

- Demonstrates **Abuse Recovery: Sexual**, as evidenced by the following indicators (specify 1–5: none, limited, moderate, substantial, or extensive):
  - Evidence of non-abusive same-sex relationships
  - Evidence of non-abusive opposite-sex relationships
  - Expressions of comfort with gender identity and sexual orientation
- Demonstrates **Self-Esteem**, as evidenced by the following indicators (specify 1–5: never, rarely, sometimes, often, or consistently positive):
  - Verbalizations of self-acceptance
  - Feelings about self-worth
  - Expected response from others

Other Examples

Patient and partner will:

- Actively participate in counseling
- Request needed information about sexuality
- Acknowledge importance of discussing sexual issues with partner

- Discuss concerns about sexuality
- Express satisfaction with sexuality
- Verbalize feelings of self-acceptance and/or self-worth

NIC Interventions

Abuse Protection Support: Identification of high-risk, dependent relationships and actions to prevent further infliction of physical or emotional harm

Body Image Enhancement: Improving a patient's conscious and unconscious perceptions and attitudes toward his body

Coping Enhancement: Assisting a patient to adapt to perceived stressors, changes, or threats that interfere with meeting life demands and roles

Counseling: Use of an interactive helping process focusing on the needs, problems, or feelings of the patient and significant others to enhance or support coping, problem solving, and interpersonal relationships

Role Enhancement: Assisting a patient, significant other, or family to improve relationships by clarifying and supplementing specific role behaviors

Self-Esteem Enhancement: Assisting a patient to increase his personal judgment of self-worth

Sexual Counseling: Use of an interactive helping process focusing on the need to make adjustments in sexual practice or to enhance coping with a sexual event or disorder

Teaching: Safe Sex: Providing instruction concerning sexual protection during sexual activity

Teaching: Sexuality: Assisting individuals to understand physical and psychosocial dimensions of sexual growth and development

Nursing Activities

Refer to Nursing Activities for the diagnosis Sexual Dysfunction, preceding.

SHOCK, RISK FOR

(2008)

Domain 11, Safety/Protection; Class 2, Physical Injury

Definition: At risk for an inadequate blood flow to the body's tissues, which may lead to life-threatening cellular dysfunction

Risk Factors

Hypotension
Hypovolemia
Hypoxemia

Hypoxia
Infection
Sepsis
Systemic inflammatory response syndrome

Suggestions for Use

The risk factors for this diagnosis represent collaborative problems, for which the primary independent nursing actions are monitoring and prevention. For example, if the risk factor is hypotension, focus would be on monitoring the blood pressure. Instead of stating a diagnosis such as Risk for shock related to hypotension, it seems preferable to write a collaborative problem (e.g., Potential Complication of hypotension: Shock).

NOC Outcomes

The primary outcome for measuring actual occurrence of shock is Tissue Perfusion: Cellular. Select other outcomes depending on the patient's unique risk factors.

Blood Loss Severity: Severity of internal or external bleeding/hemorrhage
Blood Transfusion Reaction: Severity of complications with blood transfusion reaction
Circulation Status: Unobstructed, unidirectional blood flow at an appropriate pressure through large vessels of the systemic and pulmonary circuits
Infection Severity: Severity of infection and associated symptoms
Risk Control: Personal actions to prevent, eliminate, or reduce modifiable health threats
Risk Detection: Personal actions to identify personal health threats
Tissue Perfusion: Cellular: Adequacy of blood flow through the vasculature to maintain function at the cellular level
Vital Signs: Extent to which temperature, pulse, respiration, and blood pressure are within normal range

Goals/Evaluation Criteria

Examples Using NOC Language

- Patient will not experience shock, as demonstrated by adequate Tissue Perfusion: Cellular, and Vital Signs within normal range.
- Will demonstrate normal **Tissue Perfusion: Cellular**, as evidenced by the following indicators (specify 1–5, severe, substantial, moderate, mild, or no deviation from normal range):
  - Blood pressure (systolic and diastolic)
  - Capillary refill
  - Oxygen saturation
  - Creatinine clearance

Other Examples

- Vital signs within normal range for the patient (as a rule, blood pressure at least 90 mmHg, heart rate between 60 and 100 bpm with normal rhythm, and respiratory rate of 12 to 20 breaths/minute)
- Normal urine output (0.5 mL/kg/hr)
- Fluid intake and output in balance
- Skin warm and dry

NIC Interventions

NIC interventions that focus on monitoring and preventing shock, regardless of the risk factors, are Risk Identification, Shock Prevention, and Vital Signs Monitoring. Choose other interventions depending on the patient's actual risk factors.

Bleeding Precautions: Reduction of stimuli that may induce bleeding or hemorrhage in at-risk patients

Bleeding Reduction: Limitation of the loss of blood volume during an episode of bleeding

Bleeding Reduction: Antepartum Uterus: Limitation of the amount of blood loss from the pregnant uterus during third trimester of pregnancy

Bleeding Reduction: Gastrointestinal: Limitation of the amount of blood loss from the pregnant uterus during third trimester of pregnancy

Bleeding Reduction: Nasal: Limitation of the amount of blood loss from the nasal cavity

S

Bleeding Reduction: Postpartum: Limitation of the amount of blood loss from the postpartum uterus

Bleeding Reduction: Wound: Limitation of the amount of blood loss from a wound that may be a result of trauma, incisions, or placement of a tube or catheter

Blood Products Administration: Administration of blood or blood products and monitoring of patient's response

Circulatory Care: Arterial Insufficiency: Promotion of arterial circulation

Circulatory Care: Venous Insufficiency: Promotion of venous circulation

Embolus Care: Pulmonary: Limitation of complications for a patient experiencing, or at risk for, occlusion of pulmonary circulation

Hemorrhage Control: Reduction or elimination of rapid and excessive blood loss

Hypovolemia Management: Expansion of intravascular fluid volume in a patient who is volume depleted

Infection Control: Minimizing the acquisition and transmission of infectious agents

Infection Protection: Prevention and early detection of infection in a patient at risk

Oxygen Therapy: Administration of oxygen and monitoring of its effectiveness

Respiratory Monitoring: Collection and analysis of patient data to ensure airway patency and adequate gas exchange

Risk Identification: Analysis of potential risk factors, determination of health risks, and prioritization of risk-reduction strategies for an individual or group

Shock Prevention: Detecting and treating a patient at risk for impending shock

Surveillance: Purposeful and ongoing acquisition, interpretation, and synthesis of patient data for clinical decision making

Vital Signs Monitoring: Collection and analysis of cardiovascular, respiratory, and body temperature data to determine and prevent complications

Nursing Activities

Nursing activities for this potential problem focus on monitoring for and preventing actual shock, as well as assessing for risk factors. Choose preventive measures to address your patient's risk factors (e.g., hypovolemia, infection).

Assessments

- Monitor for conditions that may lead to hypovolemia (e.g., surgery, anticoagulant therapy, prolonged diarrhea and vomiting, heavy bleeding)
- Assess for cardiac conditions (myocardial infarction, ventricular dysrhythmias, cardiac arrest, malignant hypertension, severe congestive heart failure)
- Assess for circulatory conditions (e.g., pulmonary embolus, tension pneumothorax, aortic stenosis)
- Monitor intake and output, including wounds, drains, vomiting, and diarrhea
- Monitor vital signs (TPR and BP)
- Monitor skin color and moisture

Patient/Family Teaching

- Teach patient/family about preventing infection (e.g., wound and skin care, hand hygiene, avoiding crowds if Immunocompromised)
- Teach signs and symptoms of shock (e.g., excessive bleeding, fluid loss, chest pain); teach to report these symptoms

Collaborative Activities

- Monitor invasive hemodynamic parameters, if available (e.g., central venous pressure, cardiac output, mean arterial pressure)
- Administer prescribed medicated to treat risk factors (e.g., vasoactive drugs, antimicrobials, cardiac gylcosides)
- Administer oxygen, if symptoms indicate progression to actual shock, or as needed for ongoing treatment of a risk factor
- Refer to nutritionist if special diet is needed to promote immune system health or healing

Other

- Be prepared to administer fluids, electrolytes, colloids, or blood/blood products for circulating volume problems
- Use strict aseptic methods to prevent infection (e.g., hand hygiene between clients, aseptic wound care, isolation precautions)
- Provide oral, enteral, or parenteral nutrition

SKIN INTEGRITY, IMPAIRED

(1975, 1998) **Domain 11, Safety/Protection, Class 2, Physical Injury**

Definition: Altered epidermis and dermis

Defining Characteristics

Objective

Destruction of skin layers (dermis)
Disruption of skin surface (epidermis)
Invasion of body structures

Related Factors

External [Environmental]

Chemical substance
Humidity
Hyperthermia
Hypothermia
Mechanical factors (e.g., shearing forces, pressure, restraint)
Medications
Moisture
Physical immobilization
Radiation

Internal [Somatic]

Changes in fluid status
Changes in pigmentation
Changes in turgor (changes in elasticity)
Developmental factors
Imbalanced nutritional state (e.g., obesity, emaciation)
Immunological deficit
Impaired circulation
Impaired metabolic state
Impaired sensation
Skeletal prominence

Developmental Factors

Extremes in age

Suggestions for Use

Impaired skin integrity is rather nonspecific. A disruption of the skin surface could be a surgical incision, abrasion, blisters, or decubitus ulcers. When this label is used, the type of disruption should be specified in the problem, not in the etiology. **Note**: In the following example, the dermal ulcer is a specific type of *Impaired skin integrity*, not a cause of *Impaired skin integrity*:

Correct: Impaired skin integrity: dermal ulcer related to complete immobility
Incorrect: Impaired skin integrity related to dermal ulcer

When an ulcer is deeper than the epidermis, use *Impaired tissue integrity* instead of *Impaired skin integrity*. Deeper ulcers may require a collaborative approach (i.e., surgical treatment). Do not use *Impaired skin integrity* as a label for a surgical incision, because there are no independent nursing actions to treat this type of "impairment" and the condition is usually self-limiting. The usual nursing care for a surgical incision is to prevent and detect infection; therefore, a diagnosis of *Risk for infection of surgical incision* or the collaborative problem Potential Complication of Surgery: Incision infection might be used instead of *Impaired skin integrity*.

Suggested Alternative Diagnoses

Infection, risk for
Skin integrity, risk for impaired
Tissue integrity, impaired

NOC Outcomes

Allergic Response: Localized: Severity of localized hypersensitive immune response to a specific environmental (exogenous) antigen

Burn Healing: Extent of healing of a burn site

Tissue Integrity: Skin and Mucous Membranes: Structural intactness and normal physiologic function of skin and mucous membranes

Wound Healing: Primary Intention: Extent of regeneration of cells and tissues following intentional closure

Wound Healing: Secondary Intention: Extent of regeneration of cells and tissues in an open wound

Goals/Evaluation Criteria

Examples Using NOC Language

- Demonstrates **Tissue Integrity: Skin and Mucous Membranes**, as evidenced by the following indicators (specify 1–5: severely, substantially, moderately, mildly, or not compromised):
  - Skin temperature, elasticity, hydration, and sensation
  - Tissue perfusion
  - Skin integrity
- Demonstrates **Wound Healing: Primary Intention**, as evidenced by the following indicators (specify 1–5: none, limited, moderate, substantial, or extensive):
  - Skin approximation
  - Wound edge approximation
  - Scar formation
- Demonstrates **Wound Healing: Primary Intention**, as evidenced by the following indicators (specify 1–5: extensive, substantial, moderate, limited, or none):
  - Surrounding skin erythema
  - Foul wound odor
- Demonstrates **Wound Healing: Secondary Intention**, as evidenced by the following indicators (specify 1–5: none, limited, moderate, substantial, or extensive):
  - Granulation
  - Scar formation
  - Decreased wound size

Other Examples

- Patient and family demonstrate optimal skin or wound care routine
- Purulent (or other) drainage or wound odor minimal
- Blistered or macerated skin not present
- Necrosis, sloughing, tunneling, undermining, or sinus tract formation decreased to absent
- Skin and periwound erythema limited

NIC Interventions

Medication Administration: Preparing, giving, and evaluating the effectiveness of prescription and nonprescription drugs

Incision Site Care: Cleansing, monitoring, and promotion of healing in a wound that is closed with sutures, clips, or staples

Pressure Management: Minimizing pressure to body parts

Pressure Ulcer Care: Facilitation of healing in pressure ulcers

Pruritus Management: Preventing and treating itching

Skin Care: Topical Treatments: Application of topical substances or manipulation of devices to promote skin integrity and minimize skin breakdown

Skin Surveillance: Collection and analysis of patient data to maintain skin and mucous membrane integrity

Wound Care: Prevention of wound complications and facilitation of wound healing

Nursing Activities

Also see Nursing Activities for Skin Integrity, Risk for Impaired.

Assessments

- Assess functioning of equipment such as pressure-relieving devices, including static-air mattress, low-air loss therapy, air-fluidized therapy, and water bed
- *(NIC) Incision Site Care*: Inspect the incision site for redness, swelling, or signs of dehiscence or evisceration
- *(NIC) Wound Care:*

  Inspect the wound with each dressing change

  Monitor characteristics of the wound, including drainage, color, size, and odor

  Monitor wound for:

  Location, dimensions, and depth

  Presence and character of exudate, including tenacity, color, and odor

  Presence or absence of granulation or epithelialization

  Presence or absence of necrotic tissue, describe color, odor, amount

  Presence or absence of symptoms of local wound infection (e.g., pain on palpation, edema, pruritus, induration, warmth, foul odor, eschar, exudate)

  Presence or absence of undermining or sinus-tract formation

Patient/Family Teaching

- Instruct in care of surgical incision, including signs and symptoms of infection, ways to keep incision dry during bath, and minimization of stress on the incision

Collaborative Activities

- Consult dietitian for foods high in proteins, minerals, calories, and vitamins
- Consult physician regarding implementation of enteral feedings or parenteral nutrition to increase wound healing potential
- Refer to enterostomal therapy nurse for assistance with assessment, staging, treatment, and documentation of wound care or skin breakdown
- *(NIC) Wound Care*: Apply TENS (transcutaneous electrical nerve stimulation) unit for wound healing enhancement, as appropriate

Other

- Evaluate topical dressing and treatment measures, which may include hydrocolloid dressings, hydrophilic dressings, absorbent dressings, and so forth
- Establish a wound or skin care routine, which may include the following:
- Frequently turn and reposition patient
  - Keep surrounding tissue free from excess moisture and drainage
  - Protect patient from fecal and urinary contamination
  - Protect patient from other wound and drain-tube excretions into wound
- Clean and dress surgical incision site using the following principles of sterility or medical asepsis, as appropriate:
  - Wear disposable gloves (sterile, if needed)
  - Clean incision from "clean to dirty," using one swab for each wipe
  - Clean around staples or sutures, using sterile cotton-tipped applicator
  - Clean around drain last, moving from center outward in a circular motion
  - Apply antiseptic ointment, as ordered
  - Change dressing at appropriate intervals or leave open to air according to order
- *(NIC) Wound Care:*
  - Remove dressing and adhesive tape
  - Clean with normal saline or a nontoxic cleanser, as appropriate
  - Place affected area in a whirlpool bath, as appropriate
  - Administer skin ulcer care, as needed
  - Position to avoid placing tension on the wound, as appropriate
- Administer IV site, Hickman line, or central venous line site care, as appropriate
- Massage the area around the wound to stimulate circulation

Home Care

- The preceding activities are appropriate for home care use
- Institute case management or refer to a wound or ostomy nurse as needed
- *(NIC) Skin Surveillance*: Instruct family member and caregiver about signs of skin breakdown, as appropriate
- *(NIC) Wound Care*: Instruct patient or family member(s) in wound care procedures

SKIN INTEGRITY, IMPAIRED, RISK FOR

(1975, 1998, 2010) **Domain 11, Safety/Protection; Class 2, Physical Injury**

Definition: At risk for alteration in epidermis and/or dermis
NOTE: Risk should be determined by the use of a standardized risk assessment tool (e.g., Braden Scale).

Risk Factors

External [Environmental]

Chemical substance
Excretions and secretions
Extremes of age
Humidity
Hyperthermia
Hypothermia
Mechanical factors (e.g., shearing forces, pressure, restraint)
[Medications]
Moisture
Physical immobilization
Radiation

Internal [Somatic]

Changes in pigmentation
Changes in skin turgor (i.e., changes in elasticity)
Developmental factors
Imbalanced nutritional state (e.g., obesity, emaciation)
Immunologic factors
Impaired circulation
Impaired metabolic state
Impaired sensation
Psychogenetic factors
Skeletal prominence

Suggestions for Use

Use this diagnosis for patients who have no symptoms but who are at risk of developing disruption of skin surface or destruction of skin layers if preventive measures are not instituted. The presence of more than one risk factor increases the likelihood of skin damage. When *Risk for impaired skin integrity* occurs as a result of immobility and when other body systems are also at risk for impairment, consider using *Risk for disuse syndrome*.

Suggested Alternative Diagnosis

Disuse syndrome, risk for
Skin integrity, impaired

NOC Outcomes

To assess for actual occurrence of Impaired Skin Integrity, use the following outcome:

Tissue Integrity: Skin and Mucous Membranes: Structural intactness and normal physiological function of skin and mucous membranes

The following are examples of outcomes associated with risk factors:

Immobility Consequences: Physiological: Severity of compromise in physiologic functioning due to impaired physical mobility

Nutritional Status: Extent to which nutrients are available to meet metabolic needs

Risk Control: Sun Exposure: Personal actions to prevent or reduce threats to the skin and eyes from sun exposure

Tissue Perfusion: Peripheral: Adequacy of blood flow through the small vessels of the extremities to maintain tissue function

Urinary Continence: Control of elimination of urine from the bladder

Goals/Evaluation Criteria

Examples Using NOC Language

- Demonstrates **Immobility Consequences: Physiological**, as evidenced by the following indicators (specify 1–5: severe, substantial, moderate, mild, or none): Pressure sores
- Demonstrates **Tissue Integrity: Skin and Mucous Membranes**, as evidenced by the following indicators (specify 1–5: severely, substantially, moderately, mildly, or not compromised):

    Sensation
    Elasticity
    Hydration
    Texture
    Thickness
    Skin integrity

Other Examples

- Demonstrates effective skin care routine
- Has strong and symmetric pulses
- Normal skin color
- Warm skin temperature
- Absence of pain in the extremities
- Ingests foods adequate to promote skin integrity

NIC Interventions

Bed Rest Care: Promotion of comfort and safety and prevention of complications for a patient unable to get out of bed

Bowel Incontinence Care: Promotion of bowel continence and maintenance of perianal skin integrity

Circulatory Care: Arterial Insufficiency: Promotion of arterial circulation

Circulatory Care: Venous Insufficiency: Promotion of venous circulation

Incision Site Care: Cleansing, monitoring, and promotion of healing in a wound that is closed with sutures, clips, or staples

Nutrition Management: Assisting with or providing a balanced dietary intake of foods and fluids

Pressure Management: Minimizing pressure to body parts

Pressure Ulcer Prevention: Prevention of pressure ulcers for an individual at high risk for developing them

Skin Surveillance: Collection and analysis of patient data to maintain skin and mucous membrane integrity

Nursing Activities

Nursing activities for this diagnosis are primarily for surveillance and prevention.

All Patients at Risk

Assessments

- On admission and whenever physical condition changes, assess for risk factors that may lead to skin breakdown (e.g., bed or chair confinement, inability to move, loss of bowel or bladder control, poor nutrition, and lowered mental awareness)
- Identify sources of pressure and friction (e.g., cast, bedding, clothing)
- *(NIC) Pressure Ulcer Prevention:*

  Use an established risk assessment tool to monitor patient's risk factors (e.g., Braden scale)

  Inspect skin over bony prominences and other pressure points when repositioning or at least daily

- *(NIC) Skin Surveillance:*
  - Monitor skin and mucous membranes for the following:
  - Rashes and abrasions
  - Color and temperature
  - Excessive dryness and moistness
  - Areas of discoloration, bruising, and breakdown

Collaborative Activities

- Refer to enterostomal therapy nurse for assistance with prevention, assessment, and treatment of skin breakdown or wounds

Other

- Use a pressure-reducing mattress (e.g., polyurethane foam pad)
- Avoid massage over bony prominences
- *(NIC) Pressure Ulcer Prevention:*
  - Apply elbow and heel protectors, as appropriate
  - Keep bed linens clean, dry, and wrinkle-free

Patients with Mobility/Activity Deficit

Assessments

- Assess for extent of limitations in ability to transfer or move about in bed

Other

- Pad cast edges and traction connections

For chair-bound individuals:

- Consider postural alignment; distribution of weight, balance, and stability; and pressure relief when positioning individuals in chairs or wheelchairs
- Have patient shift weight q 15 minutes if able
- Use pressure-reducing devices for seating surfaces, do not use donut-type devices

S

For bed-bound individuals:

- Avoid positioning directly on the trochanter
- Elevate the head of the bed as little and for as short a time as possible
- Use a pressure-reducing mattress or bed (e.g., foam, air, egg-crate)
- Use proper positioning, transferring, and turning techniques
- Use lifting devices to move, rather than drag, individuals during transfers and position changes
- *(NIC) Pressure Ulcer Prevention:*
  - Turn q 1–2 h, as appropriate
  - Provide trapeze to assist patient in shifting weight frequently
  - Position with pillows to elevate pressure points off the bed
  - Apply elbow and heel protectors, as appropriate

Patients with Incontinence or Presence of Moisture

Assessments

- Assess need for indwelling or condom catheter
- Check for urinary or fecal incontinence q ______________

Other

- Cleanse skin at time of soiling
- Individualize bathing schedule, avoid hot water, use mild cleansing agent
- Minimize skin exposure to moisture
- *(NIC) Pressure Ulcer Prevention:*
  Remove excessive moisture on the skin resulting from perspiration, wound drainage, and fecal or urinary incontinence
  Apply protective barriers, such as creams or moisture-absorbing pads, to remove excess moisture, as appropriate
  Avoid use of "donut" type devices to sacral area
  Avoid massaging over bony prominences
  Turn with care (e.g., avoid shearing) to prevent injury to fragile skin

Patients with Nutritional Deficit

Assessments

- Monitor nutritional status and food intake

Collaborative Activities

- Consult dietitian for foods high in protein, minerals, and vitamins
- Request physician order for serum albumin level, packed-cell volume, and transferrin levels

Other

- Compare actual weight to ideal body weight
- Investigate factors that compromise an apparently well-nourished individual's dietary intake (especially protein or calories) and offer support with eating
- *(NIC) Pressure Ulcer Prevention:* Ensure adequate dietary intake, especially protein, vitamins B and C, iron, and calories, using supplements, as appropriate

Home Care

- The preceding activities may be adapted for home care use

SLEEP DEPRIVATION

(1998)

Domain 4, Activity/Rest; Class 1, Sleep/Rest

Definition: Prolonged periods of time without sleep (sustained natural, periodic suspension of relative consciousness)

Defining Characteristics

Subjective

Anxiety
Daytime drowsiness
Fatigue
Hallucinations
Heightened sensitivity to pain
Inability to concentrate
Malaise
Perceptual disorders (e.g., disturbed body sensation, delusions, feeling afloat)

Objective

Acute confusion
Agitation
Apathy
Combativeness
Decreased ability to function
Hand tremors
Irritability
Lethargy
Listlessness
Nystagmus, fleeting
Restlessness
Slowed reaction
Transient paranoia

Related Factors

Aging-related sleep stage shifts
Dementia
Familial sleep paralysis
Idiopathic central nervous system hypersomnolence
Inadequate daytime activity
Narcolepsy
Nightmares

Nonsleep-inducing parenting practices
Periodic limb movement (e.g., restless leg syndrome, nocturnal myoclonus)
Prolonged physical discomfort
Prolonged psychologic discomfort
Prolonged use of pharmacologic or dietary antisoporifics
Sleep apnea
Sleep terror
Sleepwalking
Sleep-related enuresis
Sleep-related painful erections
Sundowner's syndrome
Sustained circadian asynchrony
Sustained environmental stimulation
Sustained inadequate sleep hygiene
Sustained [unfamiliar or] uncomfortable sleep environment

Suggestions for Use

Because *Sleep deprivation* represents a lack of sleep that continues over long periods of time, the defining characteristics are more varied and more severe than those for *Insomnia* or *Disturbed sleep pattern*, which involve a short-term lack of sleep that might occur, for example, during a brief hospitalization. Therefore, in addition to measures to promote and restore sleep, nursing activities for *Sleep deprivation* will focus on relieving symptoms, such as paranoia, restlessness, and confusion. *Sleep deprivation* can be the etiology of other nursing diagnoses, for example, *Anxiety, Acute confusion*, and *Impaired memory*.

Suggested Alternative Diagnoses

Activity intolerance
Confusion, acute
Fatigue
Insomnia
Sleep pattern, disturbed

NOC Outcomes

Acute Confusion Level: Severity of disturbance in consciousness and cognition that develops over a short period of time

Sleep: Natural periodic suspension of consciousness during which the body is restored

Symptom Severity: Severity of perceived adverse changes in physical, emotional, and social functioning

Goals/Evaluation Criteria

Examples Using NOC Language

- Demonstrates **Sleep**, as evidenced by the following indicators (specify 1–5: severely, substantially, moderately, mildly, or not compromised):
  Feelings of rejuvenation after sleep
  Sleep pattern and quality
  Sleep routine
  Observed hours of sleep
  Wakeful at appropriate times

Other Examples

The patient will:

- Report relief from symptoms of *Sleep deprivation* (e.g., confusion, anxiety, daytime drowsiness, perceptual disorders, and tiredness)
- Identify and use measures that will increase rest or sleep
- Identify factors that contribute to *Sleep deprivation* (e.g., pain, inadequate daytime activity)

NIC Interventions

Delirium Management: Provision of a safe and therapeutic environment for the patient who is experiencing an acute confusional state

Energy Management: Regulating energy use to treat or prevent fatigue and optimize function

Medication Management: Facilitation of safe and effective use of prescription and over-the-counter drugs

S

Mood Management: Providing for safety, stabilization, recovery, and maintenance of a patient who is experiencing dysfunctionally depressed or elevated mood

Reality Orientation: Promotion of patient's awareness of personal identity, time, and environment

Sleep Enhancement: Facilitation of regular sleep–wake cycles

Nursing Activities

See Nursing Activities for Insomnia, and Nursing Activities for Readiness for Enhanced Sleep.

Assessments

- Assess for symptoms of *Sleep deprivation*, such as *Acute confusion*, agitation, *Anxiety*, perceptual disorders, slowed reactions, and irritability

Patient Teaching

- Teach physiological and safety consequences of sleep apnea
- Teach patient and family about factors that interfere with sleep (e.g., stress, hectic lifestyle, shift work, room temperature too cold or too hot)

Collaborative Activities

- Confer with physician regarding need to revise medication regimen when it interferes with sleep
- Confer with physician regarding use of sleep medications that do not suppress rapid eye movement (REM) sleep
- Make referrals as needed for treatment of severe symptoms of *Sleep deprivation* (e.g., *Acute confusion*, agitation, or *Anxiety*)

Other

- Treat symptoms of *Sleep deprivation*, as needed (e.g., *Anxiety*, restlessness, transient paranoia, inability to concentrate); these will vary with individual patients

Home Care

- Provide teaching for clients learning to use continuous positive airway pressure (CPAP) machines

SLEEP PATTERN, DISTURBED

(1980, 1998, 2006) **Domain 4, Activity/Rest; Class 1, Sleep/Rest**

Definition: Time-limited interruptions of sleep amount and quality due to external factors

S

Defining Characteristics

Subjective

Dissatisfaction with sleep
Reports being awakened
Reports no difficulty falling asleep
Reports not feeling well rested

Objective

Change in normal sleep pattern
Other possible defining characteristics (non-NANDA-I)
Dark circles under the eyes
Decreased attention span
Frequent daytime napping
Frequent yawning
Restless

Related Factors

Ambient humidity
Ambient temperature
Caregiving responsibilities
Change in daylight-darkness exposure
Interruptions (e.g., for therapeutics, monitoring, lab tests)
Lack of sleep control
Lack of sleep privacy
Lighting
Noise
Noxious odors
Physical restraint
Sleep partner
Unfamiliar sleep furnishings

Suggestions for Use

Disturbed sleep pattern is used when sleep is temporarily disrupted, as is common in hospitalization. It is a general diagnosis. Etiologic factors are needed to make it specific enough to direct nursing interventions (e.g., *Disturbed sleep pattern related to frequent awakening of infant during the night*). When sleep disruption is prolonged or when symptoms are severe enough to interfere with the patient's lifestyle, diagnose either *Insomnia* or *Sleep deprivation*.

Suggested Alternative Diagnoses

Fatigue
Insomnia
Sleep Deprivation

NOC Outcomes

Sleep: Natural periodic suspension of consciousness during which the body is restored

Goals/Evaluation Criteria

Examples Using NOC Language

- Demonstrates **Sleep**, as evidenced by the following indicators (specify 1–5: severely, substantially, moderately, mildly, or not compromised):
    - Feelings of rejuvenation after sleep
    - Sleep pattern and quality
    - Sleep routine

Observed hours of sleep
Wakeful at appropriate times

Other Examples

The patient will:

- Identify measures that will increase rest or sleep
- Demonstrate physical and psychological well-being
- Report sleeping well at night

NIC Interventions

Energy Management: Regulating energy use to treat or prevent fatigue and optimize function

Environmental Management: Manipulation of the patient's surroundings for therapeutic benefit, sensory appeal, and psychological well-being

Medication Management: Facilitation of safe and effective use of prescription and over-the-counter drugs

Relaxation Therapy: Use of techniques to encourage and elicit relaxation for the purpose of decreasing undesirable signs and symptoms such as pain, muscle tension, or anxiety

Sleep Enhancement: Facilitation of regular sleep–wake cycles

Nursing Activities

Nursing activities for *Disturbed sleep pattern* focus on teaching and supporting sleep hygiene, as well as modifying external factors that interrupt sleep.

Assessments

- Assess for symptoms of *Sleep deprivation* and *Insomnia,* such as *Acute confusion*, agitation, *Anxiety*, perceptual disorders, slowed reactions, and irritability
- Identify environmental factors (e.g., noise, lights) that can interrupt sleep
- *(NIC) Sleep Enhancement:*
  Determine the effects of the patient's medications on sleep pattern
  Determine patient's sleep/activity pattern
  Monitor/record patient's sleep pattern and number of sleep hours

Patient Teaching

- *(NIC) Sleep Enhancement:*
  Instruct patient and significant others about factors (e.g., physiological, psychological, lifestyle, frequent work shift changes, rapid time zone changes, excessively long work hours, and other environmental factors) that contribute to sleep pattern disturbances

Instruct patient how to perform autogenic muscle relaxation or other nonpharmacological forms of sleep inducement

Explain the importance of adequate sleep during pregnancy, illness, psychosocial stresses, and so on

Instruct patient to avoid bedtime foods and beverages that interfere with sleep [e.g., caffeine]

Collaborative Activities

- Confer with physician regarding need to revise medication regimen when it interferes with sleep
- Confer with physician regarding use of sleep medications that do not suppress rapid eye movement (REM) sleep
- Make referrals as needed for treatment of severe symptoms of *Disturbed sleep pattern* (e.g., *Acute confusion*, agitation, or *Anxiety*)

Other

- Treat symptoms of *Disturbed sleep pattern*, as needed (e.g., drowsiness, restlessness, inability to concentrate); these will vary with individual patients
- Avoid loud noises and use of overhead lights during nighttime sleep, providing a quiet, peaceful environment and minimizing interruptions
- Find a compatible roommate for the patient, if possible
- Help patient identify possible underlying causes of sleeplessness, such as fear, unresolved problems, and conflicts
- Reassure patient that irritability and mood alterations are common consequences of interrupted sleep
- *(NIC) Sleep Enhancement*

Facilitate maintenance of patient's usual bedtime routine, presleep cues/props, and familiar objects (e.g., for children, a favorite blanket/toy, rocking, pacifier, or story; for adults, a book to read), as appropriate

Assist to eliminate stressful situations before bedtime

Initiate/implement comfort measures of massage, positioning, and affective touch

Provide for naps during the day, if indicated, to meet sleep requirements

Regulate environmental stimuli to maintain normal day–night cycles

SLEEP, READINESS FOR ENHANCED

(2002) **Domain 4, Activity/Rest; Class 1, Sleep/Rest**

Definition: A pattern of natural, periodic suspension of consciousness that provides adequate rest, sustains a desired lifestyle, and can be strengthened

Defining Characteristics

Subjective

Reports being rested after sleep
Expresses willingness to enhance sleep

Objective

Amount of sleep is congruent with developmental needs
Follows sleep routines that promote sleep habits
Occasional use of medications to induce sleep

Related Factors

This is a wellness diagnosis; an etiology is not necessary.

Suggestions for Use

If risk factors are present, use *Risk for disturbed sleep pattern, Risk for sleep deprivation*, or *Risk for insomnia*.

Suggested Alternative Diagnoses

Sleep pattern, disturbed (risk for)
Sleep deprivation (risk for)
Insomnia (risk for)

NOC Outcomes

Sleep: Natural periodic suspension of consciousness during which the body is restored

Goals/Evaluation Criteria

Refer to NOC Outcomes for the diagnosis Sleep Deprivation.

Other Examples

Patient will:

- Identify measures that will increase rest or sleep
- Demonstrate physical and psychologic well-being
- Obtain adequate sleep without use of medications

NIC Interventions

Environmental Management: Comfort: Manipulation of the patient's surroundings for promotion of optimal comfort
Sleep Enhancement: Facilitation of regular sleep–wake cycles

Nursing Activities

Assessments

- Assess for evidence of improvements in sleep
- Monitor the patient's sleep pattern
- *(NIC) Sleep Enhancement:* Determine the effects of the patient's medications on sleep pattern

Patient/Family Teaching

- *(NIC) Sleep Enhancement:*
  Instruct patient to avoid bedtime foods and beverages that interfere with sleep
  Instruct the patient and significant others about factors (e.g., physiologic, psychologic, lifestyle, frequent work-shift changes, rapid time-zone changes, excessively long work hours, and other environmental factors) that contribute to sleep pattern disturbances

Collaborative Activities

- Confer with physician regarding need to revise medication regimen when it interferes with sleep pattern
- *(NIC) Sleep Enhancement*: Encourage use of sleep medications that do not contain REM-sleep suppressors

Other

- Avoid loud noises and use of overhead lights during night time sleep, providing a quiet, peaceful environment and minimizing interruptions
- Find a compatible roommate for the patient, if possible
- Help patient identify and anticipate factors that can cause sleeplessness, such as fear, unresolved problems, and conflicts
- *(NIC) Sleep Enhancement:*
  Facilitate maintenance of patient's usual bedtime routine, presleep cues/props, and familiar objects (e.g., for children, a favorite blanket/toy, rocking, pacifier, or story; for adults, a book to read), as appropriate
  Assist patient to limit daytime sleep by providing activity that promotes wakefulness, as appropriate

S

Home Care

- The preceding activities are appropriate or can be modified for home care use

For Older Adults

- Suggest a warm bath before bedtime
- Advise client to limit fluid intake during the evening
- Advise client to take diuretics early in the morning

SOCIAL INTERACTION, IMPAIRED

(1986) **Domain 7, Role Relationships; Class 3, Role Performance**

Definition: Insufficient or excessive quantity or ineffective quality of social exchange

Defining Characteristics

Subjective

Discomfort in social situations
Inability to receive a satisfying sense of social engagement (e.g., belonging, caring, interest, or shared history)

Objective

Dysfunctional interaction with others
Family reports changes in interactions (e.g., style, pattern)
Inability to communicate a satisfying sense of social engagement (e.g., belonging, caring, interest, or shared history)
Use of unsuccessful social interaction behaviors

Related Factors

Absence of significant others
Communication barriers
Deficit about ways to enhance mutuality (e.g., knowledge, skills)
Disturbed thought processes
Environmental barriers
Limited physical mobility
Self-concept disturbance
Sociocultural dissonance
Therapeutic isolation

Other Related Factors (Non-NANDA International)

Chemical dependence
Developmental disability
Impaired cognitive abilities
Psychologic impairment (specify)

Suggestions for Use

Differentiate between *Impaired social interaction* and *Social isolation*. A diagnosis of *Impaired social interaction* focuses more on the patient's social skills and abilities, whereas *Social isolation* focuses on the patient's feelings of aloneness and may not be a result of his ineffective social skills. Compare the defining characteristics and related factors in Table 9 in Suggestions for Use for Social Isolation.

Suggested Alternative Diagnoses

Communication: verbal, impaired
Self-esteem, chronic or situational low
Social isolation

NOC Outcomes

Child Development: Middle Childhood (6–11 Years), and Adolescence (12–17 Years): Milestones of physical, cognitive, and psychosocial progression from 6 years through 11 years and from 12 years through 17 years of age [NOC lists each age as a separate outcome.]

Family Social Climate: Supportive milieu as characterized by family member relationships and goals

Leisure Participation: Use of relaxing, interesting, and enjoyable activities to promote well-being

Play Participation: Use of activities by a child from 1 year through 11 years of age to promote enjoyment, entertainment, and development

Social Interaction Skills: Personal behaviors that promote effective relationships

Social Involvement: Social interactions with persons, groups, or organizations

S

Goals/Evaluation Criteria

Examples Using NOC Language

- Demonstrates **Play Participation** (specify 1–5: never, rarely, sometimes, often, or consistently demonstrated)
- Demonstrates **Social Interaction Skills** (specify 1–5: never, rarely, sometimes, often, or consistently demonstrated)
- Demonstrates **Child Development**, as evidenced by the following indicators (specify 1–5: never, rarely, sometimes, often, or consistently demonstrated). [Refer to pediatrics text or NOC manual for age-specific indicators; an exhaustive list is beyond the scope of this text.]
  - 2 months: Shows pleasure in interactions, especially with primary caregivers
  - 4 months: Recognizes parents' voices and touch
  - 6 months: Comforts self
  - 12 months: Waves bye-bye
  - 2 years: Interacts with adults in simple games
  - 3 years: Plays interactive games with peers

4 years: Describes a recent experience
5 years: Follows simple rules of interactive games with peers
6–11 years: Plays in groups
12–17 years: Uses effective social interaction skills

- Demonstrates **Family Social Climate**, as evidenced by the following indicators (specify 1–5: never, rarely, sometimes, often, or consistently demonstrated): Participates in activities together
- Demonstrates **Social Involvement**, as evidenced by the following indicators (specify 1–5: never, rarely, sometimes, often, or consistently demonstrated): Interacts with close friends, neighbors, family members, and members of work group(s)

Other Examples

Patient will:

- Acknowledge the effect of own behavior on social interactions
- Demonstrate behaviors that may increase or improve social interactions
- Acquire/improve social interaction skills (e.g., disclosure, cooperation, sensitivity, assertiveness, genuineness, compromise)
- Express a desire for social contact with others
- Participate in and enjoy appropriate play

NIC Interventions

Behavior Modification: Social Skills: Assisting the patient to develop or improve interpersonal social skills

Developmental Enhancement: Adolescent: Facilitating optimal physical, cognitive, social, and emotional growth of individuals during the transition from childhood to adulthood

Developmental Enhancement: Child: Facilitating or teaching parents and caregivers to facilitate the optimal gross-motor, fine-motor, language, cognitive, social, and emotional growth of preschool and school-aged children

Family Integrity Promotion: Promotion of family cohesion and unity

Family Process Maintenance: Minimization of family process disruption effects

Recreation Therapy: Purposeful use of recreation to promote relaxation and enhancement of social skills

Socialization Enhancement: Facilitation of another person's ability to interact with others

Therapeutic Play: Purposeful and directive use of toys or other materials to assist children in communicating their perception and knowledge of their world and to help in gaining mastery of their environment

Nursing Activities

Assessments

- Assess established pattern of interaction between patient and others

Patient/Family Teaching

- Provide information on community resources that will assist the patient to continue with increasing social interaction after discharge

Collaborative Activities

- Confer with other disciplines and patient to establish, implement, and evaluate a plan to increase or improve the patient's interactions with others
- *(NIC) Socialization Enhancement*: Refer patient to interpersonal skills group or program in which understanding of transactions can be increased, as appropriate

Other

- Assign scheduled interactions
- Identify specific behavior change
- Identify tasks that will increase or improve social interactions
- Involve supportive peers in giving feedback to patient on social interactions
- Mediate between patient and others when patient exhibits negative behavior
- *(NIC) Socialization Enhancement:*
  - Encourage honesty in presenting oneself to others
  - Encourage respect for the rights of others
  - Encourage patience in developing relationships
  - Help patient increase awareness of strengths and limitations in communicating with others
  - Use role playing to practice improved communication skills and techniques
  - Request and expect verbal communication
  - Give positive feedback when patient reaches out to others
  - Facilitate patient input and planning of future activities

Home Care

- The preceding activities may be adapted for use in home care
- Suggest the use of the Internet for those who live alone and are homebound
- Arrange for home health aides, Meals-on-Wheels, visiting volunteers, and other care activities that provide social interaction
- Encourage the client to volunteer in the community (e.g., as a volunteer visitor)

For Older Adults

- Assess for hearing and other functional deficits that interfere with communication
- Assess for depression
- Provide adaptive devices for functional deficits
- For inpatients, provide crafts, games, music, and other small group activities
- Allow the patient to choose those with whom he wishes to socialize; provide introductions
- Provide physical activities
- Suggest participation in programs such as Foster Grandparents

SOCIAL ISOLATION

(1982) **Domain 12, Comfort; Class 3, Social Support**

Definition: Aloneness experienced by the individual and perceived as imposed by others and as a negative or threatened state

Defining Characteristics

Subjective

Developmentally inappropriate interests
Expresses feelings of aloneness imposed by others
Experiences feelings of differences from others
Expresses feelings of rejection
Reports inadequate purpose in life
Inability to meet expectations of others
Insecurity in public
Expresses values unacceptable to the dominant cultural group

Objective

Absence of supportive significant others (e.g., family, friends, group)
Developmentally inappropriate behaviors
Dull affect
Evidence of physical or mental handicap
Exists in a subculture
Illness
Meaningless actions
No eye contact
Preoccupation with own thoughts
Projects hostility [in voice or behavior]

Repetitive actions
Sad affect
Seeks to be alone
Shows behavior unacceptable to dominant cultural group
Uncommunicative
Withdrawal

Related Factors

Alterations in mental status
Alterations in physical appearance
Altered state of wellness
Factors contributing to the absence of satisfying personal relationships (e.g., delay in accomplishing developmental tasks)
Immature interests
Inability to engage in satisfying personal relationships
Inadequate personal resources
Unaccepted social behavior or values

Other Related Factors (Non-NANDA International)

Chemical dependence
Psychologic impairment (specify)
Treatment-imposed isolation

Suggestions for Use

Differentiate between *Social isolation* and *Impaired social interaction*. A diagnosis of *Impaired social interaction* focuses more on the patient's social skills and abilities, whereas *Social isolation* focuses on the patient's feelings of aloneness and may not be a result of his ineffective social skills. Table 9 compares the defining characteristics and related factors of *Impaired social interaction* to *Social isolation*.

Table 9

	Impaired Social Interaction	Social Isolation
Shared Defining Characteristics	Verbalized or observed discomfort in social situations	Verbalized or observed discomfort in social situations
Differentiating Defining Characteristics	Ineffective social behaviors Feelings of rejection	Feelings of aloneness imposed by others
Related Factors	Lack of knowledge of social skills	Mental impairment
	Communication barriers	Physical disabilities

Suggested Alternative Diagnoses

Communication, verbal, impaired
Post-trauma syndrome
Relocation stress syndrome
Social interaction, impaired

NOC Outcomes

Family Social Climate: Supportive milieu as characterized by family member relationships and goals

Leisure Participation: Use of relaxing, interesting, and enjoyable activities to promote well-being

Loneliness Severity: Severity of emotional, social, or existential isolation response

Mood Equilibrium: Appropriate adjustment of prevailing emotional tone in response to circumstances

Play Participation: Use of activities by a child from 1 year through 11 years of age to promote enjoyment, entertainment, and development

Social Interaction Skills: Personal behaviors that promote effective relationships

Social Involvement: Social interactions with persons, groups, or organizations

Social Support: Reliable assistance from others

Goals/Evaluation Criteria

Examples Using NOC Language

- Demonstrates **Social Involvement**, as evidenced by the following indicators (specify 1–5: never, rarely, sometimes, often, or consistently demonstrated):
- Interacts with close friends, neighbors, family members, and/or members of work groups
- Participates as a volunteer, in organized activity, or in active church work
- Participates in leisure activities with others

Other Examples

Patient will:

- Identify and accept personal characteristics or behaviors that contribute to social isolation
- Identify community resources that will assist in decreasing social isolation after discharge
- Verbalize fewer feelings or experiences of being excluded
- Begin to establish contact with others

- Develop a mutual relationship
- Exhibit affect appropriate to situation
- Develop social skills that decrease isolation (e.g., cooperation, compromise, consideration, warmth, and engagement)
- Report increasing social support (e.g., help from others in the form of emotional help, time, money, labor, or information)

NIC Interventions

Behavior Modification: Social Skills: Assisting the patient to develop or improve interpersonal social skills

Developmental Enhancement: Child: Facilitating or teaching parents and caregivers to facilitate the optimal gross-motor, fine-motor, language, cognitive, social, and emotional growth of preschool and school-aged children

Family Integrity Promotion: Promotion of family cohesion and unity

Family Involvement Promotion: Facilitating family participation in the emotional and physical care of the patient

Hope Inspiration: Facilitation of the development of a positive outlook in a given situation

Mood Management: Providing for safety, stabilization, recovery, and maintenance of a patient who is experiencing dysfunctionally depressed or elevated mood

Recreation Therapy: Purposeful use of recreation to promote relaxation and enhancement of social skills

Self-Awareness Enhancement: Assisting a patient to explore and understand his thoughts, feelings, motivations, and behaviors

S

Socialization Enhancement: Facilitation of another person's ability to interact with others

Support System Enhancement: Facilitation of support to patient by family, friends, and community

Therapeutic Play: Purposeful and directive use of toys or other materials to assist children in communicating their perception and knowledge of their world and to help in gaining mastery of their environment

Nursing Activities

Also see Nursing Activities for Social Interaction, Impaired.

Other

- Assist patient to distinguish reality from perceptions
- Identify with patient those factors that may be contributing to feelings of social isolation
- Reduce stigma of isolation by respecting patient's dignity
- Reduce visitor anxiety by explaining reason for isolation precautions or equipment

- Reinforce efforts by patient, family, or friends to establish interactions
- *(NIC) Socialization Enhancement:*
  Encourage enhanced involvement in already established relationships
  Allow testing of interpersonal limits
  Give feedback about improvement in care of personal appearance or other activities
  Confront patient about impaired judgment, when appropriate
  Encourage patient to change environment, such as going outside for walks and movies

Home Care

- The preceding activities can be used in or adapted for home care

SORROW, CHRONIC

(1998) **Domain 9, Coping/Stress Tolerance; Class 2, Coping Responses**

Definition: Cyclical, recurring, and potentially progressive pattern of pervasive sadness experienced (by a parent, caregiver, or individual with chronic illness or disability) in response to continual loss, throughout the trajectory of an illness or disability

Defining Characteristics

Subjective

Reports feelings of sadness (e.g., periodic, recurrent)

Reports feelings that interfere with the client's ability to reach his highest level of personal or social well-being [**Note**: Feelings vary in intensity, are periodic, may progress and intensify over time.]

Reports one or more of the following negative feelings: anger, being misunderstood, confusion, depression, disappointment, emptiness, fear, frustration, guilt or self-blame, helplessness, hopelessness, loneliness, low self-esteem, recurring loss, being overwhelmed

Expresses periodic, recurrent feelings of sadness

Related Factors

Death of a loved one

Chronic physical or mental illness or disability [such as: mental retardation, multiple sclerosis, prematurity, spina bifida or other birth defects, chronic mental illness, infertility, cancer, Parkinson disease]

Person experiences one or more trigger events (e.g., crises in management of the illness or disability, crises related to developmental stages, and missed opportunities or milestones) [that bring comparisons with developmental, social, or personal norms]
Unending caregiving [as a constant reminder of loss]

Suggestions for Use

Compared to normal grieving that occurs in response to loss, *Chronic sorrow* does not subside with time, in part, because the loss continues unabated (as it does in a chronic disability) and the condition remains as a constant reminder of loss. *Chronic sorrow* demonstrates coping that is more effective than that which occurs with *Complicated grieving*.

Several of the defining characteristics of *Chronic sorrow* are, themselves, nursing diagnoses. When more than one of the following diagnoses are present, a diagnosis of *Chronic sorrow* may be more useful: *Fear*, *Hopelessness*, *Loneliness*, *Chronic low self-esteem*, and *Powerlessness*.

Suggested Alternative Diagnoses

Death anxiety
Fear
Grieving
Grieving, complicated
Hopelessness
Loneliness, risk for
Powerlessness
Self-esteem, chronic low
Spiritual distress

NOC Outcomes

Acceptance: Health Status: Reconciliation to significant change in health circumstances
Depression Level: Severity of melancholic mood and loss of interest in life events
Depression Self-Control: Personal actions to minimize melancholy and maintain interest in life events
Grief Resolution: Adjustment to actual or impending loss
Hope: Optimism that is personally satisfying and life-supporting
Mood Equilibrium: Appropriate adjustment of prevailing emotional tone in response to circumstances
Psychosocial Adjustment: Life Change: Adaptive psychosocial response of an individual to a significant life change

Goals/Evaluation Criteria

Examples Using NOC Language

- Demonstrates **Grief Resolution**, as evidenced by the following indicators (specify 1–5: never, rarely, sometimes, often, or consistently demonstrated):

  Verbalizes acceptance of loss
  Participates in planning funeral
  Reports decreased preoccupation with loss
  Shares loss with significant others
  Progresses through stages of grief
  Maintains personal grooming and hygiene

Other Examples:

Patient will:

- Express feelings of guilt, anger, or sorrow
- Identify and use effective coping strategies
- Verbalize the impact of the loss(es)
- Seek information about illness and treatment
- Identify and use available social supports, including significant others
- Work toward acceptance of the loss(es)
- Draw upon spiritual beliefs for comfort
- Report adequate sleep and nutrition

NIC Interventions

Coping Enhancement: Assisting a patient to adapt to perceived stressors, changes, or threats that interfere with meeting life demands and roles

Grief Work Facilitation: Assistance with the resolution of a significant loss

Grief Work Facilitation: Perinatal Death: Assistance with the resolution of a perinatal loss

Hope Inspiration: Facilitation of the development of a positive outlook in a given situation

Mood Management: Providing for safety, stabilization, recovery, and maintenance of a patient who is experiencing dysfunctionally depressed or elevated mood

Spiritual Support: Assisting the patient to feel balance and connection with a greater power

Nursing Activities

Refer to Nursing Activities for Grieving and for Complicated Grieving. Also refer to Nursing Activities for Spiritual Distress.

For patients for whom *Fear* is an etiology, refer to Nursing Activities for Fear.

For patients for whom *Chronic low self-esteem* is an etiology, refer to Nursing Activities for Self-Esteem, Chronic Low.

For patients for whom *Hopelessness* is an etiology, refer to Nursing Activities for Hopelessness and Readiness for Enhanced Hope.

For patients for whom *Powerlessness* is an etiology, refer to Nursing Activities for Powerlessness.

Assessments

- Assess and document the presence and source of patient's sorrow

Patient/Family Teaching

- Discuss characteristics of normal and abnormal grieving
- Provide patient and family with information about hospital and community resources, such as self-help groups

Collaborative Activities

- Initiate a patient care conference to review patient and family needs related to their stage of the grieving process and to establish a plan of care

Other

- Acknowledge the grief reactions of patient and family while continuing necessary care activities
- Discuss with patient and family the impact of the loss on the family and its functioning
- Establish a schedule for contact with patient
- Establish a trusting relationship with patient and family
- Provide a safe, secure, and private environment to facilitate patient and family grieving process
- Recognize and reinforce the strength of each family member
- *(NIC) Grief Work Facilitation:*

    Assist the patient to identify the nature of the attachment to the lost object or person

    Include significant others in discussions and decisions, as appropriate

    Encourage patient to implement cultural, religious, and social customs associated with the loss

    Encourage expression of feelings about the loss

For Children

- *(NIC) Grief Work Facilitation:*

    Answer children's questions associated with the loss

    Assist the child to clarify misconceptions

SPIRITUAL DISTRESS

(1978, 2002) **Domain 10, Life Principles; Class 3, Value/Belief/Action Congruence**

Definition: Impaired ability to experience and integrate meaning and purpose in life through connectedness with self, others, art, music, literature, nature, or a power greater than oneself

Defining Characteristics

Connections to Self

Anger
Guilt
Coping
Expresses lack of:
Acceptance
Courage
Hope
Love
Meaning and purpose in life
Peace and serenity
Self-forgiveness

Connections with Others

Expresses alienation
Refuses interactions with significant others
Refuses interactions with spiritual leaders
Verbalizes being separated from support system

Connections with Art, Music, Literature, Nature

Disinterest in nature
Disinterest in reading spiritual literature
Inability to express previous state of creativity (singing and listening to music and writing)

Connections with Power Greater Than Oneself

Expresses being abandoned
Expresses having anger toward power greater than self
Expresses hopelessness
Expresses suffering
Inability to be introspective
Inability to experience the transcendent
Inability to participate in religious activities

S

Inability to pray
Requests to see a spiritual leader
Sudden changes in spiritual practices

Related Factors

Active dying
Anxiety
Chronic illness [of self and others]
Death [of others]
Life change
Loneliness or social alienation
Pain
Self-alienation
Sociocultural deprivation

Other Related Factors (Non-NANDA International)

Discrepancy between spiritual beliefs and prescribed treatment

Suggestions for Use

(a) Spiritual well-being should be thought of in a broad sense and not limited to religion. All people are religious in the sense that they need something to give meaning to their lives. For some it is belief in God in the traditional sense; for others, it is a feeling of harmony with the universe; for still others, it may be family and children. When the patient believes that life has no meaning or purpose, in whatever sense, then *Spiritual distress* is present. (b) Some of the following suggested alternative diagnoses may lead to *Spiritual distress*.

Suggested Alternative Diagnoses

Anxiety, death
Decisional conflict
Coping, ineffective
Sorrow, chronic
Spiritual distress, risk for

NOC Outcomes

Dignified Life Closure: Personal actions to maintain control and comfort with the approaching end of life
Hope: Optimism that is personally satisfying and life-supporting
Quality of Life: Extent of positive perception of current life circumstances
Social Involvement: Social interactions with persons, groups, or organizations

Spiritual Health: Connectedness with self, others, higher power, all life, nature, and the universe that transcends and empowers the self

Goals/Evaluation Criteria

Examples Using NOC Language

- Demonstrates **Hope**, as evidenced by the following indicators (specify 1–5: never, rarely, sometimes, often, or consistently demonstrated): Expresses faith, meaning in life, and inner peace
- Demonstrates **Spiritual Health**, as evidenced by the following indicators (specify 1–5: severely, substantially, moderately, mildly, or not compromised):

    Meaning and purpose in life
    Achievement of spiritual world view
    Ability to love and forgive
    Ability to pray and worship
    Interaction with spiritual leaders
    Connectedness with inner self

Other Examples

Patient will:

- Acknowledge that illness is a challenge to belief system
- Acknowledge that treatment conflicts with belief system
- Demonstrate coping techniques to deal with spiritual distress
- Express acceptance of limited religious or cultural ties
- Discuss spiritual practices and concerns

S

Dying patient will:

- Express acceptance or readiness for death
- Reconcile previous relationships
- Express affection toward significant others

NIC Interventions

Coping Enhancement: Assisting a patient to adapt to perceived stressors, changes, or threats that interfere with meeting life demands and roles

Decision-Making Support: Providing information and support for a patient who is making a decision regarding health care

Dying Care: Promotion of physical comfort and psychological peace in the final phase of life

Emotional Support: Provision of reassurance, acceptance, and encouragement during times of stress

Hope Inspiration: Facilitation of the development of a positive outlook in a given situation

Socialization Enhancement: Facilitation of another person's ability to interact with others

Spiritual Growth Facilitation: Facilitation of growth in patients' capacity to identify, connect with, and call upon the source of meaning, purpose, comfort, strength, and hope in their lives

Spiritual Support: Assisting the patient to feel balance and connection with a greater power

Values Clarification: Assisting another to clarify her or his own values in order to facilitate effective decision making

Nursing Activities

Assessments

- For patients who indicate a religious affiliation, assess for direct indicators of patient's spiritual status by asking questions such as the following:

  Do you feel your faith is helpful to you? In what ways is it important to you right now?

  How can I help you carry out your faith? For example, would you like me to read your prayer book to you?

  Would you like a visit from your spiritual counselor or the hospital chaplain?

  Please tell me about any particular religious practices that are important to you.

- Make indirect assessments of the patient's spiritual status by doing the following:

  Determine patient's concept of God by observing the books at the bedside or the programs he watches on television. Also note whether the patient's life seems to have meaning, value, and purpose.

  Determine the patient's source of hope and strength. Is it God in the traditional sense, a family member, or an "inner source" of strength? Note who the patient talks about most, or ask: Who is important to you?

  Observe whether the patient seems to be praying when you enter the room, before meals, or during procedures.

  Look for items such as religious literature, rosaries, and religious get-well cards at the bedside.

  Listen for patient's thoughts about the relationship between spiritual beliefs and his state of health, particularly for statements such as: Why did God let this happen to me? or If I have faith, I will get well.

Collaborative Activities

- Communicate dietary needs (e.g., kosher food, vegetarian diet, pork-free diet) to dietitian
- Request spiritual consultation to help patient and family determine posthospitalization needs and community resources for support
- *(NIC) Spiritual Support*: Refer to spiritual advisor of patient's choice

Other

- Explain limitations that hospitalization imposes on religious observances
- Make immediate changes necessary to accommodate patient's needs (e.g., encourage patient's family or friends to bring special food)
- Provide privacy and time for patient to observe religious practices
- *(NIC) Spiritual Support*:

  Be open to individual's expressions of loneliness and powerlessness

  Use values clarification techniques to help individual clarify beliefs and values, as appropriate

  Express empathy with individual's feelings

  Listen carefully to individual's communication and develop a sense of timing for prayer or spiritual rituals

  Assure individual that nurse will be available to support individual in times of suffering

  Encourage chapel service attendance, if desired

  Provide desired spiritual articles, according to individual preference

Home Care

- The preceding activities are appropriate for use in home care
- Assist patient and family to create a space in the home for meditation or prayer

For Older Adults

- Arrange for someone (e.g., a housekeeping aide) to read sacred texts to the client if he wishes and cannot do so himself

SPIRITUAL DISTRESS, RISK FOR

(1998, 2004) **Domain 10, Life Principles; Class 3, Value/Belief/Action Congruence**

Definition: At risk for an impaired ability to experience and integrate meaning and purpose in life through connectedness with self, others, art, music, literature, nature, or a power greater than oneself

Risk Factors

Developmental

Life changes

Environmental

Environmental changes
Natural disasters

Physical

Chronic illness
Physical illness
Substance abuse

Psychosocial

Anxiety
Blocks to experiencing love
Change in religious rituals
Change in spiritual practices
Cultural conflict
Depression
Inability to forgive
Loss
Low self-esteem
Poor relationships
Racial conflict
Separated support systems
Stress

Suggestions for Use

See Suggestions for Use for the diagnosis Spiritual Distress, preceding.

Suggested Alternative Diagnoses

Anxiety, death
Coping, ineffective

Decisional conflict
Grieving, complicated
Sorrow, chronic
Spiritual distress

NOC Outcomes

To evaluate occurrence of Spiritual Distress, use the following outcome:

Spiritual Health: Connectedness with self, others, higher power, all life, nature, and the universe that transcends and empowers the self

The following are examples of outcomes associated with risk factors for *Spiritual distress*:

Hope: Optimism that is personally satisfying and life-supporting

Suffering Severity: Severity of anguish associated with a distressing symptom, injury, or loss that has potential long-term effects

Goals/Evaluation Criteria

See Goals/Evaluation Criteria for the diagnosis Spiritual Distress, preceding.

NIC Interventions

Dying Care: Promotion of physical comfort and psychological peace in the final phase of life

Grief Work Facilitation: Assistance with the resolution of a significant loss

Hope Inspiration: Facilitation of the development of a positive outlook in a given situation

Religious Ritual Enhancement: Facilitating participation in religious practices

Spiritual Support: Assisting the patient to feel balance and connection with a greater power

Nursing Activities

See Nursing Activities for the diagnosis Spiritual Distress, preceding. Nursing interventions and activities focus on removing or modifying risk factors in order to prevent Spiritual Distress.

Assessments

- Assess for situations that might lead to spiritual distress (e.g., low self-esteem, anxiety, lack of supportive relationships)

Other

- Institute the following measures to promote self-esteem:
  Assist patient in identifying personal strengths
  Encourage patient to verbalize concerns about close relationships

Encourage patient and family to air feelings and to grieve
Provide care in a nonjudgmental manner, maintaining the patient's privacy and dignity

- *(NIC) Spiritual Support:*

Use values clarification techniques to help patient clarify beliefs and values, as appropriate
Listen carefully to individual's communication and develop a sense of timing for prayer or spiritual rituals

SPIRITUAL WELL-BEING, READINESS FOR ENHANCED

(1994, 2002) **Domain 10, Life Principles; Class 2, Beliefs**

Definition: A pattern of experiencing and integrating meaning and purpose in life through connectedness with self, others, art, music, literature, nature, or a power greater than oneself that is sufficient for well-being and can be strengthened

Defining Characteristics

Connections to Self

S

Expresses desire for enhanced:
Acceptance
Coping
Courage
Forgiveness of self
Hope
Joy
Love
Meaning and purpose in life
[Peace and serenity]
Satisfying philosophy of life
Surrender
Expresses lack of serenity (e.g., peace)
Meditation

Connections with Art, Music, Literature, Nature

Displays creative energy (e.g., writing, poetry, singing)
Listens to music

Reads spiritual literature
Spends time outdoors

Connections with Others

Provides service to others
Requests forgiveness of others
Requests interactions with friends, family
Requests interactions with spiritual leaders

Connections with Power Greater Than Self

Expresses reverence, awe
Participates in religious activities
Prays
Reports mystical experiences

Suggestions for Use

Because this is a wellness diagnosis, an etiology (e.g., related factors) is not needed. If situations exist that pose a risk to spiritual development, use *Risk for spiritual distress*.

Suggested Alternative Diagnosis

Spiritual distress, risk for

NOC Outcomes

Hope: Optimism that is personally satisfying and life-supporting
Personal Well-Being: Extent of positive perception of one's health status
Spiritual Health: Connectedness with self, others, higher power, all life, nature, and the universe that transcends and empowers the self

Goals/Evaluation Criteria

Examples Using NOC Language

See Examples Using NOC Language for the diagnosis Spiritual Distress, preceding.

Other Examples

Patient will:
- Continue and enhance spiritual growth
- Verbalize feelings of peace and harmony with the universe
- Verbalize satisfaction with sociocultural circumstances and interpersonal relationships
- Report satisfaction with self-concept and achievement of life goals
- Indicate happiness and satisfaction with spiritual life

NIC Interventions

Also refer to NIC Interventions for the diagnosis Spiritual Distress, Risk for, preceding.

Hope Inspiration: Facilitation of the development of a positive outlook in a given situation

Self-Awareness Enhancement: Assisting a patient to explore and understand his or her thoughts, feelings, motivations, and behaviors

Self-Esteem Enhancement: Assisting a patient to increase his personal judgment of self-worth

Spiritual Growth Facilitation: Facilitation of growth in patients' capacity to identify, connect with, and call upon the source of meaning, purpose, comfort, strength, and hope in their lives

Spiritual Support: Assisting the patient to feel balance and connection with a greater power

Values Clarification: Assisting another to clarify his own values in order to facilitate effective decision making

Nursing Activities

Also see Nursing Activities for the diagnosis Spiritual Distress, preceding.

Collaborative Activities

- *(NIC) Spiritual Support:* Encourage chapel service attendance, if desired

Other

- *(NIC) Spiritual Support:*
  - Be open to individual's feelings about illness and death
  - Assist individual to properly express and relieve anger in appropriate ways
  - Be available to listen to individual's feelings
  - Facilitate individual's use of meditation, prayer, and other religious traditions and rituals

SPONTANEOUS VENTILATION, IMPAIRED

(1992) **Domain 4, Activity/Rest; Class 4, Cardiovascular/Pulmonary Responses**

Definition: Decreased energy reserves result in an individual's inability to maintain breathing adequate to support life

Defining Characteristics

Subjective

Apprehension

Dyspnea

Objective

Decreased cooperation

Decreased SaO_2

Decreased PO_2

Decreased tidal volume

Increased heart rate

Increased metabolic rate

Increased PCO_2

Increased restlessness

Increased use of accessory muscles

Related Factors

Metabolic factors [e.g., alkalemia, hypokalemia, hypochloremia, hypophosphatemia, anemia]

Respiratory muscle fatigue

Suggestions for Use

Impaired gas exchange is one of the defining characteristics for this label. When blood gases are altered but the patient is able to breathe without mechanical assistance, a diagnosis of *Impaired gas exchange* should be made instead of *Inability to sustain spontaneous ventilation*.

The author does not recommend use of this label as a nursing diagnosis. When breathing is "inadequate to support life," an emergency exists; the interventions are physician-prescribed, including resuscitation and mechanical ventilation. The nurse is accountable for monitoring changes in the patient's condition and performing interventions according to agency protocols. Goals and interventions are included in this text only because NOC and NIC standardized language includes them.

Suggested Alternative Diagnoses

Airway clearance, ineffective

Breathing pattern, ineffective

Dysfunctional ventilatory weaning response (DVWR)

Gas exchange, impaired

NOC Outcomes

Mechanical Ventilation Response: Adult: Alveolar exchange and tissue perfusion are supported by mechanical ventilation

Respiratory Status: Gas Exchange: Alveolar exchange of CO_2 or O_2 to maintain arterial blood gas concentrations

Respiratory Status: Ventilation: Movement of air in and out of the lungs

Vital Signs: Extent to which temperature, pulse, respiration, and blood pressure within normal range

Goals/Evaluation Criteria

Examples Using NOC Language

- Demonstrates **Vital Signs**, as evidenced by the following indicators (specify 1–5: severe, substantial, moderate, mild, or no deviation from normal range): temperature, pulse, respirations, and blood pressure

Other Examples

Patient will:

- Have adequate energy level and muscle function to sustain spontaneous breathing
- Receive adequate nutrition prior to, during, and following weaning process
- Have arterial blood gases and oxygen saturation within acceptable range
- Demonstrate neurologic status adequate to sustain spontaneous breathing

NIC Interventions

Airway Management: Facilitation of patency of air passages

Artificial Airway Management: Maintenance of endotracheal and tracheostomy tubes and prevention of complications associated with their use

Aspiration Precautions: Prevention or minimization of risk factors in the patient at risk for aspiration

Emergency Care: Providing life-saving measures in life-threatening situations

Mechanical Ventilation Management: Invasive: Assisting the patient receiving artificial breathing support through a device inserted into the trachea

Medication Administration: Preparing, giving, and evaluating the effectiveness of prescription and nonprescription drugs

Oxygen Therapy: Administration of oxygen and monitoring of its effectiveness

Respiratory Monitoring: Collection and analysis of patient data to ensure airway patency and adequate gas exchange

Ventilation Assistance: Promotion of an optimal spontaneous breathing pattern that maximizes oxygen and carbon dioxide exchange in the lungs

Vital Signs Monitoring: Collection and analysis of cardiovascular, respiratory, and body temperature data to determine and prevent complications

Nursing Activities

Assessments

- For patients requiring artificial airway: monitor tube placement, check cuff inflation q4h and whenever it is deflated and reinflated
- *(NIC) Mechanical Ventilation Management: Invasive*
  - Monitor for impending respiratory failure
  - Monitor for decrease in exhaled volume and increase in inspiratory pressure
  - Monitor the effectiveness of mechanical ventilation on patient's physiologic and psychologic status
  - Monitor for adverse effects of mechanical ventilation (e.g., tracheal deviation, infection, barotraumas, volutrauma, reduced cardiac output, gastric distension, subcutaneous emphysema)
  - Monitor effects of ventilator changes on oxygenation: ABG, SaO_2, SvO_2, end-tidal CO_2, Q_{sp}/Qt, and $A\text{-}aDO_2$ levels and patient's subjective response
  - Monitor degree of shunt, vital capacity, V_d/VT, MVV, inspiratory force, FEV_1 for, and readiness to wean from mechanical ventilation, based on agency protocol
- *(NIC) Respiratory Monitoring*:
  - Note location of trachea
  - Auscultate breath sounds, noting areas of decreased or absent ventilation and presence of adventitious sounds
  - Determine the need for suctioning by auscultating for crackles and rhonchi over major airways
  - Monitor for increased restlessness, anxiety, and air hunger
  - Monitor for crepitus, as appropriate

Patient/Family Teaching

- Instruct patient and family about weaning process and goals, including the following:
  - How patient may feel as process evolves
  - Participation required by patient
  - Reasons why weaning is necessary

S

- *(NIC) Mechanical Ventilation Management: Invasive:* Instruct the patient and family about the rationale and expected sensations associated with use of mechanical ventilators

Collaborative Activities

- *(NIC) Mechanical Ventilation Management: Invasive*
  - Consult with other health care personnel in selection of a ventilator mode (initial mode usually volume control with breath rate, FIO_2 level and targeted tidal volume specified)
  - Administer muscle-paralyzing agents, sedatives, and narcotic analgesics, as appropriate

Other

- Initiate calming techniques, as appropriate
- *(NIC) Mechanical Ventilation Management: Invasive*
  - Initiate setup and application of the ventilator
  - Ensure that ventilator alarms are on
  - Provide patient with a means for communication (e.g., paper and pencil or alphabet board)
  - Perform suctioning, based on presence of adventitious breath sounds or increased inspiratory pressure
  - Provide routine oral care with soft moist swabs, antiseptic agent, and gentle suctioning

For patients requiring an artificial airway

S

- Provide artificial airway management according to agency procedures and protocols, which may include the following:
  - Provide oral care at least q4h
  - Rotate endotracheal tube from side to side daily
  - Tape endotracheal tube securely; change tapes or ties q24h
  - Administer sedation, utilize mitts or wrist restraints, if necessary, to prevent unplanned extubation
  - Clean stoma and tracheal cannula q4h (according to agency protocol)
  - Suction oropharynx, as needed

NOTE: For in-depth information about artificial airway management, refer to med/surg text, nursing techniques/skills manual, or agency protocols

For patients requiring ventilatory weaning

- Refer to Nursing Activities for the diagnosis Ventilatory Weaning Response, Dysfunctional (DVWR).

Home Care

- Assess caregivers' ability and commitment to provide care to a ventilator-dependent family member
- As a part of discharge planning, involve a case worker or social worker to help the family compare the cost of home care to that of an extended care facility
- Instruct client and caregivers about operation of the ventilator, suctioning, tracheostomy care, and respiratory medications
- Notify the electric company to place the residence on a high-risk list in the event of a power failure
- Help the family create an emergency plan, including measures to institute until medical help arrives

For Infants and Children

For neonates requiring resuscitation

- Refer to maternity or pediatric nursing text for full details of resuscitation procedure
- Have resuscitation equipment available at birth
- Calmly explain procedures to parents to minimize anxiety
- Prepare for neonatal transfer or transport

For Older Adults

- Institute early interventions to support nutrition and circulation to help prevent the rapid decline associated with mechanical ventilation in older adults

STRESS OVERLOAD

(2006) **Domain 9, Coping/Stress Tolerance; Class 2, Coping Responses**

Definition: Excessive amounts and types of demands that require action

Defining Characteristics

Demonstrates increased feelings of anger
Demonstrates increased feelings of impatience
Expresses difficulty in functioning
Expresses a feeling of pressure

Expresses a feeling of tension
Expresses increased feelings of anger
Expresses increased feelings of impatience
Expresses problems with decision making
Reports negative impact from stress (e.g., physical symptoms, psychological distress, feeling of "being sick" or of "going to get sick")
Reports excessive situational stress (e.g., rates stress level as 7 or above on a 10-point scale)

Related Factors

Inadequate resources (e.g., financial, social, education/knowledge level)
Intense or repeated stressors (e.g., family violence, chronic illness, terminal illness)
Multiple coexisting stressors (e.g., environmental threats, demands; physical threats, demands; social threats, demands)

Suggested Alternative Diagnoses

Caregiver role strain
Coping, ineffective
Therapeutic regimen management: Family, ineffective

NOC Outcomes

Agitation Level: Severity of disruptive physiological and behavioral manifestations of stress or biochemical triggers
Anxiety Level: Severity of manifested apprehension, tension, or uneasiness arising from an unidentifiable source
Coping: Personal actions to manage stressors that tax an individual's resources
Stress Level: Severity of manifested physical or mental tension resulting from factors that alter an existing equilibrium

Goals/Evaluation Criteria

Examples Using NOC Language

- Demonstrates acceptable **Stress Level**, as evidenced by the following indicators (specify 1–5: severe, substantial, moderate, mild, or none):
  - Anxiety
  - Change in food intake
  - Frequent cognitive mistakes
  - Emotional outbursts
  - Sleep disturbance
  - Tension headache

Other Examples

Patient will:

- Report anxiety at a manageable level
- Have vital signs within normal range
- Not experience muscle tension
- Not engage in maladaptive coping responses (e.g., alcohol use, self-medication, smoking)
- Perform usual roles adequately
- Describe methods to reduce stressors
- Make a plan for adaptive strategies to cope with stressors that cannot be removed

NIC Interventions

Anger Control Assistance: Facilitation of the expression of anger in an adaptive, nonviolent manner

Anxiety Reduction: Minimizing apprehension, dread, foreboding, or uneasiness related to an unidentified source of anticipated danger

Coping Enhancement: Assisting a patient to adapt to perceived stressors, changes, or threats that interfere with meeting life demands and roles.

Relaxation Therapy: Use of techniques to encourage and elicit relaxation for the purpose of decreasing undesirable signs and symptoms such as pain, muscle tension, or anxiety

Support System Enhancement: Facilitation of support to patient by family, friends, and community

Nursing Activities

Assessments

- Identify client's perceived and actual stressors
- Assess physical and emotional responses to present stressors (e.g., sleep patterns, nutrition, mood)
- Ask client to describe how he has previously coped successfully with stressors
- Identify client's unsuccessful or maladaptive coping strategies
- Assess anxiety level
- Identify client's usual family, work, and community roles
- Identify the client's support systems
- *(NIC) Coping Enhancement:*

  Evaluate the patient's decision-making ability

  Appraise the impact of the patient's life situation on roles and relationships

Patient/Family Teaching

- Teach stress management techniques such as progressive relaxation, visualization, biofeedback, listening to music, and journal writing

Collaborative Activities

- Refer to spiritual leaders, counselor, social worker, psychologist, and other professionals, as needed

Other

- Assist the client to recognize his negative focus and to restructure his thinking in more positive and realistic ways
- Encourage positive self-talk: when you hear a negative comment about self, ask the client to rephrase the statement so that it is positive
- Provide crisis intervention, if necessary
- Assist client to specifically identify stressors; then explore ways in which he/she might eliminate or minimize them.
- Help the client to recognize which of his coping strategies are successful and which are maladaptive
- Encourage client to use coping strategies that have been successful for him in the past

Home Care

- The preceding activities are appropriate for home care use

SUDDEN INFANT DEATH SYNDROME, RISK FOR

(2002) **Domain 11, Safety/Protection; Class 2, Physical Injury**

Definition: Presence of risk factors for sudden death of an infant under 1 year of age

Risk Factors

Modifiable

Delayed or lack of prenatal care
Infant overheating or overwrapping
Infant placed to sleep in the prone or side-lying position
Pre- and postnatal infant smoke exposure
Soft underlayment or loose articles in the sleep environment

Potentially Modifiable

Low birth weight
Prematurity
Young maternal age

Nonmodifiable

Ethnicity (e.g., African American or Native American)
Infant age of 2 to 4 months
Male gender
Seasonality of sudden infant death syndrome (SIDS) deaths (higher in winter and fall months)

Suggestions for Use

Use the most specific label that matches the patient's defining characteristics. This label is more specific than *Risk for injury*, for example. Note that risk factors for *Risk for SIDS* are limited to the sleep environment, except for prenatal and nonmodifiable factors; whereas *Risk for suffocation* includes risk factors throughout the entire environment; it also is applicable to children older than 1 year.

Suggested Alternative Diagnoses

Injury, risk for
Suffocation, risk for

NOC Outcomes

NOTE: The desired outcome for Risk for Sudden Infant Death Syndrome is that the infant does not experience sudden infant death. There is no such NOC outcome. The following outcomes are associated with risk factors for SIDS.

Parenting: Infant/Toddler Physical Safety: Parental actions to avoid physical injury of a child from birth through 2 years of age

Preterm Infant Organization: Extrauterine integration of physiologic and behavioral function by the infant born 24 to 37 (term) weeks' gestation

Smoking Cessation Behavior: Personal actions to eliminate tobacco use

Goals/Evaluation Criteria

Examples Using NOC Language

- Demonstrates **Parenting: Infant/Toddler Physical Safety**, as evidenced by the following indicators (specify 1–5: never, rarely, sometimes, often, or consistently demonstrated):
  - Uses crib that meets federal regulations
  - Positions on back for sleep

Other Examples

Parent will:

- Obtain early and adequate prenatal care
- Identify appropriate safety factors that protect individual or child from SIDS
- Verbalize knowledge of safe mattress and bed linens
- Avoid smoking during pregnancy; do not expose infant to secondhand smoke

NIC Interventions

Developmental Care: Structuring the environment and providing care in response to the behavioral cues and states of the preterm infant

Parent Education: Infant: Instruction on nurturing and physical care needed during the first year of life

Risk Identification: Childbearing Family: Identification of an individual or family likely to experience difficulties in parenting and prioritization of strategies to prevent parenting problems

Teaching: Infant Safety: Instruction on safety during first year of life

Nursing Activities

Assessments

- Assess sleeping arrangements for safety (e.g., no featherbed mattresses or pillows in infant crib)
- Assess prenatally for risk factors such as young maternal age, smoking
- Assess whether home cardiorespiratory monitoring is indicated

Patient/Family Teaching

- Provide educational materials related to strategies and countermeasures for preventing SIDS and to emergency resuscitation measures for dealing with it
- Provide patient with emergency phone numbers (e.g., ambulance, 911)
- Teach family to not expose infant to secondhand smoke
- Teach parents not to sleep with infant
- Teach to position infant supine for sleeping
- Teach to not use featherbed or other fluffy-type mattresses, blankets, or pillows in infant's bed

Collaborative Activities

- Refer patient to educational classes in the community (e.g., CPR)

Home Care

- The preceding activities are appropriate for home care use

SUFFOCATION, RISK FOR

(1980) **Domain 11, Safety/Protection; Class 2, Physical Injury**

Definition: At risk of accidental suffocation (i.e., inadequate air available for inhalation)

Risk Factors

External (Environmental)

Children unattended in water
Discarding refrigerators or freezers without removing doors
Eating large mouthfuls of food
Fuel-burning heaters not vented to outside
Hanging a pacifier around infant's neck
Household gas leaks
Inserting small objects into airway
Low-strung clothesline
Pillow placed in an infant's crib
Playing with plastic bags
Propped bottle in an infant's crib
Smoking in bed
Vehicle warming in closed garage

Internal (Individual)

Cognitive or emotional difficulties
Deficient knowledge regarding safe situations
Deficient knowledge regarding safety precautions
Disease or injury process
Reduced motor abilities
Reduced olfactory sensation

Suggestions for Use

Use the most specific label that matches the patient's defining characteristics. This label is more specific than *Risk for injury* or *Risk for trauma*, for example.

Suggested Alternative Diagnoses

Injury, risk for
Sudden infant death syndrome, risk for
Trauma, risk for

NOC Outcomes

Outcome to assess for occurrence of suffocation:

Respiratory Status: Ventilation: Movement of air in and out of the lungs

Outcomes associated with risk factors for suffocation:

Aspiration Prevention: Personal actions to prevent the passage of fluid and solid particles into the lung

Asthma Self-Management: Personal actions to reverse inflammatory condition resulting in bronchial constriction of the airways

Parenting: Infant/Toddler Physical Safety: Parental actions to avoid physical injury of a child from birth through 2 years of age

Goals/Evaluation Criteria

Examples Using NOC Language

- Demonstrates **Aspiration Prevention**, as evidenced by the following indicators (specify 1–5: never, rarely, sometimes, often, or consistently demonstrated):
  Identifies and avoids risk factors
  Selects foods according to swallowing abilities

Other Examples

Parent will:

- Identify appropriate safety factors that protect individual or child from suffocation
- Recognize signs of substance abuse or addiction
- Verbalize knowledge of emergency procedures
- Provide age-appropriate toys
- Remove doors from unused refrigerators and freezers

NIC Interventions

Airway Management: Facilitation of patency of air passages

Aspiration Precautions: Prevention or minimization of risk factors in the patient at risk for aspiration

Asthma Management: Identification, treatment, and prevention of reactions to inflammation or constriction in the airway passages

Environmental Management: Safety: Monitoring and manipulation of the physical environment to promote safety

Respiratory Monitoring: Collection and analysis of patient data to ensure airway patency and adequate gas exchange

Teaching: Infant Safety: Instruction on safety during first year of life

Nursing Activities

Assessments

- *(NIC) Environmental Management: Safety:* Identify safety hazards in the environment (i.e., physical, biologic, and chemical) [e.g., gas leaks, portable heaters]
- *(NIC) Respiratory Monitoring:*
  Monitor rate, rhythm, depth, and effort of respirations
  Monitor for hoarseness and voice changes every hour in patients with facial burns
  Institute resuscitation efforts, as needed

Patient/Family Teaching

- Provide educational materials related to strategies and countermeasures for preventing suffocation and to emergency measures for dealing with it
- Provide information on environmental hazards and characteristics (e.g., stairs, windows, cupboard locks, swimming pools, streets, gates)
- *(NIC) Environmental Management: Safety:* Provide patient with emergency phone numbers (e.g., health department, environmental services, EPA [Environmental Protection Agency], and police)

Collaborative Activities

- Refer parent to educational classes in the community (CPR), first aid, swimming classes
- *(NIC) Environmental Management: Safety:* Notify agencies authorized to protect the environment (e.g., health department, environmental services, EPA, and police)

S

Other

- *(NIC): Airway Management:* Position the patient to maximize ventilation potential
- *(NIC) Environmental Management: Safety:* Modify the environment to minimize hazards and risks

Home Care

- The preceding activities are appropriate for home care use
- Advise clients to install smoke detectors
- Advise to have heating systems checked periodically and install carbon monoxide detectors
- If day care is used for children or older adults, teach family to assess that environment for suffocation hazards

For Infants and Children

- Teach parents to avoid using loose bedding; blankets and sheets should be tucked in around the mattress and reach only to the infant's chest
- Advise parents to not sleep with an infant
- Advise to not smoke in bed
- Provide age-appropriate toys (e.g., do not give small cylindrical- or spherical-shaped toys to small children and infants)
- Remove doors from large appliances (e.g., refrigerators) when disposing of them
- Teach parents the foods that constitute a choking hazard for toddlers (e.g., hot dogs, nuts, popcorn, raisins, grapes, peanut butter)

For Older Adults

- Assess swallowing ability
- Have the client sit upright to eat

SUICIDE, RISK FOR

(2000) **Domain 11, Safety/Protection; Class 3, Violence**

Definition: At risk for self-inflicted, life-threatening injury

Risk Factors

Behavioral

Buying a gun
Giving away possessions
History of prior suicide attempt
Impulsiveness
Making or changing a will
Marked changes in behavior, attitude, school performance
Stockpiling medicines
Sudden euphoric recovery from major depression

Demographic

Age: elderly, young adult males, adolescents
Divorced, widowed
Gender: male
Race: White, Native American

Physical

Chronic pain
Physical illness
Terminal illness

Psychological

Abuse in childhood
Family history of suicide
Guilt
Homosexual youth
Psychiatric illness or disorder [e.g., schizophrenia, bipolar disorder]
Substance abuse

Situational

Adolescents living in nontraditional settings (e.g., juvenile detention center, prison, half-way house, group home)
Economically disadvantaged
Living alone
Loss of autonomy or independence
Presence of gun in home
Relocation, institutionalization
Retired

Social

Cluster suicides
Disciplinary problems
Disrupted family life
Grieving
Helplessness
Hopelessness
Legal problems
Loneliness
Loss of important relationship
Poor support systems
Social isolation

Verbal

States desire to die [and end it all]
Threats of killing oneself

Suggestions for Use

When risk factors for suicide (e.g., suicidal ideation, suicidal plan) are present, use *Risk for suicide* instead of *Risk for self-directed violence*, which is less specific.

Suggested Alternative Diagnoses

Risk for self-directed violence

Risk for self-mutilation

NOC Outcomes

NOTE: The following outcome can be used to measure the occurrence of the diagnosis.

Suicide Self-Restraint: Personal actions to refrain from gestures and attempts at killing self

NOTE: The following outcomes are associated with some of the risk factors for suicide.

Depression Level: Severity of melancholic mood and loss of interest in life events

Family Functioning: Capacity of the family system to meet the needs of its members during developmental transitions

Impulse Self-Control: Self-restraint of compulsive or impulsive behaviors

Mood Equilibrium: Appropriate adjustment of prevailing emotional tone in response to circumstances

Goals/Evaluation Criteria

Examples Using NOC Language

- *Risk for suicide* is diminished, as demonstrated by Mood Equilibrium, Suicide Self-Restraint, and Impulse Self-Control.
- Demonstrates **Suicide Self-Restraint**, as evidenced by the following indicators (specify 1–5: never, rarely, sometimes, often, or consistently demonstrated):

  Obtains assistance as needed
  Verbalizes suicidal ideas
  Refrains from gathering means for suicide
  Refrains from giving away possessions
  Refrains from attempting suicide
  Obtains treatment for depression or substance abuse

Other Examples

- Verbalizes the desire to live
- Verbalizes feelings of anger
- Contacts agreed-upon persons if suicidal thoughts occur

NIC Interventions

Behavior Management: Self-Harm: Assisting the patient to decrease or eliminate self-mutilating or self-abusive behaviors

Counseling: Use of an interactive helping process focusing on the needs, problems, or feelings of the patient and significant others to enhance or support coping, problem solving, and interpersonal relationships

Hope Inspiration: Facilitation of the development of a positive outlook in a given situation

Mood Management: Providing for safety, stabilization, recovery, and maintenance of a patient who is experiencing dysfunctionally depressed or elevated mood

Suicide Prevention: Reducing risk of self-inflicted harm with intent to end life

Support System Enhancement: Facilitation of support to patient by family, friends, and community

Nursing Activities

Nursing activities focus on preventing suicide and modifying risk factors.

Assessments

- As often as indicated, but at least daily, assess and document patient's potential for suicide (specify intervals)
- Assess for behaviors that signal thoughts or plans for suicide (e.g., giving away possessions)
- *(NIC) Suicide Prevention:*

  Monitor for medication side effects and desired outcomes

  Search the newly hospitalized patient and personal belongings for weapons or potential weapons during inpatient admission procedure, as appropriate

  Search environment routinely and remove dangerous items to maintain it as hazard free

  Monitor patient during use of potential weapons (e.g., razor)

  Observe, record, and report any change in mood or behavior that may signify increasing suicidal risk and document results of regular surveillance checks

  Conduct mouth checks following medication administration to ensure that patient is not "cheeking" the medications for later overdose attempt

Patient/Family Teaching

- Teach visitors about restricted items (e.g., razors, scissors, plastic bags)
- *(NIC) Suicide Prevention:*

  Explain suicide precautions and relevant safety issues to the patient, family, and significant others (e.g., purpose, duration, behavioral expectations, and behavioral consequences)

Involve family in discharge planning (e.g., illness and medication teaching, recognition of increasing suicidal risk, patient's plan for dealing with thoughts of harming self, community resources)

Collaborative Activities

- Initiate a multidisciplinary patient care conference to develop a plan of care, or when modifying suicide precautions
- *(NIC) Suicide Prevention:*

  Refer patient to mental health care provider (e.g., psychiatrist or psychiatric or mental health advanced practice nurse) for evaluation and treatment of suicide ideation and behavior, as needed

  Administer medications to decrease anxiety, agitation, or psychosis and to stabilize mood, as appropriate

  Assist patient to identify network of supportive persons and resources (e.g., clergy, family, care providers)

  Communicate risk and relevant safety issues to other care providers

Other

- Institute suicide precautions, as needed (e.g., 24-hr attendant)
- Reassure patient that you will protect him against suicidal impulses until he is able to regain control by (a) observing patient constantly (even though privacy is lost), (b) checking patient frequently, and (c) taking the suicidal ideation seriously
- Encourage patient to verbalize anger
- Discuss with patient and family the role of anger in self-harm
- Require patient to wear a hospital gown instead of own clothing if there is risk that he may leave the building
- Use restraint and seclusion, as needed, but place in least restrictive environment that still allows for the necessary level of observation
- Conduct room searches according to institutional policy
- *(NIC) Suicide Prevention:*

  Contract (verbally or in writing) with patient, as appropriate, for "no self-harm" for a specified period of time, recontracting at specified time intervals

  Interact with the patient at regular intervals to convey caring and openness and to provide an opportunity for the patient to talk about feelings

  Avoid repeated discussion of past suicide history by keeping discussions present- and future-oriented

  Limit access to windows, unless locked and shatterproof, as appropriate

  Consider strategies to decrease isolation and opportunity to act on harmful thoughts (e.g., use of a sitter)

Home Care

- Some of the preceding activities can be adapted for home care use
- Teach limit-setting techniques to family
- Teach family and significant others to recognize behaviors signaling an increase in risk (e.g., verbal expressions such as "I'm going to kill myself," or "I wish I could just be gone"; withdrawal)
- *(NIC) Suicide Prevention:* Consider hospitalization of patient who is at serious risk for suicidal behavior

For Infants and Children

- Assess for self-mutilation and eating disorders
- Encourage schools to institute suicide prevention programs

For Older Adults

- Be especially alert for suicidal ideation in older Caucasian men
- Assess for causes of depression (e.g., financial stressors, medications) and intervene appropriately
- Assess for recent, cumulative, or multiple losses
- Evaluate support system
- Encourage physical activity

SURGICAL RECOVERY, DELAYED

(1998, 2006) **Domain 11, Safety/Protection; Class 2, Physical Injury**

Definition: Extension of the number of postoperative days required to initiate and perform activities that maintain life, health, and well-being

Defining Characteristics

Difficulty in moving about
Evidence of interrupted healing of surgical area (e.g., red, indurated, draining, immobile)
Fatigue
Loss of appetite with or without nausea
Perception that more time is needed to recover
Postpones resumption of work or employment activities
Report of pain or discomfort
Requires help to complete self-care

Related Factors

Extensive surgical procedure
Obesity
Pain
Postoperative surgical site infection
Preoperative expectations
Prolonged surgical procedure

Suggestions for Use

The defining characteristics for this diagnosis represent several other nursing diagnoses: *Impaired skin integrity*, *Risk for imbalanced nutrition*, *Nausea*, *Impaired mobility*, *Self-care deficit*, *Fatigue*, and *Pain*. If only one or two of the defining characteristics are present, use those individual diagnoses. If several are present, *Delayed surgical recovery* may be used.

Suggested Alternative Diagnoses

Activity intolerance
Fatigue
Impaired mobility
Impaired skin integrity
Pain
Risk for imbalanced nutrition: less than body requirements
Self-care deficit

NOC Outcomes

Ambulation: Ability to walk from place to place independently with or without assistive device
Endurance: Capacity to sustain activity
Infection Severity: Severity of infection and associated symptoms
Nausea and Vomiting: Severity of nausea, retching, and vomiting symptoms
Pain Level: Severity of observed or reported pain
Postprocedure Recovery: Extent to which an individual returns to baseline function following a procedure(s) requiring anesthesia or sedation
Wound Healing: Primary Intention: Extent of regeneration of cells and tissue following intentional closure

Goals/Evaluation Criteria

Patient will:

- Recognize and cope effectively with surgery-related anxiety
- Regain presurgery energy level, as evidenced by rested appearance, ability to concentrate, and statements that exhaustion is not present

- Regain presurgery mobility
- Demonstrate healing of surgical incision: edges approximated and no drainage, redness, or induration
- Experience timely resolution of pain, progressing to oral analgesics by (date), and requiring no pain medications by (date)
- Meet all discharge criteria by the date of expected stay for his particular surgery

NIC Interventions

Bed Rest Care: Promotion of comfort and safety and prevention of complications for a patient unable to get out of bed

Energy Management: Regulating energy use to treat or prevent fatigue and optimize function

Exercise Promotion: Facilitation of regular physical activity to maintain or advance to a higher level of fitness and health

Exercise Therapy: Ambulation: Promotion and assistance with walking to maintain or restore autonomic and voluntary body functions during treatment and recovery from illness or injury

Fluid Management: Promotion of fluid balance and prevention of complications resulting from abnormal or undesired fluid levels

Incision Site Care: Cleansing, monitoring, and promotion of healing in a wound that is closed with sutures, clips, or staples

Infection Control: Minimizing the acquisition and transmission of infectious agents

Nausea Management: Prevention and alleviation of nausea

Nutrition Management: Assisting with or providing a balanced dietary intake of foods and fluids

Pain Management: Alleviation of pain or a reduction in pain to a level of comfort that is acceptable to the patient

Self-Care Assistance: Assisting another to perform activities of daily living

Surveillance: Purposeful and ongoing acquisition, interpretation, and synthesis of patient data for clinical decision making

Vital Signs Monitoring: Collection and analysis of cardiovascular, respiratory, and body temperature data to determine and prevent complications

Vomiting Management: Prevention and alleviation of vomiting

Wound Care: Prevention of wound complications and promotion of wound healing

Wound Care: Closed Drainage: Maintenance of a pressure drainage system at the wound site

Nursing Activities

NOTE: The following nursing activities are general because the nursing diagnosis is nonspecific. It does not specify any particular type of surgery, and it includes several different nursing diagnoses (see the preceding Suggestions for Use). For more specific nursing activities, refer to Nursing Activities for the nursing diagnoses *Activity intolerance*, *Fatigue*, *Nausea*, *Impaired mobility*, *Impaired skin integrity*, *Pain*, *Risk for imbalanced nutrition: less than body requirements*, and *Self-care deficit.*

Assessments

- Monitor nature and location of pain
- Assess patient's self-care abilities (e.g., consider mobility, sedation, and level of consciousness)
- *(NIC) Surveillance:*
  - Select appropriate patient indices for ongoing monitoring, based on patient's condition
  - Establish the frequency of data collection and interpretation, as indicated by status of the patient
  - Monitor neurologic status
  - Monitor vital signs, as appropriate
  - Monitor for signs and symptoms of fluid and electrolyte imbalance
  - Monitor tissue perfusion, as appropriate
  - Monitor for infection, as appropriate
  - Monitor nutritional status, as appropriate
  - Monitor gastrointestinal function, as appropriate
  - Monitor elimination patterns, as appropriate
  - Monitor for bleeding tendencies in high-risk patient
  - Note type and amount of drainage from tubes and orifices and notify the physician of significant changes
- *(NIC) Energy Management:*
  - Monitor cardiorespiratory response to activity (e.g., tachycardia, other dysrhythmias, dyspnea, diaphoresis, pallor, hemodynamic pressures, and respiratory rate)
  - Monitor or record patient's sleep pattern and number of sleep hours
- *(NIC) Nutrition Management:* Ascertain patient's food preferences
- *(NIC) Wound Care:* Inspect the wound with each dressing change

S

Patient Teaching

- *(NIC) Incision Site Care:* Teach the patient how to minimize stress on the incision site

Collaborative Activities

- *(NIC) Nutrition Management:* Determine—in collaboration with dietitian, as appropriate—number of calories and type of nutrients needed to meet nutrition requirements
- *(NIC) Surveillance:*
  - Analyze physician orders in conjunction with patient status to ensure safety of the patient
  - Obtain consultation from the appropriate health care worker to initiate new treatment or change existing treatments

Other

- Ensure that the patient receives appropriate analgesic care
- Consider cultural influences on pain response
- Reduce or eliminate factors that precipitate or increase the pain experience (e.g., fear, fatigue, monotony, and lack of knowledge)
- Provide assistance until patient is fully able to assume self-care
- Encourage independence but intervene when patient is unable to perform activities
- Compare current status with previous status to detect improvements and deterioration in patient's condition
- Administer IV site care, as appropriate
- *(NIC) Energy Management:*
  - Determine what and how much activity is required to build endurance
  - Use passive and active range-of-motion exercises to relieve muscle tension
  - Avoid care activities during scheduled rest periods
- *(NIC) Wound Care:*
  - Provide incision site care, as needed
  - Reinforce the dressing as needed
  - Change dressing according to amount of exudate and drainage
  - Position to avoid placing tension on the wound, as appropriate

Home Care

- *(NIC) Energy Management:* Instruct the patient and/or significant other techniques of self-care that will minimize oxygen consumption (e.g., self-monitoring and pacing techniques for performance of activities of daily living)
- *(NIC) Incision Site Care:*
  - Instruct the patient on how to care for the incision during bathing or showering
  - Teach the patient and/or family how to care for the incision, including signs and symptoms of infection

For Infants and Children

- Use distraction for pain relief

For Older Adults

- Monitor changes in the patient's baseline temperature; older adults may have subnormal body temperature
- Keep the patient well covered, use warm blankets, and do not administer cold fluids.

SWALLOWING, IMPAIRED

(1986, 1998) **Domain 2, Nutrition; Class 1, Ingestion**

Definition: Abnormal functioning of the swallowing mechanism associated with deficits in oral, pharyngeal, or esophageal structure or function

Defining Characteristics

Pharyngeal Phase Impairment

Abnormality in pharyngeal phase by swallow study
Altered head positions
Choking, coughing, or gagging
Delayed swallow
Food refusal
Gurgly voice quality
Inadequate laryngeal elevation
Multiple swallows
Nasal reflux
Recurrent pulmonary infections
Unexplained fevers

Esophageal Phase Impairment

Abnormality in esophageal phase by swallow study
Acidic-smelling breath
Bruxism
Food refusal or volume limiting
Heartburn or epigastric pain
Hematemesis
Hyperextension of head (e.g., arching during or after meals)
Nighttime coughing or awakening

Observed evidence of difficulty in swallowing (e.g., stasis of food in oral cavity, coughing or choking)
Odynophagia
Regurgitation of gastric contents or wet burps
Repetitive swallowing
Reports "something stuck"
Unexplained irritability surrounding mealtime
Vomiting
Vomitus on pillow

Oral Phase Impairment

Abnormality in oral phase of swallow study
Coughing, choking, gagging before a swallow
Food falls from mouth
Food pushed out of mouth
Inability to clear oral cavity
Incomplete lip closure
Lack of chewing
Lack of tongue action to form bolus
Long meals with little consumption
Nasal reflux
Piecemeal deglutition
Pooling in lateral sulci
Premature entry of bolus
Sialorrhea or drooling
Slow bolus formation
Weak suck, resulting in inefficient nippling

Related Factors

Congenital Deficits

Behavioral feeding problems
Conditions with significant hypotonia
Congenital heart disease
Failure to thrive or protein energy malnutrition
History of tube feeding
Mechanical obstruction (e.g., edema, tracheostomy tube, tumor)
Neuromuscular impairment (e.g., decreased or absent gag reflex, decreased strength or excursion of muscles involved in mastication, perceptual impairment, facial paralysis)
Respiratory disorders
Self-injurious behavior
Upper airway anomalies

Neurological Problems

Achalasia
Acquired anatomic defects
Cerebral palsy
Cranial nerve involvement
Developmental delay
Gastroesophageal reflux disease
Laryngeal or oropharynx abnormalities
Nasal or nasopharyngeal cavity defects
Premature infants
Tracheal, laryngeal, esophageal defects
Traumas
Traumatic head injury
Upper airway anomalies

Suggestions for Use

Impaired swallowing may be associated with a variety of medical conditions (e.g., cerebral palsy, CVA, Parkinson disease, malignancies affecting the brain, reconstructive surgery of the head and neck, and decreased consciousness from anesthesia or other causes). It may also be related to *Fatigue*.

Suggested Alternative Diagnoses

Aspiration, risk for
Infant feeding pattern, ineffective

NOC Outcomes

Aspiration Prevention: Personal actions to prevent the passage of fluid and solid particles into the lung

Swallowing Status: Safe passage of fluids or solids from the mouth to the stomach

Swallowing Status: Esophageal Phase: Safe passage of fluids or solids from the pharynx to the stomach

Swallowing Status: Oral Phase: Preparation, containment, and posterior movement of fluids or solids in the mouth

Swallowing Status: Pharyngeal Phase: Safe passage of fluids or solids from the mouth to the esophagus

Goals/Evaluation Criteria

Examples Using NOC Language

- Demonstrates **Swallowing Status**, as evidenced by the following indicators (specify 1–5: severely, substantially, moderately, mildly, or not compromised):
  - Maintains food in mouth
  - Chewing ability
  - Delivery of bolus to hypopharynx is timed with swallow reflex
  - Ability to clear oral cavity
- Demonstrates **Swallowing Status**, as evidenced by the following indicators (specify 1–5: severe, substantial, moderate, mild, or none):
  - Choking, coughing, or gagging
  - Discomfort with swallowing
  - Increased swallow effort

Other Examples

- Identifies emotional or psychologic factors that interfere with swallowing
- Tolerates food ingestion without choking or aspiration
- Has no impairment of facial and throat muscles, swallowing, tongue movement, or gag reflex

NIC Interventions

Aspiration Precautions: Prevention or minimization of risk factors in the patient at risk for aspiration

Positioning: Deliberative placement of the patient or a body part to promote physiological or psychological well-being

Swallowing Therapy: Facilitating swallowing and preventing complications of impaired swallowing

Surveillance: Purposeful and ongoing acquisition, interpretation, and synthesis of patient data for clinical decision making

Vomiting Management: Prevention and alleviation of vomiting

Nursing Activities

Assessments

- Evaluate family's comfort level
- *(NIC) Aspiration Precautions:* Monitor level of consciousness, cough reflex, gag reflex, and swallowing ability

- *(NIC) Swallowing Therapy:*
  Monitor patient's tongue movements while eating
  Monitor for signs and symptoms of aspiration
  Monitor for sealing of lips during eating, drinking, and swallowing
  Check mouth for pocketing of food after eating
  Monitor body hydration (e.g., intake, output, skin turgor, and mucous membranes)

Patient/Family Teaching

- *(NIC) Swallowing Therapy:*
  Instruct patient to reach for particles of food on lips or chin with tongue
  Instruct patient and caregiver on emergency measures for choking

Collaborative Activities

- Consult dietitian for food that can be easily swallowed
- *(NIC) Aspiration Precautions:* Request medication in elixir form
- *(NIC) Swallowing Therapy:*
  Collaborate with other members of health care team (e.g., occupational therapist, speech pathologist, and dietitian) to provide continuity in patient's rehabilitative plan
  Collaborate with speech therapist to instruct patient's family about swallowing exercise regimen

Other

- Reassure patient during episodes of choking
- *(NIC) Aspiration Precautions:*
  Position upright 90 degrees or as far as possible
  Keep tracheal cuff inflated
  Keep suction setup available
  Feed in small amounts
  Avoid liquids or use thickening agent
  Cut food into small pieces
  Break or crush pills before administration
- *(NIC) Swallowing Therapy:*
  Provide mouth care, as needed
  Provide or use assistive devices, as appropriate
  Avoid use of drinking straws
  Assist patient to position head in forward flexion in preparation for swallowing (chin tuck)
  Assist patient to place food at back of mouth and on unaffected side

Home Care

- The preceding activities can be used or adapted for home care
- *(NIC) Swallowing Therapy:*
  Instruct family or caregiver how to position, feed, and monitor patient

For Infants and Children

- Assess for structural defects (e.g., pyloric stenosis) that may interfere with swallowing; refer to a physician as needed
- For infants, support the jaw and cheeks to facilitate sucking

For Older Adults

- Recognize that dysphagia is not a normal change related to aging
- Allow adequate time for eating; do not rush the patient
- Assess dentition
- Identify medications the client is taking that might cause difficulty swallowing

THERAPEUTIC REGIMEN MANAGEMENT: FAMILY, INEFFECTIVE

(1994) **Domain 1, Health Promotion; Class 2, Health Management**

Definition: A pattern of regulating and integrating into family processes a program for the treatment of illness and its sequelae that is unsatisfactory for meeting specific health goals

Defining Characteristics

Subjective

Verbalized desire to manage the illness [and prevent sequelae]

Verbalized difficulty with prescribed regimen

Objective

Acceleration [expected or unexpected] of illness symptoms of a family member

Failure to take action to reduce risk factors

Inappropriate family activities for meeting health goals

Lack of attention to illness [and its sequelae]

Related Factors

Complexity of health care system
Complexity of therapeutic regimen
Decisional conflicts
Economic difficulties
Excessive demands [made on individual or family]
Family conflict

Suggestions for Use

Use this diagnosis for families who are motivated to follow a therapeutic regimen but who are having difficulty doing so. It is not appropriate for families who are not interested in adhering to the treatment program. This diagnosis is more narrowly focused than *Interrupted family processes* or *Compromised or Disabled family coping*, all of which include problems other than managing the family's treatment program.

Suggested Alternative Diagnoses

Coping: family, disabled
Family processes, interrupted
Health maintenance, ineffective

NOC Outcomes

Caregiver Home Care Readiness: Preparedness of a caregiver to assume responsibility for the health care of a family member in the home

Family Normalization: Capacity of the family system to maintain routines and develop strategies for optimal functioning when a member has a chronic illness or disability

Family Participation in Professional Care: Family involvement in decision-making, delivery, and evaluation of care provided by health care personnel

Family Resiliency: Positive adaptation and function of the family system following significant adversity or crisis

Goals/Evaluation Criteria

The family will:

- Indicate a desire to manage the therapeutic regimen or program
- Identify factors interfering with adhering to the therapeutic regimen
- Adjust usual activities as needed to incorporate the treatment programs of family members (e.g., diet, school activities)
- Experience a decrease in illness symptoms among family members

NIC Interventions

Caregiver Support: Provision of the necessary information, advocacy, and support to facilitate primary patient care by someone other than a health care professional

Coping Enhancement: Assisting a patient to adapt to perceived stressors, changes, or threats that interfere with meeting life demands and roles

Decision-Making Support: Providing information and support for a patient who is making a decision regarding health care

Family Integrity Promotion: Promotion of family cohesion and unity

Family Involvement Promotion: Facilitating family participation in the emotional and physical care of the patient

Family Mobilization: Utilization of family strengths to influence patient's health in a positive direction

Family Process Maintenance: Minimization of family process disruption effects

Normalization Promotion: Assisting parents and other family members of children with chronic illness or disabilities in providing normal life experiences for their children and families

Resiliency Promotion: Assisting individuals, families, and communities in development, use, and strengthening of protective factors to be used in coping with environmental and societal stressors

Self-Efficacy Enhancement: Strengthening an individual's confidence in his or her ability to perform a health behavior

Teaching: Procedure/Treatment: Preparing a patient to understand and mentally prepare for a prescribed procedure or treatment

T

Nursing Activities

Assessments

- Assess present status of family coping and processes
- Assess family members' levels of understanding of illness, complications, and recommended treatments
- Assess family members' readiness to learn
- Identify family cultural influences and health beliefs
- Interview family members to determine problem areas in integrating treatment regimen into lifestyle
- *(NIC) Family Involvement Promotion:*

  Identify family members' capabilities for involvement in care of patient

  Determine physical, emotional, and educational resources of primary caregiver

  Monitor family structure and roles

  Identify family members' expectations for the patient

Determine level of patient dependence on family, as appropriate for age or illness

Identify and respect coping mechanisms used by family members

Patient/Family Teaching

- Teach family time management and organizational skills
- Provide caregivers with skills needed for patient's therapy
- Teach strategies for maintaining or restoring patient's health
- Teach strategies for care of a dying patient
- Offer information on community resources specific to health goals of the patient
- Provide information on illness, complications, and recommended treatments
- *(NIC) Family Involvement Promotion:* Facilitate understanding of the medical aspects of the patient's condition for family members

Collaborative Activities

- Help family to identify community health care resources
- Refer family to family support groups
- Collaborate with other health care providers to determine how to modify therapeutic regimen without jeopardizing patient's health

Other

- Involve family in discussion of strengths and resources
- Assist patient and family to establish realistic goals
- Assist family members to plan and implement patient therapies and lifestyle changes
- Support maintenance of family routines and rituals in hospital (e.g., private meals together, family discussions)
- Discuss family's plans for child care when parents must be absent
- Assist the family to develop a realistic plan to achieve adherence to the therapeutic regimen
- Plan patient home care activities to decrease disruption of family routine
- Provide coaching and support to motivate continued adherence to the therapy
- *(NIC) Family Involvement Promotion:*

  Encourage care by family members during hospitalization or stay in a long-term care facility

  Encourage family members to keep or maintain family relationships, as appropriate

  Encourage family members and patient to be assertive in interactions with health care professionals

  Identify with family members the patient's coping difficulties, strengths, and abilities

Home Care

- The preceding activities can be used or adapted for home care
- Assist the family to find ways to integrate the therapeutic regimen into their activities of daily living

THERMAL INJURY, RISK FOR

(2010) **Domain 11, Safety/Protection; Class 2, Physical Injury**

Definition: At risk for damage to skin and mucous membranes due to extreme temperatures

Risk Factors

Cognitive impairment (e.g., dementia, psychoses)
Developmental level (infants, aged)
Exposure to extreme temperatures
Fatigue
Inadequate supervision
Inattentiveness
Intoxication (alcohol, drug)
Lack of knowledge (patient, caregiver)
Lack of protective clothing (e.g., flame-retardant sleepwear, gloves, ear covering)
Neuromuscular impairment (e.g., stroke, amyotrophic lateral sclerosis, multiple sclerosis)
Neuropathy
Smoking
Treatment-related side effects (e.g., pharmaceutical agents)
Unsafe environment

Suggestions for Use

This diagnosis is differentiated from *Hypothermia* and *Hyperthermia* because it is limited to skin and mucous membrane injury; it does not refer to elevation in body temperature. Risk for thermal injury is a potential problem; if damage to skin or mucous membranes occurs, use *Impaired skin integrity* or *Impaired tissue integrity*, depending on the severity of the damage. If body temperature is elevated and other defining characteristics are present, diagnose *Hyperthermia*.

Suggested Alternative Diagnoses

Hyperthermia
Skin integrity, impaired
Tissue integrity, impaired

NOC Outcomes

NOTE: NOC outcomes have not yet been linked to this diagnosis; however, the following may be useful.

Risk Control: Sun Exposure: Personal actions to prevent or reduce threats to the skin and eyes from sun exposure

Sensory Function: Extent to which an individual correctly senses skin stimulation, sounds, proprioception, taste and smell, and visual images

Tissue Integrity: Skin and Mucous Membranes: Structural intactness and normal physiological function of skin and mucous membranes

Goals/Evaluation Criteria

Examples Using NOC Language

- Thermal injury will be avoided, as evidenced by Risk Control: Sun Exposure, and Tissue Integrity: Skin and Mucous Membranes
- **Tissue Integrity: Skin and Mucous Membranes** is demonstrated, as evidenced by the following indicators (specify 1–5: severely, substantially, moderately, mildly, or not compromised): Erythema, elasticity, skin temperature

Other Examples

- Uses appropriate amount of sunscreen with recommended sun protection factor (SPF)
- Wears ultraviolet protection glasses as appropriate
- Avoids exposure to midday sun (10 A.M. to 4 P.M.)
- Protects face and head by wearing a hat with a 4-in. brim

NIC Interventions

NOTE: NIC interventions have not yet been linked to *Risk for thermal injury*; however, the following may be useful.

Health Screening: Detecting health risks or problems by means of history, examination, and other procedures

Skin Surveillance: Collection and analysis of patient data to maintain skin and mucous membrane integrity

Nursing Activities

In general, nursing activities for this diagnosis focus on identifying and modifying risk factors to prevent thermal injury.

Assessments

- Assess for cognitive impairment
- Assess for physical factors that might increase risk of thermal injury (e.g., neuropathy)
- Note skin color (pale skin burns more readily than darker skin)
- Determine developmental level
- Inquire how much time the patient spends in the sun
- Assess knowledge of measures to protect against sunburn
- Ask whether the patient or other family members smoke
- Inspect the skin for past overexposure to the sun (e.g., redness, peeling, blisters)

Patient/Family Teaching

- Teach home safety measures regarding fire and burns prevention, for example:
  - Turn pot handles toward the back of the stove when cooking
  - Do not leave burning cigarettes unattended; do not smoke in bed
  - Never wear loose-fitting clothing when cooking
- Teach the risks of sun exposure (e.g., skin cancer, eye damage)
- Teach sun protection measures, as needed, for example:
  - Wear protective clothing and sunscreen when outside (use broad-spectrum sunscreen of at least 15 or higher)
  - See a medical provider if blistering covers a large portion of your body, or if you have a high fever, severe pain, headache, confusion, nausea, or chills
  - Remember, you can get a sunburn on hazy or cloudy days
  - Do not use tanning booths (they increase the risk of skin cancer)

Home Care

- Inspect the home for fire hazards

Infants and Children

- Keep infants younger than 6 months old out of the sun. Always use sunscreen on older children

THERMOREGULATION, INEFFECTIVE

(1986) **Domain 11, Safety/Protection; Class 6, Thermoregulation**

Definition: Temperature fluctuation between hypothermia and hyperthermia

Defining Characteristics

Objective

Cool skin
Cyanotic nail beds
Fluctuations in body temperature above or below normal range
Flushed skin
Hypertension
Increased body temperature
Increased respiratory rate
Pallor (moderate)
Piloerection
Reduction in body temperature below normal range
Seizures [convulsions]
Shivering (mild)
Slow capillary refill
Tachycardia
Warm to touch

T

Related Factors

Extremes of age
Fluctuating environmental temperature
Illness
Trauma

Suggestions for Use

This label is most appropriate for patients who are especially vulnerable to environmental conditions (e.g., newborns and the elderly). If body temperature is not fluctuating, use *Hypothermia*, *Hypothermia*, or *Risk for imbalanced body temperature*.

Suggested Alternative Diagnoses

Body temperature, risk for imbalanced
Hyperthermia
Hypothermia

NOC Outcomes

Thermoregulation: Balance among heat production, heat gain, and heat loss

Thermoregulation: Newborn: Balance among heat production, heat gain, and heat loss during the first 28 days of life

Goals/Evaluation Criteria

For specific patient outcomes and evaluation criteria, refer to Goals/Evaluation Criteria for Hyperthermia, Hypothermia, and Risk for Imbalanced Body Temperature.

NIC Interventions

Newborn Monitoring: Measurement and interpretation of physiologic status of the neonate the first 24 hr after delivery

Newborn Care: Management of neonate during the transition to extrauterine life and subsequent period of stabilization

Temperature Regulation: Attaining or maintaining body temperature within a normal range

Temperature Regulation: Intraoperative: Attaining or maintaining desired intraoperative body temperature

Nursing Activities

Nursing interventions focus on teaching for prevention of *Ineffective thermoregulation* and on maintaining a normal body temperature by manipulating external factors, such as clothing and room temperature. Refer to Nursing Activities for Risk for Imbalanced Body Temperature, Hyperthermia, and Hypothermia.

TISSUE INTEGRITY, IMPAIRED

(1986, 1998) **Domain 11, Safety/Protection; Class 2, Physical Injury**

Definition: Damage to mucous membrane, corneal, integumentary, or subcutaneous tissues

Defining Characteristics

Objective

Damaged or destroyed tissue (e.g., corneal, mucous membrane, integumentary, or subcutaneous)

Related Factors

Altered circulation
Chemical irritants [e.g., body excretions and secretions, medications)]
Fluid deficit or excess
Impaired physical mobility
Knowledge deficit
Mechanical factors (e.g., pressure, shear, friction)
Nutritional factors (e.g., deficit or excess)
Radiation [including therapeutic radiation]
Temperature extremes

Suggestions for Use

1. If tissue integrity is at risk because of immobility and if other systems are also at risk, consider using *Risk for disuse syndrome*.
2. If the necessary defining characteristics are present, use the more specific problems of *Impaired oral mucous membrane* or *Impaired skin integrity*. *Impaired tissue integrity* should be used only when the damage is to tissue other than the skin and mucous membranes.
3. Do not use *Impaired tissue integrity* to rename a surgical incision or ostomy.

Suggested Alternative Diagnoses

Disuse syndrome, risk for
Oral mucous membrane, impaired
Skin integrity, impaired
Surgical recovery, delayed

NOC Outcomes

Allergic Response: Localized: Severity of localized hypersensitive immune response to a specific environmental (exogenous) antigen
Ostomy Self-Care: Personal actions to maintain ostomy for elimination
Tissue Integrity: Skin and Mucous Membranes: Structural intactness and normal physiologic function of skin and mucous membranes
Wound Healing: Primary Intention: Extent of regeneration of cells and tissue following intentional closure
Wound Healing: Secondary Intention: Extent of regeneration of cells and tissues in an open wound

Goals/Evaluation Criteria

Also refer to Goals/Evaluation Criteria for Impaired Skin Integrity.

Examples Using NOC Language

- Demonstrates **Tissue Integrity: Skin and Mucous Membranes**, as evidenced by the following indicators (specify 1–5: severely, substantially, moderately, mildly, or not compromised):
  - Skin integrity
  - Tissue texture and thickness
  - Tissue perfusion

Other Examples

- No signs or symptoms of infection
- No lesions
- No necrosis

NIC Interventions

Incision Site Care: Cleansing, monitoring, and promotion of healing in a wound that is closed with sutures, clips, or staples

Infection Protection: Prevention and early detection of infection in a patient at risk

Oral Health Maintenance: Maintenance and promotion of oral hygiene and dental health for the patient at risk for developing oral or dental lesions

Ostomy Care: Maintenance of elimination through a stoma and care of surrounding tissue

Pressure Management: Minimizing pressure to body parts

Pressure Ulcer Care: Facilitation of healing in pressure ulcers

Pressure Ulcer Prevention: Prevention of pressure ulcers for an individual at high risk for developing them

Skin Care: Topical Treatments: Application of topical substances or manipulation of devices to promote skin integrity and minimize skin breakdown

Skin Surveillance: Collection and analysis of patient data to maintain skin and mucous membrane integrity

Wound Care: Prevention of wound complications and promotion of wound healing

Nursing Activities

For specific nursing activities, refer to Nursing Activities, in the following nursing diagnoses:

Infection, risk for
Oral mucous membrane, impaired
Skin integrity, impaired
Skin integrity, risk for impaired
Tissue perfusion, ineffective (peripheral)

TISSUE PERFUSION: CARDIAC, RISK FOR DECREASED

(2008) **Domain 4, Activity/Rest; Class 4, Cardiovascular/Pulmonary Responses**

Definition: At risk for a decrease in cardiac (coronary) circulation that may compromise health

Risk Factors

Birth control pills
Cardiac surgery
Cardiac tamponade
Coronary artery spasm
Deficient knowledge of modifiable risk factors (e.g., smoking, sedentary lifestyle, obesity)
Diabetes mellitus
Elevated C-reactive protein
Family history of coronary artery disease
Hyperlipidemia
Hypertension
Hypovolemia
Hypoxemia
Hypoxia
Substance abuse

Suggestions for Use

Risk for ineffective cardiac tissue perfusion is a potential diagnosis. If it becomes an actual problem, medical care is needed. The nurse's role is to monitor and detect changes in the patient's condition; therefore, you may wish to use a collaborative problem label such as *Potential Complication of coronary artery spasm: Ineffective cardiac tissue perfusion.*

Suggested Alternative Diagnoses

Cardiac output, decreased

NOC Outcomes

NOTE: The following outcomes are used to measure occurrence of actual ineffective cardiac tissue perfusion.

Circulation Status: Unobstructed, unidirectional blood flow at an appropriate pressure through large vessels of the systemic and pulmonary circuits

Tissue Perfusion: Cardiac: Adequacy of blood flow through the coronary vasculature to maintain heart function

NOTE: The following outcomes are associated with risk factors for decreased cardiac tissue perfusion.

Cardiac Pump Effectiveness: Adequacy of blood volume ejected from the left ventricle to support systemic perfusion pressure

Knowledge: Diabetes Management: Extent of understanding conveyed about diabetes mellitus, its treatment, and the prevention of complications

Knowledge: Diet: Extent of understanding conveyed about recommended diet

Knowledge: Health Behavior: Extent of understanding conveyed about the promotion and protection of health

Smoking Cessation Behavior: Personal actions to eliminate tobacco use

Goals/Evaluation Criteria

Examples Using NOC Language

- Demonstrates satisfactory **Cardiac Pump Effectiveness** and **Cardiac Tissue Perfusion**
- Demonstrates **Circulation Status**, as evidenced by the following indicators (specify 1–5: severe, substantial, moderate, mild, or no deviation from normal range):
  - PaO_2 and $PaCO_2$ (partial pressure of oxygen or carbon dioxide in arterial blood)
  - Left and right carotid, brachial, radial, femoral, and pedal pulses
  - Systolic BP, diastolic BP, pulse pressure, mean BP, CVP, and pulmonary wedge pressure
- Demonstrates **Circulation Status**, as evidenced by the following indicators (specify 1–5: severe, substantial, moderate, mild, or none):
  - Angina
  - Adventitious breath sounds, neck vein distention, or large vessel bruits
  - Extreme fatigue
  - Peripheral edema and ascites

NIC Interventions

NOTE: Nursing interventions focus on prevention of decreased cardiac tissue perfusion.

Cardiac Precautions: Prevention of an acute episode of impaired cardiac function by minimizing myocardial oxygen consumption or increasing myocardial oxygen supply

Exercise Promotion: Facilitation of regular physical activity to maintain or advance to a higher level of fitness and health

Fluid Management: Promotion of fluid balance and prevention of complications resulting from abnormal or undesired fluid levels

Oxygen Therapy: Administration of oxygen and monitoring of its effectiveness

Smoking Cessation Assistance: Helping another to stop smoking

Substance Use Treatment: Supportive care of patient and family members with physical and psychosocial problems associated with the use of alcohol or drugs

Surveillance: Purposeful and ongoing acquisition, interpretation, and synthesis of patient data for clinical decision making

Vital Signs Monitoring: Collection and analysis of cardiovascular, respiratory, and body temperature data to determine and prevent complications

Weight Reduction Assistance: Facilitating loss of weight and/or body fat

Nursing Activities

Assessments

- Monitor chest pain (e.g., intensity, duration, and precipitating factors)
- Observe for ST changes on ECG
- Monitor cardiac rate and rhythm
- Auscultate heart and lung sounds
- Monitor coagulation studies (e.g., prothrombin time [PT], partial thromboplastin time [PTT], and platelet counts)
- Weigh patient daily
- Monitor electrolyte values associated with dysrhythmias (e.g., serum potassium and magnesium)
- Perform a comprehensive assessment of peripheral circulation (e.g., peripheral pulses, edema, capillary refill, skin color, and temperature)
- Monitor intake and output
- Monitor peripheral pulses and edema
- *(NIC) Cardiac Precautions:*

  Identify patient's readiness to learn lifestyle modifications

  Identify the patient's methods of handling stress

Patient/Family Teaching

- Instruct the patient to avoid performing Valsalva maneuver (e.g., do not strain during bowel movement)
- Explain restrictions on caffeine, sodium, cholesterol, and fat intake
- Explain rationale for eating small, frequent meals

Collaborative Activities

- Administer medications according to order or protocols (e.g., analgesics, anticoagulants, nitroglycerin, vasodilators, diuretic, and positive inotropic and contractility medications)

Other

- Reassure patient and family that call bells, lights, and pages will be answered promptly
- Promote rest (e.g., limit visitors, control environmental stimuli)
- Apply compression therapy, as appropriate (e.g., antiembolism stockings, sequential compression device)

TISSUE PERFUSION: CEREBRAL, RISK FOR INEFFECTIVE

(2008) **Domain 4, Activity/Rest; Class 4, Cardiovascular/Pulmonary Responses**

Definition: At risk for a decrease in cerebral tissue circulation that may compromise health

Risk Factors

Abnormal partial thromboplastin time
Abnormal prothrombin time
Akinetic left ventricular segment
Aortic atherosclerosis
Arterial dissection
Atrial fibrillation
Atrial myxoma
Brain tumor
Carotid stenosis
Cerebral aneurysm
Coagulopathy (e.g., sickle cell anemia)
Dilated cardiomyopathy
Disseminated intravascular coagulation
Embolism
Head trauma
Hypercholesterolemia
Hypertension
Infective endocarditis
Mechanical prosthetic valve

Mitral stenosis
Neoplasm of the brain
Recent myocardial infarction
Sick sinus syndrome
Substance abuse
Thrombolytic therapy
Treatment-related side effects (cardiopulmonary bypass, pharmaceutical agents)

Suggestions for Use

Actual ineffective cerebral tissue perfusion would represent a medical diagnoses or condition. The outcomes and interventions would be for medical/surgical treatments. The nurse's role is to monitor and detect changes in the patient's condition. Therefore, nursing care may be better directed by the use of collaborative problems (e.g., Potential Complication of recent myocardial infarction: Ineffective cerebral tissue perfusion).

Suggested Alternative Diagnoses

Cardiac output, decreased

NOC Outcomes

NOTE: The following outcome is used to assess actual occurrence of ineffective cerebral tissue perfusion:

Tissue Perfusion: Cerebral: Adequacy of blood flow through the cerebral vasculature to maintain brain function

T

NOTE: The following outcomes are associated with risk factors for *Risk for ineffective cerebral tissue perfusion.*

Blood Coagulation: Extent to which blood clots within normal period of time

Cardiac Pump Effectiveness: Adequacy of blood volume ejected from the left ventricle to support systemic perfusion pressure

Circulation Status: Unobstructed, unidirectional blood flow at an appropriate pressure through large vessels of the systemic and pulmonary circuits

Knowledge: Hypertension Management: Extent of understanding conveyed about high blood pressure, its treatment, and the prevention of complications

Neurologic Status: Ability of the peripheral and central nervous systems to receive, process, and respond to internal and external stimuli

Physical Injury Severity: Severity of injuries from accidents and trauma

Examples Using NOC Language

- Demonstrates **Circulation Status**, as evidenced by the following indicators (specify 1–5: severely, substantially, moderately, mildly, or not compromised): Systolic and diastolic BP
- Demonstrates **Cerebral Tissue Perfusion**, as evidenced by the following indicators (specify 1–5: severe, substantial, moderate, mild, or no deviation from normal range):
  - Intracranial pressure
  - Systolic and diastolic blood pressure
- Demonstrates **Cerebral Tissue Perfusion**, as evidenced by the following indicators (specify 1–5: severe, substantial, moderate, mild, or none):
  - Agitation
  - Carotid bruit
  - Impaired neurological reflexes
  - Vomiting

Other Examples

Patient will:

- Have intact central and peripheral nervous systems
- Demonstrate intact cranial sensorimotor function
- Demonstrate normal level of consciousness
- Exhibit intact autonomic functioning
- Have pupils equal and reactive
- Be free from seizure activity
- Not experience headache

NIC Interventions

T

Nursing interventions focus on assessing for and preventing ineffective cerebral tissue perfusion.

Cerebral Edema Management: Limitation of secondary cerebral injury resulting from swelling of brain tissue

Intracranial Pressure (ICP) Monitoring: Measurement and interpretation of patient data to regulate intracranial pressure

Neurologic Monitoring: Collection and analysis of patient data to prevent or minimize neurologic complications

Intracranial Pressure (ICP) Monitoring: Measurement and interpretation of patient data to regulate intracranial pressure

Nursing Activities

NOTE: Nursing activities vary depending on which risk factors are present. Only a few examples can be given here.

Assessments

- Monitor the following:
  - Vital signs: temperature, BP, pulse, and respirations
  - WBC count
  - PO_2, PCO_2, pH, and bicarbonate levels
  - $PaCO_2$, SaO_2, and hemoglobin levels to determine delivery of oxygen to tissues
  - Pupil size, shape, symmetry, and reactivity
  - Diplopia, nystagmus, blurred vision, and visual acuity
  - Headache
  - Level of consciousness and orientation
  - Memory, mood, and affect
  - Cardiac output
  - Corneal, cough, and gag reflexes
  - Muscle tone, motor movement, gait, and proprioception
- *(NIC) Intracranial Pressure (ICP) Monitoring:*
  - Monitor patient's intracranial pressure and neurological response to care activities and environmental stimuli
  - Monitor cerebral perfusion pressure
  - Monitor insertion site for infection or leakage of fluid

Collaborative Activities

- Maintain hemodynamic parameters (e.g., systemic arterial pressure) within prescribed range
- Administer medications to expand intravascular volume, as ordered
- Induce hypertension to maintain cerebral perfusion pressure, as ordered
- Administer osmotic and loop diuretics, as ordered
- Elevate head of bed from 0 to 45 degrees, depending on patient's condition and medical orders

T

Other

- Minimize environmental stimuli
- *(NIC) Intracranial Pressure (ICP) Monitoring:*
  - Maintain sterility of monitoring system
  - Space nursing care to minimize ICP elevation

TISSUE PERFUSION: PERIPHERAL, INEFFECTIVE

(2008, 2010)

Domain 4, Activity/Rest; Class 4, Cardiovascular/Pulmonary Responses

Definition: Decrease in blood circulation to the periphery that may compromise health

Table 10

Objective data	Chances that characteristics will be present in given diagnosis	Chances that characteristics will not be explained by any other diagnosis
Skin temperature: cold extremities	High	Low
Skin color: dependent blue or purple	Moderate	Low
Pale on elevation, color does not return on lowering leg	High	High
Diminished arterial pulsations	High	High
Skin quality shining	High	Low
Lack of lanugo; round scars covered with atrophied skin	High	Moderate
Gangrene	Low	High
Slow-growing, dry, brittle nails	High	Moderate
Claudication	Moderate	High
Blood pressure changes in extremities	Moderate	Moderate
Bruits	Moderate	Moderate
Slow healing of lesions	High	Low

T

Defining Characteristics

Absent pulses
Altered motor function
Altered skin characteristics (color, elasticity, hair, moisture, nails, sensation, temperature)
Ankle-brachial index < 0.90
Blood pressure changes in extremities
Capillary refill time > 3 s
Claudication
Color does not return to leg on lowering it
Delayed peripheral wound healing
Diminished pulses
Edema
Extremity pain

Femoral bruit
Shorter total distances achieved in the 6-min walk test
Shorter pain-free distance achieved in the 6-min walk test
Paresthesia
Skin color pale on elevation [of limb]

Related Factors

Deficient knowledge of aggravating factors (e.g., smoking, sedentary lifestyle, trauma, obesity, salt intake, immobility)
Deficient knowledge of disease process (e.g., diabetes, hyperlipidemia)
Diabetes mellitus
Hypertension
Sedentary lifestyle
Smoking

Suggestions for Use

Because some of the nursing interventions are different, it is usually important to determine whether *Ineffective peripheral tissue perfusion* is of arterial or venous origin.

Suggested Alternative Diagnoses

Injury, risk for
Neurovascular dysfunction: peripheral, risk for
Skin integrity, risk for impaired
Tissue integrity, risk for impaired

NOC Outcomes

Circulation Status: Unobstructed, unidirectional blood flow at an appropriate pressure through large vessels of the systemic and pulmonary circuits

Fluid Overload Severity: Severity of excess fluids in the intracellular and extracellular compartments of the body

Sensory Function: Cutaneous: Extent to which stimulation of the skin is correctly sensed

Tissue Integrity: Skin and Mucous Membranes: Structural intactness and normal physiological function of skin and mucous membranes

Tissue Perfusion: Peripheral: Adequacy of blood flow through the small vessels of the extremities to maintain tissue function

Goals/Evaluation Criteria

Examples Using NOC Language

- Demonstrates **Circulation Status**, as evidenced by the following indicators (specify 1–5: severe, substantial, moderate, mild, or no deviation from normal range):
  - PaO_2 and $PaCO_2$ or partial pressure of oxygen and carbon dioxide in arterial blood
  - Left and right carotid, brachial, radial, femoral, and pedal pulses
  - Systolic BP, diastolic BP, pulse pressure, mean BP, CVP, and pulmonary wedge pressure
- Demonstrates **Circulation Status**, as evidenced by the following indicators (specify 1–5: severe, substantial, moderate, mild, or none):
  - Adventitious breath sounds, neck vein distention, [pulmonary] edema, or large vessel bruits
  - Fatigue
  - Peripheral edema and ascites
- Demonstrates **Tissue Integrity: Skin and Mucous Membranes**, as evidenced by the following indicators (specify 1–5: severely, substantially, moderately, mildly, or not compromised):
  - Skin temperature, sensation, elasticity, hydration, intactness, and thickness
  - Tissue perfusion
- Demonstrates **Tissue Perfusion: Peripheral**, as evidenced by the following indicators (specify 1–5: severely, substantially, moderately, mildly, or not compromised):
  - Capillary refill (fingers and toes)
  - Skin color
  - Sensation
  - Skin integrity

Other Examples

Patient will:

- Exhibit intact autonomic functioning
- Report sufficient energy
- Walk 6 min with no lower extremity pain

NIC Interventions

NOTE: Interventions vary depending on the etiology. Not every possible intervention can be shown here.

Circulatory Care: Arterial Insufficiency: Promotion of arterial circulation

T

Circulatory Care: Venous Insufficiency: Promotion of venous circulation

Circulatory Precautions: Protection of a localized area with limited perfusion

Exercise Promotion: Facilitation of regular physical activity to maintain or advance to a higher level of fitness and health

Fluid/Electrolyte Management: Regulation and prevention of complications from altered fluid and/or electrolyte levels

Fluid Management: Promotion of fluid balance and prevention of complications resulting from abnormal or undesired fluid levels

Lower Extremity Monitoring: Collection, analysis, and use of patient data to categorize risk and prevent injury to the lower extremities

Peripheral Sensation Management: Prevention or minimization of injury or discomfort in the patient with altered sensation

Pressure Management: Minimizing pressure to body parts

Skin Surveillance: Collection and analysis of patient data to maintain skin and mucous membrane integrity

Smoking Cessation Assistance: Helping another to stop smoking

Teaching: Procedure/Treatment: Preparing a patient to understand and mentally prepare for a prescribed procedure or treatment

Nursing Activities

Assessments

- Assess for stasis ulcers and symptoms of cellulitis (i.e., pain, redness, and swelling in extremities)
- *(NIC) Circulatory Care (Arterial and Venous Insufficiency):*
  - Perform a comprehensive appraisal of peripheral circulation (e.g., check peripheral pulses, edema, capillary refill, color, and temperature [of extremity])
  - Monitor degree of discomfort or pain with exercise, at night, or while resting [arterial]
  - Monitor fluid status, including intake and output
- *(NIC) Peripheral Sensation Management:*
  - Monitor [peripherally] sharp or dull or hot or cold discrimination
  - Monitor for paresthesia: numbness, tingling, hyperesthesia, and hypoesthesia
  - Monitor for thrombophlebitis and deep vein thrombosis
  - Monitor fit of bracing devices, prosthesis, shoes, and clothing
- Monitor coagulation studies (e.g., prothrombin time [PT], partial thromboplastin time [PTT], and platelet counts)
- Monitor electrolyte values associated with dysrhythmias (e.g., serum potassium and magnesium)

- Perform a comprehensive assessment of peripheral circulation (e.g., peripheral pulses, edema, capillary refill, skin color, skin temperature)
- Assess peripheral skin integrity
- Assess muscle tone, motor movement, gait, and proprioception
- Monitor intake and output
- Monitor hydration status (e.g., moist mucous membranes, adequacy of pulses, and orthostatic blood pressure), as appropriate
- Monitor lab results relevant to fluid retention (e.g., increased specific gravity, increased BUN, decreased hematocrit, and increased urine osmolality levels)
- Monitor for indications of fluid overload or retention (e.g., crackles, elevated CVP or pulmonary capillary wedge pressure, edema, neck vein distention, and ascites), as appropriate

Patient/Family Teaching

- Teach the benefits of exercise to peripheral circulation
- Teach the importance of alternating exercise with rest, especially with arterial insufficiency
- Teach the effects of smoking on peripheral circulation

Instruct patient and family about:

- Avoiding extremes of temperature to extremities
- The importance of adhering to diet and medication regimen
- Reportable signs and symptoms that may require notification of physician
- The importance of prevention of venous stasis (e.g., not crossing legs, elevating feet without bending knees, and exercise)
- *(NIC) Circulatory Care (Arterial and Venous Insufficiency):* Instruct patient on proper foot care
- *(NIC) Peripheral Sensation Management:*
  - Instruct patient or family to monitor position of body parts while patient is bathing, sitting, lying, or changing position
  - Instruct patient or family to examine skin daily for alteration in skin integrity

T

Collaborative Activities

- Administer medications according to order or protocols (e.g., analgesics, anticoagulants, nitroglycerin, vasodilators, diuretic, and positive inotropic and contractility medications)
- Notify physician if pain is unrelieved
- *(NIC) Circulatory Care (Arterial and Venous Insufficiency):* Administer antiplatelet or anticoagulant medications, as appropriate

Other

- Distribute prescribed fluid intake appropriately over 24-hr period
- Maintain fluid and diet restrictions (e.g., low sodium, no salt), as ordered
- Avoid chemical, mechanical, or thermal trauma to involved extremity
- Discourage smoking and use of stimulants
- *(NIC) Circulatory Care: Arterial Insufficiency:*
  Place extremity in a dependent position, as appropriate
- *(NIC) Circulatory Care: Venous Insufficiency:*
  Apply compression therapy modalities (short-stretch or long-stretch bandages), as appropriate
  Elevate affected limb 20 degrees or greater above the level of the heart, as appropriate
  Encourage passive or active range-of-motion exercises especially of the lower extremities, during bed rest
- *(NIC) Peripheral Sensation Management:*
  Avoid or carefully monitor use of heat or cold, such as heating pads, hot-water bottles, and ice packs
  Place bed cradle over affected body parts to keep bedclothes off affected areas
  Discuss or identify causes of abnormal sensations or sensation changes

T

Home Care

- The preceding activities can be used or adapted for home care

For Older Adults

- Be especially alert for symptoms of pulmonary embolism in older adults

TISSUE PERFUSION: PERIPHERAL, RISK FOR INEFFECTIVE

(2010)

Domain 4, Activity/Rest;
Class 4, Cardiovascular/Pulmonary Responses

Definition: At risk for a decrease in blood circulation to the periphery that may compromise health

Risk Factors

Age > 60 years
Deficient knowledge of aggravating factors (e.g., smoking, sedentary lifestyle, trauma, obesity, salt intake, immobility)
Deficient knowledge of disease process (e.g., diabetes, hyperlipidemia)
Diabetes mellitus
Endovascular procedures
Hypertension
Sedentary lifestyle
Smoking

Suggestions for Use

The following Suggested Alternative Diagnoses offer alternative labels that specifically address responses to impaired perfusion of renal, cerebral, cardiopulmonary, and gastrointestinal tissue. *Ineffective tissue perfusion* can be used appropriately as an etiology for other diagnoses (e.g., *Acute confusion related to Ineffective cerebral tissue perfusion*). If specific organs are not being sufficiently perfused, use the suggested alternative diagnoses.

Suggested Alternative Diagnoses

Perfusion: Gastrointestinal, impaired
Peripheral neurovascular dysfunction, risk for
Skin integrity, risk for impaired
Tissue integrity, impaired
Tissue perfusion: Cardiac, Risk for Decreased
Tissue perfusion: Cerebral, risk for ineffective
Tissue perfusion: Peripheral, ineffective

T

NOC Outcomes

NOTE: NOC outcomes have not yet been linked to this diagnosis; however, the following may be useful in assessing for occurrence of actual *Ineffective peripheral tissue perfusion*. Other outcomes would depend on the patient's risk factors (e.g., Deficient Knowledge of disease process, diabetes mellitus, hypertension). The primary desired outcome, of course, is that peripheral tissue perfusion will be effective.

Circulation Status: Unobstructed, unidirectional blood flow at an appropriate pressure through large vessels of the systemic and pulmonary circuits

Tissue Perfusion: Peripheral: Adequacy of blood flow through the small vessels of the extremities to maintain tissue function

Examples Using NOC Language

- Demonstrates **Circulation Status**, as evidenced by the following indicators (specify 1–5: severely, substantially, moderately, mildly, or not compromised):
  - Systolic and diastolic BP
  - Urinary output
- Demonstrates **Tissue Perfusion: Peripheral**, as evidenced by the following indicators (specify 1–5: severe, substantial, moderate, mild, or no deviation from normal range):
  - Capillary refill fingers (and toes) [2–3 seconds]
  - Brachial (radial, femoral, and pedal) pulse strength (right and left)

Other Examples

- Skin of extremities warm and dry
- No dependent rubor or pallor
- Urine output within normal limits
- No edema
- No lower extremity ulcers
- No numbness or paresthesia in extremities
- Patient identifies lifestyle changes needed to improve tissue perfusion

NIC Interventions

T

NOTE: NIC interventions have not yet been linked to this diagnosis. Nursing interventions focus on (a) assessing peripheral circulation (for development of *Ineffective peripheral tissue perfusion*), (b) assessing for risk factors for *Ineffective peripheral tissue perfusion*, and (c) modifying or removing the risk factors. Many of the interventions will depend on which risk factors are present for the patient, so not every intervention can be listed here. However, the following may be useful.

Skin Surveillance: Collection and analysis of patient data to maintain skin and mucous membrane integrity

Vital Signs Monitoring: Collection and analysis of cardiovascular, respiratory, and body temperature data to determine and prevent complications

Teaching: Disease Process: Assisting the patient to understand information related to a specific disease process

Teaching: Prescribed Activity/Exercise: Preparing a patient to achieve or maintain a prescribed level of activity

Smoking Cessation Assistance: Helping another to stop smoking

Nursing Activities

Assessments

- Monitor peripheral pulses bilaterally; use a Doppler stethoscope if you are unable to find a pulse. Notify the physician if a pulse is not present.
- Assess skin color and temperature.
- Assess for ulcers, loss of hair, and dry shiny skin on the legs and feet.
- Check capillary refill.
- Assess for and describe any pain in the extremities.
- If there are symptoms of ineffective tissue perfusion, determine whether it is arterial or venous, for example:

  With venous insufficiency, the pain is relieved with exercise and leg elevation. The patient may report cramping, aching, and discomfort.

  With arterial insufficiency, pain increases when the legs are elevated, and there may be pain when walking that is relieved by rest. Patients may report that leg pain keeps them awake at night.
- Assess for risk factors (e.g., hypertension, older adults, diabetes)
- Assess the patient's level of knowledge with regard to his risk factors (e.g., diabetes)
- Assess the patient's self-care abilities, especially with regard to foot care.

Patient/Family Teaching

- Teach the benefits of regular exercise (to the patient's tolerance).
- Teach the effects of smoking on peripheral circulation.
- Explain techniques for foot care and their importance.
- Teach patients with risk factors to limit exposure to cold (e.g., wear warm clothing)

T

Collaborative Activities

Refer to counseling or support groups, as needed, for smoking cessation.

Other

- Distribute prescribed fluid intake appropriately over 24-hr period
- Maintain fluid and diet restrictions (e.g., low sodium, no salt), as ordered
- For patients with varicose veins, elevate the legs with no pressure under the knee and heels.
- For patients with risk for venous insufficiency, apply graduated compression stockings as ordered (e.g., postoperatively; when on bed rest) to help promote venous return and prevent deep-vein thrombosis.

TRANSFER ABILITY, IMPAIRED

(1998, 2006)

Domain 4, Activity/Rest; Class 2, Activity/Exercise

Definition: Limitation of independent movement between two nearby surfaces

NOTE: Specify level of independence using a standardized functional scale.

Defining Characteristics

Objective

Impaired ability to transfer:

- From bed to chair and chair to bed
- On or off a toilet or commode
- In or out of tub or shower
- Between uneven levels
- From chair to car or car to chair
- From chair to floor or floor to chair
- From standing to floor or floor to standing
- From standing to bed or bed to standing
- From chair to standing or standing to chair

Other Defining Characteristics (Non-NANDA International)

Reluctance to initiate movement
Sedentary lifestyle or disuse or deconditioning

Related Factors

Cognitive impairment
Deconditioning
Environmental constraints (e.g., bed height, inadequate space, wheelchair type, treatment equipment, restraints)
Impaired balance
Impaired vision
Insufficient muscle strength
Lack of knowledge
Musculoskeletal impairment (e.g., contractures)
Neuromuscular impairment
Obesity
Pain

Suggestions for Use

(a) Use *Impaired transfer ability* to describe individuals with limited ability for independent physical movement, such as decreased ability to move arms or legs or generalized muscle weakness, or when nursing interventions will focus on restoring mobility and function or preventing further deterioration. Do not use this label to describe temporary conditions that cannot be changed by the nurse (e.g., traction, prescribed bed rest, or permanent paralysis). When the patient's transfer ability cannot be improved, this label should be used as a related or risk factor for other nursing diagnoses, such as *Risk for falls.* (b) Specify level of mobility, using the same criteria as for *Mobility: physical, impaired.*

Level 0: Is completely independent
Level 1: Requires use of equipment or device
Level 2: Requires help from another person for assistance, supervision, or teaching
Level 3: Requires help from another person and equipment or device
Level 4: Is dependent; does not participate in activity

(3) See Suggestions for Use for Impaired Physical Mobility.

Suggested Alternative Diagnoses

Disuse syndrome, risk for
Falls, risk for
Injury, risk for
Mobility: bed, impaired
Mobility: physical, impaired
Mobility: wheelchair, impaired
Walking, impaired

T

NOC Outcomes

Balance: Ability to maintain body equilibrium
Body Positioning: Self-Initiated: Ability to change own body position independently with or without assistive device
Coordinated Movement: Ability of muscles to work together voluntarily for purposeful movement
Transfer Performance: Ability to change body location independently with or without assistive device

Goals/Evaluation Criteria

Examples Using NOC Language

- Demonstrates **Transfer Ability**, as evidenced by Balance, Body Positioning: Self-Initiated, Coordinated Movement, and Transfer Performance

Other Examples

- The patient will perform full range of motion of all joints
- The patient will transfer:
  From bed to chair or bed to standing
  To and from a toilet or commode
  From wheelchair to car or car to wheelchair
  From standing to floor or floor to standing

NIC Interventions

NOTE: The following interventions focus on improving transfer ability. Other interventions may be required to treat diagnosis-related factors (e.g., as visual deficits, dementia, unsafe environment, pain, and obesity).

Exercise Promotion: Strength Training: Facilitating regular resistive muscle training to maintain or increase muscle strength

Exercise Therapy: Ambulation: Promotion and assistance with walking to maintain or restore autonomic and voluntary body functions during treatment and recovery from illness or injury

Exercise Therapy: Balance: Use of specific activities, postures, and movements to maintain, enhance, or restore balance

Exercise Therapy: Joint Mobility: Use of active or passive body movement to maintain or restore joint flexibility

Exercise Therapy: Muscle Control: Use of specific activity or exercise protocols to enhance or restore controlled body movement

Fall Prevention: Instituting special precautions with patient at risk for injury from falling

T

Self-Care Assistance: Transfer: Assisting a person with limitation of independent movement to learn to change body location

Nursing Activities

Assessments

- Perform ongoing assessment of patient's transfer ability
- Assess need for assistance from home health agency or other placement service and assess need for durable medical equipment
- Assess vision, hearing, and proprioception
- *(NIC) Exercise Therapy: Muscle Control:*
  Determine patient's readiness to engage in activity or exercise protocol
  Determine accuracy of body image
  Monitor patient's emotional, cardiovascular, and functional responses to exercise protocol
  Monitor patient's self-exercise for correct performance

Patient/Family Teaching

- Instruct in active or passive range-of-motion exercises
- Give step-by-step directions
- Provide written information and diagrams
- Give frequent feedback to prevent formation of bad habits
- Provide information about assistive devices that may help with transfers
- Teach home caregivers how to incorporate balance and strength exercises into ADLs
- *(NIC) Exercise Therapy: Muscle Control:*

  Provide step-by-step cues for each motor activity during exercise or ADLs

  Instruct patient to recite each movement as it is being performed

Collaborative Activities

- Use occupational and physical therapy as resources in developing plan to maintain or increase transfer mobility; plan should include balance and muscle-strengthening exercises

Other

- Position call light or button within easy reach
- Provide positive reinforcement during activities
- Implement pain control measures before beginning exercises or physical therapy
- Be sure care plan includes number of personnel needed to transfer patient
- Assist patient to transfer, as needed
- *(NIC) Exercise Therapy: Muscle Control:*

  Dress patient in nonrestrictive clothing

  Assist patient to maintain trunk or proximal joint stability during motor activity

  Reorient patient to movement functions of the body

  Incorporate ADLs into exercise protocol, if appropriate

  Assist patient to prepare and maintain a progress graph or chart to motivate adherence to exercise protocol

T

Home Care

- The preceding activities can be used or adapted for home care
- Assist the family to arrange furniture to maximize the client's ability to move about

TRAUMA, RISK FOR

(1980) **Domain 11, Safety/Protection; Class 2, Physical Injury**

Definition: At risk of accidental tissue injury (e.g., wound, burn, fracture)

Risk Factors

External (Environmental)

High-crime neighborhood [and vulnerable clients]; pot handles facing toward front of stove; [use of thin or worn pot holders]; knives stored uncovered; inappropriate call-for-aid mechanisms for bedbound client; inadequately stored combustibles or corrosives (e.g., matches, oily rags, lye); flammable children's toys or clothing; obstructed passageways; high beds; large icicles hanging from the roof; [snow or ice collected on stairs, walkways]; overexposure to [sun, sunlamps], radiation; overloaded electrical outlets; overloaded fuse boxes; physical proximity to vehicle pathways (e.g., driveways, lanes, railroad tracks); playing with explosives; accessibility of guns; contact with rapidly moving machinery [industrial belts or pulleys; litter or liquid spills on floors or stairways]; defective appliances; bathing in very hot water (e.g., unsupervised bathing of young children); bathtub or shower without antislip equipment [or handgrip]; children playing with dangerous objects [matches, candles, cigarettes, sharp-edged toys]; lack of gates at the top of the stairs; delayed lighting of gas burner or oven; lack of protection from heat source; contact with intense cold; grease waste collected on stoves; children riding in the front seat in car; driving a mechanically unsafe vehicle; driving while intoxicated; nonuse or misuse of seat restraints; driving at excessive speeds; driving without necessary visual aids; entering unlighted rooms; experimenting with chemical [or gasoline]; exposure to dangerous machinery; faulty electrical plugs; frayed wires; unanchored electric wires; contact with corrosives [acids or alkalis]; inadequate stair rails; use of unsteady ladders or chairs; use of cracked dishware; wearing flowing clothes around open flame; [unscreened fires or heaters]; unsafe window protection in homes with young children; [sliding on coarse bed linen]; struggling within bed restraints; [nonuse or misuse of necessary headgear for motorized cyclists or young children carried on adult bicycles]; potential igniting gas leaks; unsafe road or walkways; slippery floors (e.g., wet or highly waxed); smoking in bed or near oxygen cylinders; throw rugs

Internal (Individual)

Weakness, poor vision, balancing difficulties, reduced sensation [temperature or tactile], reduced muscle coordination, reduced hand–eye coordination, deficient knowledge regarding safe procedures, deficient knowledge regarding safety precautions, economically disadvantaged [e.g., insufficient finances to purchase safety equipment or effect repairs], cognitive or emotional difficulties, history of previous trauma

Suggestions for Use

Use a more specific diagnosis when possible.

Suggested Alternative Diagnoses

Aspiration, risk for
Home maintenance, impaired
Falls, risk for
Injury, risk for
Perioperative positioning injury, risk for
Poisoning, risk for

NOC Outcomes

NOTE: Use the following NOC outcomes to assess for actual occurrence of the diagnosis.

Physical Injury Severity: Severity of injuries from accidents and trauma

Tissue Integrity: Skin and Mucous Membranes: Structural intactness and normal physiological function of skin and mucous membranes

NOTE: The following outcomes are some of those associated with risk factors for trauma.

Balance: Ability to maintain body equilibrium

Cognition: Ability to execute complex mental processes

Community Violence Level: Incidence of violent acts compared with local, state, or national values

Fall Prevention Behavior: Personal or family caregiver actions to minimize risk factors that might precipitate falls in the personal environment

Personal Safety Behavior: Personal actions of an adult to control behaviors that can cause physical injury

Safe Home Environment: Physical arrangements to minimize environmental factors that might cause physical harm or injury in the home

Goals/Evaluation Criteria

Examples Using NOC Language

- Demonstrates **Personal Safety Behavior**, as demonstrated by (specify 1–5: never, rarely, sometimes, often, or consistently demonstrated):
  - Stores food to minimize spoilage
  - Uses seat belt appropriately
  - Practices safe sexual behaviors

- Uses tools and machinery correctly
- Avoids high-risk behaviors
- Avoids smoking in bed

Other Examples

Patient will:

- Avoid physical injury
- Not abuse alcohol or recreational drugs
- Use sunscreen

NIC Interventions

NOTE: For this very general diagnosis, a variety of interventions may be needed to promote safety and prevent trauma. Interventions differ somewhat for well patients and patients who are institutionalized (e.g., in hospital).

Environmental Management: Safety: Monitoring and manipulation of the physical environment to promote safety

Fall Prevention: Instituting special precautions with patient at risk for injury from falling

Health Education: Developing and providing instruction and learning experiences to facilitate voluntary adaptation of behavior conducive to health in individuals, families, groups, or communities

Reality Orientation: Promotion of patient's awareness of personal identity, time, and environment

Risk Identification: Analysis of potential risk factors, determination of health risks, and prioritization of risk-reduction strategies for an individual or group

T

Surveillance: Purposeful and ongoing acquisition, interpretation, and synthesis of patient data for clinical decision making

Surveillance: Safety: Purposeful and ongoing collection and analysis of information about the patient and the environment for use in promoting and maintaining patient safety

Teaching: Infant Safety: Instruction on safety during the first year of life

Teaching: Toddler Safety: Instruction on safety during the second and third years of life

Vehicle Safety Promotion: Assisting individuals, families, and communities to increase awareness of measures to reduce unintentional injuries in motorized and nonmotorized vehicles

Nursing Activities

Assessments

- *(NIC) Environmental Management: Safety:*
  Identify the safety needs of the patient based on level of physical and cognitive function and past history of behavior

Identify safety hazards in the environment (i.e., physical, biological, and chemical)

Patient/Family Teaching

- Instruct patient and family in safety measures specific to risk area
- Provide educational materials related to strategies for prevention of trauma
- Provide information on environmental hazards and characteristics (e.g., stairs, windows, cupboard locks, swimming pools, streets, or gates)

Collaborative Activities

- Refer to educational classes in the community (e.g., CPR, first aid, or swimming)
- *(NIC) Environmental Management: Safety:* Assist patient in relocating to safer environment (e.g., referral for housing assistance)

Other

- *(NIC) Environmental Management: Safety:*
  Modify the environment to minimize hazards and risk
  Provide adaptive devices (e.g., step stools and handrails) to increase the safety of the environment
  Use protective devices (e.g., restraints, side rails, locked doors, fences, and gates) to physically limit mobility or access to harmful situations

Home Care

- The preceding activities are appropriate for home care use

For Infants and Children

- Advise parents to keep guns locked up and separated from ammunition
- Teach parents child-safety measures, such as keeping flammable or poisonous materials out of the reach of children, using properly sized infant car seats and placing them correctly in the car
- Assess older homes for lead-based paint

For Older Adults

- Encourage the client to perform muscle strengthening and balance training exercises
- Advise clients to use only slip-resistant throw rugs; use nonskid grab bars in tubs and showers; keep pan handles turned toward the back of the stove when cooking; use good lighting in halls and stairways; use a nightlight in the bedroom and bathroom
- Advise clients to store medications in their original containers or in a daily medication dispenser

UNILATERAL NEGLECT

(1986, 2006) **Domain 5, Perception/Cognition; Class 1, Attention**

Definition: Impairment in sensory and motor response, mental representation, and spatial attention of the body, and the corresponding environment, characterized by inattention to one side and overattention to the opposite side. Left-side neglect is more severe and persistent than right-side neglect

Defining Characteristics

Subjective

Difficulty remembering details of internally represented familiar scenes that are on the neglected side

Objective

Appears unaware of positioning of neglected limb
Displacement of sounds to the nonneglected side
Distortion or omission of drawing on the half of the page on the neglected side
Failure to cancel lines on the half of the page on the neglected side
Failure to dress or groom neglected side
Failure to eat food from portion of the plate on the neglected side
Failure to move eyes, head, limbs, or trunk in the neglected hemispace, despite being aware of a stimulus in that space
Failure to notice people approaching from the neglected side
Lack of safety precautions with regard to the neglected side
Marked deviation of the head, eyes, and trunk to the nonneglected side (as if drawn magnetically) to stimuli and activities on that side
Perseveration of visual motor tasks on nonneglected side
Substitution of letters to form alternative words that are similar to the original in length when reading
Transfer of pain sensation to the nonneglected side
Use of only vertical half of page when writing

Related Factors

Brain injury from cerebrovascular problems
Brain injury from neurological illness
Brain injury from trauma
Brain injury from tumor
Hemianopsia
Left hemiplegia from CVA of the right hemisphere

Other Related Factors (Non-NANDA International)

Anesthesia of one side of the body (i.e., hemianesthesia)
Real or pretended ignorance of presence of paralysis (i.e., anosognosia)
Weakness of one side of body (i.e., hemiparesis)

Suggestions for Use

Unilateral neglect may occur with medical conditions such as brain injuries, cerebral aneurysms or tumors, and cerebrovascular accidents. There are usually other nursing diagnoses associated with the pathophysiology of *Unilateral neglect:* for example, those in the following section, Suggested Alternative Diagnoses.

Suggested Alternative Diagnoses

Anxiety
Injury, risk for
Self-care deficit

NOC Outcomes

Body Positioning: Self-Initiated: Ability to change own body position independently with or without assistive device

Coordinated Movement: Ability of muscles to work together voluntarily for purposeful movement

Heedfulness of Affected Side: Personal actions to acknowledge, protect, and cognitively integrate body part(s) into self

Self-Care: Activities of Daily Living (ADLs): Ability to perform the most basic physical tasks and personal care activities independently with or without assistive device

U

Goals/Evaluation Criteria

Examples Using NOC Language

- Performs **Self-Care: Activities of Daily Living (ADLs)**, as evidenced by the following indicators (specify 1–5: severely, substantially, moderately, mildly, or not compromised): eating, dressing, toileting, bathing, grooming, hygiene, walking, wheelchair mobility, and transfer performance

Other Examples

Patient will:

- Be able to change own body positions (specify: lying to sitting, sitting to lying, kneeling to standing, and so forth)
- Acknowledge extent of deficit

- Modify behavior and environment to accommodate deficit
- Demonstrate improving perception of environment
- Not experience falls or other accidents

NIC Interventions

The following interventions address Unilateral Neglect. Other interventions may be needed to address the patient's related factors (e.g., cerebral edema).

Body Mechanics Promotion: Facilitating the use of posture and movement in daily activities to prevent fatigue and musculoskeletal strain or injury

Environmental Management: Manipulation of the patient's surroundings for therapeutic benefit, sensory appeal, and psychological well-being

Exercise Therapy: Muscle Control: Use of specific activity or exercise protocols to enhance or restore controlled body movement

Self-Care Assistance: Assisting another to perform activities of daily living

Teaching: Individual: Planning, implementation, and evaluation of a teaching program designed to address a patient's particular needs

Unilateral Neglect Management: Protecting and safely reintegrating the affected part of the body while helping the patient adapt to disturbed perceptual abilities

Nursing Activities

Assessments

U

- Assess the nature and extent of deficit
- *(NIC) Unilateral Neglect Management:* Monitor for abnormal responses to three primary types of stimuli: sensory, visual, and auditory

Patient/Family Teaching

- Explain and reinforce nature and extent of deficit to patient and family
- Provide information about community resources
- *(NIC) Unilateral Neglect Management:* Instruct caregivers on the cause, mechanisms, and treatment of unilateral neglect

Collaborative Activities

- *(NIC) Unilateral Neglect Management:* Consult with occupational and physical therapists concerning timing and strategies to facilitate reintegration of neglected body parts and function

Other

- Provide visual, olfactory, and tactile stimulation
- *(NIC) Unilateral Neglect Management:*
  Provide realistic feedback about patient's perceptual deficit
  Touch unaffected shoulder when initiating conversation
  Place food and beverages within field of vision and turn plate, as necessary
  Rearrange the environment to use the right or left visual field, such as positioning personal items, television, or reading materials within view on unaffected side
  Gradually move personal items and activity to affected side as patient demonstrates an ability to compensate for neglect
  Assist patient to bathe and groom affected side first, as patient demonstrates an ability to compensate for neglect
  Keep side rail up on affected side, as appropriate
  Ensure that affected extremities are properly and safely positioned
  Include family in rehabilitation process to support the patient's efforts and assist with care, as appropriate

Home Care

- Most of the preceding activities can be used or adapted for home care
- If possible, place the client's bed so that he can arise on the unaffected side, especially when getting up at night to go to the bathroom

URINARY ELIMINATION, IMPAIRED

(1973, 2006) **Domain 3, Elimination and Exchange; Class 1, Urinary Function**

Definition: Dysfunction in urine elimination

Defining Characteristics

Subjective

Dysuria
Urgency

Objective

Frequency
Hesitancy

Incontinence
Nocturia
Retention

Related Factors

Anatomic obstruction, sensory or motor impairment, urinary tract infection, multiple causality

Suggestions for Use

Use a more specific label when possible. For specific patient outcomes, evaluation criteria, and nursing interventions, refer to the diagnoses in the following section, Suggested Alternative Diagnoses.

Suggested Alternative Diagnoses

Urinary incontinence, functional
Urinary incontinence, overflow
Urinary incontinence, reflex
Urinary incontinence, stress
Urinary incontinence, urge
Urinary incontinence: urge, risk for
Urinary retention

NOC Outcomes

Urinary Elimination: Collection and discharge of urine

Goals/Evaluation Criteria

Examples Using NOC Language

- Demonstrates **Urinary Elimination**, as evidenced by the following indicators (specify 1–5: severely, substantially, moderately, mildly, or not compromised):
  - Elimination pattern
  - Empties bladder completely
  - Recognition of urge

Other Examples

- Urine continence
- Demonstration of adequate knowledge of medications that affect urinary function
- Urinary elimination not compromised:
  - Urine odor, amount, and color in expected range
  - No hematuria

Passes urine without pain, hesitancy, or urgency
BUN, serum creatinine, and specific gravity WNL
Urine proteins, glucose, ketones, pH, and electrolytes WNL

NIC Interventions

- **Pelvic Muscle Exercise:** Strengthening and training the levator ani and orogenital muscles through voluntary, repetitive contraction to decrease stress, urge, or mixed types of urinary incontinence
- **Prompted Voiding:** Promotion of urinary continence through the use of timed verbal toileting reminders and positive social feedback for successful toileting
- **Urinary Catheterization:** Insertion of a catheter into the bladder for temporary or permanent drainage of urine
- **Urinary Bladder Training:** Improving bladder function for those with urge incontinence by increasing the bladder's ability to hold urine and the patient's ability to suppress urination
- **Urinary Elimination Management:** Maintenance of an optimum urinary elimination pattern

Nursing Activities

Also refer to Nursing Activities for the preceding Suggested Alternative Diagnoses.

Assessments

- *(NIC) Urinary Elimination Management:*

  Monitor urinary elimination, including frequency, consistency, odor, volume, and color, as appropriate

  Obtain midstream voided specimen for urinalysis, as appropriate

U

Patient/Family Teaching

- *(NIC) Urinary Elimination Management:*

  Teach patient signs and symptoms of urinary tract infection

  Instruct patient and family to record urinary output, as appropriate

  Instruct patient to respond immediately to urge to void, as appropriate

  Teach patient to drink 8 oz of liquid with meals, between meals, and in early evening

Collaborative Activities

- *(NIC) Urinary Elimination Management:* Refer to physician if signs and symptoms of urinary tract infection occur

Home Care

- The preceding activities can be used or adapted for home care

For Older Adults

- Be aware that very old adults commonly do not exhibit the classic symptoms of urinary tract infection, and that a urinary tract infection can progress quickly to sepsis; perform urinalysis for any sudden change in urine elimination
- Advise clients to drink a glass of cranberry juice daily
- Be aware that older adults may need more time to ambulate from bed to bathroom

URINARY ELIMINATION, READINESS FOR ENHANCED

(2002) **Domain 3, Elimination and Exchange; Class 1, Urinary Function**

Definition: A pattern of urinary functions that is sufficient for meeting elimination needs and can be strengthened

Defining Characteristics

Subjective

Expresses willingness to enhance urinary elimination

Objective

Amount of output is within normal limits
Fluid intake is adequate for daily needs
Positions self for emptying of bladder
Specific gravity is within normal limits
Urine is odorless
Urine is straw colored

Suggestions for Use

None

Suggested Alternative Diagnoses

Do not use this diagnosis if problems are present (e.g., urinary tract infection, incontinence, retention).

NOC Outcomes

Urinary Elimination: Collection and discharge of urine

Goals/Evaluation Criteria

Examples Using NOC Language

- Demonstrates **Urinary Elimination**, as evidenced by the following indicators (specify 1–5: severely, substantially, moderately, mildly, or not compromised):
  - Recognition of urge [5]
  - Empties bladder completely [5]
  - Elimination pattern [5]
  - Adequate fluid intake [5]

Other Examples

Patient will:

- Describe plan for enhancing urinary function
- Have a postvoid residual of > 100–200 mL
- Remain free of urinary tract infection
- Have a balanced 24-hr intake and output
- Report normal amount and characteristics of urine
- Demonstrate adequate knowledge of medications that affect urinary function
- Experience normal urinary elimination:
  - Urine odor, amount, and color in expected range
  - No hematuria
  - Passes urine without pain, hesitancy, or urgency
  - BUN, serum creatinine, and specific gravity within normal limits
  - Urine proteins, glucose, ketones, pH, and electrolytes within normal limits

NIC Interventions

- **Fluid Management:** Promotion of fluid balance and prevention of complications resulting from abnormal or undesired fluid levels
- **Infection Protection:** Prevention and early detection of infection in a patient at risk
- **Pelvic Muscle Exercise:** Strengthening and training the levator ani and orogenital muscles through voluntary, repetitive contraction to decrease stress, urge, or mixed types of urinary incontinence
- **Urinary Elimination Management:** Maintenance of an optimum urinary elimination pattern
- **Weight Management:** Facilitating maintenance of optimal body weight and percentage of body fat

Nursing Activities

Assessments

- Identify and document patient's bladder evacuation pattern
- Inquire about use of prescription and nonprescription medications with anticholinergic or alpha agonist properties
- *(NIC) Urinary Elimination Management:* Monitor urinary elimination, including frequency, consistency, odor, volume, and color, as appropriate

Patient/Family Teaching

- Provide information about normal urinary functioning
- Provide information about fluid requirements, regular voiding, and so forth
- *(NIC) Urinary Elimination Management:*
  - Teach patient signs and symptoms of urinary tract infection
  - Instruct patient to respond immediately to urge to void, as appropriate
  - Teach patient to drink 8 oz of liquid with meals, between meals, and in early evening

Other

- Assist to make plan for improving urinary function
- Encourage oral intake of fluids: _____ mL for day; _____ mL for evening; _____ mL for night

URINARY INCONTINENCE, FUNCTIONAL

(1986, 1998) **Domain 3, Elimination and Exchange; Class 1, Urinary Function**

U

Definition: Inability of usually continent person to reach toilet in time to avoid unintentional loss of urine

Defining Characteristics

Able to completely empty bladder
Amount of time required to reach toilet exceeds length of time between sensing urge and uncontrolled voiding
Loss of urine before reaching toilet
May be incontinent only in early morning
Senses need to void

Related Factors

Altered environmental factors
Impaired cognition

Impaired vision
Neuromuscular limitations
Psychologic factors
Weakened supporting pelvic structures

Suggestions for Use

None

Suggested Alternative Diagnoses

Urinary incontinence, overflow
Urinary incontinence, reflex
Urinary incontinence, stress
Urinary incontinence, urge
Self-care deficit: toileting
Urinary elimination, impaired

NOC Outcomes

Self-Care: Toileting: Ability to toilet self independently with or without assistive device

Urinary Continence: Control of the elimination of urine from the bladder

Goals/Evaluation Criteria

Examples Using NOC Language

- Demonstrates **Urinary Continence**, as evidenced by the following indicators (specify 1–5: never, rarely, sometimes, often, or consistently demonstrated):

  Recognizes urge to void
  Responds to urge in timely manner
  Gets to toilet between urge and passage of urine
  Manages clothing independently
  Toilets independently
  Maintains predictable pattern of voiding

Other Examples

- Uses adaptive equipment to help with clothing and transfers when incontinence is related to impaired mobility

NIC Interventions

Environmental Management: Manipulation of the patient's surroundings for therapeutic benefit, sensory appeal, and psychological well-being

Pelvic Muscle Exercise: Strengthening and training the levator ani and orogenital muscles through voluntary, repetitive contraction to decrease stress, urge, or mixed types of urinary incontinence

Prompted Voiding: Promotion of urinary continence through the use of timed verbal toileting reminders and positive social feedback for successful toileting

Self-Care Assistance: Toileting: Assisting another with elimination

Urinary Habit Training: Establishing a predictable pattern of bladder emptying to prevent incontinence for persons with limited cognitive ability who have urge, stress, or functional incontinence

Urinary Incontinence Care: Assistance in promoting continence and maintaining perineal skin integrity

Nursing Activities

Assessments

- Monitor urinary elimination, including frequencyodor, volume, and color
- Obtain specimen for urinalysis
- Identify etiologies of the patient's incontinence (e.g., environmental factors)

Patient/Family Teaching

- Discuss with patient and family ways to modify environment to reduce number of wetness episodes, consider the following strategies:
  Improving environmental lighting to enhance vision
  Installing raised toilet seat and hand rails
  Providing bedside commode, bedpan, and handheld urinal
  Removing loose rugs
- Instruct patient and family in prompted voiding routine (frequent reminders) based on patient's pattern of toileting to decrease wetness episodes
- Instruct patient and family in skin care and hygiene routine to prevent skin breakdown
- Offer strategies for bladder management during activities away from home
- Teach patient and caregivers the signs and symptoms of urinary tract infection
- Explain the need to respond immediately to the urge to void
- Ask patient and caregivers to record urinary output [and pattern]
- Teach the patient not to avoid liquids in an attempt to prevent incontinence. Instruct to drink 8 oz liquid with meals, between meals, and early in the evening.

Collaborative Activities

- Consult with physical and occupational therapy for assistance with manual dexterity
- Refer to primary care provider (or instruct patient to call the provider) if signs and symptoms of urinary tract infection occur

Other

- Provide protective garments or pads, as needed
- Modify clothing that can be removed quickly and easily (e.g., use elastic or Velcro for waistbands instead of zippers, buttons, snaps, and hooks)
- *(NIC) Urinary Habit Training:*

  Establish interval of initial toileting schedule, based on voiding pattern and usual routine (e.g., eating, rising, and retiring)

  Assist patient to toilet and prompt to void at prescribed intervals

  Use power of suggestion (e.g., running water or flushing toilet) to assist patient to void

  Avoid leaving patient on toilet for more than 5 min

  Reduce toileting interval by one-half hour if more than two incontinence episodes in 24 hr

  Increase the toileting interval by one-half hour if patient has no incontinence episodes for 48 hr until optimal 4-hr interval is achieved

Home Care

- The preceding activities can be used or adapted for home care
- Teach the caregiver to cleanse the skin after incontinence episodes and the routine for daily cleansing and drying
- Recommend moisture barriers if indicated
- Assist the client and family to make changes to the home environment to improve toileting access

URINARY INCONTINENCE, OVERFLOW

(2006) **Domain 3, Elimination and Exchange; Class 1, Urinary Function**

Definition: Involuntary loss of urine associated with overdistention of the bladder

Defining Characteristics

Subjective

Reports involuntary leakage of small volumes of urine

Objective

Bladder distention
High postvoid residual volume
Nocturia
Observed involuntary leakage of small volumes of urine

Related Factors

Bladder outlet obstruction
Detrusor external sphincter dyssynergia
Detrusor hypocontractility
Fecal impaction
Severe pelvic prolapse
Side effects of anticholinergic medications
Side effects of calcium channel blockers
Side effects of decongestant medications
Urethral obstruction

Suggestions for Use

None

Suggested Alternative Diagnoses

Urinary incontinence, functional
Urinary incontinence, stress
Urinary incontinence, urge
Self-care deficit: toileting
Urinary elimination, impaired
Urinary retention

NOC Outcomes

Medication Response: Therapeutic and adverse effects of prescribed medication

Urinary Continence: Control of the elimination of urine from the bladder

Goals/Evaluation Criteria

Also see NOC examples for Urinary Incontinence, Functional (preceding).

Examples Using NOC Language

- Demonstrates **Urinary Continence**, as evidenced by the following indicators (specify 1–5: never, rarely, sometimes, often, or consistently demonstrated):
  - Empties bladder completely
  - Ingests adequate amount of fluid

- Demonstrates **Urinary Continence**, as evidenced by the following indicators (specify 1–5: consistently, often, sometimes, rarely, or never demonstrated):
  Postvoid residual > 100–200 mL
  Urinary tract infection [< 100,000 white blood cell count]
  Urine leakage between voidings

NIC Interventions

Fluid Management: Promotion of fluid balance and prevention of complications resulting from abnormal or undesired fluid levels

Teaching: Prescribed Medication: Preparing a patient to safely take prescribed medications and monitor for their effects

Urinary Catheterization: Intermittent: Regular periodic use of a catheter to empty the bladder

Urinary Elimination Management: Maintenance of an optimum urinary elimination pattern

Urinary Incontinence Care: Assistance in promoting continence and maintaining perineal skin integrity

Urinary Retention Care: Assistance in relieving bladder distention

Nursing Activities

Assessments

- Assess for ability to recognize urge to void
- Monitor intake and output
- *(NIC) Urinary Retention Care:*
  Perform a comprehensive urinary assessment focusing on incontinence (e.g., urinary output, urinary voiding pattern, cognitive function, and preexisting urinary problems)
  Use double voiding technique
  Monitor degree of bladder distention by palpation and percussion
  Catheterize for residual, as appropriate

U

Patient/Family Teaching

- Teach ways to avoid constipation and stool impaction
- Teach to cleanse after every overflow episode, as well as cleansing once a day and keeping the perineum dry

Collaborative Activities

- Refer to enterostomal therapy nurse for instruction in clean intermittent self-catheterization, as appropriate
- *(NIC) Urinary Retention Care:* Refer to urinary continence specialist, as appropriate

Other

- Maintain fluid intake of approximately 2,000 mL/day
- Provide Crede maneuver, as necessary
- Provide at least 10 min for bladder emptying
- Assist patient in maintaining adequate hygiene and skin care routine; consider the following strategies:
  - Applying moisture barrier ointment or skin sealant
  - Keeping skin dry
- *(NIC) Urinary Retention Care:* Insert urinary catheter, as appropriate

Home Care

- The preceding activities can be used or adapted for home care

URINARY INCONTINENCE, REFLEX

(1986, 1998) **Domain 3, Elimination and Exchange; Class 1, Urinary Function**

Definition: Involuntary loss of urine at somewhat predictable intervals when a specific bladder volume is reached

Defining Characteristics

Subjective

No sensation of bladder fullness
No sensation of urge to void
U
No sensation of voiding
Sensation of urgency without voluntary inhibition of bladder contraction
Sensations associated with full bladder, such as sweating, restlessness, and abdominal discomfort

Objective

Incomplete emptying with lesion above pontine micturition center
Inability to voluntarily inhibit or initiate voiding
Incomplete emptying with lesion above sacral micturition center
Predictable pattern of voiding

Related Factors

Neurological impairment above level of sacral micturition center
Neurological impairment above level of pontine micturition center
Tissue damage from radiation cystitis, inflammatory bladder conditions, or radical pelvic surgery

Suggested Alternative Diagnoses

Urinary incontinence, functional
Urinary incontinence, overflow
Urinary incontinence, stress
Urinary incontinence, urge
Self-care deficit: toileting
Urinary elimination, impaired
Urinary retention

NOC Outcomes

Tissue Integrity: Skin and Mucous Membranes: Structural intactness and normal physiological function of skin and mucous membranes

Urinary Continence: Control of the elimination of urine from the bladder

Goals/Evaluation Criteria

Also see NOC examples for Urinary Incontinence, Functional.

Examples Using NOC Language

- Demonstrates **Urinary Continence**, as evidenced by the following indicators (specify 1–5: never, rarely, sometimes, often, or consistently demonstrated):
  - Voids in appropriate receptacle
  - Voids > 150 mL each time
  - Maintains predictable pattern of voiding

Other Examples

- Remains free of skin breakdown
- Demonstrates intermittent self-catheterization procedure

NIC Interventions

- **Fluid Management:** Promotion of fluid balance and prevention of complications resulting from abnormal or undesired fluid levels
- **Perineal Care:** Maintenance of perineal skin integrity and relief of perineal discomfort
- **Tube Care: Urinary:** Management of a patient with urinary drainage equipment
- **Urinary Catheterization, Intermittent:** Regular periodic use of a catheter to empty the bladder
- **Urinary Incontinence Care:** Assistance in promoting continence and maintaining perineal skin integrity

Nursing Activities

Assessments

- Assess for ability to recognize urge to void
- Identify voiding pattern (either voiding after specified intake or voiding after a specified interval)
- Monitor technique of patient and caregivers who perform intermittent catheterization
- For patients undergoing intermittent catheterization, monitor color, odor, and clarity of urine and perform frequent urinalysis to monitor for infection
- Determine patient's readiness and ability to perform intermittent self-catheterization
- Keep a continence record for 3 days to establish voiding pattern

Patient/Family Teaching

- Teach patient and family reportable signs and symptoms of autonomic dysreflexia, such as severe hypertension, severe headache, diaphoresis above level of injury, tachycardia of sudden onset
- Teach patient, family, and caregivers technique for clean intermittent catheterization
- Teach signs and symptoms of urinary tract infection (e.g., fever, chills, flank pain, hematuria, and change in consistency and odor of urine)

Collaborative Activities

- Refer to enterostomal therapy nurse for instruction in clean intermittent self-catheterization, as appropriate
- Administer antibacterial therapy, per medical order, at initiation of intermittent catheterization

Other

- Assist patient in maintaining adequate hygiene and skin care routine, consider the following strategies:

  Applying moisture barrier ointment or skin sealant

  Keeping skin dry

  Using collection device for urine
- Consider condom catheter collection device with leg bag
- Remind the patient to try to hold urine until scheduled elimination time
- Maintain fluid intake of approximately 2,000 mL/day

For intermittent urinary catheterization:

- Provide quiet room and privacy for procedure
- Use clean or sterile technique (per protocol) for catheterization
- Determine catheterization schedule, based on assessment of voiding patterns
- If output of >300 mL is obtained (for adults), catheterize more frequently

Home Care

- The preceding activities can be used or adapted for home care
- Teach client and family the relationship of bladder fullness to autonomic dysreflexia
- Teach to recognize symptoms of complications of reflex incontinence that should alert her to call the primary care provider
- Teach client and family how to clean and store catheter supplies in the home (e.g., wash catheter with soap and water, allow to air dry)
- Assess for depression and loneliness, which may result from incontinence and loss of self-esteem

URINARY INCONTINENCE, STRESS

(1986, 2006) **Domain 3, Elimination and Exchange; Class 1, Urinary Function**

Definition: Sudden leakage of urine with activities that increase intra-abdominal pressure

Defining Characteristics

Subjective

Reports involuntary leakage of small amounts of urine:

In the absence of detrusor contraction

In the absence of an overdistended bladder

On effort or exertion or with sneezing, laughing, or coughing

Objective

Observed involuntary leakage of small amounts of urine:

In the absence of detrusor contraction

In the absence of an overdistended bladder

On exertion or with sneezing, laughing, or coughing

Related Factors

Degenerative changes in pelvic muscles
High intra-abdominal pressure (e.g., obesity, gravid uterus)
Intrinsic urethral sphincter deficiency
Weak pelvic muscles

Suggested Alternative Diagnoses

Urinary incontinence, functional
Urinary incontinence, overflow
Urinary incontinence, reflex
Urinary incontinence, urge
Self-care deficit: toileting
Urinary elimination, impaired
Urinary retention

NOC Outcomes

Urinary Continence: Control of elimination of urine from the bladder

Goals/Evaluation Criteria

Also see NOC examples for Urinary Incontinence, Functional.

Examples Using NOC Language

- Demonstrates **Urinary Continence**, as evidenced by the following indicators (specify 1–5: consistently, often, sometimes, rarely, or never demonstrated):
  - Urine leakage with increased abdominal pressure (e.g., sneezing, laughing, lifting)
  - Wets underclothing during day

U

Other Examples

- Describes a plan for treating the stress incontinence
- Maintains a voiding frequency of more than q2h

NIC Interventions

Pelvic Muscle Exercise: Strengthening and training the levator ani and urogenital muscles through voluntary, repetitive contraction to decrease stress, urge, or mixed types of urinary incontinence

Urinary Incontinence Care: Assistance in promoting continence and maintaining perineal skin integrity

Nursing Activities

Also see Nursing Activities for Urinary Incontinence, Functional.

Assessments

- Assess patient for skin breakdown and maintenance of adequate hygiene and skin care routine

Patient/Family Teaching

- Instruct patient in hygiene and skin care measures
- Teach self-administration of oral or topical estrogens to ameliorate symptoms
- Teach techniques that strengthen the sphincter and structural supports of the bladder (e.g., pelvic muscle exercises, urine stop-and-start exercises)
- Inform patient that it may require several weeks of exercising to obtain improvement
- Instruct patient and family to report signs and symptoms of urinary tract infection (e.g., fever, chills, flank pain, hematuria, and change in consistency and odor of urine)

Collaborative Activities

- Consult with physician regarding surgical or medical management of incontinent episodes

Other

- Assist patient to select appropriate garment or pad for short-term incontinence management
- Give positive feedback for doing pelvic floor exercises
- *(NIC) Urinary Incontinence Care:* Limit ingestion of bladder irritants (e.g., cola, coffee, tea, and chocolate)

URINARY INCONTINENCE, URGE

(1986, 2006) **Domain 3, Elimination and Exchange; Class 1, Urinary Function**

Definition: Involuntary passage of urine occurring soon after a strong sense of urgency to void

Defining Characteristics

Subjective

Reports urinary urgency

Reports involuntary loss of urine with bladder contractions/spasms

Reports inability to reach toilet in time to avoid urine loss

Objective

Observed inability to reach toilet in time to avoid urine loss

Related Factors

Alcohol intake
Atrophic urethritis
Atrophic vaginitis
Bladder infection
Caffeine intake
Decreased bladder capacity [e.g., history of pelvic inflammatory disease, abdominal surgery, indwelling urinary catheter]
Detrusor hyperactivity with impaired bladder contractility
Fecal impaction
Use of diuretics

Suggested Alternative Diagnoses

Self-care deficit: toileting
Urinary elimination, impaired
Urinary incontinence, functional
Urinary incontinence, overflow
Urinary incontinence, reflex
Urinary incontinence, stress
Urinary retention

NOC Outcomes

Self-Care: Toileting: Ability to toilet self independently with or without assistive device

Urinary Continence: Control of elimination of urine from the bladder

Goals/Evaluation Criteria

Examples Using NOC Language

Also see NOC examples for Urinary Incontinence, Functional.

- Demonstrates **Urinary Continence**, as evidenced by the following indicators (specify 1–5: never, rarely, sometimes, often, or consistently demonstrated):
  - Responds in timely manner to urge
  - Identifies medications that interfere with urinary control
  - Maintains environment barrier-free to independent toileting
  - [Urine passes without urgency]

Other Examples

- Describes bladder management program to restore satisfactory urinary elimination pattern
- Experiences less frequent incontinent episodes

NIC Interventions

Medication Management: Facilitation of safe and effective use of prescription and over-the-counter drugs

Prompted Voiding: Promotion of urinary continence through the use of timed verbal toileting reminders and positive social feedback for successful toileting

Self-Care Assistance: Toileting: Assisting another with elimination

Teaching: Prescribed Medication: Preparing a patient to safely take prescribed medications and monitor for their effects

Urinary Bladder Training: Improving bladder function for those with urge incontinence by increasing the bladder's ability to hold urine and the patient's ability to suppress urination

Urinary Habit Training: Establishing a predictable pattern of bladder emptying to prevent incontinence for persons with limited cognitive ability who have urge, stress, or functional incontinence

Urinary Incontinence Care: Assistance in promoting continence and maintaining perineal skin integrity

Nursing Activities

Also see Nursing Activities for Urinary Incontinence, Functional.

Patient/Family Teaching

- Instruct patient regarding techniques that will increase bladder capacity, such as initiating pelvic floor raising when feeling the urge to void and using a bladder-training schedule that lengthens the time between voids
- Monitor for effects of antispasmodic medications, such as dry mouth that interferes with the ability to speak or eat
- Instruct patient and family to report signs and symptoms of urinary tract infection (e.g., fever, chills, flank pain, hematuria, and change in consistency and odor of urine)
- *(NIC) Urinary Incontinence Care:*

  Explain etiology of problem and rationale for actions

  Discuss procedures and expected outcomes with patient

Collaborative Activities

- Consult with physical and occupational therapists for assistance with manual dexterity
- Consult with physician regarding: (a) antispasmodic and anticholinergic medications and (b) medical management (e.g., electrostimulation therapy, investigation of underlying irritative or inflammatory bladder disorders, and surgical therapy)

Other

- Assist patient to void prior to sleep and encourage nighttime voids to reduce urgency
- Provide bedpan, bedside commode, and urinal nearby to encourage frequent voiding episodes
- For skin care, consider the following measures:
  Ensure skin is adequately dried
  Apply moisture barrier, ointment, or skin sealant
- *NIC Urinary Incontinence Care:* Limit fluids for 2–3 hr before bedtime, as appropriate

Home Care

- The preceding activities can be used or adapted for home care
- Assist the client and family to remove barriers to toileting in the home; for example, have an uncluttered path to the bathroom, have the bed as near the bathroom as possible

For Older Adults

- In addition to the preceding activities, assess the client's cognitive abilities and their effects on toileting self-care
- Assess functional abilities; provide assistive devices if needed

URINARY INCONTINENCE: URGE, RISK FOR

(1998) **Domain 3, Elimination and Exchange; Class 1, Urinary Function**

Definition: At risk for involuntary loss of urine associated with a sudden, strong sensation of urinary urgency

Risk Factors

Atrophic urethritis
Atropic vaginitis
Detrusor hyperactivity with impaired bladder contractility (e.g., from cystitis, urethritis, tumors, renal calculi, central nervous system disorders above pontine micturition center)
Effects of pharmaceutical agents, caffeine, or alcohol
Fecal impaction
Impaired bladder contractility

Ineffective toileting habits
Involuntary sphincter relaxation
Small bladder capacity

Suggested Alternative Diagnoses

Urinary incontinence, urge

NOC Outcomes

Urinary Continence: Control of the elimination of urine from the bladder
NOTE: The following are some outcomes associated with risk factors for urge incontinence.
Alcohol Abuse Cessation Behavior: Personal actions to eliminate alcohol use that poses a threat to health
Infection Severity: Severity of infection and associated symptoms
Medication Response: Therapeutic and adverse effects of prescribed medication
Self-Care: Toileting: Ability to toilet self independently with or without assistive device

Goals/Evaluation Criteria

See Goals/Evaluation Criteria for Urinary Incontinence, Functional.

NIC Interventions

Nursing interventions focus on preventing urge incontinence.
Fluid Management: Promotion of fluid balance and prevention of complications resulting from abnormal or undesired fluid levels
Medication Management: Facilitation of safe and effective use of prescription and over-the-counter drugs
Pelvic Muscle Exercise: Strengthening and training the levator ani and orogenital muscles through voluntary, repetitive contraction to decrease stress, urge, or mixed types of urinary incontinence
Prompted Voiding: Promotion of urinary continence through the use of timed verbal toileting reminders and positive social feedback for successful toileting
Self-Care Assistance: Toileting: Assisting another with elimination
Urinary Elimination Management: Maintenance of an optimum urinary elimination pattern
Urinary Habit Training: Establishing a predictable pattern of bladder emptying to prevent incontinence for persons with limited cognitive ability who have urge, stress, or functional incontinence

Nursing Activities

Also see Nursing Activities for Urinary Elimination, Readiness for Enhanced.

Assessments

- Assess for risk factors (see Risk Factors above)
- Evaluate environment for barriers to timely toileting
- Assess patient's self-care abilities and mobility
- Monitor urinary frequency, consistency, odor, volume, and color

Patient/Family Teaching

- Instruct patient regarding techniques that will increase bladder capacity, such as initiating pelvic floor raising when feeling the urge to void and using a bladder-training schedule that lengthens the time between voids
- Discuss with patient and family ways to modify environment to remove obstacles and improve self-care ability, consider the following strategies:
  - Improving environmental lighting to enhance vision
  - Installing a raised toilet seat and hand rails
  - Providing a bedside commode, bedpan, and handheld urinal
  - Using assistive devices (e.g., wheelchairs, canes, walkers, and non-skid walking shoes)

Collaborative Activities

- Consult with physical and occupational therapists for assistance with manual dexterity

Other

- Obtain clothing that is easily removed
- Substitute elastic waistbands and Velcro for zippers, buttons, snap devices, and hooks, whenever feasible
- Assist patient to void prior to sleep and encourage nighttime voids to reduce urgency
- Discourage use of bladder irritants, such as caffeine, alcohol, citrus juices, carbonated drinks, cigarette smoke, and certain spicy foods

URINARY RETENTION

(1986) **Domain 3, Elimination and Exchange; Class 1, Urinary Function**

Definition: Incomplete emptying of the bladder

Defining Characteristics

Subjective

Dysuria
Sensation of bladder fullness

Objective

Absence of urine output
Bladder distention
Dribbling
Overflow incontinence
Residual urine
Small, frequent voiding or absence of urine output

Related Factors

Blockage
High urethral pressure [e.g., caused by weak detrusor]
Inhibition of reflex arc
Strong sphincter

Suggested Alternative Diagnoses

Urinary incontinence, functional
Urinary incontinence, overflow
Urinary incontinence, stress
Urinary incontinence, urge
Urinary elimination, impaired

NOC Outcomes

Urinary Elimination: Collection and discharge of urine

Goals/Evaluation Criteria

Examples Using NOC Language

- Demonstrates **Urinary Elimination**, as evidenced by the following indicators (specify 1–5: severely, substantially, moderately, mildly, or not compromised):
  Elimination pattern
  Empties bladder completely
- Demonstrates **Urinary Elimination**, as evidenced by the following indicators (specify 1–5: severe, substantial, moderate, mild, or none): Urinary retention

Other Examples

- Postvoid residual > 100–200 cc
- Demonstrates bladder evacuation by clean intermittent self-catheterization procedure
- Describes plan of care at home
- Remains free of urinary tract infection
- Reports a decrease in bladder spasms
- Has a balanced 24-hr intake and output
- Empties the bladder completely

NIC Interventions

Fluid Monitoring: Collection and analysis of patient data to regulate fluid balance

Medication Administration: Preparing, giving, and evaluating the effectiveness of prescription and nonprescription drugs

Medication Management: Facilitation of safe and effective use of prescription and over-the-counter drugs

Urinary Catheterization: Insertion of a catheter into the bladder for temporary or permanent drainage of urine

Urinary Catheterization: Intermittent: Regular periodic use of a catheter to empty the bladder

Urinary Elimination Management: Maintenance of an optimum urinary elimination pattern

Urinary Retention Care: Assistance in relieving bladder distention

Nursing Activities

U

Also see Nursing Activities for Urinary Incontinence, Overflow.

Assessments

- Identify and document patient's bladder evacuation pattern
- *(NIC) Urinary Retention Care:*
  - Monitor use of nonprescription agents with anticholinergic or alpha agonist properties
  - Monitor effects of prescribed pharmaceuticals, such as calcium channel blockers and anticholinergics
  - Monitor intake and output
  - Monitor degree of bladder distention by palpation and percussion

Patient/Family Teaching

- Instruct patient in reportable signs and symptoms of urinary tract infection (e.g., fever, chills, flank pain, hematuria, and change in consistency and odor of urine)

- *(NIC) Urinary Retention Care:* Instruct patient and family to record urinary output, as appropriate

Collaborative Activities

- Refer to enterostomal therapy nurse for instruction in clean intermittent self-catheterization q4–6h while awake.
- *(NIC) Urinary Retention Care:* Refer to urinary continence specialist, as appropriate

Other

- Establish a bladder-evacuation training program
- Space fluids throughout the day to ensure adequate intake without bladder overdistention
- Encourage oral intake of fluids: _____ mL for day; _____ mL for evening; _____ mL for nights
- *(NIC) Urinary Retention Care:*
    - Provide privacy for elimination
    - Use the power of suggestion by running water or flushing the toilet
    - Stimulate the reflex bladder by applying cold to the abdomen, stroking the inner thigh, or running water
    - Provide enough time for bladder emptying (10 min)
    - Use spirits of wintergreen in bedpan or urinal
    - Provide Crede maneuver, as necessary
    - Catheterize for residual, as appropriate
    - Insert urinary catheter, as appropriate

VASCULAR TRAUMA, RISK FOR

(2008) **Domain 11, Safety/Protection; Class 2, Physical Injury**

Definition: At risk for damage to a vein and its surrounding tissues related to the presence of a catheter and/or infused solutions

Risk Factors

Catheter type
Catheter width
Impaired ability to visualize the insertion site
Inadequate catheter fixation
Infusion rate
Insertion site
Length of insertion time
Nature of solution (e.g., concentration, chemical irritant, temperature, pH)

Suggestions for Use

This is a very specific diagnosis, to be used only when a patient has a catheter inserted through the skin (e.g., a peripheral IV, a central IV line, a hemodialysis shunt). If symptoms of vascular trauma are present, use the diagnosis *Impaired tissue integrity*.

Suggested Alternative Diagnoses

Tissue integrity, impaired

NOC Outcomes

NOC outcomes have not yet been developed for this diagnosis. However, the following may be useful.

Hemodialysis Access: Functionality of a dialysis access site

Tissue Integrity: Skin and Mucous Membranes: Structural intactness and normal physiological function of skin and mucous membranes

Goals/Evaluation Criteria

Examples Using NOC Language

- Experiences no vascular trauma, as evidenced by **Hemodialysis Access** and **Tissue Integrity: Skin and Mucous Membranes.**
- Demonstrates **Tissue Integrity: Skin and Mucous Membranes**, as evidenced by the following indicators (specify 1–5: severely, substantially, moderately, mildly, or not compromised):
  - Skin temperature
  - Sensation
  - Skin integrity
- Demonstrates **Tissue Integrity: Skin and Mucous Membranes**, as evidenced by the following indicators (specify 1–5: severe, substantial, moderate, mild, or none):
  - Erythema
  - Blanching
  - Necrosis
  - Induration

V

Other Examples

- No leaking or dampness of the dressing
- No swelling or discomfort
- Body temperature within normal limits

NIC Interventions

NIC interventions have not yet been linked to *Risk for vascular trauma*; however, the following may be useful.

Intravenous (IV) Insertion: Insertion of a needle into a peripheral vein for the purpose of administering fluids, blood, or medication

Intravenous (IV) Therapy: Administration and monitoring of intravenous (IV) fluids and medications

Medication Administration: Intravenous (IV): Preparing and giving medications via the intravenous route

Venous Access Device (VAD) Maintenance: Management of the patient with prolonged venous access via tunneled and nontunneled (percutaneous) catheters, and implanted ports

Nursing Activities

Nursing activities focus on preventing vascular trauma (e.g., from infiltration, extravasation, infection, and phlebitis) and on early identification of symptoms to prevent further complications.

Assessments

- Determine the compatibility of IV medications and fluids before administering
- Monitor for infiltration (swelling, discomfort, burning, tightness, cool skin, blanching)
- Assess for extravasation (blanching, burning, or discomfort at the IV site; swelling at or above the site; cool skin surrounding the site)
- Assess the IV site according to agency protocol
- *(NIC) Intravenous (IV) Therapy:*

  Monitor IV flow rate and IV site during infusion

  Monitor for IV patency before administration of IV medication

  Monitor vital signs

  Monitor for signs and symptoms associated with infusion phlebitis and local infection

Patient/Family Teaching

- Instruct patient and caregivers to notify a nurse if the IV is not flowing or if signs/symptoms of complications (e.g., infiltration) occur

Collaborative Activities

- Instruct patient and family about the procedure
- Follow agency protocols and/or provider prescriptions for insertion and management of IV catheters (including hemodialysis shunts and lines inserted for hemodynamic monitoring)

Other

- Perform IV site care according to agency protocol
- Record intake and output
- Observe universal precautions

- *(NIC) Intravenous (IV) Therapy:*
  - Maintain strict aseptic technique
  - Monitor IV flow rate and IV site during infusion
  - Replace IV cannula, apparatus, and infusate every 48 to 72 hr, according to agency protocol
  - Maintain occlusive dressing

VENTILATORY WEANING RESPONSE, DYSFUNCTIONAL (DVWR)

(1992) **Domain 4, Activity/Rest; Class 4, Cardiovascular/Pulmonary Responses**

Definition: Inability to adjust to lowered levels of mechanical ventilator support that interrupts and prolongs the weaning process

Defining Characteristics

Nurses have defined three levels of DVWR in which these defining characteristics occur in response to weaning (Logan & Jenny, 1991).

Mild DVWR

Subjective

Breathing discomfort
Fatigue
Queries about possible machine malfunction
Reports feelings of increased need for oxygen
Warmth

Objective

Increased concentration on breathing
Restlessness
Slight increase in respiratory rate from baseline
Warmth

Moderate DVWR

Subjective

Reports apprehension

Objective

Baseline increase in respiratory rate < 5 breaths per minute
Color changes; pale, slight cyanosis
Decreased air entry on auscultation
Diaphoresis
Hypervigilance to activities

Inability to cooperate
Inability to respond to coaching
Minimal respiratory accessory muscle use
Slight increase from baseline BP < 20 mmHg
Slight increase from baseline heart rate < 20 BPM
Wide-eyed look

Severe DVWR

Objective

Adventitious breath sounds, audible airway secretions
Agitation
Asynchronized breathing with the ventilator
Audible airway secretions
Cyanosis
Decreased level of consciousness
Deterioration in ABG from current baseline data
Full respiratory accessory muscle use
Gasping breaths
Increase from baseline BP ≤ 20 mmHg
Increase from baseline heart rate ≤ 20 BPM
Paradoxical abdominal breathing
Profuse diaphoresis
Respiratory rate increases significantly from baseline
Shallow breaths

Related Factors

Physiological

Inadequate nutrition
Ineffective airway clearance
Sleep pattern disturbance
Uncontrolled pain [or discomfort]

Psychological

Anxiety [moderate, severe]
Decreased motivation
Decreased self-esteem
Deficient knowledge of the weaning process
Fear
Hopelessness
Insufficient trust in health care providers
Patient perceived inefficacy about the ability to wean
Powerlessness

Situational

Adverse environment (e.g., noisy, active environment, negative events in the room, low nurse–patient ratio, extended nurse absence from bedside, unfamiliar nursing staff)
History of multiple unsuccessful weaning attempts
History of ventilator dependence > 4 days
Inadequate social support
Inappropriate pacing of diminished ventilator support
Uncontrolled episodic energy demands or problems

Suggestions for Use

DVWR is concerned specifically with patient responses to separation from the mechanical ventilator. Other respiratory diagnoses may also occur during weaning, for example, *Ineffective airway clearance*, *Ineffective breathing pattern*, and *Impaired gas exchange*. This diagnostic label does not include the reasons for the weaning problems. If you do not know the etiology of the *DVWR*, use "unknown etiology."

Suggested Alternative Diagnoses

Airway clearance, ineffective
Breathing pattern, ineffective
Gas exchange, impaired

NOC Outcomes

Anxiety Level: Severity of manifested apprehension, tension, or uneasiness arising from an unidentifiable source

Mechanical Ventilation Weaning Response: Adult: Respiratory and psychological adjustment to progressive removal of mechanical ventilation

Respiratory Status: Gas Exchange: Alveolar exchange of CO_2 or O_2 to maintain ABG concentrations

Respiratory Status: Ventilation: Movement of air in and out of the lungs

Vital Signs: Extent to which temperature, pulse, respiration, and BP are within normal range

V

Goals/Evaluation Criteria

Examples Using NOC Language

- Demonstrates **Vital Signs**, as evidenced by the following indicators (specify 1–5: severe, substantial, moderate, mild, or no deviation from normal range): Body temperature, apical heart and radial pulse rate, respiratory rate, and systolic and diastolic BP

- Demonstrates **Respiratory Status: Gas Exchange**, as evidenced by the following indicators (specify 1–5: severe, substantial, moderate, mild, or no deviation from normal):
  - Oxygen saturation
  - Chest X-ray findings
  - PaO_2, $PaCO_2$, and arterial pH
- Demonstrates **Respiratory Status: Ventilation**, as evidenced by the following indicators (specify 1–5: severe, substantial, moderate, mild, or none):
  - Accessory muscle use
  - Adventitious breath sounds
  - Chest retraction
  - Dyspnea (at rest or with exertion)
  - Orthopnea

Other Examples

- Achieves established weaning goals
- Physiologically stable for weaning process
- Psychologically and emotionally ready for weaning process
- Symmetrical chest expansion

NIC Interventions

Anxiety Reduction: Minimizing apprehension, dread, foreboding, or uneasiness related to an unidentified source of anticipated danger

Mechanical Ventilation Management: Invasive: Assisting the patient receiving artificial breathing support through a device inserted into the trachea

Mechanical Ventilatory Weaning: Assisting the patient to breathe without the aid of a mechanical ventilator

Preparatory Sensory Information: Describing in concrete and objective terms the typical sensory experiences and events associated with an upcoming stressful health care procedure/treatment

Respiratory Monitoring: Collection and analysis of patient data to ensure airway patency and adequate gas exchange

Ventilation Assistance: Promotion of an optimal spontaneous breathing pattern that maximizes oxygen and carbon dioxide exchange in the lungs

Vital Signs Monitoring: Collection and analysis of cardiovascular, respiratory, and body temperature data to determine and prevent complications

Nursing Activities

Assessments

- Assess patient's readiness to wean by considering the following respiratory indicators:
  - ABG stable with $PaO_2 > 60$ on 40–60% oxygen
  - Maximum inspiratory force > -20 cm H_2O so independent respiration can be initiated
  - Unassisted tidal volume > 5 mL/kg ideal body weight
  - Vital capacity > 13 mL/kg ideal body weight
  - Stable spontaneous respiratory rate < 30 breaths per minute
  - Cough effective enough to handle secretions
  - Length of time on ventilator
- Assess patient's readiness to wean by considering the following nonrespiratory indicators:
  - Absence of constipation, diarrhea, or ileus
  - Absence of fever and infection
  - Adequate nutritional status as evidenced by acceptable serum albumin and transferrin and midarm muscle circumference > 15th percentile
  - Adequate rest and sleep
  - Hemoglobin and hematocrit WNL for patient
  - Improvements in body strength and endurance
  - Normal BP for patient
  - Psychologic and emotional readiness
  - Satisfactory fluid and electrolyte balance
  - Stable heart rate and rhythm
  - Tolerable pain or discomfort level
- Determine why previous weaning attempts were unsuccessful, if applicable
- Monitor patient's response to current medications and correlate response with weaning goals
- *(NIC) Mechanical Ventilatory Weaning:*
  - Monitor predictors of ability to tolerate weaning based on agency protocol (e.g., degree of shunt, vital capacity, V_d/V_t, mandatory minute ventilation (MMV), inspiratory force, FEV_1, and negative inspiratory pressure)
  - Monitor for signs of respiratory muscle fatigue (e.g., abrupt rise in $PaCO_2$; rapid, shallow ventilation; and paradoxical abdominal wall motion), hypoxemia, and tissue hypoxia while weaning is in process

Patient/Family Teaching

- Instruct patient and family in weaning process and goals, which should include:
  - How patient may feel as process evolves
  - Participation of family
  - Participation required by patient
  - What patient can expect from nurse
  - Reasons why weaning is necessary
- *(NIC) Mechanical Ventilatory Weaning:* Assist the patient to distinguish spontaneous breaths from mechanically delivered breaths

Collaborative Activities

- Discuss weaning process and goals with physician and respiratory care practitioner, including patient's present and preexisting medical conditions
- *(NIC) Mechanical Ventilatory Weaning:* Collaborate with other health team members to optimize patient's nutritional status, ensuring that 50% of the diet's nonprotein calorie source is fat, rather than carbohydrate

Other

- Encourage self-care to increase sense of control and participation in own care
- Normalize ADLs to patient's tolerance level
- Establish a trusting relationship that instills patient's confidence in nurse to assist patient with weaning process
- Establish effective methods of communication between patient and others (e.g., writing, blinking eyes, squeezing hand)
- Initiate weaning process by:
  - Checking equipment to make sure it is attached to oxygen and that settings are correct
  - Checking for presence of bilateral breath sounds
  - Checking tubing for kinks and excessive moisture
  - Checking vital signs and patient for indicators of nontolerance or fatigue q5–15 min
  - Documenting weaning process and patient's tolerance
  - Explaining procedure to patient and family
  - Measuring and recording baseline respiratory rate, heart rate, BP, ECG rhythm, lung sounds, vital capacity, tidal volume, inspiratory force, and saturated oxygen via pulse oximeter
  - Preoxygenating, hyperinflating, suctioning, and reoxygenating patient prior to weaning
  - Providing a quiet environment during weaning time

Providing diversions such as television or radio
Sitting patient in an upright position to decrease abdominal pressure on the diaphragm and allow for better lung expansion
Starting the weaning time when patient has rested and is awake and alert
Staying with patient during weaning time to provide coaching and reassurance
Understanding the rationale for weaning orders (e.g., use of continuous positive airway pressure [CPAP], synchronized intermittent mandatory ventilation [SIMV], pressure support ventilation [PSV], and MMV, or T-piece)

- Reconnect patient to ventilator at preweaning settings if indicators of nontolerance occur
- Document in nursing care plan those strategies that promote success with weaning process to ensure consistency (e.g., communication method with patient, family participation, and coaching methods)
- *(NIC) Mechanical Ventilatory Weaning:*

Alternate periods of weaning trials with sufficient periods of rest and sleep
Avoid delaying return of patient with fatigued respiratory muscles to mechanical ventilation
Set a schedule to coordinate other patient care activities with weaning trials
Use relaxation techniques, as appropriate

Home Care

- Assess whether it is practical (e.g., financially, psychologically, physically) to wean the patient from the ventilator at home
- If weaning at home, have an emergency plan in place for temporary ventilation while reestablishing the mechanical ventilator

V

For Older Adults

- Adults over age 80 require a longer period of time to wean

VIOLENCE: OTHER-DIRECTED, RISK FOR

(1980, 1996) **Domain 11, Safety/Protection; Class 3, Violence**

Definition: At risk for behaviors in which an individual demonstrates that he or she can be physically, emotionally, and/or sexually harmful to others

Risk Factors

Objective

Availability or possession of weapon(s)

Body language: rigid posture, clenching of fists and jaw, hyperactivity, pacing, breathlessness, threatening stances

Cognitive impairment (e.g., learning disabilities, attention-deficit disorder, decreased intellectual functioning)

Cruelty to animals

Fire setting

History of childhood abuse

History of indirect violence (e.g., tearing off clothes, ripping objects off walls, writing on walls, urinating on floor, defecating on floor, stamping feet, temper tantrum, running in corridors, yelling, throwing objects, breaking a window, slamming doors, sexual advances)

History of other-directed violence (e.g., hitting someone, kicking someone, spitting at someone, scratching someone, throwing objects at someone, biting someone, attempted rape, rape, sexual molestation, urinating or defecating on a person)

History of substance abuse

History of threats of violence (e.g., verbal threats against property, verbal threats against person, social threats, cursing, threatening notes or letters, threatening gestures, sexual threats)

History of violent antisocial behavior (e.g., stealing, insistent borrowing, insistent demand for privileges, insistent interruption of meetings, refusal to eat, refusal to take medication, ignoring instructions)

History of witnessing family violence

Impulsivity

Motor vehicle offenses (e.g., frequent traffic violations, use of a motor vehicle to release anger)

Neurologic impairment (e.g., positive EEG, CAT or MRI, head trauma, positive neurologic findings, seizure disorders)

Pathological intoxication

Prenatal and perinatal complications or abnormalities

Psychotic symptomatology (e.g., auditory, visual, command hallucinations; paranoid delusions; loose, rambling, or illogical thought processes)

Suicidal behavior

Other Risk Factors (Non-NANDA International)

Arrest or conviction pattern

Catatonic excitement

History of abuse by spouse

Manic excitement

Toxic reactions to medications

Suggestions for Use

Use this diagnosis for patients who need nursing interventions for the purpose of protecting others and preventing or decreasing violent episodes. The diagnosis *Disabled family coping* may be more useful for situations in which there is domestic violence. If the need is to focus on *Anxiety* or *Low self-esteem*, consider using those suggested alternative diagnoses.

Suggested Alternative Diagnoses

Anxiety
Coping: family, compromised
Coping, ineffective
Self-esteem, chronic low
Self-esteem, situational low

NOC Outcomes

Abusive Behavior Self-Restraint: Self-restraint of abusive and neglectful behaviors toward others
Aggression Self-Control: Self-restraint of assaultive, combative, or destructive behavior toward others
Impulse Self-Control: Self-restraint of compulsive or impulsive behavior

Goals/Evaluation Criteria

Examples Using NOC Language

- Demonstrates **Aggression Self-Control**, as evidenced by the following indicators (specify 1–5: never, rarely, sometimes, often, or consistently demonstrated):
  Refrains from:
    Verbal outbursts
    Striking others
    Violating others' personal space
    Harming others; harming animals
    Destroying property
    Identifies when angry, frustrated, or feeling aggressive
    Communicates feelings appropriately
- Demonstrates **Impulse Self-Control**, as evidenced by the following indicators (specify 1–5: never, rarely, sometimes, often, or consistently demonstrated):
  Identifies feelings or behaviors that lead to impulsive actions
  Identifies consequences of impulsive actions to self or others
  Avoids high-risk environments and situations
  Obtains assistance when experiencing impulses

Other Examples

- Identifies factors that precipitate violent behaviors
- Identifies alternative ways to cope with problems
- Identifies support systems in the community
- Does not abuse others physically, emotionally, or sexually

NIC Interventions

NOTE: Nursing interventions focus on identifying and modifying risk factors and other-directed violence. Because risk factors are numerous, not all interventions can be listed.

Abuse Protection Support: Identification of high-risk, dependent relationships and actions to prevent further infliction of physical or emotional harm

Anger Control Assistance: Facilitation of the expression of anger in an adaptive nonviolent manner

Behavior Management: Helping a patient to manage negative behavior

Environmental Management: Violence Prevention: Monitoring and manipulation of the physical environment to decrease the potential for violent behavior directed toward self, others, or environment

Impulse Control Training: Assisting the patient to mediate impulsive behavior through application of problem-solving strategies to social and interpersonal situations

Nursing Activities

Assessments

- Identify behaviors that signal impending violence against others, specify behaviors
- *(NIC) Anger Control Assistance:* Monitor potential for inappropriate aggression and intervene before its expression
- *(NIC) Environmental Management: Violence Prevention:*
  Monitor the safety of items being brought to the environment by visitors
  Monitor patient during use of potential weapons (e.g., razor)

Patient/Family Teaching

- *(NIC) Anger Control Assistance:* Instruct on use of calming measures (e.g., time-outs and deep breaths)

Collaborative Activities

- Clarify use of 72-hr hold for evaluation and treatment in psychiatric unit in the event of abuse against others
- Confer with physician on use of appropriate restraining measures when necessary to prevent injury to others

V

- Follow hospital or agency policy regarding legal responsibility for reporting abuse to authorities
- Initiate a multidisciplinary patient care conference to develop a plan of care

Other

- Encourage patient to verbalize anger
- Identify situations that provoke violence, specify situations
- Provide positive feedback when patient adheres to behavior limits
- *(NIC) Anger Control Assistance:*
  - Use a calm, reassuring approach
  - Limit access to frustrating situations until patient is able to express anger in an adaptive manner
  - Encourage patient to seek assistance of nursing staff or responsible others during periods of increasing tension
  - Prevent physical harm if anger is directed at self or others (e.g., restrain and remove potential weapons)
  - Educate on methods to modulate experience of intense emotion (e.g., assertiveness training, relaxation techniques, writing in a journal, distraction)
  - Identify consequences of inappropriate expression of anger
  - Establish expectation that patient can control his behavior
  - Assist in developing appropriate methods of expressing anger to others (e.g., assertiveness and use of feeling statements)
- *(NIC) Environmental Management: Violence Prevention:*
  - Assign single room to patient with potential for violence toward others
  - Place patient in bedroom located near nursing station
  - Limit access to windows, unless locked and shatterproof, as appropriate
  - Place patient in least restrictive environment that allows for necessary level of observation
  - Maintain a designated safe area (e.g., seclusion room) for patient to be placed when violent
  - Provide plastic, rather than metal, clothes hangers, as appropriate
  - Provide paper dishes and plastic utensils at meals

Home Care

- The preceding activities can be used or adapted for home care
- Make initial and ongoing assessments for actual and potential spousal, elder, and child abuse
- Observe for verbal aggression, which may be a cue to abuse

- If you suspect abuse, implement an emergency plan to assure client safety; report to the appropriate authorities
- Assess whether the client is taking psychotropic medications as prescribed
- If you become uncomfortable with a client's aggressiveness, even if there is no overt threat, do not remain in the home
- If aggressiveness occurs, explain to client that continued aggressive behavior may cause the agency to discontinue services. Notify the agency, and make future visits with another staff member or outside the home.

For Infants and Children

- Assess for signs of abuse; report to appropriate authorities
- Refer for early childhood home visitation
- Assess adolescent girls for dating violence
- Assess pregnant adolescents for abuse, especially if the partner is four or more years older

For Older Adults

- Assess for dementia and delirium
- Assess for actual or potential elder abuse, including financial exploitation, physical abuse, and malnourishment
- If abuse is suspected, report to Adult Protective Services
- Assess for agitation, anger, irritability, changes in physiological functions, and functional abilities (e.g., decreased mobility)

VIOLENCE: SELF-DIRECTED, RISK FOR

(1994) **Domain 11, Safety/Protection; Class 3, Violence**

Definition: At risk for behaviors in which an individual demonstrates that he or she can be physically, emotionally, or sexually harmful to self

Risk Factors

Age 15–19
Age 45 or older
Behavioral clues (e.g., writing forlorn love notes, directing angry messages at a significant other who has rejected the person, giving away personal items, taking out a large life insurance policy)
Conflictual interpersonal relationships

Emotional status (e.g., hopelessness, despair, increased anxiety, panic, anger, hostility)
Employment (e.g., unemployed, recent job loss or failure)
Engagement in autoerotic sexual acts
Family background (e.g., chaotic or conflictual, history of suicide)
History of multiple suicide attempts
Lack of personal resources (e.g., poor achievement, poor insight, affect unavailable and poorly controlled)
Lack of social resources (e.g., poor rapport, socially isolated, unresponsive family)
Marital status (e.g., single, widowed, divorced)
Mental health problems (e.g., severe depression, psychosis, severe personality disorder, alcoholism, or drug abuse)
Occupation (e.g., executive, administrator or owner of business, professional semiskilled worker)
Physical health problems (e.g., is hypochondriasis, chronic, or terminal illness)
Sexual orientation (e.g., bisexual [active], homosexual [inactive])
Suicidal ideation [frequent, intense, prolonged]
Suicidal plan [clear and specific, lethality, method and availability of destructive means]
Verbal clues (e.g., talking about death, "better off without me," asking questions about lethal dosages and drugs)

Suggestions for Use

If the specific risk factors for *Risk for self-mutilation* or *Risk for suicide* are present, use those more specific nursing diagnoses instead of *Risk for self-directed violence.*

Suggested Alternative Diagnoses

Self-mutilation, risk for
Suicide, risk for

NOC Outcomes

Self-Mutilation Restraint: Personal actions to refrain from intentional self-inflicted injury (nonlethal)

Suicide Self-Restraint: Personal actions to refrain from gestures and attempts at killing self

NOTE: The following outcomes are associated with risk factors for self-directed violence:

Anxiety Level: Severity of manifested apprehension, tension, or uneasiness arising from an unidentifiable source

Distorted Thought Self-Control: Self-restraint of disruptions in perception, thought processes, and thought content

Impulse Self-Control: Self-restraint of compulsive or impulsive behavior

Mood Equilibrium: Appropriate adjustment of prevailing emotional tone in response to circumstances

Social Interaction Skills: Personal behaviors that promote effective relationships

Social Involvement: Social interactions with persons, groups, or organizations

Goals/Evaluation Criteria

Examples Using NOC Language

- Demonstrates **Impulse Self-Control**, as evidenced by the following indicators (specify 1–5: never, rarely, sometimes, often, or consistently demonstrated):

  Identifies feelings or behaviors that lead to impulsive actions
  Identifies consequences of impulsive actions to self or others
  Avoids high-risk environments and situations
  Controls impulses

Other Examples

Patient will:

- Identify alternative ways to cope with problems
- Identify support systems in the community
- Report a decrease in suicidal thoughts
- Not attempt suicide
- Not harm self

NIC Interventions

NOTE: Nursing interventions focus on monitoring for self-directed violence, as well as on identifying and modifying risk factors.

Behavior Management: Self-Harm: Assisting the patient to decrease or eliminate self-mutilating or self-abusive behaviors

Environmental Management: Violence Prevention: Monitoring and manipulation of the physical environment to decrease the potential for violent behavior directed toward self, others, or environment

Impulse Control Training: Assisting the patient to mediate impulsive behavior through application of problem-solving strategies to social and interpersonal situation

Mood Management: Providing for safety, stabilization, recovery, and maintenance of a patient who is experiencing dysfunctionally depressed or elevated mood

Patient Contracting: Negotiating an agreement with an individual, which reinforces a specific behavior change

Substance Use Treatment: Supportive care of patient and family members with physical and psychosocial problems associated with the use of alcohol or drugs

Suicide Prevention: Reducing risk of self-inflicted harm with intent to end life

Nursing Activities

Also refer to Nursing Activities for the diagnoses *Self-mutilation*, *Risk for self-mutilation*, and *Risk for suicide*.

Assessments

- Assess and document patient's potential for suicide q ____________
- Identify behaviors that signal impending violence against self, specify behaviors
- *(NIC) Environmental Management: Violence Prevention:*
  Monitor the safety of items being brought to the environment by visitors
  Monitor patient during use of potential weapons (e.g., razor)

Patient/Family Teaching

- *(NIC) Anger Control Assistance:* Instruct on use of calming measures (e.g., time-outs and deep breaths)

Collaborative Activities

- Clarify use of 72-hr hold for evaluation and treatment in psychiatric unit in the event of abuse against self
- Confer with physician on use of appropriate restraining measures when necessary to prevent injury to self
- Initiate a multidisciplinary patient care conference to develop a plan of care

Other

- Institute suicide precautions, as needed (e.g., 24-hr attendant)
- Reassure patient that you will protect him against own suicidal impulses until able to regain control by (a) constantly observing patient, (b) frequently checking patient, and (c) taking patient's suicidal ideation seriously
- Discuss with patient and family the role of anger in self-harm
- Encourage patient to verbalize anger
- *(NIC) Anger Control Assistance:*
  Use a calm, reassuring approach
  Limit access to frustrating situations until patient is able to express anger in an adaptive manner

Encourage patient to seek assistance of nursing staff or responsible others during periods of increasing tension

Prevent physical harm if anger is directed at self (e.g., restrain and remove potential weapons)

Provide physical outlets for expression of anger or tension (e.g., punching bag, sports, clay, and writing in a journal)

Establish expectation that patient can control his behavior

- *(NIC) Environmental Management: Violence Prevention:*

  Place patient with potential for self-harm with a roommate to decrease isolation and opportunity to act on self-harm thoughts, as appropriate

  Place patient in a bedroom located near nursing station

  Limit access to windows, unless locked and shatterproof, as appropriate

  Place patient in least restrictive environment that allows for necessary level of observation

  Apply mitts, splints, helmets, or restraints to limit mobility and ability to initiate self-harm, as appropriate

  Provide plastic, rather than metal, clothes hangers, as appropriate

  Provide paper dishes and plastic utensils at meals

WALKING, IMPAIRED

(1998, 2006) **Domain 4, Activity/Rest; Class 2, Activity/Exercise**

Definition: Limitation of independent movement within the environment on foot [specify level]

Defining Characteristics

Impaired ability to:

Climb stairs

Navigate curbs

Walk on an incline or decline

Walk on uneven surfaces

Walk required distances

Related Factors

Cognitive impairment

Deconditioning

Depressed mood

Environmental constraints (e.g., stairs, inclines, uneven surfaces, unsafe obstacles, distances, lack of assistive devices or person, restraints)

Fear of falling

Impaired balance
Impaired vision
Insufficient muscle strength
Lack of knowledge [e.g., regarding value of physical activity]
Limited endurance
Musculoskeletal impairment (e.g., contractures)
Neuromuscular impairment
Obesity
Pain

Non-NANDA International Related Factors

Cultural beliefs regarding age-appropriate activity
Developmental delay
Lack of physical or social environmental supports
Limited cardiovascular endurance
Medications
Reluctance to initiate movement
Selective or generalized malnutrition

Suggestions for Use

As with other mobility diagnoses, specify the patient's functional level, as follows:

Level 0: Completely independent
Level 1: Requires use of equipment or device
Level 2: Requires help from another person for assistance, supervision, or teaching
Level 3: Requires help from another person and equipment or device
Level 4: Dependent; does not participate in activity

Use *Impaired walking* to describe individuals with limited ability for independent physical movement or generalized muscle weakness or when nursing interventions will focus on restoring mobility and function or preventing further deterioration. An example of an appropriate diagnosis would be *Impaired walking related to ineffective management of Chronic pain secondary to rheumatoid arthritis*. If immobility problems in addition to *Impaired walking* exist, consider using *Impaired physical mobility*.

Do not use this label to describe temporary immobility that cannot be changed by the nurse (e.g., traction, prescribed bed rest) or permanent paralysis. *Impaired walking* may be used effectively as the etiology of a nursing diagnosis, for example, *Self-care deficit: toileting related to Impaired walking* +4.

Suggested Alternative Diagnoses

Disuse syndrome, risk for
Injury, risk for

Mobility, physical, impaired
Self-care deficit (specify)
Transfer ability, impaired

NOC Outcomes

Ambulation: Ability to walk from place to place independently with or without assistive device

Balance: Ability to maintain body equilibrium

Coordinated Movement: Ability of muscles to work together voluntarily for purposeful movement

Endurance: Capacity to sustain activity

Joint Movement: Ankle, Hip, Knee: Active range of motion of (specify joint) with self-initiated movement

Mobility: Ability to move purposefully in own environment independently with or without assistive device

Goals/Evaluation Criteria

Examples Using NOC Language

- *Will not have Impaired walking*, as demonstrated by: Ambulation: Walking; Balance; Endurance; Active Joint Movement; and Mobility.
- Demonstrates **Mobility**, as evidenced by the following indicators (specify 1–5: severely, substantially, moderately, mildly, or not compromised):
  - Balance
  - Body positioning performance
  - Coordination
  - Muscle and joint movement
  - Walking

Other Examples

- Bears weight and walk with adequate gait
- Walks a distance appropriate to his overall condition
- Demonstrates correct use of assistive devices (e.g., crutches, cane) with supervision
- Requests assistance with mobilization activities, as needed
- Performs ADLs independently with assistive devices (specify activity and device)

NIC Interventions

Energy Management: Regulating energy use to treat or prevent fatigue and optimize function

Exercise Therapy, Ambulation: Promotion and assistance with walking to maintain or restore autonomic and voluntary body functions during treatment and recovery from illness or injury

Exercise Therapy: Balance: Use of specific activities, postures, and movements to maintain, enhance, or restore balance

Exercise Therapy, Joint Mobility: Use of active or passive body movement to maintain or restore joint flexibility

Exercise Therapy: Muscle Control: Use of specific activity or exercise protocols to enhance or restore controlled body movement

Nursing Activities

Assessments

Assessment is an ongoing process to determine the performance level at which the patient's mobility is impaired.

Level 1: Nursing Activities

- Provide positive reinforcement during activities
- Collaborate with physical therapist in developing strength, balance, and flexibility exercises
- Assess need for assistance from home health agency and need for durable medical equipment
- *(NIC) Exercise Therapy: Ambulation:*
  - Monitor patient's use of crutches or other walking aids
  - Instruct patient how to position self throughout the transfer process
  - Apply or provide assistive device (e.g., cane, walker, or wheelchair) for ambulation if the patient is unsteady
  - Assist patient to use footwear that facilitates walking and prevents injury
  - Encourage independent ambulation within safe limits

Level 2: Nursing Activities

W

- Assess patient's learning needs regarding ________________ (specify)
- Assess need for assistance from home health agency and need for durable medical equipment
- Instruct and encourage patient in active or passive range-of-motion exercises
- Instruct patient regarding weight-bearing status
- Instruct patient regarding correct body alignment
- Instruct and encourage patient to use a trapeze or weights to enhance and maintain strength of upper extremities
- Use occupational and physical therapy as resources in developing a plan for maintaining or increasing mobility
- Provide positive reinforcement during activities
- Supervise all mobilization attempts

- *(NIC) Exercise Therapy: Ambulation:*
  - Instruct patient and caregiver about safe transfer and ambulation techniques
  - Assist patient to stand and ambulate specified distance with specified number of staff

Levels 3 and 4: Nursing Activities

- Use occupational and physical therapy as resources in planning patient care activities
- Encourage patient and family to view limitations realistically
- Provide positive reinforcement during activities
- Develop a plan to include the following:
  - Perform passive range-of-motion (PROM) or assisted range-of-motion (AROM) exercises, as indicated
  - Type of assistive device
  - Number of personnel needed to mobilize patient
  - Schedule of activities
  - Maximization of patient's mobility, given necessary constraints
- Assess patient motivation level for overcoming limitations
- Administer analgesics before beginning exercises or walking, as needed
- *(NIC) Exercise Therapy: Ambulation:*
  - Use a gait belt to assist with transfer and ambulation, as needed

Home Care

- The preceding activities can be used or adapted for home care
- Assess the home environment and remove potential hazards to prevent falls (e.g., highly waxed floors, throw rugs, clutter)
- Recommend a diet high in calcium and vitamin D, with supplementation as necessary
- Refer for home health aide if impaired walking affects ability to perform activities of daily living
- Check assistive devices to keep them in safe working order (e.g., replace worn rubber tips on walkers and crutches)

For Older Adults

- Monitor vital signs before and 5 min after a new activity
- Allow the client to walk as slowly as he needs to
- Assess visual acuity and balance
- Assess for fear of falling
- Use and teach fall prevention measures

WANDERING

(2000)

Domain 4, Activity/Rest; Class 3, Energy Balance

Definition: Meandering, aimless, or repetitive locomotion that exposes the individual to harm; frequently incongruent with boundaries, limits, or obstacles

Defining Characteristics

Objective

Frequent or continuous movement from place to place [often revisiting the same destinations]

Fretful locomotion or pacing

Getting lost

Haphazard locomotion

Hyperactivity

Inability to locate significant landmarks in a familiar setting

Locomotion into unauthorized or private spaces

Locomotion resulting in unintended leaving of a premise

Locomotion that cannot be easily dissuaded [or redirected]

Long periods of locomotion without an apparent destination

Periods of locomotion interspersed with periods of nonlocomotion (e.g., sitting, standing, sleeping)

Persistent locomotion in search of something

Scanning or searching behaviors

Shadowing [or following behind] a caregiver's locomotion

Trespassing

W

Related Factors

Cognitive impairment (e.g., memory and recall deficits, disorientation, poor visuoconstructive [or visuospatial] ability, language [primarily expressive] defects)

Cortical atrophy

Emotional state (e.g., frustration, anxiety, boredom, depression, agitation)

Overstimulating [social or physical] environment

Physiological state or need (e.g., hunger or thirst, pain, urination, constipation)

Premorbid behavior (e.g., outgoing, sociable personality, premorbid dementia)

Sedation

Separation from familiar environment [people and places]

Time of day

Suggestions for Use

Wandering may occur as a result of psychosocial diagnoses such as *Confusion*. If defining characteristics of *Wandering* are present, it should be used instead of broader diagnoses such as Risk for injury. Do not use this label to describe sleepwalking.

Suggested Alternative Diagnoses

Confusion, acute
Confusion, chronic
Environmental interpretation syndrome, impaired
Injury, risk for

NOC Outcomes

Elopement Occurrence: Number of times in the past 24 hr/1 week/1 month (select one) that an individual with a cognitive impairment escapes a secure area

Elopement Propensity Risk: The propensity of an individual with cognitive impairment to escape a secure area

Fall Prevention Behavior: Personal or family caregiver actions to minimize risk factors that might precipitate falls in the personal environment

Safe Home Environment: Physical arrangements to minimize environmental factors that might cause physical harm or injury in the home

Safe Wandering: Safe, socially acceptable moving about without apparent purpose in an individual with cognitive impairment

Goals/Evaluation Criteria

Examples Using NOC Language

- Demonstrates **Fall Prevention Behavior**, as evidenced by the following indicators (specify 1–5: never, rarely, sometimes, often, or consistently demonstrated):
  - Places barriers to prevent falls
  - Provides adequate lighting
  - Eliminates clutter, spills, glare from floors
  - Removes rugs
  - Arranges for removal of snow and ice from walking surfaces
  - Controls restlessness

Other Examples

Patient will:

- Not wander into unauthorized or private places
- Not become lost

- Not leave the building (if institutionalized)
- Walk only on agreed-upon safe route

NIC Interventions

Anxiety Reduction: Minimizing apprehension, dread, foreboding, or uneasiness related to an unidentified source of anticipated danger

Area Restriction: Use of least restrictive limitation of patient mobility to a specified area for purposes of safety or behavior management

Dementia Management: Provision of a modified environment for the patient who is experiencing a chronic confusional state

Elopement Precautions: Minimizing the risk of a patient leaving a treatment setting without authorization when departure presents a threat to the safety of patient or others

Environmental Management: Safety: Monitoring and manipulation of the physical environment to promote safety

Fall Prevention: Instituting special precautions with patient at risk for injury from falling

Surveillance: Safety: Purposeful and ongoing collection and analysis of information about the patient and the environment for use in promoting and maintaining patient safety

Nursing Activities

Assessments

- *Assess for factors that create the risk for Wandering* (e.g., confusion, agitation, anxiety)
- *(NIC) Environmental Management: Safety*

  Identify the safety needs of patient, based on level of physical and cognitive function and past history of behavior
- *(NIC) Elopement Precautions:*

  Monitor patient for indicators of elopement potential (e.g., verbal indicators, loitering near exits, multiple layers of clothing, disorientation, separation anxiety, and homesickness)
- *(NIC) Dementia Management:*

  Determine type and extent of cognitive deficit(s), using standardized assessment tool

W

Patient/Family Teaching

- Explain to family and friends how best to interact with a confused person or a person with delirium or dementia
- Explain to the family the purpose or precautions such as area restriction, identification bands, increased supervision, gates, physical restraints, and so forth
- Provide information about ways to make the home safe for the patient

Collaborative Activities

- *(NIC) Elopement Precautions:*
  - Clarify the legal status of patient (e.g., minor or adult and voluntary or court-ordered treatment)
  - Communicate risk to other care providers

Other

- Use locks or gates on doors and windows/electronic buzzers at property boundaries
- If available, use electronic ID bracelets linked to a national database to help locate patients. (In the near future, microchip implants may soon be available for this purpose, for patients who are unable to communicate.)
- Notify neighbors about the patient's wandering and give them instructions for notifying if they see the person wandering
- Avoid restraints, if possible; use pressure-sensitive alarms instead (e.g., chair or bed sensors)
- Provide a consistent, familiar environment (e.g., avoid room changes and unfamiliar people)
- Mark patient's boundaries clearly (e.g., with brightly colored tape on the floor, signs on the door, and so forth)
- *(NIC) Dementia Management:*
  - Provide space for safe pacing and wandering
  - Place identification bracelet on patient
- *(NIC) Elopement Precautions:*
  - Familiarize patient with environment and routine to decrease anxiety
  - Limit patient to a physically secure environment (e.g., locked or alarmed doors at exits and locked windows), as needed
  - Increase supervision or surveillance when patient is outside secure environment (e.g., hold hands and increase staff-to-patient ratio)
  - Record physical description (e.g., height, weight, eye, hair, and skin color, and any distinguishing characteristics [for reference, should patient elope])
- *(NIC) Environmental Management:* Remove environmental hazards (e.g., loose rugs and small, movable furniture)

Home Care

- The preceding activities can be used or adapted for home care

Section III

CLINICAL CONDITIONS GUIDE TO NURSING DIAGNOSES AND COLLABORATIVE PROBLEMS

Clinical Conditions Guide to Nursing Diagnoses and Collaborative Problems

Medical Conditions
Surgical Conditions
Psychiatric Conditions
Antepartum and Postpartum Conditions
Newborn Conditions
Pediatric Conditions

This section contains lists of potential complications (also called multidisciplinary problems and collaborative problems) and nursing diagnoses associated with selected conditions (e.g., medical, surgical, childbearing). However, because nursing diagnoses represent human responses, and because human beings respond in infinite ways, any nursing diagnosis could occur with any disease process or condition. In a sense, then, all nursing diagnoses on these lists are potential diagnoses. When using these lists, keep in mind that for each condition (e.g., congestive heart failure): (a) every patient with that condition must be monitored for the associated complications, (b) a patient may have nursing diagnoses that are not included in the list, and (c) the list may include many nursing diagnoses that the patient does not have.

For the nursing diagnoses in this section, the etiologies (which follow "related to") are stated in broad, general terms. Etiologies, like problems, are highly individual. Therefore, when writing a nursing diagnosis, use the list as a starting point and expand the etiology to fully describe that patient's pathophysiology, disease process, situation, or other related factors. The format used for collaborative problems is adapted from Carpenito (1997, pp. 28–29), for example, Potential Complication (PC) of burns: Hypovolemic shock.

Some patient teaching is required for every patient. Therefore, the nursing diagnosis *Deficient knowledge* is not listed for any of the clinical conditions in this section. It is assumed that all clients, regardless of disease or medical diagnosis, will be assessed for *Deficient knowledge*.

MEDICAL CONDITIONS

Acquired immune deficiency syndrome (AIDS)
Arthritis
Autoimmune disorders
Blood disorders
Burns
Cancer
Cardiac disorders (angina/coronary insufficiency, myocardial infarction, congestive heart failure, pericarditis/endocarditis)
Chest trauma
Dying patient
Endocrine disorders (Cushing disease, diabetes mellitus, hypoglycemia, hyperthyroidism, hypothyroidism)
Gastrointestinal disorders (inflammation, bleeding, ulcers, abdominal pain)
Immobilized patient
Liver disease
Neurologic disorders (cerebrovascular accident, other)
Obesity
Pancreatitis
Renal failure, acute
Renal failure, chronic
Respiratory disorders, acute (pneumonia, pulmonary edema, pulmonary embolism)
Respiratory disorders, chronic
Urologic disorders
Vascular disease

Acquired Immune Deficiency Syndrome (AIDS)

Potential Complications (Collaborative Problems)

PC of AIDS: Human immunodeficiency virus (HIV) wasting syndrome, malignancies (e.g., Kaposi sarcoma, lymphoma), meningitis, opportunistic infections (e.g., candidiasis, cytomegalovirus, herpes, *Pneumocystis carinii* pneumonia)

Nursing Diagnoses

Activity intolerance Related factors: Fatigue, weakness, medication side effects, fever, malnutrition, *Impaired gas exchange* (secondary to lung infections or malignancy)

Airway clearance, ineffective Related factors: Decreased energy or fatigue, respiratory infections, tracheobronchial secretions, pulmonary malignancy, pneumothorax

Anxiety Related factors: Uncertain future, perception of effects of disease and treatments on lifestyle

Body image, disturbed Related factors: Chronic illness, lesions of KS, alopecia, weight loss, changes in sexuality

Caregiver role strain (actual/risk for) Related and risk factors: Illness severity of the care receiver, unpredictable illness course or instability in the care receiver's health, duration of caregiving required, inadequate physical environment for providing care, lack of respite and recreation for caregiver, complexity and number of caregiving tasks

Confusion, acute or chronic Related factors: Infection of CNS (e.g., toxoplasmosis), CMV infection, KS, lymphoma, progress of HIV

Coping: family, compromised/disabled (also consider *Family processes, interrupted*) Related factors: Inadequate or incorrect information or understanding by family member or close friend, chronic illness, chronically unresolved feelings

Coping, ineffective Related factor: Personal vulnerability in a situational crisis (e.g., terminal illness)

Diarrhea Related factors: Medication, diet, infections

Diversional activity, deficient Related factors: Frequent or lengthy medical treatments, long-term hospitalization, prolonged bed rest

Falls, risk for Related factors: *Fatigue*, weakness, cognitive changes, encephalopathy, neuromuscular changes

Fatigue Related factors: Disease process, overwhelming psychologic or emotional demands

Fear Related factors: *Powerlessness*, real threat to own well-being, possibility of disclosure, possibility of death

Fluid volume, deficient Related factors: Inadequate fluid intake secondary to oral lesions, *Diarrhea*

Grieving, complicated Related factors: Impending death or impending changes in lifestyle, loss of body function, changes in appearance, abandonment by significant others

Home maintenance, impaired Related factors: Inadequate support systems, lack of knowledge, lack of familiarity with community resources

Hopelessness Related factors: Deteriorating physical condition, poor prognosis

Human dignity, compromised, risk for Risk factors: Physical effects of the disease, invasive treatments, loss of ability to care for own body

Infection, risk for Risk factor: Cellular immunodeficiency

Infection transmission, risk for (Non-NANDA International) Risk factor: Contagious nature of body fluids

Insomnia Related factors: *Pain*, night sweats, medication regimen, medication side effects, *Anxiety*, depression, drug withdrawal (e.g., heroin, cocaine)

Nutrition, imbalanced: less than body requirements Related factors: Difficulty in swallowing, loss of appetite, oral and esophageal lesions, gastrointestinal malabsorption, increased metabolic rate, *Nausea*

Oral mucous membrane, impaired Risk factors: Compromised immune system, opportunistic infections (e.g., candidiasis, herpes)

Pain, (acute) Related factors: Progression of disease process, medication side effects, lymphedema secondary to KS, headaches secondary to CNS infection, peripheral neuropathy, severe myalgias

Powerlessness Related factors: Terminal illness, treatment regimen, unpredictable nature of disease

Self-care deficit: (specify) Related factors: Decreased strength and endurance; *Activity intolerance; Confusion, acute/chronic*

Self-esteem, low (chronic, situational) Related factors: Chronic illness, situational crisis

Sexuality pattern, ineffective Related factors: Safer sex practices, fear of HIV transmission, abstinence, impotence secondary to medications

Skin integrity, impaired Related factors: Tissue and muscle wasting secondary to altered nutritional state, perineal excoriation secondary to *Diarrhea* and lesions (e.g., candidiasis, herpes), *Impaired physical mobility*, KS lesions

Social isolation Related factors: Stigma, others' fear of contracting disease, own fear of HIV transmission, cultural and religious mores, physical appearance, *Self-esteem* and *Body image, disturbed*

Spiritual distress Related factors: Challenged belief and value system, test of spiritual beliefs

Suicide, risk for Risk factors: *Hopelessness*, isolation

Arthritis

Includes but is not limited to rheumatoid arthritis, osteoarthritis, juvenile rheumatoid arthritis, gouty arthritis, and septic arthritis

Potential Complications (Collaborative Problems)

PC of arthritis: Fibrous or bony ankylosis, joint contractures, neuropathy

PC of corticosteroids (intra-articular injections): Intra-articular infection, joint degeneration

PC of corticosteroids (systemic administration): Cushing syndrome, hyperglycemia, delayed wound healing, osteoporosis, muscle wasting, hypertension, edema, congestive heart failure, hypokalemia, depressed immune response, peptic ulcers, renal failure, growth retardation (children), psychotic reactions, cataract formation, atherosclerosis, thrombophlebitis

PC of nonsteroidal anti-inflammatory medications: Gastric ulceration or bleeding, nephropathy

Nursing Diagnoses

Body image, disturbed Related factors: Chronic illness, joint deformities, *Impaired physical mobility*

Coping, ineffective Related factors: Personal vulnerability in a situational crisis (e.g., new diagnosis of illness, declining health), unpredictable exacerbations

Family processes, interrupted Related factors: Change in family roles, disability of family member, lack of support system

Fatigue Related factors: *Pain*, overwhelming psychologic or emotional demands, systemic inflammation, anemia

Home maintenance, impaired Related factors: *Impaired physical mobility*, *Fatigue*, *Pain*

Therapeutic regimen management, family, ineffective Related factors: *Deficient knowledge* of medication and therapies, forgetful about taking medications because of *Impaired memory*, reliance on quackery

Pain, acute/chronic Related factors: Progression of joint abnormalities, inflammation

Mobility: physical, impaired Related factors: Stiffness, *Pain*, joint ankylosis, contractures, decreased muscle strength

Powerlessness Related factors: Incurable nature of the disease, not feeling better even when following therapeutic regimen

Self-care deficit: (specify) Related factors: Musculoskeletal impairment, *Pain*, *Impaired physical mobility*, *Fatigue*

Sexuality pattern, ineffective Related factors: *Fatigue*, *Pain*, *Impaired physical mobility*

Insomnia Related factor: *Pain*

Social interaction, impaired Related factors: *Fatigue*, difficulty ambulating

Autoimmune Disorders

Include but are not limited to systemic lupus erythematosus (SLE), scleroderma, rheumatic fever, glomerulonephritis, and multiple sclerosis

Potential Complications (Collaborative Problems)

PC of lupus erythematosus: Vasculitis, pericarditis, pleuritis, cerebral infarction, hemolytic anemia, glomerulonephritis

PC of glomerulonephritis or renal failure: Ascites, anasarca, sepsis

PC of corticosteroid therapy: Cushing syndrome, hyperglycemia, delayed wound healing, osteoporosis, muscle wasting, hypertension, edema, congestive heart failure, hypokalemia, depressed immune response, peptic ulcers, renal failure, growth retardation (children), psychotic reactions, cataract formation, atherosclerosis, thrombophlebitis

Nursing Diagnoses

Activity intolerance Related factors: *Anxiety*, *Acute/chronic pain*, weakness, *Fatigue*

Body image, disturbed Related factors: Chronic illness, *Chronic pain*, rash, lesions, ulcers, purpura, mottling of hands, alopecia, and altered body function

Caregiver role strain Related and risk factors: Illness severity of care receiver, duration of caregiving required, lack of respite and recreation for caregiver, complexity and number of caregiving tasks

Coping: family, compromised: See *Family processes, interrupted*

Coping, ineffective Related factors: Personal vulnerability in a situational crisis (e.g., declining health), unpredictable course of disease, exacerbations

Diversional activity, deficient Related factors: Long-term hospitalization, frequent or lengthy treatments, forced inactivity

Family processes, interrupted Related factors: Chronic illness or disability, complex therapies, change in family roles, hospitalization or change in environment, disability of family member

Fatigue Related factors: Increased energy needs secondary to chronic inflammation, altered body chemistry, effects of medication therapy

Fear Related factors: Environmental stressors or hospitalization, *Powerlessness*, real or imagined threat to own well-being

Fluid volume excess Related factor: Decreased urine output secondary to sodium retention or glomerulonephritis

Grieving, complicated Related factors: Potential loss of body function, potential loss of social role, terminal illness, chronic illness

Health behavior, risk-prone Related factors: Necessity for major lifestyle or behavior change

Home maintenance, impaired Related factors: *Pain*, *Impaired physical mobility*

Hopelessness Related factors: Failing or deteriorating physical condition, long-term stress

Infection, risk for Risk factors: Immunosuppression, chronic disease, pharmaceutical agents, secondary to glomerulonephritis

Insomnia Related factors: *Pain* and discomfort, *Anxiety*, inactivity

Mobility: physical, impaired Related factors: *Pain*, medically prescribed limitations, (joint) changes, neuromuscular impairment

Noncompliance Related factors: Denial of illness, negative perception or consequences of treatment regimen, perceived benefits of continued illness

Nutrition, imbalanced: less than body requirements Related factors: Difficulty in chewing, *Impaired swallowing*, loss of appetite, *Nausea*, and vomiting

Oral mucous membrane, impaired Related factors: Pathophysiology of the disease, medication side effects

Pain Related factors: Inflammation of connective tissues, blood vessels, and mucous membranes

Powerlessness Related factors: Unpredictability of chronic, terminal disease; complex treatment regimen; physical and psychologic changes associated with the disease

Protection, ineffective Related factor: Corticosteroid therapy

Role performance, ineffective Related factors: Chronic illness, *Chronic pain*

Self-care deficit: (specify) Related factors: Decreased strength and endurance, *Pain*, *Activity intolerance*, stiffness, *Fatigue*

Self-esteem, low (chronic, situational) Related factors: Chronic illness, *Chronic pain*, *Ineffective role performance*, inability to achieve developmental tasks because of disabling condition

Self-Health management, ineffective Related factors: *Deficient knowledge* (disease process, balanced rest and exercise, symptoms of exacerbations and complications, medications and treatment, community resources)

Sexuality pattern, ineffective Related factors: *Fatigue*, *Pain*, *Impaired physical mobility*

Skin integrity, impaired (actual/risk for) Related and risk factors: Rashes, lesions, medications, altered circulation, *Impaired physical mobility*, photosensitivity, edema

Social interaction, impaired Related factors: *Self-esteem, low* (*chronic, situational*) limited physical mobility, *Fatigue*, embarrassment over appearance

Social isolation Related factor: Others' response to appearance

Urinary incontinence, functional Related factor: *Impaired physical mobility*

Blood Disorders

Include but are not limited to anemias, polycythemia, and coagulation disorders

Potential Complications (Collaborative Problems)

PC of anemias: Cardiac failure, iron overload, bleeding, infection

PC of coagulation disorders: Hemorrhage, thrombus formation, renal failure, congestive heart failure

Nursing Diagnoses

Activity intolerance Related factors: Insufficient oxygen transport secondary to low red blood cell count, pulmonary congestion, tissue hypoxia, *Acute pain*, *Fatigue*, decreased strength and endurance

Anxiety Related factors: Lack of knowledge of disease and treatments, uncertainty of outcome

Bleeding, risk for Risk factors: Abnormal blood profile, sickle cells, decreased hemoglobin, thrombocytopenia, splenomegaly

Constipation Related factors: Atrophy of mucosa, medication (iron) side effects

Diarrhea Related factors: Atrophy of mucosa

Family processes, interrupted Related factors: Hospitalization or change in environment, illness or disability of family member

Fear Related factors: Environmental stressors or hospitalization, treatments

Infection, risk for Risk factors: Decreased resistance secondary to abnormal white blood cells

Nutrition, imbalanced: less than body requirements Related factors: Loss of appetite secondary to sore mouth, *Nausea*

Oral mucous membrane, impaired Related factors: Atrophy of GI mucosa, tissue hypoxia, papillary atrophy, and inflammatory changes (pernicious anemia)

Pain Related factor: Altered body function (e.g., bleeding in joint spaces)

Protection, ineffective See *Bleeding, risk for*

Tissue perfusion: peripheral, ineffective Related factors: Deficit or malfunction of RBCs, hyperviscosity (in polycythemia)

Burns

Potential Complications (Collaborative Problems)

PC of burns: Hypovolemic shock, hypervolemia, paralytic ileus, renal failure, sepsis, stress ulcers

Nursing Diagnoses

Airway clearance, ineffective Related factors: Tracheal edema, decreased pulmonary ciliary action

Anxiety Related factors: Suddenness of injury, pain from injury and treatments, uncertainty of prognosis, immobility

Aspiration, risk for Risk factors: Presence of tracheostomy or endotracheal tube, tube feeding, *Impaired swallowing*, hindered elevation of upper body

Body image, disturbed Related factors: Physical impairment, scarring, contractures

Body temperature, risk for imbalanced Risk factor: Dehydration secondary to *Impaired skin integrity*

Breathing pattern, ineffective Related factor: *Pain*

Caregiver role strain Related factors: Illness severity of care receiver, duration of caregiving required, lack of respite and recreation for caregiver, complexity and number of caregiving tasks

Confusion, acute (or chronic) Related factors: Sensory deficit, sensory overload (environmental), stress, *Sleep deprivation*, protective isolation, enforced immobility

Constipation Related factors: Decreased activity, medications (e.g., narcotic analgesics)

Coping: family, compromised (or disabled) Related factors: See *Family processes, interrupted (or dysfunctional)*

Disuse syndrome, risk for Risk factor: Severe *Pain*

Diversional activity, deficient Related factors: Monotony of long-term hospitalization, separation from family, *Social isolation*

Family processes, interrupted Related factors: Long-term, complex therapies; long-term hospitalization; change in environment; separation from family members; critical nature of injury

Fatigue Related factors: Overwhelming psychologic or emotional demands

Fear Related factors: Environmental stressors or hospitalization, painful procedures, threat of dying, projected effects of injury on lifestyle and relationships

Fluid volume, deficient Related factor: Abnormal fluid loss (e.g., intravascular to interstitial fluid shift)

Gas exchange, impaired Related factors: Smoke inhalation, heat damage to lungs, carbon monoxide poisoning

Hypothermia Related factor: Loss of epithelial tissue

Infection, risk for Risk factors: Tissue destruction (loss of skin barrier), impaired immune response, invasive procedures, and other increased environmental exposures

Insomnia (or sleep deprivation) Related factors: *Pain*, *Anxiety*, dressings, splints, invasive lines

Management of therapeutic regimen: family, ineffective Related factors: *Deficient knowledge* of wound care, exercise and other therapies, nutrition, pain management, and signs and symptoms of complications

Mobility: physical, impaired Related factors: *Pain*, edema, dressings, splints, wound contractures

Neurovascular dysfunction: peripheral, risk for Related factors: Constriction from circumferential burns; tissue damage from burns

Nutrition, imbalanced: less than body requirements Related factors: Difficulty swallowing, high metabolic rate needed for wound healing

Pain Related factors: Burn injury, exposed nerve endings, treatments

Powerlessness Related factor: Inability to control situation (e.g., due to treatment regimen, health care environment, *Pain*)

Self-care deficit: (specify) Related factors: *Pain*, dressings, splints, enforced immobility, *Activity intolerance*, decreased strength and endurance, limited range of motion

Self-esteem, low (chronic, situational) Related factors: *Body image, disturbed*, loss of role responsibilities, loss of functional abilities, delay in achieving developmental tasks secondary to effects of injury

Self-health management, ineffective Related factors: *Deficient knowledge* of wound care, exercise and other therapies, nutrition, pain management, and signs and symptoms of complications

Social isolation Related factors: Separation from family, infection control measures, embarrassment over appearance, response of others to appearance

Tissue perfusion, ineffective (peripheral): Related factor: Constriction from circumferential burns

Cancer

NOTE: Nursing diagnoses depend greatly upon the location, type, and stage of the cancer.

Potential Complications (Collaborative Problems)

PC of cancer: Cachexia, electrolyte imbalance, pathological fractures, hemorrhage, malnutrition (negative nitrogen balance), metastasis to vital organs (e.g., brain, bones, kidneys, lungs, liver), spinal cord compression, superior vena cava syndrome

PC of chemotherapy: Anaphylactic reaction, anemia, CNS toxicity, congestive heart failure, electrolyte imbalance, hemorrhagic cystitis, leukopenia, necrosis at IV site, renal failure, thrombocytopenia

PC of narcotic medications: Depressed respiration, consciousness and blood pressure; cardiovascular collapse; profound brain damage; biliary spasm

PC of radiation therapy: Increased intracranial pressure, myelosuppression, inflammation, fluid and electrolyte imbalances

Nursing Diagnoses

Activity intolerance Related factors: See *Fatigue*

Airway clearance, ineffective Related factors: Tracheobronchial obstruction; ineffective cough secondary to decreased energy, *Fatigue*, and *Pain*; increased viscosity of secretions

Anxiety Related factors: Unfamiliar hospital environment, uncertainty of prognosis, lack of knowledge about cancer and treatment, threat of death, threat of or change in role functioning, inadequate pain relief

Body image, disturbed Related factors: Hair loss, edema, blebs and blisters, petechiae, erythema

Bowel incontinence Related factors: Decreased awareness of need to defecate, disease process, loss of rectal sphincter control

Breathing pattern, ineffective Related factors: Medications, *Chronic pain*, *Fatigue*, anemia

Caregiver role strain Related factors: Illness severity of care receiver, duration of caregiving required, lack of respite and recreation for caregiver, complexity and number of caregiving tasks

Confusion, acute/chronic Related factors: Chemotherapy, toxicity, cerebellar localization

Constipation Related factors: Decreased activity, dietary changes, medications (e.g., narcotic analgesics, chemotherapy), radiation therapy, painful defecation

Coping, ineffective Related factors: Personal vulnerability in a maturational crisis (e.g., terminal illness in childhood) or in a situational crisis (e.g., terminal illness)

Decisional conflict Related factors: Lack of relevant information, multiple or divergent sources of information, multiple treatment choices, lack of support system

Diarrhea Related factors: Dietary changes, impaction, radiation, chemotherapy (specify), antibiotics, stress

Disuse syndrome, risk for Risk factors: Severe *Pain*, altered level of consciousness

Falls, risk for Risk factors: Weakness, disturbed sensory perception, *Confusion*

Family processes, interrupted Related factors: Change in family roles, complex therapies, hospitalization or change in environment, illness or disability of family member, separation of family members, fears associated with the diagnosis, financial effects of illness

Fatigue Related factors: *Pain*, disease process, overwhelming psychologic or emotional demands, malnutrition, hypoxia/*Impaired gas exchange*

Fear Related factors: Real or imagined threat to own well-being, environmental stressors or hospitalization, impending death, fear of pain

Fluid volume, deficient Related factors: Inadequate fluid intake (e.g., altered ability to obtain fluids, weakness, *Fatigue*, anorexia, *Nausea*, depression), abnormal fluid loss (e.g., vomiting, diarrhea)

Grieving, complicated Related factors: Terminal illness, impending loss of body function, effects of cancer on lifestyle, withdrawal from or of others

Health behavior, risk-prone Related factors: Necessity for major lifestyle changes, incomplete grieving

Home maintenance, impaired Related factors: Lack of support system, inadequate finances, *Deficient knowledge* regarding community and other supports, *Acute/chronic confusion*, disturbed sensory perception

Hopelessness Related factors: Failing or deteriorating physical condition, long-term stress, lost spiritual belief, overwhelming functional losses, impending death

Infection, risk for Risk factors: Immunosuppression, neutropenia, pharmaceutical agents

Insomnia/sleep deprivation Related factors: *Anxiety*, emotional state, medical treatment regimen, *Pain*, pruritus

Mobility: physical, impaired Related factors: Decreased strength and endurance, musculoskeletal impairment, neuromuscular impairment, *Pain*, sedation, *Fatigue*, edema, enforced immobility (e.g., for chemotherapy infusions)

Nausea Related factors: Side effects of chemotherapy and other medications, stress, *Pain*, difficulty swallowing

Nutrition, imbalanced: less than body requirements Related factors: Difficulty in swallowing, *Nausea*, vomiting, loss of appetite, changes in taste, isolation, *Anxiety*, stress, *Impaired oral mucous membrane*, *Fatigue*, increased metabolic demands of the tumor

Oral mucous membrane, impaired Related factors: Chemotherapy, radiation to head and neck, *Imbalanced nutrition: less than body requirements*, inadequate hydration, immunosuppression

Pain, acute/chronic Related factors: Ongoing tissue destruction (i.e., localizations), infection, stomatitis, chemotherapy

Powerlessness Related factor: Terminal illness, feelings of inability to change the progression of events, uncertainty about prognosis and treatments

Role performance, ineffective Related factors: *Chronic pain*, treatment side effects

Self-care deficit: (specify) Related factors: Developmental disability, maturational age, *Pain*, *Activity intolerance*, *Fatigue*, depression

Sexual dysfunction/sexuality pattern, ineffective Related factors: *Pain*, change in body image, *Fear* (patient or partner), *Fatigue* from treatments or disease, lack of privacy

Skin integrity, impaired Related factors: Radiation, chemotherapy, allergic reactions to medications, loss of muscle and subcutaneous tissue secondary to poor nutritional status, immunologic deficit, *Impaired physical mobility* secondary to weakness

Social interaction, impaired Related factors: Fear of rejection, actual rejection by others, *Self-esteem, low (chronic, situational)*, therapeutic isolation (e.g., secondary to radiation or protective isolation)

Spiritual distress Related factors: Test of spiritual beliefs, challenged belief and value system, unresolved conflicts, *Complicated grieving*

Swallowing, impaired Related factors: Irritated oropharyngeal cavity, mechanical obstruction, head and neck radiation

Cardiac Disorders

Potential Complications (Collaborative Problems)

PC of angina/coronary insufficiency: Myocardial infarction

PC of congestive heart failure: Cardiogenic shock, deep-vein thrombosis, hepatic failure, acute pulmonary edema, renal failure

PC of digitalis administration: Toxicity

PC of dysrhythmias: Decreased cardiac output, causing decreased myocardial perfusion, causing heart failure; severe atrioventricular conduction blocks; thromboemboli formation; ventricular fibrillation

PC of myocardial infarction (chest pain, arrhythmias): Cardiogenic shock, dysrhythmia, thromboembolism, pulmonary edema, pulmonary embolism, pericarditis

PC of pericarditis/endocarditis: Congestive heart failure, emboli (e.g., pulmonary, cerebral, renal, spleen, coronary), cardiac tamponade, valvular stenosis

Nursing Diagnoses

Angina/Coronary Insufficiency

Activity intolerance Related factors: *Anxiety*, arrhythmias, *Pain*, lack of exercise or conditioning due to fear of pain

Anxiety Related factors: Chest pain, threat to self-concept, change in role functioning

Breathing pattern, ineffective Related factors: *Acute Pain, Anxiety*

Denial, ineffective Related factors: *Fear* of effects of diagnosis on lifestyle, *Fear* of heart attack

Falls, risk for Risk factors: Dizziness and hypotension secondary to vasodilator, calcium channel blockers, and opiate analgesic medications

Family processes, interrupted Related factors: Change in family roles, hospitalization, inability of family member to perform usual roles

Fear Related factors: Environmental stressors or hospitalization, unknown future

Insomnia Related factors: *Pain* and discomfort, *Anxiety*

Nausea Related factors: Side effects of calcium channel blockers and opiate analgesics, *Pain*

Noncompliance Related factors: Denial of illness, negative side effects of medications, negative perception of treatment regimen, perceived benefits of continued illness, dysfunctional patient or provider relationship

Pain Related factors: Myocardial ischemia, headache secondary to vasodilators

Role performance, ineffective Related factors: Chronic illness, treatment side effects, *Fear* of heart attack

Sexual dysfunction/sexuality patterns, ineffective Related factors: *Pain*, Fear of pain, *Low self-esteem (chronic, situational)*

Myocardial Infarction (Chest Pain, Arrhythmias)

Activity intolerance Related factors: *Acute Pain*, weakness/*Fatigue* because of insufficient oxygen secondary to cardiac ischemia

Anxiety Related factors: Severe *Pain*, threat to or change in health status, anticipated change in role functioning, unknown outcome, unfamiliar environment

Cardiac output, decreased Related factors: Dysfunctional electrical conduction, increased ventricular workload, ventricular ischemia, ventricular damage

Constipation Related factors: Decreased peristalsis secondary to medications (e.g., opiate analgesics), decreased activity, NPO or soft diet

Coping, ineffective Related factors: Personal vulnerability to situational crisis (e.g., new diagnosis of illness, declining health)

Death anxiety Related factors: *Fear* of dying

Denial, ineffective Related factors: *Fear* of consequences of disease on roles, lifestyle, and so forth

Family processes, interrupted Related factors: Inability of patient to assume family roles, hospitalization, separation of family members

Fear Related factors: *Pain*, unknown future, real or imagined threat to own well-being, strange (e.g., hospital) environment, *Fear* of death

Fluid volume excess Related factor: Decreased kidney perfusion secondary to heart failure

Gas exchange, impaired Related factor: Decreased cardiac output, decreased pulmonary blood supply secondary to pulmonary hypertension or congestive heart failure

Grieving, complicated Related factors: Actual or perceived losses resulting from illness

Home maintenance, impaired Related factors: *Pain*, *Fear* of pain, *Activity intolerance*, *Fear* of another heart attack

Nausea Related factors: Severe chest pain, side effect of medications

Pain Related factor: Myocardial ischemia

Powerlessness Related factors: Treatment regimen, hospital environment, anticipated lifestyle changes

Role performance, ineffective Related factors: Situational crisis, treatment side effects, *Pain*, *Fear* of pain, *Activity intolerance*

Self-care deficit: (specify) Related factors: *Pain*, *Activity intolerance*

Self-esteem, low (chronic, situational) Related factors: Treatment side effects, perceived or actual role changes

Sexual dysfunction/sexuality pattern, ineffective Related factors: *Fear* of pain, *Activity intolerance*, *Low self-esteem (chronic, situational)*, disease-related role changes

Sleep deprivation/Insomnia Related factors: Strange (e.g., hospital) environment, *Pain*, treatments

Congestive Heart Failure

Activity intolerance Related factors: Weakness due to prolonged bed rest or sedentary lifestyle, *Fatigue*, insufficient oxygenation secondary to *Decreased cardiac output*

Anxiety Related factors: Shortness of breath, dyspnea, progressive nature of disease

Anxiety, death Related factor: Possibility of dying

Family processes, interrupted Related factors: Hospitalization or change in environment, illness or disability of family member

Fatigue Related factors: Inadequate oxygenation secondary to decreased cardiac output, difficulty sleeping

Fear See *Anxiety*

Fluid volume excess Related factors: *Decreased cardiac output*; reduced glomerular filtration; increased antidiuretic hormone (ADH) production, causing sodium or water retention

Gas exchange, impaired Related factors: Alveolar capillary membrane changes, fluid in alveoli, decreased pulmonary blood supply

Health maintenance, ineffective Related factors: *Deficient knowledge* (cardiac function or disease process, diet, activity exercise, medications, signs and symptoms of complications, and self-care), *Impaired memory*, *Fatigue*

Home maintenance, impaired Related factors: *Fatigue*, shortness of breath, clouded sensorium secondary to insufficient oxygen

Hopelessness Related factors: Failing or deteriorating physical condition, lack of energy for coping

Nutrition, imbalanced: less than body requirements Related factors: *Nausea*, anorexia secondary to venous congestion of gastrointestinal tract, *Fatigue*

Powerlessness Related factors: Chronic illness, progressive nature of illness

Self-care deficit: (specify) Related factors: *Fatigue*, dyspnea

Skin integrity, impaired Related factors: *Ineffective peripheral tissue perfusion*, *Impaired physical mobility*, edema

Sleep deprivation/Insomnia Related factors: *Anxiety*, nocturia, inability to assume preferred sleep position because of nocturnal dyspnea

Pericarditis/Endocarditis

Activity intolerance Related factors: Inadequate oxygenation secondary to restriction of cardiac filling, causing reduced cardiac output

Anxiety Related factors: *Pain*, change in health status, threat of death

Breathing pattern, ineffective Related factors: *Acute Pain* secondary to inflammation

Cardiac output, decreased Related factors: Restriction of cardiac filling or ventricular contractility, effusion, dysrhythmias, increased ventricular workload

Fear See *Anxiety*

Pain Related factors: Effusion, tissue inflammation

Chest Trauma

Includes but is not limited to hemothorax and pneumothorax

Potential Complications (Collaborative Problems)

PC of chest trauma: Flail chest, hemothorax, pneumothorax, tension pneumo thorax, and mediastinal shift

Nursing Diagnoses

Breathing pattern, ineffective Related factors: *Acute pain*, *Anxiety*

Dysfunctional ventilatory weaning response (DVWR) Related factors: *Anxiety*, history of ventilator dependence >1 week, inappropriate pacing of diminished ventilatory support, uncontrolled episodic energy demands or problems

Fear Related factors: Real or imagined threat to own well-being, sudden injury, unknown extent of or prognosis for injury

Mobility: physical, impaired Related factors: *Pain*/discomfort, presence of chest tubes, IV lines

Pain Related factor: Chest injury

Self-care deficit: (specify) Related factors: *Pain*/discomfort, presence of tubes and lines

Sleep deprivation/Insomnia Related factors: *Pain* and discomfort, medical regimen

Spontaneous ventilation, impaired Related factors: Injury to thoracic cage or lung tissue, flail chest

Dying Patient

Nursing Diagnoses

Activity intolerance Related factors: *Chronic pain*, weakness, *Fatigue* secondary to disease process, medications, or inadequate intake of calories

Airway clearance, ineffective Related factors: Decreased energy, *Fatigue*, *Pain*, tracheobronchial obstruction

Anxiety, death Related factors: Imminence of death, lack of resolution

Bowel incontinence Related factors: Loss of sphincter control, decreased awareness of need to defecate

Caregiver role strain Related factors: Illness severity of the care receiver, inability to change outcome for the patient, inadequate physical environment for providing care, lack of respite and recreation for caregiver, complexity and amount of caregiving tasks

Communication: verbal, impaired Related factors: Inability to speak, inability to speak clearly

Coping: family, compromised Related factor: Family member's temporary preoccupation with own emotional conflicts and personal suffering

Coping, ineffective Related factor: Personal vulnerability to situational crisis (terminal illness)

Denial, ineffective Related factors: *Fear* of dying, *Fear* of effect on others

Family processes, interrupted Related factors: Change in family roles, hospitalization or change in environment, illness or disability of family member, separation of family members

Fatigue Related factors: Disease process, overwhelming psychologic or emotional demands, decreased intake of nutrients for energy

Fear Related factors: *Powerlessness*, environmental stressors or hospitalization, *Fear* of pain, *Fear* of the unknown, *Fear* of dying

Grieving, complicated Related factors: *Ineffective denial*, unresolved family issues, loss of faith (e.g., *Spiritual distress*), lack of support system, impending death of self

Hopelessness Related factors: Failing or deteriorating physical condition, lack of social or family support, loss of spiritual belief

Human dignity, risk for compromised Risk factors: Loss of control of bodily functions

Incontinence, urinary, functional Related factors: Disorientation, *Impaired mobility*, neurologic dysfunction

Insomnia Related factors: *Pain* and discomfort, *Anxiety*

Nutrition, imbalanced: less than body requirements Related factors: *Impaired swallowing*, loss of appetite, *Nausea* and vomiting

Oral mucous membrane, impaired Related factors: Chemotherapy, inability to perform oral hygiene or obtain fluids, radiation to head and neck

Pain Related factors: Specific to patient's cause of death

Powerlessness Related factors: Inability to change outcome of terminal illness, loss of independence, overwhelming treatment regimen

Risk-prone health behavior Related factor: Incomplete grieving over loss of physical or role function

Self-care deficit: (specify) Related factors: *Pain* and discomfort, *Activity intolerance*, decreased strength and endurance

Skin integrity, impaired Related factors: *Impaired physical mobility*, *Urinary/Bowel incontinence*, radiation therapy, poor nutritional status, dehydration

Social isolation Related factors: Medical condition, alteration in physical appearance

Sorrow, chronic Related factors: See *Grieving, anticipatory*

Spiritual distress Related factors: Challenged belief and value system, separation from religious and cultural ties, test of spiritual beliefs

Endocrine Disorders

Include but are not limited to Cushing disease, diabetes mellitus, hyperthyroidism, hypothyroidism, hypoglycemia, and pancreatic tumors

Potential Complications (Collaborative Problems)

PC of Cushing disease: Hypertension, congestive heart failure, potassium and sodium imbalance, psychosis, hyperglycemia, osteoporosis

PC of diabetes mellitus: Ketoacidosis, coma, hypoglycemia, infections, coronary artery disease, peripheral vascular disease, retinopathy, neuropathy, nephropathy

PC of hyperthyroidism: Thyroid storm, heart disease, exophthalmos

PC of hypothyroidism: Arteriosclerotic heart disease, myxedema coma, psychosis

PC of repeated or prolonged hypoglycemia: Neuropathy, retinal hemorrhage, CVAs, personality changes, intellectual damage

Nursing Diagnoses

Cushing Disease

Activity intolerance Related factors: Muscle weakness secondary to protein wasting, hyperglycemia, and potassium depletion; congestive heart failure

Blood glucose, risk for unstable Risk factors: Diabetes that is not well controlled, comorbid acute illness (e.g., influenza)

Body image, disturbed Related factors: Change in appearance (e.g., moon face, virilism in women, acne) secondary to disease process and medication therapy, changes in social involvement

Confusion Related factors: Increased levels of glucocorticoids and ACTH

Infection, risk for Risk factors: Skin and capillary fragility, negative nitrogen balance, compromised immune response, hyperglycemia, lowered resistance to stress, poor wound healing

Injury, risk for Risk factors: Fractures secondary to osteoporosis, hypertension secondary to sodium and water retention

Nutrition, imbalanced: less than body requirements Related factors: Disturbance of carbohydrate metabolism, increased resistance to insulin

Skin integrity, impaired Related factors: Decreased connective tissue, edema secondary to sodium and water retention, thinning and dryness of the skin

Self-care deficit: (specify) Related factors: *Fatigue*, generalized weakness, demineralization of bones

Self-health management, ineffective Related factors: *Deficient knowledge* (disease process, therapeutic diet, diagnostic tests, surgical treatment, self-administration of steroids, indications of need to call physician)

Sexuality pattern, ineffective Related factors: Impotence, cessation of menses, loss of libido secondary to excessive adrenocorticotropic hormone (ACTH) production

Diabetes Mellitus/Hypoglycemia

Coping: family, compromised/disabled Related factors: Complex self-care regimen, chronic disease, inability to predict future, inadequate or incomplete information/understanding, changes required in family functioning

Fear Related factors: Effects on lifestyle, need for self-injections, diabetes complications

Infection, risk for Risk factors: Decreased leukocyte function, delayed healing, impaired circulation

Injury, risk for Risk factors: Impaired vision, hypoglycemia, impaired tactile sensation

Neurovascular dysfunction: peripheral, risk for Related factors: Glucose, insulin, or electrolyte imbalance, peripheral neurovascular changes

Noncompliance Related factors: Complexity of self-care and medical regimen, chronicity of disease, denial

Nutrition, imbalanced: less than body requirements Related factors: Inability to utilize glucose, resulting in weight loss, muscle weakness, and thirst

Powerlessness Related factors: Perceived inability to prevent complications such as blindness and amputations

Self-health management, ineffective Related factors: *Deficient knowledge* (disease process, diet and exercise balance, self-monitoring and self- medication, foot care, signs and symptoms of complications, community resources)

Sexual dysfunction/sexuality pattern, ineffective Related factors: Impotence secondary to peripheral neuropathy, psychologic conflicts (male), psychologic stressors, frequent genitourinary problems (female)

Hyperthyroidism

Anxiety Related factor: CNS irritability

Comfort, impaired (heat intolerance) (non-NANDA International) Related factor: Increased metabolic rate

Diarrhea Related factor: Increased peristalsis secondary to increased metabolic rate

Fatigue Related factors: Increased energy requirements, CNS irritability

Hyperthermia, risk for: Risk factor: Inability to compensate for excess thyroid activity

Nutrition, imbalanced: less than body requirements Related factors: Hypermetabolic rate, constant activity, inability to ingest enough calories, vomiting, *Diarrhea*

Tissue integrity, impaired [corneal] Related factors: Periorbital edema, reduced ability to blink, eye dryness, corneal abrasions or ulcerations

Hypothyroidism

Activity intolerance Related factors: Apathy, weakness, inadequate oxygen and decreased energy secondary to decreased metabolic rate

Comfort, impaired (cold intolerance) Related factor: Slowed metabolic rate

Constipation Related factors: Decreased activity and decreased peristalsis secondary to decreased metabolic rate

Fatigue Related factors: See *Activity intolerance*

Hypothermia Related factor: Decreased metabolic rate

Injury, risk for Risk factors: Hypersensitivity to sedatives, narcotics, and anesthetics secondary to decreased metabolic rate

Mobility: physical, impaired Related factors: *Fatigue*, weakness, mucin deposits in joints and interstitial spaces, changes in reflexes and coordination

Nutrition, imbalanced: more than body requirements Related factor: Intake greater than body needs secondary to decreased metabolic rate

Skin integrity, impaired Related factors: Dryness and edema secondary to movement of fluid into interstitial spaces

Social interaction, impaired Related factors: Weakness, apathy, changes in appearance, depression

Gastrointestinal Disorders

Potential Complications (Collaborative Problems)

PC of GI inflammatory diseases (e.g., diverticulitis): GI bleeding, anal fissure, fluid and electrolyte imbalances, anemia, intestinal obstruction, fistula, abscess, perforation

PC of GI bleeding: Hypovolemic shock, anemia

PC of peptic ulcers: Perforation, pyloric obstruction, hemorrhage

Nursing Diagnoses

GI Inflammation (e.g., Diverticulitis, Inflammatory Bowel Disease)

Constipation Related factors: Inadequate ingestion of dietary fiber, narrowing of intestinal lumen secondary to scar tissue

Coping, ineffective Related factors: Chronic condition, no definitive treatment, *Chronic pain*, *Insomnia*, ostomy

Diarrhea Related factors: Inflammation of GI tract, malabsorption

Fluid volume, deficient Related factors: *Diarrhea*, vomiting, decreased fluid intake

Nutrition, imbalanced: less than body requirements Related factors: *Diarrhea*, *nausea* and abdominal cramping associated with eating, ulcers of the mucous membrane, decreased absorption of nutrients

Pain, chronic Related factors: Inflammation or obstruction of GI tract, hyperperistalsis

GI Bleeding

Activity intolerance Related factor: Weakness/*Fatigue* secondary to anemia or blood loss

Coping, ineffective Related factor: Personal vulnerability to situational crisis (e.g., acute illness)

Fatigue Related factors: Disease process, low hemoglobin level

Fear Related factor: Real or imagined threat to own well-being

Fluid volume, deficient Related factor: Abnormal fluid loss (e.g., emesis, diarrhea)

Nutrition, imbalanced: less than body requirements Related factors: Loss of appetite, *Nausea* and vomiting

Ulcers

Constipation Related factors: Effects of antacids and anticholinergics

Diarrhea Related factor: Effects of magnesium-containing antacids

Pain, acute/chronic Related factors: Lesions secondary to increased gastric secretions

Abdominal Pain/Irritable Bowel Syndrome

Anxiety Related factors: Necessity for frequent bowel movements, *Diarrhea*, *Pain*, chronicity of the condition

Constipation Related factors: Decreased activity, decreased fluid intake, dietary changes, medications (specify)

Diarrhea Related factors: Dietary changes, increased intestinal motility, medications (specify), alcohol intake, smoking, *Fatigue*, cold drinks

Fluid volume, deficient Related factors: Abnormal fluid loss (specify), inadequate fluid intake, abnormal blood loss (specify), excessive continuous consumption of alcohol

Nutrition, imbalanced: less than body requirements Related factors: Loss of appetite, *Nausea*, vomiting, food intolerance, fear of precipitating *Diarrhea*

Pain, acute Related factors: Injury, noxious stimulus (e.g., fruits, alcohol)

Pain, chronic Related factors: Specific to patient

Sleep deprivation/Insomnia Related factors: *Pain* and discomfort, *Anxiety*, *Diarrhea*

Immobilized Patient

Potential Complications (Collaborative Problems)

PC of immobility: Contractures; joint ankylosis; osteoporosis; thrombophlebitis, embolus; hypostatic pneumonia; renal calculi

Nursing Diagnoses

Activity intolerance Related factors: Generalized weakness, *Fatigue*, compromised circulatory or respiratory system

Constipation Related factors: Decreased activity, decreased colon motility secondary to increased adrenaline production

Coping, ineffective Related factor: Personal vulnerability to a situational crisis (specify), inability to perform usual role functions, dependence on others, *Low self-esteem* (*chronic*, *situational*)

Disuse syndrome, risk for Risk factors: Paralysis, mechanical immobilization, prescribed immobility, severe *Pain*, altered level of consciousness

Diversional activity, deficient Related factor: Prolonged bed rest

Dysreflexia, autonomic Related factor: Spinal cord injury T7 or above

Mobility: physical, impaired Related factors: Decreased strength and endurance; *Activity intolerance; Pain*; neuromuscular, musculoskeletal, and cognitive impairment; depression, severe *Anxiety*

Self-care deficit: (specify) Related factors: *Pain*, *Activity intolerance*, decreased strength and endurance, prescribed immobility

Skin integrity, impaired Related factors: *Impaired physical mobility*, atrophy of dermis and subcutaneous tissues, loss of skin turgor, impaired circulation

Insomnia Related factors: Lack of physical activity, *Pain* and discomfort, inability to change positions independently or assume usual sleep position

Urinary incontinence, functional Related factor: Neurologic impairment

Urinary retention Related factors: Decreased muscle tone of bladder, inability to relax the perineal muscles, embarrassment of using bedpan, lack of privacy, unnatural position for urination

Liver Disease

Includes but is not limited to cirrhosis and hepatitis

Potential Complications (Collaborative Problems)

PC of liver disease: Anemia; hepatic encephalopathy; glomerulonephritis, renal failure; esophageal varices; GI bleeding, hemorrhage; hypokalemia; negative nitrogen balance; disseminated intravascular coagulation (DIC)

Nursing Diagnoses

Activity intolerance Related factors: Weakness, extreme *Fatigue* secondary to bed rest, impaired respiratory function secondary to ascites

Anxiety Related factors: Unknown prognosis of the disease, uncertainty of the future, alcohol withdrawal

Body image, disturbed Related factors: Change in appearance (e.g., jaundice, ascites), chronic illness

Breathing patterns, ineffective Related factor: Pressure on diaphragm secondary to ascites

Confusion, acute Related factors: Alcohol abuse, inability of liver to detoxify certain substances, increased serum ammonia level

Coping, ineffective Related factor: Personal vulnerability to situational crisis (e.g., new diagnosis of illness, declining health)

Diarrhea Related factors: Dietary changes, inability to metabolize fats, stress

Family processes, interrupted Related factors: Change in family roles, illness or disability of family member

Fatigue Related factors: Disease process, malnutrition

Fear Related factor: Real or imagined threat to own well-being

Fluid volume excess Risk factors: Malnutrition, portal hypertension, sodium retention

Infection, risk for Risk factors: Hypoproteinemia, enlarged spleen, leukopenia

Injury, risk for Risk factors: Continued intake of hepatotoxins (e.g., alcohol), decreased prothrombin and coagulation factors

Mobility: physical, impaired Related factor: Weakness secondary to prolonged bed rest

Nutrition, imbalanced: less than body requirements Related factors: Loss of appetite; *Nausea*; vomiting; bile stasis; decreased absorption and storage of fat-soluble vitamins; impaired fat, glucose, and protein metabolism; *Diarrhea*

Pain, acute/chronic Related factors: Ascites, liver enlargement

Self-care deficit: (specify) Related factors: *Pain*, *Fatigue*, *Activity intolerance*

Self-esteem, low (chronic, situational) Related factors: Chronic illness, situational crisis, *Disturbed body image*, inability to stop drinking alcohol

Self-health management, ineffective Related factors: *Deficient knowledge* (e.g., disease process, nutritional needs, symptoms of complications, effects of alcohol), lack of motivation to stop drinking

Skin integrity, impaired Related factors: Physical immobility; itching secondary to jaundice, edema, and ascites

Neurologic Disorders

Include but not limited to CVA (stroke), multiple sclerosis, amyotrophic lateral sclerosis, brain tumors, Guillain-Barré syndrome, myasthenia gravis, seizure disorders, Alzheimer disease, coma, head injury, cerebral thrombosis, and transient ischemic attack. Associated psychiatric diagnoses include CNS infections (e.g., tertiary neurosyphilis, viral encephalitis, Jakob-Creutzfeldt disease), brain trauma, Huntington chorea, Parkinson disease, and meningitis

Potential Complications (Collaborative Problems)

PC of cerebrovascular accident (stroke): Increased intracranial pressure, respiratory infection, brain stem failure, cardiac dysrhythmias

PC of brain tumor: Increased intracranial pressure, paralysis, hyperthermia, sensorimotor changes

PC of other neurologic disorders (e.g., multiple sclerosis): Pneumonia, respiratory failure, renal failure

Nursing Diagnoses

CVA (Stroke)

NOTE: Nursing diagnoses for CVA will vary depending upon the location and severity of the lesion. CVA can have mild to severe effects.

Activity intolerance Related factors: *Anxiety*, *Fatigue*, weakness, deconditioning secondary to immobility, neuromuscular deficits

Airway clearance, ineffective Related factors: Decreased energy, *Fatigue*, decreased cough and gag reflexes, muscle paralysis

Aspiration, risk for Risk factors: Reduced level of consciousness, *Impaired swallowing*, depressed cough and gag reflexes

Body image, disturbed Related factors: Chronic illness, diminished physical function, loss of control over body

Caregiver role strain Related factors: Illness severity of care receiver, duration of caregiving required, lack of respite and recreation for caregiver, complexity and number of caregiving tasks, elderly caregiver

Communication: verbal, impaired Related factors: Aphasia, dysarthria, inability to speak, inability to speak clearly

Confusion Related factors: Altered sensory reception, transmission, or integration, secondary to hypoxia and compression or displacement of brain tissue

Constipation Related factors: Decreased activity, medications (specify), weak abdominal muscles

Disuse syndrome, risk for Risk factors: Altered level of consciousness, paralysis

Falls, risk for Risk factors: *Impaired physical mobility*, disturbed sensory perception

Family processes, interrupted Related factors: Hospitalization or change in environment, separation of family members, illness or disability of family member, change in family roles

Fluid volume, deficient Related factors: Decreased access to, intake of, or absorption of fluids secondary to weakness, impaired motor functions (e.g., swallowing), impaired cognition and level of consciousness

Grieving, complicated Related factors: Actual loss (e.g., of function), chronic illness, inability to fulfill usual roles

Home maintenance, impaired Related factors: Home environment obstacles; inadequate support system; lack of familiarity with community resources; sensorimotor or cognitive deficits; caregiver's lack of knowledge of reality orientation, skin care, and so forth

Hopelessness Related factor: Failing or deteriorating physical condition

Memory, impaired Related factor: Residual effects of CVA

Mobility: physical, impaired Related factors: Neuromuscular impairment (e.g., weakness, paresthesia, flaccid paralysis, spastic paralysis)

secondary to damage of upper motor neurons, perceptual impairment, cognitive impairment

Nutrition, imbalanced: less than body requirements Related factors: Difficulty chewing, *Impaired swallowing*, inability to prepare food secondary to mobility deficits

Powerlessness Related factors: Treatment regimen, chronic disease

Relocation stress syndrome Related factors: Change in environment or location (e.g., transfer to long-term care facility), *Anxiety*, depression

Self-care deficit: (specify) Related factors: Neuromuscular impairment, decreased strength and endurance, *Activity intolerance*, decreased range of motion, weakness secondary to disease and immobility

Tissue Perfusion: cerebral, risk for ineffective Risk factors: Interrupter circulation to the brain

Skin integrity, impaired Related factors: Altered sensation, *Impaired mobility*, incontinence of stool or urine, poor nutritional status

Social interaction, impaired Related factors: *Impaired verbal communication*, *Impaired physical mobility*, embarrassment about disabilities

Swallowing, impaired Related factors: Muscle paralysis secondary to damaged upper motor neurons, impaired perception or level of consciousness

Unilateral neglect (specify side) Related factors: Disturbed sensory perception (visual) with perceptual loss of corresponding body segment

Urinary Incontinence, functional Related factors: Cognitive impairment, inability to reach toilet secondary to *Impaired physical mobility*

Other Neurologic Disorders

Activity intolerance Related factors: *Acute/Chronic pain*, weakness and *Fatigue*

Airway clearance, ineffective Related factor: Decreased energy and *Fatigue*, neuromuscular weakness

Anxiety Related factors: Change in health status, threat to or change in role functioning, change in interaction patterns, seriousness of condition, threat to self-concept, separation from support system

Aspiration, risk for Risk factors: *Impaired swallowing*, presence of tracheostomy or endotracheal tube, reduced level of consciousness, depressed cough and gag reflexes, tube feedings, hindered elevation of upper body

Breathing pattern, ineffective Related factors: Neuromuscular paralysis or weakness, decreased energy and *Fatigue*

Caregiver role strain Related factors: Complex, long-term needs of patient

Communication: verbal, impaired Related factors: Psychologic impairment, aphasia, inability to speak, inability to speak clearly, tracheostomy, muscle weakness

Confusion Related factors: Chronic organic disorder, pressure on brain tissue

Constipation Related factors: Decreased activity, inability to ingest adequate fiber

Coping, ineffective Related factor: Personal vulnerability to situational crisis (e.g., new diagnosis of illness, declining health, terminal illness)

Disuse syndrome, risk for Risk factors: Paralysis, altered level of consciousness

Diversional activity, deficient Related factors: Forced inactivity, long-term hospitalization

Family processes, interrupted Related factors: Change in family roles; change in family structure; cognitive and emotional changes of family member; hospitalization or change in environment; *Impaired verbal communication*, secondary to CNS changes

Fatigue Related factors: Disease process, immobility

Fear Related factor: Real threat to well-being (see *Anxiety*)

Fluid volume, deficient Related factors: Inadequate fluid intake, vomiting secondary to increased intracranial pressure

Grieving, complicated Related factors: Functional losses, role changes, uncertain prognosis, inability to change outcome of disease process

Home maintenance, impaired Related factors: *Activity intolerance*, effects of debilitating disease, home environment obstacles, inadequate support system, insufficient family organization or planning, psychologic impairment, lack of familiarity with community resources

Hopelessness Related factors: Failing or deteriorating physical condition, perception of having no way to improve situation

Injury (e.g., falls), risk for Risk factors: Sensory dysfunction (e.g., visual disturbances), cognitive, and psychomotor deficits secondary to compression or displacement of brain tissue, muscular weakness, unsteady gait

Mobility: physical, impaired Related factors: Neuromuscular impairment, decreased strength and endurance, *Pain*/discomfort, medically prescribed treatment, muscle rigidity, tremors

Nutrition, imbalanced: less than body requirements Related factors: Difficulty chewing secondary to cranial nerve involvement, *Impaired swallowing*, psychologic impairment, loss of appetite, *Fatigue*

Pain, acute/chronic Related factors: Neurologic injury, headache secondary to displaced brain tissue or increased intracranial pressure

Powerlessness See *Hopelessness*

Role performance, ineffective Related factors: Chronic illness, treatment side effects, brain changes

Self-care deficit: (specify) Related factors: *Pain* (e.g., headache, joint pain), decreased strength and endurance, sensorimotor impairments, cognitive deficits, *Fatigue*, paralysis

Sexual dysfunction/sexuality pattern, ineffective Related factors: Loss of perineal sensation, *Fatigue*, decreased libido, *Low self-esteem (chronic, situational)*, *Impaired physical mobility*

Skin integrity, impaired Related factors: Physical immobilization, impaired circulation

Social interaction, impaired Related factors: Communication barriers, *Low self-esteem (chronic, situational)*, extended hospitalization, *Impaired physical mobility*, embarrassment

Spontaneous ventilation, impaired Related factors: Impaired neuromuscular function, pressure on brain stem

Swallowing, impaired Related factors: Impairment of laryngeal or pharyngeal neuromuscular function; impaired sensory transmission, reception, or integration secondary to cerebellar lesions

Urinary incontinence, functional Related factors: Cognitive impairment; *Impaired physical mobility*; *Confusion acute/chronic*; disorientation; lack of sphincter control; spastic bladder

Urinary incontinence, total Related factor: Neurologic dysfunction (see *Functional urinary incontinence*)

Urinary retention Related factor: Sensory or motor impairment

Violence: self-directed or directed at others, risk for Risk factor: Organic mental disorder

Obesity

PC of obesity: Adult-onset diabetes, sleep apnea, delayed wound healing

Nursing Diagnoses

Activity intolerance Related factors: Sedentary lifestyle, exertional discomfort (e.g., shortness of breath)

Coping, ineffective Related factors: Personal vulnerability in situational crisis, use of food to cope with stressors

Family processes, interrupted Related factor: Effects of weight-loss therapy on family relationships

Health maintenance, ineffective Related factor: Lack of ability to make deliberate and thoughtful judgments about exercise, nutrition, and so forth

Mobility: physical, impaired Related factor: Decreased strength and endurance

Nutrition, imbalanced: more than body requirements Related factors: Eating disorder, lack of physical exercise, decreased metabolic requirements, lack of basic nutritional knowledge

Self-esteem, low (chronic, situational) Related factors: Responses of peers and family to obesity, negative view of self as compared to societal ideal, *Disturbed body image*

Sexuality pattern, ineffective Related factors: *Disturbed body image*, difficulty assuming sexual positions, rejection by partner

Social interaction, impaired Related factors: Self-concept disturbance, feelings of embarrassment, actual rejection by others because of appearance

Pancreatitis

Potential Complications (Collaborative Problems)

PC of pancreatitis: Coma, delirium tremens, hemorrhage, hypovolemic shock, hypocalcemia, hyperglycemia or hypoglycemia, psychosis, pleural effusion or respiratory failure

Nursing Diagnoses

Activity intolerance Related factors: *Acute Pain*, weakness/*Fatigue*, malnutrition

Anxiety Related factors: Change in health status, unfamiliar environment, *Fear* of recurrence of *Pain*

Blood glucose, risk for unstable Risk factor: Physiological effects of disease process on the pancreas

Breathing patterns, ineffective Related factors: Abdominal distention, ascites, *Pain*, pleural effusion, respiratory failure

Coping, ineffective Related factors: Alcohol abuse, severity of illness, chronicity of illness

Denial, ineffective Related factors: Failure to acknowledge alcohol abuse or dependency (see *Ineffective coping*)

Diarrhea Related factor: Excessive fats in stools secondary to insufficient pancreatic enzymes

Family processes, dysfunctional Related factors: Hospitalization or change in environment, change in family roles, alcohol abuse by family member or patient

Fear Related factor: Real or imagined threat to own well-being (see *Anxiety*)

Fluid volume, deficient Related factors: Abnormal fluid loss (e.g., nasogastric suctioning, vomiting, fever, diaphoresis), inadequate fluid intake (e.g., NPO status), fluid shifts (e.g., into retroperitoneal space), bleeding

Infection, risk for Related factors: Stasis and shifts of body fluids (e.g., retroperitoneal effusion), change in pH of fluids, immunosuppression, chronicity of disease, *Imbalanced nutritional, less than body requirements*

Noncompliance Related factors: Negative perception of treatment regimen, dysfunctional relationship between patient and provider, poor judgment secondary to alcohol abuse

Nutrition, imbalanced: less than body requirements Related factors: Loss of appetite, *Nausea*/vomiting, decreased ability to digest foods secondary to loss of insulin and digestive enzymes, chemical dependence, NPO status, nasogastric suctioning

Pain Related factors: Inflammation of pancreas and surrounding tissue, pancreatic duct obstruction, interruption of blood supply, pleural effusion, pancreatic enzymes in peritoneal tissues, nasogastric suctioning

Self-care deficit: (specify) Related factors: *Pain*/discomfort, *Activity intolerance*, *Confusion*

Self-health management, ineffective Related factors: *Deficient knowledge* (e.g., related to disease process, treatments, therapeutic diet, follow-up care, alcohol treatment programs, signs and symptoms of addiction), impaired judgment secondary to alcohol abuse

Renal Failure, Acute

Potential Complications (Collaborative Problems)

PC of renal failure: Electrolyte imbalance, fluid overload, metabolic acidosis, pericarditis, platelet dysfunction, secondary infections

Nursing Diagnoses

Activity intolerance Related factors: Increased energy requirements (e.g., fever, inflammation), decreased energy production, inadequate nutrition, anemia

Anxiety Related factors: Unknown prognosis, severity of illness

Cardiac output, decreased Related factor: Increased ventricular workload secondary to volume overload

Confusion Related factors: Decreased cerebral perfusion, accumulation of toxic wastes

Environmental interpretation syndrome, impaired See *Thought processes, disturbed*

Fear Related factors: Environmental stressors or hospitalization, *Powerlessness*, threat to own well-being, threat to child's well-being, severity of illness, multisystem effects

Fluid volume excess Related factors: Changes in renal vascular supply resulting in ischemia, tubular necrosis, decreased glomerular filtration rate

Infection, risk for Risk factors: Invasive procedures, disease process, lowered resistance, malnutrition

Nutrition, imbalanced: less than body requirements Related factors: Anorexia, *Nausea* and vomiting, dietary restrictions, change in taste, loss of smell, stomatitis, increased metabolic needs

Oral mucous membrane, impaired Related factors: Extracellular fluid depletion, stomatitis

Skin integrity, impaired Related factors: Poor skin turgor secondary to extracellular fluid, *Diarrhea*

Renal Failure, Chronic

Potential Complications (Collaborative Problems)

PC chronic renal failure: Anemia, congestive heart failure, fluid and electrolyte imbalance, fluid overload, hyperparathyroidism, infections, medication toxicity, metabolic acidosis, GI bleeding, pericarditis, cardiac tamponade, pleural effusion, pulmonary edema, uremia

Nursing Diagnoses

Activity intolerance Related factors: Weakness or *Fatigue* secondary to anemia, inadequate oxygenation secondary to cardiac or pulmonary complications

Body image, disturbed Related factors: *Delayed growth and development*, treatment side effects, chronic illness, surgery (e.g., insertion of hemodialysis blood access or peritoneal catheter, amputations), kidney transplant

Breathing pattern, ineffective Related factors: Anemia, volume overload, pressure of dialysate on diaphragm

Caregiver role strain Related factors: Complexity, amount, and duration of caregiving tasks; illness severity; situational stressors within the family; caregiver's health, knowledge, skills, experience, competing role commitments, and coping styles; isolation, lack of opportunity for respite and recreation

Comfort, impaired Related factors: Pruritus, fluid retention, vomiting, urate or calcium phosphate crystals on skin

Confusion, acute/chronic Related factors: Uremic encephalopathy, inadequate oxygenation secondary to cardiac or respiratory complications, anemia

Constipation Related factors: Restriction of fluids and fiber-rich foods, decreased activity, presence of phosphate-binding agents, medications

Coping: family, disabled Related factors: Chronically unresolved feelings, chronic illness and uncertain future of patient, complexity of home care (e.g., home dialysis)

Coping, ineffective Related factors: Personal vulnerability in situational crisis (e.g., new diagnosis of chronic illness, declining health, terminal illness), inability to concentrate, short attention span, and impaired reasoning secondary to central nervous system involvement

Diversional activity, deficient Related factor: Frequent or lengthy medical treatments, lack of energy and mobility to participate

Falls, risk for Risk factors: Impaired mobility, sensory impairment, hypotension, weakness

Fatigue Related factors: Altered renal function, inactivity, inadequate nutrition (see *Activity intolerance*)

Fear Related factors: Environmental stressors/hospitalization, *Powerlessness*, real or imagined threat to well-being

Fluid volume, deficient Related factors: Abnormal fluid loss (e.g., vomiting), abnormal blood loss secondary to hemodialysis procedure, inadequate fluid intake, compensatory diuresis of dilute urine secondary to decreased ability to concentrate urine, inability of tubules to reabsorb sodium, shifts between blood and dialysate

Fluid volume excess Related factors: Increased fluid intake secondary to excess sodium intake, sodium retention, hyperglycemia, *Noncompliance* with fluid restriction, shifts between blood and dialysate

Grieving, complicated Related factors: Chronic illness, loss, terminal illness, separation from significant others, loss of role function

Hopelessness Related factors: Failing or deteriorating physical condition, lack of social supports, long-term stress, inability to change progression of disease

Infection, risk for Risk factors: Immunosuppression, malnutrition, invasive therapy (e.g., dialysis)

Memory, impaired Related factor: Neurologic changes

Mobility: physical, impaired Related factors: Decreased strength and endurance secondary to anemia, cardiac or respiratory complications, musculoskeletal impairment (e.g., fractures secondary to osteoporosis), neuromuscular impairment

Noncompliance Related factors: Denial of illness, dysfunctional relationship between patient and provider, negative perception or consequence of treatment regimen, perceived benefits of continued illness

Nutrition, imbalanced: less than body requirements Related factors: Loss of appetite, *Nausea* or vomiting, dietary restrictions, stomatitis, loss of taste or smell secondary to cranial nerve changes

Powerlessness Related factors: Treatment regimen, inability to change progressive course of the disease

Self-care deficit: (specify) Related factors: Depression, *Pain* and discomfort, *Activity intolerance*, neuromuscular impairment, musculoskeletal impairment

Self-esteem, low (chronic, situational): See *Body image, disturbed*

Self-health management, ineffective Related factors: *Deficient knowledge* (e.g., related to disease, dietary restrictions, medications, signs and symptoms of complications, community resources), complexity of regimen, *Acute/chronic confusion* and *Impaired memory* secondary to disease process

Sexual dysfunction Related factors: *Low self-esteem* (*chronic, situational*), impotence, loss of libido, *Activity intolerance*

Skin integrity, impaired Related factors: Edema, dry skin, pruritus, impaired venous circulation secondary to surgical creation of hemodialysis blood access, impaired arterial circulation secondary to hypertension, hyperglycemia

Respiratory Disorders, Acute

Potential Complications (Collaborative Problems)

PC of pneumonia: Lung tissue necrosis

PC of pulmonary edema: Right-sided heart failure, anasarca, multiple-organ system failure

PC of pulmonary embolism: Pulmonary infarction with necrosis

Nursing Diagnoses

Pneumonia

Activity intolerance Related factor: Weakness and *Fatigue*

Anxiety Related factors: Threat to or change to health status, dyspnea

Fluid volume, deficient Related factors: Factors affecting fluid needs (e.g., fever)

Gas exchange, impaired Related factors: Decreased functional lung tissue secondary to consolidation, increased secretions

Nutrition, imbalanced: less than body requirements Related factor: Loss of appetite

Pain Related factors: Injury, difficulty breathing

Self-care deficit: (specify) Related factors: *Pain* and discomfort, *Activity intolerance*

Sleep deprivation/Insomnia Related factors: Dyspnea, *Pain*

Pulmonary Edema

Activity intolerance Related factors: Imbalance between oxygen supply and demand, weakness and *Fatigue*

Cardiac output, decreased Related factors: Increased ventricular workload

Fatigue: See *Activity intolerance*

Fear Related factors: Environmental stressors or hospitalization

Fluid volume excess Related factor: Decreased urine output secondary to pulmonary edema

Nutrition, imbalanced: less than body requirements Related factor: Loss of appetite

Self-care deficit: (specify) Related factors: *Pain* and discomfort, *Activity intolerance*

Sleep deprivation/Insomnia Related factor: Dyspnea

Pulmonary Embolism

Activity intolerance Related factors: *Acute pain*, imbalance between oxygen supply and demand

Fear Related factor: Real or imagined threat to own well-being

Gas exchange, impaired Related factor: Decreased pulmonary blood supply secondary to pulmonary embolus

Self-care deficit: (specify) Related factors: *Pain* and discomfort, *Activity intolerance*

Respiratory Disorders, Chronic

Includes but is not limited to asthma, COPD, and chronic restrictive pulmonary disease.

Potential Complications (Collaborative Problems)

PC of chronic pulmonary disease: Hypoxemia, right-sided heart failure, respiratory infection, spontaneous pneumothorax

Nursing Diagnoses

Activity intolerance Related factors: Dyspnea, weakness and *Fatigue*, inadequate oxygenation, *Anxiety*, *Insomnia*

Airway clearance, ineffective Related factors: Tracheobronchial obstruction, excessive and tenacious secretions, ineffective cough secondary to decreased energy and *Fatigue*

Anxiety Related factors: Dyspnea, *Fear* of suffocation, smoking cessation

Caregiver role strain Related factors: Illness severity of the care receiver, unpredictable course of the illness, amount and duration of caregiving required, inadequate physical environment for providing care, lack of respite and recreation for caregiver

Communication: verbal, impaired Related factor: Dyspnea

Coping, ineffective Related factors: Personal vulnerability in situational crisis (e.g., declining health), difficulty of smoking cessation

Family processes, interrupted Related factors: Change in family roles or structure, hospitalization or change in environment, chronic illness or disability of family member

Fear: See *Anxiety*

Fluid volume, deficient Related factors: Inadequate fluid intake secondary to difficulty in breathing, fluid loss secondary to fever and diaphoresis

Health maintenance, ineffective Related factors: Health beliefs, lack of social supports, difficulty with smoking cessation

Home maintenance, impaired Related factors: *Fatigue*, *Activity intolerance*, lack of social support

Insomnia Related factors: *Anxiety*, medical regimen (e.g., pulmonary treatments), inability to assume usual sleep position because of dyspnea, unfamiliar hospital environment, cough

Nutrition, imbalanced: less than body requirements Related factors: Loss of appetite, *Nausea* and vomiting, decreased energy, dyspnea

Powerlessness Related factors: Treatment regimen, chronic illness, lifestyle changes, loss of control (e.g., "too late" to improve lung function)

Self-care deficit: (specify) Related factors: Decreased strength and endurance, *Activity intolerance*

Sexual dysfunction/sexuality pattern, ineffective Related factors: Dyspnea, lack of energy, relationship changes

Ventilatory weaning response, dysfunctional (DVWR) Related factors: *Ineffective airway clearance*, patient perceived inefficacy about the ability to wean, *Fear* of suffocation, lack of motivation, *Anxiety*, inappropriate pacing of diminished ventilator support, history of ventilator dependence >1 week, history of multiple unsuccessful weaning attempts

Urologic Disorders

Include but are not limited to cystitis, glomerulonephritis, pyelonephritis, and urolithiasis

Potential Complications (Collaborative Problems)

PC of cystitis: Renal infection, ulceration of bladder

PC of urolithiasis: Pyelonephritis, renal insufficiency

PC of pyelonephritis: Chronic pyelonephritis, bacteremia, renal insufficiency

Nursing Diagnoses

Diarrhea Related factor: Stimulation of renal or intestinal reflexes

Fluid volume, deficient Related factors: Fever, vomiting, *Diarrhea* secondary to stimulation of renal or intestinal reflexes

Hyperthermia Related factors: Inflammatory process, increased metabolic rate

Incontinence, urinary, urge Related factors: Bladder irritation, dysuria, pyuria, frequency

Nutrition, imbalanced: less than body requirements Related factors: Anorexia secondary to fever, *Nausea*, vomiting, and *Pain*

Pain Related factors: Inflammation of bladder or renal tissues; headache; muscular pain; abdominal pain; distention, trauma, and smooth-muscle spasms; and edema in renal tissue (in urolithiasis)

Vascular Disease

Includes but is not limited to deep-vein thrombosis, hypertension, stasis ulcers, varicosities, peripheral vascular disease, and thrombophlebitis

Potential Complications (Collaborative Problems)

PC of varicose veins: Vascular rupture, hemorrhage, venous stasis ulcers, cellulitis

PC of peripheral arterial disease: Arterial thrombosis, CVA, hypertension, ischemic ulcers, cellulitis

PC of deep-vein thrombosis: Chronic leg edema, stasis ulcers, pulmonary embolism

Nursing Diagnoses

Activity intolerance Related factors: *Pain*, claudication

Body image, disturbed Related factors: Chronic illness, appearance of legs

Injury, risk for Risk factors: Sensory dysfunction, *Impaired physical mobility*

Pain Related factors: Tissue ischemia secondary to decreased peripheral circulation, engorgement or distention of veins

Role performance, ineffective Related factor: *Chronic Pain*

Self-esteem, low (chronic, situational) Related factor: Chronic illness (see *Disturbed body image*)

Skin integrity, impaired Related factors: Draining wound, tissue ischemia secondary to impaired circulation, physical immobilization, ankle or leg edema, decreased sensation secondary to chronic atherosclerosis

Tissue perfusion: peripheral, ineffective Related factors: Impaired venous circulation, impaired arterial circulation

SURGICAL CONDITIONS

Abdominal surgery
Breast surgery
Chest surgery
Craniotomy
Ear surgery

Eye surgery
Musculoskeletal surgery
Neck surgery
Rectal surgery
Skin graft
Spinal surgery
Urologic surgery
Vascular surgery

Abdominal Surgery

Includes but is not limited to appendectomy, cholecystectomy, colectomy, colon resection, colostomy, gastrectomy, gastric resection, gastroenterostomy, abdominal hysterectomy with or without salpingo-oophorectomy, ileostomy, laparotomy, lysis of adhesions, Marshall-Marchetti-Krantz operation, ovarian cystectomy, salpingotomy, small bowel resection, splenectomy, vagotomy, and hiatal hernia repair

Potential Complications (Collaborative Problems)

PC of general anesthesia: Stasis pneumonia, cardiac changes

PC of surgery: Dehiscence, evisceration, fistula formation, hemorrhage, paralytic ileus, incision infection, peritonitis, sepsis, pulmonary embolism, renal failure, surgical trauma (e.g., to ureter, bladder, or rectum), thrombophlebitis, urinary retention

Nursing Diagnoses

Airway clearance, ineffective See *Breathing pattern, ineffective*

Anxiety Related factors: Surgical procedure, preoperative procedures (e.g., IV insertion, Foley catheter, fluid restrictions), postoperative procedures (e.g., coughing and deep breathing, NPO status)

Aspiration, risk for Risk factors: Decreased motility and depressed cough and gag reflexes secondary to anesthesia or analgesics, presence of endotracheal tube, incomplete lower esophageal sphincter, GI tubes, increased intragastric pressure, increased gastric residual, delayed gastric emptying, hindered elevation of upper body

Body image, disturbed Related factors: Surgery (e.g., ostomy), situational crisis, treatment side effects, cultural or spiritual factors

Breathing pattern, ineffective Related factors: *Pain*, immobility, postanesthesia state

Caregiver role strain Related factors: Illness severity of care receiver, discharge of family member with significant home care needs, past history of poor relationship between caregiver and care receiver

Constipation Related factors: Decreased activity, decreased fluid and fiber intake, lack of privacy, change in daily routine, decreased peristalsis secondary to anesthetic, narcotic analgesics

Delayed surgical recovery Related factors: Infection, ileus, poor preoperative health, chronic illnesses, poor nutritional status

Fear Related factors: Environmental stressors or hospitalization, real or imagined threat to own well-being, unpredictable outcome of surgical procedure, general anesthesia, surgical outcome, *Pain*

Fluid volume, deficient Related factors: Abnormal blood loss, abnormal fluid loss (e.g., vomiting), failure of regulatory mechanisms

Infection, risk for Risk factors: Stasis of body fluids, altered peristalsis, suppressed inflammatory response, invasive procedures and lines, surgical incision, urinary catheter

Nutrition, imbalanced: less than body requirements Related factors: Loss of appetite, *Nausea* or vomiting, diet restrictions, increased protein and vitamin requirements for healing

Oral mucous membrane, impaired Related factors: Mouth breathing and NPO status secondary to nasogastric tube

Pain Related factors: Incision, abdominal distention, immobility

Perfusion: gastrointestinal, risk for ineffective Risk factors: Possible interruption of arterial flow, exchange problems, hypervolemia, hypovolemia

Perioperative positioning injury, risk for Risk factors: Advanced age, disorientation, edema, emaciation, muscle weakness, obesity, sensory or perceptual disturbances due to anesthesia

Sexual dysfunction or Ineffective sexuality pattern Related factors: *Pain*, health-related transitions, *Disturbed body image*, altered body function or structure, reaction of partner (e.g., to ostomy or hysterectomy), physiologic impotence or inadequate vaginal lubrication secondary to the surgery

Skin integrity, impaired Related factors: Mechanical factors, *Impaired physical mobility* secondary to pain and invasive lines, excretions and secretions, poor nutritional state, altered sensation

Social isolation Related factors: Embarrassment about odors, appearance, or appliance (e.g., ostomy pouch); reaction of others to appearance and odors

Breast Surgery

Includes but is not limited to breast augmentation, mastectomy, reconstruction, lumpectomy, and biopsy

Potential Complications (Collaborative Problems)

PC of breast surgery: Cellulitis, lymphedema, hematoma, seroma

Nursing Diagnoses

Anxiety Related factors: Threat to self-concept, threat to or change in health status, threat to or change in interaction patterns with significant others, situational or maturational crisis

Body image, disturbed Related factors: Surgery, treatment side effects, cultural or spiritual factors pertaining to changes in breast and sexuality

Coping, ineffective Related factors: Changes in appearance, concern over others' reaction, loss of function, diagnosis of cancer

Family processes, interrupted Related factors: Complex therapies (e.g., radiation, chemotherapy), hospitalization or change in environment, reactions of significant others to disfigurement

Fear Related factors: Disease process or prognosis (e.g., cancer), *Powerlessness*

Grieving, complicated Related factors: Loss of body part or function, change in appearance

Mobility: physical, impaired Related factors: Decreased range of motion of shoulder or arm secondary to lymphedema, nerve or muscle damage, or *Pain*

Pain Related factors: Surgical procedure, paresthesia

Self-care deficit: dressing/grooming Related factors: *Pain* and discomfort, neuromuscular impairment

Sexuality pattern, ineffective Related factors: *Pain*, altered body function or structure, illness, medical treatment, *Disturbed body image*, *Low self-esteem* (*chronic*, *situational*), reaction of significant other

Chest Surgery

Includes but is not limited to biopsy, cardiopulmonary bypass, coronary artery bypass, lobectomy, and thoracotomy

Potential Complications (Collaborative Problems)

PC of coronary artery bypass graft: Cardiovascular insufficiency, respiratory insufficiency, renal insufficiency

PC of thoracotomy: Atelectasis, cardiac dysrhythmias, hemorrhage, pneumonia, pneumothorax, hemothorax, mediastinal shift, pulmonary edema, pulmonary embolus, subcutaneous emphysema, thrombophlebitis

PC of chest surgery: Myocardial infarction

Nursing Diagnoses

Activity intolerance Related factors: Imbalance between oxygen supply and demand, *acute Pain*, weakness and *Fatigue*, narcotic analgesics, loss of alveolar ventilation

Breathing pattern, ineffective Related factors: Ineffective cough secondary to decreased energy and *Fatigue*, *acute Pain*, increased tracheobronchial secretions

Cardiac output, decreased Related factors: Dysfunctional electrical conduction, ventricular ischemia, ventricular damage, diminished circulating volume, increased systemic vascular resistance

Communication, impaired verbal Related factor: Intubation

Coping, ineffective Related factors: Personal vulnerability in situational crisis (specify), inability to perform usual roles, loss of body function (e.g., respiratory), temporary dependence, need for changes in lifestyle

Family processes, interrupted Related factors: Fear of death or disability, disruption of family processes, stressful environment (e.g., intensive care unit, hospital)

Fear Related factors: Environmental stressors or hospitalization, threat to own well-being, *Fear* of complications after being transferred out of intensive care unit

Gas exchange, impaired Related factors: Decreased functional lung tissue secondary to pneumonia or lung resection, respiratory distress syndrome, ventilation imbalance

Infection, risk for Risk factor: Collection of fluid in thoracic cavity

Mobility, physical, impaired Related factors: Limited arm or shoulder movement secondary to muscle dissection and prescribed position restrictions, *Pain*

Noncompliance Related factors: Denial of illness, negative perception of treatment regimen, difficulty with smoking cessation

Pain Related factors: Surgical incisions, chest tubes, immobility

Role performance, ineffective Related factors: Surgery, treatment side effects, dependent role during recuperation, uncertain future

Self-care deficit: (specify) Related factors: *Pain* and discomfort, *Activity intolerance* secondary to inadequate oxygenation, *Impaired physical mobility* (arms, shoulders)

Self-esteem, low (chronic, situational) Related factors: Changes in lifestyle, symbolic meaning of the heart, inability to perform usual roles

Sleep deprivation/Insomnia Related factors: *Pain* and discomfort, unfamiliar surroundings, medically prescribed treatments (e.g., nebulizer)

Ventilatory weaning response, dysfunctional (DVWR) Related factors: Uncontrolled *Pain* and discomfort, moderate-to-severe *Anxiety*, *Fear*, history of ventilatory dependence >1 week

Craniotomy

Includes but is not limited to acoustic neuroma removal, cerebral aneurysm clipping, cerebral bleed, and cerebral trauma

Potential Complications (Collaborative Problems)

PC of craniotomy: Cardiac dysrhythmias, cerebral or cerebellar dysfunction, cerebrospinal fluid leaks, cranial nerve impairment, fluid and electrolyte imbalance, GI bleeding, hemorrhage, hematomas, hydrocephalus, hygromas, hyperthermia/hypothermia, hypoxemia, meningitis or encephalitis, seizures, residual neurologic defects

Nursing Diagnoses

Activity intolerance Related factors: Weakness and *Fatigue*, *Pain*, *Sleep deprivation*, decreased level of consciousness

Airway clearance, ineffective Related factors: Tracheobronchial secretions, increased intracranial pressure

Aspiration, risk for Risk factor: Cranial nerve dysfunction

Body image, disturbed Related factors: Surgery, treatment side effects (e.g., difficulty speaking, appearance)

Bowel incontinence Related factor: Decreased level of consciousness

Breathing pattern, ineffective Related factors: Depression of respiratory center, neuromuscular paralysis or weakness, cranial nerve dysfunction, airway obstruction secondary to neck edema

Caregiver role strain Related factors: Illness severity of care receiver, discharge of family member with significant home care needs, unpredictable illness course, psychologic or cognitive problems in care receiver

Confusion, acute/chronic Related factors: Increased intracranial pressure, *Sleep deprivation*, brain tissue loss secondary to cerebral edema, hypoxia or surgical resection

Communication, impaired verbal Related factors: Aphasia, dysarthria, *Acute confusion*, intubation

Disuse syndrome, risk for Risk factors: Paralysis, prescribed or mechanical immobilization, decreased level of consciousness

Environmental interpretation syndrome, impaired See *Thought processes, disturbed*

Fear Related factors: Environmental stressors or hospitalization, *Powerlessness*, threat to own well-being, seriousness of surgery, possibility of dying

Fluid volume, excess Related factor: Decreased urine output secondary to renal dysfunction

Injury (contractures), risk for Risk factors: Sensory dysfunction, *Impaired physical mobility*

Mobility, physical, impaired Related factors: Neuromuscular impairment, perceptual or cognitive impairment, depression, severe *Anxiety*

Nutrition, imbalanced: less than body requirements Related factor: Inability to eat secondary to decreased level of consciousness

Pain Related factors: Surgical procedure, paresthesia

Role performance, ineffective Related factors: Surgery, psychologic impairment, treatment side effects, visual and speech disturbances, seizures, memory loss

Self-care deficit: (specify) Related factors: *Activity intolerance*, neuromuscular impairment, altered level of consciousness, *Pain*, weakness

Swallowing, impaired Related factors: Cranial nerve dysfunction; altered sensory reception, transmission, or integration; neuromuscular impairment

Health maintenance, ineffective Related factors: *Acute* or *chronic confusion*; *Impaired memory* and judgment secondary to residual effects on brain tissue; lack of social support

Tissue perfusion: cerebral, risk for ineffective Related factors: Interruption of arterial blood flow, increased intracranial pressure

Urinary incontinence, functional Related factors: Cognitive impairment, disorientation, *Impaired physical mobility*

Ear Surgery

Includes but is not limited to myringotomy, reconstruction, and stapedectomy

Potential Complications (Collaborative Problems)

PC of ear surgery: Facial paralysis, hearing loss, infection

Nursing Diagnoses

Communication, impaired verbal Related factor: Hearing loss

Falls, risk for Risk factors: Vertigo, nystagmus

Infection, risk for Risk factors: Exposure to upper respiratory infections, invasive procedures

Pain Related factors: Inflammation, tissue trauma, edema, presence of surgical packing

Self-care deficit: (specify) Related factor: *Activity intolerance* secondary to dizziness and loss of balance

Sensory perception, disturbed (auditory) [non-NANDA-I] Related factors: Sensory deficit, sensory overload, surgical packing, edema, disturbance of middle-ear structures

Trauma, risk for Risk factor: Displacement of prosthesis secondary to increased middle-ear pressure

Eye Surgery

Includes but is not limited to blepharoplasty, cataract removal, cryosurgery for retinal detachment, iridectomy, iridotomy, and lens implant

Potential Complications (Collaborative Problems)

PC of eye surgery: Bleeding, endophthalmus, hyphema (i.e., blood in anterior chamber of the eye), increased intraocular pressure, infection, lens implant dislocation, macular edema, retinal detachment, secondary glaucoma

Nursing Diagnoses

Body image, disturbed Related factor: Change in appearance (enucleation)

Falls, risk for Risk factors: Unsafe ambulation secondary to limited vision, eye patches, unfamiliar environment

Fear Related factor: Real or imagined threat to own well-being (e.g., permanent loss of vision)

Mobility: physical, impaired Related factors: Medically prescribed treatment and positioning, impaired vision

Self-care deficit: (specify) Related factors: Eye patches, impaired vision

Sensory perception, disturbed (visual) (non-NANDA-I) Related factor: Sensory deficit secondary to eye patches or impaired vision

Musculoskeletal Surgery

Includes but is not limited to amputation, arthrotomy, bunionectomy, casts, hip pinning, hip prosthesis, open reduction or internal fixation of fracture, shoulder repair, total ankle replacement, total hip replacement, total knee replacement, and traction

Potential Complications (Collaborative Problems)

PC of amputation: Edema of the stump

PC of fractures: Fat embolus, nonunion of bone, reflex sympathetic dystrophy

PC of fractures and casts: Compartmental syndrome

PC of fractures and musculoskeletal surgery: Deep-vein thrombosis, nerve damage

PC of joint replacement surgery: Joint dislocation or displacement of prosthesis

PC of musculoskeletal surgery: Flexion contractures, hematoma, hemorrhage, infection, pulmonary embolism, sepsis, stress fractures, synovial herniation,

PC of total hip replacement: Femoral head necrosis

PC of regional anesthesia: Hypotension, urinary retention

Nursing Diagnoses

Activity intolerance Related factors: *Pain*, weakness, *Sleep deprivation*

Anxiety Related factors: Lack of knowledge of surgery and postoperative routines (e.g., physical therapy, walking with crutches), threat to self-concept, threat to or change in role functioning

Body image, disturbed Related factors: Surgery (e.g., loss of limb), loss of functional abilities (e.g., need to use wheelchair), fear of others' response to appearance

Confusion, acute Related factors: Hypoxemia, medications (e.g., opiate analgesics), infection, impaction

Constipation Related factors: Decreased activity, dietary changes, medication (e.g., opiates, anesthetics)

Coping, ineffective Related factors: *Pain*, *Self-care deficits*, long-term and debilitating nature of disease

Disuse syndrome, risk for Risk factor: Prescribed immobilization

Diversional activity, deficient Related factors: Prolonged bed rest, institutionalization

Falls, risk for Risk factors: Unfamiliarity of assistive devices (e.g., crutches), weakness secondary to surgery and immobility

Grieving, complicated Related factors: Loss of limb, changes in lifestyle, loss of ability to perform usual roles

Home maintenance, impaired Related factors: Barriers (e.g., stairs) and hazards (e.g., throw rugs), Activity intolerance

Infection, risk for Risk factors: Inadequate primary defense secondary to exposure of joint, broken skin

Injury (contractures), risk for Risk factors: Immobility secondary to *Pain* or weakness

Mobility: physical, impaired Related factors: *Pain*, stiffness, decreased strength

Neurovascular dysfunction: peripheral, risk for Related factors: Fractures, mechanical compression, orthopedic surgery, trauma, immobilization, casts and traction devices

Pain Related factors: Muscle cramps, paresthesia, inflammation, surgical procedure, joint destruction, phantom limb pain

Self-care deficit: (specify) Related factors: *Pain*, *Activity intolerance*, *Impaired physical mobility*, decreased strength and endurance

Skin integrity, impaired Related factors: Mechanical factors, prescribed physical immobilization, *Impaired physical mobility*, impaired circulation, altered sensation, casts and other appliances, edema (e.g., of stump)

Sleep deprivation/Insomnia Related factors: *Pain* and discomfort, unfamiliar surroundings, medically induced regimen, inability to assume usual sleep position

Self-Health management, ineffective Related factors: Lack of knowledge of disease process, surgical treatment, self-care, complex rehabilitation regimen, alterations in lifestyle, insufficient energy to perform exercises

Tissue perfusion: peripheral, ineffective Related factors: Reduced arterial or venous blood flow, trauma to blood vessels, edema, dislocation of prosthesis

Neck Surgery

Includes but is not limited to carotid endarterectomy, laryngectomy, parathyroidectomy, radical neck dissection, thyroidectomy, tonsillectomy, and tracheostomy

Potential Complications (Collaborative Problems)

PC of neck surgery: Airway obstruction, aspiration, cerebral infarction, cranial nerve damage (e.g., facial, hypoglossal, glossopharyngeal, vagus), fistula formation (e.g., between hypopharynx and skin), hemorrhage, hypertension, hypotension, infection, local nerve impairment, thyroid storm, tracheal stenosis, vocal cord paralysis

PC radical neck dissection: Flap rejection

PC thyroidectomy/parathyroidectomy: Hypoparathyroidism, causing hypocalcemia and tetany

Nursing Diagnoses

Activity intolerance Related factors: Imbalance between oxygen supply and demand, *Anxiety*, *Pain*, weakness secondary to limited mobility, *Fatigue* secondary to accelerated metabolic rate (e.g., thyroidectomy)

Airway clearance, ineffective Related factors: Decreased energy, edema, *Pain*, tracheobronchial obstruction, increased tracheobronchial secretions, edema of the glottis, tracheal compression secondary to hemorrhage, presence of tracheostomy tube

Anxiety See *Fear*

Aspiration, risk for Risk factors: Depressed cough or gag reflexes, presence of tracheostomy or endotracheal tube, *Impaired swallowing*, hindered elevation of upper body, removal of epiglottis (in partial laryngectomy), loss of normal reflexes, and excessive secretions secondary to surgery

Body image, disturbed Related factors: Changes in appearance secondary to surgery, depression, treatment side effects

Breathing pattern, ineffective Related factors: *Anxiety*, decreased energy, accidental decannulation

Communication, impaired verbal Related factors: *Acute confusion*, inability to speak, inability to speak clearly secondary to *Pain* and edema, tracheostomy, laryngectomy, weak or hoarse voice secondary to trauma to laryngeal nerve

Coping, ineffective Related factors: Personal vulnerability in situational crisis (specify), inability to speak, disfigurement, inadequate support system (see *Body image, disturbed*)

Falls, risk for Risk factors: Sensory dysfunction, integrative dysfunction, vascular insufficiency, altered mobility

Fear Related factors: Real or imagined threat to own well-being (e.g., fear of suffocation), unfamiliarity with environment and pre- and postoperative routines

Fluid volume, deficient Related factors: Loss of fluid through abnormal routes, hypermetabolic state, decreased intake secondary to *Pain* and *Impaired swallowing*

Grieving, complicated Related factors: Actual loss of function, change in appearance, threat of dying

Infection, risk for Risk factors: Tissue destruction and increased environmental exposure, loss of normal filtration systems in the mouth and nose secondary to use of artificial airway, immunosuppression secondary to chemotherapy and malignancies

Mobility: physical, impaired Related factors: Limited shoulder and head movement secondary to removal of muscles and nerves, flap graft reconstruction

Nutrition, imbalanced: less than body requirements Related factors: *Pain*, *Impaired swallowing*, loss of appetite, *Nausea* and vomiting, loss of sense of smell, cachexia secondary to malignancy, accelerated metabolic rate (e.g., from thyroidectomy)

Oral mucous membrane, impaired Related factors: Inadequate oral hygiene, tubes, surgery in oral cavity, infection, radiation therapy to head and neck

Pain Related factor: Surgical procedure, edema, tracheostomy tube irritation

Role performance, ineffective Related factors: Surgery, treatment side effects, *Impaired physical mobility*

Self-esteem, low (chronic, situational) See *Body image, disturbed*

Skin integrity, impaired Related factors: Mechanical factors, radiation, altered nutritional state

Social isolation Related factors: Difficulty communicating, embarrassment and concern over others' response to disfigurement, avoidance by others

Swallowing, impaired Related factors: Irritated oropharyngeal cavity, mechanical obstruction, edema, cranial nerve damage

Tissue integrity, impaired Related factors: Nutritional deficit, irritants, mechanical factors (e.g., tracheostomy tube), radiation

Ventilatory weaning response, dysfunctional (DVWR) Related factors: *Ineffective airway clearance*, lack of motivation secondary to malaise, moderate-to-severe *Anxiety*, *Fear*, uncontrolled episodic energy demands or problems

Rectal Surgery

Includes but is not limited to fissurectomy, hemorrhoidectomy, pilonidal cystectomy, and polypectomy

Potential Complications (Collaborative Problems)

PC of rectal surgery: Hemorrhage, infection, stricture formation

Nursing Diagnoses

Constipation Related factors: Dietary changes, decreased motility secondary to medication and inactivity, *Fear* of painful defecation

Incontinence, bowel Related factor: Loss of sphincter integrity

Infection, risk for Risk factors: Loss of primary line of defense secondary to surgery, fecal contamination

Pain Related factors: Surgical procedure, passage of stool

Skin Graft

Includes but is not limited to excision of lesion with flap, excision of lesion with full-thickness graft, excision of lesion with split-thickness graft, and excision of lesion with synthetic graft

Potential Complications (Collaborative Problems)

PC of skin graft: Edema, flap necrosis, hematoma, infection

Nursing Diagnoses

Body image, disturbed Related factor: Results of reconstructive surgery not as anticipated by patient

Constipation Related factor: Decreased activity secondary to prescribed positioning

Diversional activity, deficient Related factors: Prolonged bed rest, prescribed positioning

Fear Related factors: Real or imagined threat to own well-being, fear of flap failure, fear of others' reactions to appearance

Mobility: physical, impaired Related factors: *Pain* and discomfort, prescribed position

Neurovascular dysfunction: peripheral, risk for Risk factors: Immobilization, burns, edema

Pain Related factors: Surgical procedure, paresthesia

Tissue perfusion: ineffective, peripheral Related factors: Restricted blood flow secondary to edema, blood clot, or tension on the flap

Spinal Surgery

Includes but is not limited to Harrington rod implant, laminectomy, Luque rod implant, and spinal fusion

Potential Complications (Collaborative Problems)

PC of laminectomy/spinal fusion: Displacement of bone graft

PC of spinal surgery: Bladder and bowel dysfunction, cerebrospinal fistula, hematoma, hemorrhage, infection, nerve root injury, paralytic ileus, sensorineural impairments, spinal cord edema or injury, leakage of cerebrospinal fluid, headache

Nursing Diagnoses

Activity intolerance Related factors: *Fear* of damaging surgical site, *Pain*, weakness and *Fatigue*, sedentary lifestyle, enforced inactivity

Caregiver role strain Related factors: Premature birth and congenital defect, developmental delay or retardation of the care receiver–caregiver, duration of caregiving required

Constipation Related factors: Decreased activity, medications (e.g., opiates), inability to assume normal position for defecation, change in daily routine, temporary loss of parasympathetic function innervating the bowels

Falls, risk for Risk factors: Sensory dysfunction, loss of balance, muscle weakness secondary to recent inactivity, vertigo secondary to postural hypotension

Mobility: physical, impaired Related factors: *Pain*, neuromuscular impairment, stiffness in fused area, prescribed activity, and position limitations

Neurovascular dysfunction: peripheral, risk for Related factors: Fractures, mechanical compression, trauma, immobilization

Nutrition, imbalanced: more than body requirements Related factors: increased appetite when pain subsides, sedentary lifestyle, decreased activity

Pain, acute/chronic Related factors: Bed rest, muscle cramps, paresthesia, surgical procedure (e.g., graft site), inflammation, localized edema, muscle spasms

Self-care deficit: (specify) Related factors: Prescribed postoperative immobility, *Pain*

Skin integrity, impaired Related factors: Prescribed activity restrictions, diminished or interrupted blood flow secondary to edema, hematoma, or hypovolemia

Urinary retention Related factors: Swelling in operative area, inability to assume usual position for voiding

Urologic Surgery

Includes but is not limited to cystocele repair, rectocele repair, removal of bladder tumor, cystoscopy, nephrectomy, penile implant, percutaneous nephrostomy, retroperitoneal lymphadenotomy, prostatectomy, transurethral resection of the prostate, ureterolithotomy, urostomy, and vasectomy

Potential Complications (Collaborative Problems)

PC of prostate resection/prostatectomy: Retrograde ejaculation

PC of urologic surgery: Bladder neck constriction, bladder perforation (intraoperative), epididymitis, hemorrhage, paralytic ileus, urethral stricture, urinary tract infection

PC of urostomy/nephrostomy: Stomal necrosis, stenosis, obstruction

Nursing Diagnoses

Anxiety Related factors: Threat to self-concept, change in health status, change in body appearance or function, threat to or change in role functioning, threat to or change in interaction pattern

Body image, disturbed Related factors: Surgery, depression, treatment side effects (e.g., impotence), appearance of ostomy (e.g., urostomy)

Grieving, complicated Related factor: Potential loss of body parts or function

Incontinence, urinary, urge Related factors: Decreased bladder capacity, surgery, irritation of bladder stretch receptors causing spasms, overdistention of bladder

Infection, risk for Risk factors: Stasis of body fluids, change in pH of secretions, suppressed inflammatory response, tissue destruction and increased environmental exposure, invasive procedures and lines (e.g., catheters, irrigation, suprapubic drains)

Mobility: physical, impaired Related factor: *Pain*

Pain Related factors: Muscle cramps, surgical procedure, coughing and deep breathing (e.g., renal surgeries), bladder spasms, back and leg pain, clot in drainage devices (e.g., from transurethral resection)

Sexual dysfunction Related factors: Side effects of surgery, *Pain*, altered body function or structure, *Disturbed body image*, reaction of partner to ostomy, erectile dysfunction (male), inadequate vaginal lubrication (female)

Social isolation Related factors: Concern about others' reaction to ostomy, worry about odor and leaking from appliance

Urinary incontinence, stress Related factors: Incompetent bladder outlet, overdistention between voidings, weak pelvic muscles and structural supports

Urinary retention Related factors: Inhibition of reflex arc, blockage secondary to edema or inflammation

Vascular Surgery

Includes but is not limited to aortic aneurysm resection, aortoiliac bypass graft, embolectomy, femoroiliac bypass graft, portacaval shunt, sympathectomy, and vein ligation

Potential Complications (Collaborative Problems)

PC of aortic aneurysm resection: Renal failure, myocardial infarction, hemorrhage, emboli, spinal cord ischemia, congestive heart failure, rupture of suture line

PC of vascular surgery: Cardiac dysrhythmia, compartmental syndrome, failure of anastomosis, infection, lymphocele, occlusion of graft

Nursing Diagnoses

Activity intolerance Related factors: *Anxiety*, *Pain*, weakness secondary to inactivity, imbalance between oxygen supply and demand

Caregiver role strain Related factors: Illness severity of care receiver, unpredictable illness course or instability in the care receiver's health, complexity and amount of caregiving tasks

Fear Related factor: Real or imagined threat to own well-being (e.g., surgery, failure of graft, loss of limb, death)

Fluid volume, deficient Related factors: Loss of fluid through abnormal routes, medications, third spacing, hematoma, diuresis secondary to contrast media given for angiography

Fluid volume excess Related factor: Decreased urine output secondary to heart failure

Grieving, complicated Related factor: Potential loss of body part or function

Injury, risk for Risk factors: Tissue hypoxia, abnormal blood profile, *Impaired mobility*

Mobility: physical, impaired Related factors: *Pain*, nerve injury secondary to ischemia

Neurovascular dysfunction, peripheral, risk for Risk factors: Immobilization, vascular obstruction

Pain, acute/chronic Related factors: Surgical procedure, increased tissue perfusion to previously ischemic tissue, peripheral nerve ischemia, paresthesias

Sexual dysfunction Related factors: Impotence and retrograde ejaculation secondary to aortic aneurysm resection

Tissue integrity, impaired Related factors: Chronically compromised peripheral tissue perfusion, decreased activity postoperatively, multiple surgical procedures

Tissue perfusion, ineffective: (cardiac, cerebral, peripheral) Related factors: Interruption of venous blood flow, exchange problems, graft occlusion, edema, compartmental syndrome, inadequate anticoagulation, progressive arterial disease

PSYCHIATRIC CONDITIONS

Assaultive patient
Borderline personality
Eating disorders
Mania
Paranoia
Phobias
Psychosis
Severe depression
Substance abuse
Suicide
Withdrawn patient

Assaultive Patient

Associated psychiatric diagnoses include but are not limited to bipolar disorder, manic; disorganized schizophrenia; substance use disorders; organic mental disorders; drug-induced psychoses; personality disorders; panic disorder; and post-traumatic stress disorder

Nursing Diagnoses

Confusion Related factors: Mental disorder (specify), organic mental disorder (specify), personality disorder (specify), substance abuse

Coping: defensive Related factors: Psychologic impairment (specify), situational crisis (specify), neurologic alteration, other physical factors (specify)

Environmental Interpretation Syndrome, impaired Related factors: Alcoholism, dementia, brain infarction, depression, Huntington disease, Parkinson disease, substance abuse

Posttrauma syndrome Related factors: Abuse, incest, rape, participation in combat

Self-esteem, chronic low Related factors: Psychologic impairment (specify), repeatedly unmet expectations

Self-esteem, situational low Related factor: Situational crisis (specify)

Social interaction, impaired Related factors: Developmental disability, communication barriers, psychologic impairment (specify)

Violence: self-directed or other-directed, risk for Risk factors: Manic excitement, panic states, rage reaction, history of violence, drug or alcohol intoxication or withdrawal, temporal lobe epilepsy, paranoid ideation, organic brain syndrome, arrest or conviction pattern, toxic reaction to medications, command hallucinations

Borderline Personality

Nursing Diagnoses

Anxiety Related factors: Threat to or change in role functioning, situational crises (specify), maturational crisis (specify), unmet needs, change in environment, threat to or change in interaction patterns, unconscious conflict about values or beliefs, negative self-talk, posttraumatic experience

Coping: family, disabled Related factors: Conflicting coping styles, highly ambivalent family relationships, chronically unresolved feelings (specify), role changes, and ongoing family disorganization secondary to patient's illness

Coping, ineffective Related factors: Personal vulnerability in situational or maturational crisis (specify); procrastination, stubbornness, and inefficiency in performing social roles; unrealistic perceptions; unmet expectations; disregard for social norms; inadequate support

Eating Disorders

Associated psychiatric diagnoses are limited to anorexia nervosa and bulimia

Potential Complications (Collaborative Problems)

PC of eating disorders: Amenorrhea, anemia, dysrhythmias

Nursing Diagnoses

Activity intolerance Related factor: Weakness and *Fatigue* secondary to malnutrition

Anxiety Related factors: Threat to self-concept, worry about being overweight, change in environment, situational or maturational crises, unmet needs

Body image, disturbed Related factors: Eating disorder (see *Anxiety*), dysfunctional family system

Constipation Related factors: Less than adequate amounts of fiber and bulk-forming foods in diet, chronic use of medication and enemas, inadequate fluid intake

Coping: family, disabled Related factors: Arbitrary disregard for patient's needs, chronically unresolved feelings (specify guilt, anxiety, hostility, despair, and so forth), conflicting coping styles, highly ambivalent family relationships, effect of marital discord on family members

Coping, ineffective Related factors: Personal vulnerability in a maturational or situational crisis (specify), feelings of loss of control, inaccurate perception of weight status, *Anxiety* about maturing body

Fluid volume, deficient Related factors: Extreme weight loss, self-induced vomiting, abuse of laxatives or diuretics

Noncompliance Related factors: Denial of illness, negative perception of treatment regimen, perceived benefits of continued illness

Nutrition, imbalanced: less than body requirements Related factors: Psychologic impairment (e.g., bulimia, anorexia), refusal to eat, self-induced vomiting, laxative abuse, need for more calories because of physical exertion (e.g., excessive exercising)

Self-esteem, chronic low Related factors: Psychologic impairment (specify), repeatedly unmet expectations, perception of self as fat

Sexuality patterns, ineffective Related factors: Ineffective or absent role models, *Disturbed body image*, impaired relationship with significant other, *Chronic or situational low self-esteem*

Self-health management, ineffective Related factors: *Decisional conflict*, family conflict, mistrust of regimen or health care personnel, denial of illness, perceived lack of benefits of treatment, *Powerlessness*

Social interaction, impaired Related factor: Psychologic impairment (e.g., anorexia, bulimia), fear and mistrust of relationships

Mania

Associated psychiatric diagnoses include but are not limited to bipolar disorders (manic, mixed), schizophrenia (undifferentiated type, catatonic type), schizoaffective disorder, and substance use disorders

Potential Complications (Collaborative Problems)

PC of lithium therapy: Lithium toxicity

Nursing Diagnoses

Anxiety Related factors: Change in role functioning, change in environment, change in interaction patterns, unmet needs, threats to self-concept

Communication: verbal, impaired Related factors: Hyperactivity, pressured speech

Confusion Related factor: Mental disorder (specify), delusions, hallucinations, euphoria, flight of ideas

Coping, defensive Related factors: Ideas of grandiosity, self-importance, or abilities secondary to feelings of inferiority

Coping, ineffective Related factor: Personal vulnerability in a situational crisis (specify)

Family processes, interrupted Related factors: Illness or disability of family member, exhaustion of family members, situational crises (e.g., financial difficulty, role changes), patient's euphoria and grandiose ideas, manipulative behavior, limit testing, patient's refusal to take responsibility for own actions

Environmental Interpretation Syndrome, impaired Related factors: Mental disturbance, delusions, hallucinations, euphoria, flight of ideas

Fluid volume, deficient Related factors: Inadequate fluid intake secondary to manic behaviors, medication-induced *Diarrhea* and vomiting, polyuria

Health maintenance, ineffective Related factors: Significant alteration in communication skills, lack of ability to make deliberate and thoughtful judgments

Injury, risk for Risk factors: Orientation; drugs (e.g., alcohol, caffeine, nicotine); cognitive, affective, and psychomotor factors

Insomnia Related factors: Psychologic impairment (specify), inability to recognize *Fatigue* and need for sleep, hyperactivity, denial of need to sleep

Nutrition, imbalanced: less than body requirements Related factor: Inadequate intake to balance excessive (i.e., manic) activity

Personal identity, disturbed Related factor: Psychologic impairment (specify)

Role performance, ineffective Related factor: Psychologic impairment (specify), see *Interrupted family processes*

Stress overload Related factors: Characteristics of the disease that limit ability to cope with stressors

Social interaction, impaired Related factors: Psychologic impairment (specify), others' unwillingness to tolerate patient's behaviors

Suicide, risk for Risk factors: Impulsive behavior, delusional thinking, command hallucinations, impaired reality testing

Violence: self-directed or directed at others, risk for Risk factors: Manic excitement, rage reaction, history of violence, irritability, impulsive behavior, delusional thinking, command hallucinations, impaired reality testing

Paranoia

Associated psychiatric diagnoses include but are not limited to schizophrenia (undifferentiated type, paranoid type), mood disorders (major depression [e.g., single episode, recurrent]), bipolar disorders (e.g., mixed, manic, depressed), schizoaffective disorder, paranoid disorders, substance-abuse disorders, organic mental disorders, and personality disorders

Nursing Diagnoses

Anxiety (severe) Related factors: Failure to master developmental task of trust versus mistrust, delusions

Confusion Related factors: Mental disorder (specify), organic mental disorder (specify), personality disorder (specify), poor reality testing secondary to mistrust of others, delusions, hallucinations

Coping, defensive Related factor: Psychologic impairment (specify)

Coping, ineffective Related factors: Personal vulnerability in situational crisis, use of projection to control fears and anxieties

Family processes, interrupted Related factors: Illness or disability of family member, temporary or long-term family disorganization, exhausted family, patient's behaviors

Fear Related factor: Imagined threat to own well-being

Health maintenance, ineffective Related factors: Significant alteration in communication skills, lack of ability to make deliberate and thoughtful judgments

Insomnia Related factors: Psychologic impairment, *Fear* of danger, hypervigilance

Noncompliance Related factors: Denial of illness, negative perception of treatment regimen, mistrust of caregivers

Powerlessness Related factors: Health care environment, treatment regimen, feelings of inadequacy, maladaptive interpersonal relationships (e.g., use of force, abusive relationships), *Situational or chronic low self-esteem*, feelings that he has no control over situations

Self-esteem, low (chronic, situational) Related factors: Psychologic impairment (specify), failure of relationships, feelings of *Powerlessness*

Sexuality patterns, ineffective Related factors: Impaired relationship with significant other secondary to manipulative, violent, or other unacceptable behaviors; conflicts with sexual orientation

Social interaction, impaired Related factors: Psychologic impairment (specify), delusions, suspiciousness, *Fear,* and mistrust of others

Violence: self-directed or other-directed, risk for Risk factors: Panic states, drug or alcohol intoxication or withdrawal, delusions, feelings of *Anxiety*, perceived danger

Phobias

Associated psychiatric diagnoses include but are not limited to agoraphobia, simple phobia, and social phobia

Nursing Diagnoses

Anxiety Related factors: Threat to or change in role functioning, change in environment, threat to self-concept, threat to or change in interaction pattern, unmet needs

Coping, ineffective Related factor: Personal vulnerability in situational or maturational crisis (specify)

Diversional activity, deficient Related factors: Impaired perception of reality, fear of loss of control if dreaded object or situation is encountered

Fear Related factors: Real or imagined threat to own well-being, learned irrational response to objects or situations

Role performance, ineffective Related factors: Psychologic impairment (e.g., phobic disorder), inability to perform role behaviors secondary to irrational fears

Social interaction, impaired Related factors: Psychologic impairment (e.g., phobic disorder), *Fear* of encountering dreaded object or situation, *Fear* of loss of control

Social isolation Related factors: Psychologic impairment (e.g., phobic disorder), others' reactions to irrational behaviors

Psychosis

Associated psychiatric diagnoses include but are not limited to schizophrenia (disorganized, catatonic, paranoid, and undifferentiated types) schizophreniform disorder; bipolar disorders (mixed, manic, and depressed); organic mental disorders; substance-abuse disorders; and medical conditions

Nursing Diagnoses

Anxiety (severe, panic) Related factors: Continuation of maladaptive coping learned early in life, unconscious conflicts, unmet needs, threats to self-concept

Communication: verbal, impaired Related factors: Psychologic impairment (specify), incoherent or illogical speech, medication side effects

Confusion Related factors: Mental disorder (specify), organic mental disorder (specify), dementia, delirium

Coping: family, disabled Related factors: Long-term pattern of multiple stressors, significant others exhausted by prolonged illness

Health maintenance, ineffective Related factors: Lack of ability to make deliberate and thoughtful judgments

Home maintenance, impaired Related factors: Psychologic impairment (specify), *Disturbed thought processes*, impaired judgment or decision making

Noncompliance Related factors: Denial of illness, negative perception of treatment regimen, *Confusion, Impaired environmental interpretation syndrome*, responding to delusions and hallucinations

Personal identity, disturbed Related factors: Psychologic impairment (specify), psychologic conflicts, childhood abuse, underdeveloped ego, threats to self-concept, threats to physical integrity

Self-care deficit: (specify) Related factors: Psychologic impairment (specify), severe *Anxiety*, *Disturbed thought processes*, inability to make decisions, feelings of worthlessness, lack of energy

Self-mutilation, risk for Risk factors: Fluctuating emotions, command hallucinations, patients in psychotic state—frequently males in young adulthood

Social interaction, impaired Related factor: Psychologic impairment (specify)

Violence: self-directed or other-directed, risk for Risk factors: Paranoid ideation, suicidal ideation, history of violence, substance abuse (specify), responding to delusions and hallucinations

Severe Depression

Associated psychiatric diagnoses include but are not limited to bipolar disorder (depressed) and major depression

Nursing Diagnoses

Activity intolerance Related factors: Weakness and *Fatigue*, depression, inadequate nutrition

Anxiety Related factors: Psychologic conflicts, unmet needs, unconscious values/goals conflicts, change in role functioning, change in interaction patterns, threat to self-concept

Confusion Related factors: Mental disorder (specify), overgeneralizing, negative thinking, dichotomous thinking

Constipation Related factors: Decreased activity, lack of exercise, inadequate intake of fiber and fluids, medications (specify)

Coping: family, disabled Related factors: Role conflicts, marital discord secondary to long-term depression (see *Interrupted family processes*)

Coping, ineffective Related factors: Personal vulnerability in situational or maturational crisis, guilt, *Low self-esteem*, feelings of rejection, unconscious conflicts

Family processes, interrupted Related factors: Illness or disability of family member, changes in roles or responsibilities, family disorganization, *Impaired verbal communication*, difficulty accepting or receiving help

Grieving, complicated Related factors: Actual loss (specify), anticipated loss (specify), perceived loss (specify), unresolved grief secondary to prolonged *Ineffective denial*, repressed feelings

Health maintenance, ineffective Related factors: Lack of ability to make deliberate and thoughtful judgments, significant alteration in communication skills, lack of energy, feelings of worthlessness

Home maintenance, impaired Related factors: Psychologic impairment (specify), inability to concentrate, impaired decision making, lack of energy

Hopelessness Related factors: Long-term stress, lack of social supports, abandonment by others

Injury, risk for Risk factors: Orientation; drugs (e.g., alcohol, caffeine, nicotine); cognitive, affective, and psychomotor factors; electroconvulsive therapy and anesthesia effects on cardiovascular and respiratory systems; medication side effects such as sedation or blurred vision

Insomnia Related factors: *Anxiety*, psychologic impairment (e.g., depression), decreased serotonin, daytime inactivity, naps, difficulty falling asleep at night, hypersomnia, early awakening

Nutrition, imbalanced: less than body requirements Related factors: Psychologic impairment (specify), loss of appetite, feelings of worthlessness, emotional stress or *Anxiety*

Powerlessness Related factors: Psychologic impairment (specify), negative beliefs about own abilities, past failures, lack of energy, feelings of worthlessness

Role performance, ineffective Related factors: Psychologic impairment (specify), lack of energy, *Powerlessness*, helplessness

Self-care deficit: (specify) Related factors: Depression, lack of energy

Self-esteem, chronic low Related factors: Psychologic impairment (specify), repeatedly unmet expectations, past failures, feelings of worthlessness

Sexuality patterns, ineffective Related factors: *Chronic or situational low self-esteem*, lack of energy, loss of interest, decreased sex drive

Social interaction, impaired Related factors: Psychologic impairment (depression), failure to initiate interactions secondary to decreased energy or inertia, poor self-concept, lack of social skills, feelings of worthlessness

Social isolation Related factors: Others' responses to depressed mood, *Disturbed thought processes*, lack of social skills, feelings of unworthiness

Suicide, risk for Risk factors: Suicidal ideation or intent secondary to feelings of worthlessness and *Hopelessness*, loneliness

Violence: self-directed, risk for Risk factors: Suicidal ideation or intent secondary to feelings of worthlessness and *Hopelessness*, loneliness

Substance Abuse

Associated psychiatric diagnoses include alcohol or drug intoxication, withdrawal and dependence

Potential Complications (Collaborative Problems)

PC of alcoholism: Delirium tremens

PC of substance abuse: Hallucinations, hypertension, sepsis, toxic overdose

PC of substance abuse or withdrawal: Seizures

Nursing Diagnoses

Anxiety Related factors: Change in health status, change in role functioning, situational crisis, unmet needs, *Impaired memory*, loss of control, fear of withdrawal, legal implications

Coping: family, compromised/disabled Related factors: Temporary family disorganization and role changes, unrealistic expectations and demands, lack of mutual decision-making skills, inadequate information or understanding by family member, arbitrary disregard for patient's needs, chronically unresolved feelings (specify guilt, anxiety, hostility, despair, and so forth), conflicting coping styles, inconsistent limit setting, highly ambivalent family relationships, violence

Coping, ineffective Related factors: Personal vulnerability in situational or maturational crisis (specify), anger, denial, dependence, inability to manage stressors

Decisional conflict (specify) Related factor: Chemical dependence

Denial, ineffective Related factors: Feelings of vulnerability, ambivalence about withdrawal, inability to cope without alcohol or drugs, *Anxiety, Fear*

Diarrhea Related factors: Excessive alcohol or drug intake, withdrawal

Environmental interpretation syndrome, impaired (e.g., auditory, kinesthetic, tactile, visual disturbances) Related factors: Alcohol intoxication, substance intoxication (specify)

Family processes, dysfunctional Related factor: Alcohol or other substance abuse by a family member

Fluid volume, deficient Related factors: Excessive, continuous consumption of alcohol, vomiting, *Diarrhea*

Home maintenance, impaired Related factors: Insufficient family organization or planning, psychologic impairment (e.g., substance abuse), decreased motivation, *Confusion, Impaired environmental interpretation syndrome*, depression, severe *Anxiety*

Injury, risk for Risk factors: Orientation; affective factors; impaired judgment; *Confusion, acute/chronic*; *Impaired environmental interpretation syndrome*; delirium; substance intoxication

Insomnia Related factors: Chemical dependence (specify, e.g., stimulants), nightmares, difficulty sleeping at night secondary to sleeping during the day

Memory, impaired Related factor: Organic brain damage

Moral distress Related factor: Believing that the right thing to do is stop drinking (e.g., recognizing effects on family), but feeling (or being) unable to do it

Noncompliance Related factors: Denial of illness, negative perception of treatment regimen, inability to ask for or accept help, lack of social support, inability to cope with stressors without alcohol or drugs

Nutrition, imbalanced: less than body requirements Related factors: Chemical dependence (specify), anorexia, hypermetabolism secondary to stimulants, no money for food

Nutrition, imbalanced: more than body requirements Related factor: Increased appetite secondary to drug taking (e.g., marijuana)

Parenting, impaired Related factors: Dysfunctional relationship between parents, change in marital status, psychologic impairment (substance abuse) (see *Family coping* and *Family processes*)

Post-trauma syndrome Related factors: Abuse, accidents, assault, disaster, epidemic, incest, kidnapping, torture, terrorism, participation in combat

Powerlessness Related factors: Pattern of helplessness, failed attempts to abstain, changes in personal or social life

Role performance, ineffective Related factor: Psychologic impairment (e.g., substance abuse)

Self-esteem, chronic low Related factors: Repeatedly unmet expectations, guilt, failed withdrawal, ambivalence

Sexual dysfunction/Sexuality patterns, ineffective Related factors: *Chronic or situational low self-esteem*, impotence, loss of libido secondary to substance abuse, neurologic damage, debilitation from drug use, embarrassment about changes in appearance (e.g., testicular atrophy, spider angiomas)

Social interaction, impaired Related factors: Chemical dependence (specify), inability to focus on others, emotional immaturity, aggressiveness, *Anxiety*

Social isolation Related factors: Others' responses to impulsive behaviors, avoidance behaviors and anger, job loss, perceived difference from others

Violence: self-directed or directed at others, risk for Risk factors: Substance intoxication (specify), substance withdrawal (specify), disorientation, impaired judgment, altered perceptions, poor impulse control

Suicide

Risk for suicide actually represents a nursing diagnosis that can be associated with any of the psychiatric diagnoses (e.g., schizophrenia, substance abuse). The following nursing diagnoses may also occur for patients who are suicidal.

Nursing Diagnoses

Anxiety Related factors: Threat to self-concept, threat to or change in role functioning, situational or maturational crises, unmet needs, changes in social supports

Coping, ineffective Related factors: Personal vulnerability in situational or maturational crisis (specify)

Decisional conflict Related factors: Perceived threat to value system, lack of support system

Environmental interpretation syndrome, impaired Related factors: Mental disorders (specify), organic mental disorders (specify), personality disorders (specify), substance abuse

Hopelessness Related factors: Abandonment, lack of social supports, lost spiritual belief

Personal identity, disturbed Related factor: Situational crisis (specify)

Post-trauma syndrome Related factors: Abuse, accidents, assault, disaster, epidemic, incest, kidnapping, terrorism, torture, catastrophic illness or accident, participation in combat

Rape-trauma syndrome Related factor: Patient's biopsychosocial response to event

Self-esteem, chronic low Related factors: Psychologic impairment (specify), repeatedly unmet expectations

Self-mutilation, risk for Risk factors: Inability to cope with increased psychologic or physiologic tension in a healthy manner; feelings of depression, rejection, self-hatred, separation anxiety, guilt, and depersonalization; fluctuating emotions; drug or alcohol abuse

Spiritual distress Related factor: Challenged beliefs and values systems

Violence: self-directed, risk for Risk factors: History of suicide attempt, command hallucinations, battered women, panic states, history of abuse by others, suicidal ideation, substance abuse

Withdrawn Patient

Associated psychiatric diagnoses include but are not limited to major depression; schizophrenia: disorganized, catatonic, paranoid, and undifferentiated types; schizophreniform disorder; phobic disorders; schizoid personality disorder; avoidant personality disorder; substance use disorders; and organic mental disorders

Nursing Diagnoses

Anxiety Related factors: Threat to or change in role functioning, real or perceived threat to physical self or to self-concept, unconscious conflicts (e.g., values, beliefs), negative self-talk, feelings of apprehension and uneasiness, altered perceptions

Communication: verbal, impaired Related factors: Psychologic impairment (specify), refusal to speak or make eye contact

Coping, ineffective Related factor: Personal vulnerability in situational or maturational crisis (specify)

Diversional activity, deficient Related factors: Lack of motivation, deficit in social skills, impaired perception of reality

Family processes, interrupted Related factors: Illness or disability of family member, inability to communicate secondary to withdrawal

Fear Related factors: *Powerlessness*, real or imagined threat to own well-being

Grieving, complicated Related factors: Actual loss (specify), anticipated loss (specify), perceived loss (specify)

Health maintenance, ineffective Related factors: Lack of ability to make thoughtful and deliberate judgments, significant alteration in communication skills, lack of awareness of environment and own needs

Environmental interpretation syndrome, impaired Related factors: Mental disorders (specify), organic mental disorders (specify), personality disorders (specify)

Parenting, impaired Related factors: Psychologic impairment (specify), situational crisis (specify), see *Interrupted family processes*

Personal identity, disturbed Related factor: Psychologic impairment (specify)

Role performance, ineffective Related factor: Psychologic impairment (specify)

Self-esteem, low (chronic, situational) Related factor: Psychologic impairment (specify)

Self-mutilation, risk for Risk factors: Inability to cope with increased psychologic or physiologic tension in a healthy manner; feelings of depression, rejection, self-hatred, separation anxiety, guilt, and depersonalization; need for sensory stimuli

Social interaction, impaired Related factors: Psychologic impairment (specify), *Fear* of social situations, *Anxiety*, depression

Social isolation Related factors: Psychologic impairment (specify), others' difficulty communicating with patient

ANTEPARTUM AND POSTPARTUM CONDITIONS

Abortion, spontaneous or induced
Change in birthing plans
Gestational diabetes

Hyperemesis gravidarum
Maternal infection
Painful breast
Perinatal loss
Postpartum care, uncomplicated
Preeclampsia
Suppression of preterm labor
Uterine bleeding

Abortion, Spontaneous or Induced

Potential Complications (Collaborative Problems)

PC of abortion: Hemorrhage, infection

Nursing Diagnoses

Anxiety Related factors: Threat to health status, ambivalence, *Deficient knowledge* regarding procedures and postprocedural care, unfamiliar sights and sounds, *Fear* of implications for future pregnancies

Coping, ineffective Related factors: Unresolved feelings (e.g., guilt) about elective abortion; societal, moral, religious, and family conflicting values; unresolved feelings over loss of baby

Decisional conflict Related factors: Values conflicts, inadequate support system

Family processes, interrupted Related factors: Effects of elective procedure or spontaneous loss on relationships, inability of family members to agree on decisions, adolescent identity conflicts, preexisting personal or marital conflicts

Grieving, complicated Related factors: Perinatal loss, perceived or actual loss of cultural or religious approval

Health maintenance, ineffective Related factor: *Deficient knowledge* (e.g., of contraception, "safer sex")

Infection, risk for Risk factors: Invasive procedures, traumatized tissue, incomplete expulsion of uterine contents

Moral distress Related factor: Believing the right thing to do is to continue the pregnancy, but giving in to external pressures to have the abortion. Or, conversely, believing that it would be best to have the abortion (e.g., because of the high risk of a birth defect), but giving in to external pressure to continue the pregnancy

Pain Related factor: Strong uterine contractions

Powerlessness Related factors: Treatment regimen, inability to change the course of events or prevent the loss, perception that there are limited or no options

Self-esteem, low (chronic, situational) Related factors: Unmet expectations for pregnancy, unmet expectations for child, preexisting *Low self-esteem*

Sexual dysfunction/Sexuality patterns, ineffective Related factors: *Low Self-esteem*, fear of pregnancy, unstable relationship with significant others, *Disturbed body image*

Spiritual distress Related factors: Test of spiritual beliefs, unresolved feelings about elective abortion, inability to find meaning in spontaneous abortion

Change in Birthing Plans

May include any deviation from a couple's original birthing plans. Such a change may include but is not limited to use of analgesia, anesthesia, or forceps; limitation of visitors; episiotomy, and cesarean birth.

Nursing Diagnoses

Attachment, risk for impaired Risk factors: Unmet expectations for childbirth, separation of family members

Family processes, interrupted Related factors: Unmet expectations for childbirth, situational crisis (e.g., fetal distress), separation of family members (e.g., emergency hysterectomy secondary to uterine rupture)

Fear Related factors: Real or imagined threat to child or to own well-being, unfamiliar equipment, urgency of emergency procedures

Pain Related factors: Surgery, episiotomy, uterine contractions, invasive procedures

Powerlessness Related factors: Complication threatening pregnancy, perceived inability to effect outcome of situation, inability to cope with overwhelming uterine contractions

Self-esteem, low (chronic, situational) Related factors: Unmet expectations for childbirth (e.g., inability to "tolerate" uterine contractions, inability to deliver vaginally)

Gestational Diabetes

Potential Complications (Collaborative Problems)

PC of gestational diabetes: Anemia, dystocia, fetal morbidity or mortality, hydramnios, ketoacidosis, pregnancy-induced hypertension, pyelonephritis, diabetic retinopathy

Nursing Diagnoses

Blood glucose, risk for unstable Related factor: Physiological changes of pregnancy that decrease the sensitivity to insulin

Family processes, interrupted Related factors: Hospitalization or change in environment, illness or disability of family member, inadequate finances

Fear Related factors: Environmental stressors or hospitalization, *Powerlessness*, real or imagined threat to own well-being, real or imagined threat to child, implications for future pregnancies

Infection (urinary tract infection, vaginitis), risk for Risk factors: Favorable environment for bacterial growth secondary to glycosuria

Injury, risk for (maternal or fetal) Risk factors: Hypoglycemia, hyperglycemia

Nutrition, imbalanced: less than body requirements Related factors: Inadequate intake to support increased calorie needs of pregnancy, secondary to limited exposure to basic nutritional knowledge; *Nausea*

Nutrition, imbalanced: more than body requirements Related factors: Limited exposure to new basic nutritional knowledge, imbalance between intake and available insulin

Hyperemesis Gravidarum

Potential Complications (Collaborative Problems)

PC of hyperemesis: Bleeding secondary to hypothrombinemia, fetal death, fluid and electrolyte imbalance, hypotension, negative nitrogen balance, peripheral neuropathy

Nursing Diagnoses

Activity intolerance Related factors: Inadequate nutrition, dehydration, decreased activity

Coping, ineffective Related factors: Personal vulnerability during health crisis, projected role changes, worry about safety of fetus

Family processes, interrupted Related factors: Hospitalization or change in environment, illness or disability of family member, threats to job security (of patient or spouse), need for child care for siblings

Fatigue See *Activity intolerance*

Fear Related factor: Real or imagined threat to child

Fluid volume, deficient Related factors: Inadequate fluid intake secondary to *Nausea*, abnormal fluid loss secondary to vomiting

Nutrition, imbalanced: less than body requirements Related factors: Limited intake of nutrients secondary to *Nausea*, loss of nutrients secondary to vomiting

Parenting, risk for impaired See *Role performance, ineffective*

Powerlessness Related factors: Complications threatening pregnancy, perceived or actual inability to change the course of events

Role performance, ineffective Related factors: Unmet expectations for pregnancy, *Nausea*, hospitalization

Self-esteem, low (chronic, situational) Related factors: Unmet expectations for pregnancy, inability to meet role demands (e.g., work, mother, spouse)

Maternal Infection

Includes but is not limited to active genital herpes, amnionitis, AIDS, and hepatitis B

Potential Complications (Collaborative Problems)

PC of infection: Fetal morbidity or mortality, sepsis

Nursing Diagnoses

Activity intolerance Related factors: Disease process, malaise

Body image, disturbed Related factors: Pregnancy, odors and lesions secondary to infection, precautions regarding handwashing and spread of infection

Breastfeeding, interrupted Related factors: Maternal illness, maternal medications that are contraindicated for the infant

Diversional activity, deficient See *Risk for loneliness*

Family processes, interrupted Related factors: Change in family roles, hospitalization or change in environment, unresolved feelings about how the infection was acquired

Fear Related factor: Real or imagined threat to child

Infection, risk for Risk factor: Presence of lesions (e.g., herpes) predispose patient to secondary infections

Infection (transmission), risk for Risk factor: Contagious nature of disease (e.g., herpes, hepatitis B)

Loneliness, risk for Related factor: Therapeutic isolation

Pain Related factors: Cesarean birth, infection, lesions

Parenting, impaired Risk factor: Delayed parent–infant attachment secondary to need for infection precautions

Self-esteem, low (chronic, situational) Related factors: Cesarean birth, inability to assume new role, inability to fulfill usual role requirements (e.g., wife, mother, worker)

Social interaction, impaired Related factor: Therapeutic isolation

Painful Breast

Includes but is not limited to sore, cracked nipples, engorgement, and mastitis.

Potential Complications (Collaborative Problems)

PC of cracked nipples: engorgement: Mastitis

PC of mastitis: Abscess

Nursing Diagnoses

Attachment, risk for impaired Risk factors: *Pain*, unmet expectations

Breastfeeding, ineffective See *Interrupted breastfeeding*

Breastfeeding, interrupted Related factors: *Pain*, engorgement; sore, cracked nipples; mastitis; maternal medications that are contraindicated for the infant

Health maintenance, ineffective Related factors: Limited exposure to information about breast hygiene, care of nipples, treatments, or signs and symptoms of infection

Pain Related factors: Sore nipples, breast engorgement, edema, and inflammation of breast tissues

Role performance, ineffective Related factors: Assumption of new role, unmet expectations for childbirth, *Pain* and discomfort, Interrupted breastfeeding

Skin integrity (nipples), impaired Related factors: Inadequate breast care, improper positioning of baby at breast, incorrect sucking by infant

Perinatal Loss

Includes but is not limited to less-than-perfect baby, miscarriage, stillbirth, adoption, and elective abortion.

Nursing Diagnoses

Coping: family, compromised/disabled Related factor: Chronically unresolved feelings about loss

Coping, ineffective Related factor: Personal vulnerability in a situational crisis

Family processes, interrupted Related factors: Illness or disability of baby, fetal demise, stillbirth, lack of adequate support system, *Complicated grieving*, conflicting styles of grieving among family members, guilt, blaming

Fear Related factors: Real or imagined threat to child, environmental stressors or hospitalization, *Powerlessness*, implications for future pregnancies

Grieving, complicated Related factors: Inability to resolve feelings about actual or anticipated loss of child or of perfect child, marital discord, lack of support system

Parenting, impaired Related factors: Interruption in bonding process, unrealistic expectations of self or partner (see *Interrupted family processes*)

Powerlessness Related factors: Complication threatening pregnancy, inability to change course of events

Role performance, ineffective Related factors: *Complicated grieving* secondary to loss of child, birth of less-than-perfect baby, guilt, blame

Self-esteem, low (chronic, situational) Related factors: Unmet expectations for child, feelings of failure (e.g., to produce a perfect child)

Sexual dysfunction Related factors: Medically imposed restrictions, *Fear* of harming fetus, *Chronic or situational low self-esteem*, *Fear* of another pregnancy

Spiritual distress Related factors: Test of spiritual beliefs, intense suffering

Postpartum Care, Uncomplicated

Potential Complications (Collaborative Problems)

PC of childbirth: Hematoma; hemorrhage secondary to uterine atony, retained placental fragments, lacerations; infection or sepsis

Nursing Diagnoses

Anxiety Related factors: Changes in role functioning, inexperience

Attachment, risk for impaired See *Impaired parenting*

Body image, disturbed Related factors: Lack of or inaccurate information about body's adjustment after delivery, change in body appearance (e.g., striae)

Breastfeeding, effective Related factors: Basic breastfeeding knowledge, normal breast structure, normal infant oral structure, gestational age of more than 34 weeks, supportive resources, maternal confidence

Breastfeeding, ineffective Related factors: *Interrupted breastfeeding*, inexperience, cultural influences, breast engorgement, infant factors (e.g., inability to latch on or suck)

Constipation Related factors: *Fear* of painful defecation, decreased peristalsis after delivery, decreased activity, decreased fluid intake, effects of analgesics, decreased tone of abdominal muscles

Family processes, interrupted Related factors: Transition in family roles, change in family structure, lack of adequate support systems

Health maintenance, ineffective Related factors: *Deficient knowledge* (e.g., hygiene, contraception, nutrition, infant care, symptoms of complications), lack of support from partner

Home maintenance, impaired Related factors: Inadequate support system, lack of organizational skills, *Ineffective coping*

Insomnia Related factors: Excessive social demands, role demands (e.g., frequent breastfeeding), *Pain*, *Anxiety*, exhilaration and excitement

Nutrition, imbalanced: less than body requirements Related factor: Lack of basic nutritional knowledge concerning lactation

Pain Related factors: Episiotomy, sore nipples, breast engorgement, hemorrhoids, sore muscles, uterine contractions (afterpains)

Parenting, impaired Related factors: Lack of knowledge or skill regarding effective parenting; unrealistic expectations of self, infant, and partner; unwanted child; no role models; inexperience

Role performance, ineffective Related factor: Assumption of new role

Sexuality patterns, ineffective Related factors: *Pain*, *Fear* of pain, *Disturbed body image*, demands of infant, lack of sleep

Urinary incontinence, stress Related factor: Tissue trauma during delivery

Urinary retention Related factors: Local tissue edema, effects of medication/anesthesia, *Pain*, inability to assume normal voiding position secondary to effects of epidural anesthesia or analgesia

Preeclampsia

Preeclampsia is sometimes referred to as toxemia of pregnancy, pregnancy-induced hypertension, pregnancy-related hypertension (PRH), and eclampsia (when seizures occur).

Potential Complications (Collaborative Problems)

PC of magnesium sulfate therapy: Magnesium toxicity

PC of PRH: Cerebral edema, coma, fetal morbidity or mortality, HELLP syndrome (hemolysis, elevated liver enzymes, low platelet count), hypertension (malignant), pulmonary edema, renal insufficiency or damage, seizures

PC of malignant hypertension: Uncontrolled hypertension: cerebral hemorrhage

PC of seizures: Precipitous birth, fetal bradycardia, placental separation

Nursing Diagnoses

Activity intolerance Related factors: Imbalance between oxygen supply and demand; lethargy, weakness, and *Fatigue* secondary to prescribed bed rest and magnesium sulfate side effects; preeclampsia

Body image, disturbed Related factors: Changes in appearance related to pregnancy and edema

Breathing pattern, ineffective Related factor: Side effects of magnesium sulfate

Constipation Related factors: Side effects of magnesium sulfate, decreased activity, decreased intake of fiber

Diversional activity, deficient Related factor: Prolonged bed rest

Family processes, interrupted Related factors: Hospitalization or change in environment, illness or disability of family member, enforced bed rest, role changes

Fear Related factors: Changes in birthing plans, real or imagined threat to child (e.g., premature labor), environmental stressors or hospitalization, threat to own well-being

Fluid volume, deficient (intravascular) Related factors: Intercompartmental fluid shifts secondary to loss of plasma proteins and decreased plasma colloid osmotic pressure

Fluid volume excess (extracellular tissues) Related factors: Sodium and water retention, fluid shift into extracellular spaces secondary to decreased plasma colloid osmotic pressure

Home maintenance, impaired Related factors: Inadequate support system, *Deficient knowledge*, inability to perform usual roles

Injury, risk for (maternal and fetal) Risk factors: Seizure activity, inadequate placental perfusion, falls secondary to vertigo or postural hypotension, visual disturbances, fetal distress secondary to inadequate placental perfusion

Nausea Related factor: Side effect of magnesium sulfate

Noncompliance Related factors: Unable to comply with bed rest secondary to perceived demands of role (e.g., care of siblings), perceived negative effects of medical regimen (e.g., unpalatable diet), perception that condition is not serious secondary to having no subjectively unpleasant symptoms, *Deficient knowledge* (e.g., related to disease, treatments, symptom relief, dietary restrictions)

Nutrition, imbalanced: less than body requirements Related factors: Lack of basic nutritional knowledge, loss of appetite, *Nausea* and vomiting, drowsiness secondary to medications

Pain Related factors: Epigastric (precursor to eclampsia), headache secondary to magnesium sulfate administration

Environmental interpretation syndrome, impaired Related factor: Lack of sensory stimulation from caregiver or parents

Sensory perception, disturbed (visual) [non-NANDA-I] Related factor: Alterations precede eclampsia

Tissue perfusion, ineffective: cerebral, renal, placental Related factors: Vasospasm (spiral arteries), edema, decreased intravascular volume

Suppression of Preterm Labor

Potential Complications (Collaborative Problems)

PC of preterm labor: Preterm delivery of infant, pulmonary edema (secondary to tocolytic medications)

PC of magnesium sulfate therapy: Magnesium toxicity

Nursing Diagnoses

Anxiety Related factors: Outcome of pregnancy, side effects of tocolytics, insufficient time to prepare for labor or infant care

Diversional activity, deficient Related factor: Prolonged bed rest

Family processes, interrupted Related factors: Illness or disability of family member, change in family roles, lack of adequate support systems, enforced bed rest

Fear Related factor: Possibility of early labor and delivery

Home maintenance, impaired Related factors: Inadequate support system, enforced bed rest

Nausea Related factor: Side effects of tocolytic medications

Pain (headache) Related factor: Side effects of magnesium sulfate

Powerlessness Related factors: Complications threatening pregnancy, lack of improvement despite complying with bed rest and medication regimen

Self-esteem, low (chronic, situational) Related factors: Unmet expectations for childbirth, inability to fulfill usual roles

Self-Health management, ineffective Related factors: *Deficient knowledge*, excessive demands made on individual or family, social support deficits

Sexual dysfunction Related factors: Medically imposed restrictions, *Fear* of harming fetus, *Fear* of causing uterine contractions

Insomnia Related factors: Frequency of medication and monitoring

Uterine Bleeding

This includes but is not limited to the following conditions: (a) Antepartal bleeding may result from first trimester spotting, placenta previa, abruptio placentae, uterine rupture, or hydatidiform mole; (b) postpartal bleeding may be a consequence of postpartum hemorrhage or shock or uterine atony.

Potential Complications (Collaborative Problems)

PC of uterine bleeding: Anemia, DIC, fetal death, renal failure, sepsis, shock

Nursing Diagnoses

Breastfeeding, interrupted Related factors: Maternal illness, *Fatigue*, Activity intolerance, activities of caregivers

Cardiac output, decreased Related factor: Hypovolemia

Diversional activity, deficient Related factors: Prolonged bed rest or activity limitations

Family processes, interrupted Related factors: Change in family roles, patient's inability to assume usual role, hospitalization or change in environment

Fear Related factors: Threat to the pregnancy or baby, threat to own well-being, *Powerlessness*, environmental stressors or hospitalization, implications for future pregnancies

Grieving Related factors: Possible loss of pregnancy and expected child, possible effect on future childbearing abilities secondary to intractable postpartum hemorrhage

Home maintenance, impaired Related factors: Inadequate support system, prescribed bed rest, *Activity intolerance* secondary to blood loss and anemia

Infection, risk for Risk factors: Traumatized tissue, invasive procedures, blood loss, partial separation of placenta

Mobility: physical, impaired Related factors: Increased bleeding in response to activity, presence of lines (e.g., IV, urinary catheter, fetal monitor)

Pain Related factors: Surgical procedure, uterine contractions, collection of blood between placenta and uterine wall

Powerlessness Related factors: Complications threatening pregnancy or future pregnancies

Self-care deficit: (specify) Related factors: Medically imposed restrictions, *Activity intolerance* secondary to blood loss

Self-esteem, low (chronic, situational) Related factors: Unmet expectations for childbirth, inability to perform usual role functions

Sexual dysfunction Related factors: Medically imposed restrictions, *Fear* of harming fetus, *Fear* of starting labor or increasing bleeding

Tissue perfusion, ineffective or risk for ineffective [placental] Related factors: Imbalance between oxygen supply and demand to the fetus secondary to hypovolemia, hypotension, placental separation

NEWBORN CONDITIONS

Congenital anomalies
Drug withdrawal
Feeding problems
High-risk infant
Hyperbilirubinemia
Hypoglycemia
Hypothermia
Low birth weight/small for gestational age
Normal newborn
Respiratory distress

Congenital Anomalies

Include but are not limited to infants with serious congenital anomalies (e.g., congenital heart disease, meningomyelocele, choanal atresia, tracheo esophageal fistula)

Potential Complications (Collaborative Problems)

PC of congenital heart disease: Congestive heart failure, dysrhythmias

PC of meningomyelocele: Hydrocephalus, neurovascular deficits below lesion

PC of tracheoesophageal fistula Aspiration pneumonia, choking

Nursing Diagnoses

Activity intolerance Related factor: Imbalance between oxygen supply and demand

Aspiration, risk for Risk factor: Secondary to tracheoesophageal fistula

Breastfeeding, ineffective Related factors: Infant *Fatigue*, inadequate sucking reflex, interrupted or infrequent feeding, difficulty breathing, secondary to cardiac anomaly

Breastfeeding, interrupted Related factor: Infant illness

Breathing pattern, ineffective Related factors: Decreased energy or *Fatigue* secondary to cardiac anomaly, aspiration pneumonia

Cardiac output, decreased Related factors: Increased ventricular workload, hypovolemia, cardiac anomaly (specify)

Caregiver role strain Related factors: Illness severity of the infant; premature birth or congenital defect; unpredictable illness course; situational stressors within the family; complexity and duration of caregiving; caregiver's health; lack of developmental readiness, knowledge, skills, or experience; competing role commitments; ineffective coping styles; isolation; limited opportunity for respite and recreation

Development: delayed, risk for See *Growth and development; risk for, delayed*

Family processes, interrupted Related factors: Unmet expectations for child, separation of family members, illness or disability of infant, immaturity of parents, lack of resources, lack of social supports, lack of knowledge

Fatigue Related factor: Disease process (e.g., cardiac anomaly, aspiration pneumonia)

Fear Related factor: Real threat to child

Gas exchange, impaired Related factors: Decreased pulmonary blood supply secondary to pulmonary hypertension, congestive heart failure, respiratory distress syndrome, decreased functional lung tissue secondary to respiratory distress syndrome, atelectasis

Grieving, anticipatory Related factor: Anticipatory loss of child

Growth and development, delayed Risk factors: Congenital anomaly, fetal distress, prematurity, unhealthy maternal lifestyle during pregnancy, serious illness, delayed bonding secondary to infant's condition or parent's unmet expectations

Infant feeding pattern, ineffective Related factors: Prematurity, neurologic impairment or delay, prolonged NPO status, anatomical abnormalities (e.g., of esophagus and stomach), *Fatigue,* and difficulty breathing secondary to heart anomaly

Injury, risk for Risk factors: Meningomyelocele, omphalocele, other defects creating vulnerability

Insomnia Related factor: *Sleep deprivation* secondary to frequent therapeutic interventions

Nutrition, imbalanced: less than body requirements Related factors: Difficulty in swallowing, inadequate sucking reflex in infant, vomiting, food intolerance

Mobility: physical, impaired Related factors: *Fatigue* secondary to inadequate oxygenation, spinal cord lesions

Skin integrity, impaired Related factors: Impaired circulation, immobility (e.g., inability to move lower extremities), See *Nutrition, imbalanced*

Spontaneous ventilation, impaired Related factors: Metabolic factors, respiratory muscle fatigue, pulmonary immaturity

Tissue perfusion: peripheral, ineffective Related factors: Imbalance between oxygen supply and demand secondary to high metabolic rate, *Decreased cardiac output, Impaired gas exchange*

Urinary retention Related factor: Congenital anomaly affecting spinal cord (specify)

Ventilatory weaning response, dysfunctional (DVWR) Related factors: Pulmonary immaturity, *Impaired gas exchange, Ineffective airway clearance*, ventilator dependence >1 week

Drug Withdrawal

Potential Complications (Collaborative Problems)

PC of drug withdrawal: Dehydration, drug or alcohol withdrawal, electrolyte imbalances, respiratory distress syndrome, seizures, sepsis, tachypnea

Nursing Diagnoses

Aspiration, risk for Risk factor: Oral feeding of infant with CNS irritability

Attachment, risk for impaired See *Parenting, impaired*

Breastfeeding, ineffective Related factors: Infant *Fatigue*, poor nursing secondary to alcohol or drug exposure *in utero* and growth-deficient status at birth

Breathing pattern, ineffective Related factors: Depression of respiratory center secondary to ________________ (specify drug), meconium aspiration pneumonia

Coping: family, disabled Related factors: Arbitrary disregard for patient's needs, overwhelming needs of infant in the presence of poor coping skills and continued drug use by parent(s)

Development, delayed (e.g., failure to thrive), risk for See *Growth, disproportionate, risk for*

Diarrhea Related factor: Hyperperistalsis secondary to narcotic withdrawal

Disorganized infant behavior Related factors: Abnormal structural development and CNS dysfunction secondary to alcohol or drug exposure *in utero*, prematurity secondary to maternal drug use, fetal withdrawal *in utero*

Family processes, dysfunctional: Related factors: Alcohol use by parent(s), lack of support from others, lack of coping skills

Fluid volume, deficient Related factors: Inadequate fluid intake secondary to inadequate sucking reflex, vomiting secondary to fetal alcohol syndrome or narcotic withdrawal

Growth, disproportionate, risk for (e.g., small for gestational age) Risk factors: Unhealthy maternal lifestyle during pregnancy, intrauterine exposure to alcohol/drugs

Home maintenance, impaired Related factors: Physical or psychologic impairment of family member other than infant, inadequate support system, insufficient family organization or planning, continued substance abuse by parent(s)

Infant feeding pattern, ineffective Related factors: Neurologic impairment or delay (see *Breastfeeding, ineffective*), lethargy, failure to thrive secondary to fetal alcohol syndrome

Injury, risk for Risk factors: Psychomotor hyperactivity, seizure activity

Insomnia Related factors: Sleep deprivation secondary to ________________ (specify), effect of depressants or stimulants on CNS *in utero*, newborn withdrawal

Nutrition, imbalanced: less than body requirements Related factors: Chemical dependence or withdrawal, inadequate sucking reflex in infant, vomiting, food intolerance, failure to thrive secondary to fetal alcohol syndrome

Parenting, impaired Related factors: Psychologic or developmental impairment of infant, substance abuse by parent(s), presence of stressors (e.g., legal, financial), interrupted bonding process, difficulty interacting with a child with inability to express feelings of pleasure, anger, and so forth

Skin integrity, impaired Related factors: Excoriated buttocks, knees, elbows; facial scratches; pressure point abrasions—all secondary to intrauterine or newborn withdrawal or abstinence syndrome; diaphoresis; *Diarrhea*

Feeding Problems

Include but are not limited to food allergies or intolerances, malabsorption, or motor problems that affect the infant's ability to consume food

Potential Complications (Collaborative Problems)

PC of feeding problems: Anemia, fluid and electrolyte imbalance

Nursing Diagnoses

Breastfeeding, ineffective Related factors: Inadequate sucking reflex in infant, infant *Fatigue* secondary to illnesses such as respiratory distress syndrome or heart anomalies, inability of infant to latch on, CNS anomalies, prematurity

Diarrhea Related factor: Food intolerance

Disorganized infant behavior Related factors: Abnormal structural development and CNS dysfunction, prematurity

Family processes, interrupted Related factors: Illness or disability of family member, separation of family members

Fluid volume, deficient Related factors: Inadequate fluid intake, psychomotor immaturity (e.g., poor suck-swallow response), inadequate milk production, *Diarrhea*

Infant feeding pattern, ineffective Related factors: Prematurity, neurologic impairment or delay, oral hypersensitivity, prolonged NPO status, anatomical abnormalities

Nutrition, imbalanced: less than body requirements Related factors: Difficulty in swallowing, inadequate sucking reflex in the infant, vomiting, food intolerance, failure to thrive, insufficient maternal milk production

Swallowing, impaired Related factor: Motor problem (specify)

High-Risk Infant

Includes but is not limited to birth asphyxia, meconium aspiration, prematurity, postmaturity, large for gestational age (LGA), small for gestational age (SGA), premature rupture of membranes, maternal infection, infant of diabetic mother, intrauterine growth retardation, infant of adolescent mother, infant of chemically dependent mother, and lack of prenatal care

Potential Complications (Collaborative Problems)

PC of *in utero* infections: Anemia, cataracts, congenital heart disease, deafness, hepatosplenomegaly, hydrocephalus, hyperbilirubinemia, mental retardation, microcephaly, seizures, septicemia, thrombocytopenic purpura

PC of prematurity: Acidosis, apnea, bradycardia, cold stress, hyperbilirubinemia, hypocalcemia, hypoglycemia, pneumonia, respiratory distress syndrome, seizures, sepsis

PC of postmaturity: Birth asphyxia, birth trauma secondary to LGA status, CNS depression, cerebral edema, hypoglycemia, intestinal absorption problems, meconium aspiration, polycythemia (due to SGA status), renal tubular necrosis

Nursing Diagnoses

Activity intolerance Related factors: Inadequate oxygenation secondary to respiratory insufficiency, *Ineffective airway clearance*, respiratory distress syndrome

Airway clearance, ineffective Related factors: Meconium aspiration, tracheobronchial secretions

Aspiration, risk for Risk factors: Immobility, increased secretions, presence of enteral or tracheal tubes

Blood glucose, risk for unstable Risk factor: Prematurity, postmaturity

Body temperature, risk for imbalanced See *Thermoregulation, ineffective*

Breastfeeding, ineffective Related factors: Infant *Fatigue*, inadequate sucking reflex, interrupted or infrequent feeding

Breastfeeding, interrupted Related factors: Infant illness, prematurity, maternal obligations outside the home, abrupt weaning of infant

Breathing pattern, ineffective Related factors: Decreased energy or *Fatigue* secondary to illness (e.g., sepsis, respiratory distress syndrome), medication side effects, immature respiratory center, metabolic imbalances

Cardiac output, decreased Related factors: Increased ventricular workload, hypovolemia, cardiac anomaly (specify)

Caregiver role strain Related factors: Illness severity of the infant; premature birth or congenital defect; unpredictable illness course; situational stressors within the family; chronicity of caregiving; caregiver's health; lack of developmental readiness, knowledge, skills, or experience; competing role commitments; ineffective coping styles; isolation; limited opportunity for respite and recreation

Constipation Related factors: Decreased activity and decreased motility secondary to prematurity

Diarrhea Related factor: Increased intestinal motility secondary to inflammation

Disorganized infant behavior Related factors: Immature CNS and excess environmental stimulation

Development, risk for delayed See *Growth, disproportionate, risk for*

Family processes, interrupted Related factors: Illness or disability of family member, separation of family members

Fear (parental) Related factor: Threat to child

Fluid volume, deficient Related factors: Abnormal blood loss, abnormal fluid loss (specify, e.g., *Diarrhea*, diaphoresis), inadequate fluid intake secondary to ________________ (specify, e.g., poor sucking reflex)

Fluid volume excess Related factor: Decreased urinary output secondary to heart failure

Gas exchange, impaired Related factors: Decreased functional lung tissue secondary to pneumonia, chronic lung disease, atelectasis, alveolar capillary membrane changes secondary to inadequate surfactant, cold stress, immature CNS

Grieving, (parental) Related factor: Imminent loss of child

Growth and development, delayed See *Growth, disproportionate, risk for*

Growth, disproportionate, risk for Risk factors: Congenital anomaly, fetal distress, prematurity, unhealthy maternal lifestyle during pregnancy, serious illness

Home maintenance, impaired Related factors: Inadequate support system, insufficient family organization or planning, complex needs of infant

Infant feeding pattern, ineffective Related factors: Prematurity, neurologic impairment or delay, prolonged NPO status, anatomical abnormalities, lethargy

Infection, risk for Risk factors: Inadequate immune system; lack of normal flora; insufficient family knowledge, organization, or planning; invasive treatments or lines; open wounds (e.g., circumcision, umbilical cord), *in utero* infection

Infection (transmission), risk for Risk factor: Contagious nature of organism acquired *in utero*

Nutrition, imbalanced: less than body requirements Related factors: Inadequate sucking reflex in the infant, vomiting, food intolerance, high metabolic rate

Skin integrity, impaired Related factors: Fragility of skin, immobility, susceptibility to infections, and lack of normal skin flora secondary to prematurity; absence of vernix and prolonged exposure to amniotic fluid secondary to postmaturity and LGA status

Spontaneous ventilation, impaired Related factors: Metabolic factors, respiratory muscle fatigue, pulmonary immaturity

Thermoregulation, ineffective Related factors: Prematurity (immature CNS, decreased body mass to body-surface ratio, minimal subcutaneous fat, limited brown fat, inability to shiver or sweat), transition to extrauterine environment, exposure to environment secondary to need for frequent treatments or interventions

Ventilatory weaning response, dysfunctional (DVWR) Related factors: Pulmonary immaturity, *Impaired gas exchange*, *Ineffective airway clearance*, ventilator dependence >1 week

Hyperbilirubinemia

Potential Complications (Collaborative Problems)

PC of hyperbilirubinemia: Anemia, hepatosplenomegaly, hydrops fetalis (including hepatosplenomegaly, anasarca, hydrothorax, ascites, thrombocytopenia, hypoglycemia secondary to adrenal and pancreatic hyperplasia), kernicterus, renal failure

PC of kernicterus: Athetosis, hearing loss, intellectual deficits

PC of phototherapy: Dehydration, diarrhea, hyperthermia, hypothermia, weight loss, retinal damage, corneal abrasions

Nursing Diagnoses

Attachment, risk for impaired Risk factors: Lack of visual stimulation and contact secondary to phototherapy, *Fear* of hurting infant or displacing tubes or lines

Blood glucose, risk for unstable Risk factor: Kernicterus

Breastfeeding, ineffective Related factor: Poor sucking reflex secondary to kernicterus

Breastfeeding, interrupted Related factor: Infant illness

Diarrhea Related factors: Dietary changes, phototherapy

Family processes, interrupted Related factor: Separation of family members

Fluid volume, deficient Related factors: Abnormal fluid loss (specify, e.g., *Diarrhea* and insensible loss secondary to phototherapy), inadequate fluid intake secondary to (specify)

Injury, risk for Risk factor: Reabsorption of bilirubin secondary to decreased defecation

Insomnia Related factors: *Sleep deprivation* secondary to frequent assessment and treatment, discomfort, environmental stimuli

Liver function, risk for impaired Risk factor: Kernicterus

Nutrition, imbalanced: less than body requirements Related factors: Lethargy, inadequate sucking reflex in infant

Parenting, impaired Related factor: Interruption in bonding process

Skin integrity, impaired Related and risk factors: *Diarrhea*, drying of skin secondary to phototherapy, pruritus, excretion of bilirubin in urine and feces, exposure to phototherapy

Tissue integrity, impaired (corneal) Related factors: Phototherapy, continuous wearing of eye pads

Hypoglycemia

Potential Complications (Collaborative Problems)

PC of hypoglycemia: Apnea, CNS damage, respiratory distress, seizures, tremors, jerkiness

Nursing Diagnoses

Cardiac output, decreased Related factor: Poor cardiac contractility

Family processes, interrupted Related factors: Illness of infant, separation of family members, *Ineffective coping*, *Deficient knowledge*

Injury, risk for Risk factor: Seizure activity

Nutrition, imbalanced: less than body requirements Related factors: Inadequate sucking reflex in infant, high metabolic rate or physiologic stress, vomiting, loss of swallowing reflex

Hypothermia

Potential Complications (Collaborative Problems)

PC of hypothermia: Atelectasis, hyperbilirubinemia, hypoglycemia, hypoxemia, metabolic acidosis

Nursing Diagnoses

Breathing pattern, ineffective Related factor: Decreased energy or *Fatigue*, atelectasis

Cardiac output, decreased Related factor: Bradycardia

Family processes, interrupted Related factor: Separation of family members, *Anxiety*, *Ineffective coping*

Nutrition, imbalanced: less than body requirements Related factor: Loss of or decreased appetite

Tissue perfusion: peripheral, ineffective Related factors: Imbalance between oxygen supply and demand, hypoxemia secondary to atelectasis and pulmonary vasoconstriction

Low Birth Weight/Small for Gestational Age

Potential Complications (Collaborative Problems)

PC of SGA: Aspiration syndrome; hypocalcemia; hypoglycemia, causing CNS abnormalities, and mental retardation; hypothermia; perinatal asphyxia; polycythemia

Nursing Diagnoses

Activity intolerance Related factor: Weakness or *Fatigue*

Airway clearance, ineffective Related factors: Decreased energy or *Fatigue*, meconium aspiration

Attachment, risk for impaired Risk factors: Infant's illness, need for technologic support, long hospitalization

Body temperature, imbalanced, risk for Risk factors: Diminished subcutaneous fat, large body surface compared to body mass, decreased brown fat stores

Breastfeeding, ineffective Related factors: Infant *Fatigue*, inadequate sucking reflex, interrupted or infrequent feeding

Breastfeeding, interrupted Related factor: Illness of infant

Breathing pattern, ineffective Related factor: Decreased energy or *Fatigue*

Family processes, interrupted Related factors: Illness or disability of family member, separation of family members, feelings of guilt, blame

Fatigue Related factors: Decreased energy, high metabolic rate, poor oxygenation

Fluid volume, deficient Related factor: Inadequate fluid intake

Gas exchange, impaired Related factors: Decreased pulmonary blood supply secondary to respiratory distress syndrome; decreased functional lung tissue secondary to atelectasis, respiratory distress syndrome, and meconium aspiration

Grieving or Grieving, complicated Related factor: Anticipated or perceived loss of the perfect child

Home maintenance, impaired Related factors: Inadequate support system, insufficient family organization or planning, lack of resources, lack of support

Infant feeding pattern, ineffective See *Imbalanced nutrition: less than body requirements*

Nutrition, imbalanced: less than body requirements Related factors: Inadequate sucking reflex in infant, food intolerance, high metabolic rate, decreased glycogen stores

Parenting, impaired Related factor: Prolonged separation of newborn and parents

Skin integrity, impaired Related factors: Fragile, dry, desquamating skin; lack of subcutaneous fat

Insomnia Related factor: *Sleep deprivation* secondary to frequent therapeutic interventions

Tissue perfusion: peripheral, ineffective Related factors: Imbalance between oxygen supply and demand, increased blood viscosity

Normal Newborn

Potential Complications (Collaborative Problems)

PC of adjustment to extrauterine life: Bleeding secondary to circumcision, cold stress, hemorrhagic disease of newborn, hyperbilirubinemia, hypoglycemia, meconium aspiration pneumonia

Nursing Diagnoses

Airway clearance, ineffective Related factors: Oropharynx secretions, obligatory nose breather, apnea

Body temperature, risk for imbalanced Risk factors: Large body surface to mass ratio, inability to shiver, extrauterine transition

Fluid volume, deficient Related factors: Inadequate oral intake, increased metabolic rate secondary to excessive handling of newborn

Infection, risk for Risk factors: Lack of acquired immunity, inadequate primary defenses (e.g., open wound such as circumcision) and secondary defenses (e.g., altered phagocytosis), lack of normal flora, exposure to pathogens (e.g., *Neisseria gonorrhoeae*) during passage through birth canal

Nutrition, imbalanced: less than body requirements Related factors: *Ineffective breastfeeding*, inadequate breast milk production, inadequate glucose stores, parental *Deficient knowledge*

Pain Related factors: Circumcision, gastroesophageal reflux, colic

Parent/infant attachment, risk for impaired Risk factors: *Anxiety* about parenting, unmet expectations of parents for labor, delivery, and infant; lack of early parent–infant contact; marital discord; lack of privacy during immediate postpartum period

Parenting, impaired Related factors: *Deficient knowledge* (e.g., related to infant care, follow-up visits), *Anxiety* over new roles, lack of support, financial problems, marital problems

Skin integrity, impaired Related and risk factors: Lack of normal skin flora, inadequate primary or secondary defenses, relative fragility of skin

Thermoregulation, ineffective See *Body temperature, risk for imbalanced*

Urinary retention Related factor: Urethral obstruction secondary to postcircumcision edema

Respiratory Distress

Includes but is not limited to bronchopulmonary dysplasia, respiratory distress syndrome and hyaline membrane disease, meconium aspiration, pneumonia, pneumothorax, and transient tachypnea

Potential Complications (Collaborative Problems)

PC of respiratory distress: Acidosis, atelectasis, cardiopulmonary shunting, hypoxemia, respiratory failure

Nursing Diagnoses

Activity intolerance Related factor: Weakness and *Fatigue* secondary to inadequate oxygenation and respiratory difficulty

Airway clearance, ineffective Related factors: Decreased energy and *Fatigue*, tracheobronchial secretions

Aspiration, risk for Risk factors: Presence of enteral or tracheal tubes, increased oropharyngeal secretions

Breastfeeding, interrupted Related factors: Prematurity, infant illness

Breathing pattern, ineffective Related factors: Decreased energy and *Fatigue*, dependence on ventilator

Cardiac output, decreased Related factors: Increased ventricular workload, cardiac anomaly (specify), hypotension

Caregiver role strain Related and risk factors: Life-threatening illness, premature birth or congenital defect; unpredictable illness course; situational stressors within the family; chronicity of caregiving; caregiver's health; lack of developmental readiness, knowledge, skills, or experience; competing role commitments; ineffective coping styles; isolation; limited opportunity for respite and recreation; financial difficulties

Constipation Related factor: Decreased fluid intake

Coping: family, compromised/disabled Related factors: Life-threatening illness, ineffective communication among family members, lack of support, lack of resources (see *Caregiver role strain*)

Family processes, interrupted Related factors: Illness or disability of family member, separation of family members (see *Caregiver role strain* and *Family Coping, Compromised/disabled)*

Fatigue Related factor: Disease process

Fear (parental) Related factor: Real threat to child

Fluid volume, deficient Related factors: Inadequate fluid intake secondary to *Fatigue* with oral feedings, prescribed fluid restrictions (e.g., to treat cerebral edema), abnormal fluid loss (insensible water loss secondary to rapid respiratory rate)

Gas exchange, impaired Related factors: Decreased pulmonary blood supply secondary to pulmonary hypertension and persistent fetal circulation, respiratory distress syndrome, decreased functional lung tissue secondary to pneumonia, atelectasis, respiratory distress syndrome, diaphragmatic hernia

Grieving, anticipatory (parental) Related factor: Anticipated or perceived loss of child

Home maintenance, impaired Related factors: Inadequate support system, insufficient family planning or organization, overwhelming demands of caregiving and maintaining usual roles

Infant feeding pattern, ineffective Related factors: Prematurity, anatomical abnormalities

Infection, risk for Risk factors: Inadequate immune system, invasive procedures, break in primary defenses (e.g., circumcision, umbilical cord)

Insomnia Related factor: *Sleep deprivation* secondary to frequent therapeutic interventions

Nutrition, imbalanced: less than body requirements Related factors: Inadequate sucking reflex in infant, food intolerance, high metabolic rate of stressed infant, lethargy

Skin integrity, impaired Related and risk factors: Decreased peripheral perfusion, fragility of skin, lack of normal skin flora

Spontaneous ventilation, impaired Related factors: Metabolic factors, respiratory muscle fatigue, pulmonary immaturity

Thermoregulation, ineffective Related factors: Increased respiratory effort secondary to respiratory distress syndrome

Tissue perfusion: peripheral, ineffective Related factors: Imbalance between oxygen supply and demand, compensatory responses

Ventilatory weaning response, dysfunctional (DVWR) Related factors: Pulmonary immaturity, *Impaired gas exchange*, *Ineffective airway clearance*, ventilator dependence >1 week

PEDIATRIC CONDITIONS

Developmental problems/needs related to illness
Burns
Cancer (see *Medical conditions: Cancer*)
Casts and traction
Child abuse
Cleft lip/cleft palate: surgical repair
Coagulation disorders
Congenital malformations of the central nervous system: surgical repair
Diabetes mellitus (see *Medical conditions: Diabetes mellitus/hypoglycemia*)
Failure to thrive
Gastroenteritis
Gastrointestinal obstruction: Surgical repair
Infection of CNS
Ingestion or accidental poisoning
Juvenile rheumatoid arthritis (see *Medical conditions: Arthritis*)
Obese child
Osteomyelitis
Pregnancy in adolescence
Renal failure, Acute (see *Medical conditions: Renal failure, Acute*)
Renal failure, Chronic (see *Medical conditions: Renal failure, Chronic*)
Respiratory disorder, chronic
Respiratory infection, acute
Rheumatic fever (see *Medical conditions: Pericarditis/endocarditis*)
Seizure disorders

Sepsis
Sickle cell crisis
Suicidal adolescent (see *Psychiatric conditions: Suicide*)
Tonsillectomy

Developmental Problems/Needs Related to Illness

The following nursing diagnoses (as well as *Deficient knowledge*) should be considered for all pediatric medical/surgical conditions. For nursing diagnoses specific to a medical condition (e.g., burns, gastroenteritis), add the nursing diagnoses in that section to the following general illness and development-related diagnoses that apply.

Nursing Diagnoses

Activity intolerance Related factors: Decreased strength and endurance, weakness and *Fatigue*, imbalance between oxygen supply and demand, *Pain (acute or chronic)*, *Imbalanced nutrition: less than body requirements*, limited mobility, frail or debilitated state, chronic illness, decreased hemoglobin, dehydration

Anxiety Related factors: Threat to or change in role functioning and interaction patterns, unmet needs, separation anxiety

Caregiver role strain Related factors: Illness severity of the child, premature birth or congenital defect, developmental delay or retardation of the child or caregiver, marginal caregiver coping patterns, duration of caregiving required, caregiver's competing role commitments, complexity and amount of caregiving tasks, lack of respite and recreation for caregiver

Coping: family, compromised/disabled Related factors: Arbitrary disregard for child's needs, conflicting coping styles, highly ambivalent relationships (see *Interrupted family processes* and *Caregiver role strain*)

Decisional conflict Related factors: Necessity to make choices about treatments or interventions, weighing needs of ill child against those of healthy siblings

Development, risk for delayed See *Growth and development, delayed*

Diversional activity, deficient Related factors: Separation from school, friends, and family secondary to hospitalization or disability, *Pain*, illness

Family processes, interrupted Related factors: Change in family roles, illness or disability of family member, unmet expectations for child, inadequate support systems, overwhelming stressors, emotional and physical exhaustion, financial problems, separation of family members, prolonged illness

Fear Related factors: *Powerlessness*, threat to well-being of self/child

Grieving, and Grieving, complicated Related factors: Loss (actual or anticipated) secondary to the particular condition, chronic illness

Growth, disproportionate, risk for See *Growth and development, delayed*

Growth and development, delayed Related factors: Inability to achieve developmental tasks secondary to serious illness, prescribed dependence or limitations

Health behavior, risk prone Related factors: Incomplete grieving, *Complicated grieving*, necessity for major lifestyle or behavior change, pattern of dependence, inadequate support systems, failure to accomplish developmental tasks

Home maintenance, impaired Related factors: Home environment obstacles, inadequate support system, insufficient family organization or planning, insufficient finances, lack of familiarity with community resources, developmental disability of caregivers, physical and psychologic impairment of family member other than patient, *Deficient knowledge*

Hopelessness Related factor: Failing or deteriorating physical condition of child

Noncompliance Related factors: Denial of illness, negative consequence of treatment regimen, perceived benefits of continued illness, lack of parental supervision or support

Parenting, impaired Related factors: Interruption in bonding process; treatment-imposed separation; abuse, rejection, or overprotection secondary to inadequate coping skills; lack of knowledge or skill necessary to address the child's special needs; inadequate supports and resources

Powerlessness Related factor: Chronic illness

Role conflict, parental Related factors: Separation of family members secondary to hospitalization(s) of child, inability to maintain usual role demands (e.g., work, spouse), intimidation with invasive or technical procedures

Role performance, ineffective Related factors: Chronic illness, *Chronic pain*

Self-care deficit: (specify) Related factors: Specific to illness (e.g., depression, *Pain* and discomfort, *Activity intolerance*, decreased strength and endurance)

Self-esteem, low (chronic, situational) Related factors: Chronic illness, *Chronic pain*

Self-health management, ineffective Related factors: *Deficient knowledge* (e.g., illness or surgical procedure, signs and symptoms of complications, medications, home care and treatments, dietary modifications), complex treatments and medication regimens

Social interaction, impaired Related factors: Self-concept disturbance, limited physical mobility

Social isolation Related factors: Actual or perceived reactions of others to child's disability, intensity of caregiving demands (e.g., lack of time, energy)

Spiritual distress Related factor: Test of spiritual beliefs

Burns

Nursing Diagnoses

See *Medical conditions: Burns*, and *Pediatric conditions: Developmental problems/needs related to illness (preceding).*

Body image, disturbed Related factors: Burns, scarring

Body temperature, imbalanced, risk for Risk factors: Dehydration secondary to impairment in skin integrity, infection

Constipation Related factors: Decreased GI motility, dehydration

Coping, ineffective Related factors: Multiple stressors (e.g., severe injury, *Pain*, repeated painful procedures, *Fear* of disfigurement), prolonged treatment period

Fear Related factors: Painful therapeutic procedures, environmental stressors secondary to hospitalization, separation from family

Fluid volume, deficient Related factor: Abnormal fluid loss secondary to loss of skin integrity

Infection, risk for Risk factors: Malnutrition, loss of primary defense (i.e., *Impaired skin integrity*)

Nutrition, imbalanced: less than body requirements Related factors: High metabolic needs, loss of appetite secondary to *Fear* and *Pain*

Pain Related factors: Injury, *Fear*

Skin integrity, impaired Related factors: Burns, immobility

Social interaction, impaired Related factor: Fear of rejection

Social isolation Related factor: Reactions of others to disfigurement

Casts and Traction

Includes but is not limited to orthopedic trauma and congenital hip dysplasia. See *Surgical Conditions: Musculoskeletal Surgery;* and *Pediatric Conditions: Developmental Problems/Needs Related to Illness.*

Nursing Diagnoses

Body image, disturbed Related factors: Surgery, appliances, congenital defects

Constipation Related factors: Immobility, opioid analgesics

Infection, risk for Risk factors: *Impaired tissue integrity* secondary to trauma or surgery, broken skin (e.g., secondary to pins)

Mobility: physical, impaired Related factors: *Pain* and discomfort, medically imposed restrictions, musculoskeletal impairment, casts, traction

Neurovascular dysfunction: peripheral, risk for Risk factors: Immobilization, tissue trauma

Pain Related factors: *Pain* secondary to injury, *Pain* secondary to surgery, muscle cramps secondary to immobilization, muscle soreness (e.g., from walking with crutches)

Skin integrity, impaired Related factors: Altered circulation, prescribed immobility, *Impaired mobility* secondary to pain, broken skin (e.g., secondary to external pins)

Tissue perfusion, ineffective (peripheral) Related factors: Interruption of venous flow to ________________ (specify) secondary to constriction pressure; interruption of arterial flow to ________________ (specify) secondary to compartmental syndrome, tissue trauma

Urinary incontinence, functional Related factor: Mobility deficits

Child Abuse

Nursing Diagnoses

See *Pediatric Conditions: Developmental Problems/Needs Related to Illness*.

Coping: family, compromised/disabled Related factors: Chronically unresolved feelings (specify), lack of extended family, financial problems, highly ambivalent family relationships, unwanted child, unwanted characteristics of child (e.g., appearance, mental retardation, hyperactivity), substance-abusing family member, emotionally disturbed family member, use of violence to manage conflict, child sexual or physical abuse

Coping (abuser), ineffective Related factors: History of abuse by own family, lack of love from own family, *Social isolation*, lack of support system, *Situational low self-esteem*, mental illness, emotional immaturity, unrealistic expectations of child

Coping (child), ineffective Related factor: Personal vulnerability in situational crisis

Fear (child) Related factors: Real threat to own well-being, *Powerlessness*, possibility of placement in a foster home

Fear (parent) Related factors: Possibility that abuse will be discovered, anticipated reactions of others, loss of child, criminal prosecution

Hopelessness Related factors: Long-term stress or abuse, inability to escape

Injury, risk for Risk factors: Physical or psychologic abuse, parental neglect

Insomnia Related factors: *Anxiety*, emotional state

Nutrition, imbalanced: less than body requirements Related factor: Parental neglect

Pain Related factor: Trauma

Parenting, impaired Related factors: Absent or ineffective role model; interruption in bonding process; lack of knowledge or skill; lack of or inappropriate response of child to parent; lack of support for nurturing figure(s); psychologic impairment; physical illness; unrealistic expectations of self, child, or partner; dysfunctional relationship between parents or nurturing figures; situational crisis (specific to family)

Posttrauma syndrome Related factors: Abuse, assault, torture, accidents, and incest

Self-esteem, low (chronic, situational) Related factors: Abuse, negative feedback from family members, feelings of abandonment

Social interaction, impaired Related factors: *Chronic or situational low self-esteem*, isolation enforced by parents

Social isolation See *Social interaction, impaired*

Trauma (specify; e.g., poisoning, physical injury), risk for Risk factors: Vulnerability secondary to congenital problems or chronic illness; lack of support system for caregivers; dysfunctional family interactions

Violence: directed at others, risk for Risk factor: History of physical or mental abuse by others

Cleft Lip/Cleft Palate: Surgical Repair

See *Pediatric Conditions: Developmental Problems/Needs Related to Illness*.

Potential Complications (Collaborative Problems)

PC of cleft lip/palate: Failure to thrive, otitis media, excessive scar formation, poor cosmetic effect secondary to sloughing of sutures

PC of cleft lip/palate, surgical repair: Hypostatic pneumonia

Nursing Diagnoses

Airway clearance, ineffective Related factor: Edema secondary to surgery

Aspiration, risk for Risk factors: Aspiration of feedings through congenital defect in palate, postoperative aspiration of mucus and blood

Body image, disturbed Related factor: Obvious congenital anomaly

Communication: verbal, impaired Related factors: Incomplete palate repair, delayed muscle development, dental problems, hearing loss

Fear Related factors: Environmental stressors or hospitalization, separation from parent, parental *Fear* that child will aspirate or suture line will be harmed

Fluid volume, deficient Related factor: Deviation affecting access to or intake of fluids secondary to difficult handling of oral fluids

Infant feeding pattern, ineffective Related factors: Anatomical abnormalities, oral hypersensitivity

Infection, risk for Risk factors: Trauma secondary to surgery, aspiration of feedings, difficulty cleaning sutures

Injury, risk for (disruption of surgical site) Risk factors: Limitations of maturational age; tension on suture line secondary to crying, feeding, or cleansing the area, sucking or blowing

Nutrition, imbalanced: less than body requirements Related factors: Difficulty in chewing, difficulty in swallowing secondary to *Acute pain*, postoperative *Nausea* and vomiting, prescribed diet modifications (e.g., liquids)

Oral mucous membrane, impaired Related factor: Surgery in oral cavity

Pain Related factors: Surgical repair of cleft lip and palate, restraints

Mobility: physical, impaired Related factors: Use of restraints to protect surgical repair

Self-care deficit: feeding Related factors: Age of child and need for adapted feeding

Swallowing, impaired Related factors: *Pain*, unfamiliar method of feeding

Coagulation Disorders

These include but are not limited to hemophilia, von Willebrand disease, and idiopathic thrombocytopenic purpura. See *Pediatric Conditions: Developmental Problems/Needs Related to Illness*; and *Medical Conditions: Blood Disorders*.

Potential Complications (Collaborative Problems)

PC of coagulation disorders: Hemorrhage

Nursing Diagnoses

Coping, ineffective Related factors: Chronic illness and limitations

Fear Related factors: Risks associated with diagnosis (e.g., uncontrollable bleeding, potential joint degeneration, transfusion-acquired diseases)

Mobility: physical, impaired Related factors: Joint hemorrhage, swelling, or degenerative changes; muscle atrophy

Pain Related factors: Joint hemorrhage, swelling

Protection, ineffective Related factors: Abnormal blood profile, medication therapy (e.g., corticosteroids)

Congenital Malformations of the Central Nervous System: Surgical Repair

These include but are not limited to spina bifida, meningocele, myelomeningocele, and hydrocephalus. See *Pediatric Conditions: Developmental Problems/Needs Related to Illness*.

Potential Complications (Collaborative Problems)

PC of hydrocephalus Increased intracranial pressure

PC of myelomeningocele: Hydrocephalus

PC of congenital malformation or surgery of the CNS Neurovascular insufficiency, sepsis, urinary tract infections

Nursing Diagnoses

Bowel incontinence Related factors: Effects of spinal cord anomaly on anal sphincter

Infection, risk for Risk factor: Loss of intact skin secondary to congenital anomaly or surgery

Injury, risk for Risk factors: Increased intracranial pressure or seizures secondary to shunt malfunction in hydrocephalus, inability to support large head

Mobility: physical, impaired Related factor: Neuromuscular impairment secondary to spinal cord involvement

Nutrition, imbalanced: less than body requirements Related factor: Vomiting secondary to increased intracranial pressure

Pain Related factor: Surgery

Sensory perception, disturbed (kinesthetic, tactile) (non-NANDA-I) Related factors: Sensory deficits secondary to spinal cord involvement

Skin integrity, risk for impaired Risk factors: Immobility (e.g., related to limbs, head and neck), incontinence of stool or urine

Urinary elimination, impaired Related factors: Effects of spinal cord anomaly on bladder

Failure to Thrive

See *Pediatric Conditions: Developmental Problems/Needs Related to Illness.*

Potential Complications (Collaborative Problems)

PC of failure to thrive: Dehydration, metabolic disorders

Nursing Diagnoses

Activity intolerance Related factor: Weakness and *Fatigue* secondary to malnutrition

Environmental interpretation syndrome, impaired Related factor: Lack of sensory stimulation from caregiver or parents

Fluid volume, deficient Related factors: Inadequate fluid intake secondary to disinterest in eating or drinking, parental neglect, abnormal fluid loss (loose stools)

Infection, risk for Risk factors: Weakened defenses secondary to malnutrition, parental neglect (e.g., hygiene)

Insomnia Related factors: *Anxiety*, parental emotional deprivation

Nutrition, imbalanced: less than body requirements Related factors: Food intolerance, malabsorption, loss of appetite, parental neglect, lack of emotional and sensory stimulation, parental *Deficient knowledge*, metabolic disorders, organ dysfunction

Skin integrity, impaired Related factors: Impaired nutritional status, parental neglect (e.g., hygiene)

Social interaction, impaired Related factors: Developmental disability, limited physical mobility, *Low self-esteem*

Gastroenteritis

See *Pediatric Conditions: Developmental Problems/Needs Related to Illness.*

Potential Complications (Collaborative Problems)

PC of gastroenteritis: Fluid and electrolyte imbalance

Nursing Diagnoses

Diarrhea Related factors: Food intolerance, infection and inflammation, stress, dietary changes, increased intestinal motility

Fluid volume, deficient Related factors: Abnormal fluid loss (*Diarrhea*, vomiting) secondary to infection, food intolerance, malabsorption

Nutrition, imbalanced: less than body requirements Related factors: Loss of appetite, *Nausea* and vomiting

Oral mucous membrane, impaired Related factor: Dehydration, vomiting

Pain Related factor: *Diarrhea*, abdominal cramps secondary to inflammation, distention, and hyperperistalsis

Environmental interpretation syndrome, impaired Related factor: Electrolyte imbalance

Skin integrity, impaired Related and risk factor: Incontinence of stool secondary to *Diarrhea*

Gastrointestinal Obstruction: Surgical Repair

This includes but is not limited to gastroschisis, omphalocele, intestinal atresia, meconium ileus, imperforate anus, Hirschsprung disease, pyloric stenosis, intussusception, inguinal hernia, and hydrocele. See *Surgical Conditions, Abdominal Surgery*; and *Pediatric Conditions: Developmental Problems/Needs Related to Illness.*

Potential Complications (Collaborative Problems)

PC of GI obstruction/surgery: Hemorrhage, ileus, sepsis

Nursing Diagnoses

Activity intolerance Related factors: Dehydration, electrolyte imbalance, blood loss, inadequate food intake

Body image, disturbed Related factors: Effects of condition or surgery on body

Breathing pattern, ineffective Related factor: *Acute pain*

Fluid volume, deficient Related factors: Abnormal blood loss, abnormal fluid loss, NPO status

Nausea Related factors: *Pain*, abdominal distention, obstruction

Nutrition, imbalanced: less than body requirements Related factors: Loss of appetite, *Nausea* and vomiting, dietary changes

Pain Related factor: Surgery

Skin integrity, impaired Related and risk factors: Altered nutritional status, surgical wound

Infection of Central Nervous System (CNS)

This includes but is not limited to meningitis, encephalitis, rabies, Reye syndrome, and Guillain-Barré syndrome. See *Pediatric Conditions: Developmental Problems/Needs Related to Illness, and Medical Conditions: Neurologic Disorders.*

Potential Complications (Collaborative Problems)

PC of CNS infection: Atelectasis, coma, fluid and electrolyte imbalance, hepatic failure, increased intracranial pressure, pneumonia, renal failure, respiratory distress, seizures, sepsis

PC of Reye syndrome: Diabetes insipidus

Nursing Diagnoses

Airway clearance, ineffective Related factors: Impaired gag reflex, Impaired swallowing, Fatigue, weakness or paralysis of respiratory muscles, tracheobronchial obstruction, aspiration pneumonia

Breathing patterns, ineffective See *Airway clearance, ineffective*

Communication, impaired verbal Related factors: Inability to speak secondary to coma, dysarthrias secondary to weakness of speech muscles

Confusion, acute See *Memory, impaired*

Disuse syndrome, risk for Risk factors: Paralysis, coma

Environmental interpretation syndrome, impaired Related factors: Sensory deficits secondary to coma; sleep deprivation; altered sensory reception, transmission, and integration; electrolyte imbalance; hypoxia; emotional stress

Fluid volume, deficient Related factors: Inadequate fluid intake secondary to *Nausea*, abnormal fluid loss secondary to vomiting, failure of regulatory mechanisms (e.g., diabetes insipidus)

Hyperthermia Related factors: Illness, dehydration, increased metabolic rate secondary to infectious process

Infection, risk for (transmission) Risk factor: Contagious pathogen

Injury, risk for Risk factors: Seizure activity, generalized weakness, reduced coordination, cognitive deficits, sensory deficits, unsteady gait

Memory, impaired Related factors: Decreased cerebral tissue perfusion secondary to edema, hypovolemia, or increased intracranial pressure

Mobility: physical, impaired Related factors: Neuromuscular impairment, coma, *Pain*, partial or complete paralysis, loss of muscle strength and control, muscle rigidity or tremors

Nutrition, imbalanced: less than body requirements Related factors: *Impaired swallowing*, dysphagia or chewing difficulties secondary to cranial nerve involvement

Pain Related factors: *Nausea* and vomiting, headache secondary to meningeal irritation or inflammation, muscle spasms (neck, shoulders), paresthesia

Skin integrity, impaired Related factor: Impaired physical mobility

Suffocation, risk for Risk factors: Decreased level of consciousness, seizures, muscle weakness or paralysis

Swallowing, impaired Related factor: Cerebellar lesions

Tissue perfusion: cerebral, risk for ineffective Related factors: Cerebral edema, increased intracranial pressure, hypovolemia, acidosis

Ingestion/Accidental Poisoning

See *Pediatric Conditions: Developmental Problems/Needs Related to Illness*.

Potential Complications (Collaborative Problems)

PC of lead poisoning: Anemia, aspiration, blindness, burns (e.g., acid, alkaline), hemorrhage, metabolic acidosis, respiratory alkalosis (Carpenito 1997 p. 536)

Nursing Diagnoses

Anxiety Related factors: Emergency nature of situation, concern about parents' reactions, guilt feelings

Breathing pattern, ineffective Related factor: Depression of respiratory center secondary to ________________ (specify drug)

Confusion Related factor: Deposit of lead in brain tissue and central nervous system

Environmental interpretation syndrome, impaired Related factors: Decreased consciousness, encephalopathy

Fluid volume excess Related factors: Decreased urine output secondary to renal dysfunction, vomiting, *Diarrhea*, decreased intake

Injury (e.g., falls), risk for Risk factors: Seizures secondary to lead poisoning, aspirin toxicity, seizures, loss of coordination, decreased level of consciousness

Nutrition, imbalanced: less than body requirements Related factors: Chemically induced changes in GI, anorexia, abdominal *Pain*, anemia secondary to lead poisoning

Pain, chronic Related factor: Deposits of lead in soft tissues and bone

Obese Child

See *Pediatric Conditions: Developmental Problems/Needs Related to Illness.*

Nursing Diagnoses

Activity intolerance Related factors: Sedentary lifestyle, difficulty exercising because of extra weight, exertional discomfort

Body image, disturbed Related factors: Eating disorder (i.e., obesity), view of self in contrast to cultural values

Coping, ineffective Related factor: Use of food to cope with stressors

Family processes, interrupted Related factors: Effects of therapy (e.g., food restriction) on parent–child relationship

Health maintenance, ineffective Related factors: Cultural beliefs, lack of social supports, inability to make deliberate and thoughtful judgments secondary to maturational age, lack of exercise

Mobility: physical, impaired Related factor: Strain on muscles and joints because of weight

Nutrition, imbalanced: more than body requirements Related factors: Psychologic impairment; sedentary lifestyle; lack of basic nutritional knowledge; ethnic or cultural norms; eating as a way of coping; control, sex, or love issues

Self-esteem, low (chronic, situational) Related factors: Obesity, appearance not culturally valued, response of others to obesity

Social interaction, impaired Related factor: Inability to initiate relationships because of self-concept disturbance, embarrassment, and fear of others' negative responses

Social isolation Related factors: Obesity, reactions of others

Osteomyelitis

See *Pediatric Conditions: Developmental Problems/Needs Related to Illness.*

Potential Complications (Collaborative Problems)

PC of osteomyelitis: Infective emboli, pathologic fractures

PC of antibiotic therapy: Hematologic, hepatic, and renal problems; anaphylactic shock

Nursing Diagnoses

Constipation Related factors: Immobility, narcotic medications

Hyperthermia Related factors: Infectious process, increased metabolic rate

Injury, risk for Risk factor: Pathologic fractures related to disease process

Mobility: physical, impaired Related factors: *Pain* and discomfort, musculoskeletal impairment, prescribed immobility

Nutrition, imbalanced: less than body requirements Related factors: High metabolic rate, anorexia secondary to infectious process and *Pain*

Pain Related factors: Inflammation, swelling, hyperthermia, tissue necrosis, fractures

Skin integrity, impaired Related factors: Immobility, irritation from cast or splint

Tissue perfusion: peripheral, risk for ineffective; or **Tissue perfusion: peripheral, ineffective** Related factors: Inflammatory reaction with thrombosis of vessels, edema, abscess formation, tissue destruction

Pregnancy in Adolescence

This includes pregnancy, antepartum and postpartum periods, and parenting. See *Pediatric Conditions: Developmental Problems/Needs Related to Illness*. See also *Antepartum and Postpartum Conditions*.

Nursing Diagnoses

Attachment, risk for impaired See *Parenting, impaired*

Body image, disturbed Related factors: Pregnancy and developmental stage

Coping, ineffective Related factors: Adolescent pregnancy, adolescent parenthood

Health maintenance, ineffective Related factors: Lack of social supports, lack of material resources, cultural beliefs, lack of ability to make deliberate and thoughtful judgments secondary to maturational age

Deficient knowledge (specify) Related factors: Limited exposure to information (e.g., about birth control, parenting), limited practice of skills, information misinterpretation

Nutrition, imbalanced: less than body requirements Related factors: High metabolic needs secondary to both adolescence and pregnancy, lack of basic nutritional knowledge, limited access to food, *Nausea* and vomiting

Nutrition, imbalanced: more than body requirements Related factors: Ethnic or cultural norms, lack of basic nutritional knowledge, "fast" food, "junk" food

Parenting, impaired Related factors: Lack of knowledge or skill; lack of support for nurturing figure from own parents; alienation from own parents; unrealistic expectations of self, infant, and partner; situational crisis

Social interaction, impaired Related factors: Sociocultural conflict, self-concept disturbance, embarrassment, withdrawal from school

Social isolation Related factors: Alteration in physical appearance, life-style changes

Violence: directed at others (child), risk for Risk factors: Rage reaction, history of physical or mental abuse by others, ineffective coping skills, substance abuse

Respiratory Disorder, Chronic

This includes but is not limited to asthma, bronchopulmonary dysplasia, and cystic fibrosis. See *Pediatric Conditions: Developmental Problems/Needs Related to Illness.* See also *Medical Conditions: Acute Respiratory Disorders* (e.g., pneumonia, pulmonary edema, pulmonary embolism), and *Chronic Respiratory Disorders.*

Potential Complications (Collaborative Problems)

PC of chronic respiratory disorder: Hypoxemia, respiratory acidosis

PC of corticosteroid therapy: Hypertension, hypokalemia, hypoglycemia, immunosuppression, osteoporosis, ulcers

Nursing Diagnoses

Activity intolerance Related factors: Inadequate oxygenation secondary to bronchospasm or increased pulmonary secretions

Airway clearance, ineffective Related factors: Tracheobronchial secretions, spasms of the bronchi and bronchioles, ineffective cough secondary to *Fatigue* or weakness

Anxiety Related factors: Air hunger, difficulty breathing, *Fear* of suffocation or dying

Breathing pattern, ineffective Related factors: *Anxiety*, pulmonary infection, decreased energy or *Fatigue*

Fear Related factors: Dyspnea, fear of recurrences

Fluid volume, deficient, risk for Risk factors: Inadequate fluid intake secondary to difficulty in breathing, abnormal fluid loss secondary to increased insensible water loss from rapid respirations

Gas exchange, impaired Related factor: Decreased functional lung tissue secondary to fibrotic, nonventilated areas of lung parenchyma in bronchopulmonary dysplasia

Infection, risk for Risk factors: Malnutrition, stasis of respiratory secretions

Nutrition, imbalanced: less than body requirements Related factors: Loss of appetite with chronic illness, high metabolic needs secondary to pulmonary infection, malabsorption of nutrients secondary to cystic fibrosis

Respiratory Infection, Acute

This includes but is not limited to tonsillitis, pharyngitis, croup, laryngotracheobronchitis, epiglottitis, bronchitis, and pneumonia. See *Pediatric Conditions: Developmental Problems/Needs Related to Illness*. See also *Medical Conditions: Acute Respiratory Disorders* (e.g., pneumonia, pulmonary edema, pulmonary embolism) and *Chronic Respiratory Disorders*.

Potential Complications (Collaborative Problems)

PC of acute respiratory infection: Hypoxemia, respiratory acidosis, respiratory insufficiency, sepsis

PC of corticosteroid therapy: Hypertension, hypokalemia, hypoglycemia, immunosuppression, osteoporosis, ulcers

Nursing Diagnoses

Airway clearance, ineffective Related factors: Edema, increased or viscous tracheobronchial or pulmonary secretions, bronchospasm, tracheobronchial inflammation, pleuritic pain, ineffective cough secondary to *Fatigue*

Anxiety Related factors: *Fear* of dying, dyspnea, inadequate oxygenation

Fear Related factors: Real threat to well-being, environmental stressors or hospitalization, separation from parent, dyspnea, *Fear* of recurring attacks

Fluid volume, deficient Related factors: Inadequate fluid intake secondary to difficulty in breathing, abnormal fluid loss secondary to increased insensible water loss from rapid respirations or fever

Gas exchange, impaired Related factors: Decreased functional lung tissue secondary to pneumonia, air trapping, impaired exchange of oxygen in alveoli secondary to collected secretions, hypoventilation (see *Airway clearance, ineffective*)

Nutrition, imbalanced: less than body requirements Related factors: Loss of appetite secondary to dyspnea and malaise, high metabolic needs

Pain Related factors: Sore throat, *Pain* with inspiration, pleural *Pain*

Skin integrity, risk for impaired Risk factors: Altered nutritional status, hyperthermia, damp therapeutic environment, decreased mobility, diaphoresis

Seizure Disorders

See *Pediatric Conditions: Developmental Problems/Needs Related to Illness*. See also *Medical Conditions: Neurologic Disorders*.

Potential Complications (Collaborative Problems)

PC of seizure disorder: Status epilepticus

Nursing Diagnoses

Airway clearance, ineffective Related factors: Loss of tongue and gag reflexes during seizure activity

Injury, risk for Risk factor: Uncontrolled muscle movements during seizure activity

Self-esteem, low (chronic, situational) Related factors: Chronic illness, feelings of being out of control, stigma associated with seizures, perceived "weakness"

Social interaction, impaired Related factors: Embarrassment, fear of having a seizure in public

Suffocation, risk for Risk factors: Weakness, altered level of consciousness, cognitive limitations

Sepsis

See *Pediatric Conditions: Developmental Problems/Needs Related to Illness.*

Potential Complications (Collaborative Problems)

PC of sepsis: Anemia, edema, hemorrhage, hypotension, hypothermia or hyperthermia, meningitis, respiratory distress, seizures

Nursing Diagnoses

Cardiac output, decreased Related factors: Decreased circulating volume and venous return, increased systemic vascular resistance, effects of hypoxia

Constipation Related factor: Decreased fluid intake

Diarrhea Related factors: Increased intestinal motility, intestinal irritation secondary to infectious process

Fluid volume, deficient Related factors: Decreased fluid intake, fever, widespread vasodilation, and intercompartmental fluid shifts

Gastrointestinal perfusion, risk for ineffective See *Tissue perfusion: Peripheral*

Injury, risk for Risk factor: Seizure activity secondary to high fever

Nutrition, imbalanced: less than body requirements Related factors: Inadequate sucking reflex in infant, vomiting, food intolerance, increased metabolic rate, lethargy

Skin integrity, impaired Related factors: Decreased peripheral perfusion, hyperthermia, edema, immobility

Insomnia Related factors: Frequent therapeutic interventions, discomfort secondary to fever, difficulty breathing, diaphoresis

Tissue perfusion: peripheral (cardiac, cerebral, or renal) Related factors: Selective vasoconstriction, presence of microemboli, hypovolemia

Sickle Cell Crisis

See *Pediatric Conditions: Developmental Problems/Needs Related to Illness*

Potential Complications (Collaborative Problems)

PC of sickle cell crisis: Vaso-occlusive crisis, causing infarctions of vital organs (e.g., liver, kidneys, central nervous system); infections (e.g., pneumonia, osteomyelitis); aplastic crisis (rapidly developing severe anemia); splenic sequestration, causing circulatory collapse

PC of repeated transfusions: Hemosiderosis

Nursing Diagnoses

Body image, disturbed Related factors: Delayed onset of puberty, swelling of the hands and feet, prominence of the bones of the face and skull, *Pain*, need to avoid strenuous activities

Fluid volume, deficient Related factor: Increased need for fluid volume in blood to prevent sickling and thrombosis. (**NOTE:** This is a relative deficit. Enough fluid must be ingested to create hemodilution.)

Gas exchange, impaired Related factors: Susceptibility to pneumonia and pulmonary infarctions, decreased oxygen-carrying capacity of the blood

Infection, risk for Risk factors: Chronic illness, defects in immunologic system

Pain Related factors: Sickle cell crisis, causing tissue hypoxia and impaired peripheral circulation

Tissue perfusion: peripheral (or cardiac, cerebral, gastrointestinal, or renal), ineffective Related factors: Imbalance between oxygen supply and demand secondary to anemia, thrombosis secondary to clumping of red blood cells in sickle cell crisis, increased blood viscosity, arteriovenous shunts in peripheral and pulmonary circulation

Tonsillectomy

See *Pediatric Conditions: Developmental Problems/Needs Related to Illness*.

Potential Complications (Collaborative Problems)

PC of tonsillectomy: Airway obstruction, aspiration, hemorrhage

Nursing Diagnoses

Airway clearance, ineffective Related factors: Trauma, edema, *Pain*, tracheobronchial secretions, collection of blood in oropharynx, vomiting, sedation

Fluid volume, deficient Related factors: Blood loss secondary to surgery of highly vascular site, decreased intake secondary to painful swallowing

Nutrition, imbalanced: less than body requirements Related factors: Loss of appetite secondary to sore throat and blood swallowing

Pain Related factors: Surgery, packing, edema

BIBLIOGRAPHY

General Bibliography

Ackley, B. J., & Ladwig, G. B. (2011). *Nursing diagnosis handbook: An evidence-based guide to planning care* (9th ed.). St. Louis: Mosby.

Bulechek, G., Butcher, H., & Docterman, J. (2008). *Nursing interventions classification (NIC)* (5th ed.). St. Louis: Mosby.

Carpenito-Moyet, L. J. (1997). *Nursing diagnosis: Application to clinical practice* (7th ed.). Philadelphia: Lippincott Williams & Wilkins.

Carpenito-Moyet, L. J. (2006a). *Handbook of nursing diagnoses* (11th ed.). Philadelphia: Lippincott Williams & Wilkins.

Carpenito-Moyet, L. J. (2006b). *Nursing diagnosis: Application to clinical practice* (11th ed.). Philadelphia: Lippincott Williams & Wilkins.

Carpenito-Moyet, L. J. (2010). *Nursing diagnosis: Application to clinical practice* (13th ed.). Philadelphia: Lippincott Williams & Wilkins.

Dochterman, J., & Bulechek, G. (Eds.). (2004). *Nursing interventions classification (NIC)* (4th ed.). St. Louis: Mosby.

Doenges, M. E., Moorhouse, M. F., & Murr, A. C. (2004). *Nurse's pocket guide: Diagnoses, prioritized interventions, and rationales* (10th ed.). Philadelphia, PA: F.A. Davis.

Doenges, M. E., Moorhouse, M. F., & Murr, A. C. (2010). *Nursing diagnosis manual: Planning, individualizing, and documenting client care* (3rd ed.). Philadelphia: F.A. Davis.

Gordon, M. (1994). *Nursing diagnosis: Process and application* (3rd ed.). St. Louis: Mosby.

Johnson, M., Moorhead, S., Bulechek, G., Butcher, H., Maas, M., & Swanson, E. (2012). *NOC and NIC linkages to NANDA-I and clinical conditions* (3rd ed.). St. Louis: Mosby.

Moorhead, S., Johnson, M., Maas, M., & Swanson, E. (2008). *Nursing outcomes classification (NOC)* (4th ed.). St. Louis: Mosby.

NANDA International. (2012). *Nursing diagnoses: Definitions & classification 2012-2014*. Oxford: Wiley-Blackwell.

Activity Intolerance

Astrup, A. (2003). Is there any conclusive evidence that exercise alone reduces glucose intolerance? *British Journal of Diabetes & Vascular Disease, 3,* S18–S23.

Boyd, M. A. (2005). Psychiatric-mental health nursing interventions. In M. A. Boyd (Ed.), *Psychiatric nursing: Contemporary practice* (3rd ed., pp. 218–232). Philadelphia, PA: Lippincott Williams & Wilkins.

Buchner, D. M. (1995). Clinical assessments of physical activity in older adults. In L. Z. Rubenstein, D. Wieland, & R. Bernbei (Eds.), *Geriatric assessment technology: The state of the art* (pp. 147–159). New York: Springer.

da Silva, M., AR, A., Michel, J., & Aparecida Barosa, D. (2006). Most frequently identified nursing diagnoses in HIV/AIDS patients. *International Journal of Nursing Terminologies & Classifications, 17*(1), 53–53.

Garutti Rodrigues, F., & Barros, A. (2006). NIC interventions and NOC outcomes in patients with activity intolerance. *International Journal of Nursing Terminologies & Classifications, 17*(1), 79.

Gordon, M. (1994). *Nursing diagnosis: Process and application* (3rd ed.). St. Louis: Mosby.

Hea-Kung Hur, R. N., Park, S., So-Sun Kim, Storey, M. J., & Gi-yon Kim. (2005). Activity intolerance and impaired physical mobility in elders. *International Journal of Nursing Terminologies & Classifications, 16*(3), 47–53.

Hur, H., Park, S., Kim, S., Storey, M. J., & Kim, G. (2005). Activity intolerance and impaired physical mobility in elders. *International Journal of Nursing Terminologies & Classifications, 16*(3), 47–53.

National Guideline Clearinghouse (NGC). (2001, Revised 2007). Guideline summary: Exercise promotion: Walking in elders. In National Guideline Clearinghouse (NGC). Rockville, MD. Retrieved October 16, 2011, from http://www.guideline.gov/content.aspx?id=10948.

Oguro, V., Espíritu, D., Carmagnani, M., Silva, G., & Michel, J. (2002). Nursing diagnosis identification in hospitalized patients with coronary artery disease during the pre- and postoperative period in a cardiac surgery ward. *Classification of nursing diagnoses: Proceedings of the fourteenth conference, North American Nursing Diagnosis Association* (pp. 206–210). Glendale, CA: CINAHL Information Systems.

Rochester, C. L. (2003). Exercise training in chronic obstructive pulmonary disease. *Journal of Rehabilitation Research & Development, 40*(5), 59–80.

Tack, B. B., & Gilliss, C. L. (1990). Nurse-monitored cardiac recovery: A description of the first 8 weeks. *Heart & Lung, 19*(5), 491–499.

Tiesinga, L. J., Dassesn, T. W. N., & Halfens, R. J. G. (1996). Fatigue: A summary of the definitions, dimensions, and indicators. *Nursing Diagnosis, 7*(2), 51–62.

Tinetti, M., McAvay, G., & Claus, E. (2003). Preventing falls in elderly persons. *New England Journal of Medicine, 348,* 42–49.

Activity Intolerance, Risk for

Bauldoff, G., Hoffman, L., Sciurba, F., & Zullo, T. (1996). Home based upper arm exercises training for patients with chronic obstructive pulmonary disease. *Heart and Lung, 25*(4), 288–294.

Bo, M., Fontana, M., Mantelli, M., & Molaschi, M. (2006). Positive effects of aerobic physical activity in institutionalized older subjects complaining of dyspnea. *Archives of Gerontology & Geriatrics, 43*(1), 139–145.

Cobb, S. L., Brown, D. J., & Davis, L. L. (2006). Effective interventions for lifestyle change after myocardial infarction or coronary artery revascularization. *Journal of the American Academy of Nurse Practitioners, 18*(1), 31–39.

Cohen, J., Gorenberg, B., & Schroeder, B. (2000). A study of functional status among elders at two academic nursing centers. *Home Care Provider, 5*(3), 108–112.

Activity Planning, Ineffective

American Psychiatric Association. (2004). *Mini DSM IV-TR* (p. 384). Paris: Masson.

Noud, R. B., & Lee, K. (2005). Anxiety disorders. In M. A. Boyd (Ed.), *Psychiatric nursing: Contemporary practice* (3rd ed., pp. 374–419). Philadelphia: Lippincott Williams & Wilkins.

Riberio, K. L. (1999). The labyrinth of community mental health: In search of meaningful occupation. *Psychiatric Rehabilitation Journal, 23,* 2.

Activity Planning: Ineffective, Risk for

American Psychiatric Association. (2004). *Mini DSM IV-TR* (p. 384). Paris: Masson.

Beck, A., Rush, A., Shaw, B., & Emery, G. (1979). *Cognitive therapy of depression.* New York: Guilford Press.

Ellis, A. (1962). *Reason and emotion in psychotherapy.* New York: Secausus, Lyle Stuart.

Noud, R. B., & Lee, K. (2005). Anxiety disorders. In M. A. Boyd (Ed.), *Psychiatric nursing: Contemporary practice* (3rd ed., pp. 374–419). Philadelphia: Lippincott Williams & Wilkins.

Riberio, K. L. (1999). The labyrinth of community mental health: In search of meaningful occupation. *Psychiatric Rehabilitation Journal,* (23), 2.

Seyle, H. (1959). *The stress of life.* New York: McGraw-Hill.

Adaptive Capacity: Intracranial, Decreased

Alverzo, J. P. (2006). A review of the literature on orientation as an indicator of level of consciousness. *Journal of Nursing Scholarship, 38*(2), 159–164.

Blissitt, P. A. (2006). Care of the critically ill patient with penetrating head injury. *Critical Care Nursing Clinics of North America, 18*(3), 321–332.

Carty, R., Mooraby, R., & Paterson, J. (2006). Stroke management. Evolution of a model for the thrombolysis of acute stroke patients. *British Journal of Nursing (BJN), 15*(8), 453–457.

Cook, N. F., Deeny, P., & Thompson, K. (2004). Management of fluid and hydration in patients with acute subarachnoid haemorrhage—an action research project. *Journal of Clinical Nursing, 13*(7), 835–849.

Ewert, T., Grill, E., Bartholomeyczik, S., Finger, M., Mokrusch, T., Kostanjsek, N., et al. (2005). ICF core set for patients with neurological conditions in the acute hospital. *Disability & Rehabilitation, 27*(7), 367–373.

Fan, J. (2004). Effect of backrest position on intracranial pressure and cerebral perfusion pressure in individuals with brain injury: A systematic review. *Journal of Neuroscience Nursing, 36*(5), 278–288.

Grill, E., Ewert, T., Chatterji, S., Kostanjsek, N., & Stucki, G. (2005). ICF core sets development for the acute hospital and early post-acute rehabilitation facilities. *Disability & Rehabilitation, 27*(7), 361–366.

Hafsteinsdóttir, I. B., Algra, A., Kappelle, L. J., & Grypclonck, M. H. F. (2005). Neurodevelopmental treatment after stroke: A comparative study. *Journal of Neurology, Neurosurgery & Psychiatry, 76*(6), 788–792.

Kneafsey, R., & Gawthorpe, D. (2004). Head injury: Long-term consequences for patients and families and implications for nurses. *Journal of Clinical Nursing, 13*(5), 601–608.

March, K. (2005). Intracranial pressure monitoring: Why monitor? *AACN Clinical Issues: Advanced Practice in Acute & Critical Care, 16*(4), 456–475.

Marcoux, K. K. (2005). Management of increased intracranial pressure in the critically ill child with an acute neurological injury. *AACN Clinical Issues: Advanced Practice in Acute & Critical Care, 16*(2), 212.

Mathiesen, C., Tavianini, H. D., & Palladino, K. (2006). Best practices in stroke rapid response: A case study. *MEDSURG Nursing, 15*(6), 364–369.

National Guideline Clearinghouse (NGC). (2000, Revised 2007). Guideline Summary: Guidelines for the management of severe traumatic brain injury. Cerebral perfusion thresholds. In: National Guideline Clearinghouse (NGC) website. Rockville, MD. Retrieved October 16, 2011, from http://www.ngc.gov/content.aspx?id=10997.

Price, T., & McGloin, S. (2003). A review of cooling patients with severe cerebral insult in ICU (part 1). *Nursing in Critical Care, 8*(1), 30–36.

Stier-Jarmer, M., Grill, E., Ewert, T., Bartholomeyczik, S., Finger, M., Mokrusch, T., et al. (2005). ICF core set for patients with neurological conditions in early post-acute rehabilitation facilities. *Disability & Rehabilitation, 27*(7), 389–395.

Wojner, A. W., El-Mitwalli, A., & Alexandrov, A. V. (2002). Effect of head positioning on intracranial blood flow velocities in acute ischemic stroke: A pilot study. *Critical Care Nursing Quarterly, 24*(4), 57–66.

Yanko, J., & Mitcho, K. (2001). Acute care management of severe traumatic brain injuries. *Critical Care Nursing Quarterly, 23*(4), 1–23.

Zeitzer, M. B. (2005). Inducing hypothermia to decrease neurological deficit: Literature review. *Journal of Advanced Nursing, 52*(2), 189–199.

Airway Clearance, Ineffective

Alves Napoleão, A., & Campos de Carvalho, E. (2006). Ineffective airway clearance: Applicability of NIC priority interventions in a Brazilian pediatric intensive care unit. *International Journal of Nursing Terminologies & Classifications, 17*(1), 76.

Collard, H., Saint, S., & Matthay, M. (2003). Prevention of ventilator-associated pneumonia: An evidence-based systemic review. *Annals of Internal Medicine, 138*(6), 494.

Drakulovic, M., Torres, A., Bauer, T., Nicolas, J., Nogue, S., & Ferrer, M. (1999). Supine body position as a risk factor for nosocomial pneumonia in mechanically ventilated patients: A randomized trial. *Lancet, 354*(9193), 1851.

Elkins, M. R., Jones, A., & van der Schans, C. (2006). Positive expiratory pressure physiotherapy for airway clearance in people with cystic fibrosis. *Cochrane Library* (4). DOI: 10.1002/14651858.CD003147.pub3

Fifoot, S., Wilson, C., MacDonald, J., & Watter, P. (2005). Respiratory exacerbations in children with cystic fibrosis: Physiotherapy treatment outcomes. *Physiotherapy Theory & Practice, 21*(2), 103–111.

Marques, A., Bruton, A., & Barney, A. (2006). Clinically useful outcome measures for physiotherapy airway clearance techniques: A review. *Physical Therapy Reviews, 11*(4), 299–307.

McCool, F. D. (2006). Global physiology and pathophysiology of cough: ACCP evidence-based clinical practice guidelines. *Chest, 129,* 48S–53S.

McCool, F. D., & Rosen, M. J. (2006). Nonpharmacologic airway clearance therapies: ACCP evidence-based clinical practice guidelines. *Chest, 129,* 250S–259S.

Prasad, S. A., & Main, E. (2006). Routine airway clearance in asymptomatic infants and babies with cystic fibrosis in the UK: Obligatory or obsolete? *Physical Therapy Reviews, 11*(1), 11–20.

Pryor, J. A. (2006). Airway clearance in the spontaneously breathing adult—the evidence. *Physical Therapy Reviews, 11*(1), 5–10.

Rajkumar, A., Karmarkar, A., & Knott, J. (2006). Pulse oximetery: An overview. *Journal of Perioperative Practice, 16,* 502–504.

Smith-Sims, K. (2001). Hospital-acquired pneumonia. *American Journal of Nursing, 101*(1), 24AA.

Wilkinson, J., & Treas, L. (2011). Performing upper airway suctioning, pp. 870–873; Caring for a patient requiring mechanical ventilation, pp. 873–877; Setting up disposable chest drainage systems, pp. 877–882; Tips for obtaining accurate pulse oximetery readings, p. 887; Guidelines for preventing aspiration, p. 888. *Fundamentals of Nursing* (Vol. 2). Philadelphia: F. A. Davis Company.

Anxiety

Antall, G., & Kresevic, D. (2004). The use of guided imagery to manage pain in an elderly orthopaedic population. *Orthopaedic Nursing, 23*(5), 335–340.

Bartels, S. (2002). Patients with depression and anxiety might be contemplating suicide. *Geriatrics, 57,* 8.

Byrne, B. (2000). Relationships between anxiety, fear, self-esteem, and coping strategies in adolescence. *Adolescence, 35*(137), 201–216.

Carpenito-Moyet, L. (2006). *Nursing diagnosis: Application to clinical practice.* Philadelphia: Lippincott Williams & Wilkins.

Christie, W., & Moore, C. (2005). The impact of humor on patients with cancer. *Clinical Journal of Oncology Nursing, 9*(2), 211.

Cooke, M., Chaboyer, W., & Hiratos, M. A. (2005). Music and its effect on anxiety in short waiting periods: A critical appraisal. *Journal of Clinical Nursing, 14*(2), 145–155.

Cooke, M., Chaboyer, W., Schluter, P., & Hiratos, M. (2005). The effect of music on preoperative anxiety in day surgery. *Journal of Advanced Nursing, 52*(1), 47–55.

Deering, C. (2006). Therapeutic relationships and communication. In W. K. Mohr (Ed.), *Psychiatric-mental health nursing* (6th ed., pp. 55–78). Philadelphia: Lippincott Williams & Wilkins.

Fleet, R., Lesperance, F., Arsenault, A., Gregoire, J., Lavoie, K., Laurin, C., et al. (2005). Myocardial perfusion study of panic attacks in patients with coronary artery disease. *The American Journal of Cardiology, 96*(8), 1064–1068.

Gold, J. I., Seok Hyeon Kim, Kant, A. J., Joseph, M. H., & Rizzo, A. (2006). Effectiveness of virtual reality for pediatric pain distraction during IV placement. *CyberPsychology & Behavior, 9*(2), 207–212.

Gunnarsdottir, T. J., & Jonsdottir, H. (2007). Does the experimental design capture the effects of complementary therapy? A study using reflexology for patients undergoing coronary artery bypass graft surgery. *Journal of Clinical Nursing, 16*(4), 777–785.

Halm, M., & Alpen, M. (1993). The impact of technology on patients and families. *Nursing Clinics of North America, 33*(1), 135.

Jolley, J. (2007). Separation and psychological trauma: A paradox examined. *Paediatric Nursing, 19*(3), 22–25.

Keister, K. J. (2006). Predictors of self-assessed health, anxiety, and depressive symptoms in nursing home residents at week 1 postrelocation. *Journal of Aging & Health, 18*(5), 722–742.

Lai, H., Chen, C., Peng, T., Chang, F., Hsieh, M., Huang, H., et al. (2006). Randomized controlled trial of music during kangaroo care on maternal state anxiety and preterm infants' responses. *International Journal of Nursing Studies, 43*(2), 139–146.

Lipsky, D., & Richards, W. (2009). *Managing meltdowns: Using the S.C.A.R.E.D. calming technique with children*. Athenaeum Press: Gateshead, Tyne and Wear.

May, R. (1977). *The meaning of anxiety*. New York: W.W. Norton.

McKinley, S., Coote, K., & Stein-Parbury, J. (2003). Development and testing of a faces scale for the assessment of anxiety in critically ill patients. *Journal of Advanced Nursing, 41*(1), 73–79.

Melnyk, B., Feinstein, N., Moldenhouer, Z., & Small, L. (2001). Coping in parents of children who are chronically ill. *Pediatrics, 27*(6), 548–558.

Roffe, L., Schmidt, K., & Ernst, E. (2005). A systematic review of guided imagery as an adjuvant cancer therapy. *Psycho-Oncology, 14*(8), 607–617.

Rothrock, N. B., Matthews, A. K., Sellergren, S. A., Fleming, G., & List, M. (2004). State anxiety and cancer-specific anxiety in survivors of breast cancer. *Journal of Psychosocial Oncology, 22*(4), 93–109.

Ruiz, R. J., & Avant, K. C. (2005). Effects of maternal prenatal stress on infant outcomes: A synthesis of the literature. *Advances in Nursing Science, 28*(4), 345–355.

Stuart, G., & Sundeen, S. (Eds.). (1995). *Principles and practice of psychiatric nursing* (5th ed.). St. Louis, MO: Mosby-Year Book.

Tusaie, K., & Dyer, J. (2004). Resilience: A historical review of construct. *Holistic Nursing Practice, 18*(1), 3–8.

Vanderboom, T. (2007). Does music reduce anxiety during invasive procedures with procedural sedation? An integrative research review. *Journal of Radiology Nursing, 26*(1), 15–22.

Vaughn, F., Wichowski, H., & Bosworth, G. (2007). Does preoperative anxiety level predict postoperative pain? *AORN Journal, 85*(3), 589.

Wilkinson, J., & Treas, L. (2011). *Fundamentals of nursing* (2nd ed., Vol. 2, pp. 111, 117–119). Philadelphia: F. A. Davis.

Allergy Response, Risk for

Diaz, J. (2005). Syndromic diagnosis and management of confirmed mushroom poisonings. *Critical Care Medicine, 33*(2), 427–436.

Ellis, A., & Day, J. (2005). Clinical reactivity to insect stings. *Current Opinion in Allergy and Clinical Immunology, 5*(4), 349–354.

Friedlander, M. (2004). Objective measurement of allergic reactions in the eye. *Current Opinion in Allergy and Clinical Immunology, 4*(5), 447–453.

Gomes, E., & Demoly, P. (2005). Epidemiology of hypersensitivity drug reactions. *Current Opinion in Allergy and Clinical Immunology, 5*(4), 305–316.

Hathaway, L. (2005). Anaphylaxis. *LPN, 1*(3), 38–39.

Johansson, S., & Haahtela, T. (2004). World Allergy Organization guidelines for prevention of allergy and allergic asthma. *Allergy & Clinical Immunology International—Journal of the World Allergy Organization, 16*(5), 176–185. Retrieved December 13, 2011, from http://www.worldallergy.org/wad2007/article.pdf

McKevity, B., & Theobald, H. (2005). Common food allergies. *Nursing Standard, 19*(29), 39–42.

National Institute of Allergy and Infectious Diseases. (2010). *Food allergy: An overview*. Retrieved December 13, 2011, from http://www.niaid.nih.gov/topics/foodAllergy/Documents/foodallergy.pdf

Shovlin, J., & Corso, M. (2005). Ocular allergy: Recognizing, treating, and avoiding. *Contemporary Optometry, 3*(3), 1–7.

Weir, E. (2005). Sushi, nematodes, and allergies. *Canadian Medical Association Journal, 172*(3), 329.

Anxiety, Death

Abdel-Khalek, A., & Tomàs-Sàbado, J. (2005). Anxiety and death anxiety in Egyptian and Spanish nursing students. *Death Studies, 29,* 157–169.

Brisley, P., & Wood, L. (2004). The impact of education and experience on death anxiety in new graduate nurses. *Contemporary Nurse: A Journal for the Australian Nursing Profession, 17*(1), 102–108.

Kastenbaum, R. (1992). *The psychology of death*. New York: Guilford.

Lamb, E. H. (2002). The impact of previous perinatal loss on subsequent pregnancy and parenting. *Journal of Perinatal Education, 11*(2), 33–40.

Nelson, K. A., Walsh, D., Behrens, C., Zhukovsky, D. S., Lipnickey, V., & Brady, D. (2000). The dying cancer patient. *Seminars in Oncology, 27*(1), 84–89.

Pierce, S. (1999). Improving end-of-life care: Gathering suggestions from family members. *Nursing Forum, 34*(2), 5.

Regehr, C., Kjerulf, M., Popova, S. R., & Baker, A. J. (2004). Issues in clinical nursing trauma and tribulation: The experiences and attitudes of operating room nurses working with organ donors. *Journal of Clinical Nursing, 13*(4), 430–437.

Tarzian, A. (2000). Caring for dying patients who have air hunger. *Journal of Nursing Scholarship, 32*(2), 137–143.

Thomas, S. A., Friedmann, E., Kao, C. W., Inguito, P., Metcalf, M., Kelley, F. J., et al. (2006). Quality of life and psychological status of patients with implantable cardioverter defibrillators. *American Journal of Critical Care, 15*(4), 389–398.

Aspiration, Risk for

Bowman, A., Greiner, J. E., Doerschug, K. C., Little, S. B., Bombei, C. L., & Comried, L. M. (2005). Implementation of an evidence-based feeding protocol and aspiration risk reduction algorithm. *Critical Care Nursing Quarterly, 28*(4), 324–333.

Brady, M., Kinn, S., & Stuart, P. (2004). Review: Evidence is lacking to show that adults given fluids 1.5–3 hours preoperatively have greater risks of aspiration or regurgitation than those given a standard fast. *Evidence-Based Medicine, 9*(3), 88.

Deane, K., Whurr, R., Clarke, C. E., Playford, E. D., & Ben-Shlomo, Y. (2006). Nonpharmacological therapies for dysphagia in Parkinson's disease. *Cochrane Library* (4). DOI: 10.1002/14651858.CD002816

DiBartolo, M. C. (2006). Careful hand feeding: A reasonable alternative to PEG tube placement in individuals with dementia. *Journal of Gerontological Nursing, 32*(5), 25–35.

Johnson, J. L., & Hirsch, C. S. (2003). Aspiration pneumonia. *Postgraduate Medicine, 113*(3), 99–107.

Matsui, T., Yamaya, M., Ohrui, T., Arai, H., & Sasaki, H. (2002). Sitting position to prevent aspiration in bed-bound patients. *Gerontology, 48*(3), 194.

Metheny, N. A. (2006). Preventing respiratory complications of tube feedings: Evidence-based practice. *American Journal of Critical Care, 15*(4), 360–369.

Oh, E., Weintraub, N., & Dhanai, S. (2004). Can we prevent aspiration pneumonia in the nursing home? *Journal of the American Medical Directors Association, 6*(3, Suppl. 1), S76–S80

Oshodi, T. O. (2004). Clinical skills: An evidence-based approach to preoperative fasting. *British Journal of Nursing (BJN), 13*(16), 958–962.

Racht, E. M. (2002). 10 pitfalls in airway management: How to avoid common airway management complications. *JEMS: Journal of Emergency Medical Services, 27*(3), 28–34, 36–38, 40–42.

Ng, W. Q., & Neill, J. (2006). Evidence for early oral feeding of patients after elective open colorectal surgery: A literature review. *Journal of Clinical Nursing, 15*(6), 696–709.

Westhus, N. (2004). Methods to test feeding tube placement in children. *MCN: The American Journal of Maternal Child Nursing, 29*(5), 282.

Wilkinson, J., & Treas, L. (2011). *Fundamentals of nursing* (2nd ed.). Philadelphia: F. A. Davis Company.

Yu-Chih Chen, Shin-Shang Chou, Li-Hwa Lin, & Li-Fen Wu. (2006). The effect of intermittent nasogastric feeding on preventing aspiration pneumonia in ventilated critically ill patients. *Journal of Nursing Research, 14*(3), 167–180.

Attachment, Risk for Impaired

Ahern, N. R. (2003). Maternal–fetal attachment in African-American and Hispanic-American women. *Journal of Perinatal Education, 12*(4), 27–35.

Cannella, B. L. (2005). Maternal–fetal attachment: An integrative review. *Journal of Advanced Nursing, 50*(1), 60–68.

Denehy, J. A. (2001). Parenting promotion. In M. Craft-Rosenberg & J. Denehy (Eds.), *Nursing interventions for infants, children, and families* (pp. 99–118). Thousand Oaks, CA: Sage.

Ebersole, P., Hess, P., Touhy, T., & Jett, K. (2005). *Gerontological nursing & health aging* (2nd ed.). St. Louis, MO: Mosby.

Franck, L. S., & Spencer, C. (2003). Parent visiting and participation in infant caregiving activities in a neonatal unit. *Birth: Issues in Perinatal Care, 30*(1), 31–35.

Franklin, C. F. (2006). The neonatal nurse's role in parental attachment in the NICU. *Critical Care Nursing, 29*(1), 81–85.

Goulet, C., Bell, L., & Tribble, D. (1998). A concept analysis of parent–infant attachment. *Journal of Advanced Nursing, 28*(5), 1071–1081.

Horowitz, J. A., Logsdon, M. C., & Anderson, J. K. (2005). Measurement of maternal-infant interaction. *Journal of the American Psychiatric Nurses Association, 11*(3), 164–172.

Klossner, N. J., & Hatfield, N. (2006). *Introductory maternity and pediatric nursing* (pp. 283–284). Philadelphia: Lippincott Williams & Wilkins.

Lamb, E. H. (2002). The impact of previous perinatal loss on subsequent pregnancy and parenting. *Journal of Perinatal Education, 11*(2), 33–40.

Larsen, P. D., Lewis, P. R., & Lubkin, I. M. (2006). Illness behavior and roles. In I. M. Lubkin & P. D. Larsen (Eds.), *Chronic illness: Impact and interventions* (pp. 23–44). Sudbury, MA: Jones and Bartlett.

Leonard, L. G. (2002). Prenatal behavior of multiples: Implications for families and nurses. *JOGNN: Journal of Obstetric, Gynecologic, & Neonatal Nursing, 31*(3), 248–255.

Melnyk, B., & Feinstein, N. (2000). Mediating functions of maternal anxiety and participation in care on young children's posthospital adjustment. *Research in Nursing and Health, 24,* 18.

Mercer, R. T., & Walker, L. O. (2006). A review of nursing interventions to foster becoming a mother. *JOGNN: Journal of Obstetric, Gynecologic, & Neonatal Nursing, 35*(5), 568–582.

Pillitteri, A. (2007). The family with an infant. In *Maternal and child health nursing: Care of the childbearing and childrearing family* (5th ed., pp. 824–859). Philadelphia: Lippincott Williams & Wilkins.

Shaw, E., Levitt, C., Wong, S., & Kaczorowski, J. (2006). Systematic review of the literature on postpartum care: Effectiveness of postpartum support to improve maternal parenting, mental health, quality of life, and physical health. *Birth: Issues in Perinatal Care, 33*(3), 210–220.

Smith, E., Gomm, S., & Dickens, C. (2003). Assessing the independent contribution to quality of life from anxiety and depression in patients with advanced cancer. *Palliative Medicine, 17*(6), 509–513.

Tessier, R., Cristo, M., Velez, S., Giron, M., de Calume, Z. F., Ruiz-Palaez, J. G., et al. (1998). Kangaroo mother care and the bonding hypothesis. *Pediatrics, 102*(2), e17.

Witkowski, A., Wieck, A., & Mann, S. (2007). An evaluation of two bonding questionnaires: A comparison of the mother-to-infant bonding scale with the postpartum bonding questionnaire in a sample of primiparous mothers. *Archives of Women's Mental Health, 10*(4), 171–175.

Zahr, L. (1991). Correlates of mother–infant interaction in premature infants from low socioeconomic background. *Pediatric Nursing, 17*(3), 259–263.

Bleeding, Risk for

American College of Surgeons Committee on Trauma. (1997). *Advanced trauma life support for doctors*. Chicago: American College of Surgeons.

Baird, M. S., & Bethel, S. (2011). *Manual of critical care nursing: Nursing interventions and collaborative management* (6th ed.). St. Louis: Mosby.

Baron, B. J., Sinert, R., Zehtabchi, S., Stavile, K. L., & Scalea, T. M. (2004). Diagnostic utility of sublingual PCO2 for detecting hemorrhage in penetrating trauma patients. *Journal of Trauma, 57*(1), 69–74.

Bose, P., Regan, F., & Paterson-Brown, S. (2006). Improving the accuracy of estimated blood loss at obstetric haemorrhage using clinical reconstructions. *BJOG: An International Journal of Obstetrics & Gynaecology, 113*(8), 919–924.

Brozenec, S. A. (2007). Hepatic problems. In F. D. Monahan, J. K. Sands, M. Neighbors, J. F. Marek, & C. J. Green (Eds.), *Phipps medical-surgical nursing: Health and illness perspectives* (8th ed., pp. 1209–1212). St. Louis: Mosby Elsevier.

Callahan, L. (2004). Surgery in pregnancy. In S. Mattson & J. E. Smith (Eds.), *Core curriculum for maternal-newborn nursing* (3rd ed., pp. 727–749). St. Louis: Elsevier Saunders.

Deitch, E. A., & Dayal, S. D. (2006). Intensive care unit management of the trauma patient. *Critical Care Medicine, 34,* 2294–2301.

Erickson, J., & Field, R. (2007). Cancer. In F. D. Monahan, J. K. Sands, M. Neighbors, J. F. Marek, & C. J. Green (Eds.), *Phipps medical-surgical nursing: Health and illness perspectives* (8th ed.). St. Louis: Mosby Elsevier.

Garrigues, A. L. (2007). Hematologic problems. In F. D. Monahan, J. K. Sands, M. Neighbors, J. F. Marek, & C. J. Green (Eds.), *Phipps medical-surgical nursing: Health and illness perspectives* (8th ed., pp. 923–928). St. Louis: Mosby Elsevier.

Haney, S. (2004). Trauma in pregnancy. In S. Mattson & J. E. Smith (Eds.), *Core curriculum for maternal-newborn nursing* (3rd ed., pp. 703–726). St. Louis: Elsevier Saunders.

Higgins, P. G. (2004). Postpartum complications. In S. Mattson & J. E. Smith (Eds.), *Core curriculum for maternal-newborn nursing* (3rd ed., pp. 850–854). St. Louis: Elsevier Saunders.

Lowdermilk, D., & Perry, S. (2006). *Maternity nursing* (7th ed., pp. 599–601). St. Louis: Mosby Elsevier.

Marek, J., & Boehnlein, M. (2007). Postoperative nursing. In F. D. Monahan, J. K. Sands, M. Neighbors, J. F. Marek, & C. J. Green (Eds.), *Phipps medical-surgical nursing: Health and illness perspectives* (8th ed.). St. Louis: Mosby Elsevier.

Maxson, J. H. (2000). Management of disseminated intravascular coagulation. *Critical Care Nursing Clinics of North America, 12,* 341–352.

Maxwill-Thompson, C., & Reid, K. (2007). Vascular problems. In F. D. Monahan, J. K. Sands, M. Neighbors, J. F. Marek, & C. J. Green (Eds.), *Phipps medical-surgical nursing: Health and illness perspectives* (8th ed., pp. 1209–1212). St. Louis: Mosby Elsevier.

Sands, J. K. (2007). Stomach and duodenal problems. In F. D. Monahan, J. K. Sands, M. Neighbors, J. F. Marek, & C. J. Green (Eds.), *Phipps medical-surgical nursing: Health and illness perspectives* (8th ed.). St. Louis: Mosby Elsevier.

Sims, C., Seigne, P., Menconi, M., Monarca, J., Barlow, C., Pettit, J., et al. (2001). Skeletal muscle acidosis correlates with the severity of blood volume loss during shock and resuscitation. *Journal of Trauma, 51*(6), 1137–1146.

Smeltzer, S. C., & Bare, B. G. (2004). *Brunner & Suddarth's textbook of medical surgical nursing* (Vol. 1, 105th ed.). Philadelphia: Lippincott Williams & Wilkins.

Warshaw, M. (2007). Male reproductive problems. In F. D. Monahan, J. K. Sands, M. Neighbors, J. F. Marek, & C. J. Green (Eds.), *Phipps medical-surgical nursing: Health and illness perspectives* (8th ed.). St. Louis: Mosby Elsevier.

Blood Glucose, Risk for Unstable

Abbott, S., Burns, T., Gleadell, A., & Gunnell, C. (2007). Community nurses and self monitoring of blood glucose [cover story]. *British Journal of Community Nursing, 12*(1), 6–11.

American Diabetes Association. (2010). Standards of medical care in diabetes 2010. *Diabetes Care, 33,* S11–S61. Retrieved October 26, 2011, from http://www.ncbi.nlm.nih.gov/pmc/articles/PMC2797382/

Bierschbach, J., Cooper, L., & Liedl, J. (2004). Insulin pumps: What every school nurse needs to know. *Journal of School Nursing, 20,* 117–123.

Bindler, R. M., & Bruya, M. A. (2006). Evidence for identifying children at risk for being overweight, cardiovascular disease, and type 2 diabetes in primary care. *Journal of Pediatric Healthcare, 20*(2), 82–87.

Biuso, T. J., Butterworth, S., & Linden, A. (2007). A conceptual framework for targeting prediabetes with lifestyle, clinical, and behavioral management interventions. *Disease Management, 10*(1), 6–15.

Boucher, J. L., Swift, C. S., Franz, M. J., Kulkami, K., Schafer, R. G., Pritchett, E., et al. (2007). Inpatient management of diabetes and hyperglycemia: Implications for nutrition practice and the food and nutrition professional. *Journal of the American Dietetic Association, 107*(1), 105–111.

Brenner, Z. R. (2006). Management of hyperglycemic emergencies. *AACN Clinical Issues: Advanced Practice in Acute & Critical Care, 17*(1), 56–65.

Brien, C. A., Van Rooyen, D., & Carlson, S. (2006). National guidelines for the management of diabetes mellitus: A nursing perspective. *Health SA Gesondheid, 11*(4), 32–45.

Campbell, J., & McDowell, J. R. S. (2007). Comparative study on the effect of enteral feeding on blood glucose. *British Journal of Nursing (BJN), 16*(6), 344–349.

Crowther, C. A., Hiller, J. E., & Moss, J. R. (2005). Screening and active management reduced perinatal complications more than routine care in gestational diabetes. *Evidence-Based Medicine, 10*(6), 171–171.

Delmas, L. (2006). Best practice in the assessment and management of diabetic foot ulcers. *Rehabilitation Nursing, 31*(6), 228–234.

DePalma, J. A. (2006). Diabetes care: Evidence for community-based programs. *Home Health Care Management & Practice, 18*(4), 326–328.

Dilkhush, D., Lannigan, J., Pedroff, T., Riddle, A., & Tittle, M. (2005). Insulin infusion protocol for critical care units. *American Journal of Health-System Pharmacy, 62*(21), 2260.

Evans, J., & Chance, T. (2005). Improving patient outcomes using a diabetic foot assessment tool. *Nursing Standard, 19*(45), 65–77.

Gerard, S. O., Neary, V., Apuzzo, D., Giles, M. E., & Krinsley, J. (2006). Implementing an intensive glucose management initiative: Strategies for success. *Critical Care Nursing Clinics of North America, 18*(4), 531–543.

Ibrahem, I. A. (2006). Diabetes mellitus. In D. L. Huber (Ed.), *Disease management: A guide for case managers* (pp. 81–99). St. Louis: Saunders.

Ingersoll, S., Valente, S. M., & Roper, J. (2005). Using the best evidence to change practice. Nurse care coordination for diabetes: A literature review and synthesis. *Journal of Nursing Care Quality, 20*(3), 208–214.

Kirk, J. K., D'Agostino, R., Jr., Bell, R. A., Passmore, L. V., Bonds, D. E., Karter, A. J., et al. (2006). Disparities in HbA1c levels between African-American and non-Hispanic white adults with diabetes: A meta-analysis. *Diabetes Care, 29*(9), 2130–2136.

Lee, S. W., Im, R., & Magbual, R. (2004). Current perspectives on the use of continuous subcutaneous insulin infusion in the acute care setting and overview of therapy. *Critical Care Nursing Quarterly, 27*(2), 172–184.

Miller, D. K., & Fain, J. A. (2006). Diabetes 2000: Acute complications. *RN, 58*(8), 36–41.

Presutti, E., & Millo, J. (2006). Controlling blood glucose levels to reduce infection. *Critical Care Nursing Quarterly, 29*(2), 123–131.

Quinn, K., Hudson, P., & Dunning, T. (2006). Diabetes management in patients receiving palliative care. *Journal of Pain & Symptom Management, 32*(3), 275–286.

Scott, L. K. (2006). Insulin resistance syndrome in children. *Pediatric Nursing, 32*(2), 119–143.

Smeltzer, S. C., & Bare, B. G. (2004). Assessment and management of patients with diabetes mellitus. In *Brunner & Suddarth's textbook of medical surgical nursing* (Vol. 2, 10th ed., pp. 1150–1203). Philadelphia: Lippincott Williams & Wilkins.

U.S. Department of Health & Human Services. (2010). *Helping the student with diabetes succeed: A guide for school personnel*. Retrieved October 26, 2011, from http://ndep.nih.gov/publications/PublicationDetail.aspx?PubId=97

Whitehorn, J. L. (2007). A review of the use of insulin protocols to maintain normoglycaemia in high dependency patients. *Journal of Clinical Nursing, 16*(1), 16–27.

Wilkinson, J. M., & Treas, L. S. (2011). Chapter 24, Teaching Clients. *Fundamentals of nursing* (2nd ed.). Philadelphia: F. A. Davis Company.

Willoughby, D., Dye, C., Burriss, P., & Carr, R. (2005). Protecting the kidneys of patients with diabetes. *Clinical Nurse Specialist: The Journal for Advanced Nursing Practice, 19*(3), 150–156.

Body Image, Disturbed

Bergamasco, E. C., Rossi, L., da Amancio, C. G., & Carvalho, E. C. (2002). Body image of patients with burn sequellae. *Burns, 28,* 47–52.

Berger, K. S. (2012). *The developing person through the life span* (8th ed.). New York: Worth Publishers.

Black, P. K., & Hyde, C. (2002). Parents with colorectal cancer: "What do I tell the children?" *British Journal of Nursing (BJN), 11*(10), 679.

Carlsson, E., Berglund, B., & Norgren, S. (2001). Living with an ostomy and short bowel syndrome: Practical aspects and impact on daily life. *Journal of WOCN: Wound, Ostomy, and Continence Nursing, 28*(2), 96–105.

Dixon, J., Dixon, M., & O'Brien, P. (2002). Body image: Appearance orientation and evaluation in the severely obese. Changes with weight loss. *Obesity Surgery, 12*(1), 65–71.

Fritz, G. K. (Ed.). (2004). *Body image—tips for parents.* The Brown University Child and Adolescent Behavior Letter. Providence, RI: Manisses Communications Group.

Furness, P. J. (2005). Head and neck nursing. Exploring supportive care needs and experiences of facial surgery patients. *British Journal of Nursing (BJN), 14*(12), 641–645.

Gignac, M. A., Cott, C., & Badley, E. M. (2000). Adaptation to chronic illness and disability and its relationship to perceptions of independence and dependence. *Journal of Gerontology Series B—Psychological Sciences, 55*(6), P362–P372.

Hockenberry, M., & Wilson, D. (2009). *Wong's essentials of pediatric nursing* (8th ed.). St. Louis: Mosby.

Kater, K., Rohwer, J., & Londre, K. (2002). Evaluation of an upper elementary school program to prevent body image, eating, and weight concerns. *Journal of School Health, 72*(5), 199–204.

Key, A., George, C., Beattie, D., Stammers, K., Lacey, H., & Waller, G. (2002). Body image treatment within an inpatient program for anorexia nervosa: The role of mirror exposure in the desensitization process. *International Journal of Eating Disorders, 31*(2), 185–190.

Pillitteri, A. (2007). *Maternal and child health nursing: Care of the childbearing and child-rearing family* (5th ed.). Philadelphia: Lippincott Williams & Wilkins.

Price, B. (1990). A model for body-image care. *Journal of Advanced Nursing, 5,* 585–593.

Pym, K. (2006). Identifying and managing problem scars. *British Journal of Nursing (BJN), 15*(2), 78–82.

Riesch, S., Anderson, L., & Krueger, H. (2006). Parent–child communication processes: Preventing children's health-risk behavior. *Journal for Specialists in Pediatric Nursing, 11*(1), 41–56.

Schartau, E., Tolson, D., & Fleming, V. (2003). Parkinson's disease: The effects on womanhood. *Nursing Standard, 17*(42), 33–39.

Whall, A., & Parent, C. (1991). Self-esteem disturbance. In M. Maas, K. Buckwalter, & M. Hardy (Eds.), *Nursing diagnosis and interventions for the elderly* (pp. 480–488). Redwood City, CA: Addison-Wesley.

Body Temperature: Imbalanced, Risk for

Ainslie, P., Campbell, I., Lambert, J., MacLaren, D., & Reilly, R. (2005). Physiological and metabolic aspects of very prolonged exercise with particular reference to hill walking. *Sports Medicine, 35*(7), 619–647.

Bernthal, E. (1999). Inadvertent hypothermia prevention: The anaesthetic nurse's role. *British Journal of Nursing, 8*(1), 17–18, 20–25.

Bohnhorst, B., Heyne, T., Peter, C., & Poets, C. (2001). Skin-to-skin (kangaroo) care, respiratory control, and thermoregulation. *Journal of Pediatrics, 138*(2), 193–197.

DeFabio, D. C. (2000). Fluid and nutrient maintenance before, during and after exercise. *Journal of Sports Chiropractic and Rehabilitation, 14*(2), 21–24, 42–43.

Elliott, F. (2005). Do the prep work. *Occupational Health & Safety, 74*(11), 68, 70.

Fallis, W. (2002). Monitoring urinary bladder temperature in the intensive care unit: State of the science. *American Journal of Critical Care, 11*(1), 38–47.

Fisk, J., & Arcona, S. (2001). Comparing tympanic membrane and pulmonary artery catheter temperatures. *Dimensions of Critical Care Nursing, 20*(2), 44–49.

Fulbrook, P. (1997). Core body temperature measurement: A comparison of axilla, tympanic membrane and pulmonary artery blood temperature. *Intensive & Critical Care Nursing, 13*(5), 266–272.

Giuliano, K. K., Giuliano, A. J., Scott, S. S., MacLachlan, E., Pysznik, E., Elliot, S., et al. (2000). Temperature measurement in critically ill adults: A comparison of tympanic and oral methods. *American Journal of Critical Care, 9*(4), 254–261.

Holtzclaw, B. (2001). Risk for altered body temperature. In M. Maas, K. Buckwalter, M. Hardy, T. Tripp-Reimer, M. Titler, & J. Specht (Eds.), *Nursing care of older adults: Diagnoses, outcomes & interventions* (pp. 201–216). St. Louis: Mosby.

Howell, R., Macrae, L., Sanjines, S., Burke, J., & DeStefano, P. (1992). Effects of two types of head coverings in the rewarming of patients after coronary artery bypass graft surgery. *Heart and Lung, 21,* 1–6.

Mahoney, C. B., & Odom, J. (1999). Maintaining intra-operative normothermia: A meta-analysis of outcomes with costs. *AANA Journal, 67*(2), 155–164.

Pillitteri, A. (2007). Nursing care of a newborn and family. In *Maternal and child health nursing* (5th ed., pp. 679–721). Philadelphia: Lippincott Williams & Wilkins.

Smith, L. (2004). Temperature measurement in critical care adults: A comparison of thermometry and measurement routes. *Biological Research for Nursing, 6*(2), 117–125.

Truman, P. (2006). Jaundice in the preterm infant. *Paediatric Nursing, 18*(5), 20–22.

Watson, G., Casa, D., Fiala, K., Hile, A., Roti, M., Healey, J., et al. (2006). Creatine use and exercise heat tolerance in dehydrated men. *Journal of Athletic Training, 41*(1), 18–29.

Wilkinson, J., & Treas, L. (2011). *Fundamentals of nursing* (2nd ed.). Philadelphia: F. A. Davis Company.

Bowel Incontinence

Bywater, A., & While, A. (2006). Management of bowel dysfunction in people with multiple sclerosis. *British Journal of Community Nursing, 11*(8), 333.

Doherty, W. (2004). Managing faecal incontinence or leakage: The Peristeen Anal Plug. *British Journal of Nursing, 13*(21), 1293–1297.

Gray, M., Ratliff, C., & Donovan, A. (2002). Perineal skin care for the incontinent patient. *Advances in Skin & Wound Care, 15*(4), 170–175.

McCance, K., & Heuther, S. (2006). *Pathophysiology: The biologic basis for disease in adults and children* (5th ed.). St. Louis, MO: Mosby.

Norton, C. (2004). Nurses, bowel continence, stigma, and taboos. *Journal of Wound, Ostomy & Continence Nursing, 31*(2), 85–94.

Rao, S. S. (2004). Diagnosis and management of fecal incontinence. *American Journal of Gastroenterology, 99*(8), 1584–1604.

Slater, W. (2003). Continence care. Management of faecal incontinence of a patient with spinal cord injury. *British Journal of Nursing (BJN), 12*(12), 727–734.

Smeltzer, S., & Bare, B. (2004a). *Brunner & Suddarth's textbook of medical surgical nursing* (Vol. 1, 10th ed.). Philadelphia: Lippincott Williams & Wilkins.

Smeltzer, S., & Bare, B. (2004b). *Brunner & Suddarth's textbook of medical surgical nursing* (Vol. 2, 10th ed.). Philadelphia: Lippincott Williams & Wilkins.

Taunton, R. L., Swagerty, D. L., Lasseter, J. A., & Lee, R. H. (2005). Continent or incontinent? That is the question. *Journal of Gerontological Nursing, 31*(9), 36–44.

Urden, L., Stacy, K., & Lough, M. (2006). *Thelan's critical care nursing: Diagnosis and management* (5th ed.). St. Louis, MO: Mosby.

Weeks, S. K., Hubbartt, E., & Michaels, T. K. (2000). Keys to bowel success. *Rehabilitation Nursing, 25*(2), 66–69.

Wilkinson, J., & Treas, L. (2011). *Fundamentals of nursing* (2nd ed.). Philadelphia: F. A. Davis Company.

Breast Milk, Insufficient

Aragaki, I., Silva, I., & Santos, J. (2006). Traco e estado de ansiedade de nutrizes com indcadores de hipogalactia e nutrizes com galactia normal [Trait and state anxiety of nursing mothers with indicators of nursing mothers with insufficient and normal lactation]. *Revista Da Escola De Enfermagem Da U S P, 40*(3), 396–403.

Callahan, S., Sejourne, N., & Denis, A. (2006). Fatigue and breastfeeding—an inevitable relationship. *Journal of Human Lactation, 22*(2), 182–187.

Carpenito-Moyet, L. J. (2010). *Nursing diagnosis: Application to clinical practice* (13th ed.). Philadelphia: Lippincott Williams & Wilkins.

Hill, P., Aldag, J., Chatterton, R., & Zinaman, M. (2005). Psychological distress and milk volume in lactating mothers. *Western Journal of Nursing Research, 37*(6), 676–683; discussion 694–700.

Lowdermilk, D., Perry, S., Cashion, K., & Alden, K. (2012). *Maternity & women's health care* (10th ed.). St. Louis: Mosby.

Page-Goertz, S. (2005). Weight gain concerns in the breastfed infant. Maternal factors. *Advance for Nurse Practitioners, 13*(2), 45–48, 72.

Pérez-Escamilla, R. (2007). Evidence based breast-feeding promotion: The Baby-Friendly Hospital Initiative. *Journal of Nutrition, 137*(2), 484–487.

Pillitteri, A. (2007). The family with an infant. In *Maternal and child health nursing: Care of the childbearing and childrearing family* (5th ed., pp. 824–859). Philadelphia: Lippincott Williams & Wilkins.

Riordan, J., & Wambach, K. (2009). *Breastfeeding and human lactation* (4th ed.). Sudbury, MA: Jones & Bartlett Publishers.

Sievers, E., Haase, S., Oldigs, H., & Schaub, J. (2003). The impact of peripartum factors on the onset and duration of lactation. *Biology of the Neonate, 83*(4), 246–252.

Breastfeeding, Effective

Biancuzzo, M. (2003). *Breastfeeding the newborn* (2nd ed.). St. Louis: Mosby.

Callahan, S., Sejourne, N., & Denis, A. (2006). Fatigue and breastfeeding—an inevitable relationship. *Journal of Human Lactation, 22*(2), 182–187.

Carpenito-Moyet, L. J. (2010). *Nursing diagnosis: Application to clinical practice* (13th ed.). Philadelphia: Lippincott Williams & Wilkins.

Cricco-Lizza, R. (2006). Black non-Hispanic mother's perception about the promotion of infant feeding methods by nurses and physicians. *Journal of Obstetric, Gynecologic, and Neonatal Nursing (JOGNN), 35*(2), 173–180.

Dick, M., Evans, M., Arthurs, J., Barnes, J., Caldwell, R., Hutchins, S., et al. (2002). Predicting early breastfeeding attrition. *Journal of Human Lactation, 18*(1), 21–28.

Hellings, P., & Howe, C. (2004). Breastfeeding knowledge and practice of pediatric nurse practitioners. *Journal of Pediatric Healthcare, 18*(1), 8–14.

Hurtekant, K. M., & Spatz, D. L. (2007). Special considerations for breastfeeding the infant with spina bifida. *Journal of Perinatal & Neonatal Nursing, 21*(1), 69–75.

Leonard, L. G. (2002). Insights in practice. Breastfeeding higher order multiples: Enhancing support during the postpartum hospitalization period. *Journal of Human Lactation, 18*(4), 386–392.

Lowdermilk, D., Perry, S., Cashion, K., & Alden, K. (2012). *Maternity & women's health care* (10th ed.). St. Louis: Mosby.

Morland-Schultz, K., & Hill, P. D. (2005). Prevention of and therapies for nipple pain: A systematic review. *JOGNN: Journal of Obstetric, Gynecologic, & Neonatal Nursing, 34*(4), 428–437.

Ortiz, J., McGilligan, K., & Kelly, P. (2004). Duration of breast milk expression among working mothers enrolled in an employer-sponsored location program. *Pediatric Nursing, 30*(2), 111–119.

Pérez-Escamilla, R. (2007). Evidence based breast-feeding promotion: The Baby-Friendly Hospital Initiative. *Journal of Nutrition, 137*(2), 484–487.

Pillitteri, A. (2007). *Maternal and child health nursing: Care of the childbearing and childrearing family* (5th ed.). Philadelphia: Lippincott Williams & Wilkin.

Stevens, B., Guerriere, D., McKeever, P., Croxford, R., Miller, K., Watson-MacDonell, J., et al. (2006). Economics of home vs. hospital breastfeeding support for newborns. *Journal of Advanced Nursing, 53*(2), 233–243.

Breastfeeding, Ineffective

Chiu, S.-H., Anderson, G. C., & Burkhammer, M. D. (2005). Newborn temperature during skin to skin breastfeeding in couples having breastfeeding difficulties. *Birth, 32*(2), 115–121.

Hurtekant, K. M., & Spatz, D. L. (2007). Special considerations for breastfeeding the infant with spina bifida. *Journal of Perinatal & Neonatal Nursing, 21*(1), 69–75.

Pérez-Escamilla, R. (2007). Evidence based breast-feeding promotion: The Baby-Friendly Hospital Initiative. *Journal of Nutrition, 137*(2), 484–487.

Pillitteri, A. (2007). The family with an infant. In *Maternal and child health nursing: Care of the childbearing and childrearing family* (5th ed., pp. 824–859). Philadelphia: Lippincott Williams & Wilkins.

Rasmussen, K. M., & Kjolhede, C. L. (2004). Prepregnant overweight and obesity diminish the prolactin response to suckling in the first week postpartum. *Pediatrics, 113*(5), e465–471.

Riordan, J., & Wambach, K. (2009). *Breastfeeding and human lactation* (4th ed.). Sudbury, MA: Jones & Bartlett Publishers.

Stevens, B., Guerriere, D., McKeever, P., Croxford, R., Miller, K., Watson-MacDonell, J., et al. (2006). Economics of home vs. hospital breastfeeding support for newborns. *Journal of Advanced Nursing, 53*(2), 233–243.

Breastfeeding, Interrupted

Callahan, S., Sejourne, N., & Denis, A. (2006). Fatigue and breastfeeding—An inevitable relationship. *Journal of Human Lactation, 22*(2), 182–187.

Cricco-Lizza, R. (2006). Black non-Hispanic mother's perception about the promotion of infant feeding methods by nurses and physicians. *Journal of Obstetric, Gynecologic and Neonatal Nursing (JOGNN), 35*(2), 173–180.

Hellings, P., & Howe, C. (2004). Breastfeeding knowledge and practice of pediatric nurse practitioners. *Journal of Pediatric Healthcare, 18*(1), 8–14.

Hurtekant, K. M., & Spatz, D. L. (2007). Special considerations for breastfeeding the infant with spina bifida. *Journal of Perinatal & Neonatal Nursing, 21*(1), 69–75.

Leonard, L. G. (2002). Insights in practice. Breastfeeding higher order multiples: Enhancing support during the postpartum hospitalization period. *Journal of Human Lactation, 18*(4), 386–392.

Lewallen, L. P., Dick, M., Flowers, J., Powell, W., Zickefoose, K., Wall, Y., et al. (2006). Breastfeeding support and early cessation. *Journal of Obstetric, Gynecologic, and Neonatal Nursing (JOGNN), 35*(2), 166–172.

Morland-Schultz, K., & Hill, P. D. (2005). Prevention of and therapies for nipple pain: A systematic review. *JOGNN: Journal of Obstetric, Gynecologic, & Neonatal Nursing, 34*(4), 428–437.

Nystedt, A., Edvardsson, D., & Willman, A. (2004). Women and children epidural analgesia for pain relief in labour and childbirth—a review with a systematic approach. *Journal of Clinical Nursing, 13*(4), 455–466.

Stevens, B., Guerriere, D., McKeever, P., Croxford, R., Miller, K., Watson-MacDonell, J., et al. (2006). Economics of home vs. hospital breastfeeding support for newborns. *Journal of Advanced Nursing, 53*(2), 233–243.

Breathing Pattern, Ineffective

Allison, R. D., Ray Lewis, A., Liedtke, R., Buchmeyer, N. D., & Frank, H. (2005). Early identification of hypovolemia using total body resistance measurements in long-term care facility residents. *Gender Medicine, 2*(1), 19–34.

American Association of Critical Care Nurses. (2006). In J. G. Alspach (Ed.), *Core curriculum for critical care nursing* (6th ed.). Philadelphia: W. B. Saunders.

Bianchi, R., Gigliotti, F., Romagnoli, I., Lanini, B., Castellani, C., Grazzini, M., et al. (2004). Chest wall kinematics and breathlessness during pursed-lip breathing in patients with COPD. *Chest, 125*(2), 459–465.

Gallagher, R., & Roberts, D. (2004). Systematic review of oxygen and airflow effect on relief of dyspnea at rest in patients with advanced disease of any cause. *Journal of Pain & Palliative Care Pharmacotherapy, 18*(4), 3–15.

Goodridge, D. M. (2006). COPD as a life-limiting illness: Implications for advanced practice nurses. *Topics in Advanced Practice Nursing, 6*(4), 11p.

Jantarakupt, P., & Porock, D. (2005). Dyspnea management in lung cancer: Applying the evidence from chronic obstructive pulmonary disease. *Oncology Nursing Forum, 32*(4), 785–795.

Lewith, G. T., Prescott, P., & Davis, C. L. (2004). Can a standardized acupuncture technique palliate disabling breathlessness? *Chest, 125*(5), 1783–1790.

MacDonald, S., Yates, J., Lance, R., Giganti, N., & Chepurko, D. (2005). Are you asking the right admission questions when assessing dyspnea? *Heart & Lung, 34*(4), 260–269.

Monahan, F., Sands, J., Neighbors, M., Marek, J., & Green, C. (2007). *Phipps' medical-surgical nursing: Health and illness perspectives* (8th ed.). St. Louis, MO: Mosby.

Oh, E. (2003). The effects of home-based pulmonary rehabilitation in patients with chronic lung disease. *International Journal of Nursing Studies, 40*(8), 873.

Spector, N., Connolly, M. A., & Carlson, K. K. (2007). Dyspnea: Applying research to bedside practice. *AACN Advanced Critical Care, 18*(1), 45–60.

Tinker, R., & While, A. (2006). Promoting quality of life for patients with moderate to severe COPD. *British Journal of Community Nursing, 11*(7), 278.

Cardiac Output, Decreased

American Association of Critical Care Nurses. (2006). In J. G. Alspach (Ed.), *Core curriculum for critical care nursing* (6th ed.). Philadelphia: W. B. Saunders.

Beales, D. (2005). How accurate are automated blood pressure monitors? *British Journal of Community Nursing, 10*(7), 334–338.

Clark, A. M., Hartling, L., Vandermeer, B., & McAlister, F. A. (2005). Meta-analysis: Secondary prevention programs for patients with coronary artery disease. *Annals of Internal Medicine, 143*(9), 659–672.

Davidson, P., Macdonald, P., Paull, G., Rees, D., Howes, L., Cockburn, J., et al. (2003). Diuretic therapy in chronic heart failure: Implications for heart failure nurse specialists. *Australian Critical Care, 16*(2), 59–69.

Donohue, M. A. T. (2005). Evidence-based care for acute myocardial infarction. *Nursing Management, 36*(8), 23–27.

Drew, B. J., Califf, R. M., Funk, M., Kaufman, E. S., Krucoff, M. W., Laks, M. M., et al. (2005). Practice standards for electrocardiographs monitoring in hospital settings. *Journal of Cardiovascular Nursing, 20*(2), 76–106.

Driscoll, A., Worrall-Carter, L., & Stewart, S. (2006). Rationale and design of the national benchmarking and evidence-based national clinical guidelines for chronic heart failure management programs study. *Journal of Cardiovascular Nursing, 21*(4), 276–282.

Duffy, J. R., & Salerno, S. M. (2004). New blood test to measure heart attack risk. *Journal of Cardiovascular Nursing, 19*(6), 425–429.

Fanning, M. F. (2004). Reducing postoperative pulmonary complications in cardiac surgery patients with the use of the best evidence. *Journal of Nursing Care Quality, 19*(2), 95–99.

Gregory, J. (2005). Cardiac nursing: Using the 12-lead ECG to assess acute coronary patients. *British Journal of Nursing (BJN), 14*(21), 1135–1140.

Holst, M., Strömberg, A., Lindholm, M., Uden, G., & Willenheimer, R. (2003). Fluid restriction in heart failure patients: Is it useful? The design of a prospective, randomised study. *European Journal of Cardiovascular Nursing, 2*(3), 237.

Jonson, S. B., Galvin, C. A., Thompson, B., & Rasmussen, M. J. (2007). Optimizing therapy for heart failure patients. *Journal of Cardiovascular Nursing, 22*(2), 118–124.

Lee, G. (2007). A review of the literature on atrial fibrillation: Rate reversion or control? *Journal of Clinical Nursing, 16*(1), 77–83.

Mathiesen, C., Tavianini, H. D., & Palladino, K. (2006). Best practices in stroke rapid response: A case study. *MEDSURG Nursing, 15*(6), 364–369.

McGillion, M., Watt-Watson, J., Kim, J., & Yamada, J. (2004). A systematic review of psychoeducational intervention trials for the management of chronic stable angina. *Journal of Nursing Management, 12*(3), 174–182.

Monahan, F., Sands, J., Neighbors, M., Marek, J., & Green, C. (2007). *Phipps' medical-surgical nursing: Health and illness perspectives* (8th ed.). St. Louis, MO: Mosby.

Rosati, E., Chitano, G., Dipaola, L., De Felice, C., & Latini, G. (2005). Indications and limitations for a neonatal pulse oximetry screening of critical congenital heart disease. *Journal of Perinatal Medicine, 33*(5), 455–457.

Ruxto, C. (2004). Health benefits of omega-3 fatty acids. *Nursing Standard, 18*(48), 38–42.

Caregiver Role Strain

Bowers, B. (1987). Intergenerational caregiving: Adult caregivers and their aging parents. *Advances in Nursing Science, 9*(2), 20–31.

Carr, G. F. (2006). Vulnerability: A conceptual model for African American grandmother caregivers. *Journal of Theory Construction & Testing, 10*(1), 11–14.

Chilman, C., Nunnally, E., & Cox, F. (1988). *Chronic illness and disability* (pp. 30–31). Beverly Hills, CA: Sage Publications.

de Geest, G. (2003). The relation between the perceived role of family and the behavior of the person with dementia. *American Journal of Alzheimer's Disease & Other Dementias, 18*(3), 181–187.

Honea, N., Brintnall, R., Given, B., Sherwood, P., Colao, D., Somers, S., et al. (2008). Putting evidence into practice®: Nursing assessment and interventions to reduce family caregiver strain and burden. *Clinical Journal of Oncology Nursing, 12*(3), 507–516.

Lobchuk, M. M. (2006). Concept analysis of perspective-taking: Meeting informal caregiver needs for communication competence and accurate perception. *Journal of Advanced Nursing, 54*(3), 330–341.

McBride, K. L., White, C. L., Sourial, R., & Mayo, N. (2004). Postdischarge nursing interventions for stroke survivors and their families. *Journal of Advanced Nursing, 47*(2), 192–200.

Rabow, M. W., Hauser, J. M., & Adams, J. (2004). Supporting family caregivers at the end of life: "They don't know what they don't know." *JAMA: Journal of the American Medical Association, 291*(4), 483–491.

Stoltz, P., Udén, G., & Willman, A. (2004). Support for family carers who care for an elderly person at home—a systematic literature review. *Scandinavian Journal of Caring Sciences, 18*(2), 111–119.

Yu-Nu Wang, Yea-Ing Lotus Shyu, Min-Chi Chen, & Pei-Shan Yang. (2011). Reconciling work and family caregiving among adult–child family caregivers of older people with dementia: Effects on role strain and depressive symptoms. *Journal of Advanced Nursing, 67*(4), 829–840.

Caregiver Role Strain, Risk for

Corcaran, M. A., & Gitlin, L. N. (2001). Family caregiver acceptance and use of environmental strategies provided in an occupational therapy intervention. *Physical Occupational Therapy in Geriatrics,* 19(1): 1–20.

DiBartolo, M. C. (2002). Exploring self-efficacy and hardiness in spousal caregivers of individuals with dementia. *Journal of Gerontological Nursing, 28*(4), 24–33.

Gilmour, J. A. (2002). Disintegrated care: Family caregivers and in-hospital respite care. *Journal of Advanced Nursing, 39*(6), 546–553.

Grant, J. S., Elliott, T. R., Weaver, M., Bartolucci, A. A., & Giger, J. N. (2002). Telephone intervention with family caregivers of stroke survivors after rehabilitation. *Stroke (00392499), 33*(8), 2060–2065.

Honea, N., Brintnall, R., Given, B., Sherwood, P., Colao, D., Somers, S., et al. (2008). Putting evidence into practice®: Nursing assessment and interventions to reduce family caregiver strain and burden. *Clinical Journal of Oncology Nursing, 12*(3), 507–516.

Ingleton, C., Payne, S., Nolan, M., & Carey, I. (2003). Respite in palliative care: A review and discussion of the literature. *Palliative Medicine, 17*(7), 567.

Larson, J., Franzén-Dahlin, Å., Billing, E., Arbin, M., Murray, V., & Wredling, R. (2005). The impact of a nurse-led support and education programme for spouses of stroke patients: A randomized controlled trial. *Journal of Clinical Nursing, 14*(8), 995–1003.

Lazarus, R. S., & Folkman, S. (1984). *Stress, appraisal and coping*. New York: Springer.

Lobchuk, M. M. (2006). Concept analysis of perspective-taking: Meeting informal caregiver needs for communication competence and accurate perception. *Journal of Advanced Nursing, 54*(3), 330–341.

McBride, K. L., White, C. L., Sourial, R., & Mayo, N. (2004). Postdischarge nursing interventions for stroke survivors and their families. *Journal of Advanced Nursing, 47*(2), 192–200.

Rabow, M. W., Hauser, J. M., & Adams, J. (2004). Supporting family caregivers at the end of life: "They don't know what they don't know." *JAMA: Journal of the American Medical Association, 291*(4), 483–491.

Stoltz, P., Udén, G., & Willman, A. (2004). Support for family carers who care for an elderly person at home—a systematic literature review. *Scandinavian Journal of Caring Sciences, 18*(2), 111–119.

Tusaie, K., & Dyer, J. (2004). Resilience: A historical review of construct. *Holistic Nursing Practice, 18*(1), 3–8.

Wachterman, M. W., & Sommers, B. D. (2006). The impact of gender and marital status on end-of-life care: Evidence from the national mortality follow-back survey. *Journal of Palliative Medicine, 9*(2), 343–352.

Yu-Nu Wang, Yea-Ing Lotus Shyu, Min-Chi Chen, & Pei-Shan Yang. (2011). Reconciling work and family caregiving among adult-child family caregivers of older people with dementia: Effects on role strain and depressive symptoms. *Journal of Advanced Nursing, 67*(4), 829–840.

Childbearing Process, Ineffective

Aoki, Y. (Ed.). (1998). *Coaching, education, and counseling in maternal health* (Vol. 2). Tokyo: Life Science Co.

Aoki, Y., Kato, N., & Hirasawa, M. (Eds.). (2002). *Midwifery system, Vol. 5: Psychosociology for mother and child*. Tokyo: Japanese Nursing Association Publishing Co.

Aoki, Y., Kato, N., & Hirasawa, M. (Eds.). (2003). *Midwifery system, Vol. 8: Maternity diagnoses and techniques 2*. Tokyo: Japanese Nursing Association Publishing Co.

Association of Women's Health, Obstetric and Neonatal Nurses. (2009). *Standards for professional nursing practice in the care of women and newborns* (7th ed.). Washington, DC: Author.

Callister, L., Holt, S., & Kuhre, M. (2010). Giving birth: The voices of Australian women. *Journal of Perinatal and Neonatal Nursing, 24*(2), 128–136.

Darvill, R., Skirton, H. L., & Farrand, P. (2008). Psychological factors that impact on women's experiences of first-time motherhood: A qualitative study of the transition. *Midwifery, 26*(3), 357–366.

Davidson, M., Longon, M., & Ladewig, P. (2012). *Olds' maternal-newborn nursing & women's health across the lifespan* (9th ed.). Upper Saddle River, NJ: Prentice Hall.

Franklin, C. (2006). The neonatal nurse's role in parental attachment in the NICU. *Critical Care Nursing, 29*(1), 81–85.

Furber, C., Garrod, D., Maloney, E., Lovell, K., & McGowan, L. (2009). A qualitative study of mild to moderate psychological distress during pregnancy. *International Journal of Nursing Studies, 46*(5), 669–677.

Kabeyama, K. (Ed.). (2006). *Essentials of clinical midwifery: Caring based on life and culture* (2nd ed.). Tokyo: Igakushoin.

Kennell, J., Jerauld, R., Wolfe, H., Chesler, D., Kreger, N., McAlpine, W., et al. (1974). Maternal behavior one year after early and extended post-partum contact. *Developmental Medicine and Child Neurology, 16*(2), 172–279.

Koniak-Griffin, D. (1988). The relationship between social support, self-esteem, and maternal–fetal attachment in adolescents. *Research in Nursing and Health, 11*(4), 269–278.

Mercer, R., & Walker, L. (2006). A review of nursing interventions to foster becoming a mother. *Journal of Obstetric, Gynecologic, and Neonatal Nursing, 35*(5), 568–582.

Savage, C. (2009). A proposed framework related to the care of addicted mothers. *Journal of Addiction Nursing, 20*(3), 158–160.

Sharps, P., Laughon, K., & Giangrande, S. (2007). Intimate partner violence and the childbearing year: Maternal and infant health consequences. *Trauma Violence Abuse, 8*(2), 105–116.

Childbearing Process: Ineffective, Risk for

(See the bibliography for Childbearing Process: Ineffective.)

Childbearing Process, Readiness for Enhanced

Aoki, Y. (Ed.). (1998). *Coaching, education, and counseling in maternal health (Vol. 2).* Tokyo: Life Science Co.

Aoki, Y., Kato, N., & Hirasawa, M. (Eds.). (2002). *Midwifery system, Vol. 5: Psychosociology for mother and child.* Tokyo: Japanese Nursing Association Publishing Co.

Aoki, Y., Kato, N., & Hirasawa, M. (Eds.). (2003). *Midwifery system, Vol. 8: Maternity diagnoses and techniques 2.* Tokyo: Japanese Nursing Association Publishing Co.

Association of Women's Health, Obstetric and Neonatal Nurses. (2009). *Standards for professional nursing practice in the care of women and newborns* (7th ed.). Washington, DC: Author.

Davidson, M., Longon, M., & Ladewig, P. (2012). *Olds' maternal-newborn nursing & women's health across the lifespan* (9th ed.). Upper Saddle River, NJ: Prentice Hall.

Franklin, C. (2006). The neonatal nurse's role in parental attachment in the NICU. *Critical Care Nursing, 29*(1), 81–85.

Japan Society for Maternity Diagnoses (Ed.). (2004). *Guidebook of maternity diagnoses*. Tokyo: Igakushoin.

Kabeyama, K. (Ed.). (2006). *Essentials of clinical midwifery: Caring based on life and culture* (2nd ed.). Tokyo: Igakushoin.

Kennell, J., Jerauld, R., Wolfe, H., Chesler, D., Kreger, N., McAlpine, W., et al. (1974). Maternal behavior one year after early and extended post-partum contact. *Developmental Medicine and Child Neurology, 16*(2), 172–279.

Koniak-Griffin, D. (1988). The relationship between social support, self-esteem, and maternal-fetal attachment in adolescents.*Research in Nursing and Health, 11*(4), 269–278.

Mercer, R., & Walker, L. (2006). A review of nursing interventions to foster becoming a mother. *Journal of Obstetric, Gynecologic, and Neonatal Nursing, 35*(5), 568–582.

Nichols, F., & Humenick, S. (2000). *Childbirth education: Practice, research and theory* (2nd ed.). Philadelphia: W. B. Saunders.

Okayama National Hospital (Ed.). (2000). *Breast-feeding and newborn-care teaching manuals from a baby-friendly hospital*. Tokyo: Medica Publishing Co.

Scott-Ricci, S. (2007). *Essentials of maternity, newborn and women's health nursing*. Philadelphia: Lippincott Williams & Wilkins.

Taketani, Y., & Kabeyama, S. (Eds.). (2007). *Midwifery course* (Vol. 6). Tokyo: Igakushoin.

Comfort, Impaired

Coleman, C., Holzemer, W., Eller, L., Corless, L., Reynolds, N., Nokes, K., et al. (2006). Gender differences in use of prayer as a self-care strategy for managing symptoms in African Americans living with HIV/AIDS. *Journal of the Association of Nurses in AIDS Care, 17*(4), 16–23.

Edvardsson, J., Sandman, P., & Rasumssen, B. (2005). Sensing an atmosphere of ease: A tentative theory of supportive care settings. *Scandinavian Journal of Caring Science, 19*(4), 344–353.

Field, T., Peck, M., Hernandez-Reif, M., Krugman, S., Burman, I., & Ozment-Schenck, L. (2000). Postburn itching, pain and psychological symptoms are reduced with massage therapy. *Journal of Burn Care Rehabilitation, 21*(3), 189–193.

Fisher, K. (2006). School nurses' perception of self-efficacy in providing diabetes care. *Journal of School Nursing, 22*(4), 223–228.

Fox, H., Berquisst, K., Hong, K., & Sinha, R. (2007). Stress-induced and alcohol cue-induced craving in recently abstinent alcohol-dependent individuals. *Alcoholism: Clinical and Experimental Research, 31*(3), 395–403.

Kercsmar, C., Dearborn, D., Schluchter, M., Xue, L., Kirchner, H., Sobolewski, J., et al. (2006). Reduction in asthma morbidity in children as a result of home remediation aimed at moisture sources. *Environmental Health Perspectives, 114*(10), 1574–1580.

Kolcaba, K. (2003). *Comfort theory and practice: A vision for holistic health care and research*. New York: Springer Publishing Co.

Lau-Walker, M. (2006). A conceptual care model for individualized care approach in cardiac rehabilitation—combining both illness representation and self-efficacy. *British Journal of Health Psychology, 11,* 103–117.

Leininger, M. (1994). Culturally competent care: Visible and invisible. *Journal of Transcultural Nursing, 6*(1), 23–25.

McCaffery, M., & Pasero, C. (1999). *Pain. Clinical manual for nursing practice* (2nd ed.). St. Louis, MO: Mosby.

Pasero, C., & McCaffery, M. (2011). *Pain assessment and pharmacologic management.* St. Louis, MO: Mosby.

Segrin, T., Dorros, S., Meek, P., & Lopez, A. (2007). Depression and anxiety in women with breast cancer and their partners. *Nursing Research, 56*(1), 44–53.

Stuart, G. (2008). *Principles and practice of psychiatric nursing* (9th ed.). St. Louis: Mosby.

Thorns, A., & Edmonds, P. (2000). The management of pruritus in palliative care patients. *European Journal of Palliative Care, 7*(1), 9–12.

Van Dover, L., & Bacon, J. (2001). Spiritual care in nursing practice: A close-up view. *Nursing Forum, 36*(3), 24–27.

White, M., & Grilo, C. (2007). Symptom severity in obese women with binge eating disorder as a function of smoking history. *International Journal of Eating Disorders, 40*(1), 77–81.

Wilkinson, J., & Treas, L. (2011). *Fundamentals of nursing: Theory, concepts, and application* (2nd ed.). Philadelphia: F. A. Davis.

Williams, A., & Irurita, V. (2005). Enhancing the therapeutic potential of hospital environments by increasing the personal control and emotional comfort of hospitalized patients. *Applied Nursing Research, 18*(1), 22–28.

Williams, P., Piamjariyakul, U., Ducey, K., Badura, J., Boltz, K., Olberding, K., et al. (2006). Cancer treatment, symptom monitoring, and self-care in adults: Pilot study. *Cancer Nursing, 29*(5), 347–355.

Comfort, Readiness for Enhanced

Arruda, E., Larson, P., & Meleis, A. (1992). Immigrant Hispanic cancer patients' views. *Cancer Nursing, 15,* 387–395.

Bailey, F. A., Burgio, K. L., Woodby, L. L., Williams, B. R., Redden, D. T., Kovac, S. H., et al. (2005). Improving processes of hospital care during the last hours of life. *Archives of Internal Medicine, 165*(15), 1722–1727.

Berry, A. M., & Davidson, P. M. (2006). Beyond comfort: Oral hygiene as a critical nursing activity in the intensive care unit. *Intensive & Critical Care Nursing, 22*(6), 318–328.

Billhult, A., & Määtä, S. (2009). Light pressure massage for patients with severe anxiety. *Complementary Therapies in Clinical Practice, 15*(2), 96–101.

Cameron, B. (1993). The nature of comfort to hospitalized medical surgical patients. *Journal of Advanced Nursing, 18,* 424–436.

Couchman, B. A., Wetzig, S. M., Coyer, F. M., & Wheeler, M. K. (2007). Nursing care of the mechanically ventilated patient: What does the evidence say? Part one. *Intensive & Critical Care Nursing, 23*(1), 4–14.

Duggleby, W., & Berry, P. (2005). Transitions in shifting goals of care for palliative patients and their families. *Clinical Journal of Oncology Nursing, 9,* 425–428.

Feeley, K., & Gardner, A. (2006). Sedation and analgesia management for mechanically ventilated adults: Literature review, case study and recommendations for practice. *Australian Critical Care, 19*(2), 73–77.

Foster, R. L., Yucha, C. B., Zuk, J., & Vojir, C. P. (2003). Physiologic correlates of comfort in healthy children. *Pain Management Nursing, 4*(1), 23–30.

Gleeson, M., & Timmins, F. (2004). The use of touch to enhance nursing care of older person in long-term mental health care facilities. *Journal of Psychiatric & Mental Health Nursing, 11*(5), 541–545.

Kolcaba, K. (1994). A theory of holistic comfort for nursing. *Journal of Advanced Nursing, 19,* 1178–1184.

Malinowski, A., & Stamler, L. L. (2002). Comfort: Exploration of the concept in nursing. *Journal of Advanced Nursing, 39,* 599–606.

Minden, P. (2005). The importance of words. *Holistic Nursing Practice, 19*(6), 267–271.

Morse, J. (2000). On comfort and comforting. *American Journal of Nursing, 100*(9), 34–38.

Perrin, K., Sheehan, C., Potter, M., & Kazanowski, M. (2012). *Palliative care nursing: Caring for suffering patients*. Sudbury, MA: Jones & Bartlett Learning.

Roffe, L., Schmidt, K., & Ernst, E. (2005). A systematic review of guided imagery as an adjuvant cancer therapy. *Psycho-Oncology, 14*(8), 607–617.

Stringer, M., Shaw, V. D., & Savani, R. C. (2004). Comfort care of neonates at the end of life. *Neonatal Network, 23*(5), 41–46.

Tutton, E., & Seers, K. (2004). Comfort on a ward for older people. *Journal of Advanced Nursing, 46*(4), 380–389.

Communication, Readiness for Enhanced

Alasad, J., & Ahmad, M. (2005). Communication with critically ill patients. *Journal of Advanced Nursing, 50*(4), 356–362.

Block, L. M., & LeGrazie, B. A. (2006). Don't get lost in translation. *Nursing Management, 37*(5), 37–40.

Brach, C., Fraser, I., & Paez, K. (2005). Crossing the language chasm. *Health Affairs, 24*(2), 424–434.

Brice, A. (2000). Access to health service delivery for Hispanics: A communication issue. *Journal of Multicultural Nursing & Health (JMCNH), 6*(2), 7–17.

Edwards, N., Peterson, W. E., & Davies, B. L. (2006). Evaluation of a multiple component intervention to support the implementation of a 'therapeutic relationships' best practice guideline on nurses' communication skills. *Patient Education & Counseling, 63*(1), 3–11.

Elliott, R., Wright, L., & Elliot, R. (1999). Verbal communication: What do critical care nurses say to their unconscious or sedated patients? *Journal of Advanced Nursing, 29*(6), 1412–1420.

Knobf, M. T. (2007). Psychosocial responses in breast cancer survivors. *Seminars in Oncology Nursing, 23*(1), 71–83.

Leonard, M., Graham, S., & Bonacum, D. (2004). The human factor: The critical importance of effective teamwork and communication in providing safe care. *Quality & Safety in Health Care, 13,* i85–90.

Communication: Verbal, Impaired

Cadogan, M. P., Franzi, C., Osterweil, D., & Hill, T. (1999). Barriers to effective communication in skilled nursing facilities: Differences in perception between nurses and physicians. *Journal of the American Geriatrics Society, 47*(1), 71–75.

Haskard, K., DiMatteo, M., & Heritage, J. (2009). Affective and instrumental communication in primary care interactions: Predicting the satisfaction of nursing staff and patients. *Health Communication, 24*(1), 21–32.

Iezzoni, L. F., O'Day, B., Keleen, M. A., & Harker, H. (2004). Improving patient care: Communicating about health care: Observations from persons who are deaf or hard of hearing. *Annals of Internal Medicine, 140*(5), 356–362.

Koester, L. S., Karkowski, A. M., & Traci, M. A. (1998). How do deaf and hearing-impaired mothers regain eye contact when their infants look away? *American Annals of the Deaf, 143*(1), 5–131.

Lindeblade, P. O., & McDonald, M. (1995). Removing communication barriers for the hearing impaired elderly. *Med-Surg Nursing, 4*(5), 379–385.

Underwood, C. (2004). How can we best deliver an inclusive health service? *Primary Health Care, 14*(9), 20–21.

Vogt, A., Kappos, L., Calabrese, P., Stocklin, M., Gschwind, L., Opwis, K., et al. (2009). Working memory training in patients with multiple sclerosis—comparison of two different training schedules. *Restorative Neurology and Neuroscience, 27*(3), 225–235.

Wittenberg-Lyles, E., Goldsmith, J., & Ragan, S. (2010). The COMFORT initiative: Palliative nursing and the centrality of communication. *Journal of Hospice & Palliative Nursing, 12*(5), 282–292.

Community Health, Deficient

Edmundson, S., Stuenkel, D., & Connolly, P. (2005). Upsetting the apple cart: A community anticoagulation clinic survey of life event factors that undermine safe therapy. *Journal of Vascular Nursing, 23*(3), 105–111.

Goetzel, R., Ozminkowski, R., Bruno, J., Rutter, K., Isaac, F., & Wang, S. (2002). The long-term impact of Johnson & Johnson's Health & Wellness Program on employee health risks. *Journal of Occupational and Environmental Medicine, 44*(5), 417–424.

Hawkins, J., Catalano, R., & Aarthur, M. (2002). Promoting science-based prevention in communities. *Addictive Behaviors, 27*(6), 951–976.

Keller, L., Schaffer, M., Lia-Hoagberg, B., & Strohschein, S. (2002). Assessment, program planning, and evaluation in population-based public health practice. *Journal of Public Health Management and Practice, 8*(5), 30–43.

McGinnis, J., Williams-Russo, P., & Knickman, J. (2002). The case for more active policy attention to health promotion. *Health Affairs, 21*(2), 78–93.

Pegus, C., Bazzare, T., Brown, J., & Menzin, J. (2002). Effect of the Heart at Work program on awareness of risk factors, self-efficacy, and health behaviors. *Journal of Occupational and Environmental Medicine, 44*(3), 228–236.

Porter, H., Avery, S., Edmond, L., Straw, R., & Young, J. (2002). Program evaluation in pediatric education. *Journal for Nurses in Staff Development, 18*(5), 258–266.

Rome, S. (2002). Developing a fall-prevention program for patients. *American Journal of Nursing, 102*(6), 24A, 24C-D.

Swallow, A., & Dykes, P. (2004). Tobacco cessation at Greenwich Hospital. *American Journal of Nursing, 104*(12), 61–62.

Woodward, D. (2005). Developing a pain management program through continuous improvement strategies. *Journal of Nursing Care Quality, 20*(3), 261–267.

Confusion, Acute

Alverzo, J. P. (2006). A review of the literature on orientation as an indicator of level of consciousness. *Journal of Nursing Scholarship, 38*(2), 159–164.

Dewing, J. (2003). Sundowning in older people with dementia: Evidence base, nursing assessment and interventions. *Nursing Older People, 15*(8), 24.

Fleminger, S. (2003). Managing agitation and aggression after head injury. *BMJ: British Medical Journal, 327*(7405), 4.

Kehl, K. A. (2004). Treatment of terminal restlessness: A review of the evidence. *Journal of Pain & Palliative Care Pharmacotherapy, 18*(1), 5–30.

Korevaar, J., van Munster, B., & de Rooij, S. (2005). Risk factors for delirium in acutely admitted elderly patients: A prospective cohort study. *BMC Geriatric, 5*(1), 6.

Ludwick, R. (1999). Clinical decision making: Recognition of confusion and application of restraints. *Orthopedic Nursing, 18*(1), 65–72.

Pratico, C., Quattrone, D., Lucanto, T., Amato, A., Penna, A., Roscitano, C., et al. (2005). Drugs of anesthesia acting on central cholinergic system may cause post operative cognitive dysfunction and delirium. *Medical Hypotheses, 65,* 972–982.

Seaman, J., Schillerstrom, J., Carroll, D., & Brown, T. (2006). Impaired oxidative metabolism precipitates delirium: A study of 101 ICU patients. *Psychosomatics, 47*(1), 56–61.

Confusion, Acute, Risk for

Alasad, J., & Ahmad, M. (2005). Communication with critically ill patients. *Journal of Advanced Nursing, 50*(4), 356–362.

Dewing, J. (2003). Sundowning in older people with dementia: Evidence base, nursing assessment and interventions. *Nursing Older People, 15*(8), 24.

Fleminger, S. (2003). Managing agitation and aggression after head injury. *BMJ: British Medical Journal, 327*(7405), 4.

Gleeson, M., & Timmins, F. (2005). A review of the use and clinical effectiveness of touch as a nursing intervention. *Clinical Effectiveness in Nursing, 9*(1), 69–77.

Irving, K. (2002). Governing the conduct of conduct: Are restraints inevitable? *Journal of Advanced Nursing, 40*(4), 405–412.

Korevaar, J., van Munster, B., & de Rooij, S. (2005). Risk factors for delirium in acutely admitted elderly patients: A prospective cohort study. *BMC Geriatric, 5*(1), 6.

Poole, J. (2003). Poole's algorithm: Nursing management of disturbed behaviour in older people—the evidence. *Australian Journal of Advanced Nursing, 20*(3), 38–43.

Seaman, J., Schillerstrom, J., Carroll, D., & Brown, T. (2006). Impaired oxidative metabolism precipitates delirium: A study of 101 ICU patients. *Psychosomatics, 47*(1), 56–61.

Stickley, T., & Freshwater, D. (2006). The art of listening in the therapeutic relationship [cover story]. *Mental Health Practice, 9*(5), 12–18.

Confusion, Chronic

Alasad, J., & Ahmad, M. (2005). Communication with critically ill patients. *Journal of Advanced Nursing, 50*(4), 356–362.

Anderson, C. (1999). Delirium and confusion are not interchangeable terms [letter to editor]. *Oncology Nursing Forum, 26*(3), 497–498.

Burnside, I., & Haight, B. (1994). Reminiscence and life review: Therapeutic interventions for older people. *Nurse Practitioner, 19*(4), 55–60.

Dewing, J. (2003). Sundowning in older people with dementia: Evidence base, nursing assessment and interventions. *Nursing Older People, 15*(8), 24.

Gleeson, M., & Timmins, F. (2005). A review of the use and clinical effectiveness of touch as a nursing intervention. *Clinical Effectiveness in Nursing, 9*(1), 69–77.

Hall, G. R., & Buckwalter, K. C. (1987). Progressively lowered stress threshold: A conceptual model for care of adults with Alzheimer's disease. *Archives of Psychiatric Nursing, 1,* 399–406.

Kehl, K. A. (2004). Treatment of terminal restlessness: A review of the evidence. *Journal of Pain & Palliative Care Pharmacotherapy, 18*(1), 5–30.

Rasin, J., & Barrick, A. L. (2004). Bathing patients with dementia. *American Journal of Nursing, 104*(3), 30–33.

Roberts, B. L. (2001). Managing delirium in adult intensive care patients. *Critical Care Nurse, 21*(1), 48–55.

Smith, B. (1990). *Role of orientation therapy and reminiscence therapy: Alzheimer's disease*. St. Louis, MO: Mosby.

Spector, A., Orrell, M., & Woods, B. (2010). Cognitive stimulation therapy (CST): Effects on different areas of cognitive function for people with demential. *International Journal of Geriatric Psychiatry, 25*(12), 1253–1258.

Stickley, T., & Freshwater, D. (2006). The art of listening in the therapeutic relationship [cover story]. *Mental Health Practice, 9*(5), 12–18.

Constipation

Bosshard, W., Dreher, R., Schnegg, J., & Büla, C. J. (2004). The treatment of chronic constipation in elderly people: An update. *Drugs & Aging, 21*(14), 911–930.

Bowers, B. (2006). Evaluating the evidence for administering phosphate enemas. *British Journal of Nursing (BJN), 15*(7), 378–381.

Bywater, A., & While, A. (2006). Management of bowel dysfunction in people with multiple sclerosis. *British Journal of Community Nursing, 11*(8), 333–341.

Craft, L., & Prahlow, J. (2011). From fecal impaction to colon perforation. *American Journal of Nursing, 111*(8), 38–43.

Davies, C. (2004). Clinical. The use of phosphate enemas in the treatment of constipation. *Nursing Times, 100*(18), 32–35.

Ellins, N. (2006). Water for health—hydration best practice for older people. *Nursing & Residential Care, 8*(10), 470–472.

Emly, M., & Rochester, P. (2006). A new look at constipation management in the community. *British Journal of Community Nursing, 11*(8), 326–332.

Kyle, G. (2005). Steps to best practice in bowel care. *Nursing Times, 101*(2), 47.

Kyle, G. (2006). Assessment and treatment of older patients with constipation [cover story]. *Nursing Standard, 21*(8), 41–46.

Kyle, G., Prynn, P., & Oliver, H. (2004). An evidence-based procedure for the digital removal of faeces. *Nursing Times, 100*(48), 71.

Peate, I. (2003). Nursing role in the management of constipation: Use of laxatives. *British Journal of Nursing (BJN), 12*(19), 1130–1136.

Schnelle, J., Leung, F., Satish, S., Beuscher, L., Keeler, E., Clift, J., et al. (2010). A controlled trial of an intervention to improve urinary and fecal incontinence and constipation. *Journal of the American Geriatrics Society, 58*(8), 1504–1511.

Suares, N., & Ford, A. (2011). Systematic review: The effects of fibre in the management of chronic idiopathic constipation. *Alimentary Pharmacology & Therapeutics, 33*(8), 895–901.

Tariq, S. H. (2007). Constipation in long-term care. *Journal of the American Medical Directors Association, 8*(4), 209–218.

Constipation, Perceived

Annells, M., & Koch, T. (2002). Older people seeking solutions to constipation: The laxative mire. *Journal of Clinical Nursing, 11*(5), 603–612.

Annells, M., & Koch, T. (2003). Constipation and the preached trio: Diet, fluid intake, exercise. *International Journal of Nursing Studies, 40*(8), 843.

Bosshard, W., Dreher, R., Schnegg, J., & Büla, C. J. (2004). The treatment of chronic constipation in elderly people: An update. *Drugs & Aging, 21*(14), 911–930.

Bowers, B. (2006). Evaluating the evidence for administering phosphate enemas. *British Journal of Nursing (BJN), 15*(7), 378–381.

Ellins, N. (2006). Water for health—hydration best practice for older people. *Nursing & Residential Care, 8*(10), 470–472.

Emly, M., & Rochester, P. (2006). A new look at constipation management in the community. *British Journal of Community Nursing, 11*(8), 326–332.

Gates, A., & Bhatia, J. (2010). On my way home: Practical solutions for nutritional management of the ELBW and VLBW infant after discharge from the NICU. *Dietetic Currents, 1*(1), 1–5. Retrieved November 28, 2011, from http://abbottnutrition.com/downloads/nicu/74675%202010%20Dietetic%20Currents%206_24.pdf

Kyle, G. (2006). Assessment and treatment of older patients with constipation. [cover story]. *Nursing Standard, 21*(8), 41–46.

Peate, I. (2003). Nursing role in the management of constipation: Use of laxatives. *British Journal of Nursing (BJN), 12*(19), 1130–1136.

Constipation, Risk for

(Also see the bibliography for Constipation.)

Annells, M., & Koch, T. (2002). Older people seeking solutions to constipation: The laxative mire. *Journal of Clinical Nursing, 11*(5), 603–612.

Annells, M., & Koch, T. (2003). Constipation and the preached trio: Diet, fluid intake, exercise. *International Journal of Nursing Studies, 40*(8), 843.

Bell, S., Fowler, S., Hinkle, J., Mcilvoy, L., & Thompson, H. J. (2007). Best practices: Prevention of constipation. *Synapse (American Association of Neuroscience Nurses), 34*(2), 3.

Ellins, N. (2006). Water for health—hydration best practice for older people. *Nursing & Residential Care, 8*(10), 470–472.

Kyle, G. (2005). Steps to best practice in bowel care. *Nursing Times, 101*(2), 47.

Kyle, G. (2006). Assessment and treatment of older patients with constipation [cover story]. *Nursing Standard, 21*(8), 41–46.

Peate, I. (2003). Nursing role in the management of constipation: Use of laxatives. *British Journal of Nursing (BJN), 12*(19), 1130–1136.

Tariq, S. H. (2007). Constipation in long-term care. *Journal of the American Medical Directors Association, 8*(4), 209–218.

Weeks, S. K., Hubbartt, E., & Michaels, T. K. (2000). Keys to bowel success. *Rehabilitation Nursing, 25*(2), 66–80.

Contamination

Allen, G. (2003). Evidence for practice: Transmission of Whipple's disease via gastroscopes. *AORN Journal, 78*(2), 310–311.

Allen, G. (2004a). Evidence for practice: Comparison of hand hygiene methods and effects of ring wearing on hand contamination. *AORN Journal, 79*(1), 236.

Allen, G. (2004b). Evidence for practice: Infections associated with injections from a multiple-dose vial. *AORN Journal, 79*(1), 238–238.

Allen, G. (2005). Evidence for practice: Contamination in standard versus ultraclean ORs. *AORN Journal, 81*(4), 890.

Allen, G. (2006a). Evidence for practice: Bacterial contamination in orthopedic implant surgery. *AORN Journal, 83*(4), 968–969.

Allen, G. (2006b). Evidence for practice: Protein contamination on surgical instruments. *AORN Journal, 83*(4), 965–966.

Brown, M. J., McLaine, P., Dixon, S., & Simon, P. (2006). A randomized, community-based trial of home visiting to reduce blood lead levels in children. *Pediatrics, 117*(1), 147–153.

Centers for Disease Control and Prevention. (2005). *Third national report on human exposure to environmental chemicals: Executive summary* (NCEH Pub # 05-0725). Atlanta, GA: Author.

Chu, J. J. (2004). Sterile gloves and the repairing of uncomplicated lacerations. *American Journal of Nursing, 104*(7), 72GG–72II.

Colodner, R., Sakran, W., Miron, D., Teitler, N., Khavalevsky, E., & Kopelowitz, J. (2003). Listeria monocytogenes cross-contamination in a nursery. *American Journal of Infection Control, 31*(5), 322–324.

Hicks, J., Weinstock, C., Coleman, D., Hanfling, S., Cantrill, I., Redlener, J., et al. (2011). Health care system planning for and response to a nuclear detonation. *Disaster Medicine and Public Health Preparedness, 5*(Suppl. 1), S73–S88

Kreiss, Y., Merin, O., Peleg, K., Levy, G., Vinker, S., Sagi, R., et al. (2010). Early disaster response in Haiti: The Israeli Field Hospital experience. *Annals of Internal Medicine, 153*(1), 45–48.

Lipp, A., & Edwards, P. (2005). Disposable surgical face masks: A systematic review. *Canadian Operating Room Nursing Journal, 23*(3), 21.

McCauley, L. A., Michaels, S., Rothlein, J., Muniz, J., Lasarev, M., & Ebbert, C. (2003). Pesticide exposure and self-reported home hygiene. *AAOHN Journal, 51,* 113–119.

Sprung, C., Zimmerman, J., Christian, M., Joynt, G., Hick, J., Taylor, B., et al. (2010). Recommendations for intensive care unit and hospital preparations for an influenza epidemic or mass disaster: Summary report of the European Society of Intensive Care Medicine's Task Force for intensive care unit triage during an influenza epidemic or mass disaster. *Intensive Care Medicine, 36*(3), 428–443.

Williams, T. A., & Leslie, G. D. (2004). A review of the nursing care of enteral feeding tubes in critically ill adults: Part 1. *Intensive & Critical Care Nursing, 20*(6), 330–343.

Williams, T. A., & Leslie, G. D. (2005). A review of the nursing care of enteral feeding tubes in critically ill adults: Part II. *Intensive & Critical Care Nursing, 21*(1), 5–15.

Contamination, Risk for

Allen, G. (2006). Evidence for practice: Permanent marking pen sterility. *AORN Journal, 83*(4), 966.

Chu, J. J. (2004). Sterile gloves and the repairing of uncomplicated lacerations. *American Journal of Nursing, 104*(7), 72GG–72II.

Earsing, K. A., Hobson, D. B., & White, K. M. (2005). Best-practice protocols: Preventing central line infection. *Nursing Management, 36*(10), 18.

Hanrahan, K. S., & Lofgren, M. (2004). Evidence-based practice: Examining the risk of toys in the microenvironment of infants in the neonatal intensive care unit. *Advances in Neonatal Care, 4*(4), 184–205.

Hughes, F. (2011). Nurses' contribution following an emergency. *Kai Tiaki Nursing New Zealand, 17*(8), 33.

LaCharity, L. A., & McClure, E. R. (2003). Are plants vectors for transmission of infection in acute care? *Critical Care Nursing Clinics of North America, 15,* 119–124.

Mermel, L. A. (2002). Prevention of intravascular catheter-related infections. *CINA: Official Journal of the Canadian Intravenous Nurses Association, 18,* 40.

O'Keefe-McCarthy, S. (2006). Evidence-based nursing strategies to prevent ventilator-acquired pneumonia. *Dynamics, 17*(1), 8–11.

Powers, R., & Daily, E. (2010). *International disaster nursing*. Cambridge, NY: Cambridge University Press.

Strangeland, P. (2010). Disaster nursing: A retrospective review. *Critical Care Nursing Clinics of North America, 22*(4), 421–436.

Coping: Community, Ineffective

Allender, J., & Spradley, B. (2005). *Community health nursing* (6th ed.). Philadelphia: Lippincott Williams & Wilkins.

Barry, K. L. (1999). *Brief interventions and brief therapies for substance abuse* (Center for Substance Abuse Treatment Protocol (TIP) Series 34). Rockville, MD: Department of Health and Human Services.

Hemming, L., & Maher, D. (2005). Complementary therapies in palliative care: A summary of current evidence. *British Journal of Community Nursing, 10*(10), 448–452.

Keister, K. J. (2006). Predictors of self-assessed health, anxiety, and depressive symptoms in nursing home residents at week 1 postrelocation. *Journal of Aging & Health, 18*(5), 722–742.

Killaspy, H., Kingett, S., Bebbington, P., Blizard, R., Johnson, S., Nolan, F., et al. (2009). Randomised evaluation of assertive community treatment: 3-year outcomes. *The British Journal of Psychiatry, 195,* 81–82.

McBride, K. L., White, C. L., Sourial, R., & Mayo, N. (2004). Postdischarge nursing interventions for stroke survivors and their families. *Journal of Advanced Nursing, 47*(2), 192–200.

Sadowski, L., Kee, R., VanderWeele, T., & Buchanan, D. (2009). Effect of a housing and case management program on emergency department visits and hospitalizations among chronically ill homeless adults. *The Journal of the American Medical Association, 301*(17), 1771–1778.

Trappes-Lomax, T., Ellis, A., Fox, M., Taylor, R., Power, M., Stead, J., et al. (2006). Buying time I: A prospective, controlled trial of a joint health/social care residential rehabilitation unit for older people on discharge from hospital. *Health & Social Care in the Community, 14*(1), 49–62.

Wai Tong Chien, Chan, S., Morrissey, J., & Thompson, D. (2005). Effectiveness of a mutual support group for families of patients with schizophrenia. *Journal of Advanced Nursing, 51*(6), 595–608.

Wright, M. O., Fopma-Loy, J., & Fischer, S. (2005). Multidimensional assessment of resilience in mothers who are child sexual abuse survivors. *Child Abuse & Neglect, 29*(10), 1173–1193.

Coping: Community, Readiness for Enhanced

Barbera, J., Yeatts, D., & Macintyre, A. (2009). Challenge of hospital emergency preparedness: Analysis and recommendations. *Disaster Medicine and Public Health Preparedness, 3,* S74–S82.

Ervin, N. E., & Chen, S. C. (2005). Development of an instrument measuring family care. *Journal of Nursing Measurement, 13*(1), 39–50.

Ewing, J. A. (1984). Detecting alcoholism: The CAGE questionnaire. *Journal of the American Medical Association, 252,* 1905–1907.

Hemming, L., & Maher, D. (2005). Complementary therapies in palliative care: A summary of current evidence. *British Journal of Community Nursing, 10*(10), 448–452.

Jaramillo-Velez, D., Ospina-Munoz, D., Cabarcas-Iglesias, G., & Humphreys, J. (2005). Resilience, spirituality, distress and tactics for battered women's conflict resolution. *Rev Salud Publica, 7,* 281–291 (Spanish).

Keister, K. J. (2006). Predictors of self-assessed health, anxiety, and depressive symptoms in nursing home residents at week 1 postrelocation. *Journal of Aging & Health, 18*(5), 722–742.

Marshall, H., Ryan, P., Roberton, D., Street, J., & Watson, M. (2009). Pandemic influenza and community preparedness. *American Journal of Public Health, 99*(S2), 365–371.

Meredith, P., Strong, J., & Feeney, J. (2006). The relationship of adult attachment to emotion, catastrophizing, control, threshold and tolerance, in experimentally-induced pain. *Pain, 120*(1–2), 44–52. Epub December 13, 2005.

Sexton, K., & Linder, S. (2011). Cumulative risk assessment for combined health effects from chemical and nonchemical stressors. *American Journal of Public Health, 101*(S1), S81–S88.

Trappes-Lomax, T., Ellis, A., Fox, M., Taylor, R., Power, M., Stead, J., et al. (2006). Buying time I: A prospective, controlled trial of a joint health/social care residential rehabilitation unit for older people on discharge from hospital. *Health & Social Care in the Community, 14*(1), 49–62.

Wai Tong Chien, Chan, S., Morrissey, J., & Thompson, D. (2005). Effectiveness of a mutual support group for families of patients with schizophrenia. *Journal of Advanced Nursing, 51*(6), 595–608.

Wright, M. O., Fopma-Loy, J., & Fischer, S. (2005). Multidimensional assessment of resilience in mothers who are child sexual abuse survivors. *Child Abuse & Neglect, 29*(10), 1173–1193.

Coping, Defensive

Alasad, J., & Ahmad, M. (2005). Communication with critically ill patients. *Journal of Advanced Nursing, 50*(4), 356–362.

Arias, M., & Smith, L. N. (2007). Early mobilization of acute stroke patients. *Journal of Clinical Nursing, 16*(2), 282–288.

Beck, J. (2011). *Cognitive behavior therapy* (2nd ed.). New York: The Guilford Press.

Carney, R., Fitzsimons, D., & Dempster, M. (2002). Why people experiencing acute myocardial infarction delay seeking medical assistance. *European Journal of Cardiovascular Nursing, 1*(4), 237.

England, M. (2007). Efficacy of cognitive nursing intervention for voice hearing. *Perspectives in Psychiatric Care, 43*(2), 69–76.

Kirshbaum, M. N. (2007). A review of the benefits of whole body exercise during and after treatment for breast cancer. *Journal of Clinical Nursing, 16*(1), 104–121.

Patterson, G. (2005). The bully as victim? *Paediatric Nursing, 17*(10), 27–30.

Reichow, B., & Volkmar, F. (2010). Social skills interventions for individuals with autism: Evaluation for evidence-based practices within a best practice synthesis framework. *Journal of Autism and Developmental Disorders, 40*(2), 149–166.

Coping: Family, Compromised

Chang, B., Nitta, S., Carter, P., & Markham, Y. (2004). Technology innovations. Perceived helpfulness of telephone calls: Providing support for caregivers of family members with dementia. *Journal of Gerontological Nursing, 30*(9), 14–21.

Comfort, M., Sockloff, A., Loverro, J., & Kaltenbach, K. (2003). Multiple predictors of substance abuse, women's treatments and outcomes: A prospective longitudinal study. *Addiction Behavior, 28*(2), 199–224.

Finkelman, A. W. (2000). Self-management for psychiatric patient at home. *Home Care Provider, 5*(6), 95–101.

Hodgkinson, R., & Lester, H. (2002). Stresses and coping strategies of mothers living with a child with cystic fibrosis: Implications for nursing professionals. *Journal of Advanced Nursing, 39*(4), 377–383.

Johansson, I., Hildingh, C., Wenneberg, S., Fridlund, B., & Ahlström, G. (2006). Theoretical model of coping among relatives of patients in intensive care units: A simultaneous concept analysis. *Journal of Advanced Nursing, 56*(5), 463–471.

Long, L. E. (2003). Stress in families of children with sepsis. *Critical Care Nursing Clinics of North America, 15*(1), 47–53.

McMillan, S. C. (2005). Interventions to facilitate family caregiving at the end of life. *Journal of Palliative Medicine, 8,* S132–S139.

Nichols, L., Martindale-Adams, J., Burns, R., Graney, M., & Zuber, J. (2011). Translation of a dementia caregiver support program in a health care system—REACH VA. *Archives of Internal Medicine, 171*(4), 353–359.

O'Haire, S. E., & Blackford, J. C. (2005). Nurses' moral agency in negotiating parental participation in care. *International Journal of Nursing Practice, 11*(6), 250–256.

Scott, J. T., Prictor, M. J., Harmsen, M., Broom, A., Entwistle, V., Sowden, A., et al. (2006). Interventions for improving communication with children and adolescents about a family member's cancer. *Cochrane Library* (4).

Tak, Y. R., & McCubbin, M. (2002). Family stress, perceived social support and coping following the diagnosis of a child's congenital heart disease. *Journal of Advanced Nursing, 39*(2), 190–198.

Viegas, L., Turrini, R., & Cerullo, J. (2010). An analysis of nursing diagnoses for patients undergoing procedures in a Brazilian interventional radiology suite. *AORN, 91*(5), 544–557.

Wai Tong Chien, Chan, S., Morrissey, J., & Thompson, D. (2005). Effectiveness of a mutual support group for families of patients with schizophrenia. *Journal of Advanced Nursing, 51*(6), 595–608.

Wray, L., Shulan, M., Toseland, R., Freeman, K., Vasquez, B., & Gao, J. (2010). The effect of telephone support groups on costs of care for veterans with dementia. *The Gerontologist, 50*(5), 623–631.

Coping: Family, Disabled

Note: Also refer to references in Coping: Family, Compromised (preceding).

Comfort, M., Sockloff, A., Loverro, J., & Kaltenbach, K. (2003). Multiple predictors of substance abuse, women's treatments and outcomes: A prospective longitudinal study. *Addiction Behavior, 28*(2), 199–224.

Kovalesky, A. (2004). Women with substance abuse concerns. *Nursing Clinics of North America, 39*(1), 97–115.

Long, L. E. (2003). Stress in families of children with sepsis. *Critical Care Nursing Clinics of North America, 15*(1), 47–53.

Tak, Y. R., & McCubbin, M. (2002). Family stress, perceived social support and coping following the diagnosis of a child's congenital heart disease. *Journal of Advanced Nursing, 39*(2), 190–198.

Willis, D., & Porche, D. (2004). Male battering of intimate partners: Theoretical underpinnings, approaches and interventions. *Nursing Clinics of North America, 39*(1), 271–282.

Coping: Family, Readiness for Enhanced

Finkelman, A. W. (2000). Self-management for psychiatric patient at home. *Home Care Provider, 5*(6), 95–101.

Grant, J. S., Elliott, T. R., Weaver, M., Bartolucci, A. A., & Giger, J. N. (2002). Telephone intervention with family caregivers of stroke survivors after rehabilitation. *Stroke (00392499), 33*(8), 2060–2065.

Hodgkinson, R., & Lester, H. (2002). Stresses and coping strategies of mothers living with a child with cystic fibrosis: Implications for nursing professionals. *Journal of Advanced Nursing, 39*(4), 377–383.

Holden, J., Harrison, L., & Johnson, M. (2002). Families, nurses and intensive care patients: A review of the literature. *Journal of Clinical Nursing, 11*(2), 140–148.

Hudson, P. L. (2006). How well do family caregivers cope after caring for a relative with advanced disease and how can health professionals enhance their support? *Journal of Palliative Medicine, 9*(3), 694–703.

Johansson, I., Hildingh, C., Wenneberg, S., Fridlund, B., & Ahlström, G. (2006). Theoretical model of coping among relatives of patients in intensive care units: A simultaneous concept analysis. *Journal of Advanced Nursing, 56*(5), 463–471.

Lyon, B. L. (2002). Cognitive self-care skills: A model for managing stressful lifestyles. *Nursing Clinics of North America, 37*(2), 285–294.

McMillan, S. C. (2005). Interventions to facilitate family caregiving at the end of life. *Journal of Palliative Medicine, 8,* S132–S139.

O'Haire, S. E., & Blackford, J. C. (2005). Nurses' moral agency in negotiating parental participation in care. *International Journal of Nursing Practice, 11*(6), 250–256.

Scott, J. T., Prictor, M. J., Harmsen, M., Broom, A., Entwistle, V., Sowden, A., et al. (2006). Interventions for improving communication with children and adolescents about a family member's cancer. *Cochrane Library* (4).

Wai Tong Chien, Chan, S., Morrissey, J., & Thompson, D. (2005). Effectiveness of a mutual support group for families of patients with schizophrenia. *Journal of Advanced Nursing, 51*(6), 595–608.

Coping, Ineffective

Comfort, M., Sockloff, A., Loverro, J., & Kaltenbach, K. (2003). Multiple predictors of substance abuse, women's treatments and outcomes: A prospective longitudinal study. *Addiction Behavior, 28*(2), 199–224.

Ditre, J., Heckman, B., Butts, E., & Brandon, T. (2010). Effects of expectancies and coping on pain-induced motivation to smoke. *Journal of Abnormal Psychology, 119*(3), 524–533.

Flagler, S., Hughes, T., & Kovalesky, A. (1997). Toward understanding of addiction. *JOGNN, 26*(4), 441–448.

Folkman, S., Lazarus, R., Pimley, S., & Novacek, J. (1987). Age differences in stress and coping processes. *Psychology and Aging, 2,* 171–184.

Kovalesky, A. (2004). Women with substance abuse concerns. *Nursing Clinics of North America, 39*(1), 97–115.

Lazarus, R. (1985). The costs and benefits of denial. In A. Monat & R. Lazarus (Eds.), *Stress and coping: An anthology* (2nd ed.). New York: Columbia.

Lederman, T., Bodenmann, G., Rudaz, M., & Bradbury, T. (2010). Stress, communication, and marital quality in couples. *Family Relations, 59*(2), 195–206.

Stanley, S., Allen, E., Markman, H., Rhoades, G., & Prentice, D. (2010). Decreasing divorce in U. S. Army couples: Results from a randomized controlled trial using PREP for strong bonds. *Journal of Couple & Relationship Therapy, 9*(2), 149–160.

Coping, Readiness for Enhanced

Gaston-Johansson, F. (2000). The effectiveness of the comprehensive coping strategy program on clinical outcomes in breast cancer autologous bone marrow transplantation. *Cancer Nursing, 23*(4), 277–285.

Lazarus, R., & Folkman, S. (1984). *Stress, appraisal and coping*. New York: Springer.

Lyon, B. L. (2002). Cognitive self-care skills: A model for managing stressful lifestyles. *Nursing Clinics of North America, 37*(2), 285–294.

Potocki, E., & Everly, G. (1989). Control and the human stress response. In G. Everly (Ed.), *A clinical guide to treatment of human stress response*. New York: Plenum.

Selye, H. (1974). *Stress without distress*. Philadelphia: Lippincott Williams & Wilkins.

Stanley, S., Allen, E., Markman, H., Rhoades, G., & Prentice, D. (2010). Decreasing divorce in U. S. Army couples: Results from a randomized controlled trial using PREP for strong bonds. *Journal of Couple & Relationship Therapy, 9*(2), 149–160.

Decision Making, Readiness for Enhanced

Albano, A., & DiBartolo, P. (2007). *Cognitive-behavioral therapy for social phobia in adolescents: Stand up, speak out, therapist guide*. New York: Oxford University Press.

Evans, R., Elwyn, G., & Edwards, A. (2004). Making interactive decision support for patients a reality. *Informatics in Primary Care, 12,* 109–113.

Harkness, J. (2005). Patient involvement: A vital principle for patient-centered health care. *World Hospitals and Health Services: The Official Journal of the International Hospital Federation, 41*(2), 12–16.

Kettunen, T., Liimatainen, L., Villberg, J., & Perko, U. (2006). Developing empowering health counseling measurement: Preliminary results. *Patient Education & Counseling, 64*(1), 159–166.

O'Connor, A. M., Stacey, D., Entwistle, V., Llewllyn-Thomas, H., Rovner, D., Homes-Rovner, M., et al. (2005). *Decision aids for people facing health treatment or screening decisions. The Cochrane Library, Vol. 3, CD-ROM Computer file*. London: BMJ Publishing Group.

Paterson, B. L., Russell, C., & Thorne, S. (2001). Critical analysis of everyday self-care decision making in chronic illness. *Journal of Advanced Nursing, 35,* 335–341.

Pender, N., Murdaugh, C., & Parsons, M. (2006). *Health promotion in nursing practice* (5th ed.). Upper Saddle River, NJ: Pearson Prentice/Hall.

Raines, D. A. (1993). Values: A guiding force. *A WHONNS Clinical Issues in Perinatal and Women's Health Nursing, 4,* 531–533.

Saba, G. W., Wong, S. T., Schillinger, D., Fernandez, A., Somkin, C. P., Wilson, C. C., et al. (2006). Shared decision making and the experience of partnership in primary care. *Annals of Family Medicine, 4*(1), 54–62.

Sebern, M. (2005). Shared care, elder and family member skills used to manage burden. *Journal of Advanced Nursing, 52*(2), 170–179.

Tunis, S. R. (2005). Perspective: A clinical research strategy to support shared decision-making. *Health Affairs, 24,* 180–184.

Wiest, D. A. (2006). Application of a decision-making model in clinical practice. *Topics in Emergency Medicine, 28*(2), 149–151.

Wilson, D. (2010). Stress management for adult survivors of childhood sexual abuse: A holistic inquiry. *Western Journal of Nursing Research, 32,* 103–127.

Decisional Conflict

Arries, E. (2005). Virtue ethics: An approach to moral dilemmas in nursing. *Curationis, 28*(3), 64–72.

Beauchamp, T., & Childress, J. (2001). *Principles of biomedical ethics* (5th ed.). New York: Oxford University Press.

Cicirelli, V., & MacLean, A. P. (2000). Hastening death: A comparison of two end-of-life decisions. *Death Studies, 24*(3), 401–419.

Connor, A. M., Jacobsen, M. J., & Stacey, D. (2002). An evidence-based approach to managing women's decisional conflict. *JOGNN: Journal of Obstetric, Gynecologic, & Neonatal Nursing, 31*(5), 570–581.

Edwards, A., Evans, R., & Elwyn, G. (2003). Manufactured but not imported: New directions for research in shared decision making support and skills. *Patient Education and Counseling, 50,* 33–38.

Elwyn, G. (2009). *Shared decision making in health care: Achieving evidence-based choice*. Oxford, UK: Oxford University Press.

Elwyn, G., Laitner, S., Coulter, A., Walker, E., Watson, P., & Thomson, R. (2010). Implementing shared decision making in the NHS. *British Medical Journal, 341,* 971–973.

Hewitt, J. (2002). A critical review of the arguments debating the role of the nurse advocate. *Journal of Advanced Nursing, 37*(5), 439–445.

Hiltunen, E. (1987). Decisional conflict: A phenomenological description from the points of view of the nurse and the client. In A. M. McLane (Ed.), *Classification of nursing diagnosis: Proceedings of the seventh conference*. St. Louis, MO: Mosby.

Kopala, B., & Burkhart, L. (2005). Ethical dilemma and moral distress: Proposed new NANDA diagnoses. *International Journal of Nursing Terminologies and Classifications, 16,* 3–13.

Lawn, S., & Condon, J. (2006). Psychiatric nurses' ethical stance on cigarette smoking by patients: Determinants and dilemmas in their role in supporting cessation. *International Journal of Mental Health Nursing, 15*(2), 111–118.

O'Connor, A. M. (1995). Validation of a decisional conflict scale. *Medical Decision Making, 15*(1), 25–30.

Denial, Ineffective

Carney, R., Fitzsimons, D., & Dempster, M. (2002). Why people experiencing acute myocardial infarction delay seeking medical assistance. *European Journal of Cardiovascular Nursing, 1*(4), 237.

Duhamel, F., Dupuis, F., & Wright, L. (2009). Families' and nurses' responses to the "one question question": Reflections for clinical practice, education, and research in family nursing. *Journal of Family Nursing, 15*(4), 461–485.

Gammon, J. (1998). Analysis of the stressful effects of hospitalisation and source isolation coping and psychological constructs. *International Journal of Nursing Practice, 4*(2), 84–96.

Lazarus, R. (1985). The costs and benefits of denial. In A. Monat & R. Lazarus (Eds.), *Stress and coping: An anthology* (2nd ed.). New York: Columbia.

McKinley, S., Dracup, K., Moser, D., Riegel, B., Doering, L., Meischke, H., et al. (2009). The effect of a short one-on-one nursing intervention on knowledge, attitudes and beliefs related to response to acute coronary syndrome in people with coronary heart disease: A randomized controlled trial. *International Journal of Nursing Studies, 46*(8), 1037–1046.

Sandstrom, M. J., & Cramer, P. (2003). Defense mechanisms and psychological adjustment in childhood. *Journal of Nervous and Mental Disease, 191,* 487–495.

Dentition, Impaired

American dental hygienists' association dental hygiene diagnosis position paper. (2006). *Access, 20*(1), 23–24.

Chalmers, J., & Pearson, A. (2005). Oral hygiene care for residents with dementia: A literature review. *Journal of Advanced Nursing, 52*(4), 410–419.

Early childhood pacifier use in relation to breastfeeding, SIDS, infection and dental malocclusion. (2006). *Nursing Standard, 20*(38), 52–57.

Grap, M. J., Munro, C. L., Ashtiani, B., & Bryant, S. (2003). Oral care interventions in critical care: Frequency and documentation. *American Journal of Critical Care, 12*(2), 113–119.

O'Reilly, M. (2003). Oral care of the critically ill: A review of the literature and guidelines for practice. *Australian Critical Care, 16*(3), 101–110.

Pearson, A., & Chalmers, J. (2004). Oral hygiene care for adults with dementia in residential aged care facilities. *JBI Reports, 2*(3), 65–113.

Development: Delayed, Risk for

Bagnato, S. J., Blair, K., Slater, J., McNally, R., Mathews, J., & Minzenberg, B. (2004). Developmental healthcare partnerships in inclusive early childhood intervention. *Infants & Young Children: An Interdisciplinary Journal of Special Care Practices, 17*(4), 301–317.

Beal, J. (2005). Toward evidence-based practice. Implications of kangaroo care for growth and development in preterm infants. *MCN: The American Journal of Maternal Child Nursing, 30*(5), 338.

Bultas, M. (2011). The health care experiences of the preschool child with autism. *Journal of Pediatric Nursing*. DOI: 10. 1016/j.pedn.2011.05.005. Retrieved December 21, 2011, from http://www.sciencedirect.com/science/article/pii/S0882596311002831#FCANote

Hussey-Gardner, B., McNinch, A., Anastasi, J. M., & Miller, M. (2002). Early intervention best practice: Collaboration among an NICU, an early intervention program, and an NICU follow-up program. *Neonatal Network, 21*(3), 15–22.

Kennedy, M. S. (2002). Educational program for NICU moms helps infants develop. *American Journal of Nursing, 102*(2), 21.

Magill-Evans, J., Harrison, M. J., Rempel, G., & Slater, L. (2006). Interventions with fathers of young children: Systematic literature review. *Journal of Advanced Nursing, 55*(2), 248–264.

Nanthamongkolchai, S., Meerod, C., Munsawaengsub, C., Shuaythong, P., & Khajornchaikul, P. (2010). Effect of a training program to enhance knowledge and practice of mothers and the development of children aged one to three years. *Asia Journal of Public Health, 1*(1), 2–7.

Ohgi, S., Fukuda, M., Akiyama, T., & Gima, H. (2004). Effect of an early intervention programme on low birthweight infants with cerebral injuries. *Journal of Paediatrics & Child Health, 40*(12), 689–695.

Rick, S. L. (2006). Developmental care on newborn intensive care units: Nurses' experiences and neurodevelopmental, behavioural, and parenting outcomes. A critical review of the literature. *Journal of Neonatal Nursing, 12*(2), 56–61.

Symington, A., & Pinelli, J. M. (2002). Distilling the evidence on developmental care: A systematic review. *Advances in Neonatal Care, 2*(4), 198–221.

Symington, A., & Pinelli, J. M. (2006). Developmental care for promoting development and preventing morbidity in preterm infants. *Cochrane Library* (4). DOI: 10.1002/14651858.CD001814.pub2

Turrill, S. (2002). Focusing nursing care on quality of life: Part 1. The relevance of the developmental care model. *Journal of Neonatal Nursing, 8*(1), 15–19.

Welby, J. (2006). Using a health promotion model to promote benchmarking. *Paediatric Nursing, 18*(6), 34–36.

Diarrhea

Larson, C. E. (2000). Evidence-based practice. Safety and efficacy of oral rehydration therapy for treatment of diarrhea and gastroenteritis in pediatrics. *Pediatric Nursing, 26*(2), 177–179.

Lim, B., Manheimer, E., Lao, L., Ziea, E., Wisniewski, J., Liu, J., et al. (2008). Acupuncture for treatment of irritable bowel syndrome. *Cochrane Library* (4). Retrieved December 20, 2012, from http://www.thecochranelibrary.com/userfiles/ccoch/file/Acupuncture_ancient_traditions/CD005111.pdf

Marrs, J. A. (2006). Abdominal complaints: Diverticular disease. *Clinical Journal of Oncology Nursing, 10*(2), 155–157.

Marshall, A., & West, S. (2004). Nutritional intake in the critically ill: Improving practice through research. *Australian Critical Care, 17*(1), 6.

Sabol, V. K., & Carlson, K. K. (2007). Diarrhea: Applying research to bedside practice. *AACN Advanced Critical Care, 18*(1), 32–44.

Schaffner, A. (2010). Continence. *Journal of Wound, Ostomy & Continence Nursing, 37*(1), 91–93.

Simor, A. E., Bradley, S. F., Strausbaugh, L. J., Crossley, K., & Nicolle, L. E. (2002). SHEA position paper. Clostridium difficile in long-term-care facilities for the elderly. *Infection Control & Hospital Epidemiology, 23*(11), 696–703.

Visich, K., & Yeo, T. (2010). The prophylactic use of probiotics in the prevention of radiation therapy-induced diarrhea. *Clinical Journal of Oncology Nursing, 14*(4), 467–473.

Disuse Syndrome, Risk for

Baumgarten, M., Margolis, D. J., Localio, A. R., Kagan, S. H., Lowe, R. A., Kinosian, B., et al. (2006). Pressure ulcers among elderly patients early in the hospital stay. *Journals of Gerontology Series A: Biological Sciences & Medical Sciences, 61A*(7), 749–754.

Carpenito-Moyet, L. J. (2010). *Nursing diagnosis: Application to clinical practice* (13th ed.). Philadelphia: Lippincott Williams & Wilkins.

Mackey, D. (2005). Support surfaces: Beds, mattresses, overlays—oh my! *Nursing Clinics of North America, 40*(2), 251–265.

McKinley, W. O., Jackson, A. B., Cardenas, D. D., & Devivo, M. J. (1999). Long-term medical complications after traumatic spinal cord injury. *Archives of Physical Medical Rehabilitation, 80*(11), 1402–1410.

Tyler, M. (1984). The respiratory effects of body positioning and immobilization. *Respiratory Care, 29,* 472–481.

Willock, J., & Maylor, M. (2004). Pressure ulcers in infants and children. *Nursing Standard, 18*(24), 56–62.

Yamaguchi, H., Maki, Y., & Takahashi, K. (2010). Rehabilitation for dementia using enjoyable video-sports games. *International Psychogeriatrics, 23*(04). DOI: 10.1017/S1041610210001912. Retrieved December 21, 2011, from http://journals.cambridge.org/action/displayAbstract?romPage=online&aid=8235004

Zubek, J. P., & McNeil, M. (1967). Perceptual deprivation phenomena: Role of the recumbent position. *Journal of Abnormal Psychology, 72,* 147.

Diversional Activity, Deficient

Buettner, L., & Kolanowski, A. (2003). Practice guidelines for recreation therapy in the care of people with dementia. *Geriatric Nursing, 24*(1), 25.

Çinar, Y., Eşer, I., Kocaçal, G., & Khorshid, L. (2011). Nursing diagnoses in patients having mechanical ventilation support in a respiratory intensive care unit in Turkey. *International Journal of Nursing Practice, 17*(5), 502–508.

Cutting, A., & Dunn, J. (2006). Conversations with siblings and with friends: Links between relationship quality and social understanding. *British Journal of Developmental Psychology, 24*(1), 73–87.

Davidson, M., & de Morton, N. (2007). A systematic review of the human activity profile. *Clinical Rehabilitation, 21*(2), 151–162.

Gerstorf, D., Lövdén, M., Röcke, C., Smith, J., & Lindenberger, U. (2007). Well-being affects changes in perceptual speed in advanced old age: Longitudinal evidence for a dynamic link. *Developmental Psychology, 43*(3), 705–718.

Redmond, G. M. (2006). Developing programs for older adults in a faith community. *Journal of Psychosocial Nursing & Mental Health Services, 44*(11), 15–18.

Richeson, N. E., & McCullough, W. T. (2003). A therapeutic recreation intervention using animal-assisted therapy: Effects on the subjective well-being of older adults. *Annual in Therapeutic Recreation, 12,* 1.

Stuart, G., & Laraia, M. (2005). *Principles and practice of psychiatric nursing* (8th ed.). St. Louis, MO: Mosby.

Dry Eye, Risk for

Dawson, D. (2005). Development of a new eye care guideline for critically ill patients. *Intensive and Critical Care Nursing, 21*(2), 119–122.

Ezra, D., Chan, M., Solebo, L., Malik, A., Crane, E., Coombes, A., et al. (2009). Randomised trial comparing ocular lubricants and polyacrylamide hydrogel dressings in the prevention of exposure keratopathy in the critically ill. *Intensive Care Medicine, 35*(3), 455–461.

Ezra, D., Lewis, G., Healy, M., & Coombs, A. (2005). Preventing exposure keratopathy in the critically ill: A prospective study comparing eye care regimes. *British Journal of Ophthalmology, 89*(8), 1068–1069.

Germano, E., Mello, M., Sena, D., Correia, J., & Amorim, M. (2009). Incidence and risk factors of corneal epithelial defects in mechanically ventilated children. *Critical Care Medicine, 37*(3), 1097–1100.

Joyce, N. (2002). Eye care for the intensive care patient: A systematic review. *Best Practice, 6*(1), 1–6. Joanna Briggs Institute for Evidence Based Nursing and Midwifery, North Terrace, South Australia.

Kanski, J. (2007). *Clinical ophthalmology: A systematic approach* (6th ed.). London, UK: Butterworth-Heinemann.

Latkany, R. (2008). Dry eyes: Etiology and management. *Current Opinion in Ophthalmology, 19*(4), 287–291.

Latkany, R., Lock, B., & Speaker, M. (2006). Eye care for patients receiving neuromuscular blocking agents or propofol during mechanical ventilation. *American Journal of Critical Care, 9*(3), 188–191.

Moss, S., Klein, R., & Klein, B. (2000). Prevalence of and risk factors for dry eye syndrome. *Archives of Ophthalmology, 122*(3), 369–373.

Rao, S. (2008). Progression: The new approach to dry eye. *Review of Ophthalmology*. Retrieved December 23, 2011, from http://www.revophth.com/index.asp?page=1_14035.htm

Rosenberg, J., & Eisen, L. (2008). Eye care in the intensive care unit: Narrative review and meta-analysis. *Critical Care Medicine, 36*(12), 3151–3155.

So, H., Lee, C., Lleung, A., Lim, J., Chan, C., & Yan, W. (2008). Comparing the effectiveness of polyethylene covers with lanolin eye ointment to prevent corneal abrasions in critically ill patients. A randomized controlled study. *International Journal of Nursing Studies, 45*(11), 1565–1571.

Dysreflexia, Autonomic

Note: Also see Dysreflexia, Autonomic, Risk for.

Caliri, M. (2005). Spinal cord injury and pressure ulcers. *Nursing Clinics of North America, 40*(2), 337–347.

Carpenito-Moyet, L. J. (2006b). *Nursing diagnosis: Application to clinical practice* (11th ed.). Philadelphia: Lippincott Williams & Wilkins.

Fries, J. M. (2005). Critical rehabilitation of the patient with spinal cord injury. *Critical Care Nursing Quarterly, 28*(2), 179–187.

Kavchak-Keyes, M. A. (2000). Autonomic hyperreflexia. *Rehabilitation Nursing, 25*(1), 31–35.

Lehman, C. (2009). APN knowledge, self-efficacy, and practices in providing women's healthcare services to women with disabilities. *Rehabilitation Nursing, 34*(5), 186–194.

McClain, W., Shields, C., & Sixsmith, D. (1999). Autonomic dysreflexia presenting as a severe headache. *American Journal of Emergency Medicine, 17*(3), 238–240.

Nayduch, D. (2010). Back to basics: Identifying and managing acute spinal cord injury. *Nursing, 40*(9), 24–31.

Perks, D. H. (2005). Issues in pediatrics. Transient spinal cord injuries in the young athlete. *Journal of Trauma Nursing, 12*(4), 127–133.

Safaz, I., Kesikburun, S., Omac, O., Tugcu, I., & Alaca, R. (2010). Autonomic dysreflexia as a complication of a fecal management system in a man with tetraplegia. *Journal of Spinal Cord Medicine, 33*(3), 266–267.

Silver, J. R. (2000). Early autonomic dysreflexia. *Spinal Cord, 38,* 229–233.

Thompson, H. J., & Bourbonniere, M. (2006). Traumatic injury in the older adult from head to toe. *Critical Care Nursing Clinics of North America, 18*(3), 419–431.

Travers, P. (1999). Autonomic dysreflexia: A clinical rehabilitation problem. *Rehabilitation Nursing, 24*(1), 9–23.

Dysreflexia, Autonomic, Risk for

Note: Also see Dysreflexia, Autonomic (preceding)

Caliri, M. (2005). Spinal cord injury and pressure ulcers. *Nursing Clinics of North America, 40*(2), 337–347.

Fries, J. M. (2005). Critical rehabilitation of the patient with spinal cord injury. *Critical Care Nursing Quarterly, 28*(2), 179–187.

Perks, D. H. (2005). Issues in pediatrics. Transient spinal cord injuries in the young athlete. *Journal of Trauma Nursing, 12*(4), 127–133.

Thompson, H. J., & Bourbonniere, M. (2006). Traumatic injury in the older adult from head to toe. *Critical Care Nursing Clinics of North America, 18*(3), 419–431.

Electrolyte Imbalance, Risk for

American Association of Critical Care Nurses. (2006). In J. G. Alspach (Ed.), *Core curriculum for critical care nursing* (6th ed.). Philadelphia: W. B. Saunders.

Elgart, H. (2004). Assessment of fluids and electrolytes. *ACCN Clinical Issues, 15*(4), 607–621.

Mendez-Eastman, S. (2005). Burn injuries. *Plastic Surgical Nursing, 25*(3), 133–139.

Nowlin, A. (2006). The delicate business of burn care. *RN, 69*(1), 52–58.

Timby, B., & Smith, N. (2006). Caring for clients with fluid, electrolyte, and acid-base imbalances. In *Introductory medical-surgical nursing* (9th ed., pp. 204–223). Philadelphia: Lippincott Williams & Wilkins.

Weglicki, W., Quamme, G., Tucker, K., Haigney, M., & Resnick, L. (2005). Potassium, magnesium, and electrolyte imbalance and complications in disease management. *Clinical and Experimental Hypertension, 27*(1), 95–112.

Energy Field, Disturbed

Aveyard, B., Sykes, M., & Doherty, D. (2002). Therapeutic touch in dementia care. *Nursing Older People, 14*(6), 20–21.

Bradley, D. B. (1987). Energy fields: Implications for nurses. *Journal of Holistic Nursing, 5*(1), 32–35.

Denison, B. (2004). Touch the pain away. *Holistic Nursing Practice, 18*(3), 142–151.

Gleeson, M., & Timmins, F. (2005). A review of the use and clinical effectiveness of touch as a nursing intervention. *Clinical Effectiveness in Nursing, 9*(1), 69–77.

Krieger, D. (1979). *The therapeutic touch: How to use your hands to help or to heal.* Englewood Cliffs, NJ: Prentice Hall.

Krieger, D. (1981). *Foundations of holistic health nursing practices: The Renaissance nurse.* Philadelphia: Lippincott Williams & Wilkins.

Krieger, D. (1987). *Living the therapeutic touch: Healing as a lifestyle.* New York: Dodd, Mead.

Larden, C. N., Palmer, L., & Janssen, P. (2004). Efficacy of therapeutic touch in treating pregnant inpatients who have a chemical dependency. *Journal of Holistic Nursing, 22*(4), 320–332.

Mathuna, D. P., & Ashford, R. L. (2006). Therapeutic touch for healing acute wounds. *Cochrane Library* (4).

Meehan, T. C. (1991). Therapeutic touch. In G. Bulechek & J. McCloskey (Eds.), *Nursing interventions: Essential nursing treatments*. Philadelphia: Saunders.

Meehan, T. C. (1998). Therapeutic touch as nursing intervention. *Journal of Advanced Nursing, 28*(1), 117–125.

O'Mathúna, D. P., Pryjmachuk, S., Spencer, W., Stanwick, M., & Matthiesen, S. (2002). A critical evaluation of the theory and practice of therapeutic touch. *Nursing Philosophy, 3*(2), 163–176.

Smith, M. C., Reeder, F., Daniel, L., Baramee, J., & Hagman, J. (2003). Outcomes of touch therapies during bone marrow transplant. *Alternative Therapies in Health & Medicine, 9*(1), 40–49.

Tavernier, S. S. (2006). An evidence-based conceptual analysis of presence. *Holistic Nursing Practice, 20*(3), 152–156.

Umbreit, A. W. (2000). Healing touch: Applications in the acute care setting. *ACCN Clinical Issues of Advanced Practice in Acute Critical Care, 11*(1), 105–119.

Vitale, A. (2006). The use of selected energy touch modalities as supportive nursing interventions: Are we there yet? *Holistic Nursing Practice, 20*(4), 191–196.

Wendler, M. C. (2002). Tellington touch before venipuncture: An exploratory descriptive study. *Holistic Nursing Practice, 16*(4), 51–64.

Woods, D. L., Craven, R. F., & Whitney, J. (2005). The effect of therapeutic touch on behavioral symptoms of persons with dementia. *Alternative Therapies in Health & Medicine, 11*(1), 66–74.

Woods, D. L., & Dimond, M. (2002). The effect of therapeutic touch on agitated behavior and cortisol in persons with Alzheimer's disease. *Biological Research for Nursing, 4*(2), 104–114.

Environmental Interpretation Syndrome, Impaired

Algase, D. L., Beattie, E., Song, J., Milke, D., Duffield, C., & Cowan, B. (2004). Validation of the Algase wandering scale (version 2) in a cross cultural sample. *Aging & Mental Health, 8*(2), 133–142.

Shalek, M., Richeson, N. E., & Buettner, L. L. (2004). Air mat therapy for treatment of agitated wandering: An evidence-based recreational therapy intervention. *American Journal of Recreation Therapy, 3*(2), 18–26.

Woods, D. L., Rapp, C. G., & Beck, C. (2004). Special section—behavioral symptoms of dementia: Their measurement and intervention. *Aging & Mental Health, 8*(2), 126–132.

Failure to Thrive, Adult

Bergland, A. (2001). Thriving—a useful theoretical perspective to capture the experience of well-being among frail elderly in nursing homes? *Journal of Advanced Nursing, 36*(3), 426–432.

Diehr, P., Williamson, J., Burke, G. L., & Psaty, B. M. (2002). The aging and dying processes and the health of older adults. *Journal of Clinical Epidemiology, 55*(3), 269.

Haight, Barbara, K. (2002). Thriving: A life span theory. *Journal of Gerontological Nursing, 28,* 14–22.

Higgins, P. A., & Daly, B. J. (2005). Adult failure to thrive in the older rehabilitation patient. *Rehabilitation Nursing, 30*(4), 152–159.

Murray, J., & Sullivan, P. A. (2006). Frail elders and the failure to thrive [cover story]. *ASHA Leader, 11*(14), 14–16.

Falls, Risk for

Brown, J. S., Vittinghoff, E., Wyman, J. F., Stone, K. L., Nevitt, M. C., Ensrud, K. E., et al. (2000). Urinary incontinence: Does it increase risk for falls and fractures? Study of Osteoporotic Fractures Research Group. *Journal of the American Geriatric Society, 48*(7), 721.

Cameron, I., Murray, G., Gillespie, L., Robertson, M., Hill, K., Cumming, R., et al. (2010). Interventions for preventing falls in older people in nursing care facilities and hospitals. *Cochrane Database of Systematic Reviews* (1), Art No: CD005465. DOI: 10.1002/14651858.CD005465.pub2. Retrieved December 27, 2011, from http://onlinelibrary.wiley.com/doi/10.1002/14651858.CD005465.pub2/abstract

Capezuti, E. (2004). Minimizing the use of restrictive devices in dementia patients at risk for falling. *Nursing Clinics of North America, 39*(3), 625–647.

Capezuti, E., Taylor, J., Brown, H., Strothers, H., & Ouslander, J. G. (2007). Challenges to implementing an APN-facilitated falls management program in long-term care. *Applied Nursing Research, 20*(1), 2–9.

Colón-Emeric, C., Schenck, A., Gorospe, J., McArdle, J., Dobson, L., DePorter, C., et al. (2006). Translating evidence-based falls prevention into clinical practice in nursing facilities: Results and lessons from a quality improvement collaborative. *Journal of the American Geriatrics Society, 54*(9), 1414–1418.

Cooper, C. L., & Nolt, J. D. (2007). Development of an evidence-based pediatric fall prevention program. *Journal of Nursing Care Quality, 22*(2), 107–112.

Currie, L. M. (2006). Fall and injury prevention. *Annual Review of Nursing Research, 24,* 39–74.

Dykes, P., Carroll, D., Hurley, A., Lipsitz, S., Benoit, A., Chang, F., et al. (2010). Fall prevention in acute care hospitals: A randomized trial. *The Journal of the American Medical Association, 304*(17), 1912–1918. DOI: 10.1001/jama.2010.1567. Retrieved December 27, 2011, from http://jama.ama-assn.org/content/304/17/1912.full

Fortinsky, R. H., Lannuzzi-Sucich, M., Baker, T. I., Gottschalk, M., King, M. B., Brown, C. J., et al. (2004). Fall-risk assessment and management in clinical practice: Views from healthcare providers. *Journal of the American Geriatrics Society, 52*(9), 1522–1526.

Härlein, J., Dassen, T., Halfens, R., & Heinze, C. (2009). Fall risk factors in older people with dementia or cognitive impairment: A systematic review. *Journal of Advanced Nursing, 65*(5), 922–933.

Hayes, N. (2004). Prevention of falls among older patients in the hospital environment. *British Journal of Nursing (BJN), 13*(15), 896–901.

Hook, M. L., & Winchel, S. (2006). Fall-related injuries in acute care: Reducing the risk of harm. *MEDSURG Nursing, 15*(6), 370–381.

Kalyani, R., Stein, B., Valiyil, R., Manno, R., Maynard, J., & Crews, D. (2010). Vitamin D treatment for the prevention of falls in older adults: Systematic review and meta-analysis. *Journal of the American Geriatrics Society, 58*(7), 1299–1310.

Lake, E. T., & Cheung, R. B. (2006). Are patient falls and pressure ulcers sensitive to nurse staffing? *Western Journal of Nursing Research, 28*(6), 654–677.

McClure, R., Nixon, J., Spinks, A., & Turner, C. (2005). Community-based programmes to prevent falls in children: A systematic review. *Journal of Paediatrics & Child Health, 41*(9), 465–470.

Miceli, D. L., Strumpf, N. E., Johnson, J., Draganescu, M., & Ratcliffe, S. J. (2006). Psychometric properties of the post-fall index. *Clinical Nursing Research, 15*(3), 157–176.

Oliver, D., Connelly, J. B., Victor, C. R., Shaw, F. E., Whitehead, A., Genc, Y., et al. (2007). Strategies to prevent falls and fractures in hospitals and care homes and effect of cognitive impairment: Systematic review and meta-analyses. *BMJ: British Medical Journal, 334*(7584), 82–85.

Poe, S. S., Cvach, M. M., Gartrell, D. G., Radzik, B. R., & Joy, T. L. (2005). An evidence-based approach to fall risk assessment, prevention, and management. *Journal of Nursing Care Quality, 20*(2), 107–116.

Pynoos, J., Rose, D., Rubenstein, L., Choi, I. H., & Sabata, D. (2006). Evidence-based interventions in fall prevention. *Home Health Care Services Quarterly, 25*(1), 55–73.

Quigley, P., Bulat, T., Kurtzman, E., Olney, R., Powell-Cope, G., & Rubenstein, L. (2010). Fall prevention and injury protection for nursing home residents. *Journal of the American Medical Directors Association, 11*(4), 284–293.

Wang, W., & Moyle, W. (2005). Physical restraint use on people with dementia: A review of the literature. *Australian Journal of Advanced Nursing, 22*(4), 46–52.

Family Processes, Dysfunctional

Boyle, A. R., & Davis, H. (2006). Early screening and assessment of alcohol and substance abuse in the elderly: Clinical implications. *Journal of Addictions Nursing, 17*(2), 95–103.

Corte, C., & Farchaus Stein, K. (2007). Self-cognitions in antisocial alcohol dependence and recovery. *Western Journal of Nursing Research, 29*(1), 80–99.

Crumpler, J., & Ross, A. (2005). Development of an alcohol withdrawal protocol. *Journal of Nursing Care Quality, 20*(4), 297–301.

Keiffer-Kristensen, R., & Teasdale, T. (2011). Parental stress and marital relationships among patients with brain injury and their spouses. *NeuroRehavilitation, 28*(4), 321–330.

Kellett, S. K. (2000). Do women carry more emotional baggage? Gender difference in contact length to a community alcohol treatment alcohol treatment service. *Journal of Substance Use, 5*(3), 211–217.

Lock, C. A., Kaner, E., Heather, N., Doughty, J., Crawshaw, A., McNamee, P., et al. (2006). Effectiveness of nurse-led brief alcohol intervention: A cluster randomized controlled trial. *Journal of Advanced Nursing, 54*(4), 426–439.

Pagani, L., Japel, C., Vaillancourt, T., & Tremblay, R. (2010). Links between middle-childhood trajectories of family dysfunction and indirect aggression. *Journal of Interpersonal Violence, 25,* 2175–2196.

Sexton, T., & Turner, C. (2010). The effectiveness of functional family therapy for youth with behavioral problems in a community practice setting. *Journal of Family Psychology, 24*(3), 339–348.

Family Processes, Interrupted

Clark, J., & Gwin, R. (2001). Psychological responses of the family. In S. Groenwald, M. Frogge, M. Goodman, & C. Yarbo (Eds.), *Cancer nursing: Principles and practice* (3rd ed.). Boston, MA: Jones and Bartlett.

Davidson, K. M. (2003). Evidence-based protocol: Family bereavement support before and after death of a nursing home resident. *Journal of Gerontological Nursing, 29*(1), 10–18.

Hudson, P. L., Kristjanson, L. J., Ashby, M., Kelly, B., Schofield, P., Hudson, R., et al. (2006). Desire for hastened death in patients with advanced disease and the evidence base of clinical guidelines: A systematic review. *Palliative Medicine, 20*(7), 693–701.

Hughes, F., Bryan, K., & Robbins, I. (2005). Relatives' experiences of critical care. *Nursing in Critical Care, 10*(1), 23–30.

Keiffer-Kristensen, R., & Teasdale, T. (2011). Parental stress and marital relationships among patients with brain injury and their spouses. *NeuroRehavilitation, 28*(4), 321–330.

Pagani, L., Japel, C., Vaillancourt, T., & Tremblay, R. (2010). Links between middle-childhood trajectories of family dysfunction and indirect aggression. *Journal of Interpersonal Violence, 25,* 2175–2196.

Reiss, J. G., Gibson, R. W., & Walker, L. R. (2005). Health care transition: Youth, family, and provider perspectives. *Pediatrics, 115*(1), 112–120.

Sexton, T., & Turner, C. (2010). The effectiveness of functional family therapy for youth with behavioral problems in a community practice setting. *Journal of Family Psychology, 24*(3), 339–348.

Wilson, D., McBride-Henry, K., & Huntington, A. (2005). Family violence: Walking the tight rope between maternal alienation and child safety. In P. Darbyshire & D. Jackson (Eds.), *Advances in contemporary child and family health care* (pp. 85–96). Palo Alto, CA: eContent Management Pty Ltd.

Family Processes, Readiness for Enhanced

Kienmtz, J., Arriaga, R., & Abowd, G. (2009). Baby steps: Evaluation of a system to support record-keeping for parents of young children. *Proceedings of the 27th International Conference on Human Factors in Computing Systems.* DOI: 10.1145/1518701.1518965. Retrieved (purchased) January 1, 2012, from https://dl.acm.org/purchase.cfm?id=1518965& CFID=60381814&CFTOKEN=15469494

Kratochwill, T., McDonald, L., Levin, J., Scalia, P., & Coover, G. (2009). Families and schools together: An experimental study of multi-family support groups for children at risk. *Journal of School Psychology, 47*(4), 245–265.

Kumakech, E., Cantor-Graae, E., Maling, S., & Bajunirwe, F. (2009). Peer-group support intervention improves the psychosocial well-being of AIDS orphans: Cluster randomized trial. *Social Science & Medicine, 68*(6), 1038–1043.

Lewis, M., & Noyes, J. (2007). Discharge management for children with complex needs. *Paediatric Nursing, 19*(4), 26–30.

Nugent, K., Hughes, R., Ball, B., & Davis, K. (1992). A practice model for pediatric support groups. *Pediatric Nursing, 18*(1), 11–16.

Sin, J., Moone, N., & Newell, J. (2007). Developing services for the carers of young adults with early-onset psychosis—implementing evidence-based practice on psycho-educational family intervention. *Journal of Psychiatric & Mental Health Nursing, 14*(3), 282–290.

While, A., Forbes, A., Ullman, R., Lewis, S., Mathes, L., & Griffiths, P. (2004). Good practices that address continuity during transition from child to adult care: Synthesis of the evidence. *Child: Care, Health & Development, 30*(5), 439–452.

Fatigue

Aaronson, L. S., Teel, C. S., Cassmeyer, V., Neuberger, G. B., Pallikkathayil, L., Pierce, J., et al. (1999). Defining and measuring fatigue. *Image: Journal of Nursing Scholarship, 31*(1), 45–50.

Borneman, T., Sun, V., Ferrell, B., Piper, B., Koczywas, M., & Uman, G. (2007). Evidence based fatigue management. *Oncology Nursing Forum, 34*(1), 218–219.

Brown, T. R., & Kraft, G. H. (2005). Exercise and rehabilitation for individuals with multiple sclerosis. *Physical Medicine & Rehabilitation Clinics of North America, 16*(2), 513–555.

Crosby, L. (1991). Factors which contribute to fatigue associated with rheumatoid arthritis. *Journal of Advanced Nursing, 16,* 974–981.

Edwards, J. L., Gibson, F., Richardson, A., Sepion, B., & Ream, E. (2003). Fatigue in adolescents with and following a cancer diagnosis: Developing an evidence base for practice. *European Journal of Cancer, 39*(18), 2671.

Escalante, C., & Manzullo, E. (2009). Cancer-related fatigue: The approach and treatment. *Journal of General Internal Medicine, 24*(S2), 412–416.

Hinds, P. S., Hockenberry, M., Rai, S. N., Lijun Zhang, Razzouk, B. I., McCarthy, K., et al. (2007). Nocturnal awakenings, sleep environment interruptions, and fatigue in hospitalized children with cancer. *Oncology Nursing Forum, 34*(2), 393–402.

Jenkin, P., Koch, T., & Kralik, D. (2006). The experience of fatigue for adults living with HIV. *Journal of Clinical Nursing, 15*(9), 1123–1131.

Kirshbaum, M. N. (2007). A review of the benefits of whole body exercise during and after treatment for breast cancer. *Journal of Clinical Nursing, 16*(1), 104–121.

Lavdaniti, M., Patiraki, E., Dafni, U., Katapodi, M., Papathanasoglou, E., & Sotiropoulou, A. (2006). Prospective assessment of fatigue and health status in Greek patients with breast cancer undergoing adjuvant radiotherapy. *Oncology Nursing Forum, 33*(3), 603–610.

Mitchell, S. A., Beck, S. L., Hood, L. E., Moore, K., & Tanner, E. R. (2007). Putting evidence into practice: Evidence-based interventions for fatigue during and following cancer and its treatment. *Clinical Journal of Oncology Nursing, 11*(1), 99–113.

Mitchell, S. A., & Berger, A. M. (2006). Cancer-related fatigue: The evidence base for assessment and management. *Cancer Journal, 12*(5), 374–387.

Perkins, H., Baum, G., Taylor, C., & Basen-Engquist, K. (2009). Effects of treatment factors, comorbidities and health-related quality of life on self-efficacy for physical activity in cancer survivors. *Psycho-Oncology, 18*(4), 405–411.

Pires, G., Andersen, M., Giovernadi, M., & Tufik, S. (2010). Sleep impairment during pregnancy: Possible implications on mother-infant relationship. *Medical Hypotheses, 75*(6), 578–582.

Ream, E., Richardson, A., & Evison, M. (2005). A feasibility study to evaluate a group intervention for people with cancer experiencing fatigue following treatment. *Clinical Effectiveness in Nursing, 9*(3), 178–187.

Ward, N., & Winters, S. (2003). Multiple sclerosis. Results of a fatigue management programme in multiple sclerosis. *British Journal of Nursing (BJN), 12*(18), 1075–1080.

Fear

Broome, M. E., Bates, T. A., Lillis, P. P., & McGahee, T. W. (1990). Children's medical fears, coping behaviors, and pain perceptions during a lumbar puncture. *Oncology Nursing Forum, 17,* 361–367.

Cesarone, D. (1991). Fear. In M. Maas, K. Buckwalter, & M. Hardy (Eds.), *Nursing diagnoses and interventions for the elderly*. Redwood City, CA: Addison-Wesley Nursing.

Neuhäuser, C., Wagner, B., Heckmann, M., Weigand, M., & Zimmer, K.-P. (2010). Analgesia and sedation for painful interventions in children and adolescents. *Deutsches Ärzteblatt International, 107*(14), 241–227.

Nicastro, E., & Whetsell, M. V. (1999). Children's fears. *Journal of Pediatric Nursing, 14*(6), 392–402.

Wade, J. (2006). "Crying alone with my child": Parenting a school age child diagnosed with bipolar disorder. *Issues in Mental Health Nursing, 27*(8), 885–903.

Wagley, L., & Newton, S. (2010). Emergency nurses' use of psychosocial nursing interventions for management of ED patient fear and anxiety. *Journal of Emergency Nursing, 36*(5), 415–419.

Yip, P., Middleton, P., Cyna, A., & Carlyle, A. (2011). Cochrane review: Non-pharmacological interventions for assisting the induction of anaesthesia in children. *Evidence-Based Child Health: A Cochrane Review Journal, 6*(1), 71–134.

Yuenyong, S., Jirapaet, V., & O'Brien, B. (2008). Support from a close female relative in labour: The ideal maternity nursing intervention in Thailand. *Journal of the Medical Association of Thailand, 91*(2), 253–260.

Fluid Balance, Readiness for Enhanced

Anderson, M., & Comrie, R. (2009). Adopting preoperative fasting guidelines. *AORN Journal, 90*(1), 73–80.

Baraz, S., Parvardeh, S., Mohammadi, E., & Broumand, B. (2010). Dietary and fluid compliance: An educational intervention for patients having haemodialysis. *Journal of Advanced Nursing, 66*(1), 60–68.

Holte, K. (2010). Pathophysiology and clinical implications of perioperative fluid management in elective surgery. *Danish Medical Bulletin, 57*(7), 1–17.

House, N. (1992). The hydration question: Hydration or dehydration for terminally ill patients. *Professional Nurse, 8*(1), 10–23.

Maughan, R., Leiper, J., & Shirreffs, S. (1997). Factors influencing the restoration of fluid and electrolyte balance after exercise in the heat. *British Journal of Sports Medicine, 31*(3), 175–182.

Parkash, R., & Burge, F. (1997). The family's perspective on issues of hydration in terminal care. *Journal of Palliative Care, 13*(4), 23–27.

Redolfi, S., Yumino, D., Ruttanaumpaway, P., Yau, B., Su, M.-C., Lam, J., et al. (2009). Relationship between overnight rostral fluid shift and obstructive sleep apnea in nonobese men. *American Journal of Respiratory and Critical Care Medicine, 179*(3), 241–246.

Sansevero, A. (1997). Dehydration in the elderly: Strategies for prevention and management. *Nurse Practitioner: American Journal of Primary Health Care, 22*(4), 41-42, 51-52, 54-57.

Smith, K., Coston, M., Glock, K., Elasy, T., Wallston, K., Ikizler, A., et al. (2010). Patient perspectives on fluid management in chronic hemodialysis. *Journal of Renal Nutrition, 20*(5), 334–341

Steiner, N., & Bruera, E. (1998). Methods of hydration in palliative care patients. *Journal of Palliative Care, 14*(2), 6–18.

Wilkinson, J., & Treas, L. (2011). *Preventing fluid and electrolyte imbalances.* In *Fundamentals of nursing* (Vol. 1, p. 931). Philadelphia: F. A. Davis.

Fluid Volume, Deficient

(Also see Bibliography for Fluid Volume, Readiness for Enhanced.)

Allison, R. D., Ray Lewis, A., Liedtke, R., Buchmeyer, N. D., & Frank, H. (2005). Early identification of hypovolemia using total body resistance measurements in long-term care facility residents. *Gender Medicine, 2*(1), 19–34.

American Association of Critical Care Nurses. (2006). In J. G. Alspach (Ed.), *Core curriculum for critical care nursing* (6th ed.). Philadelphia: W. B. Saunders.

Gershan, J. (1990). Fluid volume deficit: Validating indicators. *Heart and Lung, 19,* 152–156.

Greenfield, E. (2010, September). The pivotal role of nursing personnel in burn care. *Indian Journal of Plastic Surgery, 43*(Suppl.), S94–S100.

Hodgkinson, B., Evans, D., & Wood, J. (2003). Maintaining oral hydration in older adults: A systematic review. *International Journal of Nursing Practice, 9*(3), S19–S28.

Makic, M., VonRueden, K., Rauen, C., & Chadwick, J. (2010). Evidence-based practice habits: Putting more sacred cows out to pasture. *Critical Care Nurse, 31*(2), 38–62.

Marchiondo, K. (2010). Emergency: Recognizing and treating vasovagal syncope. *American Journal of Nursing, 110*(4), 50–53.

Maughan, R., Leiper, J., & Shirreffs, S. (1997). Factors influencing the restoration of fluid and electrolyte balance after exercise in the heat. *British Journal of Sports Medicine, 31*(3), 175–182.

Maxwell, L. (2005). Purposeful dehydration in a terminally ill cancer patient. *British Journal of Nursing (BJN), 14*(21), 1117–1119.

Sansevero, A. (1997). Dehydration in the elderly: Strategies for prevention and management. *Nurse Practitioner: American Journal of Primary Health Care, 22*(4), 41–42, 51–52, 54–57.

Wilmot, L. (2010). Shock: Early recognition and management. *Journal of Emergency Nursing, 36*(2), 134–139.

Fluid Volume, Excess

Albert, N. M., Eastwood, C. A., & Edwards, M. L. (2004). Evidence-based practice for acute decompensated heart failure. *Critical Care Nurse, 24*(6), 14.

Bongi, S., Del Rosso, A., Passalacqua, M., Miccio, S., & Cerinic, M. (2011). Manual lymph drainage improving upper extremity edema and hand function in patients with systemic sclerosis in edematous phase. *Arthritis Care & Research, 63*(8), 1134–1141.

Devoogdt, N., Christiaens, M.-R., Geraerts, I., Truijen, S., Smeets, A., Leunen, K., et al. (2011). Effect of manual lymph drainage in addition to guidelines and exercise therapy on arm lymphoedema related to breast cancer: Randomised controlled trial. *British Medical Journal, 343*. DOI: 10.1136/gmj.d5326. Retrieved December 3, 2012, from http://www.bmj.com/content/343/bmj.d5326?tab=full

DiPasquale, L. R., & Lynett, K. (2003). The use of water immersion for treatment of massive labial edema during pregnancy. *MCN: The American Journal of Maternal Child Nursing, 28*(4), 242–245.

House, N. (1992). The hydration question: Hydration or dehydration for terminally ill patients. *Professional Nurse, 8*(1), 10–23.

Lopes, J., Leite de Barros, A., & Michel, J. (2009). A pilot study to validate the priority nursing interventions classification interventions and nursing outcomes classification outcomes for the nursing diagnosis "excess fluid volume" in cardiac patients. *International Journal of Nursing Terminologies and Classifications, 20*(2), 76–88.

Terry, M., O'Brien, S., & Derstein, M. (1998). Lower-extremity edema: Evaluation and diagnoses. *Wounds: A Compendium of Clinical Research and Practice, 10*(4), 118–124.

Fluid Volume, Risk for Deficient

(Also see the Bibliography for Fluid Volume, Readiness for Enhanced and Fluid Volume, Deficient.)

Cook, N. F., Deeny, P., & Thompson, K. (2004). Management of fluid and hydration in patients with acute subarachnoid haemorrhage—an action research project. *Journal of Clinical Nursing, 13*(7), 835–849.

Hodgkinson, B., Evans, D., & Wood, J. (2003). Maintaining oral hydration in older adults: A systematic review. *International Journal of Nursing Practice, 9*(3), S19–S28.

Maughan, R., Leiper, J., & Shirreffs, S. (1997). Factors influencing the restoration of fluid and electrolyte balance after exercise in the heat. *British Journal of Sports Medicine, 31*(3), 175–182.

Sansevero, A. (1997). Dehydration in the elderly: Strategies for prevention and management. *Nurse Practitioner: American Journal of Primary Health Care, 22*(4), 41–42, 51–52, 54–57.

Speksnijder, H., Mank, A., & Achterberg, T. (2011). Nursing diagnoses (NANDA-I) in hematology-oncology: A Delphi-study. *International Journal of Nursing Terminologies and Classifications, 22*(2), 77–91.

Sumnall, R. (2007). Fluid management and diuretic therapy in acute renal failure. *Nursing in Critical Care, 12*(1), 27–33.

Fluid Volume, Risk for Imbalanced

(Also see the Bibliography for Fluid Volume, Readiness for Enhanced; Fluid Volume, Risk for Deficient; and Fluid Volume, Excess.)

Batts, E., & Lazarus, H. (2007). Diagnosis and treatment of transplantation-associated thrombotic microangiopathy: Real progress or are we still waiting? *Bone Marrow Transplant, 40*(8), 79–719 [Review].

DeFabio, D. C. (2000). Fluid and nutrient maintenance before, during and after exercise. *Journal of Sports Chiropractic and Rehabilitation, 14*(2), 21–24, 42–43.

Fortenberry, J., & Paden, M. (2006). Extracorporeal therapies in the treatment of sepsis: Experience and promise. *Seminars in Pediatric Infectious Diseases, 17*(2), 72–79.

Gershan, J. (1990). Fluid volume deficit: Validating indicators. *Heart and Lung, 19,* 152–156.

House, N. (1992). The hydration question: Hydration or dehydration for terminally ill patients. *Professional Nurse, 8*(1), 10–23.

Maughan, R., Leiper, J., & Shirreffs, S. (1997). Factors influencing the restoration of fluid and electrolyte balance after exercise in the heat. *British Journal of Sports Medicine, 31*(3), 175–182.

Sansevero, A. (1997). Dehydration in the elderly: Strategies for prevention and management. *Nurse Practitioner: American Journal of Primary Health Care, 22*(4), 41–42, 51–52, 54–57.

Steiner, N., & Bruera, E. (1998). Methods of hydration in palliative care patients. *Journal of Palliative Care, 14*(2), 6–18.

Gas Exchange, Impaired

Caldwell, C. D. (2003). Incidence and effects of premedication for intubation in neonates in a level III NICU: An observational study. *Neonatal Intensive Care, 16*(3), 16–24.

Celik, S. A., & Kanan, N. (2006). A current conflict: Use of isotonic sodium chloride solution on endotracheal suctioning in critically ill patients. *Dimensions of Critical Care Nursing, 25*(1), 11–14.

Cook, N. (2003). Respiratory care in spinal cord injury with associated traumatic brain injury: Bridging the gap in critical care nursing interventions. *Intensive & Critical Care Nursing, 19*(3), 143–153.

Corbridge, S. J., & Corbridge, T. C. (2004). Severe exacerbations of asthma. *Critical Care Nursing Quarterly, 27*(3), 207–230.

Corff, K. E., & McCann, D. L. (2005). Room air resuscitation versus oxygen resuscitation in the delivery room. *Journal of Perinatal & Neonatal Nursing, 19*(4), 379–390.

Diaz, J., Brower, R., Calfee, C., & Matthay, M. (2010). Therapeutic strategies for severe acute lung injury. *Critical Care Medicine, 38*(8), 1644–1650.

Gallagher, R., & Roberts, D. (2004). Systematic review of oxygen and airflow effect on relief of dyspnea at rest in patients with advanced disease of any cause. *Journal of Pain & Palliative Care Pharmacotherapy, 18*(4), 3–15.

Gronkiewicz, C., & Borkgren-Okonek, M. (2004). Acute exacerbation of COPD: Nursing application of evidence-based guidelines. *Critical Care Nursing Quarterly, 27*(4), 336–352.

Jantarakupt, P., & Porock, D. (2005). Dyspnea management in lung cancer: Applying the evidence from chronic obstructive pulmonary disease. *Oncology Nursing Forum, 32*(4), 785–795.

Malkoç, M., Didem, K., & Yücel, Y. (2009). The effect of physiotherapy on ventilatory dependency and the length of stay in an intensive care unit. *International Journal of Rehabilitation Research, 33*(1), 85–88.

Marklew, A. (2006). Body positioning and its effect on oxygenation—a literature review. *Nursing in Critical Care, 11*(1), 16–22.

Nicholson, C. (2004). A systematic review of the effectiveness of oxygen in reducing acute myocardial ischaemia. *Journal of Clinical Nursing, 13*(8), 996–1007.

Pease, P. (2006). Oxygen administration: Is practice based on evidence? [cover story]. *Paediatric Nursing, 18*(8), 14–18.

Pruitt, B., & Lawson, R. (2011). Assessing and managing asthma: A global initiative for asthma update. *Nursing, 41*(5), 46–52.

Rosati, E., Chitano, G., Dipaola, L., De Felice, C., & Latini, G. (2005). Indications and limitations for a neonatal pulse oximetry screening of critical congenital heart disease. *Journal of Perinatal Medicine, 33*(5), 455–457.

Ryerson, C., Berkeley, J., Carrieri-Kohlman, V., Pantilat, S., Landefeld, C., & Collard, H. (2011). Depression and functional status are strongly associated with dyspnea in interstitial lung disease. *CHEST, 139*(3), 609–616.

Vollman, K. M. (2004). Prone positioning in the patient who has acute respiratory distress syndrome: The art and science. *Critical Care Nursing Clinics of North America, 16*(3), 319–336.

Wilkinson, J., & Treas, L. (2011). *Fundamentals of nursing*, Chapter 35. Philadelphia: F. A. Davis Company.

Gastrointestinal Motility, Dysfunctional

Note: Also refer to the Bibliographies for Constipation and Diarrhea.

Chial, H., & Camilleri, M. (2003). Motility disorders of the stomach and small intestine. In S. Friedman, K. McQuaid, & J. Grendell (Eds.), *Current diagnosis & treatment in gastroenterology* (pp. 355–367). New York: Lange Medical Books/McGraw-Hill.

Chiantri, T., & Prabhakar, K. (2007). Diarrheal diseases in the elderly. *Clinics in geriatric medicine, 23*(4), 833–856.

Holmes, H., Henry, K., Bilotta, K., Comerford, K., & Weinstock, D. (Eds.). (2007). *Professional guide to signs & symptoms* (5th ed., pp. 112–118). Philadelphia: Lippincott Williams & Wilkins.

Kahrilas, P. (2005). Esophageal motility disorders. In W. Weinstein, C. Hawkey, & J. Bosch (Eds.), *Clinical gastroenterology and hepatology* (pp. 253–259). St. Louis: Elsevier Mosby.

Madsen, D., Sebolt, T., Cullen, L., Folkedahl B., Mueller T., Richardson C., et al. (2005). Listening to bowel sounds: An evidence-based practice project. *American Journal of Nursing, 105*(12), 40–49.

Perry, S., Hockenberry, M., Lowdermilk, D., & Wilson, D. (2012). *Maternal–child nursing care* (4th ed.). St. Louis: Elsevier.

Tursi, A. (2004). Gastrointestinal disorders. In M. Verklan & M. Walden (Eds.), *Core curriculum for neonatal intensive care nursing* (3rd ed., pp. 654–683). St. Louis: Elsevier Saunders.

Visich, K., & Yeo, T. (2010). The prophylactic use of probiotics in the prevention of radiation therapy-induced diarrhea. *Clinical Journal of Oncology Nursing, 14*(4), 467–473.

Wilkinson, J., & Treas, L. (2011). *Fundamentals of nursing* (Chapter 28). Philadelphia: F. A. Davis Company.

Wong, D., Hockenberry, M., Perry, S., Lowdermilk, D., & Wilson, D. (2006). *Maternal–child nursing care* (4th ed.). St. Louis: Mosby.

Gastrointestinal Motility: Dysfunctional, Risk for

Note: Refer to the Bibliographies for Gastrointestinal Motility, Dysfunctional; Constipation; and Diarrhea.

Grieving

Center for the Advancement of Health. (2004a). Report on bereavement and grief research: Outcomes of bereavement. *Death Studies, 28*(1), 520–542.

Center for the Advancement of Health. (2004b). Report on bereavement and grief research: Themes in research on bereavement. *Death Studies, 28*(6), 498–505.

Haidinyak, G., & Walker, G. C. (2005). Don't let the grievance process cause grief. *Nurse Educator, 30*(2), 73–75.

Harrington, C., & Sprowl, B. (2011-2012). Family members' experiences with viewing in the wake of sudden death. *OMEGA—Journal of Death and Dying, 64*(1), 65–82.

Haylor, M. (1987). Human response to loss. *Nurse Practitioner, 12*(5), 63.

Hendry, C. (2009). Incarceration and the tasks of grief: A narrative review. *Journal of Advanced Nursing, 65*(2), 270–278.

Hentz, P. (2010). Chapter 13, Exemplar: The body grieves. In P. Munhall (Ed.), *Nursing research: A qualitative perspective* (5th ed.). Sudbury, MA: Jones & Bartlett Publishers.

Kehl, K. A. (2005). Recognition and support of anticipatory mourning. *Journal of Hospice & Palliative Nursing, 7*(4), 206–211.

Knapp, C., Madden, V., Button, D., Brown, R., & Hastie, B. (2011). Partnerships between pediatric palliative care and psychiatry. *Pediatric Clinics of North America, 58*(4), 1025–1039.

Kübler-Ross, E. (1975). *Death: The final stage of growth*. Englewood Cliffs, NJ: Prentice Hall.

Kübler-Ross, E. (1983). *On children and death*. New York: Macmillan.

Paris, M., Carter, B., Day, S., & Armsworth, M. (2009). Grief and trauma in children after the death of a sibling. *Journal of Child & Adolescent Trauma, 2*(2), 71–80.

Rabow, M. W., Hauser, J. M., & Adams, J. (2004). Supporting family caregivers at the end of life: "They don't know what they don't know." *JAMA: Journal of the American Medical Association, 291*(4), 483–491.

Reed, K. S. (2003). Grief is more than tears. *Nursing Science Quarterly, 16*(1), 77–81.

Rowland, A., & Goodnight, W. (2009). Fetal loss: Addressing the evaluation and supporting the emotional needs of parents. *Journal of Midwifery & Women's Health, 54*(3), 241–248.

Sjöblom, L., Pejlert, A., & Asplund, K. (2005). Nurses' view of the family in psychiatric care. *Journal of Clinical Nursing, 14*(5), 562–569.

Todd, M., Welsh, J., & Moriarty, D. (2002). Do interventions make a difference to bereaved parents? A systematic review of controlled studies. *International Journal of Palliative Nursing, 8*(9), 452.

Tschetter, L., & Hildreth, M. (2005). Grief enriched us: A model of perinatal loss support. *Journal of Perinatal Education, 14*(4), 3–4.

Walter, C., & McCoyd, J. (2009). *Grief and loss across the lifespan*. New York: Springer Publishing Co.

Worden, W. (2002). *Grief counseling and grief therapy* (3rd ed.). New York: Springer.

Grieving, Complicated

Burke, L., Neimeyer, R., & McDevitt-Murphy, M. (2010). African American homicide bereavement: Aspects of social support that predict complicated grief, PTSD, and depression. *OMEGA—Journal of Death and Dying, 61*(1), 1–24.

Center for the Advancement of Health. (2004). Report on bereavement and grief research. *Death Studies, 28,* 498–505.

Cutcliffe, J. R. (2004). The inspiration of hope in bereavement counseling. *Issues in Mental Health Nursing, 25*(2), 165–190.

Hogan, N., Worden, J., & Schmidt, L. (2004). An empirical study of the proposed complicated grief disorder criteria. *OMEGA—Journal of Death and Dying, 48,* 263–277.

Kent, H., & McDowell, J. (2004). Sudden bereavement in acute care settings. *Nursing Standard, 19*(6), 38–42.

Kidby, J. (2003). Family-witnessed cardiopulmonary resuscitation. *Nursing Standard, 17*(51), 33–36.

Lichtenthal, W., & Cruess, D. (2010). Effects of directed written disclosure on grief and distress symptoms among bereaved individuals. *Death Studies, 34*(6), 475–499.

Mallinson, R. K. (1999). The lived experiences of AIDS-related multiple losses by HIV-negative gay men. *Journal of the Association of Nurses in AIDS Care, 10*(5), 22–31.

Matthews, L., & Marwit, S. (2004). Complicated grief and the trend toward cognitive-behavioral therapy. *Death Studies, 28*(9), 849–863.

Mccallum, F., & Bryant, R. (2010). Impaired autobiographical memory in complicated grief. *Behaviour Research and Therapy, 48*(4), 328–334.

Niemeyer, R., Burke, L., Mackay, M., & Stringer, J. (2010). Grief therapy and the reconstruction of meaning: From principles to practice. *Journal of Contemporary Psychotherapy, 40*(2), 73–83.

O'Connor, M., Lasgaard, M., Shevlin, M., & Guidin, M.-B. (2010). A confirmatory factor analysis of combined models of the Harvard Trauma Questionnaire and the Inventory of Complicated Grief-Revised: Are we measuring complicated grief or posttraumatic stress? *Journal of Anxiety Disorders, 24*(7), 672–679.

Ott, C. (2003). The impact of complicated grief on mental and physical health at various points in the bereavement process. *Death Studies, 27,* 249–272.

Pallikkathayil, L., & Flood, M. (1991). Adolescent suicide. *Nursing Clinics of North America, 26*(3), 623–630.

Ransohoff-Adler, M., & Berger, C. S. (1989). When newborns die: Do we practice what we preach? *Journal of Perinatology, 9,* 311–316.

Rosner, R., Kruse, J., & Hagi, M. (2010). A meta-analysis of interventions for bereaved children and adolescents. *Death Studies, 34*(2), 99–136.

Shear, M., Simmon, N., Wall, M., Zisook, S., Neimeyer, M., Duan, N., et al. (2011). Complicated grief and related bereavement issues for DSM-5. *Depression and Anxiety, 28*(2), 103–117.

Strada, E. (2011). Complicated grief. In S. Qualls & J. Kasl-Godley (Eds.), *End-of-life issues, grief, and bereavement: What clinicians need to know*. Hoboken, NJ: John Wiley & Sons, Inc.

Vanezis, M., & McGee, A. (1999). Mediating factors in the grieving process of the suddenly bereaved. *British Journal of Nursing, 8*(14), 932–937.

Vickers, J. L., & Carlisle, C. (2000). Choices and control: Parental experiences in pediatric terminal home care. *Journal of Pediatric Oncology Nursing, 17*(1), 12–21.

Walter, C., & McCoyd, J. (2009). *Grief and loss across the lifespan*. New York: Springer Publishing Co.

Grieving, Complicated, Risk for

Note: Also see Bibliography for Grieving and Grieving, Complicated.

Andrews, M., & Hansen, P. (2004). Religious beliefs: Implications for nursing practice. In M. Andrews & J. Boye (Eds.), *Transcultural concepts in nursing* (4th ed.). Philadelphia: Lippincott Williams & Wilkins.

Cutcliffe, J. R. (2004). The inspiration of hope in bereavement counseling. *Issues in Mental Health Nursing, 25*(2), 165–190.

Lamb, E. H. (2002). The impact of previous perinatal loss on subsequent pregnancy and parenting. *Journal of Perinatal Education, 11*(2), 33–40.

Mallinson, R. K. (1999). The lived experiences of AIDS-related multiple losses by HIV-negative gay men. *Journal of the Association of Nurses in AIDS Care, 10*(5), 22–31.

Ott, C. (2003). The impact of complicated grief on mental and physical health at various points in the bereavement process. *Death Studies, 27,* 249–272.

Ransohoff-Adler, M., & Berger, C. S. (1989). When newborns die: Do we practice what we preach? *Journal of Perinatology, 9,* 311–316.

Vanezis, M., & McGee, A. (1999). Mediating factors in the grieving process of the suddenly bereaved. *British Journal of Nursing, 8*(14), 932–937.

Vickers, J. L., & Carlisle, C. (2000). Choices and control: Parental experiences in pediatric terminal home care. *Journal of Pediatric Oncology Nursing, 17*(1), 12–21.

Walter, C., & McCoyd, J. (2009). *Grief and loss across the lifespan*. New York: Springer Publishing Co.

Growth, Disproportionate, Risk for

Abrams, S. E., & Wells, M. E. (2005). Feeding better food habits in mid-20th-century America. *Public Health Nursing, 22*(6), 529–534.

Beal, J. (2005). Toward evidence-based practice. Implications of kangaroo care for growth and development in preterm infants. *MCN: The American Journal of Maternal Child Nursing, 30*(5), 338.

Carlsson, E., Ehrenberg, A., & Ehnfors, M. (2004). Stroke and eating difficulties: Long-term experiences. *Journal of Clinical Nursing, 13*(7), 825–834.

Craig, D., Fayter, D., Stirk, L., & Crott, R. (2011,). Growth monitoring for short stature: Update of a systematic review and economic model. *Health Technology Assessment, 15*(11). DOI: 10.3310/hta15110. Retrieved January 6, 2012, from http://www.hta.ac.uk/fullmono/mon1511.pdf

Eberhardie, C. (2002). Continuing professional development: Nutrition. Nutrition and the older adult. *Nursing Older People, 14*(2), 22–28.

Hatfield, L., Schwoebel, A., & Lynyak, C. (2011). Caring for the infant of a diabetic mother. *MCN, American Journal of Maternal Child Nursing, 36*(1), 10–16.

Healthy eating and activity together (HEAT) clinical practice guideline: Identifying and preventing overweight in childhood. (2006). *Journal of Pediatric Healthcare, 20*(2), S1–S63.

Hossain, S., Begum, J., & Akhter, Z. (2011). Measurement of stature from arm-span: An anthropometric study on Garo tribal Bangladeshi females. *Bangladesh Journal of Anatomy, 9*(1), 5–9.

Krulewitch, C. J. (2005). Alcohol consumption during pregnancy. *Annual Review of Nursing Research, 23,* 101–134.

Luke, B. (2005). The evidence linking maternal nutrition and prematurity. *Journal of Perinatal Medicine, 33*(6), 500–505.

Mcalpine, D. E., Schroder, K., Pankratz, V. S., & Maurer, M. (2004). Survey of regional health care providers on selection of treatment for bulimia nervosa. *International Journal of Eating Disorders, 35*(1), 27–32.

Moyer, V. A., Klein, J. D., Ockene, J. K., Teutsch, S. M., Johnson, M. S., & Allan, J. D. (2005). Screening for overweight in children and adolescents: Where is the evidence? A commentary by the childhood obesity working group of the U.S. preventive services task force. *Pediatrics, 116*(1), 235–238.

Nassar, A. H., Usta, I. M., Khalil, A. M., Aswad, N. A., & Seoud, M. A.-F. (2003). Neonatal outcome of growth discordant twin gestations. *Journal of Perinatal Medicine, 31*(4), 330–336.

Pinelli, J., Symington, A., & Ciliska, D. (2002). Nonnutritive sucking in high-risk infants: Benign intervention or legitimate therapy? *JOGNN: Journal of Obstetric, Gynecologic, & Neonatal Nursing, 31*(5), 582–591.

Pullen, C. H., Walker, S. N., Hageman, P. A., Boeckner, L. S., & Oberdorfer, M. K. (2005). Differences in eating and activity markers among normal weight, overweight, and obese rural women. *Women's Health Issues, 15*(5), 209–215.

Symington, A., & Pinelli, J. (2006). Developmental care for promoting development and preventing morbidity in preterm infants. *Cochrane Library* (4). DOI: 10.1002/14651858.CD001814.pub2

Ter Goon, D., Toriola, A., Musa, D., & Akusu, S. (2011). The relationship between arm span and stature in Nigerian adults. *Kinesiology, 43*(1), 38–43.

Growth and Development, Delayed

Bujia-Couso, P., O'Rourke, A., & Cerezo, M. (2010). Criteria based case review: The parent child psychological support program. *Irish Journal of Applied Social Studies, 10*(1), 6–19.

Diesel, H., & Ercole, P. (2011, October 13). Soothability and growth in preterm infants. *Journal of Holistic Nursing.* DOI: 10.1177/0898010111417875. Retrieved January 7,

2012, from http://jhn.sagepub.com/content/early/2011/10/13/0898010111417875.abstract

Gregory, K. (2005). Update on nutrition for preterm and full-term infants. *JOGNN: Journal of Obstetric, Gynecologic, & Neonatal Nursing, 34*(1), 98–108.

Grieve, A., Tluczek, A., Racine-Gilles, C., Laxova, A., Albers, C., & Farrell, P. (2011). Associations between academic achievement and psychosocial variables in adolescents with cystic fibrosis. *Journal of School Health, 81*(11), 713–720.

Kennedy, M. S. (2002). Educational program for NICU moms helps infants develop. *American Journal of Nursing, 102*(2), 21.

McCain, G. C. (2003). An evidence-based guideline for introducing oral feeding to healthy preterm infants. *Neonatal Network, 22*(5), 45–50.

Okumakpeyi, P. (2010). Case study: Child with global developmental delay. *International Journal of Nursing Terminologies and Classifications, 21*(3), 134–136.

Pillitteri, A. (2007). *Maternal and child health nursing: Care of the childbearing and childrearing family* (5th ed.). Philadelphia: Lippincott Williams & Wilkins.

Symington, A., & Pinelli, J. M. (2002). Distilling the evidence on developmental care: A systematic review. *Advances in Neonatal Care, 2*(4), 198–221.

Symington, A., & Pinelli, J. M. (2006). Developmental care for promoting development and preventing morbidity in preterm infants. *Cochrane Library* (4). DOI: 10.1002/14651858.CD001814.pub2

Vickers, A., Ohlsson, A., Lacy, J. B., & Horsley, A. (2006). Massage for promoting growth and development of preterm and/or low birth-weight infants. *Cochrane Library* (4). Retrieved December 20, 2012, from http://summaries.cochrane.org/CD000390/massage-for-promoting-growth-and-development-of-premature-and-low-birth-weight-infants

Wright, C. M., & Parkinson, K. N. (2004). Postnatal weight loss in term infants: What is "normal" and do growth charts allow for it? *Archives of Disease in Childhood—Fetal & Neonatal Edition, 89*(3), F254–F257.

Health Behavior, Risk Prone

Ahern, N. R., & Kiehl, E. (2006). Adolescent sexual health & practice—a review of the literature: Implications for healthcare providers, educators, and policy makers. *Journal of Family and Community Health, 29*(4), 299–313.

Bartlett, R., Holditch-Davis, D., & Belyea, M. (2007). Problem behaviors in adolescents. *Pediatric Nursing, 33*(1), 13–18.

Bassuk, S. S., Albert, C. M., Cook, N. R., Zaharris, E., MacFadyen, J. G., Danielson, E., et al. (2004). The women's antioxidant cardiovascular study: Design and baseline characteristics of participants. *Journal of Women's Health, 13*(1), 99–117.

Bick, D. (2003). Strategies to reduce postnatal psychological morbidity: The role of midwifery services. *Disease Management & Health Outcomes, 11*(1), 11–20.

Birchfield, P. C. (2003). Identifying women at risk for coronary artery disease. *AAOHN Journal, 51*(1), 15–22.

Biuso, T. J., Butterworth, S., & Linden, A. (2007). A conceptual framework for targeting prediabetes with lifestyle, clinical, and behavioral management interventions. *Disease Management, 10*(1), 6–15.

Bosworth, H. B., Olsen, M. K., Dudley, T., Orr, M., Neary, A., Harrelson, M., et al. (2007). The take control of your blood pressure (TCYB) study: Study design and methodology. *Contemporary Clinical Trials, 28*(1), 33–47.

Busen, N. H., Marcus, M. T., & Sternberg, K. L. (2006). What African-American middle school youth report about risk-taking behaviors. *Journal of Pediatric Healthcare, 20*(6), 393–400.

Cleaver, K. (2007). Adolescent nursing: Characteristics and trends of self-harming behaviour in young people. *British Journal of Nursing (BJN), 16*(3), 148–152.

Cook, L. J. (2004). Educating women about the hidden dangers of alcohol. *Journal of Psychosocial Nursing & Mental Health Services, 42*(6), 24.

Corte, C. M., & Sommers, M. S. (2005). Alcohol and risky behaviors. *Annual Review of Nursing Research, 23,* 327–360.

Etzioni, D. A., Yano, E. M., Rubenstein, L. V., Lee, M. L., Ko, C. Y., Brook, R. H., et al. (2006). Measuring the quality of colorectal cancer screening: The importance of follow-up. *Diseases of the Colon & Rectum, 49*(7), 1002–1010.

Feroli, K. L., & Burstein, G. R. (2003). Adolescent sexually transmitted diseases: New recommendations for diagnosis, treatment, and prevention. *MCN: The American Journal of Maternal Child Nursing, 28*(2), 113–118.

Glazebrook, C., Garrud, P., Avery, A., Coupland, C., & Williams, H. (2006). Impact of a multimedia intervention "Skinsafe" on patients' knowledge and protective behaviors. *Preventive Medicine, 42*(6), 449–454.

Guiao, I. Z., Blakemore, N. M., & Wise, A. B. (2004). Predictors of teen substance use and risky sexual behaviors: Implications for advanced nursing practice. *Clinical Excellence for Nurse Practitioners, 8*(2), 52–59.

Hart, P. L. (2005). Women's perceptions of coronary heart disease. *Journal of Cardiovascular Nursing, 20*(3), 170–176.

Kashdan, T., & McKnight, P. (2010). The darker side of social anxiety: When aggressive impulsivity prevails over shy inhibition. *Current Directions in Psychological Science, 19*(1), 47–50.

Koenigsberg, M., Barlett, D., & Carmer, J. (2004). Facilitating treatment adherence with lifestyle changes in diabetes. *American Family Physician, 69,* 309–316, 319–320, 323–324.

Krulewitch, C. J. (2005). Alcohol consumption during pregnancy. *Annual Review of Nursing Research, 23,* 101–134.

Lang, A., & Froelicher, E. S. (2006). Management of overweight and obesity in adults: Behavioral intervention for long-term weight loss and maintenance. *European Journal of Cardiovascular Nursing, 5*(2), 102–114.

Mallory, C., & Gabrielson, M. (2005). Preventing HIV infection among women who trade sex. *Clinical Excellence for Nurse Practitioners, 9*(1), 17–22.

McFarlane, J. M., Groff, J. Y., Brien, J. A., & Watson, K. (2006). Secondary prevention of intimate partner violence: A randomized controlled. *Nursing Research, 55*(1), 52–61.

Morrison-Beedy, D., Nelson, L. E., & Volpe, E. (2005). Evidence-based practice. HIV risk behaviors and testing rates in adolescent girls: Evidence to guide clinical practice. *Pediatric Nursing, 31*(6), 508–512.

Newsom, J., Kaplan, M., Huguet, N., & McFarland, B. (2004). Health behaviors in a representative sample of older Canadians: Prevalences, reported change, motivation to change, and perceived barriers. *Gerontologist, 44*(92), 193–205.

Pearlstein, I. (2005). Evidence-based practice: A theory-based tobacco dependence treatment at an adolescent health clinic. *New Jersey Nurse, 35*(1), 15.

Reagan, P. B., & Salsberry, P. J. (2005). Race and ethnic differences in determinants of preterm birth in the USA: Broadening the social context. *Social Science & Medicine, 60*(10), 2217–2228.

Rooney, M., & Wald, A. (2007). Interventions for the management of weight and body composition changes in women with breast cancer. *Clinical Journal of Oncology Nursing, 11*(1), 41–52.

Sawatzky, J. V., & Naimark, B. J. (2005). Cardiovascular health promotion in aging women: Validating a population health approach. *Public Health Nursing, 22*(5), 379–388.

Schettler, A. E., & Gustafson, E. M. (2004). Osteoporosis prevention starts in adolescence. *Journal of the American Academy of Nurse Practitioners, 16*(7), 274–282.

Shemesh, E. (2004). Non-adherence to medications following pediatric liver transplantation. *Pediatric Transplantation, 8*(6), 600–605.

Sieck, C. J., Heirich, M., & Major, C. (2004). Alcohol counseling as part of general wellness counseling. *Public Health Nursing, 21*(2), 137–143.

Vaughn, K., & Waldrop, J. (2007). Parent education key to beating early childhood obesity [cover story]. *Nurse Practitioner, 32*(3), 36–41.

Von Ah, D., Ebert, S., Ngamvitroj, A., Park, N., & Kang, D.-H. (2004). Predictors of health behaviours in college students. *Journal of Advanced Nursing, 48*(5), 463–474.

Zwane, I. T., Mngadi, P. T., & Nxumalo, M. P. (2004). Adolescents' views on decision-making regarding risky sexual behaviour. *International Nursing Review, 51*(1), 15–22.

Health Maintenance, Ineffective

Berra, K. (2011). Does nurse case management improve implementation of guidelines for cardiovascular disease risk reduction? *Journal of Cardiovascular Nursing, 26*(2), 145–167.

Chow, S., & Wong, F. (2010). Health-related quality of life in patients undergoing peritoneal dialysis: Effects of a nurse-led case management programme. *Journal of Advanced Nursing, 66*(8), 1780–1792.

Eden, L., & Callister, L. (2010). Parent involvement in end-of-life care and decision making in the newborn intensive care unit: An integrative review. *Perinatal Education, 19*(1), 29–39.

Leon, L. (2002). Smoking cessation—developing a workable program. *Nursing Spectrum, FL9*(18), 12–13.

Manworren, R. C. B., & Woodring, B. (1998). Evaluating children's literature as a source for patient education. *Pediatric Nursing, 24*(6), 548–553.

Moti, R., McAuley, E., Snook, E., & Gliottoni, R. (2009). Physical activity and quality of life in multiple sclerosis: Intermediary roles of disability, fatigue, mood, pain, self-efficacy and social support. *Psychology, Health & Medicine, 14*(1), 111–124.

Woodhead, G. (1996). The management of cholesterol in coronary heart disease. *Nurse Practitioner, 21*(9), 45, 48, 51, 53.

Home Maintenance, Impaired

Bottari, C., Dassa, C., Rainville, C., & Dutil, E. (2009). The factorial validity and internal consistency of the Instrumental Activities of Daily Living Profile in individuals with a traumatic brain injury. *Neuropsychological Rehabilitation, 19*(2), 177–207.

Gitlin, L., Winter, L., Dennis, M., Hodgson, N., & Hauck, W. (2010). A biobehavioral home-based intervention and the well-being of patients with dementia and their caregivers: The COPE randomized trial. *The Journal of the American Medical Association, 304*(9), 983–991.

Green, K. (1998). *Home care survival guide*. Philadelphia: Lippincott Williams & Wilkins.

Hébert, R., Raîche, M., Dubois, M.-F., Gueye, N., Dubuc, N., & Tousignant, M. (2010). Impact of PRISMA, a coordination-type integrated service delivery system for frail older people in Quebec (Canada): A quasi-experimental study. *The Journals of Gerontology Series B: Psychological Sciences and Social Sciences, 65B*(1), 107–118.

Liebel, D., Friedman, B., Watson, N., & Powers, B. (2009). Review: Review of nurse home visiting interventions for community-dwelling older persons with existing disability. *Medical Care Research and Review, 66*(2), 119–146.

Salter, A., & Cutter, G. (2009). Impact of loss of mobility on instrumental activities of daily living and socioeconomic status in patients with MS. *Current Medical Research and Opinion, 26*(2), 493–500.

Sato, D., Kaneda, K., Wakabayashi, H., & Nomura, T. (2009). Comparison of 2-year effects of once and twice weekly water exercise on activities of daily living ability of community dwelling frail elderly. *Archives of Gerontology and Geriatrics, 49*(1), 123–128.

Schank, M. J., & Lough, M. A. (1990). Profile: Frail elderly women, maintaining independence. *Journal of Advanced Nursing, 15,* 674–682.

Spillman, B., & Long, S. (2009). Does high caregiver stress predict nursing home entry? *Inquiry, 46*(2), 140–161.

Wong, D. L. (1991). Transition from hospital to home for children with complex medical care. *Journal of Pediatric Oncology Nursing, 8*(1), 3–9.

Hope, Readiness for Enhanced

Benzein, E., & Saveman, B.-L. (1998). One step towards the understanding of hope: A concept analysis. *International Journal of Nursing Studies, 35,* 322–329.

Benzein, E. G. (2005). The level of and relation between hope, hopelessness and fatigue in patients and family members in palliative care. *Palliative Medicine, 19,* 234–240.

Borneman, T., Stahl, C., Ferrell, B. R., & Smith, D. (2002). The concept of hope in family caregivers of cancer patients at home. *Journal of Hospice and Palliative Nursing, 4*(1), 21–33.

Burkes, N. (2004). Spirit matters: Evidence of things hoped for. *Neonatal Network, 23*(6), 73.

Casarett, D. J., & Quill, T. E. (2007). "I'm not ready for hospice": Strategies for timely and effective hospice discussions. *Annals of Internal Medicine, 146*(6), 443–449.

Davis, B. (2005). Mediators of the relationship between hope and well-being in older adults. *Clinical Nursing Research, 14,* 253–272.

Folkman, S. (2010). Stress, coping, and hope. *Psycho-Oncology, 19*(9), 901–908.

Fromm, E. (1968). *The evolution of hope*. New York: Harper.

Hickey, S. S. (1986). Enabling hope. *Cancer Nursing, 9,* 133–137.

Kylmä, J., Juvakka, T., Nikkonen, M., Korhonen, T., & Isohanni, M. (2006). Hope and schizophrenia: An integrative review. *Journal of Psychiatric & Mental Health Nursing, 13*(6), 651–664.

Leininger, M. (1978). *Transcultural nursing: Concepts, theories, and practices*. New York: Wiley.

Parse, R. R. (1990). Parse's research methodology within an illustration of the lived experience of hope. *Nursing Science Quarterly, 3*(3), 9–17.

Smith, T., Dow, L., Virago, E., Khatcheressian, J., Lyckholm, L., & Matsuyama, R. (2010). Giving honest information to patients with advanced cancer maintains hope. *Oncology, 24*(6). Retrieved January 8, 2012, from http://www.psychiatrictimes.com/display/article/10165/1568753?p_p_id=EXT_4&p_p_action=1&p_p_state=normal&p_p_mode=view&p_p_col_id=column-2&p_p_col_count=1&_EXT_4_struts_action=%2Farticles_display%2Fview_article&_EXT_4_showComments=true&_EXT_4_curCommentPage=0#

Stotland, E. (1969). *The psychology of hope*. San Francisco, CA: Jossey-Bass.

Hopelessness

Drew, B. L. (1990). Differentiation of hopelessness, helplessness and powerlessness using Erikson's "Roots of Virtue." *Archives of Psychiatric Nursing, 14,* 332–337.

Engel, G. (1989). A life setting conductive to illness: The giving up–given up complex. *Annals of Internal Medicine, 69,* 293–300.

Fallowfield, L. J., Jenkins, V. A., & Beveridge, H. A. (2002). Truth may hurt but deceit hurts more: Communication in palliative care. *Palliative Medicine, 16*(4), 297–303.

Folkman, S. (2010). Stress, coping, and hope. *Psycho-Oncology, 19*(9), 901–908.

Johnson, J., Gooding, P. A., Wood, A. M., Taylor P. J., Pratt, D., & Tarrier, N. (2010). Resilience to suicidal ideation in psychosis: Positive self-appraisals buffer the impact of hopelessness. *Behavior Research and Therapy, 48*(9), 883–889.

Klotz, L. (2010). Hope in relation to nursing interventions for HIV-infected patients and their significant others. *Journal of the Association of Nurses in AIDS Care, 21*(4), 345–355.

Lin, Y., Dai, Y., & Hwang, S. (2003). The effect of reminiscence on the elderly population: A systematic review. *Public Health Nursing, 20*(4), 297–306.

Schmale, A. H., & Iher, H. P. (1966). The affect of hopelessness and the development of cancer. *Psychosomatic Medicine, 28,* 714–721.

Smith, T., Dow, L., Virago, E., Khatcheressian, J., Lyckholm, L., & Matsuyama, R. (2010). Giving honest information to patients with advanced cancer maintains hope. *Oncology, 24*(6). Retrieved January 8, 2012, from http://www.psychiatrictimes.com/display/article/10165/1568753?p_p_id=EXT_4&p_p_action=1&p_p_state=normal&p_p_mode=view&p_p_col_id=column-2&p_p_col_count=1&_EXT_4_struts_action=%2Farticles_display%2Fview_article&_EXT_4_showComments=true&_EXT_4_curCommentPage=0#

Van Laahoven, H., Schilderman, J., Bleijenberg, G., Donders, R., Verhagen, C., & Prins, J. (2011). Coping, quality of life, depression, and hopelessness in cancer patients in a curative and palliative, end-of-life setting. *Cancer Nursing, 34*(4), 302–314.

Yağmur, Y., & Oltuluoğlu, H. (2011). Social support and hopelessness in women undergoing infertility treatment in Eastern Turkey. *Public Health Nursing.* DOI: 10.1111/j.1525-1446.2011.00976.x. Retrieved January 8, 2012, from http://onlinelibrary.wiley.com/doi/10.1111/j.1525-1446.2011.00976.x/full

Human Dignity, Risk for Compromised

Fahrenwald, N. L., Bassett, S. D., Tschetter, L., Carson, P. P., White, L., & Winterboer, V. J. (2005). Teaching core nursing values. *Journal of Professional Nursing, 21*(1), 46–51.

Gibson, R., & Ferrini, R. (2010). You let them do what??!! Decision-making capacity and the exercise of patient autonomy in LTC. *Annals of Long-Term Care*, 25–30. Retrieved January 8, 2012, from http://www.annalsoflongtermcare.com/content/you-let-them-do-what-decision-making-capacity-and-exercise-patient-autonomy-ltc

Hanks, R. (2010). The medical-surgical nurse perspective of advocate role. *Nursing Forum, 45*(2), 97–107.

Mairis, E. (1994). Concept clarification of professional practice-dignity. *Journal of Advanced Nursing, 19,* 924–931.

Matiti, M. R., & Trorey, G. (2004). Perceptual adjustment levels: Patients' perception of their dignity in the hospital setting. *International Journal of Nursing Studies, 41*(7), 735–744.

Mayers, P., Keet, N., Winkler, G., & Flisher, A. (2010). Mental health service users' perceptions and experiences of sedation, seclusion and restraint. *International Journal of Social Psychiatry, 56*(1), 60–73.

Milton, C. (2011). Human dignity: Scenarios with doing the right thing. *Nursing Science Quarterly, 24*(1), 16–19.

Pellatt, G. C. (2005). Safe handling. The safety and dignity of patients and nurses during patient handling. *British Journal of Nursing (BJN), 14*(21), 1150–1156.

Robinson, E. M. (2002). An ethical analysis of cardiopulmonary resuscitation for elders in acute care. *AACN Clinical Issues: Advanced Practice in Acute & Critical Care, 13*(1), 132–144.

Shottom, L., & Seedhouse, D. (1998). Practical dignity in caring. *Nursing Ethics, 5,* 246–255.

Walsh, K., & Kowanko, I. (2002). Nurses' and patients' perceptions of dignity. *International Journal of Nursing Practice, 8,* 143–151.

Hyperthermia

Biddle, C. (2006). AANA journal course 1: Update for nurse anesthetists: The neurobiology of the human febrile response. *AANA Journal, 74*(2), 145–160.

Carson, S. M. (2003). Alternating acetaminophen and ibuprofen in the febrile child: Examination of the evidence regarding efficacy and safety. *Pediatric Nursing, 29*(5), 379–382.

Christie, J. (2002). Managing febrile children: When and how to treat. *Kai Tiaki Nursing New Zealand, 8*(4), 15–17.

Considine, J. (2006). Paediatric fever education for emergency nurses. *Australian Nursing Journal, 14*(6), 39.

Considine, J., & Brennan, D. (2006). Emergency nurses' opinions regarding paediatric fever: The effect of an evidence-based education program. *Australasian Emergency Nursing Journal, 9*(3), 101–111.

Edwards, H., Walsh, A., Courtney, M., Monaghan, S., Wilson, J., & Young, J. (2007). Improving paediatric nurses' knowledge and attitudes in childhood fever management. *Journal of Advanced Nursing, 57*(3), 257–269.

Gray, S. (2002). Nursing management of a febrile critically ill patient. *Nursing in Critical Care, 7*(1), 37–40.

Hendrik, D., Martens, P., Müller, N., Casier, I., Mulier, J., & Heytens, L. (2010). The use of emergency medical cooling system pads in the treatment of malignant hyperthermia. *European Journal of Anesthesiology, 27*(1), 83–85.

Henker, R., & Carlson, K. K. (2007). Fever: Applying research to bedside practice. *AACN Advanced Critical Care, 18*(1), 76–87.

Holtzclaw, B. J. (2004). Shivering in acutely ill vulnerable populations. *AACN Clinical Issues: Advanced Practice in Acute & Critical Care, 15*(2), 267–279.

Hunt, J. (2007). Fever management. *Paediatric Nursing, 19*(4), 10–10.

Johnston, N. J., King, A. T., Protheroe, R., & Childs, C. (2006). Body temperature management after severe traumatic brain injury: Methods and protocols used in the United Kingdom and Ireland. *Resuscitation, 70*(2), 254–262.

Larach, M., Gronert, G., Allen, G., Brandom, B., & Lehman, E. (2010). Clinical presentation, treatment, and complications of malignant hyperthermia in North America from 1987 to 2006. *Anesthesia & Analgesia, 110*(2), 498–507.

McAllen, K., & Schwartz, D. (2010). Adverse drug reactions resulting in hyperthermia in the intensive care unit. *Critical Care Medicine, 38,* S244–S252.

Mcilvoy, L. H. (2005). The effect of hypothermia and hyperthermia on acute brain injury. *AACN Clinical Issues: Advanced Practice in Acute & Critical Care, 16*(4), 488–500.

Purssell, E. (2002). Treating fever in children: Paracetamol or ibuprofen? *British Journal of Community Nursing, 7*(6), 316.

Sarrell, E. M., Horev, Z., Cohen, Z., & Cohen, H. A. (2005). Parents' and medical personnel's beliefs about infant teething. *Patient Education & Counseling, 57*(1), 122–125.

Taylor, C. (2006). Primary care nursing. Managing infants with pyrexia. *Nursing Times, 102*(39), 42–43.

Thompson, H. J. (2005). Fever: A concept analysis. *Journal of Advanced Nursing, 51*(5), 484–492.

Walsh, A. M., Edwards, H. E., Courtney, M. D., Wilson, J. E., & Monaghan, S. J. (2005). Fever management: Paediatric nurses' knowledge, attitudes and influencing factors. *Journal of Advanced Nursing, 49*(5), 453–464.

Walsh, A. M., Edwards, H. E., Courtney, M. D., Wilson, J. E., & Monaghan, S. J. (2006). Paediatric fever management: Continuing education for clinical nurses. *Nurse Education Today, 26*(1), 71–77.

Watts, R., Robertson, J., & Thomas, G. (2003). Nursing management of fever in children: A systematic review. *International Journal of Nursing Practice, 9*(1), S1–S8.

White, M., Greiner, J., & McDonald, P. (2011). Point: Humans do demonstrate selective brain cooling during hyperthermia. *Journal of Applied Physiology, 110*(2), 569–571.

Wilkinson, J., & Treas, L. (2011). *Fundamentals of nursing* (2nd ed., Vol. 1, pp. 322, 328–329). Philadelphia: F.A. Davis.

Hypothermia

Allen, G. (2003). Evidence for practice: Use of water warming garments. *AORN Journal, 78*(1), 138.

Allen, G. (2006a). Evidence for practice: Forced-air warming blankets and surgical fires. *AORN Journal, 84*(1), 116.

Allen, G. (2006b). Evidence for practice: Preoperative warming to prevent redistribution hypothermia. *AORN Journal, 84*(2), 303–304.

Beal, J. (2005). Toward evidence-based practice. Getting to know you: Mothers' experiences of kangaroo care. *MCN: The American Journal of Maternal Child Nursing, 30*(5), 338–338.

Burger, L., & Fitzpatrick, J. (2009). Prevention of inadvertent perioperative hypothermia. *British Journal of Nursing, 18*(18), 1114–1119.

Burns, S., Wojnakowski, M., Piotrowski, K., & Caraffa, G. (2009). Unintentional hypothermia: Implications or perianesthesia nurses. *Journal of Perianesthesia Nursing, 24*(3), 167–176.

Chwo, M., Anderson, G. C., Good, M., Dowling, D. A., Shiau, S. H., & Chu, D. (2002). A randomized controlled trial of early kangaroo care for preterm infants: Effects on temperature, weight, behavior, and acuity. *Journal of Nursing Research, 10*(2), 129–142.

DeWitte, J., Demeyer, C., & Vandemaele, E. (2010). Resistive-heating or forced-air warming for the prevention of redistribution hypothermia. *Anesthesia & Analgesia, 110*(3), 829–833.

DiMenna, L. (2006). Considerations for implementation of a neonatal kangaroo care protocol. *Neonatal Network, 25*(6), 405–412.

Ellis, J. (2005). Neonatal hypothermia. *Journal of Neonatal Nursing, 11*(2), 76–82.

Farnell, S., Maxwell, L., Tan, S., Rhodes, A., & Philips, B. (2005). Temperature measurement: Comparison of non-invasive methods used in adult critical care. *Journal of Clinical Nursing, 14*(5), 632–639.

Galligan, M. (2006). Proposed guidelines for skin-to-skin treatment of neonatal hypothermia. *MCN: The American Journal of Maternal Child Nursing, 31*(5), 298–306.

Galvão, C., Marck, P., Sawada, N., & Clark, A. M. (2009). A systematic review of the effectiveness of cutaneous warming systems to prevent hypothermia. *Journal of Clinical Nursing, 18*(5), 627–636.

Holden, M., & Makic, M. (2006). Clinically induced hypothermia: Why chill your patient. *AACN Advanced Critical Care, 17*(2), 125–132.

Howell, R., Macrae, L., Sanjines, S., Burke, J., & DeStefano, P. (1992). Effects of two types of head coverings in the rewarming of patients after coronary artery bypass graft surgery. *Heart and Lung, 21,* 1–6.

Ibrahim, C., & Yoxall, C. (2009). Use of plastic bags to prevent hypothermia at birth in preterm infants: Do they work at lower gestations? *Acta Paediatrica, 98*(2), 256–260.

Keresztes, P. A., & Brick, K. (2006). Therapeutic hypothermia after cardiac arrest [cover story]. *Dimensions of Critical Care Nursing, 25*(2), 71–76.

Knobel, R. B., Vohra, S., & Lehmann, C. U. (2005). Heat loss prevention in the delivery room for preterm infants: A national survey of newborn intensive care units. *Journal of Perinatology, 25*(8), 514–518.

Kobbe, P., Lichte, P., Wellman, M., Hildebrand, F., Nast-Kolb, D., Waydhas, C., et al. (2009). Impact of hypothermia on the severely injured patient. *Unfallchirurg, 112*(12), 1055–1061.

Peng, Y., Zheng, M., Ye, Q., Chen, X., Yu, B., & Liu, B. (2009). Heated and humidified CO2 prevents hypothermia, peritoneal injury, and intra-abdominal adhesions during prolonged laparoscopic insufflations. *Journal of Surgical Research, 151*(1), 40–47.

Polderman, K. (2009). Mechanisms of action, physiological effects, and complications of hypothermia. *Critical Care Medicine, 37*(7), S186–S202.

Qadan, M., Gardner, S., Vitale, D., Lominadze, D., Joshua, I., & Polk, H. (2009). Hypothermia and surgery: Immunologic mechanisms for current practice. *Annals of Surgery, 250*(1), 134–140.

Wilkinson, J., & Treas, L. (2011). *Fundamentals of nursing* (2nd ed., Vol. 1, pp. 322, 328–330). Philadelphia: F. A. Davis.

Withers, J. (2005). The elective re-warming of postoperative cardiac patients. *Nursing Times, 101*(24), 30–33.

Wright, J. E. (2005). Therapeutic hypothermia in traumatic brain injury. *Critical Care Nursing Quarterly, 28*(2), 150–161.

Zeitzer, M. B. (2005). Inducing hypothermia to decrease neurological deficit: Literature review. *Journal of Advanced Nursing, 52*(2), 189–199.

Identity: Personal, Disturbed

Bates, J., Boote, J., & Beverley, C. (2004). Psychosocial interventions for people with a milder dementing illness: A systematic review. *Journal of Advanced Nursing, 45*(6), 644–658.

Bender, D., & Skodol, A. (2007). Borderline personality as a self-other representational disturbance. *Journal of Personality Disorders, 21*(5), 500–517.

Bergh, S., & Erling, A. (2005). Adolescent identity formation: A Swedish study of identity status using the EOM-EIS-II. *Adolescence, 40*(158), 377–396.

Dammann, G., Hügli, C., Selinger, J., Gremaud-Heitz, D., Sollberger, D., Wiesbeck, G., et al. (2011). The self-image in borderline personality disorder: An in-depth qualitative research study. *Journal of Personality Disorders, 25*(4), 517–527.

Fuchs, T. (2007). Fragmented selves: Temporality and identity in borderline personality disorder. *Psychopathology, 40*(6), 379–388.

Jørgensen, C. (2010). Invited essay: Identity and borderline personality disorder. *Journal of Personality Disorders, 24*(3), 344–364.

Kearney, M. H., & O'Sullivan, J. (2003). Identity shifts as turning points in health behavior change. *Western Journal of Nursing Research, 25*(2), 134.

Lee, S., & Harris, M. (2010). The development of an effective occupational therapy assessment and treatment pathway for women with a diagnosis of borderline personality disorder in an inpatient setting: Implementing the Model of Human Occupation. *The British Journal of Occupational Therapy, 73*(11), 559–563.

McAndrew, S., & Warne, T. (2004). Ignoring the evidence dictating the practice: Sexual orientation, suicidality and the dichotomy of the mental health nurse. *Journal of Psychiatric & Mental Health Nursing, 11*(4), 428–434.

Miers, M. (2002). Developing an understanding of gender sensitive care: Exploring concepts and knowledge. *Journal of Advanced Nursing, 40*(1), 69–77.

Moritz, S., Veckenstedt, R., Randjbar, S., Vitzthum, F., & Woodward, T. (2011). Antipsychotic treatment beyond antipsychotics: Metacognitive intervention for schizophrenia patients improves delusional symptoms. *Psychological Medicine, 41*(9), 1823–1832.

Myers, E., Startup, H., & Freeman, D. (2011). Cognitive behavioural treatment of insomnia in individuals with persistent persecutory delusions: A pilot trial. *Journal of Behavior Therapy and Experimental Psychiatry, 42*(3), 330–336.

Wilkinson, J., & Treas, L. (2011). *Fundamentals of nursing* (2nd ed.). Philadelphia: F. A. Davis.

Identity: Personal, Risk for Disturbed

Refer to the bibliography for Identity: Personal, Disturbed, preceding.

Immunization Status, Readiness for Enhanced

Baker, D., Dang, M., Ly, M., & Diaz, R. (2010). Perception of barriers to immunization among parents of Hmong origin in California. *American Journal of Public Health, 100*(5), 839–845.

Bardenheier, B. H., Shefer, A., McKibben, L., Roberts, H., Rhew, D., & Bratzler, D. (2005). Factors predictive of increased influenza and pneumococcal vaccination coverage in long-term care facilities: The CMS-CDC standing orders program project. *Journal of the American Medical Directors Association, 6*(5), 291–299.

Bardenheier, B. H., Wortley, P., Ahmed, F., Hales, C., & Shefer, A. (2010). Influenza immunization coverage among residents of long-term care facilities certified by CMS, 2005-2006: The newest MDS quality indicator. *JAMDA (Journal of the American Medical Directors Association), 11*(1), 59–69.

Bernstein, H., Starke, J., & Committee on Infectious Diseases, American Academy of Pediatrics. (2010). Policy statement: Recommendation for mandatory influenza immunization of all health care personnel. *Pediatrics, 126*(4), 809–815.

Britto, M. T., Pandzik, G. M., Meeks, C. S., & Kotagal, U. R. (2006). Performance improvement. Combining evidence and diffusion of innovation theory to enhance influenza immunization. *Joint Commission Journal on Quality & Patient Safety, 32*(8), 426–432.

Bundt, T., & Hu, H. (2004). National examination of compliance predictors and the immunization status of children: Precursor to a developmental model for health systems. *Military Medicine, 169,* 740–745.

Centers for Disease Control and Prevention (CDC). (2011a). *2011 Child & adolescent immunization schedules*. Department of Health and Human Services. Retrieved January 7, 2012, from http://www.cdc.gov/vaccines/recs/schedules/child-schedule.htm#printable

Centers for Disease Control and Prevention (CDC). (2011b). *Recommended adult immunization schedule United States 2011*. Department of Health and Human Services. Retrieved January 7, 2012, from http://www.cdc.gov/vaccines/recs/schedules/downloads/adult/adult-schedule.pdf

Davis, T. C., Frederickson, D. D., Kennen, E. M., Arnold, C., Shoup, E., Sugar, M., et al. (2004). Childhood vaccine risk/benefit communication among public health clinics: A time motion study. *Public Health Nursing, 21,* 228–236.

Fiore, A., Uyeki, T., Broder, K., Finelli, L., Euler, G., Singleton, J., et al. (2010). Prevention and control of influenza with vaccines: Recommendations of the Advisory Committee on Immunization Practices (ACIP), 2010. *MMWR Recommendation Report, 59*(RR-8), 1–62. Retrieved January 9, 2012, from http://www.ncbi.nlm.nih.gov/pubmed/20689501

Hammer, L., Curry, E., Harlor, A., Laughlin, J., Leeds, A., Lessin, H., et al. (2010). Increasing immunization coverage. *Pediatrics, 125*(6), 1295–1304.

Hoveyda, N., McDonald, P., & Behrens, R. H. (2004). A description of travel medicine in general practice: A postal questionnaire survey. *Journal of Travel Medicine, 11*(5), 295–299.

Hutt, E., Reznickova, N., Morgenstern, N., Frederickson, E., & Kramer, A. M. (2004). Improving care for nursing home-acquired pneumonia in a managed care environment. *American Journal of Managed Care, 10*(10), 681–686.

Jedrychowski, W., Maugeri, U., & Jedrychowska-Bianchi, I. (2004). Prospective epidemiologic study on respiratory diseases in children and immunization against measles. *International Journal of Occupational Medicine & Environmental Health, 17*(2), 255–261.

Keller, S., Daley, K., Hyde, J., Greif, R. S., & Church, D. R. (2005). Hepatitis C prevention with nurses. *Nursing & Health Sciences, 7*(2), 99–106.

Lugo, N. R. (2006). Wise to immunize. What works? Improving immunization coverage with evidence-based strategies. *American Journal for Nurse Practitioners, 10*(5), 17.

MacDonald, M. (2005). Parents' decisions on MMR vaccination for their children were based on personal experience rather than scientific evidence. *Evidence-Based Nursing, 8*(2), 60.

Marin, M., Broder, K., Temte, J., Snider, D., & Seward, J.; Centers for Disease Control and Prevention (CDC). (2010). Use of combination measles, mumps, rubella, and varicella vaccine: Recommendations of the Advisory Committee on Immunization Practices (ACIP). *MMWR Recommendations Report, 59*(RR-3), 1–12.

McRee, A.-L., Brewer, N., Reiter, P., Gottlieb, S., & Smith, J. (2010). The Carolina HPV Immunization Attitudes and Beliefs Scale (CHIAS): Scale development and associations with intentions to vaccinate. *Sexually Transmitted Diseases, 37*(4), 234–239.

Mouzoon, M., Munoz, F., Greisinger, A., Brehm, B., Wehman, O., Smith, F., et al. (2010). Improving influenza immunization in pregnant women and healthcare workers. *American Journal of Managed Care, 16*(3), 209–216.

Pearson, M. L., Bridges, C. B., & Harper, S. A. (2006). Influenza vaccination of health-care personnel: Recommendations of the Healthcare Infection Control Practices Advisory Committee (HICPAC) and the Advisory Committee on Immunization Practices (ACIP). *MMWR: Morbidity & Mortality Weekly Report, 55,* 1–15.

Pediatric immunization and asthma guideline updates from Colorado Clinical Guidelines Collaborative (CCGC). (2005). *Colorado Nurse, 105*(4), 21–21.

Purssell, E. (2004). Exploring the evidence surrounding the debate on MMR and autism. *British Journal of Nursing (BJN), 13*(14), 834–838.

Recommended immunization schedules for persons aged 0–18 years—United States, 2008. (2008). *Morbidity and Mortality Weekly Report, 57,* Q1. Retrieved January 9, 2012, from http://www.cdc.gov/mmwr/preview/mmwrhtml/mm5701a8.htm

Russell, M. L., Thurston, W. E., & Henderson, E. A. (2003). Theory and models for planning and evaluating institutional influenza prevention and control programs. *American Journal of Infection Control, 31*(6), 336–341.

Shui, L., Kennedy, A., Wooten, K., Schwartz, B., & Gust, D. (2005). Factors influencing African-American mothers' concerns about immunization safety: A summary of focus group findings. *Journal of the National Medical Association, 97*(5), 657–666.

Sloan, K., & Summers, A. (2006). Tetanus vaccination: The issue of 'just in case' vaccinations in emergency departments. *Australasian Emergency Nursing Journal, 9*(1), 35–38.

Thomas, R. E., Jefferson, T. O., Demicheli, V., & Rivetti, D. (2006). Influenza vaccination for health-care workers who work with elderly people in institutions: A systematic review. *Lancet Infectious Diseases, 6*(5), 273–279.

Top, K., Halperin, B., Baxendale, D., MacKinnon-Cameron, D., & Halperin, S. (2010). Pertussis immunization in paediatric healthcare workers: Knowledge, attitudes, beliefs, and behaviour. *Vaccine, 28*(10), 2169–2173.

Washington, M. L., Mason, J., & Meltzer, M. I. (2005). Maxi-Vac: Planning mass smallpox vaccination clinics. *Journal of Public Health Management & Practice, 11*(6), 542–549.

Impulse Control, Ineffective

American Psychiatric Association. (2000). *Diagnostic and statistical manual of mental disorders* (4th ed., text revision). Washington, DC: Author.

Barkley, R., Edwards, G., Laneri, M., Fletcher, K., & Metevia, L. (2001). Executive functioning, temporal discounting, and sense of time in adolescents with attention deficit hyperactivity disorder (ADHD) and oppositional defiant disorder (ODD). *Journal of Abnormal Child Psychology, 29*(6), 541–556.

Baron-Cohen, S. (1988). An assessment of violence in young man with Asperger's syndrome. *Journal of Child Psychology and Psychiatry, 29*(3), 351–360.

Bradley, E., & Isaacs, B. (2006). Inattention hyperactivity, and impulsivity in teenagers with intellectual disabilities, with and without autism. *Canadian Journal of Psychiatry, 51*(9), 598–606.

Butler, T., Schofield, P., Greenberg, D., Allnutt, S., Indig, D., Carr, V., et al. (2010). Reducing impulsivity in repeat violent offenders: An open label trial of a selective serotonin reuptake inhibitor. *Australian and New Zealand Journal of Psychiatry, 44*(12), 1137–1143.

Byun, S., Ruffini, C., Mills, J., Douglas, A., Niang, M., Stepchenkova, S., et al. (2009). Internet addiction: Metasynthesis of 1996-2006 quantitative research. *CyberPsychology & Behavior, 12*(2), 203–207.

Cloninger, C. (1987). A systematic method for clinical description and classification of personality variants: A proposal. *Archives of General Psychiatry, 44*(6), 573–588.

Coffey, S., Gudleski, G., Saladin, M., & Brady, K. (2003). Impulsivity and rapid discounting of delayed hypothetical rewards in cocaine-dependent individuals. *Experimental and Clinical Psychopharmacology, 11*(1), 18–25.

Conner, K., & Duberstein, P. (2004). Predisposing and precipitating factors for suicide among alcoholics: Empirical review and conceptual integration. *Alcoholism, Clinical and Experimental Research, 28*(5, Suppl.), 6S–17S.

DeLisi, M., & Vaughn, M. (2011). The importance of neuropsychological deficits relating to self-control and temperament to the prevention of serious antisocial behavior. *International Journal of Child, Youth, & Family Studies, 2*(1/2), 12–35.

Falissard, B., Coghill, D., Rothenberger, A., & Lorenzo, M. (2009). Short-term effectiveness of medication and psychosocial intervention in a cohort of newly diagnosed patients with inattention, impulsivity, and hyperactivity problems. *Journal of Attention Disorders, 14*(2), 147–156.

Francis, L., & Susman, E. (2009). Self-regulation and rapid weight gain in children from age 3 to 12 years. *Archives of Pediatrics and Adolescent Medicine, 163*(4), 297–302.

Grant, J., & Potenza, M. (Eds.). (2012). *The oxford handbook of impulse control disorders.* New York: Oxford University Press, Inc.

Hare, R. (2008). Hare psychopathy checklist—revised (PCL-R). In B. Cutler (Ed.), *Encyclopedia of psychology and law* (2nd ed.). Thousand Oaks, CA: Sage Publications.

Madden, G., Petry, N., Bader, G., & Bickel, W. (1997). Impulsive and self-control choices in opioid-dependent patients and non-drug-using control participants: Drug and monetary rewards. *Experimental and Clinical Psychopharmacology, 5*(3), 256–262.

Moeller, F., Barratt, E., Dougherty, D., Schmitz, J., & Swann, A. (2001). Psychiatric aspects of impulsivity. *American Journal of Psychiatry, 158*(11), 1783–1793.

Petry, N., & Casarella, T. (1999). Excessive discounting of delayed rewards in substance abusers with gambling problem. *Drug and Alcohol Dependency, 56*(1), 25–32.

Raymond, N., & Coleman, E. (2010). Augmentation with naltrexone to treat compulsive sexual behavior: A case series. *Annals of Clinical Psychiatry, 22*(1), 56–62.

Reynolds, B., Karraker, K., Horn, K., & Richards, J. (2003). Delay and probability discounting as related to different stages of adolescent smoking and non-smoking. *Behavioural Processes, 64*(3), 333–344.

Romer, D. (2010). Adolescent risk taking, impulsivity, and brain development: Implications for prevention. *Developmental Psychobiology, 52*(3), 263–276.

Thomas, A., Bonanni, L., Gambi, F., Di Iorio, A., & Onofrj, M. (2010). Pathological gambling in Parkinson diseases is reduced by amantadine. *Annals of Neurology, 68*(3), 400–404.

Verdejo-Garcia, A., Bechara, A., Recknor, E., & Perez-Garcia, M. (2007). Negative emotion-driven impulsivity predicts substance dependence problems. *Drug and Alcohol Dependence, 91*(2–3), 213–219.

Vuchinich, R., & Simpson, C. (1998). Hyperbolic temporal discounting in social drinkers and problem drinkers. *Experimental and Clinical Psychopharmacology, 6*(3), 292–305.

Infant Behavior, Disorganized

Als, H. (1986). A synactive model of neonatal behavioral organization: Framework for the assessment of neurobehavioral development in the premature infant and for the support of infants and parents in the neonatal intensive care environment. *Physical and Occupational Therapy in Pediatrics, 6,* 3–53.

Aris, C., Stevens, T. P., LeMura, C., Lipke, B., McMullen, S., Côté-Arsenault, D., et al. (2006). NICU nurses' knowledge and discharge teaching related to infant sleep position and risk of SIDS. *Advances in Neonatal Care, 6*(5), 281–294.

Blackburn, S., & Vandenberg, K. (1993). Assessment and management of neonatal neurobehavioral development. In C. Kenner, A. Brueggemeyer, & L. Gunderson (Eds.), *Comprehensive neonatal nursing*. Philadelphia: Saunders.

Broome, M. E., & Tanzillo, H. (1990). Differentiating between pain and agitation in premature neonates. *Journal of Perinatal and Neonatal Nursing, 4*(1), 33–62.

Chwo, M., Anderson, G. C., Good, M., Dowling, D. A., Shiau, S. H., & Chu, D. (2002). A randomized controlled trial of early kangaroo care for preterm infants: Effects on temperature, weight, behavior, and acuity. *Journal of Nursing Research, 10*(2), 129–142.

Cole, J., & Frappier, P. (1985). Infant stimulation reassessed. *Journal of Obstetrical, Gynecological, and Neonatal Nursing, 14,* 471–477.

Flandermyer, A. A. (1993). The drug-exposed neonate. In C. Kenner, A. Brueggemeyer, & L. Gunderson (Eds.), *Comprehensive neonatal nursing*. Philadelphia: Saunders.

Henry, S. M. (2004). Discerning differences: Gastroesophageal reflux and gastroesophageal reflux disease in infants. *Advances in Neonatal Care, 4*(4), 235–247.

Moos, M. (2006). The prevention chronicles. Responding to the newest evidence about SIDS. *A WHONN Lifelines, 10*(2), 163–166.

Solomon, J., & George, C. (2011). *Disorganized attachment and caregiving*. New York: The Guilford Press.

Symington, A., & Pinelli, J. M. (2002). Distilling the evidence on developmental care: A systematic review. *Advances in Neonatal Care, 2*(4), 198–221.

Symington, A., & Pinelli, J. M. (2006). Developmental care for promoting development and preventing morbidity in preterm infants. *Cochrane Library* (4). DOI: 10.1002/14651858.CD001814.pub2

Vickers, A., Ohlsson, A., Lacy, J. B., & Horsley, A. (2006). Massage for promoting growth and development of preterm and/or low birth-weight infants. *Cochrane Library* (4). Retrieved December 20, 2012, from http://summaries.cochrane.org/CD000390/massage-for-promoting-growth-and-development-of-premature-and-low-birth-weight-infants

Weber, J. (2010). *Nurses' handbook of health assessment* (7th ed.). Philadelphia: Wolters Kluwer Health/Lippincott Williams & Wilkins.

Yecco, G. J. (1993). Neurobehavioral development and developmental support of premature infants. *Journal of Perinatal and Neonatal Nursing, 7*(1), 56–65.

Infant Behavior: Disorganized, Risk for

Blackburn, S. (1993). Assessment and management of neurologic dysfunction. In C. Kenner, A. Brueggemeyer, & L. Gunderson (Eds.), *Comprehensive neonatal nursing*. Philadelphia: Saunders.

Blackburn, S., & Vandenberg, K. (1993). Assessment and management of neonatal neurobehavioral development. In C. Kenner, A. Brueggemeyer, & L. Gunderson (Eds.), *Comprehensive neonatal nursing*. Philadelphia: Saunders.

Bozzette, M. (1993). Observations of pain behavior in the NICU: An exploratory study. *Journal of Perinatal and Neonatal Nursing, 7*(1), 76–87.

Grunau, R., & Craig, K. (1987). Pain expression in neonates: Facial action and cry. *Pain, 28,* 395–410.

Yecco, G. J. (1993). Neurobehavioral development and developmental support of premature infants. *Journal of Perinatal and Neonatal Nursing, 7*(1), 56–65.

Infant Behavior: Organized, Readiness for Enhanced

Aspin, A. (2004). The concept of snoezelen: Sensory stimulation and relaxation for neonates. *Journal of Neonatal Nursing, 10*(2), 47–51.

Beaumont, B. (2005). Baby massage—a loving touch: Visual evidence of the benefits. *Community Practitioner, 78*(3), 93–97.

Ferber, S. G., Makhoul, I. R., & Weller, A. (2006). Does sympathetic activity contribute to growth of preterm infants? *Early Human Development, 82*(3), 205–210.

Solomon, J., & George, C. (2011). *Disorganized attachment and caregiving*. New York: The Guilford Press.

Symington, A., & Pinelli, J. M. (2002). Distilling the evidence on developmental care: A systematic review. *Advances in Neonatal Care, 2*(4), 198–221.

Symington, A., & Pinelli, J. M. (2006). Developmental care for promoting development and preventing morbidity in preterm infants. *Cochrane Library* (4). Retrieved December 20, 2012, from http://summaries.cochrane.org/CD000390/massage-for-promoting-growth-and-development-of-premature-and-low-birth-weight-infants

Vickers, A., Ohlsson, A., Lacy, J. B., & Horsley, A. (2006). Massage for promoting growth and development of preterm and/or low birth-weight infants. *Cochrane Library* (4).

Weber, J. (2010). *Nurses' handbook of health assessment* (7th ed.). Philadelphia: Wolters Kluwer Health/Lippincott Williams & Wilkins.

Infant Feeding Pattern, Ineffective

Aksu, H., Küçük, M., & Düzgün, G. (2011). The effect of postnatal breastfeeding education/support offered at home 3 days after delivery on breastfeeding duration and knowledge: A randomized trial. *Journal of Maternal-Fetal and Neonatal Medicine, 24*(2), 354–361.

Ansari, F., Ferring, V., Schulz-Weidner, N., & Wetzel, W. (2006). Concomitant oral findings in children after cardiac transplant. *Pediatric Transplantation, 10*(2), 215–219.

Arvedson, J., & Brodsky, L. (Eds.). (2002). *Pediatric swallowing and feeding: Assessment and management* (2nd ed.). San Diego, CA: Singular Publishing Group.

Beal, J. A. (2005). Evidence for best practices in the neonatal period. *MCN: The American Journal of Maternal Child Nursing, 30*(6), 397–405.

Cho, S., Cho, H., Lee, H., & Lee, K. (2010). Factors related to success in relactation. *Journal of the Korean Society of Neonatology, 17*(2), 232–238.

Collins, B., DiSantis, K., & Nair, U. (2011). Longer previous smoking abstinence relates to successful breastfeeding initiation among underserved smokers. *Breastfeeding Medicine, 6*(6), 385–391.

Dowling, D. A. (2005). Lessons from the past: A brief history of the influence of social, economic, and scientific factors on infant feeding. *Newborn & Infant Nursing Reviews, 5*(1), 2–9.

Holm, P. A. (2004). Early enteral feeding in the preterm infant: An exploration of differences in views and policies. *Journal of Neonatal Nursing, 10*(2), 41–44.

Hurtekant, K. M., & Spatz, D. L. (2007). Special considerations for breastfeeding the infant with spina bifida. *Journal of Perinatal & Neonatal Nursing, 21*(1), 69–75.

Kitsantas, P., & Pawloski, L. (2010). Maternal obesity, health status during pregnancy, and breastfeeding initiation and duration. *Journal of Maternal-Fetal and Neonatal Medicine, 23*(2), 135–141.

Lawson, M. (2003). Gastro-oesophageal reflux in infants: An evidence-based approach. *British Journal of Community Nursing, 8*(7), 296.

Leonard, L. G. (2002). Insights in practice. Breastfeeding higher order multiples: Enhancing support during the postpartum hospitalization period. *Journal of Human Lactation, 18*(4), 386–392.

Leonard, L. G., & Denton, J. (2006). Preparation for parenting multiple birth children. *Early Human Development, 82*(6), 371–378.

Meyer, R. (2006). Special feature: Preventing allergies through good maternal and infant nutrition. *British Journal of Midwifery, 14*(7), 401–402.

Minnie, C. S., & Greeff, M. (2006). The choice of baby feeding mode within the reality of the HIV/AIDS epidemic: Health education implications. *Curationis, 29*(4), 19–27.

Miracle, D. J., Meier, P. P., & Bennett, P. A. (2004). Mothers' decisions to change from formula to mothers' milk for very-low-birth-weight infants. *JOGNN: Journal of Obstetric, Gynecologic, & Neonatal Nursing, 33*(6), 692–703.

Morland-Schultz, K., & Hill, P. D. (2005). Prevention of and therapies for nipple pain: A systematic review. *JOGNN: Journal of Obstetric, Gynecologic, & Neonatal Nursing, 34*(4), 428–437.

Pickler, R. H., Chiaranai, C., & Reyna, B. A. (2006). Relationship of the first suck burst to feeding outcomes in preterm infants. *Journal of Perinatal & Neonatal Nursing, 20*(2), 157–162.

Premji, S. S. (2005). Enteral feeding for high-risk neonates. *Journal of Perinatal & Neonatal Nursing, 19*(1), 59–71.

Richardson, D. S., Branowicki, P. A., Zeidman-Rogers, L., Mahoney, J., & MacPhee, M. (2006). Clinical practice column. An evidence-based approach to nasogastric tube management: Special considerations. *Journal of Pediatric Nursing, 21*(5), 388–393.

Rodriguez, N. A., Miracle, D. J., & Meier, P. P. (2005). Sharing the science on human milk feedings with mothers of very-low-birth-weight infants. *JOGNN: Journal of Obstetric, Gynecologic, & Neonatal Nursing, 34*(1), 109–119.

Smith, J. R. (2005). Early enteral feeding for the very low birth weight infant: The development and impact of a research-based guideline. *Neonatal Network, 24*(4), 9–19.

Spatz, D. L. (2006). State of the science: Use of human milk and breast-feeding for vulnerable infants. *Journal of Perinatal & Neonatal Nursing, 20*(1), 51–55.

Taveras, E. M., Li, R., Grummer-Strawn, L., Richardson, M., Marshall, R., Rêgo, V. H., et al. (2004). Opinions and practices of clinicians associated with continuation of exclusive breastfeeding. *Pediatrics, 113*(4), e283–e290.

Usher, K., & Foster, K. (2006). The use of psychotropic medications with breastfeeding women: Applying the available evidence. *Contemporary Nurse: A Journal for the Australian Nursing Profession, 21*(1), 94–102.

Wright, C. M., & Parkinson, K. N. (2004). Postnatal weight loss in term infants: What is "normal" and do growth charts allow for it? *Archives of Disease in Childhood—Fetal & Neonatal Edition, 89*(3), F254–F257.

Zanardo, V., Gambina, I., Beglely, C., Litta, P., Cosmi, E., Guistardi, A., et al. (2011). Psychological distress and early lactation performance in mothers of late preterm infants. *Early Human Development, 87*(4), 321–323.

Infection, Risk for

Abbott, C. A., Dremsa, T., Stewart, D. W., Mark, D. D., & Swift, C. C. (2006). Adoption of a ventilator-associated pneumonia clinical practice guideline. *Worldviews on Evidence-Based Nursing, 3*(4), 139–152.

Alexander, M. (Ed.). (2006). Infusion nursing: Standards of practice. *Journal of Infusion Nursing, 29*(1S, Suppl.), S1–S92.

Allen, G. (2005). Evidence for practice: Endogenous flora in development of surgical site infections. *AORN Journal, 81*(6), 1338.

Allen, G. (2006). Evidence for practice: Transfusion and postoperative infection risk. *AORN Journal, 83*(5), 1137–1138.

Allen, U., & Green, M. (2010). Prevention and treatment of infectious complications after solid organ transplantation in children. *Pediatric Clinics of North America, 57,* 459–479.

Altman, M. R., & Lydon-Rochelle, M. T. (2006). Prolonged second stage of labor and risk of adverse maternal and perinatal outcomes: A systematic review. *Birth: Issues in Perinatal Care, 33*(4), 315–322.

Aragon, D., & Sole, M. L. (2006). Implementing best practice strategies to prevent infection in the ICU. *Critical Care Nursing Clinics of North America, 18*(4), 441–452.

Ata, A., Lee, J., Bestle, S., Desemone, J., & Stain, S. (2010). Postoperative hyperglycemia and surgical site infection in general surgery patients. *Archives of Surgery, 145,* 858–864.

Ata, A., Valerian, B., Lee, E., Bestle, S., Elmendorf, S., & Stain, S. (2010). The effect of diabetes mellitus on surgical site infections after colorectal and non colorectal general surgical operations. *American Surgeon, 76,* 697–702.

Balentine, C., Wilks, J., Robinson, C., Marshall, C., Anaya, D., Albo, D., et al. (2010). Obesity increased wound complications in rectal cancer surgery. *Journal of Surgical Research, 163*(1), 35–39.

Banning, M. (2005a). Influenza: Incidence, symptoms and treatment. *British Journal of Nursing (BJN), 14*(22), 1192–1197.

Banning, M. (2005b). Transmission and epidemiology of MRSA: Current perspectives. *British Journal of Nursing (BJN), 14*(10), 548–554.

Beam, J. W., & Buckley, B. (2006). Community-acquired methicillin-resistant *Staphylococcus* aureus: Prevalence and risk factors. *Journal of Athletic Training, 41*(3), 337–340.

Bissett, L. (2005). Controlling the risk of MRSA infection: Screening and isolating patients. *British Journal of Nursing (BJN), 14*(7), 386–390.

Bleasdale, S., Trick, W., Gonzales, I., Lyles, R., Hayden, M., & Weinstein, R. (2007). Effectiveness of chlorhexidine bathing to reduce catheter-associated bloodstream infections in medical intensive care unit patients. *Archives of Internal Medicine, 167,* 2073–2079.

Bochicchio, G., Bochicchio, K., Joshi, M., Hathi, O., & Scalea, T. (2010). Acute glucose elevation is highly predictive of infection and outcome in critically injured trauma patients. *Annals of Surgery, 252,* 597–602.

Brodie, S. J., Biley, F. C., & Shewring, M. (2002). An exploration of the potential risks associated with using pet therapy in healthcare settings. *Journal of Clinical Nursing, 11*(4), 444–456.

Chan, E. D., & Chmura, K. (2004). Diagnosis and treatment of latent tuberculosis infection. *Journal of Clinical Outcomes Management, 11*(3), 180–188.

Chee, Y., Teoh, K., Sabnis, B., Ballantyne, J., & Brenkel, I. (2010). Total hip replacement in morbidly obese patients with osteoarthritis: Results of a prospectively matched study. *Journal of Bone and Joint Surgery Br, 92,* 1066–1071.

Coia, J. E., Duckworth, G. J., Edwards, D. I., Farrington, M., Fry, C., Humphreys, H., et al. (2006). Guidelines for the control and prevention of methicillin-resistant *Staphylococcus* aureus (MRSA) in healthcare facilities. *Journal of Hospital Infection, 63,* S1–S44.

Cooper, A. C., Banasiak, N. C., & Allen, P. J. (2003). Management and prevention strategies for respiratory syncytial virus (RSV) bronchiolitis in infants and young children: A review of evidence-based practice interventions. *Pediatric Nursing, 29*(6), 452–456.

Cousens, S., Blencowe, H., Gravett, M., & Lawn, J. (2010). Antibiotic for pre-term pre-labour rupture of membranes: Prevention of neonatal deaths due to complications of pre-term birth and infection. *International Journal of Epidemiology, 39,* 134–143.

Craft, A. P., Finer, N. N., & Barrington, K. J. (2006). Vancomycin for prophylaxis against sepsis in preterm neonates. *Cochrane Library* (4).

Cutter, J., & Gammon, J. (2007). Infection control. Review of standard precautions and sharps management in the community. *British Journal of Community Nursing, 12*(2), 54.

Dorner, T., Schwarz, F., Kranz, A., Freidl, W., Reider, A., & Gisinger, C. (2010). Body mass index and the risk of infections in institutionalized geriatric patients. *British Journal of Nutrition, 103,* 1830–1835.

Duffy, J. R. (2002). Nosocomial infections: Important acute care nursing-sensitive outcomes indicators. *AACN Clinical Issues: Advanced Practice in Acute & Critical Care, 13*(3), 358–366.

Evans, B. (2005). Best-practice protocols: VAP prevention. *Nursing Management, 36*(12), 10–16.

Falsey, A. R., & Walsh, E. E. (2005). Respiratory syncytial virus infection in elderly adults. *Drugs & Aging, 22*(7), 577–587.

Gould, D., Gammon, J., Salem, R. B., Chudleigh, J., & Fontenla, M. (2004). Flowers in the clinical setting: Infection risk or workload issue? *NT Research, 9*(5), 366–377.

Grap, M. J., & Munro, C. L. (2004). Preventing ventilator-associated pneumonia: Evidence-based care. *Critical Care Nursing Clinics of North America, 16*(3), 349–358.

Grap, M. J., Munro, C. L., Hummel, R., Elswick, R. K., McKinney, J. L., & Sessler, C. N. (2005). Effect of backrest elevation on the development of ventilator-associated pneumonia. *American Journal of Critical Care, 14*(4), 325–333.

Gravante, G., Araco, A., Sorge, R., Araco, F., Delogu, D., & Cervelli, V. (2007). Wound infections in body contouring mastopexy with breast reduction after laparoscopic adjustable gastric banding: The role of smoking. *Obesity Surgery, 18,* 721–727.

Hampton, S. (2004). Nursing management of urinary tract infections for catheterized patients. *British Journal of Nursing (BJN), 13*(20), 1180–1184.

Hanrahan, K. S., & Lofgren, M. (2004). Evidence-based practice: Examining the risk of toys in the microenvironment of infants in the neonatal intensive care unit. *Advances in Neonatal Care, 4*(4), 184–205.

Ho, L., Wang, H., Chiang, C., Hung, K., & Wu, K. (2010). Malnutrition-inflammation scores independently determined cardiovascular and infection risk in peritoneal dialysis patients. *Blood Purification, 29,* 308–316.

Hsiu-fang Hsieh, Hua-hsien Chiu, & Feng-ping Lee. (2006). Surgical hand scrubs in relation to microbial counts: Systematic literature review. *Journal of Advanced Nursing, 55*(1), 68–78.

Hugonnet, S., Chevrolet, J., & Pittet, D. (2007). The effect of workload on infection risk in critically ill patients. *Critical Care Medicine, 35*(1), 76–81.

Jamsen, E., Nevalainen, P., Kalliovalkama, J., & Moilanen, T. (2010). Preoperative hyperglycemia predicts infected total knee replacement. *European Journal of Internal Medicine, 21,* 196–201.

Jenkinson, H., Wright, D., Jones, M., Dias, E., Pronyszyn, A., Hughes, K., et al. (2006). Prevention and control of infection in non-acute healthcare settings. *Nursing Standard, 20*(40), 56.

LaMar, K., & Dowling, D. A. (2006). Incidence of infection for preterm twins cared for in cobedding in the neonatal intensive-care unit. *JOGNN: Journal of Obstetric, Gynecologic, & Neonatal Nursing, 35*(2), 193–198.

Len, O., & Pahissa, A. (2007). Donor-transmitted infections. *Enfermedades Infecciosas y Microbiologia Clinica, 25,* 204–212.

Mallory, C., & Gabrielson, M. (2005). Preventing HIV infection among women who trade sex. *Clinical Excellence for Nurse Practitioners, 9*(1), 17–22.

Mayr, F., Yende, S., Linde-Zwirbie, W., Peck-Palmer, O., Barnato, A., Weissfeld, L., et al. (2010). Infection rate and acute organ dysfunction risk as explanations for racial differences in severe sepsis. *JAMA, 303,* 2495–2503.

McMillan, M., & Davis, J. (2010). Acute hospital admission for sepsis: An important but under-utilized opportunity for smoking cessation interventions. *Australian and New Zealand Journal of Public Health, 34,* 432–433.

Morris, C. G. (2005). Is sputum evaluation useful for patients with community-acquired pneumonia? *Journal of Family Practice, 54*(3), 279–281.

Morrison-Beedy, D., Nelson, L. E., & Volpe, E. (2005). HIV risk behaviors and testing rates in adolescent girls: Evidence to guide clinical practice. *Pediatric Nursing, 31*(6), 508–512.

Morritt, M. L., Harrod, M. E., Crisp, J., Senner, A., Galway, R., Petty, S., et al. (2006). Handwashing practice and policy variability when caring for central venous catheters in paediatric intensive care. *Australian Critical Care, 19*(1), 15–21.

Nazarko, L. (2007). Avoiding the pitfalls and perils of catheter care. *British Journal of Nursing (BJN), 16*(8), 468–472.

Oestreicher, P. (2007). Put evidence into practice to prevent infection in patients with cancer. *ONS Connect, 22*(2), 26–27.

Roe, V. A. (2004). Living with genital herpes. How effective is antiviral therapy? *Journal of Perinatal & Neonatal Nursing, 18*(3), 206–215.

Roodhouse, A., & Wellsted, A. (2006). Safety in urine sampling: Maintaining an infection-free environment. *British Journal of Nursing (BJN), 15*(16), 870–872.

Rupp, M., Jourdan, M., Tyner, L., Iwen, P., & Anderson, J. (2007). Outbreak of bloodstream infections temporally associated with the use of an intravascular positive displacement needleless valve. *Clinical Infectious Diseases, 44,* 1408–1414.

Simon, A., Schildgen, O., Eis-Hübinger, A. M., Hasan, C., Bode, U., Buderus, S., et al. (2006). Norovirus outbreak in a pediatric oncology unit. *Scandinavian Journal of Gastroenterology, 41*(6), 693–699.

Sole, M. L. (2005). Overcoming the barriers: A concerted effort to prevent ventilator-associated pneumonia. *Australian Critical Care, 18*(3), 92–94.

Sparse evidence to prove cranberries help in UTIs. (2005). *Practice Nurse, 29*(5), 10.

Stringer, M., Miesnik, S. R., Brown, L., Martz, A. H., & Macones, G. (2004). Nursing care of the patient with preterm premature rupture of membranes. *MCN: The American Journal of Maternal Child Nursing, 29*(3), 144–150.

Waisbren, E., Rosen, H., Bader, A., Lipsitz, S., Rogers, S., & Eriksson, E. (2010). Percent body fat and prediction of surgical site infection. *Journal of the American College of Surgeons, 210,* 381–389.

Webster, J., & Pritchard, M. A. (2006). Gowning by attendants and visitors in newborn nurseries for prevention of neonatal morbidity and mortality. *Cochrane Library* (4). Retrieved December 20, 2012, from http://www.nichd.nih.gov/cochrane_data/webster/webster.htm

Injury, Risk for

Bodin, S. (2007). Evidence and nursing informatics to improve safely and outcomes. *Nephrology Nursing Journal, 34*(2), 135–136.

Cohen, S., Gerding, D., Johnson, S., Kelly, C., Loo, V., McDonald, C., et al. (2010). Clinical practice guidelines for *Clostridium* difficile infection in adults: 2010 update by the Society for Healthcare Epidemiology of America (SHEA) and the Infectious Diseases Society of America (IDSA). *Infection Control and Hospital Epidemiology, 31*(5), 431–455.

Currie, L. M. (2006). Fall and injury prevention. *Annual Review of Nursing Research, 24,* 39–74.

Cutter, J., & Gammon, J. (2007). Review of standard precautions and sharps management in the community. *British Journal of Community Nursing, 12*(2), 54–60.

Dennision, R. D. (2006). High-alert drugs: Strategies for safe I.V. infusions. *American Nurse Today, 1*(2), 28–34.

Doughty, A., & Kane, L. (2010). Teaching abuse-protection skills to people with intellectual disabilities: A review of the literature. *Research in Developmental Disabilities, 31*(2), 331–337.

Evans, D., Wood, J., & Lambert, L. (2003). Patient injury and physical restraint devices: A systematic review. *Journal of Advanced Nursing, 41*(3), 274–282.

Garzon, D. L. (2005). Contributing factors to preschool unintentional injury. *Journal of Pediatric Nursing, 20*(6), 441–447.

Ghanizadeh, A., & Jafari, P. (2010). Risk factors of abuse of parents by their ADHD children. *European Child & Adolescent Psychiatry, 19*(1), 75–81.

Harris, G. M., & Verklan, M. T. (2005). Maximizing patient safety: Filter needle use with glass ampules. *Journal of Perinatal & Neonatal Nursing, 19*(1), 74–81.

Hayes, N. (2004). Prevention of falls among older patients in the hospital environment. *British Journal of Nursing (BJN), 13*(15), 896–901.

Hazell, L., & Shakir, S. A. W. (2006). Under-reporting of adverse drug reactions: A systematic review. *Drug Safety, 29*(5), 385.

Hignett, S., & Masud, T. (2006). A review of environmental hazards associated with in-patient falls. *Ergonomics, 49*(5), 605–616.

Hook, M. L., & Winchel, S. (2006). Fall-related injuries in acute care: Reducing the risk of harm. *MEDSURG Nursing, 15*(6), 370–381.

Howard, P. K. (2005). Parents' beliefs about children and gun safety. *Pediatric Nursing, 31*(5), 374–379.

Johnson, F., Hogg, J., & Daniel, B. (2010). Abuse and protection issues across the lifespan: Reviewing the literature. *Social Policy and Society, 9,* 291–304.

Kendig, S., Adkins-Bley, K., Carson-Smith, W., & Nelson, K. J. (2006). Patient safety: Expert roundtable discussion. *AWHONN Lifelines, 10*(3), 218–224.

Kim, T., & Nemergut, M. (2011). Preparation of modern anesthesia workstations for malignant hyperthermia-susceptible patients: A review of past and present practice. *Anesthesiology, 114*(1), 205–212.

May, S. (2007). Testing nasogastric tube positioning in the critically ill: Exploring the evidence. *British Journal of Nursing (BJN), 16*(7), 414–418.

McCartney, P. R. (2006). Using technology to promote perinatal patient safety. *JOGNN: Journal of Obstetric, Gynecologic, & Neonatal Nursing, 35*(3), 424–431.

Mercurio, J. (2011). Creating a latex-safe perioperative environment. *OR Nurse, 5*(6), 18–25.

Needleman, J., Buerhaus, P., Pankratz, S., Leibson, C., Stevens, S., & Harris, M. (2011). Nurse staffing and inpatient hospital mortality. *The New England Journal of Medicine, 364,* 1037–1045.

Nelson, A., & Baptiste, A. S. (2006). Evidence-based practices for safe patient handling and movement. *Orthopaedic Nursing, 25*(6), 366–379.

Oliver, D., Connelly, J. B., Victor, C. R., Shaw, F. E., Whitehead, A., Genc, Y., et al. (2007). Strategies to prevent falls and fractures in hospitals and care homes and effect of cognitive impairment: Systematic review and meta-analyses. *BMJ: British Medical Journal, 334*(7584), 82–85.

Page, A. E. K. (2004). Transforming nurses' work environments to improve patient safety: The institute of medicine recommendations. *Policy, Politics & Nursing Practice, 5*(4), 250–258.

Park, M., & Tang, J. H. (2007). Evidence-based guideline changing the practice of physical restraint use in acute care. *Journal of Gerontological Nursing, 33*(2), 9–16.

Polovich, M. (2004). Safe handling of hazardous drugs. *Online Journal of Issues in Nursing, 9*(3), 153–168.

Pynoos, J., Rose, D., Rubenstein, L., Choi, I. H., & Sabata, D. (2006). Evidence-based interventions in fall prevention. *Home Health Care Services Quarterly, 25*(1), 55–73.

Rossi, J., Swan, M., & Isaacs, E. (2010). The violent or agitated patient. *Emergency Medicine Clinics of North America, 28*(1), 235–256.

Stein, H. G. (2006). Best practice. Glass ampules and filter needles: An example of implementing the sixth "R" in medication administration. *MEDSURG Nursing, 15*(5), 290–294.

Thompson, M. R. (2003). The three Rs of fire safety, emergency action, and fire prevention planning: Promoting safety at the worksite. *AAOHN Journal, 51*(4), 169–179.

Wanzer, L. J., & Hicks, R. W. (2006). Medication safety within the perioperative environment. *Annual Review of Nursing Research, 24,* 127–155.

Waters, T., Collins, J., Galinsky, T., & Caruso, C. (2006). NIOSH research efforts to prevent musculoskeletal disorders in the healthcare industry. *Orthopaedic Nursing, 25*(6), 380–389.

Weir, V. L. (2005). Best practice protocols: Preventing adverse drug events. *Nursing Management, 36*(9), 24–30.

Wilburn, S. Q. (2004). Needlestick and sharps injury prevention. *Online Journal of Issues in Nursing, 9*(3), 141–153.

Wilkinson, J., & Treas, L. (2011). Chapter 21, Promoting safety; and chapter 23, Administering medication. In *Fundamentals of nursing* (2nd ed.). Philadelphia: F. A. Davis.

Woods, A. J. (2006). The role of health professionals in childhood injury prevention: A systematic review of the literature. *Patient Education & Counseling, 64*(1), 35–42.

Insomnia

Alessi, C. A., Martin, J. L., & Webber, A. P. (2005). A multidimensional non-drug intervention reduced daytime sleep in nursing home residents with sleep problems. *Evidence-Based Medicine, 10*(6), 178.

Berger, A. M., Parker, K. P., Young-McCaughan, S., Mallory, G. A., Barsevick, A. M., Beck, S. L., et al. (2005). Sleep/wake disturbances in people with cancer and their caregivers: State of the science. *Oncology Nursing Forum, 32*(6), E98–E126.

Clark, J., Cunningham, M., McMillan, S., Vena, C., & Parker, K. (2004). Sleep-wake disturbances in people with cancer part II: Evaluating the evidence for clinical decision making. *Oncology Nursing Forum, 31*(4), 747–768.

Conn, D. K., & Madan, R. (2006). Use of sleep-promoting medications in nursing home residents: Risks versus benefits. *Drugs & Aging, 23*(4), 271.

Haesler, E. J. (2004). Effectiveness of strategies to manage sleep in residents of aged care facilities. *JBI Reports, 2*(4), 115–183.

Hinds, P. S., Hockenberry, M., Rai, S. N., Lijun Zhang, Razzouk, B. I., McCarthy, K., et al. (2007). Nocturnal awakenings, sleep environment interruptions, and fatigue in hospitalized children with cancer. *Oncology Nursing Forum, 34*(2), 393–402.

Hui-Ling Lai, & Good, M. (2006). Music improves sleep quality in older adults. *Journal of Advanced Nursing, 53*(1), 134–144.

Koch, S., Haesler, E., Tiziani, A., & Wilson, J. (2006). Effectiveness of sleep management strategies for residents of aged care facilities: Findings of a systematic review. *Journal of Clinical Nursing, 15*(10), 1267–1275.

McCavey, B., & Neal-Perry, G. (2010). Evaluating and treating insomnia in menopausal women. *Menopausal Medicine, 18*(3), S1–S12.

O'Brien, L. (2011). The neurocognitive effects of sleep disruption in children and adolescents. *Sleep Medicine Clinics, 6*(1), 109–116.

Page, M. S., Berger, A. M., & Johnson, L. B. (2006). Putting evidence into practice: Evidence-based interventions for sleep-wake disturbances. *Clinical Journal of Oncology Nursing, 10*(6), 753–676.

Perlis, M. L., Smith, L. J., Lyness, J. M., Matteson, S. R., Pigeon, W. R., Jungquist, C. R., et al. (2006). Insomnia as a risk factor for onset of depression in the elderly. *Behavioral Sleep Medicine, 4*(2), 104–113.

Phillips, K. D., Mock, K. S., Bopp, C. M., Dudgeon, W. A., & Hand, G. A. (2006). Spiritual well-being, sleep disturbance, and mental and physical health status in HIV-infected individuals. *Issues in Mental Health Nursing, 27*(2), 125–139.

Shin, C., Kim, J., Yi, H., Lee, H., Lee, J., & Shin, K. (2005). Relationship between trait-anger and sleep disturbances in middle-aged men and women. *Journal of Psychosomatic Research, 58*(2), 183–189.

Tsara, V., Amfilochiou, A., Papagrigorakis, J., Georgopoulos, D., Liolios, E., Kadiths, A., et al. (2010). Guidelines for diagnosing and treating sleep related breathing disorders in adults and children (part 3: Obstructive sleep apnea in children, diagnosis and treatment). *Hippokratia, 14*(1), 57–62.

Wang, M., Wang, S., & Tsai, P. (2005). Cognitive behavioural therapy for primary insomnia: A systematic review. *Journal of Advanced Nursing, 50*(5), 553–564.

Ward, T., Archbold, K., Lentz, M., Ringold, S., Wallace, C., & Landis, C. (2010). Sleep disturbance, daytime sleepiness, and neurocognitive performance in children with juvenile idiopathic arthritis. *Sleep, 33*(2), 252–259.

Wilkinson, J., & Treas, L. (2011). Chapter 33, Sleep and rest. In *Fundamentals of nursing* (2nd ed.). Philadelphia: F. A. Davis.

Wilson, S., Nutt, D., Alford, C., Argyropoulos, S., Baldwin, D., & Bateson, A. (2010). British Association for Psychopharmacology consensus statement on evidence-based treatment of insomnia, parasomnias and circadian rhythm disorders. *Journal of Psychopharmacology, 24*(11), 1577–1601.

Iodinated Contrast Media, Risk for Adverse Reaction to

American College of Radiology. (2008). *Manual on contrast media* (version 6). Reston, VA: Author.

Bellin, M., Jakobsen, J., Tomassin, I., Thomsen, H., & Morcos, S. (2002). Contrast medium extravasation injury: Guidelines for prevention and management. *European Radiology, 12*(11), 2807–2812.

Bettmann, M. (2004). Frequently asked questions: Iodinated contrast agents. *Radiographics, 24*(Special Issue), S3–S10.

Briguori, C., Quintavalle, C., De Micco, F., & Condorelli, G. (2011). Nephrotoxicity of contrast media and protective effects of acetylcysteine. *Archives of Toxicology, 85*(3), 165–173.

Brockow, K., Christiansen, C., Kanny, G., Clément, O., Barbaud, A., Bircher, A., et al. ENDA EAACI Interest Group on Drug Hypersensitivity. (2005). Management of hypersensitivity reactions to iodinated contrast media. *Allergy, 60*(2), 150–158.

Bueschen, A., & Lockhart, M. (2011). Evolution of urological imaging. *International Journal of Urology, 18*(2), 102–112.

Costa, N. (2004). Understanding contrast media. *Journal of Infusion Nursing, 27*(5), 302–312.

European Society of Urogenital Radiology. (2007). *ESUR guidelines on contrast media* (version 6). Heidelberg: Springer-Verlag.

Goksel, O., Aydin, O., Atasoy, C., Akyar, S., Demirel, Y., Misirligil, Z., et al. (2011). Hypersensitivity reactions to contrast media: Prevalence, risk factors and the role of skin tests in diagnosis—a cross-sectional survey. *International Archives of Allergy and Immunology, 155*(3), 297–305.

Juchem, B., & Dall'Agnol, C. (2007). Immediate adverse reactions to intravenous iodinated contrast media in computed tomography. *Revista Latino-Americana de Enfermagem, 15*(1), 78–83.

Namasivayam, S., Kaira, M., Torres, W., & Small, W. (2006). Adverse reactions to intravenous iodinated contrast media: A primer for radiologists. *Emergency Radiology, 12*(5), 210–215.

Reddan, D. (2007). Patients at high risk of adverse events from intravenous contrast media after computed tomography examination. *European Journal of Radiology, 62*(1), 26–32.

Riedl, M., & Casillas, A. (2003). Adverse drug reactions: Types and treatment options. *American Family Physician, 68*(9), 1781–1790.

Schild, H., Kuhl, C., Hübner-Steiner, U., Böhm, I., & Speck, U. (2006). Adverse events after unenhanced and monomeric and dimeric contrast-enhanced CT: A prospective randomized controlled trial. *Radiology, 240*(1), 56–64.

Segal, A., & Bush, W. (2011). Avoidable errors in dealing with anaphylactoid reactions to iodinated contrast media. *Investigative Radiology, 46*(3), 147–151.

Siddiqi, N. (2008). Contrast medium reactions, recognition and treatment. *Emedicine*. Retrieved January 12, 2012, from http://emedicine.medscape.com/article/422855-overview

Singh, J., & Daftary, A. (2008). Iodinated contrast media and their adverse reactions. *Journal of Nuclear Medicine Technology, 36*(2), 69–74.

Stacul, F. (2007). Managing the risk associated with use of contrast media for computed tomography. *European Journal of Radiology, 62*(1), 33–37.

Thomsen, H., & Morcos, S. (2004). Management of acute adverse reactions to contrast media. *European Radiology, 14*(3), 476–481.

Webb, J., Stacul, F., Thompssen, H., & Morcos, S. D. (2003). Late adverse reactions to intravascular iodinated contrast media. *European Radiology, 13*(1), 181–184.

Jaundice, Neonatal

American Academy of Pediatrics. (2004). Management of hyperbilirubinemia in the newborn infant 35 or more weeks of gestation. *Pediatrics, 114*(1), 297–316.

Beachy, J. (2007). Investigating jaundice in the newborn. *Neonatal Network, 26*(5), 327–333.

Bhutani, V., Johnson, L., Schwoebel, A., & Gennaro, S. (2006). A systems approach for neonatal hyperbilirubinemia in term and near-term newborns. *Journal of Obstetric, Gynecologic and Neonatal Nursing, 35*(5), 444–455.

Boyd, S. (2004). Treatment of physiological neonatal jaundice. *Nursing Times, 100*(13), 40–43.

Brethauer, M., & Carey, L. (2010). Maternal experience with neonatal jaundice. *MCN. The American Journal of Maternal/Child Nursing, 35*(1), 8–14.

Canadian Paediatric Society Position Statement. (2007). Guidelines for detection, management and prevention of hyperbilirubinemia in term and late preterm newborn infants (35 or more weeks' gestation). *Paediatric and Child Health, 12*(Suppl. B), 1B–12B.

Chen, J., Sadakata, M., Ishida, M., Sekizuka, N., & Sayama, M. (2011). Baby massage ameliorates neonatal jaundice in full-term newborn infants. *Tohoku Journal of Experimental Medicine, 223*(2), 97–102.

Cohen, S. (2006). Jaundice in the full-term newborn. *Pediatric Nursing, 32*(3), 202–207.

Deshpande, P. (2008). *Breast milk jaundice*. Retrieved January 13, 2012, from http://emedicine.medscape.com/article/973629-overview

Donneborg, M., Knudsen, K., & Ebbesen, F. (2010). Effect of infants' position on serum bilirubin level during conventional phototherapy. *Acta Paediatrica, 99*(8), 1131–1134.

Hansen, T. (2007). *Neonatal jaundice*. Retrieved January 13, 2012, from http://emedicine.medscape.com/article/974786-overview

Hillman, N. (2007). Hyperbilirubinemia in the late preterm infant. *Newborn and Infant Nursing Reviews, 7*(2), 91–94.

Lease, M., & Whalen, B. (2010). Assessing jaundice in infants of 35-week gestation and greater. *Current Opinion in Pediatrics, 22*(3), 352–365.

Porter, M., & Dennis, B. (2003). Hyperbilirubinemia in the term newborn. *American Family Physician, 65*, 599–606, 613–615.

Saluia, S., Aqarwal, A., Kler, N., & Amin, S. (2010). Auditory neuropathy spectrum disorder in later preterm and term infants with severe jaundice. *International Journal of Pediatric Otorhinolaryngology, 74*(11), 1292–1297.

Walsh, S., & Murphy, J. (2010). Neonatal jaundice—are we over-treating? *Irish Medical Journal, 103*(1), 28–29.

Jaundice: Neonatal, Risk for

American Academy of Pediatrics. (2004). Management of hyperbilirubinemia in the newborn infant 35 or more weeks of gestation. *Pediatrics, 114*(1), 297–316.

Beachy, J. (2007). Investigating jaundice in the newborn. *Neonatal Network, 26*(5), 327–333.

Bhutani, V., Johnson, L., Schwoebel, A., & Gennaro, S. (2006). A systems approach for neonatal hyperbilirubinemia in term and near-term newborns. *Journal of Obstetric, Gynecologic and Neonatal Nursing, 35*(5), 444–455.

Boyd, S. (2004). Treatment of physiological neonatal jaundice. *Nursing Times, 100*(13), 40–43.

Brethauer, M., & Carey, L. (2010). Maternal experience with neonatal jaundice. *MCN: The American Journal of Maternal/Child Nursing, 35*(1), 8–14.

Canadian Paediatric Society Position Statement. (2007). Guidelines for detection, management and prevention of hyperbilirubinemia in term and late preterm newborn infants (35 or more weeks' gestation). *Paediatric and Child Health, 12*(Suppl. B), 1B–12B.

Chen, J., Sadakata, M., Ishida, M., Sekizuka, N., & Sayama, M. (2011). Baby massage ameliorates neonatal jaundice in full-term newborn infants. *Tohoku Journal of Experimental Medicine, 223*(2), 97–102.

Cohen, S. (2006). Jaundice in the full-term newborn. *Pediatric Nursing, 32*(3), 202–207.

Deshpande, P. (2008). *Breast milk jaundice*. Retrieved January 13, 2012, from http://emedicine.medscape.com/article/973629-overview

Donneborg, M., Knudsen, K., & Ebbesen, F. (2010). Effect of infants' position on serum bilirubin level during conventional phototherapy. *Acta Paediatrica, 99*(8), 1131–1134.

Hansen, T. (2007). *Neonatal jaundice.* Retrieved January 13, 2012, from http://emedicine.medscape.com/article/974786-overview

Hillman, N. (2007). Hyperbilirubinemia in the late preterm infant. *Newborn and Infant Nursing Reviews, 7*(2), 91–94.

Lease, M., & Whalen, B. (2010). Assessing jaundice in infants of 35-week gestation and greater. *Current Opinion in Pediatrics, 22*(3), 352–365.

Porter, M., & Dennis, B. (2003). Hyperbilirubinemia in the term newborn. *American Family Physician, 65,* 599–606, 613–615.

Saluia, S., Aqarwal, A., Kler, N., & Amin, S. (2010). Auditory neuropathy spectrum disorder in later preterm and term infants with severe jaundice. *International Journal of Pediatric Otorhinolaryngology, 74*(11), 1292–1297.

Walsh, S., & Murphy, J. (2010). Neonatal jaundice—are we over-treating? *Irish Medical Journal, 103*(1), 28–29.

Knowledge, Deficient (Specify)

Bowman, K. G. (2005). Postpartum learning needs. *JOGNN: Journal of Obstetric, Gynecologic, & Neonatal Nursing, 34*(4), 438–443.

Conley, V. (1998). Beyond *Knowledge Deficit* to a proposal for *Information-Seeking Behaviors. Nursing Diagnosis, 9*(4), 129–135.

Dorresteijn, J., Kriegsman, D., Assendelft, W., & Valik, D. (2010). Patient education for preventing diabetic foot ulceration. *Cochrane Database of Systematic Reviews, 5,* Art No: CD001488. DOI: 10.1002/14661858.CD001488.pub3.

Gordon, M. (1985). Practice based data set for a nursing information system. *Journal of Medical Systems, 9,* 43–55.

Gruman, J., Rovner, M., French, M., Jeffress, D., Sofaer, S., Shaller, D., et al. (2010). From patient education to patient engagement: Implications for the field of patient education. *Patient Education and Counseling, 78*(3), 350–356.

Howarth, M., Holland, K., & Grant, M. J. (2006). Education needs for integrated care: A literature review. *Journal of Advanced Nursing, 56*(2), 144–156.

Jenny, J. (1987). Knowledge deficit: Not a nursing diagnosis. *Image, 19*(4), 184–185.

Johansson, K., Salanterä, S., Heikkinen, K., Kuusisto, A., Virtanen, H., & Leino-Kilpi, H. (2004). Surgical patient education: Assessing the interventions and exploring the outcomes from experimental and quasiexperimental studies from 1990 to 2003. *Clinical Effectiveness in Nursing, 8*(2), 81–92.

Krau, S. (2011). Creating educational objectives for patient education using the New Bloom's Taxonomy. *Nursing Clinics of North America, 46*(3), 299–312.

Lagger, G., Pataky, Z., & Golay, A. (2010). Efficacy of therapeutic patient education in chronic diseases and obesity. *Patient Education and Counseling, 79*(3), 283–286.

Lambert, M. A., & Jones, P. E. (1989). Nursing diagnoses recorded in nursing situations encountered in a department of public health. In R. M. Carroll-Johnson (Ed.), *Classification of nursing diagnoses: Proceedings of the eighth conference.* Philadelphia: Lippincott Williams & Wilkins.

Mason, T. M. (2005). Information needs of wives of men following prostatectomy. *Oncology Nursing Forum, 32*(3), 557–563.

Nettles, A. T. (2005). Patient education in the hospital. *Diabetes Spectrum, 18*(1), 44–48.

Newall, F., Monagle, P., & Johnston, L. (2005). Patient understanding of warfarin therapy: A review of education strategies. *Hematology, 10*(6), 437–442.

Patterson, P., Whittington, R., & Bogg, J. (2007). Testing the effectiveness of an educational intervention aimed at changing attitudes to self-harm. *Journal of Psychiatric & Mental Health Nursing, 14*(1), 100–105.

Rakel, B. A., & Bulechek, G. M. (1990). Development of alterations in learning: Situational learning disabilities. *Nursing Diagnosis, 1*(4), 134–136.

Ringström, G., Störsrud, S., Posserud, I., Lundqvist, S., Westman, B., & Simrén, M. (2010). Structured patient education is superior to written information in the management of patients with irritable bowel syndrome: A randomized controlled study. *European Journal of Gastroenterology & Hepatology, 22*(4), 420–428.

Ryhänen, A., Siekkinen, M., Rankinen, S., Korvenranta, H., & Leino-Kilpi, H. (2010). The effects of Internet or interactive computer-based patient education in the field of breast cancer: A systematic literature review. *Patient Education and Counseling, 79*(1), 5–13.

Knowledge (Specify), Readiness for Enhanced

Albrecht, S. A., Maloni, J. A., Thomas, K. K., Jones, R., Halleran, J., & Osborne, J. (2004). Smoking cessation counseling for pregnant women who smoke: Scientific basis for practice for AWHONN's SUCCESS project. *JOGNN: Journal of Obstetric, Gynecologic, & Neonatal Nursing, 33*(3), 298–305.

Bowman, K. G. (2005). Postpartum learning needs. *JOGNN: Journal of Obstetric, Gynecologic, & Neonatal Nursing, 34*(4), 438–443.

Conley, V. (1998). Beyond *Knowledge Deficit* to a proposal for *Information-Seeking Behaviors. Nursing Diagnosis, 9*(4), 129–135.

Gibson, T. (2007). Training opportunities in mental health and learning disabilities. *Learning Disability Practice, 10*(1), 34–38.

Gruman, J., Rovner, M., French, M., Jeffress, D., Sofaer, S., Shaller, D., et al. (2010). From patient education to patient engagement: Implications for the field of patient education. *Patient Education and Counseling, 78*(3), 350–356.

Howarth, M., Holland, K., & Grant, M. J. (2006). Education needs for integrated care: A literature review. *Journal of Advanced Nursing, 56*(2), 144–156.

Krau, S. (2011). Creating educational objectives for patient education using the New Bloom's Taxonomy. *Nursing Clinics of North America, 46*(3), 299–312.

May, L., Day, R., & Warren, S. (2006). Perceptions of patient education in spinal cord injury rehabilitation. *Disability & Rehabilitation, 28*(17), 1041–1049.

Nettles, A. T. (2005). Patient education in the hospital. *Diabetes Spectrum, 18*(1), 44–48.

Olinzock, B. J. (2004). A model for assessing learning readiness for self-direction of care in individuals with spinal cord injuries: A qualitative study. *SCI Nursing, 21*(2), 69–74.

Patterson, P., Whittington, R., & Bogg, J. (2007). Testing the effectiveness of an educational intervention aimed at changing attitudes to self-harm. *Journal of Psychiatric & Mental Health Nursing, 14*(1), 100–105.

Ryhänen, A., Siekkinen, M., Rankinen, S., Korvenranta, H., & Leino-Kilpi, H. (2010). The effects of Internet or interactive computer-based patient education in the field of breast cancer: A systematic literature review. *Patient Education and Counseling, 79*(1), 5–13.

Shaw, E., Levitt, C., Wong, S., & Kaczorowski, J. (2006). Systematic review of the literature on postpartum care: Effectiveness of postpartum support to improve maternal parenting, mental health, quality of life, and physical health. *Birth: Issues in Perinatal Care, 33*(3), 210–220.

Templeton, H., & Coates, V. (2004). Evaluation of an evidence-based education package for men with prostate cancer on hormonal manipulation therapy. *Patient Education & Counseling, 55*(1), 55–61.

Whitehead, D., Keast, J., Montgomery, V., & Hayman, S. (2004). A preventative health education programme for osteoporosis. *Journal of Advanced Nursing, 47*(1), 15–24.

Latex Allergy Response

American Society of Anesthesiologists. (2005). *Natural rubber latex allergy: Considerations for anesthesiologists (a practice guideline)*. Park Ridge, IL: Author.

AORN. (2004). AORN latex guideline. In *AORN standards, recommended practices and guidelines* (pp. 103–118). Denver, CO: Author.

Draisci, G., Zanfini, B., Nucera, E., Catarci, S., Sangregorio, R., Schiavino, D., et al. (2011). Latex sensitization: A special risk for the obstetric population? *Anesthesiology, 114*(3), 565–569.

Gawchik, S. (2011). Latex allergy. *Mount Sinai Journal of Medicine, 78*(5), 759–772.

Heitz, J., & Bader, S. (2010). An evidence-based approach to medication preparation for the surgical patient at risk for latex allergy: Is it time to stop being stopper poppers? *Journal of Clinical Anesthesia, 22*(6), 477–483.

Lucas, J., du Toit, G., Lloyd, K., Sinnott, L., Forster, D., Austin, M., et al. (2011). The RCPCH care pathway for children with latex allergies: An evidence- and consensus-based national approach. *Archives of Disease in Childhood, 96*(Suppl. 2), i30–i33.

Sampathi, V., & Lerman, J. (2011). Case scenario: Perioperative latex allergy in children. *Anesthesiology, 114*(3), 673–680.

Sussman, G. L. (2000). Latex allergy: An overview. *Canadian Journal of Allergy and Clinical Immunology, 5,* 317–321.

Tarlo, S. (1998). Latex allergy: A problem for both health care professionals and patients. *Ostomy/Wound Management, 14*(8), 80–88.

Latex Allergy Response, Risk for

Altman, G. B., & Keller, K. M. (2003). Practice powder-free and latex safe. *Nurse Practitioner, 28*(8), 55.

American Society of Anesthesiologists. (2005). *Natural rubber latex allergy: Considerations for anesthesiologists (a practice guideline)*. Park Ridge, IL: Author.

AORN. (2004). Latex guideline. In *AORN standards, recommended practices and guidelines* (pp. 103–118). Denver, CO: Author.

Boyd, S. (2005). Latex sensitivity—avoiding allergic reactions in clinical settings. *Infant, 1*(2), 63–65.

Dehlink, E., Prandstetter, C., Eiwegger, T., Putschögl, B., Urbanek, R., & Szépfalusi, Z. (2004). Increased prevalence of latex-sensitization among children with chronic renal failure. *Allergy, 59*(7), 734–738.

Dore Geraghty, C., & Keoghan, M. T. (2007). Exposure to latex in schools. *Archives of Disease in Childhood, 92*(1), 89–90.

Draisci, G., Zanfini, B., Nucera, E., Catarci, S., Sangregorio, R., Schiavino, D., et al. (2011). Latex sensitization: A special risk for the obstetric population? *Anesthesiology, 114*(3), 565–569.

Gawchik, S. (2011). Latex allergy. *Mount Sinai Journal of Medicine, 78*(5), 759–772.

Hampton, S. (2003). Nurses' inappropriate use of gloves in caring for patients. *British Journal of Nursing (BJN), 12*(17), 1024.

Heitz, J., & Bader, S. (2010). An evidence-based approach to medication preparation for the surgical patient at risk for latex allergy: Is it time to stop being stopper poppers? *Journal of Clinical Anesthesia, 22*(6), 477–483.

Kimata, H. (2004). Latex allergy in infants younger than 1 year. *Clinical & Experimental Allergy, 34*(12), 1910–1915.

Lewis, V. J., Chowdhury, M. M. U., & Statham, B. N. (2004). Natural rubber latex allergy: The impact on lifestyle and quality of life. *Contact Dermatitis, 51*(5), 317–318.

Lucas, J., du Toit, G., Lloyd, K., Sinnott, L., Forster, D., Austin, M., et al. (2011). The RCPCH care pathway for children with latex allergies: An evidence- and consensus-based national approach. *Archives of Disease in Childhood, 96*(Suppl. 2), i30–i33.

Martin, J. A., Hughes, T. M., & Stone, N. M. (2005). 'Black henna' tattoos: An occult source of natural rubber latex allergy? *Contact Dermatitis, 52*(3), 145–146.

Pamies, R., Oliver, F., Raulf-Heimsoth, M., Rihs, H., Barber, D., Boquete, M., et al. (2006). Patterns of latex allergen recognition in children sensitized to natural rubber latex. *Pediatric Allergy & Immunology, 17*(1), 55–59.

Pereira, C., Tavares, B., Loureiro, G., Lundberg, M., & Chieira, C. (2007). Turnip and zucchini: New foods in the latex-fruit syndrome. *Allergy, 62*(4), 452–453.

Sampathi, V., & Lerman, J. (2011). Case scenario: Perioperative latex allergy in children. *Anesthesiology, 114*(3), 673–680.

Sussman, G. L. (2000). Latex allergy: An overview. *Canadian Journal of Allergy and Clinical Immunology, 5,* 317–321.

Tarlo, S. (1998). Latex allergy: A problem for both health care professionals and patients. *Ostomy/Wound Management, 14*(8), 80–88.

Waseem, M., Ganti, S., & Hipp, A. (2006). Latex-induced anaphylactic reaction in a child with spina bifida. *Pediatric Emergency Care, 22*(6), 441–442.

Liver Function, Risk for Impaired

AASLD Practice Guideline. (2004). *Diagnosis, management, and treatment of hepatitis C.* Alexandria, VA: American Association for the Study of Liver Diseases.

Christensen, T. (2004). The treatment of esophageal varices using a Sengstaken-Blakemore tube: Considerations for nursing practice. *Nursing in Critical Care, 9*(2), 58–63.

Drent, G., Haagsma, E. B., Geest, S. D., van den Berg, A., P., Ten Vergert, E. M., et al. (2005). Prevalence of prednisolone (non)compliance in adult liver transplant recipients. *Transplant International, 18*(8), 960–966.

El-Sayed, M. S., Ali, N., & Ali, Z. E. (2005). Interaction between alcohol and exercise: Physiological and haematological implications. *Sports Medicine, 35*(3), 257–269.

Faint, V. (2006). The pathophysiology of hepatic encephalopathy. *Nursing in Critical Care, 11*(2), 69–74.

Fierz, K., Steiger, J. U., Denhaerynck, K., Dobbels, F., Bock, A., & De Geest, S. (2006). Prevalence, degree and correlates of alcohol use in adult renal transplant recipients. Clinical Transplantation, 20(2), 171–178.

Fontana, R., & Lok, S. (2002). Noninvasive monitoring of patients with chronic hepatitis C. *Hepatology, 36* (Suppl. 5), S57–S64.

Gabe, S., & Culkin, A. (2010). Abnormal liver function tests in the parenteral nutrition fed patient. *Frontline Gastroenterology, 1,* 98–104.

Hunfeld, N., ten Berge, R., LeBrun, P., Smith, S., & Melief, P. (2010). Hepatotoxicity related to citalopram intake: A case report. *Risk & Safety in Medicine, 22*(1): 1–5.

National lipid association releases a special report on statin safety. (2006). *Journal of Cardiovascular Nursing, 21*(5), 336.

Nichols, A. A. (2005). Cholestasis of pregnancy. *Journal of Perinatal & Neonatal Nursing, 19*(3), 217–225.

O'Neal, H., Olds, J., & Webster, N. (2006). Managing patients with acute liver failure: Developing a tool for practitioners. *Nursing in Critical Care, 11*(2), 63–68.

Seccull, A., Richmond, J., Thomas, B., & Herrman, H. (2006). Hepatitis C in people with mental illness: How big is the problem and how do we respond? *Australasian Psychiatry, 14*(4), 374–378.

Loneliness, Risk for

Beebe, L. H. (2007). Beyond the prescription pad: Psychosocial treatments for individuals with schizophrenia. *Journal of Psychosocial Nursing & Mental Health Services, 45*(3), 35.

Bergman-Evans, B. (2004). Beyond the basics: Effects of the Eden Alternative model on quality of life issues. *Journal of Gerontological Nursing, 30*(6), 27–34.

Blomqvist, L., Pitkälä, K., & Routasalo, P. (2007). Images of loneliness: Using art as an educational method in professional training. *Journal of Continuing Education in Nursing, 38*(2), 89–93.

Brume, K. (2011). Culture change in long term care services: Eden-Greenhouse-Aging in the community. *Educational Gerontology, 37*(6), 506–525.

George, D. (2011). Intergenerational volunteering and quality of life: Mixed methods evaluation of a randomized control trial involving persons with mild to moderate dementia. *Quality of Life Research, 20*(7), 987–995.

Hawkley, L., & Cacioppo, J. (2010). Loneliness matters: A theoretical and empirical review of consequences and mechanisms. *Annals of Behavioral Medicine, 40*(2), 218–227.

Lasgaard, M., Nielsen, A., Eriksen, M., & Goossens, L. (2010). Loneliness and social support in adolescent boys with autism spectrum disorders. *Journal of Autism and Developmental Disorders, 40*(2), 218–226.

Leiderman, P. H. (1969). Loneliness: A psychodynamic interpretation. In E. S. Scheidman & M. J. Ortega (Eds.), *Aspects of depression: International psychiatric clinics*. Boston, MA: Little, Brown.

Lien-Gieschen, T. (1993). Validation of social isolation related to maturational age: Elderly. *Nursing Diagnosis, 4*(1), 37–44.

Mallinson, R. K. (1999). The lived experience of AIDS-related multiple losses by HIV-negative gay men. *Journal of Association of Nurses in AIDS Care, 10*(5), 22–31.

Maslow, A. H. (1968). *Towards a psychology of being* (2nd ed.). New York: Van Nostrand.

Ryan, M. C., & Patterson, J. (1987). Loneliness in the elderly. *Journal of Gerontological Nursing, 13*(5), 6–12.

Stange, M., Tutarel, O., Pischke, S., Schneider, A., Strassburg, C., Becker, T., et al. (2010). Fulminant hepatic failure due to chemotherapy-induced hepatitis B reactivation: Role of rituximab. *Zeitschrift Für Gastroenterology, 48*(2), 258–263.

Stepanikova, I., Nie, N., & He, X. (2010). Time on the Internet at home, loneliness, and life satisfaction: Evidence from panel time-diary data. *Computers in Human Behavior, 26*(3), 329–338.

Warren, B. J. (1993). Explaining social isolation through concept analysis. *Archives of Psychiatric Nursing, 7*, 270–276.

Weiss, R. S. (1973). *Loneliness: The experience of emotional and social isolation*. Cambridge, MA: MIT Press.

Wu, F., Ukomadu, C., Odze, R., Valente, A., Mayer, J., & Earing, M. (2011). Liver disease in the patient with Fontan circulation. *Congenital Heart Disease, 6*(3), 190–201.

Maternal-Fetal Dyad, Risk for Disturbed

Barclay, L., & Vega, C. (2009). *Severe adverse effects of smoking may be reversible if mothers quit early in pregnancy*. Retrieved January 21, 2012, from http://cme.medscape.com/viewarticle/590543?src=cmemp

Berg, M. (2005). Pregnancy and diabetes: How women handle the challenges. *Journal of Perinatal Education, 14*(3), 23–32.

Centers for Disease Control and Prevention. (2008). *STDs and pregnancy. CDC fact sheet*. Retrieved January 21, 2012, from http://www.cdc.gov/std/pregnancy/STDFact-Pregnancy.htm

Centers for Disease Control and Prevention. (2009). *Violence and reproductive health*. Retrieved January 21, 2012, from www.cdc.gov/reproductivehealth/violence/index.htm

Complications and high-risk conditions of the prenatal period. (2008). *Straight A's in maternal-neonatal nursing* (2nd ed.). Philadelphia: Lippincott Williams & Wilkins.

Curran, C. (2003). Intrapartum emergencies. *Journal of Obstetric, Gynecologic, and Neonatal Nursing, 32*(6), 802–813.

Ehrenberg, H., et al. (2009). Maternal obesity, uterine activity, and the risk of spontaneous preterm birth. *Obstetrics and Gynecology, 113*(1), 48–52.

Gibson, P., & Carson, M. (2011). *Hypertension and pregnancy*. Retrieved January 21, 2012, from http://emedicine.medscape.com/article/261435-overview

Higgins, L., & Hawkins, J. (2005). Screening for abuse during pregnancy: Implementing a multisite program. *American Journal of Maternal/Child Nursing, 30*(2), 109–114.

Holloway, B., Moredich, C., & Aduddell, K. (2006). *OB peds women's health notes: Nurse's clinical pocket guide*. Philadelphia: F. A. Davis.

Lange, S., & Jenner, M. (2004). Myocardial infarction in the obstetric patient. *Critical Care Nursing Clinics of North America: Obstetric and Neonatal Intensive Care, 16*(2), 211–219.

McCarter-Spaulding, D. (2005). Medications in pregnancy and lactation. *American Journal of Maternal/Child Nursing, 30*(1), 10–17.

Miller, D. (2005). Is advanced maternal age an independent risk factor for uteroplacental insufficiency? *American Journal of Obstetrics and Gynecology, 195*(6), 1974–1982.

National Heart, Lung, and Blood Institute. (2008). *Rh incompatibility*. Retrieved January 21, 2012, from www.nhlbi.nih.gov/health/dci/Diseases/rh/rh_what.html

National Institute of Child Health and Human Development. (2006). *High-risk pregnancy*. Retrieved January 21, 2012, from www.nichd.nih.gov/health/topics/high_risk_pregnancy.cfm

National Institute of Child Health and Human Development. (2009). *Care before and during pregnancy—Prenatal care*. Retrieved January 21, 2012, from www.nichd.nih.gov/womenshealth/research/pregbirth/prenatal_care.cfm

Poole, J. (2004). Multiorgan dysfunction in the perinatal patient. *Critical Care Nursing Clinics of North America: Obstetric and Neonatal Intensive Care, 16*(2), 193–204.

Ross, M., & Eden, R. (2009). *Preterm labor*. Retrieved January 21, 2012, from http://emedicine.medscape.com/article/260998-overview

Rudisill, P. (2004). Amniotic fluid embolism. *Critical Care Nursing Clinics of North America: Obstetric and Neonatal Intensive Care, 36*(2), 221–225.

Shannon, M., King, T., & Kennedy, H. (2007). Allostasis: A theoretical framework for understanding and evaluating perinatal health outcomes. *Critical Care Nursing Clinics of North America: Obstetric and Neonatal Intensive Care, 36*(2), 125–134.

Simpson, K. (2004). Monitoring the preterm fetus during labor. *American Journal of Maternal/Child Nursing, 29*(6), 380–388.

Stark, C., & Stepans, M. (2004). A comparison of blood pressure in term, low birth weight infants of smoking and nonsmoking mothers. *Journal of Perinatal Education, 13*(4), 17–26.

Stringer, M., Miesnik, S., Brown, L., Martz, A., & Macones, G. (2004). Nursing care of the patient with premature rupture of membranes. *American Journal of Maternal/Child Nursing, 29*(3), 144–150.

Torgerson, K., & Curran, C. (2006). A systematic approach to the physiologic adaptations of pregnancy. *Critical Care Nursing Quarterly, 29*(1), 2–19.

U.S. Department of Health and Human Services. (2010). *HIV and pregnancy*. Retrieved January 21, 2012, from http://aidsinfo.nih.gov/ContentFiles/Perinatal_FS_en.pdf

Wolfe, B. (2005). Reproductive health in women with eating disorders. *Journal of Obstetric, Gynecologic, and Neonatal Nursing, 34*(2), 255–263.

Yale Medical Group. (2012a). *High-risk pregnancy: Hyperemesis gravidarum*. Retrieved January 21, 2012, from http://ymghealthinfo.org/content.asp?pageid=P02457

Yale Medical Group. (2012b). *High-risk pregnancy: Maternal and fetal testing*. Retrieved January 21, 2012, from http://ymghealthinfo.org/content.asp?pageid=P02483

Yale Medical Group. (2012c). *High-risk pregnancy: Prenatal counseling*. Retrieved January 21, 2012, from http://ymghealthinfo.org/content.asp?pageid=P02493

Memory, Impaired

Bates, J., Boote, J., & Beverley, C. (2004). Psychosocial interventions for people with a milder dementing illness: A systematic review. *Journal of Advanced Nursing, 45*(6), 644–658.

Bauer, L., & Pozehl, B. (2011). Measurement of cognitive function in chronic heart failure: A feasibility study. *Applied Nursing Research, 24*(4), 223–228.

Feinstein, J., Duff, M., & Tranel. (2010). Sustained experience of emotion after loss of memory in patients with amnesia. *PNAS, 107*(17), 7674–7679. Retrieved February 5, 2012, from http://www.pnas.org/content/107/17/7674.full

Franks, V. (2004). Evidence-based uncertainty in mental health nursing. *Journal of Psychiatric & Mental Health Nursing, 11*(1), 99–105.

Harrison, B., Son, G.-R., Kin, J., & Whall, A. (2007). Preserved implicit memory in dementia: A potential model for care. *American Journal of Alzheimer's Disease & Other Dementias, 22*(4), w86–w293.

Herrmann, N. (2005). Some psychosocial therapies may reduce depression, aggression, or apathy in people with dementia. *Evidence-Based Mental Health, 8*(4), 104.

McDougall, G., Becker, H., Pituch, K., Acee, T., Vaughan, P., & Delville, C. (2010). Differential benefits of memory training for minority older adults in the SeniorWISE study. *The Gerontologist, 50*(5), 632–645.

Oulette, R., & Ouellette, S. (2010). Understanding postoperative cognitive dysfunction and delirium. *OR Nurse, 4*(4), 40–46.

Simmons, N., Budson, A., & Ally, G. (2010). Music as a memory enhancer in patients with Alzheimer's disease. *Neuropsychologia, 48*(10), 3164–3167.

Son, G., Therrien, B., & Whall, A. (2002). Implicit memory and familiarity among elders with dementia. *Journal of Nursing Scholarship, 34*(3), 263–267.

Mobility: Bed, Impaired

Brouwer, K., Nysseknabm, J., & Culham, E. (2004). Physical function and health status among seniors with and without fear of falling. *Gerontology, 50,* 15–141.

Davis, D., Rockwood, M., Mitnitski, A., & Rockwood, M. (2011). Impairments in mobility and balance in relation to frailty. *Archives of Gerontology and Geriatrics, 53*(1), 79–83.

Lepistö, M., Eriksson, E., Hietanen, H., Lepistö, J., & Lauri, S. (2006). Developing a pressure ulcer risk assessment scale for patients in long-term care. *Ostomy Wound Management, 52*(2), 34.

Lewis, C. L., Moutoux, M., Slaughter, M., & Bailey, S. P. (2004). Characteristics of individuals who fell while receiving home health services. *Physical Therapy, 84*(1), 23–32.

Liu, C., & Fielding, R. (2011). Exercise as an intervention for frailty. *Clinics in Geriatric Medicine, 27*(1), 101–110.

Tinetti, M. E., & Ginter, S. F. (1988). Identifying mobility dysfunction in elderly persons. *Journal of the American Medical Association, 259,* 1190–1193.

Wert, D., D., Brach, J., Perera, S., & VanSwearingen, J. (2010). Gait biomechanics, spatial and temporal characteristics, and the energy cost of walking in older adults with impaired mobility. *Physical Therapy, 90*(7), 977–985.

Wilkinson, J., & Treas, L. (2011). Chapter 31. In *Fundamentals of nursing* (2nd ed.). Philadelphia: F. A. Davis.

Mobility: Physical, Impaired

Ainsworth, R., & Lewis, J. S. (2007). Exercise therapy for the conservative management of full thickness tears of the rotator cuff: A systematic review. *British Journal of Sports Medicine, 41*(4), 200–210.

Appleton, B. (2004). The role of exercise training in patients with chronic heart failure. *British Journal of Nursing (BJN), 13*(8), 452–456.

Arias, M., & Smith, L. N. (2007). Early mobilization of acute stroke patients. *Journal of Clinical Nursing, 16*(2), 282–288.

Benton, M. J., & White, A. (2006). Osteoporosis: Recommendations for resistance exercise and supplementation with calcium and vitamin D to promote bone health. *Journal of Community Health Nursing, 23*(4), 201–211.

Bo, M., Fontana, M., Mantelli, M., & Molaschi, M. (2006). Positive effects of aerobic physical activity in institutionalized older subjects complaining of dyspnea. *Archives of Gerontology & Geriatrics, 43*(1), 139–145.

Brown, T. R., & Kraft, G. H. (2005). Exercise and rehabilitation for individuals with multiple sclerosis. *Physical Medicine & Rehabilitation Clinics of North America, 16*(2), 513–555.

Capezuti, E. (2004). Minimizing the use of restrictive devices in dementia patients at risk for falling. *Nursing Clinics of North America, 39*(3), 625–647.

Conn, V. S., Isaramalai, S., Banks-Wallace, J., Ulbrich, S., & Cochran, J. (2002). Evidence-based interventions to increase physical activity among older adults. *Activities, Adaptation & Aging, 27*(2), 39–52.

Davis, D., Rockwood, M., Mitnitski, A., & Rockwood, M. (2011). Impairments in mobility and balance in relation to frailty. *Archives of Gerontology and Geriatrics, 53*(1), 79–83.

Dugdill, L., Graham, R. C., & Mcnair, F. (2005). Exercise referral: The public health panacea for physical activity promotion? A critical perspective of exercise referral schemes; their development and evaluation. *Ergonomics, 48*(11), 1390–1410.

Edwards, N., Danseco, E., Heslin, K., Ploeg, J., Santos, J., Stansfield, M., et al. (2006). Development and testing of tools to assess physical restraint use. *Worldviews on Evidence-Based Nursing, 3*(2), 73–85.

Evangelista, L. S., Doering, L. V., Lennie, T., Moser, D. K., Hamilton, M. A., Fonarow, G. C., et al. (2006). Usefulness of a home-based exercise program for overweight and obese patients with advanced heart failure. *American Journal of Cardiology, 97*(6), 886–890.

Faulkner, G., & Biddle, S. (2002). Mental health nursing and the promotion of physical activity. *Journal of Psychiatric & Mental Health Nursing, 9*(6), 659–665.

Feskanich, D., Willett, W., & Colditz, G. (2002). Walking and leisure-time activity and risk of hip fracture in postmenopausal women. *JAMA: Journal of the American Medical Association, 288*(18), 2300.

Fries, J. M. (2005). Critical rehabilitation of the patient with spinal cord injury. *Critical Care Nursing Quarterly, 28*(2), 179–187.

Gallinagh, R., Nevin, R., Mc Ilroy, D., Mitchell, F., Campbell, L., Ludwick, R., et al. (2002). The use of physical restraints as a safety measure in the care of older people in four rehabilitation wards: Findings from an exploratory study. *International Journal of Nursing Studies, 39*(2), 147–156.

Gilbey, H. J., Ackland, T. R., Tapper, J., & Wang, A. W. (2003). Perioperative exercise improves function following total hip arthroplasty: A randomized controlled trial. *Journal of Musculoskeletal Research, 7*(2), 111–123.

Hayes, N. (2004). Prevention of falls among older patients in the hospital environment. *British Journal of Nursing (BJN), 13*(15), 896–901.

Heinen, M. M., van Achterberg, T., Reimer, W. S., van den Kerkhof, Peter, C. M., & de Laat, E. (2004). Venous leg ulcer patients: A review of the literature on lifestyle and pain-related interventions. *Journal of Clinical Nursing, 13*(3), 355–366.

Jette, D. U., Warren, R. L., & Wirtalla, C. (2005). Functional independence domains in patients receiving rehabilitation in skilled nursing facilities: Evaluation of psychometric properties. *Archives of Physical Medicine & Rehabilitation, 86*(6), 1089.

Kehl-Pruett, W. (2006). Deep vein thrombosis in hospitalized patients: A review of evidence-based guidelines for prevention. *Dimensions of Critical Care Nursing, 25*(2), 53–61.

Killey, B., & Watt, E. (2006). The effect of extra walking on the mobility, independence and exercise self-efficacy of elderly hospital in-patients: A pilot study. *Contemporary Nurse: A Journal for the Australian Nursing Profession, 22*(1), 120–133.

Liu, C., & Fielding, R. (2011). Exercise as an intervention for frailty. *Clinics in Geriatric Medicine, 27*(1), 101–110.

Mondoa, C. T. (2004). Literature review the implications of physical activity in patients with chronic heart failure. *Nursing in Critical Care, 9*(1), 13–20.

Nabkasorn, C., Miyai, N., Sootmongkol, A., Junprasert, S., Yamamoto, H., Arita, M., et al. (2006). Effects of physical exercise on depression, neuroendocrine stress hormones and physiological fitness in adolescent females with depressive symptoms. *European Journal of Public Health, 16*(2), 179–184.

Oliver, D., Connelly, J. B., Victor, C. R., Shaw, F. E., Whitehead, A., Genc, Y., et al. (2007). Strategies to prevent falls and fractures in hospitals and care homes and effect of cognitive impairment: Systematic review and meta-analyses. *BMJ: British Medical Journal, 334*(7584), 82–85.

Taggart, H. M., Arslanian, C. L., Bae, S., & Singh, K. (2003). Effects of t'ai chi exercise on fibromyalgia symptoms and health-related quality of life. *Orthopaedic Nursing, 22*(5), 353.

Unsworth, J., & Mode, A. (2003). Preventing falls in older people: Risk factors and primary prevention through physical activity. *British Journal of Community Nursing, 8*(5), 214–220.

Wert, D., Brach, J., Perera, S., & VanSwearingen, J. (2010). Gait biomechanics, spatial and temporal characteristics, and the energy cost of walking in older adults with impaired mobility. *Physical Therapy, 90*(7), 977–985.

Wilkinson, J., & Treas, L. (2011). Chapter 31. In *Fundamentals of nursing* (2nd ed.). Philadelphia: F. A. Davis.

Williams, A., & Jester, R. (2005). Delayed surgical fixation of fractured hips in older people: Impact on mortality. *Journal of Advanced Nursing, 52*(1), 63–69.

Mobility: Wheelchair, Impaired

Baptiste, A., McCleerey, M., Matz, M., & Evitt, C. P. (2008). Proper sling selection and application while using client lifts. *Rehabilitation Nursing, 33*(1), 22–32.

Batavia, M. (2010). *The wheelchair evaluation: A clinician's guide*. Sudbury, MA: Jones and Bartlett.

Brouwer, K., Nysseknabm, J., & Culham, E. (2004). Physical function and health status among seniors with and without fear of falling. *Gerontology, 50,* 15–141.

DiFazio, R. (2003). Evidence-based practice in action. Creating a halo traction wheelchair resource manual: Using the EBP approach. *Journal of Pediatric Nursing, 18*(2), 148–152.

Fliess-Douer, O., Vanlandewijck, Y., Manor, G., & Van Der Woude, L. (2010). A systematic review of wheelchair skills tests for manual wheelchair users with a spinal cord injury: Towards a standardized outcome measure. *Clinical Rehabilitation, 24*(10), 867–886.

Frank, A., Neophytou, C., Frank, J., & de Souza, L. (2010). Electric-powered indoor/outdoor wheelchairs (EPIOCs): Users' views of influence on family, friends, and carers. *Disability and Rehabilitation: Assistive Technology, 5*(5), 327–338.

Gavin-Dreschnack, D. (2004). Effects of wheelchair posture on patient safety. *Rehabilitation Nursing, 29*(6), 221–226.

Gavin-Dreschnack, D., Schonfeld, L., Nelson, A., & Luther, S. (2004). Development of a screening tool for safe wheelchair seating. In agency for healthcare research and quality (AHRQ), department o defense (DoD)—health affairs. *Advances in Patient Safety: From Research to Implementation*. Retrieved February 6, 2012, from http://www.ncbi.nlm.nih.gov/books/NBK20593/

Hettinga, F., Valent, L., Groen, W., van Drongelen, S., de Groot, S., & van der Woude, L. (2010). Hand-cycling: An active form of wheeled mobility, recreation, and sports. *Physical Medicine and Rehabilitation Clinics of North America, 21*(1), 127–140.

Lewis, C. L., Moutoux, M., Slaughter, M., & Bailey, S. P. (2004). Characteristics of individuals who fell while receiving home health services. *Physical Therapy, 84*(1), 23–32.

Matsouka, O., Harahousou, Y., Kabiatis, C., & Trigonis, I. (2003). Effects of a physical activity program: The study of selected physical abilities among elderly women. *Journal of Gerontological Nursing, 29*(7), 50–55.

McCullagh, M. (2006). Home modification. *American Journal of Nursing, 106*(10), 54–63.

Montesano, L., Diaz, M., Bhaskar, S., & Minguez, J. (2010). Towards an intelligent wheelchair system for users with cerebral palsy. *Neural Systems and Rehabilitation Engineering, 18*(2), 193–202.

Ouslander, J., Griffiths, P., McConnell, E., Riolo, L., Kutner, M., & Schnelle, J. (2005). Functional incidental training: A randomized, controlled, crossover trial in Veterans Affairs nursing homes. *Journal of the American Geriatrics Society, 53*(7), 1091–1100.

Smith, R. (2008). Devising a system: New tools help therapists find seating solutions. *Rehab Management, 21*(3), 10, 12–15.

Tinetti, M. E., & Ginter, S. F. (1988). Identifying mobility dysfunction in elderly persons. *Journal of the American Medical Association, 259,* 1190–1193.

Walker, K., Morgan, K., Morris, C., DeGroot, K., Hollingsworth, H., & Gray, D. (2010). Development of a community mobility skills course for people who use mobility devices. *The American Journal of Occupational Therapy, 64*(4), 547–554.

Waugh, K. (2005). Measuring the right angle. *Rehab Manager, 18*(1), 40–49.

Moral Distress

Ahern, N. R., & Malvey, D. (2006). Decisions regarding infant resuscitation: A case study applying an ethical decision-making model. *Journal of Health Administration Ethics, 1*(1), 16–25.

Corley, M., Elswick, R., Gorman, M., & Clor, T. (2001). Development and evaluation of a moral distress scale. *Journal of Advanced Nursing, 33,* 250–256.

Epstein, E., & Delgado, S. (2010). Understanding and addressing moral distress. *OJIN: The Online Journal of Issues in Nursing, 15*(3). Retrieved February 6, 2012, from http://www.medscape.com/viewarticle/737893

Gaeta, S., & Price, K. (2010). End-of-life issues in critically ill cancer patients. *Critical Care Clinics, 26*(1), 219–227.

Jameton, A. (1993). Dilemmas of moral distress: Moral responsibility and nursing practice. *AWHONN's Clinical Issues in Perinatal & Women's Health Nursing, 4,* 542–551.

Kirk, T. W. (2007). Managing pain, managing ethics. *Pain Management Nursing, 8*(1), 25–34.

Kopala, B., & Burkhart, L. (2005). Ethical dilemma and moral distress: Proposed new NANDA diagnoses. *International Journal of Nursing Terminologies and Classifications, 16,* 3–13.

O'Haire, S. E., & Blackford, J. C. (2005). Nurses' moral agency in negotiating parental participation in care. *International Journal of Nursing Practice, 11*(6), 250–256.

Purdy, I. B., & Wadhwani, R. T. (2006). Embracing bioethics in neonatal intensive care, part II: Case histories in neonatal ethics. *Neonatal Network, 25*(1), 43.

Wilkinson, J. M. (1987/1988). Moral distress in nursing practice: Experience and effect. *Nursing Forum, 23,* 16–29.

Nausea

Allen, G. (2005). Evidence for practice. Preventing postoperative nausea and vomiting. *AORN Journal, 82*(2), 287.

Aurora, S., Silberstein, S., Kori, S., Tepper, S., Borland, S., Wang, M., et al. (2011). MAP0004, orally inhaled DHE: A randomized, controlled study in the acute treatment of migraine. *Headache: The Journal of Head and Face Pain, 51*(4), 507–517.

Cope, D. (2003). Oncology patient evidence-based notes: Antiemetics for chemotherapy-induced nausea and vomiting. *Clinical Journal of Oncology Nursing, 7*(4), 461–462.

Davis, M. (2004). Nausea and vomiting of pregnancy: An evidence-based review. *Journal of Perinatal & Neonatal Nursing, 18*(4), 312–328.

Fellowes, D., Barnes, K., & Wilkinson, S. (2006). Aromatherapy and massage for symptom relief in patients with cancer. *Cochrane Library* (4).

Ferrell, B., & Coyle, N. (Eds.). (2010). Chapter 10, Nausea and vomiting. *Oxford textbook of palliative nursing*. New York: Oxford University Press.

Hickman, A. G., Bell, D. M., & Preston, J. C. (2005). Update for nurse anesthetists: Acupressure and postoperative nausea and vomiting. *AANA Journal, 73*(5), 379–385.

Hooper, V. D., & Murphy, M. (2006). An introduction to the ASPAN evidence-based clinical practice guideline for the prevention and/or management of PONV/PDNV. *Journal of PeriAnesthesia Nursing, 21*(4), 228–229.

Isbir, G., & Mete, S. (2010). Nursing care of nausea and vomiting in pregnancy: Roy adaptation model. *Nursing Science Quarterly, 23*(2), 148–155.

Kaiser, R. (2005). Antiemetic guidelines: Are they being used? *Lancet Oncology, 6*(8), 622–625.

Kitzler, R., & Nolan, S. (2011). *The role of aromatherapy in postoperative nausea and vomiting*. (Presentation at Oncology Nursing Society). Virginia Henderson International Nursing Library, Retrieved February 7, 2012, from http://hdl.handle.net/10755/165002

Klein, J., & Griffiths, P. (2004). Acupressure for nausea and vomiting in cancer patients receiving chemotherapy. *British Journal of Community Nursing, 9*(9), 383–388.

Konno, R. (2010). Cochrane review summary for cancer nursing: Acupuncture-point stimulation for chemotherapy-induced nausea or vomiting. *Cancer Nursing, 33*(6), 479–480.

Kris, M., Urba, S., & Schwartzberg, L. (2011). Clinical roundtable monograph. Treatment of chemotherapy-induced nausea and vomiting: A post-MASCC 2010 discussion. *Clinical Advances in Hematology & Oncology, 9*(1, Suppl.), 1–15.

Matthews, A., Dowswell, T., Haas, D., Doyle, M., & O'Mathuna, D. (2010). Interventions for nausea and vomiting in early pregnancy. *Cochrane Database of Systematic Reviews* (9), Art No: CD007575. DOI: 1002/14651858.CD007575.pub2.

Miller, M., & Kearney, N. (2004). Chemotherapy-related nausea and vomiting—past reflections, present practice and future management. *European Journal of Cancer Care, 13*(1), 71–81.

Ng, W. Q., & Neill, J. (2006). Evidence for early oral feeding of patients after elective open colorectal surgery: A literature review. *Journal of Clinical Nursing, 15*(6), 696–709.

Rheingans, J. I. (2007). A systematic review of nonpharmacologic adjunctive therapies for symptom management in children with cancer. *Journal of Pediatric Oncology Nursing, 24*(2), 81–94.

Snively, A. (2005). Challenging practice norms: Implementing evidence to manage CINV. *ONS News, 20*(8), 45–46.

Steele, A., & Carlson, K. K. (2007). Nausea: Applying research to bedside practice. *AACN Advanced Critical Care, 18*(1), 61–75.

Sussanne, B., Arweström, C., Baker, A., & Berterö, B. (2010). Nurses' experiences in the relief of postoperative nausea and vomiting. *Journal of Clinical Nursing, 19*(13–14), 1865–1872.

Tipton, J. M., McDaniel, R. W., Barbour, L., Johnston, M. P., Kayne, M., LeRoy, P., et al. (2007). Putting evidence into practice: Evidence-based interventions to prevent, manage, and treat chemotherapy-induced nausea and vomiting. *Clinical Journal of Oncology Nursing, 11*(1), 69–78.

Walker, G. M., Neilson, A., Young, D., & Raine, P. A. M. (2006). Colour of bile vomiting in intestinal obstruction in the newborn: Questionnaire study. *BMJ: British Medical Journal, 332*(7554), 1363–1365.

Wilkinson, J., & Treas, L. (2011). *Fundamentals of nursing* (2nd ed., Vol. 2, p. 584). Philadelphia: F. A. Davis Company.

Williams, B., Orebaugh, S., & Kentor, M. (2011). Post-operative nausea and vomiting prevention with perphenazine: Long overdue. *European Journal of Anaesthesiology, 28*(2), 141–142.

Wujcik, D., Noonan, K., & Schwartz, R. (2004). Effective interventions for CINV: NCCN antiemesis clinical practice guidelines in oncology…chemotherapy-induced nausea and vomiting.National comprehensive cancer network. *ONS News, 19*(9), 17–18.

Neurovascular Dysfunction: Peripheral, Risk for

Ageno, W., Manfredi, E., Dentali, F., Silingardi, M., Ghezzi, F., Camporese, G., et al. (2007). The incidence of venous thromboembolism following gynecologic laparoscopy: A multicenter, prospective cohort study. *Journal of Thrombosis & Haemostasis, 5*(3), 503–506.

AORN guidelines for prevention of venous stasis. (2007). *AORN Journal, 85*(3), 607.

Autar, R. (2006). Evidence for the prevention of venous thromboembolism [cover story]. *British Journal of Nursing (BJN), 15*(18), 980–986.

Chen, M.-Y., Huang, W.-C., Peng, Y.-S., Jong, M.-C., Chen, C.-Y., & Lin, H.-C. (2011). Health status and health-related behaviors among Type 2 diabetes community residents. *Journal of Nursing Research, 19*(1), 35–43.

Clark, A. M., Hartling, L., Vandermeer, B., & McAlister, F. A. (2005). Meta-analysis: Secondary prevention programs for patients with coronary artery disease. *Annals of Internal Medicine, 143*(9), 659–672.

Dorgan, S. (2004). Management options for patients with intermittent claudication. *British Journal of Nursing (BJN), 13*(8), 448–451.

Fletcher, L. (2006). Management of patients with intermittent claudication. *Nursing Standard, 20*(31), 59–65.

Goodacre, S., Sutton, A. J., & Sampson, F. C. (2005). Meta-analysis: The value of clinical assessment in the diagnosis of deep venous thrombosis. *Annals of Internal Medicine, 143*(2), 129–139.

Gorski, L. A. (2007). Venous thromboembolism: A common and preventable condition: Implications for the home care nurse. *Home Healthcare Nurse, 25*(2), 94–100.

Harvey, C., & Runner, M. (2011). Venous thromboembolism after fibula fracture: A patient's perspective. *Orthopaedic Nursing, 30*(3), 182–191.

Hsieh, H. F., & Lee, F. P. (2006). Review: Wearing graduated compression stockings during air travel reduces the risk of deep venous thromboembolism. *Evidence-Based Medicine, 11*(2), 55.

Kehl-Pruett, W. (2006). Deep vein thrombosis in hospitalized patients: A review of evidence-based guidelines for prevention. *Dimensions of Critical Care Nursing, 25*(2), 53–61.

Ramzi, D. W., & Leeper, K. V. (2004). DVT and pulmonary embolism: Part I. Diagnosis. *American Family Physician, 69*(12), 2829–2836.

Shrubb, D., & Mason, W. (2006). The management of deep vein thrombosis in lymphoedema: A review. *British Journal of Community Nursing, 11*(7), 292–297.

Yang, X., Sun, L., Xu, P., Gong, L., Qiang, G., Zhang, L., et al. (2011). Effects of salvianolic acid A on plantar microcirculation and peripheral nerve function in diabetic rats. *European Journal of Pharmacology, 665*(1–3), 40–46.

Yücel, S., Eser, I., Güler, E., & Khorshid, L. (2011). Nursing diagnoses in patients having mechanical ventilation support in a respiratory intensive care unit in Turkey. *International Journal of Nursing Practice, 17*(5), 502–508.

Noncompliance (Specify)

Allen, D., Wainwright, M., & Hutchinson, T. (2011). "Non-compliance" as illness management: Hemodialysis patients' descriptions of adversarial patient–clinician interactions. *Social Science & Medicine, 73,* 129–134.

Beswick, A. D., Rees, K., West, R. R., Taylor, F. C., Burke, M., & Griebsch, I. (2005). Improving uptake and adherence in cardiac rehabilitation: Literature review. *Journal of Advanced Nursing, 49*(5), 538–555.

Burcher, P. (2012). The noncompliant patient: A Kantian and Levinasian response. *The Journal of Medicine & Philosophy, 37*(1), 74–89.

Burra, P., Germani, G., Gnoato, F., Lazzaro, S., Russo, F., Cillo, U., et al. (2011). Adherence in liver transplant patients. *Liver Transplantation, 17*(7), 760–770.

Charonko, C. (1992). Cultural influences in "noncompliant" behavior and decision making. *Holistic Nursing Practice, 6*(3), 73–78.

Coleman, C., & Lohan, M. (2007). Sexually acquired infections: Do lay experiences of partner notification challenge practice? *Journal of Advanced Nursing, 58*(1), 35–43.

Denhaerynck, K., Dobbels, F., Cleemput, I., Desmyttere, A., Schäfer-Keller, P., Schaub, S., et al. (2005). Prevalence, consequences, and determinants of nonadherence in adult renal transplant patients: A literature review. *Transplant International, 18*(10), 1121–1133.

Dobbels, F., De Geest, S., van Cleemput, J., Droogne, W., & Vanhaecke, J. (2004). Effect of late medication non-compliance on outcome after heart transplantation: A 5-year follow-up. *Journal of Heart & Lung Transplantation, 23*(11), 1245–1251.

Dracup, K. A., & Meleis, A. I. (1982). Compliance: An interactionist approach. *Nursing Research, 31,* 32–35.

Drent, G., Haagsma, E. B., Geest, S. D., van den Berg, Aad, P., Ten Vergert, E. M., et al. (2005). Prevalence of prednisolone (non)compliance in adult liver transplant recipients. *Transplant International, 18*(8), 960–966.

Dumbleton, K., Woods, C., Jones, L., & Fonn, D. (2011). The relationship between compliance with lens replacement and contact lens-related problems in silicone hydrogel wearers. *Contact Lens & Anterior Eye, 34*(5), 216–222.

Escalada, P., & Griffiths, P. (2006). Do people with cancer comply with oral chemotherapy treatments? *British Journal of Community Nursing, 11*(12), 532–536.

Forrester, S. (2011). Efficacy of the patient advocate component in a behavioral intervention to improve treatment adherence in the HIV positive population: A systematic review. *School of Physician Assistant Studies.* Paper 253. Retrieved February 7, 2012, from http://commons.pacificu.edu/pa/253

Geissler, E. (1991). Transcultural nursing and nursing diagnoses. *Nursing and Health Care, 12*(4), 190–192, 203.

Holzemer, W. L., Bakken, S., Portillo, C. J., Grimes, R., Welch, J., Wantland, D., et al. (2006). Testing a nurse-tailored HIV medication adherence intervention. *Nursing Research, 55*(3), 189–197.

Hussey, L., & Gilliland, K. (1989). Compliance, low literacy and locus of control. *Nursing Clinics of North America, 24,* 605–611.

Ilott, R. (2005). Does compliance therapy improve use of antipsychotic medication? *British Journal of Community Nursing, 10*(11), 514–519.

Lamba, S., Nagurka, R., Desai, K., Chun, S., Holland, B., & Koneru, B. (2011). Self-reported non-adherence to immune-suppressant therapy in liver transplant recipients: Demographic, interpersonal, and intrapersonal factors. *Clinical Transplantation.* DOI: 10.1111/j.1399-0012.2011.01489.x. © 2011 John Wiley & Sons A/S. Retrieved February 7, 2012, from http://onlinelibrary.wiley.com/doi/10.1111/j.1399-0012.2011.01489.x/full

Petrilla, A. A., Benner, J. S., Battleman, D. S., Tierce, J. C., & Hazard, E. H. (2005). Evidence-based interventions to improve patient compliance with antihypertensive and lipid-lowering medications. *International Journal of Clinical Practice, 59*(12), 1441–1451.

Redman, B. K. (2005). The ethics of self-management preparation for chronic illness. *Nursing Ethics, 12*(4), 360–369.

Robin, A., & Grover, D. (2011). Compliance and adherence in glaucoma management. *Indian Journal of Ophthalmology, 59*(Suppl. 1), S93–S96.

Sandman, L., Granger, B., Ekman, I., & Munthe, C. (2011). Adherence, shared decision-making and patient autonomy. *Medicine, Health Care and Philosophy.* DOI: 10.1007/s11019-011-9336-x.. Retrieved February 7, 2012, from http://www.springerlink.com/content/p420410823746627/

Theofilou, P. (2011). Noncompliance with medical regimen in haemodialysis treatment: A case study. *Case Reports in Nephrology.* DOI: 10.1155/2011/476038. Retrieved February 7, 2012, from http://www.hindawi.com/crim/nephrology/2011/476038/

Welch, J. L., & Thomas-Hawkins, C. (2005). Psycho-educational strategies to promote fluid adherence in adult hemodialysis patients: A review of intervention studies. *International Journal of Nursing Studies, 42*(5), 597–608.

Young, M. S. (2004). Tackling noncompliance. *Dermatology Nursing, 16*(1), 64.

Nutrition, Imbalanced: Less Than Body Requirements

Azam, P. (2007). Managing under-nutrition in a nursing home setting. *Nursing Older People, 19*(3), 33–36.

Bakker, R., van Meijel, B., Beukers, L., van Ommen, J., Meerwijk, E., & van Elburg, A. (2011). Recovery of normal body weight in adolescents with anorexia nervosa: The nurses' perspective on effective interventions. *Journal of Child and Adolescent Psychiatric Nursing, 24*(1), 16–22.

Benton, M. J., & White, A. (2006). Osteoporosis: Recommendations for resistance exercise and supplementation with calcium and vitamin D to promote bone health. *Journal of Community Health Nursing, 23*(4), 201–211.

Booth, J., Leadbetter, A., Francis, M., & Tolson, D. (2005a). Implementing a best practice statement in nutrition for frail older people: Part 1. *Nursing Older People, 16*(10), 26–28.

Booth, J., Leadbetter, A., Francis, M., & Tolson, D. (2005b). Implementing a best practice statement in nutrition for frail older people: Part 2. *Nursing Older People, 17*(1), 22–24.

Breiner, S. (2003). Evidence-based practice in action. An evidence-based eating disorder program. *Journal of Pediatric Nursing, 18*(1), 75–80.

Brown, J. K. (2002). A systematic review of the evidence on symptom management of cancer-related anorexia and cachexia. *Oncology Nursing Forum, 29*(3), 517–530.

Campbell, K. L., Ash, S., Bauer, J., & Davies, P. S. W. (2007). Critical review of nutrition assessment tools to measure malnutrition in chronic kidney disease. *Nutrition & Dietetics, 64*(1), 23–30.

Carlsson, E., Ehrenberg, A., & Ehnfors, M. (2004). Stroke and eating difficulties: Long-term experiences. *Journal of Clinical Nursing, 13*(7), 825–834.

Cereda, E., Pedrolli, C., Zagami, A., Vanotti, A., Piffer, S., Opizzi, A., et al. (2011). Body mass index and mortality in institutionalized elderly. *JAMDA, 12*(3), 174–178.

DiBartolo, M. C. (2006). Careful hand feeding: A reasonable alternative to PEG tube placement in individuals with dementia. *Journal of Gerontological Nursing, 32*(5), 25–35.

Dichter, J. R., Cohen, J., & Connolly, P. M. (2002). Research. Bulimia nervosa: Knowledge, awareness, and skill levels among advanced practice nurses. *Journal of the American Academy of Nurse Practitioners, 14*(6), 269–275.

Doig, G., Heighes, P., Simpson, F., & Sweetman, E. (2011). Early enteral nutrition reduces mortality in trauma patients requiring intensive care: A meta-analysis of randomised controlled trials. *Injury, 42*(1), 50–56.

Elia, M., Zellipour, L., & Stratton, R. J. (2005). To screen or not to screen for adult malnutrition? *Clinical Nutrition, 24*(6), 867–884.

Fox, V. J., Miller, J., & McClung, M. (2004). Nutritional support in the critically injured. *Critical Care Nursing Clinics of North America, 16*(4), 559–569.

Gee, C. (2006). Does alcohol stimulate appetite and energy intake? *British Journal of Community Nursing, 11*(7), 298–302.

Green, S. M., & Watson, R. (2005). Nutritional screening and assessment tools for use by nurses: Literature review. *Journal of Advanced Nursing, 50*(1), 69–83.

Mosier, M., Pham, T., Klein, M., Gibran, N., Arnoldo, B., Gamelli, R., et al. (2011). Early enteral nutrition in burns: Compliance with guidelines and associated outcomes in a multicenter study. *Journal of Burn Care & Research, 32*(1), 104–109.

Neelemaat, F., Bosmans, J., Thijs, A., Seidell, J., & van der Schueren, M. (2011). Post-discharge nutritional support in malnourished elderly individuals improves functional limitations. *JAMDA, 12*(4), 295–301.

Premji, S. S. (2005). Enteral feeding for high-risk neonates. *Journal of Perinatal & Neonatal Nursing, 19*(1), 59–71.

Sabol, V. K. (2004). Nutrition assessment of the critically ill adult. *AACN Clinical Issues: Advanced Practice in Acute & Critical Care, 15*(4), 595–606.

Schneider, P. J. (2006). Nutrition support teams: An evidence-based practice. *Nutrition in Clinical Practice, 21*(1), 62–67.

Simpson, K. J. (2002). Anorexia nervosa and culture. *Journal of Psychiatric & Mental Health Nursing, 9*(1), 65–71.

Singer, P., Anbar, R., Cohen, J., Shapiro, H., Shalita-Chesner, M., Grozovski, E., et al. (2011). The tight calorie control study (TICACOS): A prospective, randomized, controlled pilot study of nutritional support in critically ill patients. *Intensive Care Medicine, 37*(4), 601–609.

Spatz, D. L. (2006). State of the science: Use of human milk and breast-feeding for vulnerable infants. *Journal of Perinatal & Neonatal Nursing, 20*(1), 51–55.

Stuart, W. P., Broome, M. E., Smith, B. A., & Weaver, M. (2005). An integrative review of interventions for adolescent weight loss. *Journal of School Nursing, 21*(2), 77–85.

Todorovic, V. (2004). Nutritional screening in the community: Developing strategies. *British Journal of Community Nursing, 9*(11), 464–470.

Todorovic, V. (2005). Evidence-based strategies for the use of oral nutritional supplements. *British Journal of Community Nursing, 10*(4), 158–164.

Vivanti, A., Ward, N., & Haines, T. (2011). Nutritional status and associations with falls, balance, mobility and functionality during hospital admission. *The Journal of Nutrition, Health & Aging, 15*(5), 388–391.

Vizzini, A., & Aranda-Michel, J. (2011). Nutritional support in head injury. *Nutrition, 27*(2), 129–132.

Westergren, A. (2006). Detection of eating difficulties after stroke: A systematic review. *International Nursing Review, 53*(2), 143–149.

Williams, T. A., & Leslie, G. D. (2004). A review of the nursing care of enteral feeding tubes in critically ill adults: Part 1. *Intensive & Critical Care Nursing, 20*(6), 330–343.

Williams, T. A., & Leslie, G. D. (2005). A review of the nursing care of enteral feeding tubes in critically ill adults: Part II. *Intensive & Critical Care Nursing, 21*(1), 5–15.

Nutrition, Imbalanced: More Than Body Requirements

Aldrich, N., Reicks, M., Sibley, S., Redmon, B., Thomas, W., & Raatz, S. (2011). Varying protein source and quantity do not significantly improve weight loss, fat loss, or satiety in reduced energy diets among midlife adults. *Nutrition Research, 31*(2), 104–112.

Budd, G. M., & Hayman, L. L. (2006). Childhood obesity: Determinants, prevention, and treatment. *Journal of Cardiovascular Nursing, 21*(6), 437–441.

Budd, G. M., & Volpe, S. L. (2006). School-based obesity prevention: Research, challenges, and recommendations. *Journal of School Health, 76*(10), 485–495.

Cameron, A., Crawford, D., Salmon, J., Campbell, K., McNaughton, S., Mishra, G., et al. (2011). Clustering of obesity-related risk behaviors in children and their mothers. *Annals of Epidemiology, 21*(2), 95–102.

Cassidy, A. (2005). Diet and menopausal health. *Nursing Standard, 19*(29), 44–52.

Clancy, C. (2011). As obesity epidemic escalates, need for more screening and counseling grows. *Journal of Nursing Care Quality, 26*(1), 1–3.

Evangelista, L. S., Doering, L. V., Lennie, T., Moser, D. K., Hamilton, M. A., Fonarow, G. C., et al. (2006). Usefulness of a home-based exercise program for overweight and obese patients with advanced heart failure. *American Journal of Cardiology, 97*(6), 886–890.

Grabowski, D. C., Campbell, C. M., Ellis, J. E., & Morley, J. E. (2005). Obesity and mortality in elderly nursing home residents. *Journals of Gerontology Series A: Biological Sciences & Medical Sciences, 60A*(9), 1184–1189.

Green, S. M., & Watson, R. (2005). Nutritional screening and assessment tools for use by nurses: Literature review. *Journal of Advanced Nursing, 50*(1), 69–83.

Ingram, C., Courneya, K. S., & Kingston, D. (2006). The effects of exercise on body weight and composition in breast cancer survivors: An integrative systematic review. *Oncology Nursing Forum, 33*(5), 937–950.

Kitzmann, K., & Beech, B. (2011). Family-based interventions for pediatric obesity: Methodological and conceptual challenges from family psychology. *Couple and Family Psychology: Research and Practice, 1*(Suppl.), 45–62.

Lang, A., & Froelicher, E. S. (2006). Management of overweight and obesity in adults: Behavioral intervention for long-term weight loss and maintenance. *European Journal of Cardiovascular Nursing, 5*(2), 102–114.

Li, Z., & Heber, D. (2012). Sarcopenic obesity in the elderly and strategies for weight management. *Nutrition Reviews, 70*(1), 57–64.

Monasta, L., Batty, G., Macaluso, A., Ronfani, L., Lutje, V., Bavcar, A., et al. (2011). Interventions for the prevention of overweight and obesity in preschool children: A systematic review of randomized controlled trials. *Obesity Reviews, 12*(5), e107–e118.

Morrison-Sandberg, L., Kubik, M., & Johnson, K. (2011). Obesity prevention practices of elementary school nurses in Minnesota: Findings from interviews with licensed school nurses. *The Journal of School Nursing, 27*(1), 13–21.

Moyer, V. A., Klein, J. D., Ockene, J. K., Teutsch, S. M., Johnson, M. S., & Allan, J. D. (2005). Screening for overweight in children and adolescents: Where is the evidence? A commentary by the childhood obesity working group of the US preventive services task force. *Pediatrics, 116*(1), 235–238.

O'Gorman, D., & Krook, A. (2011). Exercise and the treatment of diabetes and obesity. *Medical Clinics of North America, 95*(5), 953–969.

Park, M.-J., & Kim, H.-S. (2012,). Evaluation of mobile phone and Internet intervention on waist circumference and blood pressure in post-menopausal women with abdominal obesity. *International Journal of Medical Informatics.*

Retrieved February 8, 2012, from http://www.sciencedirect.com/science/article/pii/S1386505611002711

Prevention and early treatment of overweight and obesity in young children: A critical review and appraisal of the evidence. (2007). *Pediatric Nursing, 33*(2), 149–127.

Quinn, M. (2011). Introduction of active video gaming into the middle school curriculum as a school-based childhood obesity intervention. *Journal of Pediatric Health Care.* DOI 10.1016/j.pedhc.2011.03.011. Retrieved February 8, 2012, from http://www.sciencedirect.com/science/article/pii/S0891524511001313

Rains, T., Agarwal, S., & Maki, K. (2011). Antiobesity effects of green tea catechins: A mechanistic review. *The Journal of Nutritional Biochemistry, 22*(1), 1–7.

Rasmussen, K. M., & Kjolhede, C. L. (2004). Prepregnant overweight and obesity diminish the prolactin response to suckling in the first week postpartum. *Pediatrics, 113*(5), e465–e471.

Vorona, R. D., Winn, M. P., Babineau, T. W., Eng, B. P., Feldman, H. R., & Ware, J. C. (2005). Overweight and obese patients in a primary care population report less sleep than patients with a normal body mass index. *Archives of Internal Medicine, 165*(1), 25–30.

Weinstein, P. K. (2006). A review of weight loss programs delivered via the internet. *Journal of Cardiovascular Nursing, 21*(4), 251–260.

Nutrition, Imbalanced: More Than Body Requirements, Risk for

Bindler, R. M., & Bruya, M. A. (2006). Evidence for identifying children at risk for being overweight, cardiovascular disease, and type 2 diabetes in primary care. *Journal of Pediatric Healthcare, 20*(2), 82–87.

Budd, G. M., & Hayman, L. L. (2006). Childhood obesity: Determinants, prevention, and treatment. *Journal of Cardiovascular Nursing, 21*(6), 437–441.

Budd, G. M., & Volpe, S. L. (2006). School-based obesity prevention: Research, challenges, and recommendations. *Journal of School Health, 76*(10), 485–495.

Booth, D. A., Blair, A. J., Lewis, V. J., & Baek, S. H. (2004). Patterns of eating and movement that best maintain reduction in overweight. *Appetite, 43*(3), 277–283.

Kumanyika, S., Parker, L., & Sim, L. (Eds.). (2010). *Bridging the evidence gap in obesity prevention: A framework to inform decision making.* Washington, DC: The National Academies Press.

Pullen, C. H., Walker, S. N., Hageman, P. A., Boeckner, L. S., & Oberdorfer, M. K. (2005). Differences in eating and activity markers among normal weight, overweight, and obese rural women. *Women's Health Issues, 15*(5), 209–215.

Skouteris, H., McCabe, M., Swinburn, B., Newgreen, V., Sacher, P., & Chadwick, P. (2011). Parental influence and obesity prevention in preschoolers: A systematic review of interventions. *Obesity Reviews, 12*(5), 315–328.

Teufel-Shone, N. I. (2006). Promising strategies for obesity prevention and treatment within American Indian communities. *Journal of Transcultural Nursing, 17*(3), 224–229.

Nutrition, Readiness for Enhanced

Abrams, S. E., & Wells, M. E. (2005). Feeding better food habits in mid-20th- century America. *Public Health Nursing, 22*(6), 529–534.

Banning, M. (2005). The carcinogenic and protective effects of food. *British Journal of Nursing (BJN), 14*(20), 1070–1074.

Berry, D., Sheehan, R., Heschel, R., Knafl, K., Melkus, G., & Grey, M. (2004). Family-based interventions for childhood obesity: A review. *Journal of Family Nursing, 10*(4), 429–449.

Blonde, L., Dempster, J., Gallivan, J. M., & Warren-Boulton, E. (2006). Reducing cardiovascular disease risk in patients with diabetes: A message from the national diabetes education program. *Journal of the American Academy of Nurse Practitioners, 18*(11), 524–533.

Booth, J., Leadbetter, A., Francis, M., & Tolson, D. (2005). Implementing a best practice statement in nutrition for frail older people: Part 2. *Nursing Older People, 17*(1), 22–24.

DeMille, D., Deming, P., Lupinacci, P., & Jacobs, L. A. (2006). The effect of the neutropenic diet in the outpatient setting: A pilot study. *Oncology Nursing Forum, 33*(2), 337–343.

Goldberg, G. (2005). Maternal nutrition in pregnancy and the first postnatal year—1. Pre-pregnancy and pregnancy. *Journal of Family Health Care, 15*(4), 113.

Hunt, P., Strong, M., & Poulter, J. (2004). Evaluating a new food selection guide. *Nutrition Bulletin, 29*(1), 19–25.

Janssen, J. (2006). Fat simple—a nursing tool for client education. *Nursing Praxis in New Zealand, 22*(2), 21–32.

Laws, R. (2004). A new evidence-based model for weight management in primary care: The counterweight programme. *Journal of Human Nutrition & Dietetics, 17*(3), 191–208.

Thompson, J. (2005). Breastfeeding: Benefits and implications. Part two. *Community Practitioner, 78*(6), 218–219.

Thompson, R. L., Summerbell, C. D., Hooper, L., Higgins, J., Little, P. S., Talbot, D., et al. (2006). Dietary advice given by a dietitian versus other health professional or self-help resources to reduce blood cholesterol. *Cochrane Library* (4).

Oral Mucous Membrane, Impaired

Aragon, D., & Sole, M. L. (2006). Implementing best practice strategies to prevent infection in the ICU. *Critical Care Nursing Clinics of North America, 18*(4), 441–452.

Berenholtz, S., Pham, J., Thompson, D., Needham, D., Lubomski, L., Hyzy, R., et al. (2011). Collaborative cohort study of an intervention to reduce ventilator-associated pneumonia in the intensive care unit. *Infection Control and Hospital Epidemiology, 32*(4), 305–314.

Berry, A., Davidson, P., Nicholson, L., Pasqualotto, C., & Rolls, K. (2011). Consensus based clinical guideline for oral hygiene in the critically ill. *Intensive and Critical Care Nursing, 27*(4), 180–185.

Brady, M., Furlanetto, D., Hunter, R. V., Lewis, S., & Milne, V. (2006). Staff-led interventions for improving oral hygiene in patients following stroke. *Cochrane Library* (4).

Chalmers, J., & Johnson, V. (2004). Evidence-based protocol: Oral hygiene care for functionally dependent and cognitively impaired older adults. *Journal of Gerontological Nursing, 30*(11), 5–12.

Chalmers, J., & Pearson, A. (2005). Oral hygiene care for residents with dementia: A literature review. *Journal of Advanced Nursing, 52*(4), 410–419.

Cohn, J. L., & Fulton, J. S. (2006). Nursing staff perspectives on oral care for neuroscience patients. *Journal of Neuroscience Nursing, 38*(1), 22–30.

Cutler, C. J., & Davis, N. (2005). Improving oral care in patients receiving mechanical ventilation. *American Journal of Critical Care, 14*(5), 389–394.

Garcia, R. (2005). A review of the possible role of oral and dental colonization on the occurrence of health care-associated pneumonia: Underappreciated risk and a call for interventions. *American Journal of Infection Control, 33*(9), 527–541.

Jablonski, R., Therrien, T., Mahoney, E., Kolanowski, A., Gabello, M., & Brock, A. (2011). An intervention to reduce care-resistant behavior in persons with dementia during oral hygiene: A pilot study. *Special Care in Dentistry, 31*(3), 77–87.

Kunnen, A., Blaauw, J., van Doormaal, J. J., van Pampus, M. G., van der Schans, Cees, P., Aarnoudse, J. G., et al. (2007). Women with a recent history of early-onset pre-eclampsia have a worse periodontal condition. *Journal of Clinical Periodontology, 34*(3), 202–207.

Nikoletti, S., Hyde, S., Shaw, T., Myers, H., & Kristjanson, L. J. (2005). Comparison of plain ice and flavoured ice for preventing oral mucositis associated with the use of 5-fluorouracil. *Journal of Clinical Nursing, 14*(6), 750–753.

Rutledge, D. (2005). Oncology nurses look to the latest evidence to treat mucositis. *ONS News, 20*(2), 1–6.

Santos, P., Coracin, F., Barros, J., Dulley, F., Nunes, F., & Magalhães, M. (2011). Impact of oral care prior to HSCT on the severity and clinical outcomes of oral mucositis. *Clinical Transplantation, 25*(2), 325–328.

Worthington, H., Clarkson, J., Bryan, G., Furness, S., Glenny, A., Littlewood, A., et al. (2011). Interventions for preventing oral mucositis for patients with cancer receiving treatment. *Cochrane Database of Systematic Reviews* (4), Art No: CD000978. DOI: 10.1002/14651858.CD000978.pub5.

Pain, Acute

Bergh, L., Stener-Victorin, E., Wallin, G., & Mårtensson, L. (2011). Comparison of the PainMatcher and the Visual Analogue Scale for assessment of labour pain following administered pain relief treatment. *Midwifery, 27*(1), e134–e139.

Brown, D., & McCormack, B. (2005). Developing postoperative pain management: Utilising the promoting action on research implementation in health services (PARIHS) framework. *Worldviews on Evidence-Based Nursing, 2*(3), 131–141.

Brown, D., O'Neill, O., & Beck, A. (2007). Post-operative pain management: Transition from epidural to oral analgesia [cover story]. *Nursing Standard, 21*(21), 35–40.

Chin-Mei Huang, Wan-Shu Tung, Li-Lin Kuo, & Ying-Ju Chang. (2004). Comparison of pain responses of premature infants to the heelstick between containment and swaddling. *Journal of Nursing Research, 12*(1), 31–39.

Garbez, R., & Puntillo, K. (2005). Acute musculoskeletal pain in the emergency department: A review of the literature and implications for the advanced practice nurse. *AACN Clinical Issues: Advanced Practice in Acute & Critical Care, 16*(3), 310–319.

Gold, J. I., Seok Hyeon Kim, Kant, A. J., Joseph, M. H., & Rizzo, A. (2006). Effectiveness of virtual reality for pediatric pain distraction during IV placement. *CyberPsychology & Behavior, 9*(2), 207–212.

Gordon, D. B., Dahl, J. L., Miaskowski, C., McCarberg, B., Todd, K. H., Paice, J. A., et al. (2005). American Pain Society recommendations for improving the quality of acute and cancer pain management: American Pain Society quality of care task force. *Archives of Internal Medicine, 165*(14), 1574–1580.

Johnson, L. (2003). Sickle cell disease patients and patient-controlled analgesia. *British Journal of Nursing (BJN), 12*(3), 144–153.

Kerns, R., Sellinger, J., & Goodin, B. (2011). Psychological treatment of chronic pain. *Annual Review of Clinical Psychology, 7,* 411–434.

Kovach, C. (2012). Assessing pain and unmet need in patients with advanced dementia: The role of the serial trial intervention (STI). *Handbook of Pain and Palliative Care, Part 2,* 131–144.

Lord, B., & Woollard, M. (2011). The reliability of vital signs in estimating pain severity among adult patients treated by paramedics. *Emergency Medicine Journal, 28*(2), 147–150.

Mann, C., Ouro-Bang'na, F., & Eledjam, J. J. (2005). Patient-controlled analgesia. *Current Drug Targets, 6*(7), 815–819.

McCreaddie, M., & Davison, S. (2002). Pain management in drug users. *Nursing Standard, 16*(19), 45.

Moore, A., Costello, J., Wieczorek, P., Shah, V., Taddio, A., & Carvalho, J. (2011). Gabapentin improves postcesarean delivery pain management: A randomized, placebo-controlled trial. *Anesthesia & Analgesia, 112*(1), 167–173.

Ragsdale, L., & Southerland, L. (2011). Acute abdominal pain in the older adult. *Emergency Medicine Clinics of North America, 29*(2), 429–448.

Reagan, M., DeBaun, M., & Frei-Jones, M. (2011). Multi-modal intervention for the inpatient management of sickle cell pain significantly decreases the rate of acute chest syndrome. *Pediatric Blood & Cancer, 56*(2), 262–266.

Sarrell, E. M., Cohen, H. A., & Kahan, E. (2003). Naturopathic treatment for ear pain in children. *Pediatrics, 111*(5), e574–e579.

Sharp, B., Taylor, D. L., Thomas, K. K., Killen, M. B., & Dawood, M. Y. (2002). Cyclic perimenstrual pain and discomfort: The scientific basis for practice. *JOGNN: Journal of Obstetric, Gynecologic, & Neonatal Nursing, 31*(6), 637–649.

Sobralske, M., & Katz, J. (2005). Culturally competent care of patients with acute chest pain. *Journal of the American Academy of Nurse Practitioners, 17*(9), 342–349.

Stewart, M. W. (2005). Research news. Evidence-based assessment of acute pain in older adults: Current nursing practices and perceived barriers. *Journal of PeriAnesthesia Nursing, 20*(1), 59.

Tough, J. (2006). Primary percutaneous coronary intervention in patients with acute myocardial infarction [cover story]. *Nursing Standard, 21*(2), 47–56.

Tracy, S., Dufault, M., Kogut, S., Martin, V., Rossi, S., & Willey-Temkin, C. (2006). Translating best practices in nondrug postoperative pain management. *Nursing Research, 55*(2), S57–67.

Vaajoki, A., Pietilä, A.-M., Kankkunen, P., & Vehviläinen-Julkunen, K. (2011,). Effects of listening to music on pain intensity and pain distress after surgery: An intervention. *Journal of Clinical Nursing.* Retrieved February 10, 2012, from http://onlinelibrary.wiley.com/doi/10.1111/j.1365-2702.2011.03829.x/full

Wylie, K., & Nebauer, M. (2011). The fragmented story of pain: A saga of economic discourse, confusion and lack of holistic assessment in the residential care of older people. *Collegian, 18*(1), 11–18.

Pain, Chronic

Becker, W., Starrels, J., Heo, M., Li, X., Weiner, M., & Turner, B. (2011). Racial differences in primary care opioid risk reduction strategies. *Annals of Family Medicine, 9*(3), 219–225.

Bennell, K., & Hinman, R. (2011). A review of the clinical evidence for exercise in osteoarthritis of the hip and knee. *Journal of Science and Medicine in Sport, 14*(1), 4–9.

Briggs, M. (2006). The prevalence of pain in chronic wounds and nurses' awareness of the problem. *British Journal of Nursing (BJN), 15*(21), 5–9.

Christo, P., Manchikanti, L., Ruan, X., Bottros, M., Hansen, H., Solanki, D., et al. (2011). Urine drug testing in chronic pain. *Pain Physician, 14,* 123–143.

Chronic pain [cover story]. (2006). *Nursing Standard, 20*(36), 67.

Cowan, D. (2005). Is morphine for chronic pain addictive? *British Journal of Community Nursing, 10*(3), 127.

Cowan, D. T. (2002). Chronic non-cancer pain in older people: Current evidence for prescribing. *British Journal of Community Nursing, 7*(8), 420.

Drwecki, B., Moore, C., Warrd, S., & Prkachin, K. (2011). Reducing racial disparities in pain treatment: The role of empathy and perspective-taking. *Pain, 152*(5), 1001–1006.

Eccleston, C., Bruce, E., & Carter, B. (2006). Chronic pain in children and adolescents. *Paediatric Nursing, 18*(10), 30–33.

Edrington, J. M., Paul, S., Dodd, M., West, C., Facione, N., Tripathy, D. et al. (2004). No evidence for sex differences in the severity and treatment of cancer pain. *Journal of Pain & Symptom Management, 28*(3), 225–232.

Ernst, E., Lee, M., & Choi, T.-Y. (2011). Acupuncture: Does it alleviate pain and are there serious risks? A review of reviews. *Pain, 152*(4), 755–764.

Ersek, M., Cherrier, M. M., Overman, S. S., & Irving, G. A. (2004). The cognitive effects of opioids. *Pain Management Nursing, 5*(2), 75–93.

Eshkevari, L., & Heath, J. (2005). Use of acupuncture for chronic pain. *Holistic Nursing Practice, 19*(5), 217–221.

Henderson, H. (2002). Acupuncture: Evidence for its use in chronic low back pain. *British Journal of Nursing (BJN), 11*(21), 1395.

Jensen, M., Moore, M., Bockow, T., Ehde, D., & Engel, J. (2011). Psychosocial factors and adjustment to chronic pain in persons with physical disabilities: A systematic review. *Archives of Physical Medicine and Rehabilitation, 92*(1), 146–160.

Jerzak, L. A., & Smith, S. K. (2006). Vulvodynia: Diagnosis and treatment of a chronic pain syndrome. *Women's Health Care: A Practical Journal for Nurse Practitioners, 5*(4), 29.

Kim, E. J., & Buschmann, M. T. (2006). Reliability and validity of the faces pain scale with older adults. *International Journal of Nursing Studies, 43*(4), 447–456.

Landis, C. A., Lentz, M. J., Tsuji, J., Buchwald, D., & Shaver, J. L. F. (2004). Pain, psychological variables, sleep quality, and natural killer cell activity in midlife women with and without fibromyalgia. *Brain, Behavior & Immunity, 18*(4), 304–313.

Lewandowski, W. (2004). Psychological factors in chronic pain: A worthwhile undertaking for nursing? *Archives of Psychiatric Nursing, 18*(3), 97–105.

Longley, K. (2006). Chronic pain. Fibromyalgia: Aetiology, diagnosis, symptoms and management. *British Journal of Nursing (BJN), 15*(13), 729–733.

Lynch, M., & Campbell, F. (2011). Cannabinoids for treatment of chronic non-cancer pain; a systematic review of randomized trials. *British Journal of Clinical Pharmacology, 72*(5), 735–744.

Nicholas, M., Linton, S., Watson, P., & Main, C., and the "Decade of the Flags" Working Group. (2011). Early identification and management of psychological risk factors ("yellow flags") in patients with low back pain: A reappraisal. *Physical Therapy, 91*(5), 737–753.

Passik, S., Messina, J., Golsorkhi, A., & Xie, F. (2011). Aberrant drug-related behavior observed during clinical studies involving patients taking chronic opioid therapy for persistent pain and Fentanyl buccal tablet for breakthrough pain. *Journal of Pain and Symptom Management, 41*(1), 116–125.

Ransom, S., Pearman, T., Philip, E., & Anwar, D. (2012). Adult cancer-related pain. *Handbook of Pain and Palliative Care, Part 3,* 1247–1270.

Seminowicz, D., Wideman, T., Naso, L., Hatami-Khoroushahi, Z., Fallatah, S., Ware, M., et al. (2011). Effective treatment of chronic low back pain in humans reverses abnormal brain anatomy and function. *The Journal of Neuroscience, 18,* 7540–7550.

Shaw, S. M. (2006). Nursing and supporting patients with chronic pain. *Nursing Standard, 20*(19), 60–65.

Taylor, D. (2005). Perimenstrual symptoms and syndromes: Guidelines for symptom management and self care. *Advanced Studies in Medicine, 5*(5), 228.

Veehof, M., Oskam, M.-J., Schreurs, K., & Bohlmeijer, E. (2011). Acceptance-based interventions for the treatment of chronic pain: A systematic review and meta-analysis. *Pain, 152*(3), 533–542.

Wamboldt, C., & Kapustin, J. (2006). Evidence-based treatment of diabetic peripheral neuropathy. *Journal for Nurse Practitioners, 2*(6), 370–379.

White, S. (2004). Neuroscience nursing. Assessment of chronic neuropathic pain and the use of pain tools. *British Journal of Nursing (BJN), 13*(7), 372.

Parenting, Impaired

Akesson, B., Smyth, J., Mandell, D., Doan, T., Donina, K., & Hoven, C. (2012). Parental involvement with the criminal justice system and the effects on their children: A collaborative model for researching vulnerable families. *Social Work in Public Health, 27*(1–2), 148–164.

Arria, A., Mericle, A., Meyers, K., & Winters, K. (2011). Parental substance use impairment, parenting and substance use disorder risk. *Journal of Substance Abuse Treatment.* DOI: http://dx.doi.org/10.1016/j.jsat.2011.10.001. Retrieved February 11, 2011, from http://www.sciencedirect.com/science/article/pii/S0740547211001991#FCANote

Bakewell-Sachs, C. (2002). Toward evidence-based practice. Effectiveness of a home intervention for perceived child behavioral problems and parenting stress in children with in utero drug exposure. *MCN: The American Journal of Maternal Child Nursing, 27*(2), 124.

Bensley, L., Wynkoop Simmons, K., Ruggles, D., Putvin, T., Harris, C., Allen, M., et al. (2004). Community responses and perceived barriers to responding to child maltreatment. *Journal of Community Health, 29*(2), 141–153.

Chao, C., Chen, S., Wang, C., Wu, Y., & Yeh, C. (2003). Psychosocial adjustment among pediatric cancer patients and their parents. *Psychiatry & Clinical Neurosciences, 57*(1), 75–81.

Chronis-Tuscano, A., O'Brien, K., Johnston, C., Jones, H., Clarke, T., Raggi, V., et al. (2011). The relation between maternal ADHD symptoms & improvement in child behavior following brief behavioral parent training is mediated by change in negative parenting. *Journal of Abnormal Child Psychology, 39*(7), 1047–1057.

Davies, E., Rowe, E., & Hassall, I. (2011, October). Preventing neglect of children in their early years: Some thoughts on action. *Social Work Now*, 3–9.

Drummond, J., Fleming, D., McDonald, L., & Kysela, G. M. (2005). Randomized controlled trial of a family problem-solving intervention. *Clinical Nursing Research, 14*(1), 57–80.

Fernandes, C., Muller, R., & Rodin, G. (2012). Predictors of parenting stress in patients with haematological cancer. *Journal of Psychosocial Oncology, 30*(1), 81–86.

Gewirtz, A., Erbes, C., Polusny, M., Forgatch, M., & DeGarmo, D. (2011). Helping military families through the deployment process: Strategies to support parenting. *Professional Psychology: Research and Practice, 42*(1), 56–62.

Hazen, A. L., Connelly, C. D., Kelleher, K. J., Barth, R. P., & Landsverk, J. A. (2006). Female caregivers' experiences with intimate partner violence and behavior problems in children investigated as victims of maltreatment. *Pediatrics, 117*(1), 99–109.

Humenick, S. S., & Howell, O. S. (2003). Perinatal experiences: The association of stress, childbearing, breastfeeding, and early mothering. *Journal of Perinatal Education, 12*(3), 16–41.

Kearney, J. A. (2004). Early reactions to frustration: Developmental trends in anger, individual response styles, and caregiving risk implications in infancy. *Journal of Child & Adolescent Psychiatric Nursing, 17*(3), 105–112.

Lee, C. Y., Lee, J., & August, G. (2011). Financial stress, parental depressive symptoms, parenting practices, and children's externalizing problem behaviors: Underlying processes. *Family Relations, 60*(4), 476–490.

Palusci, V., Crum, P., Bliss, R., & Bavolek, S. (2008). Changes in parenting attitudes and knowledge among inmates and other at-risk populations after a family nurturing program. *Children and Youth Services Review, 30*(1), 79–89.

Scott, L. (2003). Vulnerability, need and significant harm: An analysis tool. *Community Practitioner, 76*(12), 468–473.

Shapiro, A., Nahm, E., Gottman, J., & Content, K. (2011). Bringing baby home together: Examining the impact of a couple-focused intervention on the dynamics within family play. *American Journal of Orthopsychiatry, 81*(3), 337–350.

Swartz, M. K. (2005). Parenting preterm infants: A meta-synthesis. *MCN: The American Journal of Maternal Child Nursing, 30*(2), 115–120.

Tucker, S., Klotzbach, L., Olsen, G., Voss, J., Huus, B., Olsen, R., et al. (2006). Lessons learned in translating research evidence on early intervention programs into clinical care. *MCN: The American Journal of Maternal Child Nursing, 31*(5), 325–331.

Velez, M., Jansson, L., Montoya, I., Schweitzer, W., Golden, A., & Svikis, D. (2004). Parenting knowledge among substance abusing women in treatment. *Journal of Substance Abuse Treatment, 27*(3), 215–222.

Vuijk, P., VanLier, P., Huizink, A., Verhulst, F., & Crijnen, A. (2006). Prenatal smoking predicts non-responsiveness to an intervention targeting attention-deficit/hyperactivity symptoms in elementary schoolchildren. *The Journal of Child Psychology and Psychiatry, 47*(9), 891–901.

Wade, J. (2006). "Crying alone with my child": Parenting a school age child diagnosed with bipolar disorder. *Issues in Mental Health Nursing, 27*(8), 885–903.

Wright, M. O., Fopma-Loy, J., & Fischer, S. (2005). Multidimensional assessment of resilience in mothers who are child sexual abuse survivors. *Child Abuse & Neglect, 29*(10), 1173–1193.

Parenting, Impaired, Risk for

Akesson, B., Smyth, J., Mandell, D., Doan, T., Donina, K., & Hoven, C. (2012). Parental involvement with the criminal justice system and the effects on their children: A collaborative model for researching vulnerable families. *Social Work in Public Health, 27*(1–2), 148–164.

Bakewell-Sachs, S., & Gennaro, S. (2004). Parenting the post-NICU premature infant. *MCN: The American Journal of Maternal Child Nursing, 29*(6), 398–403.

Beeber, L. S., & Miles, M. S. (2003). Maternal mental health and parenting in poverty. *Annual Review of Nursing Research, 21,* 303–331.

Crespo-Fierro, M. (2011). Supporting breast-feeding when a woman is homeless. *International Journal of Nursing Knowledge, 22*(2), 103–107.

Gewirtz, A., Erbes, C., Polusny, M., Forgatch, M., & DeGarmo, D. (2011). Helping military families through the deployment process: Strategies to support parenting. *Professional Psychology: Research and Practice, 42*(1), 56–62.

Leonard, L. G. (2002). Prenatal behavior of multiples: Implications for families and nurses. *JOGNN: Journal of Obstetric, Gynecologic, & Neonatal Nursing, 31*(3), 248–255.

Leonard, L. G., & Denton, J. (2006). Preparation for parenting multiple birth children. *Early Human Development, 82*(6), 371–378.

Saltzman, W., Lester, P., Beardslee, W., Layne, C., Woodward, K., & Nash, W. (2011). Mechanisms of risk and resilience in military families: Theoretical and empirical basis of a family-focused resilience enhancement program. *Clinical Child and Family Psychology Review, 14*(3), 213–230.

Shapiro, A., Krysik, J., & Pennar, A. (2011). Who are the fathers in healthy families Arizona? An examination of father data in at-risk families. *American Journal of Orthopsychiatry, 81*(3), 327–336.

Parenting, Readiness for Enhanced

Alexander, D., Powell, G. M., Williams, P., White, M., & Conlon, M. (1988). Anxiety levels of rooming-in and non-rooming-in parents of young hospitalized children. *Maternal-Child Nursing Journal, 17*(2), 79–98.

Cooley, M. (2011). Short-term home visiting for parents. *Journal of Family Social Work, 14*(2), 179–188.

Forde, H., Lane, H., McCloskey, D., McManus, V., & Tierney, E. (2004). Link family support—an evaluation of an in-home support service. *Journal of Psychiatric & Mental Health Nursing, 11*(6), 698–704.

Franck, L. S., & Spencer, C. (2003). Parent visiting and participation in infant caregiving activities in a neonatal unit. *Birth: Issues in Perinatal Care, 30*(1), 31–35.

Horowitz, J. A., Logsdon, M. C., & Anderson, J. K. (2005). Measurement of maternal-infant interaction. *Journal of the American Psychiatric Nurses Association, 11*(3), 164–172.

Kendall, S., & Bloomfield, L. (2005). Developing and validating a tool to measure parenting self-efficacy. *Journal of Advanced Nursing, 51*(2), 174–181.

Klaus, M., & Kennell, J. (1976). *Maternal–infant bonding.* St. Louis, MO: Mosby.

McCartney, P. (2012). Social networking safety for children and adolescents. *MCN, American Journal of Maternal Child Nursing, 37*(1), 65.

Meadows, S. (2011). The association between perceptions of social support and maternal mental health: A cumulative perspective. *Journal of Family Issues, 32*(2), 181–208.

Shokoohi-Yekta, M., Parand, A., Zamani, N., Lotfi, S., & Ayazi, M. (2011). Teaching problem-solving for parents: Effects on children's misbehavior. *Procedia — Social and Behavioral Sciences, 30,* 163–166.

Perfusion: Gastrointestinal, Risk for Ineffective

Albert, N. (2012). Fluid heart management strategies in heart failure. *Critical Care Nurse, 32*(2), 20–32.

Fournell, A., Scheeren, T., Picker, O., & Schwarte, L. (2012). Pharmacologic interventions to improve splanchnic oxygenation during ventilation with positive end-expiratory pressure. *Oxygen Transport to Tissue XXXIII. Advances in Experimental Medicine and Biology, 737*(P. 4), 235–238.

McSweeney, M., Garwood, S., Levin, J., Marino, M., Wang, S., Kardatzke, D., et al., Investigators of the Ischemic Research and Education Foundation of the Multicenter Study of Perioperative Ischemia Research Group. (2004). Adverse gastrointestinal complications after cardiopulmonary bypass: Can outcome be predicted from preoperative risk factors? *Anesthesia and Analgesia, 98*(6), 1610–1617.

Muller, L., Jaber, S., Molinari, N., Favier, L., Larché, J., Motte, G., et al. (2012). Fluid management and risk factors for renal dysfunction in patients with severe sepsis and/or septic shock. *Critical Car, 16*(R34). Retrieved from http://ccforum.com/content/pdf/cc11213.pdf

Seller-Pérez, G., Herrera-Gutiérrez, M., Aragón-González, C., Granados, M., Dominguez, J., Navarrete, R., et al. (2012). Bladder mucosal CO_2 compared with gastric mucosal CO_2 as a marker for low perfusion states in septic shock. *The Scientific World Journal, Volume 2012.* Article ID 360378. DOI: 10.1100/2012/360378.

Perioperative Positioning Injury, Risk for

Ali, A., Breslin, D., Hardman, H., & Martin, G. (2003). Unusual presentation and complication of the prone position for spinal surgery. *Journal of Clinical Anesthesia, 15,* 471–473.

Connolly, M., & Grench, A. (2011). Special considerations in the perioperative preparation of the obese child: An evidence-based review. *Bariatric Nursing and Surgical Patient Care, 6*(2), 91–94.

Dority, J., Hassan, Z.-U., & Chau, D. (2011). Anesthetic implications of obesity in the surgical patient. *Clinics in Colon and Rectal Surgery, 24*(4), 222–228.

Facaros, Z., Stapleton, J., Polyzois, V., & Zgonis, T. (2011). Management of foot and ankle trauma. *Perioperative Nursing Clinics, 6*(1), 35–43.

Grover, V., & Jangra, K. (2012). Perioperative vision loss: A complication to watch out. *Journal of Anaesthesiology Clinical Pharmacology, 28*(1), 11–16.

Harker, R., McLauchlan, R., MacDonald, H., Waterman, C., & Waterman, H. (2002). Endless nights: Patients' experiences of posturing face down following vitreoretinal surgery. *Ophthalmic Nursing: International Journal of Ophthalmic Nursing, 6*(2), 11–15.

Iyer, U., Koh, K., Chia, N., Macachor, J., & Cheng, A. (2011). Perioperative risk factors in obese patients for bariatric surgery: A Singapore experience. *Singapore Medical Journal, 52*(2), 91–94.

Lalkhen, A., & Bhatia, K. (2012). Perioperative peripheral nerve injuries. *Continuing Education in Anaesthesia, Critical Care & Pain, 12*(1), 38–42.

Li, W., Lee, T., & Yim, A. (2004). Shoulder function after thoracic surgery. *Thoracic Surgery Clinics, 14*(3), 331–343.

Litwiller, J., Wells, R., Jr., Halliwill, J., Carmichael, S., & Warner, M. (2004). Effect of lithotomy positions on strain of the obturator and lateral femoral cutaneous nerves. *Clinical Anatomy, 17,* 45–49.

Middlebrooks, B., & Winters, T. (2011). Common perioperative complications in the pediatric day surgery setting of a patient with an elevated BMI: A resource guide to the literature on the care of the obese pediatric surgical patient. *Bariatric Nursing and Surgical Patient Care, 6*(3), 155–157.

Murphy, E. (2004). Negligence cases concerning positioning injuries. *AORN Journal, 80*(2), 311–312, 314.

Pandey, R., Garg, R., Darlong, V., Punj, J., & Chandralekha. (2011). *Journal of Robotic Surgery*. SpringerLink, DOI: 10.1007/s11701-011-030207. Retrieved February 11, 2012, from http://www.springerlink.com/content/p051x482n6029402/

Sherman, C., Rose, P., Pierce, L., Yaszemski, M., & Sim, F. (2012). Prospective assessment of patient morbidity from prone sacral positioning. *Journal of Neurosurgery: Spine, 16*(1), 51–56.

Stremler, R., Hodnett, E., Petryshen, P., Stevens, B., Weston, J., & Willan, A. R. (2005). Randomized controlled trial of hands-and-knees positioning for occipitoposterior position in labor. *Birth: Issues in Perinatal Care, 32*(4), 243–251.

Waters, T., Short, M., Lloyd, J., Baptiste, A., Butler, L., Petersen, C., et al. (2011). AORN ergonomic tool 2: Positioning and repositioning the supine patient on the OR bed. *AORN Journal, 93*(4), 445–449.

Poisoning, Risk for

American Academy of Pediatrics. (2012). *Poison prevention*. Retrieved February 13, 2012, from http://www.healthychildren.org/English/safety-prevention/all-around/Pages/Poison-Prevention.aspx

Bond, G., Woodward, R., & Ho, M. (2012). The growing impact of pediatric pharmaceutical poisoning. *The Journal of Pediatrics, 160*(2), 265–270.

Bradberry, S., & Vale, A. (2012). Management of poisoning: Antidotes. *Medicine, 40*(2), 69–70.

Brooks, D., Levine, M., O'Connor, A., French, R., & Curry, S. (2011). Toxicology in the ICU. Part 2: Specific toxing. *Chest, 140*(4), 1072–1085.

Brown, M. J., McLaine, P., Dixon, S., & Simon, P. (2006). A randomized, community-based trial of home visiting to reduce blood lead levels in children. *Pediatrics, 117*(1), 147–153.

Centers for Disease Control & Prevention. (2005). *Third national report on human exposure to environmental chemicals: Executive summary* (NCEH Pub # 05–0725). Atlanta, GA: Author.

Erickson, L., & Thompson, T. (2005). A review of a preventable poison: Pediatric lead poisoning. *Journal for Specialists in Pediatric Nursing, 10*(4), 171–182.

Gutierrez, J., Negrón, J., & García-Fragoso, L. (2011). Parental practices for prevention of home poisoning in children 1-6 years of age. *Journal of Community Health, 36*(5), 845–848.

Hamson, N., & Weaver, L. (2011). Residential carbon monoxide alarm use: Opportunities for poisoning prevention. *Journal of Environmental Health, 73*(6), 30–33.

Hawkins, L. (2006). Managing poisoning by over-the-counter analgesics. *Practice Nurse, 32*(1), 20–21.

Khan, F. (2011). Take home lead exposure in children of oil field workers. *Journal of the Oklahoma State Medical Association, 104*(6), 252–253.

Kuehn, B. (2012). Panel advises tougher limits on lead exposure. *The Journal of the American Medical Association, 307*(5), 445.

Osterhoudt, K. C., Alpern, E. R., Durbin, D., Nadel, F., & Henretig, F. M. (2004). Activated charcoal administration in a pediatric emergency department. *Pediatric Emergency Care, 20*(8), 493–498.

Poręba, R., Poręba, M., Gać, P., Steinmetz-Beck, A., Beck, B., Pilecki, W., et al. (2011). Electrocardiographic changes in workers occupationally exposed to lead. *Annals of Noninvasive Electrocardiology, 16*(1), 33–40.

Smithson, J., Garside, R., & Pearson, M. (2011). Barriers to, and facilitators of, the prevention of unintentional injury in children in the home: A systematic review and synthesis of qualitative research. *Injury Prevention, 17*(2), 119–126.

Vale, A., & Bradberry, S. (2012). Management of poisoning: Initial management and need for admission. *Medicine, 40*(2), 65–66.

Valler-Jones, T., & Wedgbury, K. (2005). Clinical skills. Measuring blood pressure using the mercury sphygmomanometer. *British Journal of Nursing (BJN), 14*(3), 145–150.

Post-Trauma Syndrome

Andreasen, N. (2011). What is post-traumatic stress disorder? *Dialogues in Clinical Neuroscience, 13*(3), 240–243.

Bender, S. (1995). Crisis intervention. In G. Stuart & S. Sundeen (Eds.), *Principles and practice of psychiatric nursing* (5th ed.). St. Louis, MO: Mosby-Year Book.

Berkowitz, S., Stover, C., & Marans, S. (2011). The child and family traumatic stress intervention: Secondary prevention for youth at risk of developing PTSD. *The Journal of Child Psychology and Psychiatry, 52*(6), 676–685.

Brennaman, L. (2012). Crisis emergencies for individuals with severe, persistent mental illnesses: A situation-specific theory. *Archives of Psychiatric Nursing.*

DOI: http://dx.doi.org/10.1016/j.apnu.2011.11.001. Retrieved February 13, 2012, from http://www.sciencedirect.com/science/article/pii/S0883941711001579

DeVoe, E., Klein, T., Bannon, W., & Miranda-Julian, C. (2011). Young children in the aftermath of the World Trade Center attacks. *Psychological Trauma: Theory, Research, Practice, and Policy, 3*(1), 1–7.

Ellis, H. (2011). The crisis intervention team: A revolutionary tool for law enforcement: The psychiatric-mental health nursing perspective. *Journal of Psychosocial Nursing and Mental Health Services, 49*(11), 37–43.

Fehler-Cabral, G., Campbell, R., & Patterson, D. (2012). Adult sexual assault survivors' experiences with sexual assault nurse examiners (SANEs). *Journal of Interpersonal Violence*. DOI: 10.1177/0886260511403761. Retrieved February 13, 2012, from http://jiv.sagepub.com/content/early/2011/05/10/0886260511403761.abstract

Green, B. L., & Lindy, J. D. (1994). Post-traumatic stress disorder in victims of disasters. *Psychiatric Clinics of North America, 17,* 301–309.

Hudson, P. (2011). Effective treatments for PTSD: Practice guidelines from the international society for traumatic stress studies. *British Journal of Guidance & Counselling, 39*(2), 194–195.

Kanel, K. (2010). *A guide to crisis intervention*. Belmont, CA: Brooks/Cole, Cengage Learning.

Lasiuk, G. C., & Hegadoren, K. M. (2006a). Posttraumatic stress disorder part I: Historical development of the concept. *Perspectives in Psychiatric Care, 42*(1), 13–20.

Lasiuk, G. C., & Hegadoren, K. M. (2006b). Posttraumatic stress disorder part II: Development of the construct within the North American psychiatric taxonomy. *Perspectives in Psychiatric Care, 42*(2), 72–81.

Margolin, G., & Vickerman, K. (2011). Posttraumatic stress in children and adolescents exposed to family violence: I. Overview and issues. *Couple and Family Psychology: Research and Practice, 1*(S), 63–73.

Martsolf, D. S., & Draucker, C. B. (2005). Psychotherapy approaches for adult survivors of childhood sexual abuse: An integrative review of outcomes research. *Issues in Mental Health Nursing, 26*(8), 801–825.

Palompon, D., Lapa, M., Caneda, H., & Gonzoga, J. (2011). The caregiver's and nurse therapist's experiences on Gestalt therapy. *Asian Journal of Health, 1*(1), 46–57.

Parent, R. (2011). The police use of deadly force in British Columbia: Mental illness and crisis intervention. *Journal of Police Crisis Negotiations, 11*(1), 57–71.

Senneseth, M., Alsaker, K., & Natvig, K. (2012). Health-related quality of life and post-traumatic stress disorder symptoms in accident and emergency attenders suffering from psychosocial crises: A longitudinal study. *Journal of Advanced Nursing, 68*(2), 402–413.

Post-Trauma Syndrome, Risk for

Note: Also see the preceding bibliography for Post-Trauma Syndrome.

Frauenfelder, F., Müller-Staub, M., Needham, K., & Van Achterberg, T. (2011). Nursing phenomena in inpatient psychiatry. *Journal of Psychiatric and Mental Health Nursing, 18*(3), 221–235.

Hafstad, G., Haavind, H., & Jensen, T. (2011). Parenting after a natural disaster: A qualitative study of Norwegian families surviving the 2004 tsunami in Southeast Asia. *Journal of Child and Family Studies*. DOI: 10.1007/s10826-011-94764-z. Retrieved February 13, 2012, from http://www.springerlink.com/content/mlt52p7617675p71/

Hagenaara, M., & Arntz, A. (2012). Reduced intrusion development after post-trauma imagery rescripting; an experimental study. *Journal of Behavior Therapy and Experimental Psychiatry, 43*(2), 808–814.

Lasiuk, G. C., & Hegadoren, K. M. (2006a). Posttraumatic stress disorder part I: Historical development of the concept. *Perspectives in Psychiatric Care, 42*(1), 13–20.

Lasiuk, G. C., & Hegadoren, K. M. (2006b). Posttraumatic stress disorder part II: Development of the construct within the North American psychiatric taxonomy. *Perspectives in Psychiatric Care, 42*(2), 72–81.

Martsolf, D. S., & Draucker, C. B. (2005). Psychotherapy approaches for adult survivors of childhood sexual abuse: An integrative review of outcomes research. *Issues in Mental Health Nursing, 26*(8), 801–825.

Renshaw, K. (2011). An integrated model of risk and protective factors for post-deployment PTSD symptoms in OEF/OIF era combat veterans. *Journal of Affective Disorders, 128*(3), 321–326.

Power, Readiness for Enhanced

Anderson, R., & Funnell, M. (2005). Patient empowerment: Reflections on the challenge of fostering the adoption of a new paradigm. *Patient Education and Counseling, 57*(2), 153–157.

Harkness, J. (2005). Patient involvement: A vital principle for patient-centered health care. *World Hospitals and Health Services, 41*(2), 12–16, 40–43.

Jeng, C., Yang, S., Chang, P., & Tsao, L. (2004). Menopausal women: Perceiving continuous power through the experience of regular exercise. *Journal of Clinical Nursing, 13,* 447–454.

Kettunen, T., Liimatainen, L., Villberg, J., & Perko, U. (2006). Developing empowering health counseling measurement: Preliminary results. *Patient Education & Counseling, 64*(1), 159–166.

McGuckin, M., Storr, J., Longtin, Y., Allegranzi, B., & Pittet, D. (2011). Patient empowerment and multimodal hand hygiene promotion: A win-win strategy. *American Journal of Medical Quality, 26*(1), 10–17.

Messias, D. K. H., Fore, E. M., McLoughlin, K., & Parra-Medina, D. (2005). Adult roles in community-based youth empowerment programs. *Family & Community Health, 28*(4), 320–337.

Oh, H., & Lee, B. (2012). The effect of computer-mediated social support in online communities on patient empowerment and doctor-patient communication. *Health Communication, 27*(1), 30–41.

Pender, N., Murdaugh, C., & Parsons, M. (2006). *Health promotion in nursing practice* (5th ed.). Stamford, CT: Appleton & Lange.

Shearer, N., & Reed, P. (2004). Empowerment: Reformulation of a non-Rogerian concept. *Nursing Science Quarterly, 17,* 253–259.

Suter, P., Suter, W., & Johnston, D. (2011). Theory-based telehealth and patient empowerment. *Population Health Management, 14*(2), 87–92.

Tang, T., Funnell, M., Gillard, M., Nwankwo, R., & Heisler, M. (2011). The development of a pilot training program for peer leaders in diabetes: Process and content. *The Diabetes Educator, 37*(1), 67–77.

Wright, B. (2004). Trust and power in adults: An investigation using Rogers' science of unitary human beings. *Nursing Science Quarterly, 17,* 139–146.

Powerlessness

(Also see the bibliography for Powerlessness, Readiness for Enhanced, preceding.)

Altman, M. R., & Lydon-Rochelle, M. T. (2006). Prolonged second stage of labor and risk of adverse maternal and perinatal outcomes: A systematic review. *Birth: Issues in Perinatal Care, 33*(4), 315–322.

Bartlett, Y., & Coulson, N. (2011). An investigation into the empowerment effects of using online support groups and how this affects health professional/patient communication. *Patient Education and Counseling, 83*(1), 113–119.

Jones, P., Winslow, B., Lee, J., Burns, M., & Zhang, X. (2011). Development of a caregiver empowerment model to promote positive outcomes. *Journal of Family Nursing, 17*(1), 11–28.

Lambert, V. A., & Lambert, C. E. (1981). Role theory and the concept of powerlessness. *Journal of Psychosocial Nursing and Mental Health Services, 19*(9), 11–14.

Milberg, A., & Strang, P. (2011). Protection against perceptions of powerlessness and helplessness during palliative care: The family members' perspective. *Palliative and Supportive Care, 9*(3), 251–262.

Miller, J. (1983). *Powerlessness: Coping with chronic illness*. Philadelphia, PA: FA Davis.

Miller, J. F. (1985). Concept development of powerlessness: A nursing diagnosis. In J. F. Miller (Ed.), *Coping with chronic illness, overcoming powerlessness*. Philadelphia, PA: FA Davis.

Mottram, A. (2011). Patients' experiences of day surgery: A Parsonian analysis. *Journal of Advanced Nursing, 67*(1), 140–148.

Mutchler, M., Wagner, G., Cowgill, B., McKay, T., Risley, B., & Bogart, L. (2011). AIDS care: Psychological and socio-medical aspects of AIDS/HIV. *AIDS Care, 23*(1), 79–90.

Nygårdh, A., Malm, D., Wikby, K., & Ahlström, G. (2012). The experience of empowerment in the patient–staff encounter: The patient's perspective. *Journal of Clinical Nursing, 21*(5–6), 897–904.

O'Heath, K. (1991). Powerlessness. In M. Maas, K. Buckwalter, & M. Hardy (Eds.), *Nursing diagnoses and interventions for the elderly*. Redwood City, CA: Addison-Wesley Nursing.

Richmond, T. S., Metcalf, J., Daly, M., & Kish, J. R. (1992). Powerlessness in acute spinal cord injury patients: A descriptive study. *Journal of Neuroscience Nursing, 24*(3), 146–152.

Staples, P., Baruth, P., Jefferies, M., & Warder, L. (1994). Empowering the angry patient. *Canadian Nurse, 90*(4), 28–30.

Vanwesenbeeck, I. (2005). Burnout among female indoor sex workers. *Archives of Sexual Behavior, 34*(6), 627–639.

Wang, L.-M., & Chiou, C.-P. (2011). Effectiveness of interactive multimedia CD on self-care and powerlessness in hemodialysis patients. *Journal of Nursing Research, 19*(2), 102–111.

Powerlessness, Risk for

(Also see the bibliography for the diagnosis, Powerlessness, Readiness for Enhanced.)

Andershed, B., & Harstäde, C. (2007). Next of kin's feelings of guilt and shame in end-of-life care. *Contemporary Nurse: A Journal of the Australian Nursing Profession, 27*(1), 61–72.

Fisker, T., & Strandmark, M. (2007). Experiences of surviving spouse of terminally ill spouse: A phenomenological study of an altruistic perspective. *Scandinavian Journal of Caring Science, 21*(2), 274–281.

Fuller, S. (1978). Inhibiting helplessness in elderly people. *Journal of Gerontological Nursing, 4,* 18–21.

Hägglund, D., & Ahlström, G. (2007). The meaning of women's experience of living with long-term urinary incontinence is powerlessness. *Journal of Clinical Nursing, 16*(10), 1946–1954.

Kain, V. (2007). Moral distress and providing care to dying babies in neonatal nursing. *International Journal of Palliative Nursing, 13*(5), 243–248.

Kersten, L. (1990). Changes in self concept during pulmonary rehabilitation; Part 1 and 2. *Heart and Lung, 19,* 456–470.

Larsson, I., Sahlsten, M., Segesten, K., & Plos, K. (2011). Patients' perceptions of barriers for participation in nursing care. *Scandinavian Journal of Caring Sciences, 25*(3), 575–582.

Stephenson, C. A. (1979). Powerlessness and chronic illness: Implications for nursing. *Baylor Nursing Educator, 1*(1), 17–28.

Thomas, S., & Gonzalez-Prendes, A. (2009). Powerlessness, anger, and stress in African American women: Implications for physical and emotional health. *Health Care for Women International, 30*(1–2), 93–113.

Van Den Tillaart, S., Kurtz, D., & Cash, P. (2009). Powerlessness, marginalized identity, and silencing of health concerns: Voiced realities of women living with a mental health diagnosis. *International Journal of Mental Health Nursing, 18*(3), 153–163.

Protection, Ineffective

Adams, D., & Elliott, T. S. J. (2007). Skin antiseptics used prior to intravascular catheter insertion. *British Journal of Nursing (BJN), 16*(5), 278–280.

Altaf, S., Oppenheimer, C., Shaw, R., Waugh, J., & Dixon-Woods, M. (2006). Practices and views on fetal heart monitoring: A structured observation and interview study. *BJOG: An International Journal of Obstetrics & Gynaecology, 113*(4), 409–418.

Altman, M. R., & Lydon-Rochelle, M. T. (2006). Prolonged second stage of labor and risk of adverse maternal and perinatal outcomes: A systematic review. *Birth: Issues in Perinatal Care, 33*(4), 315–322.

American Association of Critical-Care Nurses (AACN). (2008). *AACN practice alert. Ventilator associated pneumonia.* Retrieved February 14, 2012, from http://www.aacn.org/WD/Practice/Docs/Ventilator_Associated_Pneumonia_1-2008.pdf

Aragon, D., & Sole, M. L. (2006). Implementing best practice strategies to prevent infection in the ICU. *Critical Care Nursing Clinics of North America, 18*(4), 441–452.

Arrowsmith, V. A., Maunder, J. A., Sargent, R. J., & Taylor, R. (2006). Removal of nail polish and finger rings to prevent surgical infection. *Cochrane Library* (4).

Belkin, N. L. (2006). Opinion. Masks, barriers, laundering, and gloving: Where is the evidence? *AORN Journal, 84*(4), 655.

Betsy Lehman Center for Patient Safety and Medical Error Reduction, JSI Research and Training Institute, Inc. (2008, January 31). *Prevention and control of healthcare-associated infections in Massachusetts. Part 1: Final recommendations of the Expert Panel.* Boston, MA: Massachusetts Department of Public Health; pp. 69–82. National Guideline Clearinghouse Brief Summary. Prevention of bloodstream infections. Retrieved February 14, 2012, from http://www.guideline.gov/summary/summary.aspx?doc_id=12922&nbr=006636&string=intravenous+AND+administ ration

Britto, M. T., Pandzik, G. M., Meeks, C. S., & Kotagal, U. R. (2006). Performance improvement. Combining evidence and diffusion of innovation theory to enhance influenza immunization. *Joint Commission Journal on Quality & Patient Safety, 32*(8), 426–432.

Camp-Sorrell, D. (Ed.). (2011). *Access device guidelines: Recommendations for nursing practice and education* (3rd ed.). Pittsburgh, PA: Oncology Nursing Society.

Centers for Disease Control and Prevention (CDC). (2008). *Using over-the-counter cough and cold products in children.* Atlanta, GA. Retrieved February 14, 2012, from http://www.fda.gov/ForConsumers/ConsumerUpdates/ucm048515.htm#TipsforPa rentsandCaregivers

Coffin, W., Klompas, M., Classen, D., Arias, K. M., Podgorny, K., Anderson, D. J., et al., & the Healthcare-Associated Infections Task Force. (2008). Guideline summary: Strategies to prevent ventilator-associated pneumonia in acute care hospitals. *Infection Control and Hospital Epidemiology, 29*(Suppl. 1), S31–S40. National Guideline Clearinghouse (NGC) [Web site]. Rockville, MD. Retrieved February 14, 2012, from http://www.guideline.gov/content.aspx?d=13396

Coia, J. E., Duckworth, G. J., Edwards, D. I., Farrington, M., Fry, C., Humphreys, H., et al. (2006). Guidelines for the control and prevention of meticillin-resistant staphylococcus aureus (MRSA) in healthcare facilities. *Journal of Hospital Infection, 63,* S1–44.

Cutter, J., & Gammon, J. (2007). Review of standard precautions and sharps management in the community. *British Journal of Community Nursing, 12*(2), 54–60.

Institute for Healthcare Improvement (IHI). (n.d.). *Implement the Central line bundle* IHI.org [Web site]. Retrieved February 14, 2012, from http://www.ihi.org/IHI/Topics/CriticalCare/IntensiveCare/Changes/ImplementtheCentralLineBundle.htm

Jones, C. A. (2006). Central venous catheter infection in adults in acute hospital settings. *British Journal of Nursing (BJN), 15*(7), 362–368.

Keller, S., Daley, K., Hyde, J., Greif, R. S., & Church, D. R. (2005). Hepatitis C prevention with nurses. *Nursing & Health Sciences, 7*(2), 99–106.

Kennedy, R. D., & Cullamar, K. (2006). Immunizations for older adults. *Annals of Long Term Care, 14*(12), 19–20.

Marschall, J., Mermel, L., Classen, D., Arias, K. M., Podgorny, K., Anderson, D. J., et al. (2008, October). Guideline summary. Strategies to prevent central line-associated bloodstream infections in acute care hospitals. *Infection Control and Hospital Epidemiology, 29*(Suppl. 1), S22–S30. National Guideline Clearinghouse (NGC) [Web site]. Rockville, MD. Retrieved February 14, 2012, from http://www.guideline.gov/summary/summary.aspx?view_id=1&doc_id=13395

Maselli, D., & Restrepo, M. (2011). Strategies in the prevention of ventilator-associated pneumonia. *Therapeutic Advances in Respiratory Disease, 5*(2), 131–141.

Mateoso, J., Gonzalez, N., Sadaba, M., et al. (2011). Nursing care in the prevention of ventilator-associated pneumonia. *Enferm Intensive, 22*(1), 22–30.

Nirenberg, A., Bush, A. P., Davis, A., Friese, C. R., Gillespie, T. W., & Rice, R. D. (2006a). Neutropenia: State of the knowledge part I. *Oncology Nursing Forum, 33*(6), 1193–1201.

Nirenberg, A., Bush, A. P., Davis, A., Friese, C. R., Gillespie, T. W., & Rice, R. D. (2006b). Neutropenia: State of the knowledge part II. *Oncology Nursing Forum, 33*(6), 1202–1208.

O'Grady, N. P., Alexander, M., Burns, L. A., Dellinger, E. P., Garland, J., Heard, S. O., et al., & Healthcare Infection Control Practices Advisory Committee (HICPAC). (2011). *Guidelines for the prevention of intravascular catheter-related infections, 2011.* Atlanta, GA: Centers for Disease Control and Prevention (CDC).

O'Keefe-McCarthy, S. (2006). Evidence-based nursing strategies to prevent ventilator-acquired pneumonia. *Dynamics, 17*(1), 8–11.

Parer, J. T., King, T., Flanders, S., Fox, M., & Kilpatrick, S. J. (2006). Fetal acidemia and electronic fetal heart rate patterns: Is there evidence of an association? *Journal of Maternal-Fetal & Neonatal Medicine, 19*(5), 289–294.

Polovich, M., White, J., & Kelleher, L. (Eds.) (2006). Chemotherapy and biotherapy guidelines and recommendations for practice. *Journal of Infusion Nursing, 29* (Suppl. 1), S1–S92.

Reading, R. (2006). Impact of adverse publicity on MMR vaccine uptake: A population based analysis of vaccine uptake records for one million children, born 1987–2004. *Child: Care, Health & Development, 32*(5), 608–609.

Thomas, R. E., Jefferson, T. O., Demicheli, V., & Rivetti, D. (2006). Influenza vaccination for health-care workers who work with elderly people in institutions: A systematic review. *Lancet Infectious Diseases, 6*(5), 273–279.

U.S. Department of Agriculture (USDA), Center for Nutrition Policy and Promotion. (2011, January, 31). *2010 Dietary guidelines for Americans*. Retrieved February 14, 2012, from http://www.cnpp.usda.gov/DGAs2010-PolicyDocument.htm

Webster, J., & Pritchard, M. A. (2006). Gowning by attendants and visitors in newborn nurseries for prevention of neonatal morbidity and mortality. *Cochrane Library* (4).

Rape-Trauma Syndrome

Anderson, S., McClain, N., & Riviello, R. J. (2006). Genital findings of women after consensual and nonconsensual intercourse. *Journal of Forensic Nursing, 2*(2), 59–65.

Badmaeva, V. (2011). Consequences of sexual abuse in children and adolescents. *Neuroscience and Behavioral Physiology, 41*(3), 259–262.

Botello, S., King, D., & Ratner, E. (2003). The SANE approach to care of the adult sexual assault survivor. *Topics in Emergency Medicine, 25*(3), 199–228.

Brown, K., Streubert, G. E., & Burgess, A. W. (2004). Effectively detect and manage elder abuse. *Nurse Practitioner, 29*(8), 22

Burgess, A. W., Brown, K., Bell, K., Ledray, L. E., & Poarch, J. C. (2005). Forensic nursing files. Sexual abuse of older adults: Assessing for signs of a serious crime—and reporting it. *American Journal of Nursing, 105*(10), 66–71.

Burgess, A. W., Hanrahan, N. P., & Baker, T. (2005). Forensic markers in elder female sexual abuse cases. *Clinics in Geriatric Medicine, 21*(2), 399–412.

Burgess, A. W., Watt, M. E., Brown, K. M., & Petrozzi, D. (2006). Management of elder sexual abuse cases in critical care settings. *Critical Care Nursing Clinics of North America, 18*(3), 313–319.

Campbell, R., Bybee, D., Kelley, K., Dworkin, E., & Paatterson, D. (2011). The impact of sexual assault nurse examiner (SANE) program services on law enforcement investigational practices: A meditational analysis. *Criminal Justice and Behavior, 39,* 169–184.

Campbell, R., Townsend, S. M., Long, S. M., Kinnison, K. E., Pulley, E. M., Adames, S. B., et al. (2006). Responding to sexual assault victims' medical and emotional needs: A national study of the services provided by SANE programs. *Research in Nursing & Health, 29*(5), 384–398.

Du Mont, J., & Parnis, D. (2003). Forensic nursing in the context of sexual assault: Comparing the opinions and practices of nurse examiners and nurses. *Applied Nursing Research, 16*(3), 173–183.

Enns, C. (2011). Feminist counseling as a pathway to recovery (Chapter 12). In T. Bryant-Davis (Ed.), *Surviving sexual violence: A guide to recovery and empowerment.* Plymouth, United Kingdom: Rowman & Littlefield.

Flowers, D. (2007). Clinical nurses forum. Providing forensic care "outside of the (evidence) box": One nurse's journey. *Journal of Emergency Nursing, 33*(1), 50–52.

Gavey, N., & Schmidt, J. (2011). "Trauma of rape" discourse: A double-edged template for everyday understandings of the impact of rape? *Violence Against Women, 27*(4), 433–456.

Jenny, C. (2011). Emergency evaluation of children when sexual assault is suspected. *Pediatrics, 128*(2), 374–375.

Lasiuk, G. C., & Hegadoren, K. M. (2006). Posttraumatic stress disorder part II: Development of the construct within the North American psychiatric taxonomy. *Perspectives in Psychiatric Care, 42*(2), 72–81.

Lopez-Bonasso, D., & Smith, T. (2006). Sexual assault kit tracking application (SAKiTA): Technology at work in West Virginia. *Journal of Forensic Nursing, 2*(2), 92–95.

Martin, S. L., Young, S. K., Billings, D. L., & Bross, C. C. (2007). Health care-based interventions for women who have experienced sexual violence. *Trauma, Violence & Abuse, 8*(1), 3–18.

McKenzie-Mohr, S., & Lafrance, M. (2011). Telling stories without the words: 'Tightrope talk' in women's accounts of coming to live well after rape or depression. *Feminism & Psychology, 21*(1), 49–73.

McKibben, W., Shackelford, T., Miner, E., Bates, V., & Liddle, J. (2011). Individual differences in women's rape avoidance behaviors. *Archives of Sexual Behavior, 40*(2), 343–349.

Mahon, S. (2011). Rape myth beliefs and bystander attitudes among incoming college students. *Journal of American College Health, 59*(1), 3–11.

Moor, A., & Farchi, M. (2011). Is rape-related self blame distinct from other post traumatic attributions of blame? A comparison of severity and implications for treatment. *Women & Therapy, 34*(4), 447–460.

Orzeck, T., & Rokach, A. (2011). Relationship trauma: Assessing the criteria of trauma in adult intimate abusive relationships. *International Journal of Psychology and Counselling, 3*(3), 55–61.

Parnis, D., & Du Mont, J. (2002). Examining the standardized application of rape kits: An exploratory study of post-sexual assault professional practices. *Health Care for Women International, 23*(8), 846–853.

Resick, P., Williams, L., Suvak, M., Monson, C., & Gradus, J. (2011, December 19). Long-term outcomes of cognitive–behavioral treatments for posttraumatic stress disorder among female rape survivors. *Journal of Consulting and Clinical Psychology*. DOI: 10.1037/a0026602. Retrieved February 14, 2012, from http://psycnet.apa.org/index.cfm?fa=search.displayRecord&id=7EDFAF90-EEA5-8163-A319-04D83C36FB4C&resultID=1&page=1&dbTab=pa

Sandmoe, A., & Kirkevold, M. (2011). Nurses' clinical assessments of older clients who are suspected victims of abuse: An exploratory study in community care in Norway. *Journal of Clinical Nursing, 20*(1–2), 94–102.

Schofield, S. (2006). Body of evidence. *Emergency Nurse, 13*(9), 9–11.

Senn, C., Gee, S., & Thanke, J. (2011). Emancipatory sexuality education and sexual assault resistance: Does the former enhance the latter? *Psychology of Women Quarterly, 35*(1), 72–91.

Smith, E., Schuler, P., Cosio-Lima, L., & Rotunda, R. (2011). A treatment for rape victims with posttraumatic stress disorder utilizing therapy and aerobic exercise: 2886: Board #185. *Medicine & Science in Sports & Exercise, 43*(5), 818.

Sommers, M. S., Fisher, B. S., & Karjane, H. M. (2005). Using colposcopy in the rape exam: Health care, forensic, and criminal justice issues. *Journal of Forensic Nursing, 1*(1), 28.

Use these tips to collect evidence of sexual assault: Your evidence can make or break a conviction. (2003). *ED Nursing, 6*(3), 34–37.

Relationship, Ineffective

Chandola, T., Marmot, M., & Siegrist, J. (2007). Failed reciprocity in close social relationships and health: Findings from the Whitehall II study. *Journal of Psychosomatic Research, 63*(4), 403–411.

Gearhart, C., & Bodie, G. (2011). Active-empathic listening as a general social skill: Evidence from bivariate and canonical correlations. *Communication Reports, 24*(2), 86–98.

Kouros, C., & Cummings, E. (2011). Transactional relations between marital functioning and depressive symptoms. *American Journal of Orthopsychiatry, 81*(1), 128–138.

McNulty, J., & Fincham, F. (2012). Beyond positive psychology? Toward a contextual view of psychological processes and well-being. *American Psychologist, 67*(2), 101–110.

Morrill, M., Eubanks-Fleming, C., Harp, A., Sollenberger, J., Darling, E., & Cördova, J. (2011). The marriage checkup: Increasing access to marital health care. *Family Process, 50*(4), 471–485.

Murry, V., Harrell, A., Brody, G., Chen, Y., Simons, R., Black, A., et al. (2008). Long-term effects of stressors on relationship well-being and parenting among rural African American women. *Family Relations, 57*(2), 117–127.

Pritchett, R., Kemp, J., Wilson, P., Minnis, H., Bryce, G., & Gillberg, C. (2011). Quick, simple measures of family relationships for use in clinical practice and research. A systematic review. *Family Practice, 28*(2), 172–187.

Sautter, F., Armelie, A., Glynn, S., & Wielt, D. (2011). The development of a couple-based treatment for PTSD in returning veterans. *Professional Psychology: Research and Practice, 42*(1), 63–69.

Starratt, V., Goetz, A., Shackelford, T., McKibbin, W., & Stewart-Williams, S. (2008). Men's partner-directed insults and sexual coercion in intimate relationships. *Journal of Family Violence, 23*(5), 315–323.

Strawbridge, W., Wallhagen, M., & Shema, S. (2010). Spousal interrelations in self-reports of cognition in the context of marital problems. *Gerontology, 57*(2), 148–152.

Relationship, Ineffective, Risk for

Chandola, T., Marmot, M., & Siegrist, J. (2007). Failed reciprocity in close social relationships and health: Findings from the Whitehall II study. *Journal of Psychosomatic Research, 63*(4), 403–411.

Gearhart, C., & Bodie, G. (2011). Active-empathic listening as a general social skill: Evidence from bivariate and canonical correlations. *Communication Reports, 24*(2), 86–98.

Kouros, C., & Cummings, E. (2011). Transactional relations between marital functioning and depressive symptoms. *American Journal of Orthpsychoatry, 81*(1), 128–138.

McNulty, J., & Fincham, F. (2012). Beyond positive psychology? Toward a contextual view of psychological processes and well-being. *American Psychologist, 67*(2), 101–110.

Morrill, M., Eubanks-Fleming, C., Harp, A., Sollenberger, J., Darling, E., & Cördova, J. (2011). The marriage checkup: Increasing access to marital health care. *Family Process, 50*(4), 471–485.

Murry, V., Harrell, A., Brody, G., Chen, Y., Simons, R., Black, A., et al. (2008). Long-term effects of stressors on relationship well-being and parenting among rural African American women. *Family Relations, 57*(2), 117–127.

Pritchett, R., Kemp, J., Wilson, P., Minnis, H., Bryce, G., & Gillberg, C. (2011). Quick, simple measures of family relationships for use in clinical practice and research. A systematic review. *Family Practice, 28*(2), 172–187.

Sautter, F., Armelie, A., Glynn, S., & Wielt, D. (2011). The development of a couple-based treatment for PTSD in returning veterans. *Professional Psychology: Research and Practice, 42*(1), 63–69.

Starratt, V., Goetz, A., Shackelford, T., McKibbin, W., & Stewart-Williams, S. (2008). Men's partner-directed insults and sexual coercion in intimate relationships. *Journal of Family Violence, 23*(5), 315–323.

Strawbridge, W., Wallhagen, M., & Shema, S. (2010). Spousal interrelations in self-reports of cognition in the context of marital problems. *Gerontology, 57*(2), 148–152.

Relationship, Readiness for Enhanced

Casquarelli, E., & Fallon, K. (2011). Nurturing the relationships of all couples: Integrating lesbian, gay, and bisexual concerns into premarital education and counseling programs. *The Journal of Humanistic Counseling, 50*(2), 149–160.

Eldén, S. (2012). Scripts for the 'good couple': Individualization and the reproduction of gender inequality. *Acta Sociologica, 55*(1), 3–18.

Gearhart, C., & Bodie, G. (2011). Active-empathic listening as a general social skill: Evidence from bivariate and canonical correlations. *Communication Reports, 24*(2), 86–98.

Halford, W. (2011). *Marriage and relationship education: What works and how to provide it.* New York: The Guilford Press.

Lambert, N., Fincham, F., LaVallee, D., & Brantley, C. (2012). Praying together and staying together: Couple prayer and trust. *Psychology of Religion and Spirituality, 4*(1), 1–9.

McNulty, J., & Fincham, F. (2012). Beyond positive psychology? Toward a contextual view of psychological processes and well-being. *American Psychologist, 67*(2), 101–110.

Morrill, M., Eubanks-Fleming, C., Harp, A., Sollenberger, J., Darling, E., & Cördova, J. (2011). The marriage checkup: Increasing access to marital health care. *Family Process, 50*(4), 471–485.

Owen, J., Rhoades, G., Stanley, S., & Markman, H. (2011). The role of leaders' working alliance in premarital education. *Journal of Family Psychology, 25*(1), 49–57.

Pritchett, R., Kemp, J., Wilson, P., Minnis, H., Bryce, G., & Gillberg, C. (2011). Quick, simple measures of family relationships for use in clinical practice and research. A systematic review. *Family Practice, 28*(2), 172–187.

Vohs, K., Finkenauer, C., & Baumeister, R. (2011). The sum of friends' and lovers' self-control scores predicts relationship quality. *Social Psychological & Personality Science, 2*(2), 138–145.

Religiosity, Impaired

Burkhart, L., & Solari-Twadell, A. (2001). Spirituality and religiousness: Differentiating the diagnoses through a review of the nursing diagnosis. *Nursing Diagnosis, 12*(2), 44–54.

Burkhart, M. A. (1994). Becoming and connecting: Elements of spirituality for women. *Holistic Nursing Practice, 8,* 12–21.

Corbett, K. (1998). Patterns of spirituality in persons with advanced HIV disease. *Research in Nursing and Health, 21*(2), 143–153.

Cowchock, F., Lasker, J., Toedter, L., Skumanich, S., & Koenig, H. (2009). Religious beliefs affect grieving after pregnancy loss. *Journal of Religion and Health, 49*(4), 485–497.

Guzman, A. B., Dalay, N., Guzman, A. J., de Jesus, L., de Mesa, B., & Flores, J. (2009). Spirituality in nursing: Filipino elderly's concept of, distance from, and involvement with god. *Educational Gerontology, 35*(10), 929–944.

Herrera, A., Lee, J., Nanyonjo, R., Laufman, L., & Torres-Vigil, I. (2009). Religious coping and caregiver well-being in Mexican-American families. *Aging & Mental Health, 13*(1), 84–91.

Hinton, J. (1999). The progress of awareness and acceptance of dying assessed in cancer patients and their caring relatives. *Palliative Medicine, 13*(1), 19–35.

Nelson, C., Jacobson, C., Weinberger, M., Bhaskaran, V., Rosenfeld, B., Breitbart, W., et al. (2009). The role of spirituality in the relationship between religiosity and depression in prostate cancer patients. *Annals of Behavioral Medicine, 38*(2), 105–114.

Quintero, C. (1993). Blood administration in pediatric Jehovah's witness. *Pediatric Nursing, 19*(1), 46–48.

Sessanna, L., Finnell, D., & Jezewski, M. (2007). Spirituality in nursing and health-related literature: A concept analysis. *Journal of Holistic Nursing, 25*(4), 252–262.

Sulmasy, D. (2009). Spirituality, religion, and clinical care. *Chest, 135*(6), 1634–1642.

Wald, F. S., & Bailey, C. (1990). Nurturing the spiritual component in care for the terminally ill. *CARING Magazine, 9*(11), 64–68.

Wong, Y. J., Rew, L., & Slaikeu, K. D. (2006). A systematic review of recent research on adolescent religiosity/spirituality and mental health. *Issues in Mental Health Nursing, 27*(2), 161–183.

Religiosity, Impaired, Risk for

(Also refer to the preceding bibliography for Religiosity, Impaired.)

Emblen, J. D., & Halstead, L. (1993). Spiritual needs and interventions: Comparing the views of patients, nurses and chaplains. *Clinical Nurse Specialist, 7,* 175–182.

Goggin, K., Murray, T. S., Malcarne, V. L., Brown, S. A., & Wallston, K. A. (2007). Do religious and control cognitions predict risky behavior? I. Development and validation of the alcohol-related god locus of control scale for adolescents (AGLOC-A). *Cognitive Therapy & Research, 31*(1), 111–122.

Kendrick, K. D., & Robinson, S. (2000). Spirituality: Its relevance and purpose for clinical nursing in the new millennium. *Journal of Clinical Nursing, 9*(5), 701–705.

Taylor, E. J. (2000). Spiritual and ethical end-of-life concerns. In M. Goodman, C. H. Yarbo, & S. L. Groenwald (Eds.), *Cancer nursing: Principles and practice* (5th ed.). Boston, MA: Jones and Bartlett.

Religiosity, Readiness for Enhanced

Bearon, L., & Koenig, H. (1990). Religious cognitions and use of prayer in health and illness. *The Gerontologist, 30,* 249–253.

Burkhart, L., & Solari-Twadell, A. (2001). Spirituality and religiousness: Differentiating the diagnoses through a review of the nursing diagnosis. *Nursing Diagnosis, 12*(2), 44–54.

Burkhart, M. A. (1994). Becoming and connecting: Elements of spirituality for women. *Holistic Nursing Practice, 8,* 12–21.

Carson, V. B., & Green, H. (1992). Spiritual well-being: A predictor of hardiness in patients with acquired immunodeficiency syndrome. *Journal of Professional Nursing, 8,* 209–220.

Gall, T., Charbonneau, C., & Florack, P. (2011). The relationship between religious/spiritual factors and perceived growth following a diagnosis of breast cancer. *Psychology & Health, 26*(3), 287–305.

Hall, D., Meador, K., & Koenig, H. (2011). Measuring religiousness in health research: Review and critique. *Journal of Religion and Health, 47*(2), 134–163.

Hayley, W., & Olver, I. (2011). Prayer as a complementary therapy. *Cancer Forum, 35*(1), 27–30.

Herrera, A., Lee, J., Nanyonjo, R., Laufman, L., & Torres-Vigil, I. (2009). Religious coping and caregiver well-being in Mexican-American families. *Aging & Mental Health, 13*(1), 84–91.

Jana, A. (2011). How prayer works. *Indian Journal of Psychiatry, 53*(1), 79.

Kendrick, K. D., & Robinson, S. (2000). Spirituality: Its relevance and purpose for clinical nursing in the new millennium. *Journal of Clinical Nursing, 9*(5), 701–705.

Pargament, K., & Sweeney, P. (2011). Building spiritual fitness in the army: An innovative approach to a vital aspect of human development. *American Psychologist, 66*(1), 58–64.

Stiles, M. K. (1990). The shining stranger: Nurse–family spiritual relationship. *Cancer Nursing, 13,* 235–245.

Taubman-Ben-Ari, O., Shlomo, S., & Findler, L. (2011). Personal growth and meaning in life among first-time mothers and grandmothers. *Journal of Happiness Studies*. DOI: 10.1007/s10902-011-9291-5. Retrieved February 15, 2012, from http://www.springerlink.com/content/r3000401j4856rvu/

VanHeukelem, J. (1982). Assessing the spiritual needs of children and their families. In J. A. Shelley (Ed.), *The spiritual needs of children*. Downers Grove, IL: Intervarsity Press.

Wald, F. S., & Bailey, C. (1990). Nurturing the spiritual component in care for the terminally ill. *CARING Magazine, 9*(11), 64–68.

Relocation Stress Syndrome

Barnhouse, A. H., Brugler, C. J., & Harkulich, J. T. (1992). Relocation stress syndrome. *Nursing Diagnosis, 3*(4), 166–167.

Beard, H. (2005). Does intermediate care minimize relocation stress for patients leaving the ICU? *Nursing in Critical Care, 10*(6), 272–278.

Brugler, C., Titus, M., & Nypaver, J. (1993). Relocation stress syndrome: A patient and staff approach. *Journal of Nursing Administration, 23*(1), 45–50.

Castle, N., & Engberg, J. (2011). The health consequences of relocation for nursing home residents following Hurricane Katrina. *Research on Aging, 33*(6), 661–687.

Cutler, L., & Garner, M. (1995). Reducing relocation stress after discharge from the intensive therapy unit. *Intensive and Critical Care Nursing, 11*(6), 333–335.

Digby, R., Moss, C., & Bloomer, M. (2011). Transferring from an acute hospital and settling into a subacute facility: The experience of patients with dementia. *International Journal of Older People Nursing*. DOI: 10.1111/j.1748-3743.2011.00282.x. Retrieved February 16, 2012, from http://onlinelibrary.wiley.com/doi/10.1111/j.1748-3743.2011.00282.x/full

Ellis, J. (2010). Psychological transition into a residential care facility: Older people's experiences. *Journal of Advanced Nursing, 66*(5), 1159–1168.

Grenenger, R. (2003). Relocation stress syndrome in rehabilitation transfers: A review of the literature. *Journal of the Australasian Rehabilitation Nurses' Association (JARNA), 6*(1), 8–13.

Hutchings, D., Wells, J., O'Brien, K., Wells, C., Alteen, A., & Cake, L. (2011). From institution to "home": Family perspectives on a unique relocation process. *Canadian Journal on Aging, 30*(2), 223–232.

Johnson, R., Popejoy, L., & Radina, M. (2010). Older adults' participation in nursing home placement decisions. *Clinical Nursing Research, 19*(4), 358–375.

McDonald Gibbins, S. A., & Chapman, J. S. (1996). Holding on: Perceptions of premature infants' transfers. *Journal of Obstetric, Gynecologic, and Neonatal Nursing, 25*(2), 147–153.

Sitter, M., & Lengyel, C. (2011). Nutritional status and eating habits of older Manitobans after relocating to a personal care home. *Canadian Journal of Dietetic Practice and Research, 72*(2), e134–e139.

Smider, N. A., Essex, M. J., & Ryff, C. D. (1996). Adaptation to community relocation: The interactive influence of psychological resources and contextual factors. *Psychology of Aging, 11*(2), 362–372.

Vernberg, E. M. (1990). Experiences with peers following relocation during early adolescence. *American Journal of Orthopsychiatry, 60,* 466–472.

Washburn, A. M. (2005). Relocation puts elderly nursing home residents at risk of stress, although the stress is short lived. *Evidence-Based Mental Health, 8*(2), 49.

Relocation Stress Syndrome, Risk for

Armer, J. M. (1996). An exploration of factors influencing adjustment among relocating rural elders. *Image, 28*(1), 35–39.

Castle, N., & Engberg, J. (2011). The health consequences of relocation for nursing home residents following Hurricane Katrina. *Research on Aging, 33*(6), 661–687.

Cutler, L., & Garner, M. (1995). Reducing relocation stress after discharge from the intensive therapy unit. *Intensive and Critical Care Nursing, 11*(6), 333–335.

Digby, R., Moss, C., & Bloomer, M. (2011). Transferring from an acute hospital and settling into a subacute facility: The experience of patients with dementia. *International Journal of Older People Nursing*. DOI: 10.1111/j.1748-3743.2011.00282.x. Retrieved February 16, 2012, from http://onlinelibrary.wiley.com/doi/10.1111/j.1748-3743.2011.00282.x/full

Ellis, J. (2010). Psychological transition into a residential care facility: Older people's experiences. *Journal of Advanced Nursing, 66*(5), 1159–1168.

Hutchings, D., Wells, J., O'Brien, K., Wells, C., Alteen, A., & Cake, L. (2011). From institution to "home": Family perspectives on a unique relocation process. *Canadian Journal on Agine, 30*(2), 223–232.

Johnson, R., Popejoy, L., & Radina, M. (2010). Older adults' participation in nursing home placement decisions. *Clinical Nursing Research, 19*(4), 358–375.

Kaisik, B. H., & Ceslowitz, S. B. (1996). Easing the fear of nursing home placements: The value of stress inoculation. *Geriatric Nursing, 17*(4), 1–186.

Miles, M. S. (1999). Parents who received transfer preparation had lower anxiety about their children's transfer from the pediatric intensive care unit to a general pediatric ward. *Applied Nursing Research, 12*(3), 114–120.

Paul, F., Hendry, C., & Cabrelli, L. (2004). Meeting patient and relatives' information needs upon transfer from an intensive care unit: The development and evaluation of an information booklet. *Journal of Clinical Nursing, 13*(3), 396–405.

Puskar, K. R. (1986). The usefulness of Mahler's phases of the separation-individuation process in providing a theoretical framework for understanding relocation. *Maternal-Child Nursing Journal, 15*(1), 15–22.

Puskar, K. R., & Rohay, J. M. (1999). School relocation and stress in teens. *Journal of School Nursing, 15*(1), 16–22.

Raviv, A., Keinan, G., Abazoh, Y., & Raviv, A. (1990). Moving as a stressful life event for adolescents. *Journal of Community Psychology, 18,* 130–140.

Reed, J., Roskell Payton, V., & Bond, S. (1998). The importance of place for older people moving into care homes. *Social Science in Medicine, 46*(7), 859–867.

Smider, N. A., Essex, M. J., & Ryff, C. D. (1996). Adaptation to community relocation: The interactive influence of psychological resources and contextual factors. *Psychology of Aging, 11*(2), 362–372.

Renal Perfusion: Risk, for Ineffective

Broscious, S., & Castagnola, J. (2006). Chronic kidney disease: Acute manifestations and role of critical care nurses. *Critical Care Nurse, 26*(4), 17–28.

Erkens, P., & Prins, M. (2010). Fixed dose subcutaneous low molecular weight heparins versus adjusted dose unfractionated heparin for venous thromboembolism. *Cochrane Database of Systematic Reviews 2010*(9). Art. No.: CD001100. DOI: 10.1002/14651858.CD001100.pub3

Harrison, E., Burton, T., Steele, L., Nesbitt, R., Dell, V., Ravestein, A., et al. (2006). Care of the diabetic nephrology patient—reaching best practices. *CANNT Journal, 16*(3), 23–23.

Havel, C., Arrich, J., Losert, H., Gamper, G., Müllner, M., & Herkner, H. (2011). Vasopressors for hypotensive shock. *Cochrane Database of Systematic Reviews 2011,* Issue 5. Art. No.: CD003709. DOI: 10.1002/14651858.CD003709.pub3.

Murtagh, F. E., Hall, J. M., Donohoe, P., & Higginson, I. J. (2006). Symptom management in patients with established renal failure managed without dialysis. *EDTNA/ERCA Journal of Renal Care, 32*(2), 93–98.

Nabhan, A., & Elsedawy, M. (2011). Tight control of mild-moderate pre-existing or non-proteinuric gestational hypertension. *Cochrane Database of Systematic Reviews 2011,* Issue 76, Art. No.: CD006907. DOI: 10.1002/14651858.CD006907.pub2.

Perel, P., & Roberts, I. (2011). Colloids versus crystalloids for fluid resuscitation in critically ill patients. *Cochrane Database of Systematic Reviews 2011*(3). Art. No.: CD000567. DOI: 10.1002/14651858.CD000567.pub4

Roberts, I., Blackhall, K., Alderson, P., Bunn, F., & Schierhout, G. (2011). Human albumin solution for resuscitation and volume expansion in critically ill patients. *Cochrane Database of Systematic Reviews 2011,* Issue 11. Art. No.: CD001208. DOI: 10.1002/14651858.CD001208.pub4

Sumnall, R. (2007). Fluid management and diuretic therapy in acute renal failure. *Nursing in Critical Care, 12*(1), 27–33.

Toomtong, P., & Suksompong, S. (2010). Intravenous fluids for abdominal aortic surgery. *Cochrane Database of Systematic Reviews 2010*(1). Art. No.: CD000991. DOI: 10.1002/14651858.CD000991.pub2

Wilkinson, J., & Treas, L. (2011). *Fundamentals of nursing* (2nd ed.). Philadelphia, PA: F. A. Davis.

Resilience, Impaired Individual; Resilience, Readiness for Enhanced; Resilience, Risk for Compromised

Note: References for all three Resilience diagnoses are found together here.

Aléx, A., & Lundman, B. (2011). Lack of resilience among very old men and women: A qualitative gender analysis. *Research and Theory for Nursing Practice, 25*(4), 302–316.

Armstrong, M., Birnie-Lefcovitch, S., & Ungar, M. (2005). Pathways between social support, family well-being, quality of parenting, and child resilience: What we know. *Journal of Child and Family Studies, 14*(2), 269–281.

Bolger, K., & Patterson, C. (2003). Sequelae of child maltreatment: Vulnerability and resilience. In S. Luthar (Ed.), *Resilience and vulnerability: Adaptation in the context of childhood adversities* (pp. 156–181). Cambridge: Cambridge University Press.

Bonnano, G. (2005). Clarifying and extending the construct of adult resilience. *American Psychologist, 60,* 265–267.

Bonnano, G., Galea, S., Bucciarelli, A., & Vlahov, D (2007). What predicts psychological resilience after disaster? The role of demographics, resources, and life stress. *Journal of Consulting and Clinical Psychology, 75*(5), 671–682.

Calamaro, C., & Waite, R. (2008). Cultural proficiency, research, and evidence-based practice: Implications for the nurse practitioner. *Journal of Pediatric Health Care, 23*(1), 69–72.

Cho, E., & Oh, H. (2011). Effects of laughter therapy on depression, quality of life, resilience and immune responses in breast cancer survivors. *Journal of Korean Academy of Nursing, 41*(3), 285–293.

Crosnoe, R., & Elder, G. (2004). Family dynamics, supportive relationships, and educational resilience during adolescence. *Journal of Family Issues, 25*(5), 571–602.

Eldar-Avidan, D., Haj-Yahia, M., & Greenbaum, C. (2009). Divorce is a part of my life. . . Resilience survival, and vulnerability: Young adults' perception of the implications of parental divorce. *Journal of Marital and Family Therapy, 35*(1), 30–46.

Fergus, S., & Zimmerman, M. (2005). Adolescent resilience: A framework for understanding healthy development in the face of risk. *Annual Review of Public Health, 26,* 399–419.

Goleman, D. (1995). *Emotional intelligence*. New York: Bantam Books.

Gorman, C., Dale, S., Grossman, W., Klarreich, K., McDowell, J., & Whitaker, L. (2005). The importance of resilience. *Time, 165*(3), A52–A55.

Greef, A., & Ritman, I. (2005). Individual characteristics associated with resilience in single-parent families. *Psychological Reports, 96*(1), 36–42.

Halloran, L. (2011). Risky business: Working with high-risk teens to foster resilience. *The Journal for Nurse Practitioners, 7*(5), 426–427.

Haskett, M., & Willoughby, M. (2007). Paths to child social adjustment: Parenting quality and children's processing of social information. *Child: Care, Health and Development, 33*(1), 67–77.

Jenkins, S. (2011). Trauma, transience, and resilience in chronic illness: A perspective on the physician-patient relationship. *International Journal of Psychoanalytic Self Psychology, 6*(4), 572–577.

Kelly, T. (2005). Natural resilience and innate mental health. *American Psychologist, 60*(3), 265.

Lamblass, M. (2008). Treating pediatric overweight through reductions in sedentary behavior: A review of the literature. *Journal of Pediatric Health Care, 23*(1), 29–36.

Martin, A., & Marsh, H. (2006). Academic resilience and its psychological and educational correlates: A construct validity approach. *Psychology in the Schools, 43*(3), 267–281.

Resnick, R., & Inquito, P. (2011). The resilience scale: Psychometric properties and clinical applicability in older adults. *Archives of Psychiatric Nursing, 25*(1), 11–20.

Townsend, M. (2012). *Psychiatric mental health nursing: Concepts of care in evidence-based practice* (7th ed.). Philadelphia, PA: F. A. Davis.

West, C. (2011). Family resilience: Towards a new model of chronic pain management. *Collegian, 18*(1), 3–10.

Wu, H.-C. (2011). The protective effects of resilience and hope on quality of life of the families coping with the criminal traumatisation of one of its members. *Journal of Clinical Nursing, 20*(13–14), 1906–1915.

Role Conflict, Parental

Clements, D., Copeland, L., & Loftus, M. (1990). Critical times for families with a chronically ill child. *Pediatric Nursing, 16*(2), 157–161.

Jay, S., & Youngblut, J. (1991). Parent stress associated with pediatric critical care nursing: Linking research and practice. *AACN Clinical Issues, 2,* 278–283.

Melnyk, B. (1991). Changes in parent–child relationships following divorce. *Pediatric Nursing, 17,* 337–340.

Melnyk, B., Feinstein, N., Moldenhouer, Z., & Small, L. (2001). Coping in parents of children who are chronically ill. *Pediatrics, 27*(6), 548–558.

Newton, M. S. (2000). Family-centered care: Current realities in parent participation. *Pediatric Nursing, 26*(2), 164–168.

Ogunsiji, O., & Wilkes, L. (2005). Managing family life while studying: Single mothers' lived experience of being students in a nursing program. In P. Darbyshire & D. Jackson (Eds.), *Advances in contemporary child and family health care* (pp. 108–123). Sydney, Australia: eContent Management Pty Ltd.

Rennick, J., Lambert, S., Childerhoses, J., Campbell-Yeo, M., Filion, F., & Johnston, C. (2011). Mothers' experiences of a *Touch and Talk* nursing intervention to optimise pain management in the PICU: A qualitative descriptive study. *Intensive and Critical Care Nursing, 27*(3), 151–157.

Robinson, O. (2011). A definition of gender role conflict among Black professional fathers. *The Qualitative Report, 16*(5), 1389–1406.

Smith, L. (1999). Family-centered decision-making: A model for parent participation. *Journal of Neonatal Nursing, 5*(6), 31–33.

Steca, P., Bassi, M., Caprara, G., & Fave, A. (2011). Parents' self-efficacy beliefs and their children's psychosocial adaptation during adolescence. *Journal of Youth and Adolescence, 40*(3), 320–331.

Yu, H. (2011). Parental communication style's impact on children's attitudes toward obesity and food advertising. *The Journal of Consumer Affairs, 45*(1), 87–107.

Role Performance, Ineffective

Felicilda, R. (2011). Pictures of a client's silent distress. *Creative Nursing, 17*(4), 180–183.

Frank, D. I., & Lang, A. R. (1990). Disturbances in sexual role performance of chronic alcoholics: An analysis using Roy's adaptation model. *Issues in Mental Health Nursing, 11*(3), 243–254.

Messias, D. K. H., Fore, E. M., McLoughlin, K., & Parra-Medina, D. (2005). Adult roles in community-based youth empowerment programs. *Family & Community Health, 28*(4), 320–337.

Muller, Z., & Litwin, H. (2011). Grandparenting and psychological well-being: How important is grandparent role centrality? *European Journal of Ageing, 8*(2), 109–118.

Sheely, A. (2010). Work characteristics and family routines in low-wage families. *Journal of Sociology & Social Welfare, 37*(3), 59–77.

Small, L. (2010). Quality-of-life experiences from the perspective of patients receiving haemodialysis for chronic renal failure. *Health SA Gesonheid, 15*(1), Art. #521, 7 pages. DOI:10.4102/hsag.v15i1.521. Retrieved February 23, 2012, from http://hsag.co.za/index.php/HSAG/article/view/521

Strauss, J. (2011). The baby boomers meet menopause: Fertility, attractiveness, and affective response to the menopausal transition. *Sex Roles*. DOI: 10.1007/s11199-011-0001-9. Retrieved February 23, 2012, from https://springerlink3.metapress.com/content/m73m63587410k827/resource-secured/?target=fulltext.pdf&sid=whwttuuiigsayeoppxpgfi5h&sh=www.springerlink.com

Utz, R., Lund, D., Caserta, M., & Wright, S. (2011). The benefits of respites time-use: A comparison of employed and nonemployed caregivers. *Journal of Applied Gerontology*. DOI 10.1177/0633464810389607. Retrieved February 23, 2012, from http://jag.sagepub.com/content/early/2011/02/28/0733464810389607.full.pdf+html

Zettel-Watson, L., Rakovski, C., Levine, B., Rutledge, D., & Jones, J. (2011). Impact of employment and caregiving roles on the well-being of people with fibromyalgia syndrome. *Journal of Musculoskeletal Pain, 19*(1), 8–17.

Sedentary Lifestyle

Appleton, B. (2004). Cardiovascular nursing: The role of exercise training in patients with chronic heart failure. *British Journal of Nursing (BJN), 13*(8), 452–456.

Biuso, T. J., Butterworth, S., & Linden, A. (2007). A conceptual framework for targeting prediabetes with lifestyle, clinical, and behavioral management interventions. *Disease Management, 10*(1), 6–15.

Blackburn, G., Wollner, S., & Heymsfield, S. (2010). Lifestyle interventions for the treatment of class III obesity: A primary target for nutrition medicine in the obesity epidemic. *The American Journal of Clinical Nutrition, 91*(1), 289S–292S.

Bryan, A., Magnan, R., Nilsson, R., Marcus, B., Tompkins, S., & Hutchison, K. (2011). The big picture of individual differences in physical activity behavior change: A transdisciplinary approach. *Psychology of Sport and Exercise, 12*(1), 20–26.

Charansonney, O., & Després, J.-P. (2010). Disease prevention—should we target obesity or sedentary lifestyle? *Nature Reviews Cardiology, 7,* 468–472.

Cobb, S. L., Brown, D. J., & Davis, L. L. (2006). Effective interventions for lifestyle change after myocardial infarction or coronary artery revascularization. *Journal of the American Academy of Nurse Practitioners, 18*(1), 31–39.

Jackson, C., Coe, A., Cheater, F. M., & Wroe, S. (2007). Specialist health visitor-led weight management intervention in primary care: Exploratory evaluation. *Journal of Advanced Nursing, 58*(1), 23–34.

Kehl-Pruett, W. (2006). Deep vein thrombosis in hospitalized patients: A review of evidence-based guidelines for prevention. *Dimensions of Critical Care Nursing, 25*(2), 53–61.

Little, P., Dorward, M., Gralton, S., Hammerton, L., Pillinger, J., White, P., et al. (2004). A randomised controlled trial of three pragmatic approaches to initiate increased physical activity in sedentary patients with risk factors for cardiovascular disease. *British Journal of General Practice, 54*(500), 189–195.

Mooney, M., Fitzsimons, D., & Richardson, G. (2007). "No more couch-potato!" patients' experiences of a pre-operative programme of cardiac rehabilitation for those awaiting coronary artery bypass surgery. *European Journal of Cardiovascular Nursing, 6*(1), 77–83.

Silva, M., Markland, D., Carraça, E., Viera, P., Coutinho, S., Minderico, C., et al. (2011). Exercise autonomous motivation predicts 3-yr weight loss in women. *Medicine & Science in Sports & Exercise, 43*(4), 728–737.

Stull, V. B., Snyder, D. C., & Demark-Wahnefried, W. (2007). Lifestyle interventions in cancer survivors: Designing programs that meet the needs of this vulnerable and growing population. *Journal of Nutrition, 137,* 243S–248S.

Swenson, K. K., Henly, S. J., Shapiro, A. C., & Schroeder, L. M. (2005). Interventions to prevent loss of bone mineral density in women receiving chemotherapy for breast cancer. *Clinical Journal of Oncology Nursing, 9*(2), 177.

Teychenne, M., Ball, K., & Salmon, J. (2011). Sedentary behavior and depression among adults: A review. *International Journal of Behavioral Medicine, 17*(4), 246–254.

Self-Care, Readiness for Enhanced

Akyol, A. D., Çetinkaya, Y., Bakan, G., Yaral, S., & Akkus, S. (2007). Self-care agency and factors related to this agency among patients with hypertension. *Journal of Clinical Nursing, 16*(4), 679–687.

Armer, J., Brooks, C., & Stewart, B. (2011). Limitations of self-care in reducing the risk of lymphedema: Supportive-educative systems. *Nursing Science Quarterly, 24*(1), 57–63.

Becker, G., Gates, R. J., & Newsom, E. (2004). Self-care among chronically ill African Americans: Culture, health disparities, and health insurance status. *American Journal of Public Health, 94,* 2066–2073.

Callaghan, D. (2006). Basic conditioning factors' influences on adolescents' healthy behaviors, self-efficacy, and self-care. *Issues in Comprehensive Pediatric Nursing, 29*(4), 191–204.

Callaghan, D. M. (2003). Health-promoting self-care behaviors, self-care self-efficacy, and self-care agency. *Nursing Science Quarterly, 16*(3), 247.

Callaghan, D. M. (2005). The influence of spiritual growth on adolescents' initiative and responsibility for self-care. *Pediatric Nursing, 31*(2), 91–97.

Cutler, C. (2003). Assessing patients' perception of self-care agency in psychiatric care. *Issues in Mental Health Nursing, 24*(2), 199.

Dashiff, C., Bartolucci, A., Wallander, J., & Abdullatif, H. (2005). The relationship of family structure, maternal employment, and family conflict with self-care adherence of adolescents with type 1 diabetes. *Families, Systems, & Health, 23*(1), 66–79.

Desbiens, J.-F., Gagnon, J., & Fillion, L. (2011). Development of a shared theory in palliative care to enhance nursing competence. *Journal of Advanced Nursing*. DOI: 10.1111/j.1365-2648.2011.05917.x. Retrieved February 23, 2012, from http://onlinelibrary.wiley.com/doi/10.1111/j.1365-2648.2011.05917.x/full

DeSocio, J., Kitzman, H., & Cole, R. (2003). Testing the relationship between self-agency and enactment of health behaviors. *Research in Nursing & Health, 26*(1), 20–29.

Hines, S. H., Sampselle, C. M., Ronis, D. L., SeonAe Yeo, Fredrickson, B. L., & Boyd, C. J. (2007). Women's self-care agency to manage urinary incontinence. *Advances in Nursing Science, 30*(2), 175–188.

Kim, H. (2011). Development and evaluation of self-care agency promoting programme for prostatectomy patients. *International Journal of Urological Nursing, 5*(1), 34–44.

Mullen, K. (2011). An older adult man who is unable to sleep: Advocating self-care in home healthcare. *Home Healthcare Nurse, 29*(1), 22–25.

Orem, D. E. (2001). *Nursing: Concepts and practice* (6th ed.). St. Louis, MO: Mosby.

Ovayolu, O., Ovayolu, N., & Karadag, G. (2012). The relationship between self-care agency, disability levels and factors regarding these situations among patients with rheumatoid arthritis. *Journal of Clinical Nursing, 21*(1–2), 101–110.

Parissopoulos, S., & Kotzabassaki, S. (2004). Orem's self-care theory, transactional analysis and the management of elderly rehabilitation. *ICUs & Nursing Web Journal, 17,* 11.

Sousa, V. D., Zauszniewski, J. A., Musil, C. M., Lea, P., & Davis, S. A. (2005). Relationships among self-care agency, self-efficacy, self-care, and glycemic control. *Research & Theory for Nursing Practice, 19*(3), 217–230.

Self-Care Deficit: Bathing/Hygiene

Adams, J., Cheng, P., Deonarain, L., Frank, C., Mayers, A., Smith, B., et al. (2011). Extinction of care-induced vocalizations by a desensitization routine on a palliative care unit. *American Journal of Hospice & Palliative Medicine*. DOI: 10.1177/1049909111420701. Retrieved February 23, 2012, from http://ajh.sagepub.com/content/early/2011/08/25/1049909111420701.abstract?patientinform-links=yes&legid=spajh;1049909111420701v1

Chalmers, J., & Pearson, A. (2005). Oral hygiene care for residents with dementia: A literature review. *Journal of Advanced Nursing, 52*(4), 410–419.

Cohn, J. L., & Fulton, J. S. (2006). Nursing staff perspectives on oral care for neuroscience patients. *Journal of Neuroscience Nursing, 38*(1), 22–30.

Coyer, F., O'Sullivan, J., & Cadman, N. (2011). The provision of patient personal hygiene in the intensive care unit: A descriptive exploratory study of bed-bathing practice. *Australian Critical Care, 24*(3), 198–209.

Eigsti, J. (2011). Innovative solutions: Beds, baths, and bottoms: A quality improvement initiative to standardize use of beds, bathing techniques, and skin care in a general critical-care unit. *Dimensions of Critical Care Nursing, 30*(3), 169–176.

Hampton, S. (2004). Promoting good hygiene among older residents. *Nursing & Residential Care, 6*(4), 172.

Jury, L., Guerrero, D., Burant, C., Cadnum, J., & Donskey, C. (2011). Effectiveness of routine patient bathing to decrease the burden of spores on the skin of patients with *Clostridium* difficile infection. *Infection Control and Hospital Epidemiology, 32*(1), 181–184.

Nix, D., & Ermer-Seltun, J. (2004). A review of perineal skin care protocols and skin barrier product use. *Ostomy Wound Management, 50*(12), 59–67.

Pearson, A., & Chalmers, J. (2004). Oral hygiene care for adults with dementia in residential aged care facilities. *JBI Reports, 2*(3), 65–113.

Peck, R. L. (2002). Best-practice design for the bathing facility. [cover story]. *Nursing Homes: Long Term Care Management, 51*(1), 46.

Rader, J., Barrick, A. L., Hoeffer, B., Sloane, P. D., McKenzie, D., Talerico, K. A., et al. (2006). The bathing of older adults with dementia: Easing the unnecessarily unpleasant aspects of assisted bathing. *American Journal of Nursing, 106*(4), 40–49.

Rader, J., & Semradek, J. (2003). Organizational culture and bathing practice: Ending the battle in one facility. *Journal of Social Work in Long-Term Care, 2*(3), 269–283.

Voegeli, D. (2005). Skin hygiene practices, emollient therapy and skin vulnerability. *Nursing Times, 101*(4), 57–58.

Walker, L., Downe, S., & Gomez, L. (2005). A survey of soap and skin care product provision for well term neonates. *British Journal of Midwifery, 13*(12), 768.

Wilkinson, J., & Treas, L. (2011). *Fundamentals of nursing* (2nd ed.). Chapter 22. Philadelphia, PA: F. A. Davis.

Zingmarak, M., & Bernspång, B. (2011). Meeting the needs of elderly with bathing disability. *Australian Occupational Therapy Journal, 58*(3), 164–171.

Self-Care Deficit: Dressing/Grooming

Ashurst, A. (2003). Maintaining client hygiene and appearance. *Nursing & Residential Care, 5*(3), 104–109.

Christie, L., Bedford, R., & McCluskey, A. (2011). Task-specific practice of dressing tasks in a hospital setting improved dressing performance post-stroke: A feasibility study. *Australian Occupational Therapy Journal, 58*(5), 364–369.

Cruz, J., Marques, A., Barbosa, A., Figueiredo, D., & Sousa, L. (2011). Effects of a motor and multisensory-based approach on residents with moderate-to-severe dementia. *American Journal of Alzheimer's Disease & Other Dementias, 26*(4), 282–289.

Randall, J., & Ream, E. (2005). Hair loss with chemotherapy: At a loss over its management? *European Journal of Cancer Care, 14*(3), 223–231.

Sidani, S., Streiner, D., & LeClerc, C. (2012). Evaluating the effectiveness of the abilities-focused approach to morning care of people with dementia. *International Journal of Older People Nursing, 7*(1), 37–45.

Self-Care Deficit: Feeding

Aselage, M., Amella, E., & Watson, R. (2011). State of the science: Alleviating mealtime difficulties in nursing home residents with dementia. *Nursing Outlook, 59*(4), 210–214.

Bond, P., & Moss, D. (2003). Best practice in nasogastric and gastrostomy feeding in children. *Nursing Times, 99*(33), 28–30.

Booth, J., Leadbetter, A., Francis, M., & Tolson, D. (2005). Implementing a best practice statement in nutrition for frail older people: Part 2. *Nursing Older People, 17*(1), 22–24.

Campbell, J., & McDowell, J. R. S. (2007). Comparative study on the effect of enteral feeding on blood glucose. *British Journal of Nursing (BJN), 16*(6), 344–349.

Cullen, S. (2011). Gastrostomy tube feeding in adults: The risks, benefits and alternatives. *Proceedings of the Nutrition Society, 70*, 293–298. DOI:10.1017/S002966511100053X. Retrieved February 24, 2012, from http://journals.cambridge.org/action/displayAbstract?fromPage=online&aid=8331196

Deane, K., Whurr, R., Clarke, C. E., Playford, E. D., & Ben-Shlomo, Y. (2006). Non-pharmacological therapies for dysphagia in Parkinson's disease. *Cochrane Library* (4).

DiBartolo, M. C. (2006). Careful hand feeding: A reasonable alternative to PEG tube placement in individuals with dementia. *Journal of Gerontological Nursing, 32*(5), 25–35.

Ellett, M. L. C., Beckstrand, J., Flueckiger, J., Perkins, S. M., & Johnson, C. S. (2005). Predicting the insertion distance for placing gastric tubes. *Clinical Nursing Research, 14*(1), 11–27.

Finucane, T. E., Christmas, C., & Leff, B. A. (2007). Tube feeding in dementia: How incentives undermine health care quality and patient safety. *Journal of the American Medical Directors Association, 8*(4), 205–208.

Grady, P. (2011). Advancing the health of our aging population: A lead role for nursing science. *Nursing Outlook, 59*(4), 207–209.

Green, S. M., & Watson, R. (2005). Nutritional screening and assessment tools for use by nurses: Literature review. *Journal of Advanced Nursing, 50*(1), 69–83.

Hurtekant, K. M., & Spatz, D. L. (2007). Special considerations for breastfeeding the infant with spina bifida. *Journal of Perinatal & Neonatal Nursing, 21*(1), 69–75.

Katzberg, H., & Benatar, M. (2011). Enteral tube feeding for amyotrophic lateral sclerosis/motor neuron disease. *Cochrane Database of Systematic Reviews 2011* (1). Art. No.: CD004030. DOI: 10.1002/14651858.CD004030.pub3. Retrieved February 24, 2012, from http://onlinelibrary.wiley.com/doi/10.1002/14651858.CD004030.pub3/full

Lee, T., & Kolasa, K. (2011). Feeding the person with late-stage Alzheimer's disease. *Nutrition Today, 46*(2), 75–79.

Lin, L., Wang, S., Chen, S. H., Wang, T., Chen, M., & Wu, S. (2003). Issues and innovations in nursing practice efficacy of swallowing training for residents following stroke. *Journal of Advanced Nursing, 44*(5), 469–478.

Marshall, A., & West, S. (2004). Nutritional intake in the critically ill: Improving practice through research. *Australian Critical Care, 17*(1), 6.

Ng, W. Q., & Neill, J. (2006). Evidence for early oral feeding of patients after elective open colorectal surgery: A literature review. *Journal of Clinical Nursing, 15*(6), 696–709.

Nguyen, N., Grgurinovich, N., Bryant, L., Burgstad, C., Chapman, M., Holloway, R., et al. (2011). Plasma erythromycin concentrations predict feeding outcomes in critically ill patients with feed intolerance. *Critical Care Medicine, 39*(4), 868–871.

Pearson, A., Fitzgerald, M., & Nay, R. (2003). Mealtimes in nursing homes: The role of nursing staff. *Journal of Gerontological Nursing, 29*(6), 40–47.

Pelletier, C. A. (2004). Why do CNAs feed as they do? *ASHA Leader, 9*(7), 17–25.

Premji, S. S. (2005). Enteral feeding for high-risk neonates. *Journal of Perinatal & Neonatal Nursing, 19*(1), 59–71.

Schueren, M., der. (2005). Nutritional support strategies for malnourished cancer patients. *European Journal of Oncology Nursing, 9,* S74–83.

Smith, J. R. (2005). Early enteral feeding for the very low birth weight infant: The development and impact of a research-based guideline. *Neonatal Network, 24*(4), 9–19.

Westergren, A. (2006). Detection of eating difficulties after stroke: A systematic review. *International Nursing Review, 53*(2), 143–149.

Williams, T. A., & Leslie, G. D. (2005). A review of the nursing care of enteral feeding tubes in critically ill adults: Part II. *Intensive & Critical Care Nursing, 21*(1), 5–15.

Wilkinson, J., & Treas, L. (2011). *Fundamentals of nursing* (2nd ed.), Chapter 22. Philadelphia, PA: F. A. Davis. Self-Care Deficit: Toileting

Bayliss, V., & Salter, L. (2004). Pathways for evidence-based continence care. *Nursing Standard, 19*(9), 45–52.

Brooks, W. (2004). The use of practice guidelines for urinary incontinence following stroke. *British Journal of Nursing (BJN), 13*(20), 1176–1179.

Bywater, A., & While, A. (2006). Management of bowel dysfunction in people with multiple sclerosis. *British Journal of Community Nursing, 11*(8), 333.

Chapple, C., Khullar, V., Gabriel, Z., & Dooley, J. A. (2005). The effects of antimuscarinic treatments in overactive bladder: A systematic review and meta-analysis.*European Urology, 48*(1), 5–26.

Cotton, J. A. (2004). Essence of care: Implementing continence benchmarks in primary care. *British Journal of Community Nursing, 9*(6), 251–256.

Du Moulin, M. F. M. T., Hamers, J. P. H., Paulus, A., Berendsen, C., & Halfens, R. (2005). The role of the nurse in community continence care: A systematic review. *International Journal of Nursing Studies, 42*(4), 479–492.

Emr, K., & Ryan, R. (2004). Best practice for indwelling catheters in the home setting. *Home Healthcare Nurse, 22*(12), 820–830.

Fader, M., Clarke-O'Neill, S., Cook, D., Dean, G., Brooks, R., Cottenden, A., et al. (2003). Management of night-time urinary incontinence in residential settings for older people: An investigation into the effects of different pad changing regimes on skin health. *Journal of Clinical Nursing, 12*(3), 374–386.

Flynn, D. (2005). Improving continence care: Searching the evidence. *Journal of Community Nursing, 19*(3), 18.

Garman, K., & Ficca, M. (2011, December 1). Managing encopresis in the elementary school setting: The school nurse's role. *The Journal of School Nursing.* DOI: 10.1177/1059840511429685. Retrieved February 24, 2012, from http://jsn.sagepub.com/content/early/2011/11/30/1059840511429685.abstract

Glazener, C., Evans, J., & Peto, R. E. (2004). Treating nocturnal enuresis in children: Review of evidence. *Journal of Wound, Ostomy & Continence Nursing, 31*(4), 223–234.

Karon, S. (2005). A team approach to bladder retraining: A pilot study. *Urologic Nursing, 25*(4), 269–276.

Klimach, V., & Williams-Jones, A. (2006). Continence problems in children attending special schools. *Learning Disability Practice, 9*(8), 30–33.

Lee, E., & Malatt, C. (2011). Making the hospital safer for older adult patients: A focus on the indwelling urinary catheter. *The Permanente Journal, 15*(1), 49–52.

Matson, J., Neal, D., Hess, J., & Kozlowski, A. (2011). Assessment of toileting difficulties in adults with intellectual disabilities: An examination using the profile of toileting issues (POTI). *Research in Developmental Disabilities, 32*(1), 176–179.

Moore, K. N., & Gray, M. (2004). Urinary incontinence in men: Current status and future directions. *Nursing Research, 53*(6), S36–41.

Nahon, I., Dorey, G., Waddington, G., & Adams, R. (2006). Systematic review of the treatment of post-prostatectomy incontinence. *Urologic Nursing, 26*(6), 461–482.

Ostaszkiewicz, J., Roe, B., & Johnston, L. (2005). Effects of timed voiding for the management of urinary incontinence in adults: Systematic review. *Journal of Advanced Nursing, 52*(4), 420–431.

Resnick, B., Keilman, L. J., Calabrese, B., Parmelee, P., Lawhorne, L., Pailet, J., et al. (2006). Continence care. Nursing staff beliefs and expectations about continence care in nursing homes. *Journal of Wound, Ostomy & Continence Nursing, 33*(6), 610–618.

Roe, B., Milne, J., Ostaszkiewicz, J., & Wallace, S. (2007). Systematic reviews of bladder training and voiding programmes in adults: A synopsis of findings from data analysis and outcomes using metastudy techniques. *Journal of Advanced Nursing, 57*(1), 15–31.

Slater, W. (2003). Continence care. Management of faecal incontinence of a patient with spinal cord injury. *British Journal of Nursing (BJN), 12*(12), 727–734.

Wilkinson, J., & Treas, L. (2011). Chapter 22. In *Fundamentals of nursing* (2nd ed.). Philadelphia, PA: F. A. Davis.

Wright, J., McCormack, B., Coffey, A., & McCarthy, G. (2006). Developing a tool to assess person-centred continence care. *Nursing Older People, 18*(6), 23–28.

Zhang, A. Y., Strauss, G. J., & Siminoff, L. A. (2007). Effects of combined pelvic floor muscle exercise and a support group on urinary incontinence and quality of life of postprostatectomy patients. *Oncology Nursing Forum, 34*(1), 47–53.

Self-Concept, Readiness for Enhanced

Ahn, S., & Fedewa, A. (2011). A meta-analysis of the relationship between children's physical activity and mental health. *Journal of Pediatric Psychology, 36*(4), 385–397.

Aswathy, M., Blessy, P., & Flavia, C. (2011). Effectiveness of self enhancement programme on self esteem of institutionalized elderly. *Indian Journal of Gerontology, 25*(2), 200–207.

Bergamasco, E. C., Rossi, L., da Amancio, C. G., & Carvalho, E. C. (2002). Body image of patients with burn sequellae. *Burns, 28,* 47–52.

Corte, C. M. (2002). *The impoverished self and alcoholism: Content and structure of self-cognitions in alcohol dependence and recovery.* Ann Arbor, MI: University of Michigan.

Davis, K., & Taylor, B. (2006a). Stories of resistance and healing in the process of leaving abusive relationships. *Contemporary Nurse: A Journal for the Australian Nursing Profession, 21*(2), 199–208.

Davis, K., & Taylor, B. (2006b). Stories of resistance and healing in the process of leaving abusive relationships. In A. McMurray & D. Jackson (Eds.), *Advances in contemporary nursing and interpersonal violence* (pp. 199–208). Sydney, Australia: eContent Management Pty Ltd.

Delaney, C. (2005). The spirituality scale: Development and psychometric testing of a holistic instrument to assess the human spiritual dimension. *Journal of Holistic Nursing, 23*(2), 145–167.

Gibson, L. M., & Hendricks, C. S. (2006). Integrative review of spirituality in African American breast cancer survivors. *ABNF Journal, 17*(2), 67–72.

Lin, Y., Dai, Y., & Hwang, S. (2003). The effect of reminiscence on the elderly population: A systematic review. *Public Health Nursing, 20*(4), 297–306.

Matiti, M. R., & Trorey, G. (2004). Perceptual adjustment levels: Patients' perception of their dignity in the hospital setting. *International Journal of Nursing Studies, 41*(7), 735–744.

Pizzignacco, T., & de Lima, R. (2006). Socialization of children and adolescents with cystic fibrosis: Support for nursing care. *Revista Latino-Americana de Enfermagem, 14*(4), 569–577.

White, R. (2012). A sociocultural investigation of the efficacy of outdoor education to improve learner engagement. *Emotional and Behavioural Difficulties, 17*(1), 13–23.

Wilkinson, J., & Treas, L. (2011). *Fundamentals of nursing* (2nd ed.). Chapter 22. Philadelphia, PA: F. A. Davis. Winkelstein, M. L. (1989). Fostering positive self-concept in the school-age child. *Pediatric Nursing, 15*, 229–233.

Yuen, H., Mueller, K., Mayor, E., & Azuero, A. (2011). Impact of participation in a theatre programme on quality of life among older adults with chronic conditions: A pilot study. *Occupational Therapy International, 18*(4), 201–208.

Self-Esteem, Chronic Low

Buckner, J., Beardslee, W., Bassuk, E., & Ray, S. (2004). Exposure to violence and low-income children's mental health: Direct, moderated, and mediated relations. *American Journal of Orthopsychiatry, 74*(4), 413–423.

Callaghan, P. (2004). Exercise: A neglected intervention in mental health care? *Journal of Psychiatric & Mental Health Nursing, 11*(4), 476–483.

Crowe, M. (2004). Never good enough. II. Clinical implications. *Journal of Psychiatric Mental Health Nursing, 11*(3), 335–340.

Dennis, C., & Boyce, P. (2004). Further psychometric testing of a brief personality scale to measure vulnerability to postpartum depression. *Journal of Psychosomatic Obstetrics & Gynecology, 25*(3), 305–311.

Essler, V., Arthur, A., & Stickley, T. (2006). Using a school-based intervention to challenge stigmatizing attitudes and promote mental health in teenagers. *Journal of Mental Health, 15*(2), 243–250.

Fauchald, S. K. (2006). Community-based research to explore safer sex behaviors among women: Implications for CNS practice. *Clinical Nurse Specialist: The Journal for Advanced Nursing Practice, 20*(2), 68–74.

Gary, F., Baker, M., & Grandbois, D. (2005). Perspectives on suicide prevention among American Indian and Alaska native children and adolescents: A call for help. *Online Journal of Issues in Nursing, 10*(2), 170–211.

Gonzales, A., & Hancock, J. (2011). Mirror, mirror on my Facebook wall: Effects of exposure to Facebook on self-esteem. *Cyberpsychology, Behavior, and Social Networking, 14*(1–2), 79–83.

Harris, P. B., & Keady, J. (2004). Living with early onset dementia. *Alzheimer's Care Quarterly, 5*(2), 111–122.

Korrelboom, K., Marissen, M., & van Assendelft, T. (2011). Competitive memory training (COMET) for low self-esteem in patients with personality disorders: A randomized effectiveness study. *Behavioural and Cognitive Psychotherapy, 39*(1), 1–19.

Kort-Butler, L., & Hagewen, K. (2011). School-based extracurricular activity involvement and adolescent self-esteem: A growth-curve analysis. *Journal of Youth and Adolescence, 40*(5), 568–581.

Lin, Y., Dai, Y., & Hwang, S. (2003). The effect of reminiscence on the elderly population: A systematic review. *Public Health Nursing, 20*(4), 297–306.

Maslow, A. (1970). *Motivation and personality* (2nd ed.). New York: Harper & Row.

Matiti, M. R., & Trorey, G. (2004). Perceptual adjustment levels: Patients' perception of their dignity in the hospital setting. *International Journal of Nursing Studies, 41*(7), 735–744.

Meredith, P., Strong, J., & Feeney, J. (2006). The relationship of adult attachment to emotion, catastrophizing, control, threshold and intolerance, in experimentally-induced pain. *Pain, 120*(1–2), 44–52.

Nishina, A., & Juvonen, J. (2005). Daily reports of witnessing and experiencing peer harassment in middle school. *Child Development, 76*(2), 435–450.

Ogunsiji, O., & Wilkes, L. (2005). Managing family life while studying: Single mothers' lived experience of being students in a nursing program. In P. Darbyshire & D. Jackson (Eds.), *Advances in contemporary child and family health care* (pp. 108–123). Sydney, Australia: eContent Management Pty Ltd.

Pierce, J., & Wardle, J. (1997). Cause and effect beliefs and self esteem' of overweight children. *Journal of Child Psychology and Psychiatry and Allied Disciplines, 38*(6), 645–650.

Räty, L., & Gustafsson, B. (2002). The influence of confirming and disconfirming healthcare encounters on the self-relation and quality of life of persons with epilepsy. *Journal of Neuroscience Nursing, 34*(5), 261–272.

Ross, J., & Gowers, S. (2011). Body dysmorphic disorder. *Advances in Psychiatric Treatment, 17,* 142–149.

Self-Esteem, Risk for Chronic Low

Buckner, J., Beardslee, W., Bassuk, E., & Ray, S. (2004). Exposure to violence and low-income children's mental health: Direct, moderated, and mediated relations. *American Journal of Orthopsychiatry, 74*(4), 413–423.

Crowe, M. (2004). Never good enough. II. Clinical implications. *Journal of Psychiatric Mental Health Nursing, 11*(3), 335–340.

Davis, M., & Wosinski, N. (2011). Cognitive errors as predictors of adaptive and maladaptive perfectionism in children. *Journal of Rational-Emotive &*

Cognitive-Behavior Therapy, DOI: 10.1007/s10942-011-0129-1. Retrieved March 3, 2012, from https://springerlink3.metapress.com/content/k407073169414j40/resource-secured/?target=fulltext.html&sid=021nxcqwzkjv03pwcvpp2kkk&sh=www.springerlink.com

Dennis, C., & Boyce, P. (2004). Further psychometric testing of a brief personality scale to measure vulnerability to postpartum depression. *Journal of Psychosomatic Obstetrics & Gynecology, 25*(3), 305–311.

Fauchald, S. K. (2006). Community-based research to explore safer sex behaviors among women: Implications for CNS practice. *Clinical Nurse Specialist: The Journal for Advanced Nursing Practice, 20*(2), 68–74.

Harris, P. B., & Keady, J. (2004). Living with early onset dementia. *Alzheimer's Care Quarterly, 5*(2), 111–122.

Maslow, A. (1970). *Motivation and personality* (2nd ed.). New York: Harper & Row.

Matiti, M. R., & Trorey, G. (2004). Perceptual adjustment levels: Patients' perception of their dignity in the hospital setting. *International Journal of Nursing Studies, 41*(7), 735–744.

Meredith, P., Strong, J., & Feeney, J. (2006). The relationship of adult attachment to emotion, catastrophizing, control, threshold and intolerance, in experimentally-induced pain. *Pain, 120*(1–2), 44–52.

Nishina, A., & Juvonen, J. (2005). Daily reports of witnessing and experiencing peer harassment in middle school. *Child Development, 76*(2), 435–450.

Räty, L., & Gustafsson, B. (2002). The influence of confirming and disconfirming healthcare encounters on the self-relation and quality of life of persons with epilepsy. *Journal of Neuroscience Nursing, 34*(5), 261–272.

Ross, J., & Gowers, S. (2011). Body dysmorphic disorder. *Advances in Psychiatric Treatment, 17,* 142–149.

Self-Esteem, Risk for Situational Low

Baumeister, R. F., Smart, L., & Boden, J. M. (1996). Relation of threatened egotism to violence and aggression: The dark side of high self-esteem. *Psychological Review, 103*(l), 5–33.

Bonadonna, R. (2003). Mediation's impact on chronic illness. *Holistic Nursing Practice, 17*(6), 309–319.

Callaghan, P. (2004). Exercise: A neglected intervention in mental health care? *Journal of Psychiatric & Mental Health Nursing, 11*(4), 476–483.

Essler, V., Arthur, A., & Stickley, T. (2006). Using a school-based intervention to challenge stigmatizing attitudes and promote mental health in teenagers. *Journal of Mental Health, 15*(2), 243–250.

Fauchald, S. K. (2006). Community-based research to explore safer sex behaviors among women: Implications for CNS practice. *Clinical Nurse Specialist: The Journal for Advanced Nursing Practice, 20*(2), 68–74.

Fleitas, J. (2003). The power of words: Examining the linguistic landscape of pediatric nursing. *MCN: The American Journal of Maternal Child Nursing, 28*(6), 384–390.

Gary, F. A. (2005). Perspectives on suicide prevention among American Indian and Alaska native children and adolescents: A call for help. *Online Journal of Issues in Nursing, 10*(2), 170–211.

Harris, P. B., & Keady, J. (2004). Living with early onset dementia. *Alzheimer's Care Quarterly, 5*(2), 111–122.

Matiti, M. R., & Trorey, G. (2004). Perceptual adjustment levels: Patients' perception of their dignity in the hospital setting. *International Journal of Nursing Studies, 41*(7), 735–744.

Murray, M. F. (2000). Coping with change: Self-talk. *Hospital Practice, 31*(5), 118–120.

Self-Esteem, Situational Low

(Also see Self-Esteem, Chronic Low.)

Alessandra, Z., Silla, A., & Marlisa, C. (2011). A retrospective study of nursing diagnoses, outcomes, and interventions for patients admitted to a cardiology rehabilitation unit. *International Journal of Nursing Terminologies and Classifications, 22*(4), 148–156.

Armitage, C., & Rowe, R. (2011). Testing multiple means of self-affirmation. *British Journal of Psychology, 102*(3), 535–545.

Barton, J., Griffin, M., & Pretty, J. (2011, April 7). Exercise, nature and socially interactive based initiatives improve mood and self-esteem in the clinical population. *Perspectives in Public Health*. DOI: 10.1177/1757913910393862. Retrieved March 4, 2012, from http://rsh.sagepub.com/content/early/2011/02/06/1757913910393862.abstract

Dennis, C., & Boyce, P. (2004). Further psychometric testing of a brief personality scale to measure vulnerability to postpartum depression. *Journal of Psychosomatic Obstetrics & Gynecology, 25*(3), 305–311.

Essler, V., Arthur, A., & Stickley, T. (2006). Using a school-based intervention to challenge stigmatizing attitudes and promote mental health in teenagers. *Journal of Mental Health, 15*(2), 243–250.

Fauchald, S. K. (2006). Community-based research to explore safer sex behaviors among women: Implications for CNS practice. *Clinical Nurse Specialist: The Journal for Advanced Nursing Practice, 20*(2), 68–74.

Klym, L. M., & Colling, J. (2003). Quality of life after radical prostatectomy. *Oncology Nursing Forum, 30*(2), E24–32.

Martin, C., Keswick, J., Crayton, D., & LeVeck, P. (2012). Perceptions of self-esteem in a welfare-to-wellness-to-work program. *Public Health Nursing, 29*(1), 19–26.

Matiti, M. R., & Trorey, G. (2004). Perceptual adjustment levels: Patients' perception of their dignity in the hospital setting. *International Journal of Nursing Studies, 41*(7), 735–744.

Muehrer, R. J., Keller, M. L., Powwattana, A., & Pornchaikate, A. (2006). Sexuality among women recipients of a pancreas and kidney transplant. *Western Journal of Nursing Research, 28*(2), 137–150.

Stapel, D., & van der Linde, L. (2011). What drives self-affirmation effects? On the importance of differentiating value affirmation and attribute affirmation. *Journal of Personality and Social Psychology, 101*(1), 34–45.

Wu, Y., Prout, K., Roberts, M., Parikshak, S., & Amylon, M. (2011). Assessing experiences of children who attended a camp for children with cancer and their siblings: A preliminary study. *Child and Youth Care Forum, 40*(2), 121–133.

Yoon, H., Kim, G.-H., & Kim, J. (2011). Effectiveness of an interpersonal relationship program on interpersonal relationships, self-esteem, and depression in nursing students. *Journal of Korean Academy of Nursing, 41*(6), 805–813.

Self-Health Management, Ineffective

Banister, N., Jastrow, S., Hodges, V., Loop, R., & Gillham, M. (2004). Diabetes self-management training program in a community clinic improves patient outcomes at modest cost. *Journal of the American Dietetic Association, 104*(5), 807–810.

Benavides-Vaello, S., Garcia, A., Brown, S., & Winchell, M. (2004). Using focus groups to plan and evaluate diabetes self-management interventions for Mexican Americans. *Diabetes Educator, 30*(2), 238, 242–244, 247–250.

Bloomfield, H., Krause, A., Greer, N., Taylor, B., MacDonald, R., Rutks, I., et al. (2011). Meta-analysis: Effect of patient self-testing and self-management of long-term anticoagulation on major clinical outcomes. *Annals of Internal Medicine, 154*(7), 472–482.

Blyth, F., March, L., Nicholas, M., & Cousins, M. (2005). Self-management of chronic pain: A population-based study. *Pain, 113*(3), 285–292.

Fortier, P., Puntin, B., & Aljaroudi, O. (2011). Improved patient outcomes through collaborative monitoring and management of subtle behavioral and physiological health changes. In *System Sciences (HICSS), 2011 44th Hawaii International Conference* on January, 2011, pp. 1–10. DOI: 10.1109/HICSS.2011.236.

Grey, M., Knafl, K., & McCorkle, R. (2006). A framework for the study of self- and family management of chronic conditions. *Nursing Outlook, 54*(5), 278–286.

Haidet, P., Kroll, T., & Sharf, B. (2006). The complexity of patient participation: Lessons learned from patients' illness narratives. *Patient Education and Counseling, 62*(3), 323–329.

Harvey, I. (2006). Self management of a chronic illness: An exploratory study on the role of spirituality among older African American women. *Journal of Women and Aging, 18*(3), 75–88.

Kennedy, M. (2005). Education benefits women with IBS: Nurses teach self management techniques. *American Journal of Nursing, 105*(1), 22.

Krein, S., Heisler, M., Piette, J., Makki, F., & Kerr, E. (2005). The effect of chronic pain on diabetes patients' self-management. *Diabetes Care, 28*(1), 65–70.

McCahon, D., Murray, E., Murray, K., Holder, R., & Fitzmaurice, D. (2011). Does self-management of oral anticoagulation therapy improve quality of life and anxiety? *Family Practice, 28*(2), 134–140.

Millard, L., Hallett, C., & Luker, K. (2006). Nurse–patient interaction and decision making in care: Patient involvement in community nursing. *Journal of Advanced Nursing, 55*(2), 142–150.

Munir, F., Leka, S., & Griffiths, A. (2005). Dealing with self-management of chronic illness at work: Predictors for self-disclosure. *Social Science Medicine, 60*(6), 1397–1407.

Murray, G., Suto, M., Hole, R., Hale, S., Amari, E., & Michalak, E. (2011). Self-management strategies used by â€˜high functioning' individuals with bipolar disorder: From research to clinical practice. *Clinical Psychology & Psychotherapy, 18*(2), 95–109.

Nguyen, H., Carrieri-Kohlman, V., Rankin, S., Slaughter, R., & Stulberg, M. (2005). Is Internet-based support for dyspnea self-management in patients with chronic obstructive pulmonary disease possible? Results of a pilot study. *Heart and Lung, 34*(1), 51–62.

Rogers, A., Kennedy, A., Nelson, E., & Robinson, A. (2005). Uncovering the limits of patient centeredness: Implementing a self management trail for chronic illness. *Qualitative Health Research, 15*(2), 224–239.

Seçkin, G. (2011). I am proud and hopeful: Age-based comparisons in positive coping affect among women who use online peer-support. *Journal of Psychosocial Oncology, 29*(5), 573–591.

Stevens, S., & Sin, J. (2005). Implementing a self-management model of relapse prevention for psychosis into routine clinical practice. *Journal of Psychiatric Mental Health Nursing, 12*(4), 495–501.

Vassilev, I., Rogers, A., Sanders, C., Kennedy, A., Blickem, C., Protheroe, J., et al. (2011). Social networks, social capital and chronic illness self-management: A realist review. *Chronic Illness, 7*(1), 60–86.

Whittemore, R., Melkus, G., & Grey, M. (2005). Metabolic control, self management and psychosocial adjustment in women with type 2 diabetes. *Journal of Clinical Nursing, 14*(2), 195–203.

Zhou, Q., Li, X., Zou, F., Wu, L., Chen, H., & Liu, Z. (2011). Effect of systematic self-management education on quality of life, anxiety and depression of patients with Type 2 diabetes in communities. *Zhong Nan Da Xue Xue Bao Yi Xue Ban, 36*(2), 133–137.

Self-Health Management, Readiness for Enhanced

Note: Refer to Self-Health Management, Ineffective.

Self-Mutilation

Barr, W., Leitner, M., & Thomas, J. (2005). Psychosocial assessment of patients who attend an accident and emergency department with self-harm. *Journal of Psychiatric & Mental Health Nursing, 12*(2), 130–138.

Choate, L. (2012). Counseling adolescents who engage in nonsuicidal self-injury: A dialectical behavior therapy approach. *Journal of Mental Health Counseling, 34*(1), 56–71.

Curran, J. (2006). Cognitive behavioural therapy for patients with anxiety and depression. [cover story]. *Nursing Standard, 21*(7), 44–52.

Delion, P. (2011). Towards a dialogue between psychoanalysis and neuroscience: Connections that are both possible and necessary. *Journal of Physiology–Paris, 105*(4–6), 220–222.

Derouin, A., & Bravender, T. (2004). Living on the edge: The current phenomenon of self-mutilation in adolescents. *MCN: The American Journal of Maternal Child Nursing, 29*(1), 12–20.

Evren, C., Dalbudaak, E., Evren, B., Cetin, R., & Durkaya, M. (2011). Self-mutilative behaviours in male alcohol-dependent inpatients and relationship with posttraumatic stress disorder. *Psychiatry Research, 186*(1), 91–96.

Fikke, L., Melinder, A., & Landrø, N. (2011). Executive functions are impaired in adolescents engaging in non-suicidal self-injury. *Psychological Medicine, 41*(3), 601–610.

Flett, G., Godlstein, A., Hewitt, P., & Wekerle, C. (2012). Predictors of deliberate self-harm behavior among emerging adolescents: An initial test of a self-punitiveness model. *Current Psychology, 31*(1), 49–64.

Gough, K. (2005). Guideline for managing self-harm in a forensic setting. *British Journal of Forensic Practice, 7*(2), 10–14.

Gratz, K., Hepworth, C., Tull, M., Paulson, A., Clarke, S., Remington, B., et al. (2011). An experimental investigation of emotional willingness and physical pain tolerance in deliberate self-harm: The moderating role of interpersonal distress. *Comprehensive Psychiatry, 52*(1), 63–74.

Lang, C., & Sharma-Patel, K. (2011). The relation between childhood maltreatment and self-injury: A review of the literature on conceptualization and intervention. *Trauma, Violence, & Abuse, 12*(1), 23–37.

Poustie, A., & Neville, R. G. (2004). Deliberate self-harm cases: A primary care perspective. *Nursing Standard, 18*(48), 33–36.

Sharp, D., Liebenau, A., Stocks, N., Bennewith, O., Evans, M., Jones, W. B., et al. (2003). Locally developed guidelines for the aftercare of deliberate self-harm patients in general practice. *Primary Health Care Research & Development, 4*(1), 21–28.

Wachtel, L., Jaffe, R., & Kellner, C. (2011). Electroconvulsive therapy for psychotropic-refractory bipolar affective disorder and severe self-injury and aggression in an 11-year-old autistic boy. *European Child & Adolescent Psychiatry, 20*(3), 147–152.

Wilkinson, B. (2011). Current trends in remediating adolescent self-injury: An integrative review. *The Journal of School Nursing, 27*(2), 120–128.

Self-Mutilation, Risk for

(Also see Bibliography for the diagnosis Self-Mutilation, preceding.)

Anderson, M., Woodward, L., & Armstrong, M. (2004). Self-harm in young people: A perspective for mental health nursing care. *International Nursing Review, 51*(4), 222–228.

Angelkovska, A., Houghton, S., & Hopkins, S. (2012). Differential profiles of risk of self-harm among clinically referred primary school aged children. *School Psychology International*, DOI: 10.1177/0143034311427434. Retrieved March 4, 2012, from http://spi.sagepub.com/content/early/2012/02/07/0143034311427434.abstract

Arbuthnot, L., & Gillespie, M. (2005). Self-harm: Reviewing psychological assessment in emergency departments. *Emergency Nurse, 12*(10), 20–24.

Barr, W., Leitner, M., & Thomas, J. (2005). Psychosocial assessment of patients who attend an accident and emergency department with self-harm. *Journal of Psychiatric & Mental Health Nursing, 12*(2), 130–138.

Cleaver, K. (2007). Characteristics and trends of self-harming behaviour in young people. *British Journal of Nursing (BJN), 16*(3), 148–152.

Curran, J. (2006). Cognitive behavioural therapy for patients with anxiety and depression. [cover story]. *Nursing Standard, 21*(7), 44–52.

Duncan, E. A. S., Nicol, M. M., Ager, A., & Dalgleish, L. (2006). A systematic review of structured group interventions with mentally disordered offenders. *Criminal Behaviour & Mental Health, 16*(4), 217–241.

Goth subculture linked to self-harm and suicide. (2006). *Nursing Standard, 20*(36), 20.

Hawton, K., & O-Connor, R. (2012). Self-harm in adolescence and future mental health. *The Lancet, 379*(9812), 198–199.

Hoch, J. S., Reilly, R. L., & Carscadden, J. (2006). Best practices. Relationship management therapy for patients with borderline personality disorder. *Psychiatric Services, 57*(2), 179.

Hyldahl, R., & Richardson, B. (2011). Key considerations for using no-harm contracts with clients who self-injure. *Journal of Counseling & Development, 89*(1), 121–126.

Kumar, P., & Bhojraj, N. (2011). Successful prevention of oral self-mutilation using a lip guard: A case report. *Special Care in Dentistry, 31*(3), 114–118.

Liu, R., & Mustanski, B. (2012). Suicidal ideation and self-harm in lesbian, gay, bisexual, and transgender youth. *American Journal of Preventive Medicine, 42*(3), 221–228.

Meekings, C., & O'Brien, L. (2004). Borderline pathology in children and adolescents. *International Journal of Mental Health Nursing, 13*(3), 152–163.

Patterson, P., Whittington, R., & Bogg, J. (2007). Testing the effectiveness of an educational intervention aimed at changing attitudes to self-harm. *Journal of Psychiatric & Mental Health Nursing, 14*(1), 100–105.

Slaven, J., & Kisely, S. (2002). Staff perceptions of care for deliberate self-harm patients in rural Western Australia: A qualitative study. *Australian Journal of Rural Health, 10*(5), 233–238.

Support group for mutilated women. (2007). *Nursing Standard, 21*(26), 11–11.

Wu, C.-Y., Whitley, R., Stewart, R., & Liu, S.-I. (2012). Pathways to care and help-seeking experience prior to self-harm: A qualitative study in Taiwan. *Journal of Nursing Research, 20*(1), 32–42.

Yearwood, E., Pearson, G., & Newland, J. (2012). *Child and adolescent behavioral health: A resource for advanced practice psychiatric and primary care practitioners in nursing*. West Sussex, UK: John Wiley & Sons, Ltd.

Self-Neglect

Barocka, A., Seehuber, D., & Schone, D. (2004). Messy house syndrome. *MMW Fortschritte der Medizin, 146*(45), 36–39.

Gibbons, S. (2007). *Characteristics and behaviors of self-neglect in community-dwelling older adults*. Doctoral dissertation. Retrieved from Dissertation Abstracts International, UMI No. 3246949.

Gibbons, S., Lauder, W., & Ludwick, R. (2006). Self-neglect: A proposed new NANDA diagnosis. *International Journal of Nursing Terminologies and Classification, 17*(1), 10–18.

Greve, K., Curtis, K., Bianchini, K., & Collins, B. (2004). Personality disorder masquerading as dementia: A case of apparent Diogenes syndrome. *International Journal of Geriatric Psychiatry, 19*(7), 703–705.

Lauder, W., Anderson, I., & Barclay, A. (2005). A framework for good practice in interagency interventions with cases of self-neglect. *Journal of Psychiatric and Mental Health Nursing, 12*(2), 192–198.

Lauder, W., Anderson, I., & Barclay, A. (2005). Guidelines for good practice in self-neglect. *Journal of Psychiatric and Mental Health Nursing, 12*(2), 192–198.

Mosqueda, L. (2011). Elder abuse and self-neglect. *The Journal of the American Medical Association, 306*(5), 532–540.

Sauvageau, A., & Hunter, B. (2011). Self-neglect: Adaptation of a clinical tool to the practice of the medical examiner. *The American Journal of Forensic Medicine and Pathology,* 33(3), 289–292.

Smith, S., Oliver, S., Zwart, S., Kala, G., Kelly, A., Goodwin, J., et al. (2006). Nutritional status is altered in the self-neglecting elderly. *The Journal of Nutrition, 136*(10), 2534–2541.

Tierney, M., Charles, J., Naglie, G., Jaglal, S., Kiss, A., & Fisher, R. (2004). Risk for harm in cognitively impaired seniors who live alone: A prospective study. *Journal of the American Geriatrics Society, 52*(9), 1576–1577.

Sexual Dysfunction

Banning, M. (2007). Women's health. Advanced breast cancer: Aetiology, treatment and psychosocial features. *British Journal of Nursing (BJN), 16*(2), 86–90.

Barton, D., Wilwerding, M., Carpenter, L., & Loprinzi, C. (2004). Libido as part of sexuality in female cancer survivors. *Oncology Nursing Forum, 31*(3), 599–607.

Bond, D., Wing, R., Vithiananthan, S., Sax, H., Roye, G., Ryder, B., et al. (2011). Significant resolution of female sexual dysfunction after bariatric surgery. *Surgery for Obesity and Related Diseases, 7*(1), 1–7.

Corte, C. M., & Sommers, M. S. (2005). Alcohol and risky behaviors. *Annual Review of Nursing Research, 23,* 327–360.

Duncan, M. K. W., & Sanger, M. (2004). Coping with the pediatric anogenital exam. *Journal of Child & Adolescent Psychiatric Nursing, 17*(3), 126–136.

Guiao, I. Z., Blakemore, N. M., & Wise, A. B. (2004). Predictors of teen substance use and risky sexual behaviors: Implications for advanced nursing practice. *Clinical Excellence for Nurse Practitioners, 8*(2), 52–59.

Higgins, A., Barker, P., & Begley, C. M. (2006a). Iatrogenic sexual dysfunction and the protective withholding of information: In whose best interest? *Journal of Psychiatric & Mental Health Nursing, 13*(4), 437–446.

Higgins, A., Barker, P., & Begley, C. M. (2006b). Sexuality: The challenge to espoused holistic care. *International Journal of Nursing Practice, 12*(6), 345–351.

Indhavivadhana, S., Leerasiri, P., Rattanachaiyanont, M., Laiwejpithaya, S., Tanmahasamut, P., Techatraisak, K., et al. (2010). Vaginal atrophy and sexual dysfunction in current users of systemic postmenopausal hormone therapy. *Journal of the Medical Association of Thailand, 93*(6), 667–675.

Lund-Nielsen, B., Müller, K., & Adamsen, L. (2005). Malignant wounds in women with breast cancer: Feminine and sexual perspectives. *Journal of Clinical Nursing, 14*(1), 56–64.

Magnan, M. A., Reynolds, K. E., & Galvin, E. A. (2005). Barriers to addressing patient sexuality in nursing practice. *MEDSURG Nursing, 14*(5), 282–289.

Magnan, M. A., Reynolds, K. E., & Galvin, E. A. (2006). Barriers to addressing patient sexuality in nursing practice. *Dermatology Nursing, 18*(5), 448–454.

Martsolf, D. S., & Draucker, C. B. (2005). Psychotherapy approaches for adult survivors of childhood sexual abuse: An integrative review of outcomes research. *Issues in Mental Health Nursing, 26*(8), 801–825.

Miers, M. (2002). Developing an understanding of gender sensitive care: Exploring concepts and knowledge. *Journal of Advanced Nursing, 40*(1), 69–77.

Muehrer, R. J., Keller, M. L., Powwattana, A., & Pornchaikate, A. (2006). Sexuality among women recipients of a pancreas and kidney transplant. *Western Journal of Nursing Research, 28*(2), 137–150.

Rellini, A., & Meston, C. (2011). Sexual self-schemas, sexual dysfunction, and the sexual responses of women with a history of childhood sexual abuse. *Archives of Sexual Behavior, 40*(2), 351–362.

Reynolds, K. E., & Magnan, M. A. (2005). Nursing attitudes and beliefs toward human sexuality: Collaborative research promoting evidence-based practice. *Clinical Nurse Specialist: The Journal for Advanced Nursing Practice, 19*(5), 255–259.

Röndahl G., Innala, S., & Carlsson, M. (2004). Nurses' attitudes towards lesbians and gay men. *Journal of Advanced Nursing, 47*(4), 386–392.

Safarinejad, M. (2011). Reversal of SSRI-induced female sexual dysfunction by adjunctive bupropion in menstruating women: A double-blind, placebo-controlled and randomized study. *Journal of Psychopharmacology, 25*(3), 370–378.

Serretti, A., & Chiesa, A. (2011). A meta-analysis of sexual dysfunction in psychiatric patients taking antipsychotics. *International Clinical Psychopharmacology, 26*(3), 130–140.

Shell, J. A. (2002). Evidence-based practice for symptom management in adults with cancer: Sexual dysfunction. *Oncology Nursing Forum, 29*(1), 53–69.

Sublett, C. M. (2007). Translating evidence into clinical practice. Critique of 'effects of advanced practice nursing on patient and spouse depressive symptoms, sexual function, and marital interaction after radical prostatectomy'. *Urologic Nursing, 27*(1), 78–80.

Williams, S. S., Norris, A. E., & Bedor, M. M. (2003). Sexual relationships, condom use, and concerns about pregnancy, HIV/AIDS, and other sexually transmitted diseases. *Clinical Nurse Specialist: The Journal for Advanced Nursing Practice, 17*(2), 89–94.

Sexuality Pattern, Ineffective

Alteneder, R., & Hartzekk, D. (1999). Addressing couples' sexuality concerns during the childbearing period: Use of the PLISSIT model. *Journal of Obstetric, Gynecologic, and Neonatal Nursing, 26*(6), 651–658.

Banning, M. (2007). Advanced breast cancer: Aetiology, treatment and psychosocial features. *British Journal of Nursing (BJN), 16*(2), 86–90.

Barton, D., Wilwerding, M., Carpenter, L., & Loprinzi, C. (2004). Libido as part of sexuality in female cancer survivors. *Oncology Nursing Forum, 31*(3), 599–607.

Guiao, I. Z., Blakemore, N. M., & Wise, A. B. (2004). Predictors of teen substance use and risky sexual behaviors: Implications for advanced nursing practice. *Clinical Excellence for Nurse Practitioners, 8*(2), 52–59.

Higgins, A., Barker, P., & Begley, C. M. (2006). Sexuality: The challenge to espoused holistic care. *International Journal of Nursing Practice, 12*(6), 345–351.

Lever, K. A. (2005). Emergency contraception: Nurses can empower women. *AWHONN Lifelines, 9*(3), 218–227.

Magnan, M. A., Reynolds, K. E., & Galvin, E. A. (2005). Barriers to addressing patient sexuality in nursing practice. *MEDSURG Nursing, 14*(5), 282–289.

McAndrew, S., & Warne, T. (2004). Ignoring the evidence dictating the practice: Sexual orientation, suicidality and the dichotomy of the mental health nurse. *Journal of Psychiatric & Mental Health Nursing, 11*(4), 428–434.

Miers, M. (2002). Developing an understanding of gender sensitive care: Exploring concepts and knowledge. *Journal of Advanced Nursing, 40*(1), 69–77.

Reynolds, K. E., & Magnan, M. A. (2005). Nursing attitudes and beliefs toward human sexuality: Collaborative research promoting evidence-based practice. *Clinical Nurse Specialist: The Journal for Advanced Nursing Practice, 19*(5), 255–259.

Röndahl, G., Innala, S., & Carlsson, M. (2004). Nurses' attitudes towards lesbians and gay men. *Journal of Advanced Nursing, 47*(4), 386–392.

Williams, S. S., Norris, A. E., & Bedor, M. M. (2003). Sexual relationships, condom use, and concerns about pregnancy, HIV/AIDS, and other sexually transmitted diseases. *Clinical Nurse Specialist: The Journal for Advanced Nursing Practice, 17*(2), 89–94.

Shock, Risk for

Bridges, E., & Dukes, M. (2005). Cardiovascular aspects of septic shock: Pathophysiology, monitoring, and treatment. *Critical Care Nurse, 25*(2), 14–16, 18–20, 22–24.

Cunha, J., & Shiel, W. (2007). *Medical shock*. Retrieved April 2, 12, from http://www.medicinenet.com/shock/article.htm

Dellnger, R., Levy, M., Carlet, J., Bion, J., Parker, M., Jaeschke, R., et al. (2008). Surviving sepsis campaign: International guidelines for management of severe sepsis and septic shock. *Intensive Care Medicine, 34*(1), 17–60.

Goodrich, C. (2006). Endpoints of resuscitation: What should we be monitoring? *AACN Advanced Critical Care, 17*(3), 306–316.

Gorman, D., Calhoun, K., Carassco, M., Niclaus, D., Neron, M., Nally, L., et al. (2008). Take a rapid treatment approach to cardiogenic shock. *Nursing Critical Care, 3*(4), 18–27.

Longo, D., Fauci, A., Kasper, D., Hauser, S., Jameson, J., & Loscalzo, J. (2012). *Harrison's principles of internal medicine* (18th ed.). New York: McGraw-Hill.

Nelson, D., Lemaster, T., Plost, G., & Zahner, M. (2009). Recognizing sepsis in the adult patient. *American Journal of Nursing, 109*(3), 40–45.

Sommers, M. (2011). *Diseases and disorders: A nursing therapeutics manual* (4th ed.). Philadelphia, PA: F. A. Davis.

Spaniol, J., Knight, A., Zebley, J., Anderson, M., & Pierce, J. (2007). Fluid resuscitation therapy for hemorrhagic shock. *Journal of Trauma Nursing, 14*(13), 152–160.

Workman, M. (2012). Interventions for clients with shock. In D. Ignatavicius & M. Workman (Eds.), *Medical-surgical nursing: Critical thinking for collaborative care* (7th ed.). St. Louis, MO: Elsevier Saunders.

Skin Integrity, Impaired

Bevis, P., & Earnshaw, J. (2011, March 3). Venous ulcer review. *Clinical, Cosmetic, and Investigational Dermatology, 4*, 1–13. Dove Press.

Birchall, L., & Taylor, S. (2003). Surgical wound benchmark tool and best practice guidelines. *British Journal of Nursing (BJN), 12*(17), 1013.

Bolton, L. (2007). Operational definition of moist wound healing. *Journal of Wound, Ostomy & Continence Nursing, 34*(1), 23–29.

Briggs, M. (2006). The prevalence of pain in chronic wounds and nurses' awareness of the problem. *British Journal of Nursing (BJN), 15*(21), 5–9.

Clifton-Koeppel, R. (2006). Wound care after peripheral intravenous extravasation: What is the evidence? *Newborn & Infant Nursing Reviews, 6*(4), 202–212.

Delmas, L. (2006). Best practice in the assessment and management of diabetic foot ulcers. *Rehabilitation Nursing, 31*(6), 228–234.

D'haese, S., Van Roy, M., Bate, T., Bijdekerke, P., & Vinh-Hung, V. (2010). Management of skin reactions during radiotherapy in Flanders (Belgium): A study of nursing practice before and after the introduction of a skin care protocol. *European Journal of Oncology Nursing, 14*(5), 367–372.

Doughty, D. (2005). Dressings and more: Guidelines for topical wound management. *Nursing Clinics of North America, 40*(2), 217–231.

Erwin-Toth, P., Stricker, L., & Rijswijk, L. (2010). Wound wise: Peristomal skin complications. *American Journal of Nursing, 110*(2), 43–48.

Evans, E., & Gray, M. (2005). Do topical analgesics reduce pain associated with wound dressing changes or debridement of chronic wounds? *Journal of Wound, Ostomy & Continence Nursing, 32*(5), 287–290.

Frykberg, R. G. (2005). A summary of guidelines for managing the diabetic foot. *Advances in Skin & Wound Care, 18*(4), 209.

Gannon, R. (2007). Chronic wound management. Wound cleansing: Sterile water or saline? *Nursing Times, 103*(9), 44–46.

Groom, M., Shannon, R., Chakravarthy, D., & Fleck, C. (2010). An evaluation of costs and effects of a nutrient-based skin care program as a component of prevention of skin tears in an extended convalescent center. *Journal of Wound, Ostomy and Continence Nursing, 37*(1), 46–51.

Gwynne, B., & Newton, M. (2006). An overview of the common methods of wound debridement. *British Journal of Nursing (BJN), 15*(19), S4.

Hartmann, K., Viswanathan, M., Palmieri, R., Gartlehner, G., Thorp, J., & Lohr, K. N. (2005). Outcomes of routine episiotomy: A systematic review. *JAMA: Journal of the American Medical Association, 293*(17), 2141–2148.

Helberg, D., Mertens, E., Halfens, R., & Dassen, T. (2006). Treatment of pressure ulcers: Results of a study comparing evidence and practice. *Ostomy Wound Management, 52*(8), 60.

Hermans, M. H. (2006). Silver-containing dressings and the need for evidence. *American Journal of Nursing, 106*(12), 60–68.

Kaitani, T., Tokunaga, K., Matsui, N., & Sanada, H. (2010). Risk factors related to the development of pressure ulcers in the critical care setting. *Journal of Clinical Nursing, 19*(3–4), 414–421.

McIsaac, C. (2005). Managing wound care outcomes. *Ostomy Wound Management, 51*(4), 54.

McQuestion, M. (2011). Evidence-based skin care management in radiation therapy: Clinical update. *Seminars in Oncology Nursing, 27*(2), e1–e17.

Moore, Z. (2007). Evidence-based wound management. *Journal of Clinical Nursing, 16*(2), 428–428.

Nix, D., & Ermer-Seltun, J. (2004). A review of perineal skin care protocols and skin barrier product use. *Ostomy Wound Management, 50*(12), 59–67.

Nixon, J., Thorpe, H., Barrow, H., Phillips, A., Nelson, E. A., & Mason, S. A. (2005). Reliability of pressure ulcer classification and diagnosis. *Journal of Advanced Nursing, 50*(6), 613–623.

Ratliff, C. (2010). Early peristomal skin complications reported by WOC nurses. *Journal of Wound, Ostomy & Continence Nursing, 37*(5), 505–510.

Ratliff, C. R. (2005). WOCN's evidence-based pressure ulcer guideline. *Advances in Skin & Wound Care, 18*(4), 204.

Roberson, S., Ayello, E., & Levine, J. (2010). Clarification of pressure ulcer staging in long-term care under MDS 2.0. *Advances in Skin & Wound Care, 23*(5), 206–210.

Ruth-Sahd, L., & Gonzales, M. (2006). Multiple dimensions of caring for a patient with acute necrotizing fasciitis. *Dimensions of Critical Care Nursing, 25*(1), 15–21.

Sibbald, R., Krasner, D., & Lutz, J. (2010). SCALE: Skin changes at life's end: Final consensus statement: October 1, 2009(c). *Advances in Skin & Wound Care, 23*(5), 225–236.

Thomas, D. (2010). Does pressure cause pressure ulcers? An inquiry into the etiology of pressure ulcers. *Journal of the American Medical Directors Association (JAMDA), 11*(6), 397–405.

Vermeulin, H., Ubbink, D. T., Goossens, A., de Vos, R., & Legemate, D. A. (2005). Systematic review of dressings and topical agents for surgical wounds healing by secondary intention. *British Journal of Surgery, 92*(6), 665–672.

Wilkinson, J., & Treas, L. (2011). Chapter 34, Skin integrity and wound healing. In *Fundamentals of nursing* (2nd ed.). Philadelphia: F. A. Davis.

Willock, J., & Maylor, M. (2004). Pressure ulcers in infants and children. *Nursing Standard, 18*(24), 56–62.

Yilmaz, M., & Ozsoy, S. (2010). Effectiveness of a discharge-planning program and home visits for meeting the physical care needs of children with cancer. *Supportive Care in Cancer, 18*(2), 243–253.

Skin Integrity, Readiness for Enhanced

See references for Skin Integrity, Risk for Impaired.

Skin Integrity, Risk for Impaired

Adderley, U. Factors that influence the frequency of rebandaging. *EWMA Journal, 6*(1), 9–11.

Allen, G. (2006). Evidence for practice. Paint-only versus scrub-and-paint surgical skin prep. *AORN Journal, 83*(3), 752–753.

Anthony, T., Murray, B., Sum-Ping, J., Lenkovsky, F., Vornik, V., Parker, B., et al. (2011). Evaluating an evidence-based bundle for preventing surgical site infection. A randomized trial. *Archives of Surgery, 146*(3), 263–269.

Arrowsmith, V. A., Maunder, J. A., Sargent, R. J., & Taylor, R. (2006). Removal of nail polish and finger rings to prevent surgical infection. *Cochrane Library* (4).

Ayello, E. A., Baranoski, S., & Salati, D. S. (2006). Best practices in wound care prevention and treatment. *Nursing Management, 37*(9), 42–48.

Birchall, L., & Taylor, S. (2003). Surgical wound benchmark tool and best practice guidelines. *British Journal of Nursing (BJN), 12*(17), 1013.

Bliss, D., Savik, K., Thorson, M., Ehman, S., Lebak, K., & Beilman, G. (2011). Incontinence-associated dermatitis in critically ill adults: Time to development, severity, and risk factors. *Journal of Wound, Ostomy and Continence Nursing, 38*(4), 433–445.

Doughty, D. (2005). Dressings and more: Guidelines for topical wound management. *Nursing Clinics of North America, 40*(2), 217–231.

Evans, D., Wood, J., & Lambert, L. (2003). Patient injury and physical restraint devices: A systematic review. *Journal of Advanced Nursing, 41*(3), 274–282.

Evans, J., & Chance, T. (2005). Improving patient outcomes using a diabetic foot assessment tool. *Nursing Standard, 19*(45), 65.

Fader, M., Clarke-O'Neill, S., Cook, D., Dean, G., Brooks, R., Cottenden, A., et al. (2003). Management of night-time urinary incontinence in residential settings for older people: An investigation into the effects of different pad changing regimes on skin health. *Journal of Clinical Nursing, 12*(3), 374–386.

Frykberg, R. G. (2005). A summary of guidelines for managing the diabetic foot. *Advances in Skin & Wound Care, 18*(4), 209.

Griffin, F. A. (2005). Best-practice protocols: Preventing surgical site infection. *Nursing Management, 36*(11), 20–26.

Groom, M., Shannon, R., Chakravarthy, D., & Fleck, C. (2010). An evaluation of costs and effects of a nutrient-based skin care program as a component of prevention of skin tears in an extended convalescent center. *Journal of Wound, Ostomy and Continence Nursing, 37*(1), 46–51.

Hughes, S. (2002). Do incontinence aids help to maintain skin integrity? *Journal of Wound Care, 11*(6), 235–239.

Kaitani, T., Tokunaga, K., Matsui, N., & Sanada, H. (2010). Risk factors related to the development of pressure ulcers in the critical care setting. *Journal of Clinical Nursing, 19*(3–4), 414–421.

Nix, D., & Ermer-Seltun, J. (2004). A review of perineal skin care protocols and skin barrier product use. *Ostomy Wound Management, 50*(12), 59–67.

Nixon, J., Nelson, E. A., Cranny, G., Iglesias, C. P., Hawkins, K., & Cullum, N. A. (2006). Pressure relieving support surfaces: A randomised evaluation. *Health Technology Assessment, 10*(22), 1–180.

Odom-Forren, J. (2006). Preventing surgical site infections [cover story]. *Nursing, 36*(6), 58–64.

Ratliff, C. (2010). Early peristomal skin complications reported by WOC nurses. *Journal of Wound, Ostomy & Continence Nursing, 37*(5), 505–510.

Sarkar, R., Basu, S., Agrawal, R., & Gupta, P. (2010). Skin care for the newborn. *Indian Pediatrics, 47*(7), 593–598.

Sibbald, R., Krasner, D., & Lutz, J. (2010). SCALE: Skin changes at life's end: Final consensus statement: October 1, 2009(c). *Advances in Skin & Wound Care, 23*(5), 225–236.

Thomas, D. (2010). Does pressure cause pressure ulcers? An inquiry into the etiology of pressure ulcers. *Journal of the American Medical Directors Association (JAMDA), 11*(6), 397–405.

Voegeli, D. (2005). Skin hygiene practices, emollient therapy and skin vulnerability. *Nursing Times, 101*(4), 57–58.

Williams, H., & Griffiths, P. (2004). The effectiveness of pin site care for patients with external fixators. *British Journal of Community Nursing, 9*(5), 206–210.

Wilkinson, J., & Treas, L. (2011). Chapter 34, Skin integrity and wound healing. *Fundamentals of nursing* (2nd ed.). Philadelphia: F. A. Davis.

Wipke-Tevis, D. D., Williams, D. A., Rantz, M. J., Popejoy, L. L., Madsen, R. W., & Petroski, G. F. (2004). Nursing home quality and pressure ulcer prevention and management practices. *Journal of the American Geriatrics Society, 52*(4), 583–588.

Woods, A. J. (2006). The role of health professionals in childhood injury prevention: A systematic review of the literature. *Patient Education & Counseling, 64*(1), 35–42.

Yilmaz, M., & Ozsoy, S. (2010). Effectiveness of a discharge-planning program and home visits for meeting the physical care needs of children with cancer. *Supportive Care in Cancer, 18*(2), 243–253.

Sleep Deprivation

Ancoli-Israel, S., Bliwise, D., & NØrgaard, J. (2011). The effect of nocturia on sleep. *Sleep Medicine Reviews, 15*(2), 91–97.

Arne, F., & Arvid, S. (2003). Bright light treatment improves sleep in institutionalised elderly—an open trial. *International Journal of Geriatric Psychiatry, 18*(6), 520.

Berger, A. M., Parker, K. P., Young-McCaughan, S., Mallory, G. A., Barsevick, A. M., & Beck, S. L. (2005). Sleep/wake disturbances in people with cancer and their caregivers: State of the science. *Oncology Nursing Forum, 32,* 98–E126.

Berger, A. M., Sankaranarayanan, J., & Watanabe-Galloway, S. (2006). Current methodological approaches to the study of sleep disturbances and quality of life in adults with cancer: A systematic review. *PsychoOncology, 16*(5), 401–420.

Clark, J., Cunningham, M., McMillan, S., Vena, C., & Parker, K. (2004). Sleep-wake disturbances in people with cancer part II: Evaluating the evidence for clinical decision making. *Oncology Nursing Forum, 31*(4), 747–768.

Conn, D. K., & Madan, R. (2006). Use of sleep-promoting medications in nursing home residents: Risks versus benefits. *Drugs & Aging, 23*(4), 271.

Crowley, K. (2011). Sleep and sleep disorders in older adults. *Neuropsychology Review, 21*(1), 41–53.

Eliassen, K., & Hopstock, L. (2011). Sleep promotion in the intensive care unit—a survey of nurses' interventions. *Intensive and Critical Care Nursing, 27*(3), 138–142.

Everhart, E. (2011). Sleep disorders in children: Collaboration for school-based intervention. *Journal of Educational and Psychological Consultation, 21*(2), 133–148.

Golbidi, S., Badran, M., Ayas, N., & Laher, I. (2012). Cardiovascular consequences of sleep apnea. *Lung, 190,* 113–132.

Hellström, A., Fagerström, C., & Willman, A. (2011). Promoting sleep by nursing interventions in health care settings: A systematic review. *Worldviews on Evidence-Based Nursing, 8*(3), 128–142.

Kamdar, B., Needham, D., & Collop, N. (2012). Sleep deprivation in critical illness: Its role in physical and psychological recovery. *Journal of Intensive Care Medicine, 27*(2), 97–111.

Koch, S., Haesler, E., Tiziani, A., & Wilson, J. (2006). Effectiveness of sleep management strategies for residents of aged care facilities: Findings of a systematic review. *Journal of Clinical Nursing, 15*(10), 1267–1275.

Li, S.-Y., Wanmg, T.-J., Wu, S., Liang, S.-Y., & Tung, H.-H. (2011). Efficacy of controlling night-time noise and activities to improve patients' sleep quality in a surgical intensive care unit. *Journal of Clinical Nursing, 20*(3–4), 396–407.

Lieverse, R., Van Somedren, E., Nielen, M., Uitdehaag, B., Smit, J., & Hoogendijk, W. (2011). Bright light treatment in elderly patients with nonseasonal major depressive disorder. A randomized placebo-controlled trial. *Archives of General Psychiatry, 68*(1), 61–70.

Page, M. S., Berger, A. M., & Johnson, L. B. (2006). Putting evidence into practice: Evidence-based interventions for sleep-wake disturbances. *Clinical Journal of Oncology Nursing, 10*(6), 753–676.

Phillips, K. D., Mock, K. S., Bopp, C. M., Dudgeon, W. A., & Hand, G. A. (2006). Spiritual well-being, sleep disturbance, and mental and physical health status in HIV-infected individuals. *Issues in Mental Health Nursing, 27*(2), 125–139.

Richards, K., Lambert, C., Beck, C., Bliwise, D., Evans, W., Kaira, G., et al. (2011). Strength training, walking, and social activity improve sleep in nursing home and assisted living residents: Randomized controlled trial. *Journal of the American Geriatrics Society, 59*(2), 214–223.

Sateia, M. J., & Nowell, P. D. (2004). Insomnia. *Lancet, 364*(9449), 1959–1973.

Shin, C., Kim, J., Yi, H., Lee, H., Lee, J., & Shin, K. (2005). Relationship between trait-anger and sleep disturbances in middle-aged men and women. *Journal of Psychosomatic Research, 58*(2), 183–189.

Wilkinson, J., & Treas, L. (2011). Chapter 34, Skin integrity and wound healing. In *Fundamentals of nursing* (2nd ed.). Philadelphia: F. A. Davis.

Sleep Pattern, Disturbed

Alessi, C. A., Martin, J. L., & Webber, A. P. (2005). A multidimensional non-drug intervention reduced daytime sleep in nursing home residents with sleep problems. *Evidence-Based Medicine, 10*(6), 178.

Berger, A. M., Parker, K. P., Young-McCaughan, S., Mallory, G. A., Barsevick, A. M., & Beck, S. L. (2005). Sleep/wake disturbances in people with cancer and their caregivers: State of the science. *Oncology Nursing Forum, 32*(6), E98–E126.

Clark, J., Cunningham, M., McMillan, S., Vena, C., & Parker, K. (2004). Sleep-wake disturbances in people with cancer part II: Evaluating the evidence for clinical decision making.*Oncology Nursing Forum, 31*(4), 747–768.

Conn, D. K., & Madan, R. (2006). Use of sleep-promoting medications in nursing home residents: Risks versus benefits. *Drugs & Aging, 23*(4), 271.

Haesler, E. J. (2004). Effectiveness of strategies to manage sleep in residents of aged care facilities. *JBI Reports, 2*(4), 115–183.

Hinds, P. S., Hockenberry, M., Rai, S. N., Lijun, Z., Razzouk, B. I., McCarthy, K., et al. (2007). Nocturnal awakenings, sleep environment interruptions, and fatigue in hospitalized children with cancer. *Oncology Nursing Forum, 34*(2), 393–402.

Hui-Ling, L., & Good, M. (2006). Music improves sleep quality in older adults. *Journal of Advanced Nursing, 53*(1), 134–144.

Koch, S., Haesler, E., Tiziani, A., & Wilson, J. (2006). Effectiveness of sleep management strategies for residents of aged care facilities: Findings of a systematic review. *Journal of Clinical Nursing, 15*(10), 1267–1275.

McCavey, B., & Neal-Perry, G. (2010). Evaluating and treating insomnia in menopausal women. *Menopausal Medicine, 18*(3), S1–S12.

O'Brien, L. (2011). The neurocognitive effects of sleep disruption in children and adolescents. *Sleep Medicine Clinics, 6*(1), 109–116.

Page, M. S., Berger, A. M., & Johnson, L. B. (2006). Putting evidence into practice: Evidence-based interventions for sleep-wake disturbances. *Clinical Journal of Oncology Nursing, 10*(6), 753–676.

Perlis, M. L., Smith, L. J., Lyness, J. M., Matteson, S. R., Pigeon, W. R., & Jungquist, C. R. (2006). Insomnia as a risk factor for onset of depression in the elderly. *Behavioral Sleep Medicine, 4*(2), 104–113.

Phillips, K. D., Mock, K. S., Bopp, C. M., Dudgeon, W. A., & Hand, G. A. (2006). Spiritual well-being, sleep disturbance, and mental and physical health status in HIV-infected individuals. *Issues in Mental Health Nursing, 27*(2), 125–139.

Shin, C., Kim, J., Yi, H., Lee, H., Lee, J., & Shin, K. (2005). Relationship between trait-anger and sleep disturbances in middle-aged men and women. *Journal of Psychosomatic Research, 58*(2), 183–189.

Ward, T., Archbold, K., Lentz, M., Ringold, S., Wallace, C., & Landis, C. (2010). Sleep disturbance, daytime sleepiness, and neurocognitive performance in children with juvenile idiopathic arthritis. *Sleep, 33*(2), 252–259.

Wilkinson, J., & Treas, L. (2011). Chapter 33, Sleep and rest. In *Fundamentals of nursing* (2nd ed.). Philadelphia: F. A. Davis.

Wilson, S., Nutt, D., Alford, C., Argyropoulos, S., Baldwin, D., & Bateson, A. (2010). British association for psychopharmacology consensus statement on evidence-based treatment of insomnia, parasomnias and circadian rhythm disorders. *Journal of Psychopharmacology, 24*(11), 1577–1601.

Sleep, Readiness for Enhanced

Alexander, I. M., & Moore, A. (2007). Treating vasomotor symptoms of menopause: The nurse practitioner's perspective. *Journal of the American Academy of Nurse Practitioners, 19*(3), 152–163.

Conn, D. K., & Madan, R. (2006). Use of sleep-promoting medications in nursing home residents: Risks versus benefits. *Drugs & Aging, 23*(4), 271.

Hinds, P. S., Hockenberry, M., Rai, S. N., Lijun, Z., Razzouk, B. I., McCarthy, K., et al. (2007). Nocturnal awakenings, sleep environment interruptions, and fatigue in hospitalized children with cancer. *Oncology Nursing Forum, 34*(2), 393–402.
Kohyama, J. (2011). Sleep health and asynchronization. *Brain and Development, 33*(3), 252–259.

Kor, K., & Mullan, B. (2011). Sleep hygiene behaviours: An application of the theory of planned behaviour and the investigation of perceived autonomy support, past behaviour and response inhibition. *Psychology & Health, 26*(9), 1208–1224.

Landis, C., & Moe, K. (2004). Sleep and menopause. *Nursing Clinics of North America, 39*(1), 97–115.

Redeker, N., & McEnany, G. (2011). *Sleep disorders and sleep promotion in nursing practice*. New York: Springer Publishing Co.

Richards, K., Lambert, C., Beck, C., Bliwise, D., Evans, W., Kaira, G., et al. (2011). Strength training, walking, and social activity improve sleep in nursing home and assisted living residents: Randomized controlled trial. *Journal of the American Geriatrics Society, 59*(2), 214–223.

Shochat, T., Martin, J., Marler, M., & Ancoli-Israel, S. (2000). Illumination levels in nursing home patients: Effects on sleep and activity rhythms. *Journal of Sleep Research, 9*(4), 373–379.

Spruyt, K., & Gozal, D. (2011). Pediatric sleep questionnaires as diagnostic or epidemiological tools: A review of currently available instruments. *Sleep Medicine Reviews, 15*(1), 19–32.

Wilkinson, J., & Treas, L. (2011). Chapter 33, sleep and rest. In *Fundamentals of nursing* (2nd ed.). Philadelphia: F. A. Davis.

Social Interaction, Impaired

Adamsen, L., & Rasmussen, J. M. (2003). Exploring and encouraging through social interaction: A qualitative study of nurses' participation in self-help groups for cancer patients. *Cancer Nursing, 26*(1), 28–36.

Bengtsson-Tops, A., & Hansson, L. (2003). Clinical and social changes in severely mentally ill individuals admitted to an outpatient psychosis team: An 18-month follow-up study. *Scandinavian Journal of Caring Sciences, 17*(1), 3–11.

Darbyshire, P., Muir-Cochrane, E., Fereday, J., Jureidini, J., & Drummond, A. (2006). Engagement with health and social care services: Perceptions of homeless young people with mental health problems. *Health & Social Care in the Community, 14*(6), 553–562.

Davis, L., Mohay, H., & Edwards, H. (2003). Mothers' involvement in caring for their premature infants: An historical overview. *Journal of Advanced Nursing, 42*(6), 578–586.

Eisenegger, C., Haushofer, J., & Fehr, E. (2011). The role of testosterone in social interaction. *Trends in Cognitive Sciences, 15*(6), 263–271.

Forde, H., Lane, H., McCloskey, D., McManus, V., & Tierney, E. (2004). Link family support—an evaluation of an in-home support service. *Journal of Psychiatric & Mental Health Nursing, 11*(6), 698–704.

Granerud, A., & Severinsson, E. (2007). Knowledge about social networks and integration: A co-operative research project. *Journal of Advanced Nursing, 58*(4), 348–357.

Hari, R., & Kujala, M. (2009). Brain basis of human social interaction: From concepts to brain imaging. *Physiological Reviews, 89*(2), 453–479.

Richeson, N. E. (2003). Effects of animal-assisted therapy on agitated behaviors and social interactions of older adults with dementia: An evidence-based therapeutic recreation intervention. *American Journal of Recreation Therapy, 2*(4), 9–16.

Stichter, J., O'Connor, K., Herzog, M., Lierheimer, K., & McGhee, S. (2012). Social competence intervention for elementary students with Aspergers syndrome and high functioning autism. *Journal of Autism and Developmental Disorders, 42*(3), 354–366.

Taylor, J., & Seltzer, M. (2011). Employment and post-secondary educational activities for young adults with autism spectrum disorders during the transition to adulthood. *Journal of Autism and Developmental Disorders, 41*(5), 566–574.

Vanwesenbeeck, I. (2005). Burnout among female indoor sex workers. *Archives of Sexual Behavior, 34*(6), 627–639.

Social Isolation

Arthur, H. M. (2006). Depression, isolation, social support, and cardiovascular, disease in older adults. *Journal of Cardiovascular Nursing, 21,* S2–S7.

Beebe, L. H. (2007). Beyond the prescription pad: Psychosocial treatments for individuals with schizophrenia. *Journal of Psychosocial Nursing & Mental Health Services, 45*(3), 35.

Blomqvist, L., Pitkälä, K., & Routasalo, P. (2007). Images of loneliness: Using art as an educational method in professional training. *Journal of Continuing Education in Nursing, 38*(2), 89–93.

Cutting, A., & Dunn, J. (2006). Conversations with siblings and with friends: Links between relationship quality and social understanding. *British Journal of Developmental Psychology, 24*(1), 73–87.

Elliott, I. M., Lach, L., & Smith, M. L. (2005). I just want to be normal: A qualitative study exploring how children and adolescents view the impact of intractable epilepsy on their quality of life. *Epilepsy & Behavior, 7*(4), 664–678.

Greenslade, M. V., & House, C. J. (2006). Living with lymphedema: A qualitative study of women's perspectives on prevention and management following breast cancer-related treatment. *Canadian Oncology Nursing Journal, 16*(3), 165–171.

Hawton, A., Green, C., Dickens, A., Richards, S., Taylor, R., Edwards, R., et al. (2011). The impact of social isolation on the health status and health-related quality of life of older people. *Quality of Life Research, 20*(1), 57–67.

Lubkin, P. (2011). *Chronic illness: Impact and intervention* (10th ed.). Burlington, MA: Jones & Bartlett Publishers.

Umberson, D., & Montez, J. (2010). Social relationships and health a flashpoint for health policy. *Journal of Health and Social Behavior, 51*(1), S54–S56.

Wang, K. K., & Barnard, A. (2004). Integrative literature reviews and meta-analyses technology-dependent children and their families: A review. *Journal of Advanced Nursing, 45*(1), 36–46.

Sorrow, Chronic

Andershed, B. (2006). Relatives in end-of-life care—part 1: A systematic review of the literature the five last years, January 1999–February 2004. *Journal of Clinical Nursing, 15*(9), 1158–1169.

Chuang, Y., & Huang, H. (2007). Nurses' feelings and thoughts about using physical restraints on hospitalized older patients. *Journal of Clinical Nursing, 16*(3), 486–494.

Eggenberger, S., Meiers, S., Krumwiede, N., Bliesmer, M., & Earle, P. (2011). Reintegration within families in the context of chronic illness: A family health promoting process. *Journal of Nursing and Healthcare of Chronic Illness, 3*(3), 283–292.

Kearney, P. M., & Griffin, T. (2001). Between joy and sorrow: Being a parent of a child with developmental disability. *Journal of Advanced Nursing, 34*(5), 582–592.

Lindgren, C. L., Burke, M. L., Hainsworth, M. A., & Eakes, G. G. (1992). Chronic sorrow: A life span concept. *Scholarly Inquiry for Nursing Practice, 24*(6), 27–42.

McAdams, C., Dewell, J., & Holman, A. (2011). Children and chronic sorrow: Reconceptualizing the emotional impact of parental rejection and its treatment. *The Journal of Humanistic Counseling, 50*(1), 27–41.

Melnyk, B., Feinstein, N., Moldenhouer, Z., & Small, L. (2001). Coping of parents of children who are chronically ill. *Pediatric Nursing, 27*(6), 548–558.

Moules, N. J., Simonson, K., Fleiszer, A. R., Prins, M., & Glasgow, B. (2007). The soul of sorrow work. *Journal of Family Nursing, 13*(1), 117–141.

Northington, L. (2000). Chronic sorrow in caregivers of school age children with sickle cell disease: A grounded theory approach. *Issues in Comprehensive Pediatric Nursing, 23*(3), 141–154.

Perrin, K., Sheehan, C., Potter, M., & Kazanowski, M. (2011). *Palliative care nursing: Caring for suffering patients*. Boston, MA: Jones & Bartlett.

Richardson, M., Cobham, V., Murray, J., & McDermott, B. (2011). Parents' grief in the context of adult child mental illness: A qualitative review. *Clinical Child and Family Psychology Review, 14*(1), 28–43.

Sjöblom, L., Pejlert, A., & Asplund, K. (2005). Nurses' view of the family in psychiatric care. *Journal of Clinical Nursing, 14*(5), 562–569.

Spiritual Distress

Note: Also see the bibliography for Risk for Spiritual Distress, following.

Abrahm, J. L., & Hansen-Flaschen, J. (2002). Hospice care for patients with advanced lung disease. *Chest, 121*(1), 220.

Aminoff, B. Z., & Adunsky, A. (2005). Dying dementia patients: Too much suffering, too little palliation. *American Journal of Hospice & Palliative Medicine, 22*(5), 344–348.

Balk, D., Zaengle, D., & Corr, C. (2011). Strengthening grief support for adolescents coping with a peer's death. *School Psychology International, 32*(2), 144–162.

Brayne, S., Farnham, C., & Fenwick, P. (2006). Deathbed phenomena and their effect on a palliative care team: A pilot study. *American Journal of Hospice & Palliative Medicine, 23*(1), 17–24.

Jerome, A. (2011). Comforting children and families who grieve: Incorporating spiritual support. *School Psychology International, 32*(2), 194–209.

Mitchell, G., Murray, J., Wilson, P., Hutch, R., & Meredith, P. (2010). "Diagnosing" and "managing" spiritual distress in palliative care: Creating an intellectual framework for spirituality useable in clinical practice. *Australasian Medical Journal, 3*(6), 364–369.

Murdaugh, C., Moneyham, L., Jackson, K., Phillips, K., & Tavakoli, A. (2006). Predictors of quality of life in HIV-infected rural women: Psychometric test of the chronic illness quality of life ladder. *Quality of Life Research, 15*(5), 777–789.

O'Mahony, S., Goulet, J., Kornblith, A., Abbatiello, G., Clarke, B., & Kless-Siegel, S. (2005). Desire for hastened death, cancer pain and depression: Report of a longitudinal observational study. *Journal of Pain & Symptom Management, 29*(5), 446–457.

Phillips, K. D., Mock, K. S., Bopp, C. M., Dudgeon, W. A., & Hand, G. A. (2006). Spiritual well-being, sleep disturbance, and mental and physical health status in hiv-infected individuals. *Issues in Mental Health Nursing, 27*(2), 125–139.

Rosenbaum, J., Smith, J., & Zollfrank, B. (2011). Neonatal end-of-life spiritual support care. *Journal of Perinatal & Neonatal Nursing, 25*(1), 61–69.

Spiritual Distress, Risk for

Note: Also see bibliography for Spiritual Distress, preceding.

Adegbola, M. (2006). Spirituality and quality of life in chronic illness. *Journal of Theory Construction & Testing, 10*(2), 42–46.

Belcher, A., & Griffiths, M. (2005). The spiritual care perspectives and practices of hospice nurses. *Journal of Hospice & Palliative Nursing, 7*(5), 271–279.

Boston, P., Bruce, A., & Schreiber, R. (2011). Existential suffering in the palliative care setting: An integrated literature review. *Journal of Pain and Symptom Management, 41*(3), 604–618.

Chochinov, H., Kristjanson, L., Brietbart, W., McClement, H. T., et al. (2011). Effect of dignity therapy on distress and end-of-life experience in terminally ill patients: A randomised controlled trial. *The Lancet Oncology, 12*(8), 753–762.

Finfgeld, D. L. (2002). Feminist spirituality and alcohol treatment. *Journal of Holistic Nursing, 20*(2), 113–132.

Gaskamp, C., Sutter, R., & Meraviglia, M. (2006). Evidence-based guideline: Promoting spirituality in the older adult. *Journal of Gerontological Nursing, 32*(11), 8–13.

Gibson, L. M., & Hendricks, C. S. (2006). Integrative review of spirituality in African American breast cancer survivors. *ABNF Journal, 17*(2), 67–72.

Kandasamy, A., Chaturvedi, S., & Desai, G. (2011). Spirituality, distress, depression, anxiety, and quality of life in patients with advanced cancer. *Indian Journal of Cancer, 48*(1), 55–59.

Kim, S. (2005). Mind and body in spiritual perspectives. *Nursing & Health Sciences, 7*(1), 77.

Lake, J. (2004). The integrative management of depressed mood. *Integrative Medicine: A Clinician's Journal, 3*(3), 34–43.

Mahlungulu, S. N., & Uys, L. R. (2004). Spirituality in nursing: An analysis of the concept. *Curationis, 27*(2), 15–26.

McBrien, B. (2006). Spirituality. A concept analysis of spirituality. *British Journal of Nursing (BJN), 15*(1), 42–45.

McCorkle, R., Ercolano, E., Lazenby, M., Schulman-Green, D., Schilling, L., Lorig, K., et al. (2011). Self-management: Enabling and empowering patients living with cancer as a chronic illness. *CA: A Cancer Journal for Clinicians, 61*(1), 50–62.

Narayanasamy, A., Clissett, P., Parumal, L., Thompson, D., Annasamy, S., & Edge, R. (2004). Responses to the spiritual needs of older people. *Journal of Advanced Nursing, 48*(1), 6–16.

Ramey, S. L. (2005). Assessment of health perception, spirituality and prevalence of cardiovascular disease risk factors within a private college cohort. *Pediatric Nursing, 31*(3), 222–231.

Taylor, E. J., & Mamier, I. (2005). Spiritual care nursing: What cancer patients and family caregivers want. *Journal of Advanced Nursing, 49*(3), 260–267.

Wong, Y. J., Rew, L., & Slaikeu, K. D. (2006). A systematic review of recent research on adolescent religiosity/spirituality and mental health. *Issues in Mental Health Nursing, 27*(2), 161–183.

Spiritual Well-Being, Readiness for Enhanced

Note: Also see bibliographies for Spiritual Distress and Risk for Spiritual Distress, preceding.

Coyle, J. (2002). Spirituality and health: Towards a framework for exploring the relationship between spirituality and health. *Journal of Advanced Nursing, 37*(6), 589–597.

Delaney, C. (2005). The spirituality scale: Development and psychometric testing of a holistic instrument to assess the human spiritual dimension. *Journal of Holistic Nursing, 23*(2), 145–167.

Fawcett, T. N., & Noble, A. (2004). The challenge of spiritual care in a multifaith society experienced as a Christian nurse. *Journal of Clinical Nursing, 13*(2), 136–142.

Ledger, S. D. (2005). The duty of nurses to meet patients' spiritual and/or religious needs. *British Journal of Nursing (BJN), 14*(4), 220–225.

Mahlungulu, S. N., & Uys, L. R. (2004). Spirituality in nursing: An analysis of the concept. *Curationis, 27*(2), 15–26.

McBrien, B. (2006). Spirituality. A concept analysis of spirituality. *British Journal of Nursing (BJN), 15*(1), 42–45.

Narayanasamy, A. (2004). The puzzle of spirituality for nursing: A guide to practical assessment. *British Journal of Nursing (BJN), 13*(19), 1140–1144.

Narayanasamy, A., Clissett, P., Parumal, L., Thompson, D., Annasamy, S., & Edge, R. (2004). Responses to the spiritual needs of older people. *Journal of Advanced Nursing, 48*(1), 6–16.

Phillips, K. D., Mock, K. S., Bopp, C. M., Dudgeon, W. A., & Hand, G. A. (2006). Spiritual well-being, sleep disturbance, and mental and physical health status in hiv-infected individuals. *Issues in Mental Health Nursing, 27*(2), 125–139.

Ramey, S. L. (2005). Assessment of health perception, spirituality and prevalence of cardiovascular disease risk factors within a private college cohort. *Pediatric Nursing, 31*(3), 222–231.

Smith, J., & McSherry, W. (2004). Spirituality and child development: A concept analysis. *Journal of Advanced Nursing, 45*(3), 307–315.

Spirit matters: Evidence of things hoped for. (2004). *Neonatal Network, 23*(6), 73.

Spontaneous Ventilation, Impaired

Blackwood, B., Alderdice, F., Burns, K., Cardwell, C., Lavery, G., & O'Halloran, P. (2011). Use of weaning protocols for reducing duration of mechanical ventilation in critically ill adult patients: Cochrane systematic review and meta-analysis. *BMJ: British Medical Journal, 342*, c7237. DOI: 10.1136/bmj/c7237. Retrieved May 11, 2012, from http://www.ncbi.nlm.nih.gov/pmc/articles/PMC3020589/

Buckmaster, A. G., Arnolda, G. R., Wright, I. M., & Henderson-Smart, D. J. (2007). CPAP use in babies with respiratory distress in Australian special care nurseries. *Journal of Paediatrics & Child Health, 43*(5), 376–382.

Burns, S. M. (2005). Mechanical ventilation of patients with acute respiratory distress syndrome and patients requiring weaning. *Critical Care Nurse, 25*(4), 14–24.

Carnevale, F. A., Troini, R., Rennick, J., Davis, M., & Alexander, E. (2005). To keep alive or let die: Parental experiences with ventilatory decisions for their critically ill children. *Pediatric Intensive Care Nursing, 6*(2), 12–15.

Cason, C. L., Tyner, T., Saunders, S., & Broome, L. (2007). Nurses' implementation of guidelines for ventilator-associated pneumonia from the centers for disease control and prevention. *American Journal of Critical Care, 16*(1), 28–38.

Chmielewski, C., & Snyder-Clickett, S. (2004). The use of laryngeal mask airway with mechanical positive pressure ventilation. *AANA Journal, 72*(5), 347–351.

Clifton-Koeppel, R. (2006). Endotracheal tube suctioning in the newborn: A review of the literature. *Newborn & Infant Nursing Reviews, 6*(2), 94–99.

Corff, K. E., & McCann, D. L. (2005). Room air resuscitation versus oxygen resuscitation in the delivery room. *Journal of Perinatal & Neonatal Nursing, 19*(4), 379–390.

Crunden, E., Boyce, C., Woodman, H., & Bray, B. (2005). An evaluation of the impact of the ventilator care bundle. *Nursing in Critical Care, 10*(5), 242–246.

Feeley, K., & Gardner, A. (2006). Sedation and analgesia management for mechanically ventilated adults: Literature review, case study and recommendations for practice. *Australian Critical Care, 19*(2), 73–77.

Grap, M., Munro, C., Wetzel, P., Best, A., Ketchum, J., Hamilton, A., et al. (2012). Sedation in adults receiving mechanical ventilation: Physiological and comfort outcomes. *American Journal of Critical Care, 21*(3), e53–e64.

Grap, M. J., & Munro, C. L. (2004). Preventing ventilator-associated pneumonia: Evidence-based care. *Critical Care Nursing Clinics of North America, 16*(3), 349–358.

Greiner, J., & Greiner, J. A. (2004). Sedation management for the adult mechanically ventilated patient. *Evidence-Based Nursing, 7*(4), 101–102.

Gronkiewicz, C., & Borkgren-Okonek, M. (2004). Acute exacerbation of COPD: Nursing application of evidence-based guidelines. *Critical Care Nursing Quarterly, 27*(4), 336–352.

Grossbach, I., Stranberg, S., & Chlan, L. (2011). Promoting effective communication for patients receiving mechanical ventilation. *Critical Care Nurse, 31*(3), 46–60.

Hampton, D. C., Griffith, D., & Howard, A. (2005). Evidence-based clinical improvement for mechanically ventilated patients. *Rehabilitation Nursing, 30*(4), 160–165.

Johnson, P., St. John, W., & Moyle, W. (2006). Long-term mechanical ventilation in a critical care unit: Existing in an uneveryday world. *Journal of Advanced Nursing, 53*(5), 551–558.

Kiekkas, P., & Diamanto, A. (2011). Psychiatric long-term complications of intensive care unit survivors. *Critical Care Medicine, 39*(7), 1852–1853.

MacIntyre, N. R. (2004). Evidence-based ventilator weaning and discontinuation. *Respiratory Care, 49*(7), 830–836.

Morandi, A., Brummel, N., & Ely, E. (2011). Sedation, delirium and mechanical ventilation: The 'ABCDE' approach. *Current Opinion in Critical Care, 17*(1), 43–49.

Munro, N. (2006). Weaning smokers from mechanical ventilation. *Critical Care Nursing Clinics of North America, 18*(1), 21–28.

O'Keefe-McCarthy, S. (2006). Evidence-based nursing strategies to prevent ventilator-acquired pneumonia. *Dynamics, 17*(1), 8–11.

Pollock, T. R., & Franklin, C. (2004). Use of evidence-based practice in the neonatal intensive care unit. *Critical Care Nursing Clinics of North America, 16*(2), 243–248.

Powers, J. (2007). The five P's spell positive outcomes for ARDS patients: Use these evidence-based interventions to avoid the dangers of ARDS, its complications, and its therapy. *American Nurse Today, 2*(3), 34–39.

Sarin-Gulian, A., Heliker, B., & Gawlinski, A. (2006). The effects of music twice daily on various outcomes in intensive care patients receiving mechanical ventilation: Improving umbilical venous catheter care by implementing an evidence-based practice guideline in the neonatal intensive care unit. *American Journal of Critical Care, 15*(3), 328–329.

Tracy, F., & Chlan, L. (2011). Nonpharmacological interventions to manage common symptoms in patients receiving mechanical ventilation. *Critical Care Nurse, 31*(3), 19–28.

Stress Overload

Alasad, J., & Ahmad, M. (2005). Communication with critically ill patients. *Journal of Advanced Nursing, 50*(4), 356–362.

Barksdale, P., & Backer, J. (2005). Health-related stressors experienced by patients who underwent total knee replacement seven days after being discharged home. *Orthopaedic Nursing, 24*(5), 336–342.

Beard, H. (2005). Does intermediate care minimize relocation stress for patients leaving the ICU? *Nursing in Critical Care, 10*(6), 272–278.

Bonadonna, R. (2003). Mediation's impact on chronic illness. *Holistic Nursing Practice, 17*(6), 309–319.

Bormann, J., Thorp, S., Wetherell, J., Golshan, S., & Lang, A. (2012, March 12). Mediation-based mantram intervention for veterans with posttraumatic stress disorder: A randomized trial. *Psychological Trauma: Theory, Research, Practice, and Policy*. DOI: 10.1037/a0027522. Retrieved May 11, 2012, from http://psycnet.apa.org/index.cfm?fa=buy.optionToBuy&id=2012-06372-001

Brien, M. C., Langberg, J., Valderrama, A. L., Kirkendoll, K., Romeiko, N., & Dunbar, S. B. (2005). Implantable cardioverter defibrillator storm: Nursing care issues for patients and families. *Critical Care Nursing Clinics of North America, 17*(1), 9–16.

Dettenborn, L., James, G. D., Berge-Landry, H. V., Valdimarsdottir, H. B., Montgomery, G. H., & Bovbjerg, D. H. (2005). Heightened cortisol responses to daily stress in working women at familial risk for breast cancer. *Biological Psychology, 69*(2), 167–179.

Dewing, J. (2003). Sundowning in older people with dementia: Evidence base, nursing assessment and interventions. *Nursing Older People, 15*(8), 24.

Fellowes, D., Barnes, K., & Wilkinson, S. (2006). Aromatherapy and massage for symptom relief in patients with cancer. DOI: 10.1002/14651858.CD002287.pub3. Retrieved November 21, 2012, from http://onlinelibrary.wiley.com/doi/10.1002/14651858.CD002287.pub3/full

Gurfein, B., Stamm, A., Bacchetti, P., Dallman, M., Nadkarni, N., Milush, J., et al. (2012, February 29). The calm mouse: An animal model of stress reduction. *Mol Med.* DOI: 10.2119/molmed.2012.00053. [Epub ahead of print]

Hodgkinson, R., & Lester, H. (2002). Stresses and coping strategies of mothers living with a child with cystic fibrosis: Implications for nursing professionals. *Journal of Advanced Nursing, 39*(4), 377–383.

Hoffman, C., Ersser, S., Hopkinson, J., Nicholls, P., Harrington, J., & Thomas, P. (2012). Effectiveness of mindfulness-based stress reduction in mood, breast- and endocrine-related quality of life, and well-being in stage 0 to III breast cancer: A randomized, controlled trial. *Journal of Clinical Oncology, 30*(12), 1335–1342.

Humenick, S. S., & Howell, O. S. (2003). Perinatal experiences: The association of stress, childbearing, breastfeeding, and early mothering. *Journal of Perinatal Education, 12*(3), 16–41.

Jellesma, F., & Cornelis, J. (2012). Mind magic: A pilot study of preventive mind-body-based stress reduction in behaviorally inhibited and activated children. *Journal of Holistic Nursing, 30*(1), 55–62.

Keil, R. M. K. (2004). Coping and stress: A conceptual analysis. *Journal of Advanced Nursing, 45,* 659–665.

Lai, H.-L., Li, Y.-M., & Lee, L.-H. (2012). Effects of music intervention with nursing presence and recorded music on psycho-physiological indices of cancer patient caregivers. *Journal of Clinical Nursing, 21*(5–6), 745–756.

Mertin, S., Sawatzky, J. V., Jones, W. L., & Lee, T. (2007). Roadblock to recovery: The surgical stress response. *Dynamics, 18*(1), 14–22.

Motzer, S. A., & Hertig, V. (2004). Stress, stress response and health. *Nursing Clinics of North America, 39,* 1–17.

Ryan-Wenger, N. A., Sharrer, V. W., & Campbell, K. K. (2005). Changes in children's stressors over the past 30 years. *Pediatric Nursing, 31,* 282–291.

Shankarapillai, R., Nair, M., & George, R. (2012). The effect of yoga in stress reduction for dental students performing their first periodontal surgery: A randomized controlled study. *International Journal of Yoga, 5*(1), 48–51.

Smith, J. E., Richardson, J., Hoffman, C., & Pilkington, K. (2005). Mindfulness-based stress reduction as supportive therapy in cancer care: Systematic review. *Journal of Advanced Nursing, 52*(3), 315–327.

Tomlinson, P., Peden-McAlpine, C., & Sherman, S. (2012). A family systems nursing intervention model for paediatric health crisis. *Journal of Advanced Nursing, 68*(3), 705–714.

Sudden Infant Death Syndrome, Risk for

American Academy of Pediatrics. (2011). Policy statement. SIDS and other sleep-related infant deaths: Expansion of recommendations for a safe infant sleeping environment. *Pediatrics, 105*(3), 650–656. Published online October 17, 2011. DOI: 10.1542/peds.2011-2284. Retrieved March 11, 2012, from http://pediatrics.aappublications.org/content/early/2011/10/12/peds.2011-2284

Anderson, J. E. (2000). Co-sleeping: Can we ever put the issue to rest? *Contemporary Pediatrics, 17*(6), 98–102, 109–110, 113–114.

Aris, C., Stevens, T. P., LeMura, C., Lipke, B., McMullen, S., & Côté-Arsenault, D. (2006). NICU nurses' knowledge and discharge teaching related to infant sleep position and risk of SIDS. *Advances in Neonatal Care, 6*(5), 281–294.

Baker, N. (2011). Sudden unexpected infant death—no more "stunned amazement"! *The New Zealand Medical Journal, 124*(1345), 9–12.

Ball, H., Moya, E., Fairley, L., Westman, J., Oddie, S., & Wright, J. (2012). Infant care practices related to sudden infant death syndrome in South Asian and White British families in the UK. *Paediatric and Perinatal Epidemiology, 26*(1), 3–12.

Becher, J.-C., Bhushan, S., & Lyon, A. (2012). Unexpected collapse in apparently healthy newborns – a prospective national study of a missing cohort of neonatal deaths and near-death events. *Archives of Diseases in Childhood. Fetal and Neonatal Ed, 97*(1), F30–F34.

Behm, I., Kabir, Z., Connolly, G., & Alpert, H. (2012). Increasing prevalence of smoke-free homes and decreasing rates of sudden infant death syndrome in the United States: An ecological association study. *Tobacco Control, 21,* 6–11.

Bredemeyer, S. L. (2004). Implementation of the SIDS guidelines in midwifery practice. *Australian Midwifery, 17*(4), 17–21.

Gurbutt, D., & Gurbutt, R. (2007). Risk reduction and sudden infant death syndrome. *Community Practitioner, 80*(1), 24–27.

Hauck, F., Thompson, J., Tanabe, K., Moon, R., & Vennemann, M. (2011). Breastfeeding and reduced risk of sudden infant death syndrome: A meta-analysis. *Pediatrics, 128*(1), 103–110.

Jeffery, H. E. (2004). SIDS guidelines and the importance of nurses as role models. *Neonatal, Paediatric & Child Health Nursing, 7*(1), 4–8.

Moos, M. (2006). The prevention chronicles. Responding to the newest evidence about SIDS. *AWHONN Lifelines, 10*(2), 163–166.

Phillips, D., Brewer, K., & Wadensweiler, P. (2011). Alcohol as a risk factor for sudden infant death syndrome (SIDS). *Addiction, 106*(3), 516–525.

Policy statement: Apnea, sudden infant death syndrome, and home monitoring. (2003). *Pediatrics, 111*(4), 914–917.

Trachtenberg, F., Haas, E., Kinney, H., Stanley, C., & Krous, H. (2012). Risk factor changes for sudden infant death syndrome after initiation of back-to-sleep campaign. *Pediatrics, 129*(4), 630–638.

Young, J., & O'Rourke, P. (2003). Improving attitudes and practice relating to sudden infant death syndrome and reduce the risk messages: The effectiveness of an educational intervention in a group of nurses and midwives. *Neonatal, Paediatric & Child Health Nursing, 6*(2), 4–14.

Suffocation, Risk for

Garros, D., Klassen, T. P., King, W. J., & Brady-Fryer, B. (2003). Strangulation with intravenous tubing: A previously undescribed adverse advent in children. *Pediatrics, 111*(6), e732.

Morrongiello, B. A., Corbett, M., Lasenby, J., Johnston, N., & McCourt, M. (2006). Factors influencing young children's risk of unintentional injury: Parenting style and strategies for teaching about home safety. *Journal of Applied Developmental Psychology, 27*(6), 560–570.

Paluszynska, D. A., Harris, K. A., & Thach, B. T. (2004). Influence of sleep position experience on ability of prone-sleeping infants to escape from asphyxiating microenvironments by changing head position. *Pediatrics, 114*(6), 1634–1639.

Scheers, N. J., Rutherford, G. W., & Kemp, J. S. (2003). Where should infants sleep? A comparison of risk for suffocation of infants sleeping in cribs, adult beds, and other sleeping locations. *Pediatrics, 112*(4), 883–889.

Souheil, M., Audrey, F., Anny, G., Sebastien, R., & Bertrand, L. (2011). Fatal accidental hanging by a high-chair waist strap in a 2-year-old girl. *Journal of Forensic Sciences, 56*(2), 534–536.

Truman, T. L., & Ayoub, C. C. (2002). Considering suffocatory abuse and Munchausen by proxy in the evaluation of children experiencing apparent life-threatening events and sudden infant death syndrome. *Child Maltreatment, 7*(2), 138.

Yeh, E., Rochette, L., McKenzie, L., & Smith, G. (2011). Injuries associated with cribs, playpens, and bassinets among young children in the US, 1990–2008. *Pediatrics, 127*(3), 479–486.

Suicide, Risk for

Anderson, M., & Jenkins, R. (2006). The national suicide prevention strategy for England: The reality of a national strategy for the nursing profession. *Journal of Psychiatric & Mental Health Nursing, 13*(6), 641–650.

Bennett, S., Daly, J., Kirkwood, J., McKain, C., & Swope, J. (2006). Establishing evidence-based standards of practice for suicidal patients in emergency medicine. *Topics in Emergency Medicine, 28*(2), 138–143.

Chen, Y.-L., Tzeng, D.-S., Cheng, T.-S., & Lin, C.-H. (2012). Sentinel events and predictors of suicide among inpatients at psychiatric hospitals. *Annals of General Psychiatry, 11*, 4. DOI:10.1186/11744-859X-11-4. Retrieved May 12, 2012, from http://www.annals-general-psychiatry.com/content/pdf/1744-859X-11-4.pdf

Cleaver, K. (2007). Adolescent nursing. Characteristics and trends of self-harming behaviour in young people. *British Journal of Nursing (BJN), 16*(3), 148–152.

Cutcliffe, J. R., & Barker, P. (2004). The nurses' global assessment of suicide risk (NGASR): Developing a tool for clinical practice. *Journal of Psychiatric & Mental Health Nursing, 11*(4), 393–400.

Diamond, G., O'Malley, A., Wintersteen, M., Peters, S., Yunghans, S., Biddle, V., et al. (2012). Attitudes, practices, and barriers to adolescent suicide and mental health screening. A survey of Pennsylvania primary care providers. *Journal of Primary & Community Health, 3*(1), 29–35.

Gary, F. A. (2005). Perspectives on suicide prevention among American Indian and Alaska native children and adolescents: A call for help. *Online Journal of Issues in Nursing, 10*(2), 170–211.

Gask, L., Dixon, C., Morriss, R., Appleby, L., & Green, G. (2006). Evaluating STORM skills training for managing people at risk of suicide. *Journal of Advanced Nursing, 54*(6), 739–750.

Goth subculture linked to self-harm and suicide. (2006). *Nursing Standard, 20*(36), 20.

Holkup, P. A. (2003). Evidence-based protocol: Elderly suicide—secondary prevention. *Journal of Gerontological Nursing, 29*(6), 6–17.

Hudson, P. L., Schofield, P., Kelly, B., Hudson, R., Street, A., & O'Connor, M. (2006). Responding to desire to die statements from patients with advanced disease: Recommendations for health professionals. *Palliative Medicine, 20*(7), 703–710.

Janelidze, S., Mattei, D., Westrin, Å., Träskman-Bendz, L., & Brundin, L. (2011). Cytokine levels in the blood may distinguish suicide attempters from depressed patients. *Brain, Behavior, and Immunity, 25*(2), 335–339.

Kaslow, N., Garcia-Williams, A., Moffitt, L., McLeod, M., Zesiger, H., Ammirati, R., et al. (2012). Building and maintaining an effective campus-wide coalition for suicide prevention. *Journal of College Student Psychotherapy, 26*(2), 121–139.

McAndrew, S., & Warne, T. (2004). Ignoring the evidence dictating the practice: Sexual orientation, suicidality and the dichotomy of the mental health nurse. *Journal of Psychiatric and Mental Health Nursing, 11*(4), 428–434.

Mulder, R. (2011). Problems with suicide risk assessment. *Australian & New Zealand Journal of Psychiatry, 45*(8), 605–607.

Park, H. S., Koo, H. Y., Schepp, K. G., & Jang, E. H. (2006). Predictors of suicidal ideation among high school students by gender in South Korea. *Journal of School Health, 76*(5), 181–188.

Pinikahana, J., Happell, B., & Keks, N. A. (2003). Suicide and schizophrenia: A review of literature for the decade (1990-1999) and implications for mental health nursing. *Issues in Mental Health Nursing, 24*(1), 27.

Pompili, M., Mancinelli, I., Girardi, P., Ruberto, A., & Tatarelli, R. (2005). Childhood suicide: A major issue in pediatric health care. *Issues in Comprehensive Pediatric Nursing, 28*(1), 63–68.

Posner, K., Brown, G., Stanley, B., Brent, D., Yershova, K., et al. (2011). The Columbia-suicide severity rating scale: Initial validity and internal consistency findings from three multisite studies with adolescents and adults. *The American Journal of Psychiatry, 168*(12), 1266–1277.

Screening for suicide risk: Recommendation and rationale. (2005). *American Journal for Nurse Practitioners, 9*(3), 46.

Singh, J., Subhashni, D., & Rosenberg, K. (2012). Targeted program helps reduce suicidal behaviors. *American Journal of Nursing, 112*(1), 69.

Sullivan, A., Barron, C., Bezmen, J., Rivera, J., & Zapata-Vega, M. (2005). The safe treatment of the suicidal patient in an adult inpatient setting: A proactive preventive approach. *Psychiatric Quarterly, 76*(1), 67–83.

Surgical Recovery, Delayed

Allen, G. (2006). Evidence for practice. Transfusion and postoperative infection risk. *AORN Journal, 83*(5), 1137–1138.

Aragon, D., Ring, C. A., & Covelli, M. (2003). The influence of diabetes mellitus on postoperative infections. *Critical Care Nursing Clinics of North America, 15*(1), 125–135.

Baratee, F., Dabirian, A., Yoldashkhan, M., Zaree, F., & Rasouli, M. (2011). Effect of therapeutic play on postoperative pain of hospitalized school age children in pediatric surgical ward. *Journal of Nursing and Midwifery, 21*(72), 1–6.

Bastable, A., & Rushforth, H. (2005). Parents' management of their child's postoperative pain. *Paediatric Nursing, 17*(10), 14–17.

Börjeson, S., Arweström, C., Baker, A., & Berterö, C. (2012). Nurses' experiences in the relief of postoperative nausea and vomiting. *Journal of Clinical Nursing, 19*(13–14), 1865–1872.

Clinical practice guideline series update. (2012). *Journal of Neuroscience Nursing, 44*(2), 111.

El Solh, A. (Ed.). (2012). *Critical care management of the obese patient*. Oxford, UK: Wiley-Blackwell.

Fanning, M. F. (2004). Reducing postoperative pulmonary complications in cardiac surgery patients with the use of the best evidence. *Journal of Nursing Care Quality, 19*(2), 95–99.

Ghanem, H., & El-khayat, R. (2012). Chronic subdural hematoma: Effect of developing and implementing postoperative nursing care standards on nurses performance for reduction or prevention of postoperative complications. *Journal of American Science, 8*(2), 686–697.

Golembiewski, J. A., & O'Brien, D. (2002). A systematic approach to the management of postoperative nausea and vomiting. *Journal of PeriAnesthesia Nursing, 17*(6), 364–376.

Haycock, C., Laser, C., Keuth, J., Montefour, K., Wilson, M., & Austin, K. (2005). Implementing evidence-based practice findings to decrease postoperative sternal wound infections following open heart surgery. *Journal of Cardiovascular Nursing, 20*(5), 299–305.

Hickman, A. G., Bell, D. M., & Preston, J. C. (2005). Acupressure and postoperative nausea and vomiting. *AANA Journal, 73*(5), 379–385.

Lee, S., Lim, K.-C., Jeon, M.-K., Kim, I., Jeong, J., Hong, J., et al. (2011). Postoperative pain and influencing factors among living liver donors. *Transplantation Proceedings, 44*(2), 363–365.

McWhinnie, D., & Jackson, I. (Eds.). (2012). *Day case surgery*. Oxford, NY: Oxford University Press.

Mertin, S., Sawatzky, J. V., Jones, W. L., & Lee, T. (2007). Roadblock to recovery: The surgical stress response. *Dynamics, 18*(1), 14–22.

Moran, W. P., Chen, G. J., Watters, C., Poehling, G., & Millman, F. (2006). Using a collaborative approach to reduce postoperative complications for hip-fracture patients: A three-year follow-up. *Joint Commission Journal on Quality & Patient Safety, 32*(1), 16–23.

Nworah, U. (2012). From documentation to the problem: Controlling postoperative pain. *Nursing Forum, 47*(2), 91–99.

Parkman, S. E., & Woods, S. L. (2005). Infants who have undergone cardiac surgery: What can we learn about lengths of stay in the hospital and presence of complications? *Journal of Pediatric Nursing, 20*(6), 430–440.

Whitney, J. D. (2003). Supplemental perioperative oxygen and fluids to improve surgical wound outcomes: Translating evidence into practice. *Wound Repair & Regeneration, 11*(6), 462.

Wilkinson, J., & Treas, L. (2011). Chapter 21, Safety. In *Fundamentals of nursing* (2nd ed.). Philadelphia: F. A. Davis.

Zalon, M. (2004). Correlates of recovery among older adults after major abdominal surgery. *Nursing Research, 53,* 99–106.

Zhang, C.-Y., Jiang, Y., Yin, Q.-Y., Chen, F.-J., Ma, L.-L., & Wang, L.-X. (2012). Impact of nurse-initiated preoperative education on postoperative anxiety symptoms and complications after coronary artery bypass grafting. *Journal of Cardiovascular Nursing, 27*(1), 84–88.

Swallowing, Impaired

Boczko, F. (2004). Managing dysphagia in dementia: A timed snack protocol. *Nursing Homes: Long Term Care Management, 53*(9), 64–67.

Burton, C., Pennington, L., Roddam, H., Russell, I., Russell, D., & Krawczyk, K. (2006). Assessing adherence to the evidence base in the management of post-stroke dysphagia. *Clinical Rehabilitation, 20*(1), 46–51.

Deane, K., Whurr, R., Clarke, C. E., Playford, E. D., & Ben-Shlomo, Y. (2006). Non-pharmacological therapies for dysphagia in Parkinson's disease. *Cochrane Library* (4).

DiBartolo, M. C. (2006). Careful hand feeding: A reasonable alternative to PEG tube placement in individuals with dementia. *Journal of Gerontological Nursing, 32*(5), 25–35.

Garcia, J., & Chambers, E. (2012). Perspectives of registered dietitians about thickened beverages in nutrition management of dysphagia. *Topics in Clinical Nutrition, 27*(2), 105–113.

Leder, S., Suiter, D., Warner, H., Acton, L., & Siegel, M. (2012). Safe initiation of oral diets in hospitalized patients based on passing a 3-ounce (90 cc) water swallow challenge protocol. *QJM, 105*(3), 257–263.

Lin, L., Wang, S., Chen, S. H., Wang, T., Chen, M., & Wu, S. (2003). Issues and innovations in nursing practice efficacy of swallowing training for residents following stroke. *Journal of Advanced Nursing, 44*(5), 469–478.

Morris, H. (2005). Dysphagia in a general practice population. *Nursing Older People, 17*(8), 20–28.

Smith, P. A. (2006). Nutrition, hydration, and dysphagia in long-term care: Differing opinions on the effects of aspiration. *Journal of the American Medical Directors Association, 7*(9), 545–549.

Stegemann, S., Gosch, M., & Breitkreutz, J. (2012). Swallowing dysfunction and dysphagia is an unrecognized challenge for oral drug therapy. *International Journal of Pharmaceutics, 430*(1–2), 197–206.

Tobochnik, A., & Bitely, F. (2012). Why does this person have dysphagia? *Perspectives on Gerontology, 17*(1), 4–10.

Voytas, J., Rifai, A., & Voytas, M. (2012). The use of electrical stimulation in treatment of dysphagia: A skilled nursing facility experience. *JAMDA, 13*(3), B23.

Westergren, A. (2006). Detection of eating difficulties after stroke: A systematic review. *International Nursing Review, 53*(2), 143–149.

Therapeutic Regimen Management: Family, Ineffective

Innes, A., Morgan, D., & Kostineuk, J. (2011). Dementia care in rural and remote settings: A systematic review of informal/family caregiving. *Maturitas, 68*(1), 34–46.

McCann, E. (2001). Recent developments in psychosocial interventions for people with psychosis. *Issues in Mental Health Nursing, 22*(1), 99–107.

Muhlbauer, S. A. (1999). *The experience of living with and caring for a family member with a mental illness: It always means something*. Lincoln: University of Nebraska.

Seymour, J. E. (2000). Negotiating natural death in intensive care. *Social Science & Medicine, 51*(8), 1241–1252.

Sörensen, S., & Yeates, C. (2011). Issues in dementia caregiving: Effects on mental and physical health, intervention strategies, and research needs. *American Journal of Geriatric Psychiatry, 19*(6), 491–496.

Van Ryn, M., Sanders, S., Kahn, K., van Houtven, C., Griffin, J., Martin, M., et al. (2011). Objective burden, resources, and other stressors among informal cancer caregivers: A hidden quality issue? *Psycho-Oncology, 20*(1), 44–52.

Wang, Y.-N., Shyu, Y.-I., Chen, M.-C., & Yang, P.-S. (2011). Reconciling work and family caregiving among adult-child family caregivers of older people with dementia: Effects on role strain and depressive symptoms. *Journal of Advanced Nursing, 67*(4), 829–840.

Wuest, J., & Hodgins, M. (2011). Reflections on methodological approaches and conceptual contributions in a program of caregiving research: Development and testing of Wuest's theory of family caregiving. *Qualitative Health Research, 21*(2), 151–161.

Thermal Injury, Risk for

Centers for Disease Control. (2006). *Injury fact book 2006*. Retrieved from http://www.cdc.gov/Injury/publications/FactBook/InjuryBook2006.pdf

Christoffel, T., & Gallagher, S. (2006). *Injury prevention and public health* (2nd ed.). Sudbury, MA: Jones & Bartlett.

DiGuiseppi, C., Edwards, P., Godward, C., Roberts, I., & Wade, A. (2000). Urban residential fire and flame injuries: A population based study. *Injury Prevention, 6*(4), 249–254.

Dusza, S., Halpern, A., Satagopan, J., Oliveria, S., Weinstock, M., Scope, A., et al. (2012). Prospective study of sunburn and sun behavior patterns during adolescence. *Pediatrics, 129*(2), 309–317.

Fonseca, B., dos Santos, B., Martins, P., Bonorino, C., Corte, T., da Silva, V., et al. (2012). Neuroprotective effects of a new skin care formulation following ultraviolet exposure. *Cell Proliferation, 45*(1), 48–52.

Moyer, V. (2012). Clinical guidelines. Behavioral counseling to prevent skin cancer: U.S. Preventive Services Task Force recommendation statement. *Annals of Internal Medicine*. Retrieved from http://www.annals.org/content/early/2012/05/02/0003-4819-157-1-201207030-00442.full

Murray, R., Zentner, J., & Yakimo, R. (2009). *Health promotion strategies through the life span* (8th ed.). Upper Saddle River, NJ: Pearson.

Pickett, W., Streight, S., Simpson, K., & Brison, R. (2003). Injuries experienced by infant children: A population based epidemiological analysis. *Pediatrics, 111*(4), 365–370.

Sommers, M. (2006). Injury as a global phenomenon of concern in nursing science. *Image: Journal of Nursing Scholarship, 38*(4), 314–320.

Wilkinson, J., & Treas, L. (2011). Chapter 21, Safety. In *Fundamentals of nursing* (2nd ed.). Philadelphia: F. A. Davis.

Thermoregulation, Ineffective

Benson, E., McMillan, D., & Ong, B. (2012). Original research: The effects of active warming on patient temperature and pain after total knee arthroplasty. *American Journal of Nursing, 112*(5), 26–33.

Block, J., Lilienthal, M., Cullen, L., & White, A. (2012). Evidence-based thermoregulation for adult trauma patients. *Critical Care Nursing Quarterly, 35*(1), 50–63.

Ellis, J. (2005). Neonatal hypothermia. *Journal of Neonatal Nursing, 11*(2), 76–82.

Galligan, M. (2006). Proposed guidelines for skin-to-skin treatment of neonatal hypothermia. *MCN: The American Journal of Maternal Child Nursing, 31*(5), 298–306.

Henker, R., & Carlson, K. K. (2007). Fever: Applying research to bedside practice. *AACN Advanced Critical Care, 18*(1), 76–87.

Johnston, N. J., King, A. T., Protheroe, R., & Childs, C. (2006). Body temperature management after severe traumatic brain injury: Methods and protocols used in the United Kingdom and Ireland. *Resuscitation, 70*(2), 254–262.

Loring, C., Gregory, K., Gargan, B., LeBlanc, V., Lundgren, D., Reilly, J., et al. (2012). Tub bathing improves thermoregulation of the late preterm infant. *Journal of Obstetric, Gynecologic, & Neonatal Nursing, 41*(2), 171–179.

Mcilvoy, L. H. (2005). The effect of hypothermia and hyperthermia on acute brain injury. *AACN Clinical Issues: Advanced Practice in Acute & Critical Care, 16*(4), 488–500.

Olson, M., McNett, S., Livesay, S., Le Roux, P., Suarez, J., & Bautista, C. (2012). Neurocritical care nursing research priorities. *Neurocritical Care, 16*(1), 55–62.

Roberge, R., Kim, J.-H., & Coca, A. (2012). Protective facemask impact on human thermoregulation: An overview. *The Annals of Occupational Hygiene, 56*(1), 102–112.

Rodway, G. (2012). Mountain clothing and thermoregulation: A look back. *Wilderness Environmental Medicine, 23*(1), 91–94.

Saely, C., Geiger, K., & Drexel, H. (2012). Brown versus white adipose tissue: A mini-review. *Gerontology, 58*(1). DOI: 10.1159/000321319. Retrieved from http://content.karger.com/produktedb/produkte.asp?doi=321319

Thompson, H. J. (2005). Fever: A concept analysis. *Journal of Advanced Nursing, 51*(5), 484–492.

Wilkinson, J., & Treas, L. (2011). Chapter 21, Safety. In *Fundamentals of nursing* (2nd ed.). Philadelphia: F. A. Davis.

Zeitzer, M. B. (2005). Inducing hypothermia to decrease neurological deficit: Literature review. *Journal of Advanced Nursing, 52*(2), 189–199.

Tissue Integrity, Impaired

Aistars, J. (2006). The validity of skin care protocols followed by women with breast cancer receiving external radiation. *Clinical Journal of Oncology Nursing, 10*(4), 487–492.

Ashton, J. (2004). Managing leg and foot ulcers: The role of kerraboot®. *British Journal of Community Nursing, 9*(9), S26–S30.

Ayello, E. A., Baranoski, S., & Salati, D. S. (2006). Best practices in wound care prevention and treatment. *Nursing Management, 37*(9), 42–48.

Burbridge, N., & Kiernan, S. (2005). Pressure ulcer benchmarking within a primary care setting. *British Journal of Nursing (BJN), 14*(6), S22–S29.

Davies, C. E., Turton, G., Woolfrey, G., Elley, R., & Taylor, M. (2005). Leg ulcers. Exploring debridement options for chronic venous leg ulcers. *British Journal of Nursing (BJN), 14*(7), 393–397.

Dowsett, C. (2004). The use of silver-based dressings in wound care. *Nursing Standard, 19*(7), 56–60.

Eigsti, J. (2011). Innovative solutions: Beds, baths, and bottoms: A quality improvement initiative to standardize use of beds, bathing techniques, and skin care in a general critical-care unit. *Dimensions of Critical Care Nursing, 30*(3), 169–176.

Ersser, S. J., Getliffe, K., Voegeli, D., & Regan, S. (2005). A critical review of the inter-relationship between skin vulnerability and urinary incontinence and related nursing intervention. *International Journal of Nursing Studies, 42*(7), 823–835.

Gray, M., Beeckman, D., Bliss, D., Fader, M., Logan, S., Junkin, J., et al. (2012). Incontinence-associated dermatitis: A comprehensive review and update. *Journal of Wound, Ostomy & Continence Nursing, 39*(1), 61–74.

Ho, C., Bensitel, T., Wang, X., & Bogie, K. (2011). Pulsatile lavage for the enhancement of pressure ulcer healing: A randomized controlled trial. *Physical Therapy, 92*(1), 38–48.

Johnson, A., & Porrett, T. (2005). Developing an evidence base for the management of stoma granulomas. *Gastrointestinal Nursing, 3*(8), 26–28.

Lepistö, M., Eriksson, E., Hietanen, H., Lepistö, J., & Lauri, S. (2006). Developing a pressure ulcer risk assessment scale for patients in long-term care. *Ostomy Wound Management, 52*(2), 34.

McQuestion, M. (2011). Evidence-based skin care management in radiation therapy: Clinical update. *Seminars in Oncology Nursing, 27*(2), e1–e17.

Nixon, J., Thorpe, H., Barrow, H., Phillips, A., Nelson, E. A., & Mason, S. A. (2005). Reliability of pressure ulcer classification and diagnosis. *Journal of Advanced Nursing, 50*(6), 613–623.

Pym, K. (2006). Wound care. Identifying and managing problem scars. *British Journal of Nursing (BJN), 15*(2), 78.

Sopata, M., Tomaszewska, E., Machynska-Bucko, Z., & Kotlinsska-Lemieszek, A. (2012). Modern methods of conservative treatment of pressure ulcers. *Advances in Dermatology and Allergology, XXIX*(1), 40–46.

Thompson, D. (2005). Tissue viability. An evaluation of the waterlow pressure ulcer risk-assessment tool. *British Journal of Nursing (BJN), 14*(8), 455–459.

Tyler, P., Hollinworth, H., & Osborne, R. (2005). Tissue viability. The wearing of compression hosiery for leg problems other than leg ulcers. *British Journal of Nursing (BJN), 14*(11), S21.

Wilkinson, J., & Treas, L. (2011). Chapter 34, Skin integrity & wound healing; and Chapter 28, Bowel elimination. In *Fundamentals of nursing* (2nd ed.). Philadelphia: F. A. Davis.

Tissue Perfusion: Cardiac, Risk for Decreased

Abay, M. C., Delos Reyes, J., Everts, K., & Wisser, J. (2007). Current literature questions the routine use of low-dose dopamine. *AANA Journal, 75*(1), 57–63.

Abdelmoneim, S., Basu, A., Basu, R., Hagan, M., Mendrick, E., Pattan, V., et al. (2011). Acute hyperglycemia in nondiabetic women reduces coronary flow reserve: Novel observations during noninvasive assessment of myocardial perfusion using rapid-acquisition bedside contrast echocardiography. *Journal of the American College of Cardiology, 57*(14), E810.

Albert, N. M., Eastwood, C. A., & Edwards, M. L. (2004). Evidence-based practice for acute decompensated heart failure. *Critical Care Nurse, 24*(6), 14.

Alzamora, M., Baena-Diez, J., Sorribes, M., Forés, R., Toran, P., Vicheto, M., et al. (2007). PERART study. Peripheral Arterial Disease study (PERART): Prevalence and predictive values of asymptomatic peripheral arterial occlusive disease related to cardiovascular morbidity and mortality. *BMC Public Health, 7*, 348. DOI:10.1186/1471-2458-7-348

Bucci, M., Joutsiniemi, E., Saraste, A., Kajander, S., Ukkonen, H., Saraste, M., et al. (2011). Intrapericardial, but not extrapericardial, fat is an independent predictor of impaired hyperemic coronary perfusion in coronary artery disease. *Arteriosclerosis, Thrombosis, and Vascular Biology, 31,* 211–218.

Dogan, A., Ozgul, M., Ozaydin, M., Aslan, S., Gedikli, O., & Altinbas, A. (2005). Effect of clopidogrel plus aspirin on tissue perfusion and coronary flow in patients with ST-segment elevation myocardial infarction: A new reperfusion strategy. *American Heart Journal, 149*(6), 1037–1042.

Gentilcore, D., Jones, K. L., O'Donovan, D. G., & Horowitz, M. (2006). Postprandial hypotension - novel insights into pathophysiology and therapeutic implications. *Current Vascular Pharmacology, 4*(2), 161–171.

Hung, J., Knuiman, M., Divitini, M., Davis, T., & Beiby, J. (2008). Prevalence and risk factor correlates of elevated C-reactive protein in adult Australian population. *American Journal of Cardiology, 101*(3), 193–198.

Sehgal, A., Ramsden, C., & McNamara, P. (2012). Indomethacin impairs coronary perfusion in infants with hemodynamically significant ductus arteriosus. *Neonatology, 101*(1), 20–27.

Steen, H., Lehrke, S., Wiegand, U., Merten, C., Schuster, L., Richardt, G., et al. (2005). Very early cardiac magnetic resonance imaging for quantification of myocardial tissue perfusion in patients receiving tirofiban before percutaneous coronary intervention for ST-elevation myocardial infarction. *American Heart Journal, 149*(3), 564e1–564e7.

Tissue Perfusion: Cerebral, Risk for Ineffective

Alverzo, J. P. (2006). A review of the literature on orientation as an indicator of level of consciousness. *Journal of Nursing Scholarship, 38*(2), 159–164.

Asante-Siaw, J., Tyrrell, J., & Hoschtitzky, A. (2006). Does the use of a centrifugal pump offer any additional benefit for patients having open heart surgery? *Best BETS,* Record 01148. Retrieved from http://www.bestbets.org/cgi-bin/bets.pl?record=01148

Bader, M. K. (2004). Changing team practice: Applying evidence-based brain injury guidelines to clinical practice. *Worldviews on Evidence-Based Nursing, 1*(4), 227.

Barnard, J., Musleh, G., & Bitta, M. (2004). In aortic arch surgery is there any benefit in using antegrade cerebral perfusion or retrograde cerebral perfusion as an adjunct to hypothermic circulatory arrest? *BestBETS,* Record 00690. Retrieved from http://www.bestbets.org/cgi-bin/bets.pl?record=00690

Barrow, A., Ndikum, J., & Harris, T. (2011). Late presentations of minor head injury. *Emergency Medicine Journal.* DOI: 10.1136/emermed-22011-200523.

Bay, E., & McLean, S. A. (2007). Mild traumatic brain injury: An update for advanced practice nurses. *Journal of Neuroscience Nursing, 39*(1), 43–51.

Bush, T. (2007). Use of cognitive assessment with Alzheimer's disease. *Nursing Times, 103*(2), 31–32.

Fan, J. (2004). Effect of backrest position on intracranial pressure and cerebral perfusion pressure in individuals with brain injury: A systematic review. *Journal of Neuroscience Nursing, 36*(5), 278–288.

Griffin, L., & Hickey, J. (2012). Penetrating head injury. *Critical Care Nursing Quarterly, 35*(2), 144–150.

Hofmeijer, J., & van Putten, M. (2012). Ischemic cerebral damage: An appraisal of synaptic failure. *Stroke, 43,* 607–615.

Jia-Ching, C., & Shaw, F. (2006). Recent progress in physical therapy of the upper-limb rehabilitation after stroke. *Journal of Cardiovascular Nursing, 21*(6), 469–473.

March, K. (2005). Intracranial pressure monitoring: Why monitor? *AACN Clinical Issues: Advanced Practice in Acute & Critical Care, 16*(4), 456–475.

Marcoux, K. K. (2005). Management of increased intracranial pressure in the critically ill child with an acute neurological injury. *AACN Clinical Issues: Advanced Practice in Acute & Critical Care, 16*(2), 212.

Mathiesen, C., Tavianini, H. D., & Palladino, K. (2006). Best practices in stroke rapid response: A case study. *MEDSURG Nursing, 15*(6), 364–369.

Routhieaux, J., Sarcone, S., & Stegenga, K. (2005). Neurocognitive sequelae of sickle cell disease: Current issues and future directions. *Journal of Pediatric Oncology Nursing, 22*(3), 160–167.

Sharma, M., Clark, H., Armour, T., Stotts, G., Cote, R., Hill, M., et al. (2005). *Acute stroke: Evaluation and treatment.* Evidence Report/Technology Assessment No. 127. Rockville, MD: Agency for Healthcare Research and Quality.

Walter, S., Kostopoulos, P., Haass, A., Keller, I., Lesmeister, M., Schlechtriemen, T., et al. (2012). Diagnosis and treatment of patients with stroke in a mobile stroke unit versus in hospital: A randomised controlled trial. *The Lancet Neurology, 11*(5), 397–404.

Wojner, A. W., El-Mitwalli, A., & Alexandrov, A. V. (2002). Effect of head positioning on intracranial blood flow velocities in acute ischemic stroke: A pilot study. *Critical Care Nursing Quarterly, 24*(4), 57–66.

Zeitzer, M. B. (2005). Inducing hypothermia to decrease neurological deficit: Literature review. *Journal of Advanced Nursing, 52*(2), 189–199.

Tissue Perfusion: Peripheral, Ineffective

Byrne, B. (2002). Deep vein thrombosis prophylaxis. *Journal of Vascular Nursing, 20*(2), 53–59.

Clifton-Koeppel, R. (2006). Wound care after peripheral intravenous extravasation: What is the evidence? *Newborn & Infant Nursing Reviews, 6*(4), 202–212.

Cournot, M., Boccalon, H., Cambou, J.-P., Guilloux, J., Tarazkiewicz, D., Hanaire-Brouton, H., et al. (2007). Accuracy of the screening physical examination to identify subclinical atherosclerosis and peripheral arterial disease in asymptomatic subjects. *Journal of Vascular Surgery, 46*(6), 1215–1221. DOI: 10.1016/j.jvs.2007.08.022.

Davies, C. E., Turton, G., Woolfrey, G., Elley, R., & Taylor, M. (2005). Exploring debridement options for chronic venous leg ulcers. *British Journal of Nursing (BJN), 14*(7), 393–397.

Delmas, L. (2006). Best practice in the assessment and management of diabetic foot ulcers. *Rehabilitation Nursing, 31*(6), 228–234.

Evans, J., & Chance, T. (2005). Improving patient outcomes using a diabetic foot assessment tool. *Nursing Standard, 19*(45), 65.

Gorski, L. A. (2007). Venous thromboembolism: A common and preventable condition: Implications for the home care nurse. *Home Healthcare Nurse, 25*(2), 94–100.

Harrison, M. B., Graham, I. D., Lorimer, K., Friedberg, E., Pierscianowski, T., & Brandys, T. (2005). Leg-ulcer care in the community, before and after implementation of an evidence-based service. *CMAJ: Canadian Medical Association Journal, 172*(11), 1447–1452.

Harvey, D. (2006). New, improved kerraboot: A tool for leg ulcer healing. *British Journal of Community Nursing, 11*(6), S26–S30.

Heinen, M. M., van Achterberg, T., Reimer, W. S. O., van den Kerkhof Peter, C. M., & de Laat, E. (2004). Venous leg ulcer patients: A review of the literature on lifestyle and pain-related interventions. *Journal of Clinical Nursing, 13*(3), 355–366.

Hernando, F., & Conejero, A. (2007). Enfermedad arterial periferica: Aspectos fisiopatologicos, clinicos y terapeuticos. *Revista Española de Cardiologia, 60*(9), 969–982.

Khan, H. N., Rahim, S., Anand, S., Simel, D., & Panju, A. (2006). Does the clinical examination predict lower extremity peripheral arterial disease? *Journal of the American Medical Association, 295*(5), 536–546.

Kruidenier, L., Nicolaï, S., Willengendael, E., de Bie, R., Prins, M., & Tejink, J. (2009). Functional claudication distance: A reliable and valid measurement to assess functional limitation in patients with intermittent claudication. *BMC Cardiovascular Disorders, 9*(9). DOI: 10.1186/1471-2261-9-9.

Ma, K. K., Chan, M. F., & Pang, S. M. C. (2006). The effectiveness of using a lipidocolloid dressing for patients with traumatic digital wounds. *Clinical Nursing Research, 15*(2), 119–134.

McDermott, M., Ades, P., Dyer, A., Guralnik, J., Kibbe, M., & Criqui, M. (2008). Corridor-based functional performance measures correlate better with physical activity during daily life than treadmill measures in persons with peripheral arterial disease. *Journal of Vascular Surgery, 48*(5), 1231–1237.e1. DOI: 10.1016/j.jvs.2008.06.050.

McQuestion, M. (2006). Evidence-based skin care management in radiation therapy. *Seminars in Oncology Nursing, 22*(3), 163–173.

Nehler, M. R., McDermott, M. M., Treat-Jacobson, D., Chetter, I., & Regensteiner, J. G. (2003). Functional outcomes and quality of life in peripheral arterial disease: Current status. *Vascular Medicine, 8*(2), 115.

Shrubb, D., & Mason, W. (2006). The management of deep vein thrombosis in lymphoedema: A review. *British Journal of Community Nursing, 11*(7), 292–297.

Tyler, P., Hollinworth, H., & Osborne, R. (2005). The wearing of compression hosiery for leg problems other than leg ulcers. *British Journal of Nursing (BJN), 14*(11), S21–S27.

Velmahos, G. (2006). Posttraumatic thromboprophylaxis revisited: An argument against the current methods of DVT and PE prophylaxis after injury. *World Journal of Surgery, 30*(4), 483–487.

Wilkinson, J., & Treas, L. (2011). Chapter 36, Oxygenation. *Fundamentals of nursing* (2nd ed.). Philadelphia: F. A. Davis.

Tissue Perfusion: Peripheral, Risk for Ineffective

(See bibliography for Tissue Perfusion: Peripheral, Ineffective, preceding.)

Transfer Ability, Impaired

Auger, C., Demers, L., Gélinas, I., Miller, W., Juytai, J., & Noreau, L. (2010). Life-space mobility of middle-aged and older adults at various stages of usage of power mobility devices. *Archives of Physical Medicine and Rehabilitation, 91*(5), 765–773.

Brouwer, K., Nysseknabm, J., & Culham, E. (2004). Physical function and health status among seniors with and without fear of falling. *Gerontology, 50,* 15–141.

Guthrie, P. F., Westphal, L., Dahlman, B., Berg, M., Behnam, K., & Ferrell, D. (2004). A patient lifting intervention for preventing the work-related injuries of nurses. *Work, 22*(2), 79–88.

Hakim, R., Kotroba, E., Cours, J., Teel, S., & Leininger, P. (2010). A cross-sectional study of balance-related measures with older adults who participated in Tai Chi, yoga, or no exercise. *Physical & Occupational Therapy in Geriatrics, 28*(1), 63–74.

Holm, B., Kristensen, M., Myhrmann, L., Husted, H., Andersen, L., Iristensen, B., et al. (2010). The role of pain for early rehabilitation in fast track total knee arthroplasty. *Disability and Rehabilitation, 32*(4), 300–306.

Hignett, S. (2003). Intervention strategies to reduce musculoskeletal injuries associated with handling patients: A systematic review. *Occupational & Environmental Medicine, 60*(9), 8p.

Hignett, S., & Crumpton, E. (2005). Development of a patient handling assessment tool. *International Journal of Therapy & Rehabilitation, 12*(4), 178–181.

Hignett, S., Crumpton, E., Ruszala, S., Alexander, P., Fray, M., & Fletcher, B. (2003). Evidence-based patient handling: Systematic review. *Nursing Standard, 17*(33), 33–36.

Jolley, S. (2006). Manual handling. *Paediatric Nursing, 18*(7), 18.

Lewis, C. L., Moutoux, M., Slaughter, M., & Bailey, S. P. (2004). Characteristics of individuals who fell while receiving home health services. *Physical Therapy, 84*(1), 23–32.

Mukai, T., Hirano, S., Nakashima, H., Kato, Y., Sakaida, Y., Guo, S., et al. (2010). Development of a nursing-care assistant robot RIBA that can lift a human in its arms. *Intelligent Robots and Systems (IROS)* 2010 IEEE/RSJ International Conference, pp. 5996–6001, October 18–22, 2010. DOI: 10.1109/IROS.2010.5651735. Retrieved May 19, 2012, from http://ieeexplore.ieee.org/stamp/stamp.jsp?tp=&arnumber=5651735&isnumber=5648787

Nathenson, P. (2004). Adapting OSHA ergonomic guidelines to the rehabilitation setting. *Rehabilitation Nursing, 29*(4), 127–130.

Nelson, A., & Baptiste, A. S. (2004). Evidence-based practices for safe patient handling and movement. *Online Journal of Issues in Nursing, 9*(3), 24p.

Nelson, A., & Baptiste, A. S. (2006a). Evidence-based practices for safe patient handling and movement. Reprinted with permission from the online journal of issues in nursing, September 2004, 9(3). *Orthopaedic Nursing, 25*(6), 366–379.

Nelson, A., & Baptiste, A. S. (2006b). Update on evidence-based practices for safe patient handling and movement. *Orthopaedic Nursing, 25*(6), 367–368.

Nelson, A., Matz, M., Chen, F., Siddharthan, K., Lloyd, J., & Fragala, G. (2006). Development and evaluation of a multifaceted ergonomics program to prevent injuries associated with patient handling tasks. *International Journal of Nursing Studies, 43*(6), 717–733.

Pellatt, G. C. (2005). Safe handling. The safety and dignity of patients and nurses during patient handling. *British Journal of Nursing (BJN), 14*(21), 1150–1156.

Rabadi, M. (2011). Review of the randomized clinical stroke rehabilitation trials in 2009. *Medical Science Monitor, 17*(2), RA25–43.

Trauma, Risk for

Albers, L. L., Sedler, K. D., Bedrick, E. J., Teaf, D., & Peralta, P. (2005). Midwifery care measures in the second stage of labor and reduction of genital tract trauma at birth: A randomized trial. *Journal of Midwifery & Women's Health, 50*(5), 365–372.

Albers, L. L., Sedler, K. D., Bedrick, E. J., Teaf, D., & Peralta, P. (2006). Factors related to genital tract trauma in normal spontaneous vaginal births. *Birth: Issues in Perinatal Care, 33*(2), 94–100.

Baroni, S., & Richmond, T. S. (2006). Firearm violence in America: A growing health problem. *Critical Care Nursing Clinics of North America, 18*(3), 297–303.

Bond, A. E., Draeger, C., Mandleco, B., & Donnelly, M. (2003). Trauma. Needs of family members of patients with severe traumatic brain injury: Implications for evidence-based practice. *Critical Care Nurse, 23*(4), 63–72.

Bower, F. L., McCullough, C. S., & Timmons, M. E. (2003). A synthesis of what we know about the use of physical restraints and seclusion with patients in psychiatric and acute care settings: 2003 update. *Online Journal of Knowledge Synthesis for Nursing, 10,* 29p.

Brink, M., Visscher, C., Arends, S., Zwerver, J., Post, W., & Lemmink, K. (2010). Monitoring stress and recovery: New insights for the prevention of injuries and illnesses in elite youth soccer players. *British Journal of Sports Medicine, 44*(11), 809–815.

Clifton-Koeppel, R. (2006). Endotracheal tube suctioning in the newborn: A review of the literature. *Newborn & Infant Nursing Reviews, 6*(2), 94–99.

Corrigan, J., Selassie, A., & Orman, J. (2010). The epidemiology of traumatic brain injury. *Journal of Head Trauma Rehabilitation, 25*(2), 72–80.

Gustafsson, M., & Ahlström, G. (2004). Problems experienced during the first year of an acute traumatic hand injury—a prospective study. *Journal of Clinical Nursing, 13*(8), 986–995.

Hauret, K., Jones, B., Bullock, S., Canhan-Chervak, M., & Canada, S. (2010). Musculoskeletal injuries: Description of an under-recognized injury problem among military personnel. *American Journal of Preventive Medicine, 38*(1), S61–S70.

Jolley, J. (2007). Separation and psychological trauma: A paradox examined. *Paediatric Nursing, 19*(3), 22–25.

Kneafsey, R., & Gawthorpe, D. (2004). Head injury: Long-term consequences for patients and families and implications for nurses. *Journal of Clinical Nursing, 13*(5), 601–608.

McKinlay, A., Kyonka, E., Grace, R., Horwood, L., Fergusson, D., & MacFarlane, M. (2010). An investigation of the pre-injury risk factors associated with children who experience traumatic brain injury. *Injury Prevention, 16*(1), 31–35.

Metnitz, P. G. H., Reiter, A., Jordan, B., & Lang, T. (2004). More interventions do not necessarily improve outcome in critically ill patients. *Intensive Care Medicine, 30*(8), 1586–1593.

Minei, J., Schmicker, R., Kerby, J., Stiell, I., Schreiber, M., Bulger, E., et al. (2010). Severe traumatic injury: Regional variation in incidence and outcome. *Annals of Surgery, 252*(1), 149–157.

Parker, M. J., Gillespie, W. J., & Gillespie, L. D. (2006). Effectiveness of hip protectors for preventing hip fractures in elderly people: Systematic review. *BMJ: British Medical Journal, 332*(7541), 571–573.

Perks, D. H. (2005). Issues in pediatrics. Transient spinal cord injuries in the young athlete. *Journal of Trauma Nursing, 12*(4), 127–133.

Thompson, H. J., & Bourbonniere, M. (2006). Traumatic injury in the older adult from head to toe. *Critical Care Nursing Clinics of North America, 18*(3), 419–431.

Wilkinson, J., & Treas, L. (2011). *Fundamentals of nursing* (2nd ed.). Philadelphia: F. A. Davis.

Unilateral Neglect

Jones, A., Tilling, K., Wilson-Barnett, J., Newham, D. J., & Wolfe, C. D. A. (2005). Effect of recommended positioning on stroke outcome at six months: A randomized controlled trial. *Clinical Rehabilitation, 19*(2), 138–145.

Kalbach, L. R. (1991). Unilateral neglect: Mechanisms and nursing care. *Journal of Neuroscience Nursing, 23*(2), 125–129.

Leibovitch, F., Vasquez, B., Ebert, P., Beresford, K., & Black, S. (2012). A short bedside battery for visuoconstructive hemispatial neglect: Sunnybrook Neglect Assessment Procedure (SNAP). *Journal of Clinical and Experimental Neuropsychology, 34*(4), 359–368.

Medin, J., Windahl, J., von Arbin, M., Tham, K., & Wredling, R. (2012). Eating difficulties among patients 3 months after stroke in relation to the acute phase. *Journal of Advanced Nursing, 68*(3), 580–589.

O'Connell, A. (2002). Development of an integrated care pathway for the management of hemiplegic shoulder pain. *Disability & Rehabilitation, 24*(7), 390–398.

Rabipour, S., & Raz, A. (2012). Training the brain: Fact and fad in cognitive and behavioral remediation. *Brain and Cognition, 79*(2), 159–179.

Rickelman, B. L. (2004). Anosognosia in individuals with schizophrenia: Toward recovery of insight. *Issues in Mental Health Nursing, 25*(3), 227–242.

Rusconi, M. L., Maravita, A., Bottini, G., & Vallar, G. (2002). Is the intact side really intact? Perseverative responses in patients with unilateral neglect: A productive manifestation. *Neuropsychologia, 40,* 594–604.

Silveri, M., Ciccarelli, N., & Cappa, A. (2011). Unilateral spatial neglect in degenerative brain pathology. *Neuropsychology, 25*(5), 554–566.

Swan, L. (2001). Unilateral spatial neglect. *Physical Therapy, 81,* 1572–1580.

Ting, D., Pollock, A., Dutton, G., Doubal, F., Ting, D., Thompson, M., et al. Visual neglect following stroke: Current concepts and future focus. *Survey of Ophthalmology, 56*(2), 114–134.

Weitzel, E. A. (2001). Unilateral neglect. In M. Maas, K. Buckwalter, M. Hardy, T. Tripp-Reimer, M. Titler, & J. Specht (Eds.), *Nursing care of older adults: Diagnosis, outcomes, and interventions* (pp. 492–502). St. Louis, MO: Mosby.

Urinary Elimination, Impaired

(Also see the bibliographies for: Urinary Elimination, Readiness for Enhanced; Urinary Incontinence, Functional; Urinary Incontinence, Overflow; Urinary Incontinence, Reflex; Urinary Incontinence, Stress; Urinary Incontinence, Urge; Urinary Incontinence, Risk for Urge; and Urinary Retention.)

Dingwall, L., & McLafferty, E. (2006). Nurses' perceptions of indwelling urinary catheters in older people. *Nursing Standard, 21*(14), 35–42.

Gray, M. (2003). The importance of screening, assessing, and managing urinary incontinence in primary care. *Journal of the American Academy of Nurse Practitioners, 15*(3), 102–107.

Klym, L. M., & Colling, J. (2003). Quality of life after radical prostatectomy. *Oncology Nursing Forum, 30*(2), E24–32.

Morrow, L. (2002). Continence for adults with urinary dysfunction. *Nursing Times, 98*(29), 38–40.

Newman, D. K., Gaines, T., & Snare, E. (2005). Innovation in bladder assessment: Use of technology in extended care. *Journal of Gerontological Nursing, 31*(12), 33–43.

Schirm, V., Baumgardner, J., Dowd, T., Gregor, S., & Kolcaba, K. (2004). NGNA. Development of a healthy bladder education program for older adults. *Geriatric Nursing, 25*(5), 301–306.

Thomas, L. H., Barrett, J., Cross, S., French, B., Leathley, M., Sutton, C., et al. (2006). Prevention and treatment of urinary incontinence after stroke in adults. *Cochrane Library* (4).

Wilkinson, J., & Treas, L. (2011). Chapter 21, Safety. In *Fundamentals of nursing* (2nd ed.). Philadelphia: F. A. Davis.

Urinary Elimination, Readiness for Enhanced

Note: Also see the bibliographies for: Urinary Elimination, Impaired; Urinary Incontinence, Functional; Urinary Incontinence, Overflow; Urinary Incontinence, Reflex; Urinary Incontinence, Stress; Urinary Incontinence, Urge; Urinary Incontinence, Risk for Urge; and Urinary Retention.

Bee, T. S. (2006). Review: Determining the volume of urine by portable ultrasonography for the neurological patients. *Singapore Nursing Journal, 33*(1), 7–13.

Burns, P. A. (2006). A nurse led continence service reduced symptoms of incontinence, frequency, urgency, and nocturia. *Evidence-Based Nursing, 9*(3), 85.

Chaperon, C. (2010). Sleep deprivation impairs 12-hr urine volume excretion in old rats. *Biological Research for Nursing, 11*(3), 236–244.

Clark, W., Sontrop, J., Macnab, J., Suri, R., Moist, L., Salvadori, M., et al. (2011). Urine volume and change in estimated GFR in a community-based cohort study. *Clinical Journal of the American Society of Nephrology, 6*(11), 2634–2641.

Eustice, S., Roe, B., & Paterson, J. (2006). Prompted voiding for the management of urinary incontinence in adults. *Cochrane Library* (4).

Griffiths, R., & Fernandez, R. (2006). Policies for the removal of short-term indwelling urethral catheters. *Cochrane Library* (4).

Harper, G. M. (2005). Managing urinary incontinence in older patients. *Advanced Studies in Medicine, 5*(10), 537.

Hirayama, A., Torimoto, K., Yamada, A., Tanaka, N., Fujimoto, K., Yoshida, K., et al. (2011). Relationship between nocturnal urine volume, leg edema, and urinary antidiuretic hormone in older men. *Urology, 77*(6), 1426–1431.

Karon, S. (2005). A team approach to bladder retraining: A pilot study. *Urologic Nursing, 25*(4), 269–276.

Moore, K. N., & Gray, M. (2004). Urinary incontinence in men: Current status and future directions. *Nursing Research, 53*(6), S36–41.

Ostaszkiewicz, J., Roe, B., & Johnston, L. (2005). Effects of timed voiding for the management of urinary incontinence in adults: Systematic review. *Journal of Advanced Nursing, 52*(4), 420–431.

Thomas, L. H., Barrett, J., Cross, S., French, B., Leathley, M., Sutton, C., et al. (2006). Prevention and treatment of urinary incontinence after stroke in adults. *Cochrane Library* (4).

Wilkinson, J., & Treas, L. (2011).Chapter 27, Urinary elimination. In *Fundamentals of nursing* (2nd ed.). Philadelphia: F. A. Davis.

Urinary Incontinence, Functional

Note: Also see the bibliographies for: Urinary Elimination, Impaired; Urinary Elimination, Readiness for Enhanced; Urinary Incontinence, Functional; Urinary Incontinence, Overflow; Urinary Incontinence, Reflex; Urinary Incontinence, Stress; Urinary Incontinence, Urge; Urinary Incontinence, Risk for Urge; and Urinary Retention.

Braekken, I., Majida, M., Ellstrøm-Engh, M., Dietz, H., Umek, W., et al. (2008). Test–retest and intra-observer repeatability of two-, three- and four-dimensional perineal ultrasound of pelvic floor muscle anatomy and function. *International Urogynecology Journal, 19*(2), 227–235.

Brown, M., Pope, A., & Brown, E. (2011). Treatment of primary nocturnal enuresis in children: A review. *Child: Care, Health and Development, 37*(2), 153–160.

Chen, R., Song, Y., Jiang, L., Hong, X., & Ye, P. (2011). The assessment of voluntary pelvic floor muscle contraction by three-dimensional transperineal ultrasonography. *Archives of Gynecology and Obstetrics, 224*(4), 931–936.

Friedman, B., Friedmen, B., & Ran, D. (2011). Oxybutynin for treatment of nocturnal enuresis in children. *Canadian Family Physician, 57*(5), 559–561.

Ko, P., Liang, C., Chang, S., Lee, J., Chao, A., & Cheng, P. (2011). A randomized controlled trial of antenatal pelvic floor exercises to prevent and treat urinary incontinence. *International Urogynecology Journal Including Pelvic Floor Dysfunction, 22*(1), 17–22.

Longstaffe, S., Mofatt, M., & Whalen, J. C. (2000). Behavioral and self-concept changes after six months of enuresis treatment: A randomized, controlled trial. *Pediatrics, 105*(Suppl.), 935–940.

Macauley, M., Pettersen, L., Fader, M., Brooks, R., & Cottenden. (2004). A multicenter evaluation of absorbent products for children with incontinence and disabilities. *Journal of WOCH, 31*(4), 235–244.

Sampselle, C., & DeLancey, J. (1998). Anatomy of female continence. *Journal of Wound, Ostomy and Continence Nursing, 25*(3), 63–74.

Steeman, E., & Defever, M. (1998). Urinary incontinence among elderly persons who live at home. *Nursing Clinics of North America, 33*(3), 441–455.

Walle, J., Rittig, S., Bauer, S., Eggert, P., Marschall-Kehrel, D., & Tekgul, S. (2012). Practical consensus guidelines for the management of enuresis. *European Journal of Pediatrics*, DOI: 10.1007/s00431-012-1687.7. Retrieved from http://www.springerlink.com/content/430648g360t11781/

Wilkinson, J., & Treas, L. (2011). Chapter 21, Safety. In *Fundamentals of nursing* (2nd ed.). Philadelphia: F. A. Davis.

Urinary Incontinence, Overflow

(Also see the bibliographies for: Urinary Elimination, Impaired; Urinary Elimination, Readiness for Enhanced; Urinary Incontinence, Functional; Urinary Incontinence, Reflex; Urinary Incontinence, Stress; Urinary Incontinence, Urge; Urinary Incontinence, Risk for Urge; and Urinary Retention.)

Browning, J., Zaheer, Z., Orzechowska, A., & Mistri, A. (2012). Continence aids in the management of urinary incontinence. *Reviews in Clinical Gerontology, 22*(2), 85–98.

Mirza, M., Griebling, T., & Kazer, M. (2011). Erectile dysfunction and urinary incontinence after prostate cancer treatment. *Seminars in Oncology Nursing, 27*(4), 278–289.

National Kidney and Urologic Diseases Information Clearing House. (2004). *Urinary incontinence in women*. Bethesda, MD: Author.

Roe, B., Flanagan, L., Jack, B., Barrett, J., Chung, A., Shaw, C., et al. (2011). Systematic review of the management of incontinence and promotion of continence in older people in care homes: Descriptive studies with urinary incontinence as primary focus. *Journal of Advanced Nursing, 67*(2), 228–250.

Van Leijsen, X., Hoogstad-van Evert, J., Mol, B., Vierhout, M., Milani, A., Heesakkers, J., et al. (2011). The correlation between clinical and urodynamic diagnosis in classifying the type of urinary incontinence in women. A systematic review of the literature. *Neurology and Urodynamics, 30*(4), 495–502.

Walsh, P. (Ed.). (2002). *Campbell's urology* (8th ed.). Philadelphia: Saunders.

Wilkinson, J., & Treas, L. (2011). Chapter 21, Safety. In *Fundamentals of nursing* (2nd ed.). Philadelphia: F. A. Davis.

Urinary Incontinence, Reflex

(Also see the bibliographies for: Urinary Elimination, Impaired; Urinary Elimination, Readiness for Enhanced; Urinary Incontinence, Functional; Urinary Incontinence, Overflow; Urinary Incontinence, Stress; Urinary Incontinence, Urge; Urinary Incontinence, Risk for Urge; and Urinary Retention.)

Callsen-Cencic, P., & Mense, S. (1999). Mechanisms underlying the pathogenesis of urinary bladder instability—new perspectives for the treatment of reflex incontinence. *Restorative Neurology & Neuroscience, 14*(2), 115.

Cruz, F. (2003). Mechanisms involved in new therapies for overactive bladder. *Urology, 63,* 65.

Fernandez, B., Gaydecki, P., Jowitt, F., & van den Heuvel, E. (2011). Urinary incontinence: A vibration alert system for detecting pad overflow. *Assistive Technology: The Official Journal of RESNA, 23*(4), 218–224.

Hagen, E., Faerestrand, S., Hoff, J., Rekand, T., & Gronning, M. (2011). Cardiovascular and urological dysfunction in spinal cord injury. *Acta Neurologica Scandinavica, 124*(Suppl. s191), 71–78.

Saba, V. K. & McCormick, K. (2006). Reflex urinary incontinence. In *Essentials of nursing informatics (appendix)* New York: McGraw-Hill.

Sanders, C., Driver, C. P., & Rickwood, A. M. K. (2002). The anocutaneous reflex and urinary continence in children with myelomeningocele. *BJU International, 89*(7), 720–721.

Wilkinson, J., & Treas, L. (2011). Chapter 21, Safety. In *Fundamentals of nursing* (2nd ed.). Philadelphia: F. A. Davis.

Wyndaele, J., Kovindha, A., Madersbacher, H., Radziszewski, P., Ruffion, A., Schurch, B., et al. (2010). Neurologic urinary incontinence. *Neurourology and Urodynamics, 29*(1), 159–164.

Urinary Incontinence, Stress

(Also see the bibliographies for: Urinary Elimination, Impaired; Urinary Elimination, Readiness for Enhanced; Urinary Incontinence, Functional; Urinary Incontinence, Overflow; Urinary Incontinence, Reflex; Urinary Incontinence, Urge; Urinary Incontinence, Risk for Urge; and Urinary Retention.)

DeLancey, J. (2010). Why do women have stress urinary incontinence? *Neurology and Urodynamics, 29*(S1), S13–S17.

Dmochowski, R., Blaivas, J., Gormley, E., Juma, S., Karram, M., Lightner, D., et al. (2010). Update of AUA guideline on the surgical management of female stress urinary incontinence. *The Journal of Urology, 183*(5), 1906–1914.

Flynn, D. (2005). Improving continence care: Searching the evidence. *Journal of Community Nursing, 19*(3), 18.

Haslam, J. (2003). Continuing professional development: Stress urinary incontinence. Stress urinary incontinence. *Primary Health Care, 13*(4), 43–50.

Herschorn, S., Bruschini, H., Comiter, C., Grise, P., Hanus, T., Kirschner-Hermanns, R., et al. (2010). Surgical treatment of stress incontinence in men. *Neurology and Urodynamics, 29*(1), 179–190.

Huebner, M., Riegel, K., Hinninghofen, H., Wallwiener, D., Tunn, R., & Reisenauer, C. (2011). Pelvic floor muscle training for stress urinary incontinence: A randomized, controlled trial comparing different conservative therapies. *Physiotherapy Research International, 16*(3), 133–140.

Lewthwaite, B., & Girouard, L. (2006). Urinary drainage following continence surgery: Development of Canadian best practice guidelines. *Urologic Nursing, 26*(1), 33–39.

Richter, H., Albo, M., Zyczynski, H., Kenton, K., Norton, P., Sirls, L., et al. (2010). Retropubic versus transobturator midurethral slings for stress incontinence. *The New England Journal of Medicine, 362,* 2066–2076.

Richter, H., Burgio, K., Brubaker, L., Nygaard, I., Ye, W., Weidner, A., et al. (2010). A trial of continence pessary vs. Behavioral therapy vs. Combined therapy for stress incontinence. *Obstetrics and Gynecology, 115*(3), 619–617.

Sakala, C. (2004, September/October). Resources for evidence-based practice. *JOGNN: Journal of Obstetric, Gynecologic, & Neonatal Nursing, 33*(5), 622–625.

Sherburn, M., Bird, M., Carey, M., Bø, K., & Galea, M. (2011). Incontinence improves in older women after intensive pelvic floor muscle training: An assessor-blinded randomized controlled trial. *Neurourology and Urodynamics, 30*(3), 317–324.

Wilkinson, J., & Treas, L. (2011). Chapter 21, Safety. In *Fundamentals of nursing* (2nd ed). Philadelphia: F. A. Davis.

Urinary Incontinence, Urge

(Also see the bibliographies for: Urinary Elimination, Impaired; Urinary Elimination, Readiness for Enhanced; Urinary Incontinence, Functional; Urinary Incontinence, Overflow; Urinary Incontinence, Stress; and Urinary Retention.)

Baker, J., Costa, D., & Nygaard, I. (2012). Mindfulness-based stress reduction for treatment of urinary urge incontinence: A pilot study. *Female Pelvic Medicine & Reconstructive Surgery, 18*(1), 46–49.

Bromley, R., & Cook, T. (2011). Case report. Efficacy of behavioural training in treating symptoms of urinary urgency and urge urinary incontinence. *Journal of the Association of Chartered Physiotherapists in Women's Health, 109,* 14–19.

Groen, J., Blok, B., & Bosch, J. (2011). Sacral neuromodulation as treatment for refractory idiopathic urge urinary incontinence: 5-year results of a longitudinal study in 60 women. *The Journal of Urology, 186*(3), 954–959.

Karon, S. (2005). A team approach to bladder retraining: A pilot study. *Urologic Nursing, 25*(4), 269–276.

Kim, H., Yoshida, H., & Suzuki, T. (2011). The effects of multidimensional exercise treatment on community-dwelling elderly Japanese women with stress, urge, and mixed urinary incontinence: A randomized controlled trial. *International Journal of Nursing Studies, 48*(10), 1165–1172.

Lee, J.-S., Dwyer, P., Rosamilia, A., Lim, Y., Polyakov, A., & Stav, K. (2011). Persistence of urgency and urge urinary incontinence in women with mixed urinary symptoms after midurethral slings: A multivariate analysis. *BJOG: An International Journal of Obstetrics & Gynaecology, 118*(7), 798–805.

Marinkovic, S., Rovner, E., Moldwin, R., Stanton, S., Gillen, L., & Marinkovic, C. (2012). The management of overactive bladder syndrome. *BMJ, 344*, e2365. DOI: 10.1136/bmj.e2365. Retrieved from http://www.bmj.com/content/344/bmj.e2365?ga=w_ga_mpopular

Morgan, D., Lewicky-Gaupp, C., Dunn, R., Jayaraman, G., Fenner, D., DeLancey, J., et al. (2011). Factors associated with urge urinary incontinence after surgery for stress urinary incontinence. *Female Pelvic Medicine & Reconstructive Surgery, 17*(3), 120–124.

National Kidney and Urologic Diseases Information Clearinghouse. (2004). *Urinary incontinence in women*. Retrieved May 21, 2012, from http://kidney.niddk.nih.gov/kudiseases/pubs/uiwomen/

Sampselle, C. (2003). State of the science on urinary incontinence: Behavioral interventions in young and middle-age women. *American Journal of Nursing, 103*(3), 9–19.

Sanders, S., Bern-Klug, M., Specht, J., Mobily, P., & Bossen, A. (2012). Expanding the role of long-term care social workers: Assessment and intervention related to urinary incontinence. *Journal of Gerontological Social Work, 55*(3), 2626–2281.

Wooldridge, L. S. (2003). Behavioural training plus biofeedback or verbal feedback did not differ from self administered behavioural training in urge incontinence. *Evidence-Based Nursing, 6*(3), 87.

Wilkinson, J., & Treas, L. (2011). Chapter 21, Safety. In *Fundamentals of nursing* (2nd ed.). Philadelphia: F. A. Davis.

Urinary Incontinence, Urge, Risk for

(Refer to the bibliographies for: Urinary Elimination, Impaired; Urinary Elimination, Readiness for Enhanced; Urinary Incontinence, Functional; Urinary Incontinence, Overflow; Urinary Incontinence, Stress; Urinary Incontinence, Urge; and Urinary Retention.)

Urinary Retention

Also see the bibliography for Urinary Elimination, Impaired.

Chartier-Kastler, E., & Denys, P. (2011). Intermittent catheterization with hydrophilic catheters as a treatment of chronic neurogenic urinary retention. *Neurology and Urodynamics, 30*(1), 21–31.

Cutright, J. (2011). The effect of the bladder scanner policy on the number of urinary catheters inserted. *Journal of Wound, Ostomy & Continence Nursing, 38*(1), 71–76.

Donohue, D. R. (2004). Evidence-based literature review: Identification, assessment and management of the stroke patient with urinary retention. *Australian & New Zealand Continence Journal, 10*(3), 66–67.

Dupuis, O. (2011). Postpartum haemorrhage and postpartum urinary retention: Could voiding be the best way of avoiding postpartum haemorrhage? *BJOG: An International Journal of Obstetrics & Gynaecology, 118*(8), 1023–1024.

Emr, K., & Ryan, R. (2004). Best practice for indwelling catheters in the home setting. *Home Healthcare Nurse, 22*(12), 820–830.

Griesdale, D., Neufeld, J., Dhillon, D., Joo, J., Sandhu, S., Swinton, F., et al. (2011). Risk factors for urinary retention after hip or knee replacement: A cohort study. *Canadian Journal of Anesthesia, 58*(12), 1097–1104.

Griffiths, R., & Fernandez, R. (2006). Policies for the removal of short-term indwelling urethral catheters. *Cochrane Library* (4).

Hansen, B., SØreide, E., Warland, A., & Nilsen, O. (2011). Risk factors of postoperative urinary retention in hospitalised patients. *Acta Anaesthesiologica Scandinavica, 55*(5), 545–548.

Humburg, J., Troeger, C., Holzgreve, W., & Hoesli, I. (2011). Risk factors in prolonged postpartum urinary retention: An analysis of six cases. *Archives of Gynecology and Obstetrics, 283*(2), 179–183.

Kuppuysamy, S., & Gillatt, D. (2011). Managing patients with acute urinary retention. *Practitioner, 255*(1739), 2–3, 21–23.

Leach, S. (2011). 'Have you had a wee yet?' Postpartum urinary retention. *The Practising Midwife, 14*(1), 23–25.

Newman, D. K., Gaines, T., & Snare, E. (2005). Innovation in bladder assessment: Use of technology in extended care. *Journal of Gerontological Nursing, 31*(12), 33–43.

Ostaszkiewicz, J., O'Connell, B., & Ski, C. (2008). A guideline for the nursing assessment and management of urinary retention in elderly hospitalized patients. *Australian and New Zealand Continence, 14*(3, Spring), 76–83.

Ribby, K. J. (2006). Decreasing urinary tract infections through staff development, outcomes, and nursing process. *Journal of Nursing Care Quality, 21*(3), 272–276.

Wilkinson, J., & Treas, L. (2011). Chapter 21, Safety. In *Fundamentals of nursing* (2nd ed.). Philadelphia: F. A. Davis.

Williamson, J. (2005). Continence. Management of postoperative urinary retention. *Nursing Times, 101*(29), 53–54.

Vascular Trauma, Risk for

Adami, N., Gutierrez, M., da Fonseca, S., & de Almeida, E. (2005). Risk management of extravasation of cytostatic drugs at the adult chemotherapy outpatient clinic of a university hospital. *Journal of Clinical Nursing, 14*(7), 876–882.

The Joanna Briggs Institute. (2008). Management of peripheral intravascular devices. *Best Practice. Evidence Based Information Sheets for Health Professionals, 12*(5). ISSN: 1329-1874. Retrieved May 22, 2012, from http://connect.jbiconnectplus.org/ViewSourceFile.aspx?0=439

Koutzavekiaris, I., Vouloumanou, E., Goumi, M., Rafailidis, P., Michalopoulos, A., & Falagas, M. (2011). Knowledge and practices regarding prevention of infections associated with central venous catheters: A survey of intensive care unit medical and nursing staff. *American Journal of Infection Control, 39*(7), 542–547.

Phillips, L. (2005). *Manual of IV therapeutics* (4th ed.). Philadelphia, PA: F. A. Davis.

Segreti, J., Garcia-Houchins, S., Gorski, L., Moureau, N., Shomo, J., Zack, J., et al. (2011). Consensus conference on prevention of central line-associated bloodstream infections: 2009. *Journal of Infusion Nursing, 34*(2), 126–133.

Wilkinson, J., & Treas, L. (2011). Chapter 36, Fluids, electrolytes, and acid-Base balance; and chapter 23, administering medication. In *Fundamentals of nursing* (2nd ed.). Philadelphia: F. A. Davis.

Ventilatory Weaning Response, Dysfunctional

Bisset, B., Leditschke, I., & Green, M. (2012). Specific inspiratory muscle training is safe in selected patients who are ventilator-dependent: A case series. *Intensive and Critical Care Nursing, 28*(2), 98–104.

Blackwood, B., Wilson-Barnett, J., & Trinder, J. (2004). Protocolized weaning from mechanical ventilation: ICU physician's views. *Journal of Advanced Nursing, 48*(1), 26–34.

Burns, S., Fisher, C., Tribble, S., Lewis, R., Merrel, P., Conaway, M., et al. (2012). The relationship of 26 clinical factors to weaning outcome. *American Journal of Critical Care, 21*(1), 52–59.

Carasa, M. (2003). *Weaning the chronically critically ill patient: The meaning of the weaning experience as perceived by nurse practitioners and patients in a respiratory care unit.* (Columbia University Teachers College.)

Epstein, S. K. (2002). Weaning from mechanical ventilation. *Respiratory Care, 47*(4), 454–468.

Fulbrook, P., Delaney, N., Rigby, J., Sowden, A., Trevett, M., & Turner, L. (2004). Developing a network protocol: Nurse-led weaning from ventilation. *Connect: The World of Critical Care Nursing, 3*(2), 28–37.

Grap, M. J., Strickland, D., Tormey, L., Keane, K., Lubin, S., & Emerson, J. (2003). Collaborative practice: Development, implementation, and evaluation of a weaning protocol for patients receiving mechanical ventilation. *American Journal of Critical Care, 12*(5), 454–460.

Hampton, D. C., Griffith, D., & Howard, A. (2005). Evidence-based clinical improvement for mechanically ventilated patients. *Rehabilitation Nursing, 30*(4), 160–165.

Hancock, H. C., & Easen, P. R. (2006). The decision-making processes of nurses when extubating patients following cardiac surgery: An ethnographic study. *International Journal of Nursing Studies, 43*(6), 693–705.

Keogh, S. J. (2004). Weaning from mechanical ventilation: A national survey of Australian paediatric intensive care units. *Neonatal, Paediatric & Child Health Nursing, 7*(3), 13–19.

Laux, L., & Herbert, C. (2006). Decreasing ventilator-associated pneumonia: Getting on board. *Critical Care Nursing Quarterly, 29*(3), 253–258.

Linda, O. B., Kathryn, V. R., & Fern, M. (2002). Evaluating ventilator weaning best practice: A long-term acute care hospital system-wide quality initiative. *AACN Clinical Issues: Advanced Practice in Acute & Critical Care, 13*(4), 567–576.

Lindgren, V. A., & Ames, N. J. (2005). Caring for patients on mechanical ventilation: What research indicates is best practice. *American Journal of Nursing, 105*(5), 50–61.

Logan, J., & Jenny, J. (1991). Interventions for the nursing diagnosis "dysfunctional ventilatory weaning response": A qualitative study. In R. M. Carroll-Johnson (Ed.), *Classification of nursing diagnoses: Proceedings of the ninth conference* (pp. 141–147). Philadelphia: Lippincott.

MacIntyre, N. R. (2004). Evidence-based ventilator weaning and discontinuation. *Respiratory Care, 49*(7), 830–836 Williams & Wilkins.

Munro, N. (2006). Weaning smokers from mechanical ventilation. *Critical Care Nursing Clinics of North America, 18*(1), 21–28.

Plost, G., & Nelson, D. P. (2007). Empowering critical care nurses to improve compliance with protocols in the intensive care unit. *American Journal of Critical Care, 16*(2), 153–157.

Schädler, D., Engel, C., Elke, G., Pulletz, S., Haake, N., Frerichs, I., et al. (2012, January 20). Automatic control of pressure support for ventilator weaning in surgical intensive care patients. *American Journal of Respiratory and Critical Care Medicine*. DOI: 10.1164/rccm.201106-1127OC. Retrieved May 22, 2012, from http://ajrccm.atsjournals.org/content/early/2012/01/18/rccm.201106-1127OC.short

Violence: Other-Directed, Risk for

Antle, B., Sullivan, D., Dryden, A., Karam, E., & Barbee, A. (2011). Healthy relationship education for dating violence prevention among high-risk youth. *Children and Youth Services Review, 33*(1), 173–179.

Anglin, D., & Sachs, C. (2003). Preventive care in the emergency department: Screening for domestic violence in the emergency department. *Academic Emergency Medicine, 10*(10), 1118–1127.

Archer-Gift, C. (2003). Violence towards the caregiver: A growing crisis for professional nursing. *Michigan Nurse, 76*(1), 11–12.

Baroni, S., & Richmond, T. S. (2006). Firearm violence in America: A growing health problem. *Critical Care Nursing Clinics of North America, 18*(3), 297–303.

Bechtel, K., Le, K., Martin, K., Shah, N., Leventhal, J., & Colson, E. (2011). Impact of an educational intervention on caregivers' beliefs about infant crying and knowledge of shaken baby syndrome. *Academic Pediatrics, 11*(6), 481–486.

Cowin, L., Davies, R., Estall, G., Berlin, T., Fitzgerald, M., & Hoot, S. (2003). De-escalating aggression and violence in the mental health setting. *International Journal of Mental Health Nursing, 12*(1), 64–73.

Delaney, K., Esparza, D., Hinderliter, D., Lamb, K., & Mohr, W. (2006). Violence and abuse within the community. In W. K. Mohr (Ed.), *Psychiatric-mental health nursing* (6th ed., pp. 353–376). Philadelphia: Lippincott Williams & Wilkins.

Gómez, A. (2011). Testing the cycle of violence hypothesis: Child abuse and adolescent dating violence as predictors of intimate partner violence in young adulthood. *Youth and Society, 43*(1), 171–192.

Johnson, M. E. (2004). Violence on inpatient psychiatric units: State of the science. *Journal of the American Psychiatric Nurses Association, 10*(3), 113–121.

McGill, A. (2006). Evidence-based strategies to decrease psychiatric patient assaults. *Nursing Management, 37*(11), 41–44.

Nelson, H. W., & Cox, D. M. (2004). The causes and consequences of conflict and violence in nursing homes: Working toward a collaborative work culture. *Health Care Manager, 23*(1), 85–96.

Ornstein, A., & Dipenta, J. (2011). Abusive head trauma in infants and why we CAN afford to prevent it. *Paediatrics & Child Health, 16*(2), e9–e10.

Sadeh, N., Shabnam, J., Finy, M., & Verona, E. (2011). Gender differences in emotional risk for self- and other-directed violence among externalizing adults. *Journal of Consulting and Clinical Psychology, 79*(1), 106–117. DOI: 10.1037/a0022197.

Sousa, C., Herrenkohl, T., Moylan, C., Tajima, E., Klika, J., Herrenkohl, R., et al. (2011). Longitudinal study on the effects of child abuse and children's exposure to domestic violence, parent–child attachments, and antisocial behavior in adolescence. *Journal of Interpersonal Violence, 26*(1), 111–136.

Swogger, M., Walsh, Z., Homaifar, B., Caine, E., & Conner, K. (2012). Predicting self- and other-directed violence among discharged psychiatric patients: The roles of anger and psychopathic traits. *Psychological Medicine, 42*(2), 371–379.

Vaaler, A., Iversen, V., Morken, G., Fløvig, J., Palmstierna, T., & Linaker, O. (2011). Short-term prediction of threatening and violent behaviour in an acute psychiatric intensive care unit based on patient and environment characteristics. *BMC Psychiatry, 1*, 44. DOI: 10.1186/1471-244X-11-44. Retrieved from http://www.biomedcentral.com/1471-244X/11/44

Wilk, N. C. (2005). *The lived experience of adolescent dating violence: Walking between two worlds*. State University of New York at Buffalo. Retrieved from http://hdl.handle.net/10755/148817

Wilson, D., McBride-Henry, K., & Huntington, A. (2005). Family violence: Walking the tight rope between maternal alienation and child safety. In P. Darbyshire & D. Jackson (Eds.), *Advances in contemporary child and family health care* (pp. 85–96). Sydney, Australia: eContent Management Pty Ltd.

Violence: Self-Directed, Risk for

Barr, W., Leitner, M., & Thomas, J. (2005). Psychosocial assessment of patients who attend an accident and emergency department with self-harm. *Journal of Psychiatric & Mental Health Nursing, 12*(2), 130–138.

Cutcliffe, J. R. (2003). Mental health nursing. Research endeavours into suicide: A need to shift the emphasis. *British Journal of Nursing (BJN), 12*(2), 92–99.

Gask, L., Dixon, C., Morriss, R., Appleby, L., & Green, G. (2006). Evaluating STORM skills training for managing people at risk of suicide. *Journal of Advanced Nursing, 54*(6), 739–750.

Lanstedt, E., & Gådin, K. (2011). Deliberate self-harm and associated factors in 17-year-old Swedish students. *Scandinavian Journal of Public Health, 39*(1), 17–25.

Ougrin, D., Zundel, T., Ng, A., Banarsee, R., Bottle, A., & Taylor. (2011). Trial of therapeutic assessment (TA) in London: Randomised controlled trial of therapeutic assessment versus standard psychosocial assessment in adolescents presenting with self-harm. *Archives of Disease in Childhood, 96*(2), 148–153.

Pompili, M., Mancinelli, I., Girardi, P., Ruberto, A., & Tatarelli, R. (2005). Childhood suicide: A major issue in pediatric health care. *Issues in Comprehensive Pediatric Nursing, 28*(1), 63–68.

Sullivan, A., Barron, C., Bezmen, J., Rivera, J., & Zapata-Vega, M. (2005). The safe treatment of the suicidal patient in an adult inpatient setting: A proactive preventive approach. *Psychiatric Quarterly, 76*(1), 67–83.

Taylor, L., Oldershaw, A., Richards, C., Davidson, K., Schmidt, U., & Simic, M. (2011). Development and pilot evaluation of a manualized cognitive-behavioural treatment package for adolescent self-harm. *Behavioural and Cognitive Psychotherapy, 39*(5), 619–625.

Wilkinson, P., Kelvin, R., Roberts, C., Dubicka, B., & Goodyer, I. (2011). Clinical and psychosocial predictors of suicide attempts and nonsuicidal self-injury in the adolescent depression antidepressants and psychotherapy trial (ADAPT). *The American Journal of Psychiatry, 168*(5). Retrieved May 29, 2012, from http://ajp.psychiatryonline.org/article.aspx?articleid=106947

Walking, Impaired

Arias, M., & Smith, L. N. (2007). Early mobilization of acute stroke patients. *Journal of Clinical Nursing, 16*(2), 282–288.

Brouwer, K., Nysseknabm, J., & Culham, E. (2004). Physical function and health status among seniors with and without fear of falling. *Gerontology, 50,* 15–141.

Deep vein thrombosis: Court stresses importance of post-op ambulation by nurses. (2004). *Legal Eagle Eye Newsletter for the Nursing Profession, 12*(8), 4.

Field-Fote, E., & Roach, K. (2011). Influence of a locomotor training approach on walking speed and distance in people with chronic spinal cord injury: A randomized clinical trial. *Physical Therapy, 91*(1), 48–60.

Griffin, H., Greenlaw, R., Limousin, P., Bhatia, K., Quinn, N., & Jahanshahi, M. (2011). The effect of real and virtual visual cues on walking in Parkinson's disease. *Journal of Neurology, 258*(6), 991–1000.

Hamburg, N., & Balady, G. (2011). Exercise rehabilitation in peripheral artery disease. Functional impact and mechanisms of benefits. *Circulation, 128,* 87–97.

Killey, B., & Watt, E. (2006). The effect of extra walking on the mobility, independence and exercise self-efficacy of elderly hospital in-patients: A pilot study. *Contemporary Nurse: A Journal for the Australian Nursing Profession, 22*(1), 120–133.

Lewis, C. L., Moutoux, M., Slaughter, M., & Bailey, S. P. (2004). Characteristics of individuals who fell while receiving home health services. *Physical Therapy, 84*(1), 23–32.

Taraldsen, K., Askin, T., Sletvold, O., Einarsen, E., Bjåstad, K., Indredavik, B., et al. (2011). Evaluation of a body-worn sensor system to measure physical activity in older people with impaired function. *Physical Therapy, 91*(1), 277–285.

Wandering

Algase, D. L. (1999). Wandering in dementia. *Annual Review in Nursing Research, 17*(2), 185–217.

Algase, D. L., Beattie, E., Song, J., Milke, D., Duffield, C., & Cowan, B. (2004). Validation of the algase wandering scale (version 2) in a cross cultural sample. *Aging & Mental Health, 8*(2), 133–142.

Altus, D. E., Mathews, R. M., Xaverius, P. K., Engelman, K. K., & Nolan, B. D. (2000). Evaluation of an electronic monitoring system for people who wander. *American Journal of Alzheimer's Disease, 15*(2), 121–125.

Cook, E., Swift, K., James, I., Malouf, R., De Vugt, M., & Verhey, F. (2012). Functional analysis-based interventions for challenging behaviour in dementia. *Cochrane Database of Systematic Reviews 2012,* Issue 2. Art. No.: CD006929. DOI: 10.1002/14651858.CD006929.pub2. Retrieved May 30, 2012, from http://onlinelibrary.wiley.com/doi/10.1002/14651858.CD006929.pub2/full

Douglas, A., Letta, L., & Richardson, J. (2011). A systematic review of accidental injury from fire, wandering and medication self-administration errors for older adults with and without dementia. *Archives of Gerontology and Geriatrics, 52*(1), e1–e10.

Futrell, M., & Melillo, K. D. (2002). Evidence-based protocol: Wandering. *Journal of Gerontological Nursing, 28*(11), 14–22.

Halek, M., & Bartholomeyczik, S. (2012). Description of the behaviour of wandering in people with dementia living in nursing homes—a review of the literature. *Scandinavian Journal of Caring Sciences, 26*(2), 404–413.

Meiner, S. E. (2000). Wandering problems need ongoing nursing planning: A case study. *Geriatric Nursing, 21*(2), 101–106.

Pack, R. (2000). The "ins and outs" of wandering. *Nursing Homes, 49*(8), 55–59.

Padilla, R. (2011). Effectiveness of environment-based interventions for people with Alzheimer's disease and related dementias. *American Journal of Occupational Therapy, 65*(5), 514–522.

Rowe, M., Vandeveer, S., Greenblum, C., List, C., Fernandez, R., Mixson, N., et al. (2011). Persons with dementia missing in the community: Is it wandering or something unique? *BMC Geriatrics, 11*, 28. DOI: 10.1186/1471-2318-11-28. Retrieved May 30, 2012, from http://www.biomedcentral.com/1471-2318/11/28/

Turner, S. (2005). Behavioural symptoms of dementia in residential settings: A selective review of non-pharmacological interventions. *Aging & Mental Health, 9*(2), 93–104.

APPENDIX A

2012–2014 NANDA International-Approved Nursing Diagnoses

Grouped by Gordon's Functional Health Patterns

Nutritional/Metabolic

Bleeding, risk for
Blood glucose, risk for unstable
Body temperature, risk for imbalanced
Breast milk, insufficient
Breastfeeding, ineffective
Breastfeeding, interrupted
Breastfeeding, readiness for enhanced
Dentition, impaired
Dry eye, risk for
Dysreflexia, autonomic
Dysreflexia, autonomic, risk for
Electrolyte imbalance, risk for
Failure to thrive, adult
Fluid balance, readiness for enhanced
Fluid volume, deficient
Fluid volume, deficient, risk for
Fluid volume excess
Fluid volume, risk for imbalanced
Gastrointestinal motility, dysfunctional
Gastrointestinal motility, dysfunctional, risk for
Growth, risk for disproportionate
Growth and development, delayed
Hyperthermia
Hypothermia
Infant feeding pattern, ineffective
Jaundice, neonatal
Jaundice, neonatal, risk for
Nutrition, imbalanced: less than body requirements
Nutrition, imbalanced: more than body requirements
Nutrition, imbalanced: more than body requirements, risk for
Nutrition, readiness for enhanced
Oral mucous membrane, impaired
Perfusion: gastrointestinal, risk for ineffective
Shock, risk for
Skin integrity, impaired
Skin integrity, risk for impaired

Sudden infant death syndrome, risk for
Swallowing, impaired
Thermoregulation, ineffective
Tissue integrity, impaired
Vascular trauma, risk for

Health-Perception/Health Management

Allergy response, risk for
Aspiration, risk for
Community health, deficient
Contamination
Contamination, risk for
Denial, ineffective
Falls, risk for
Health behavior, risk prone
Health maintenance, ineffective
Health seeking behaviors (specify)
Immunization status, readiness for enhanced
Infection, risk for
Injury, risk for
Latex allergy response
Latex allergy response, risk for
Iodinated contrast media, risk for adverse reaction to
Management of therapeutic regimen: family, ineffective
Noncompliance (specify)
Poisoning, risk for
Protection, ineffective
Self-health management, ineffective
Self-health management, readiness for enhanced
Sudden infant death syndrome, risk for
Suffocation, risk for
Surgical recovery, delayed
Thermal injury, risk for
Trauma, risk for

Sleep/Rest

Insomnia
Sleep deprivation
Sleep pattern, disturbed
Sleep, readiness for enhanced

Activity/Exercise

Activity intolerance
Activity intolerance, risk for

Adaptive capacity: intracranial, decreased
Airway clearance, ineffective
Breathing pattern, ineffective
Cardiac output, decreased
Development, risk for delayed
Disorganized infant behavior
Disorganized infant behavior, risk for
Disuse syndrome, risk for
Diversional activity, deficient
Energy field disturbed
Fatigue
Gas exchange, impaired
Home maintenance, impaired
Mobility: bed, impaired
Mobility: physical, impaired
Mobility: wheelchair, impaired
Organized infant behavior, readiness for enhanced
Perioperative positioning injury, risk for
Peripheral neurovascular dysfunction, risk for
Renal perfusion, risk for ineffective
Sedentary lifestyle
Self-care deficit: bathing, dressing, feeding, toileting (specify)
Self-care, readiness for enhanced
Spontaneous ventilation, impaired
Tissue perfusion: cardiac, risk for decreased
Tissue perfusion: cerebral, risk for ineffective
Tissue perfusion: peripheral, ineffective
Tissue perfusion: peripheral, risk for ineffective
Transfer ability, impaired
Ventilatory weaning response, dysfunctional
Walking, impaired

Elimination

Constipation
Constipation, perceived
Constipation, risk for
Diarrhea
Incontinence: bowel
Incontinence: urinary, functional
Incontinence: urinary, overflow
Incontinence: urinary, reflex
Incontinence: urinary, stress
Incontinence: urinary, urge
Incontinence: urinary, urge, risk for

Liver function, risk for impaired
Urinary elimination, impaired
Urinary elimination, readiness for enhanced
Urinary retention

Value/Belief

Decision making, readiness for enhanced
Decisional conflict (specify)
Grieving
Grieving, complicated
Grieving, complicated, risk for
Human dignity, risk for compromised
Moral distress
Religiosity, impaired
Religiosity, impaired, risk for
Religiosity, readiness for enhanced
Sorrow, chronic
Spiritual distress
Spiritual distress, risk for
Spiritual well-being, readiness for enhanced

Sexuality/Reproductivity

Childbearing process, ineffective
Childbearing process: ineffective, risk for
Childbearing process, readiness for enhanced
Sexual dysfunction
Sexuality pattern, ineffective

Self-Perception/Self-Concept

Anxiety
Anxiety, death
Body image, disturbed
Environmental interpretation syndrome, impaired
Fear
Hope, readiness for enhanced
Hopelessness
Personal identity, disturbed
Personal identity, disturbed, risk for
Power, readiness for enhanced
Powerlessness
Powerlessness, risk for
Self-concept, readiness for enhanced
Self-esteem, chronic low
Self-esteem, risk for chronic low

Self-esteem, risk for situational low
Self-esteem, situational low

Cognitive/Perceptual

Comfort, impaired
Comfort, readiness for enhanced
Communication, impaired verbal
Communication, readiness for enhanced
Confusion, acute
Confusion, acute, risk for
Confusion, chronic
Knowledge, deficient (specify)
Knowledge of (specify), readiness for enhanced
Memory, impaired
Nausea
Pain, acute
Pain, chronic
Unilateral neglect
Wandering

Coping/Stress Tolerance

Activity planning, ineffective
Coping: community, ineffective
Coping: community, readiness for enhanced
Coping, defensive
Coping: family, compromised
Coping: family, disabled
Coping: family, readiness for enhanced
Coping, ineffective
Denial, ineffective
Impulse control, ineffective
Posttrauma syndrome
Posttrauma syndrome, risk for
Rape-trauma syndrome
Relocation stress syndrome
Relocation stress syndrome, risk for
Resilience, impaired individual
Resilience, readiness for enhanced
Resilience, risk for compromised
Self-mutilation
Self-mutilation, risk for
Self-neglect
Stress overload

Suicide, risk for
Violence, risk for self-directed

Role/Relationship

Attachment, risk for impaired
Caregiver role strain
Caregiver role strain, risk for
Family processes, dysfunctional
Family processes, interrupted
Family processes, readiness for enhanced
Home maintenance, impaired
Loneliness, risk for
Maternal/fetal dyad, risk for disturbed
Parenting, impaired
Parenting, readiness for enhanced
Parenting, risk for impaired
Relationship, ineffective
Relationship, ineffective, risk for
Relationship, readiness for enhanced
Role conflict, parental
Role performance, ineffective
Social interaction, impaired
Social isolation
Violence, risk for other-directed

Note: The diagnoses *Risk for delayed development*, *Delayed growth and development*, and *Risk for disproportionate growth* can occur in any of the Functional Health Patterns.

Used by permission of NANDA International.

Adapted from Functional Health Patterns, Gordon, M. (1994). *Nursing diagnosis: Process and application*, 3rd ed. St. Louis: Mosby.

APPENDIX B

NANDA International-Approved Nursing Diagnoses (2012–2014), Taxonomy II: Domains, Classes, and Diagnoses

This taxonomically organized list represents the NANDA International nursing diagnoses approved for clinical use and testing.

Domain 1. Health Promotion

The awareness of well-being or normality of function and the strategies used to maintain control of and enhance that well-being or normality of function

Class 1. Health Awareness. Recognition of normal function and well-being

00097	Deficient diversional activity
00168	Sedentary lifestyle

Class 2. Health Management. Identifying, controlling, performing, and integrating activities to maintain health and well-being

Approved Diagnoses

00215	Deficient community health
00188	Risk-prone health behavior
00099	Ineffective health maintenance
00186	Readiness for enhanced immunization status
00043	Ineffective protection
00078	Ineffective self-health management
00162	Readiness for enhanced self-health management
00080	Ineffective family therapeutic regimen management

Domain 2. Nutrition

The activities of taking in, assimilating, and using nutrients for the purposes of tissue maintenance, tissue repair, and the production of energy

Class 1. Ingestion. Taking food or nutrients into the body

Approved Diagnoses

00216	Insufficient breast milk
00107	Ineffective infant-feeding pattern
00002	Imbalanced nutrition: less than body requirements
00001	Imbalanced nutrition: more than body requirements
00003	Risk for imbalanced nutrition: more than body requirements
00163	Readiness for enhanced nutrition
00103	Impaired swallowing

Class 2. Digestion. The physical and chemical activities that convert foodstuffs into substances suitable for absorption and assimilation

Class 3. Absorption. The act of taking up nutrients through body tissues

Class 4. Metabolism. The chemical and physical processes occurring in living organisms and cells for the development and use of protoplasm and production of waste and energy, with the release of energy for all vital processes

Approved Diagnoses

00179	Risk for unstable blood glucose level
00194	Neonatal jaundice
00230	Risk for neonatal jaundice
00178	Risk for impaired liver function

Class 5. Hydration. The taking in and absorption of fluids and electrolytes

Approved Diagnoses

00195	Risk for electrolyte imbalance
00160	Readiness for enhanced fluid balance
00027	Deficient fluid volume
00026	Excess fluid volume
00026	Risk for deficient fluid volume
00025	Risk for imbalanced fluid volume

Domain 3. Elimination and Exchange

Secretion and excretion of waste products from the body

Class 1. Urinary Function. The process of secretion, reabsorption, and excretion of urine

Approved Diagnoses

00020	Functional urinary incontinence
00176	Overflow urinary incontinence
00018	Reflex urinary incontinence
00017	Stress urinary incontinence
00019	Urge urinary incontinence
00022	Risk for urge urinary incontinence
00016	Impaired urinary elimination
00166	Readiness for enhanced urinary elimination
00023	Urinary retention

Class 2. Gastrointestinal Function. The process of absorption and excretion of the end products of digestion

Approved Diagnoses

00011	Constipation
00012	Perceived constipation
00015	Risk for constipation
00013	Diarrhea
00196	Dysfunctional gastrointestinal motility
00196	Risk for dysfunctional gastrointestinal motility
00014	Bowel incontinence

Class 3. Integumentary Function. The process of secretion and excretion through the skin

Class 4. Respiratory Function. The process of exchange of gases and removal of the end products of metabolism

Approved Diagnoses

00030	Impaired gas exchange

Domain 4. Activity/Rest

The production, conservation, expenditure, or balance of energy resources

Class 1. Sleep/Rest. Slumber, repose, ease, relaxation, or inactivity

Approved Diagnoses

00095	Insomnia
00096	Sleep deprivation
00165	Readiness for enhanced sleep
00198	Disturbed sleep pattern

Class 2. Activity/Exercise. Moving parts of the body (mobility), doing work, or performing actions often (but not always) against resistance

Approved Diagnoses

00040	Risk for disuse syndrome
00091	Impaired bed mobility
00085	Impaired physical mobility
00089	Impaired wheelchair mobility
00090	Impaired transfer ability
00088	Impaired walking

Class 3. Energy Balance. A dynamic state of harmony between intake and expenditure of resources

Approved Diagnoses

00050	Disturbed energy field
00093	Fatigue
00154	Wandering

Class 4. Cardiovascular/Pulmonary Responses. Cardiopulmonary mechanisms that support activity or rest

Approved Diagnoses

00092	Activity intolerance
00094	Risk for activity intolerance
00032	Ineffective breathing pattern
00029	Decreased cardiac output
00202	Risk for ineffective gastrointestinal perfusion
00203	Risk for ineffective renal perfusion
00033	Impaired spontaneous ventilation
00204	Ineffective peripheral tissue perfusion
00200	Risk for decreased cardiac tissue perfusion
00201	Risk for ineffective cerebral tissue perfusion
00238	Risk for ineffective peripheral tissue perfusion
00034	Dysfunctional ventilatory weaning response

Class 5. Self-Care. Ability to perform activities to care for one's body and bodily functions

Approved Diagnoses

00098	Impaired home maintenance
00182	Readiness for enhanced self-care

00108	Bathing self-care deficit
00109	Dressing self-care deficit
00102	Feeding self-care deficit
00110	Toileting self-care deficit
00193	Self-neglect

Domain 5. Perception/Cognition

The human information-processing system, including attention, orientation, sensation, perception, cognition, and communication

Class 1. Attention. Mental readiness to notice or observe

Approved Diagnoses

00123	Unilateral neglect

Class 2. Orientation. Awareness of time, place, and person

Approved Diagnoses

00127	Impaired environmental interpretation syndrome

Class 3. Sensation/Perception. Receiving information through the senses of touch, taste, smell, vision, hearing, and kinesthesia and the comprehension of sense data resulting in naming, associating, or pattern recognition

Approved Diagnoses

Class 4. Cognition. Use of memory, learning, thinking, problem solving, abstraction, judgment, insight, intellectual capacity, calculation, and language

Approved Diagnoses

00128	Acute confusion
00129	Chronic confusion
00173	Risk for acute confusion
00222	Ineffective impulse control
00126	Deficient knowledge
00161	Readiness for enhanced knowledge
00131	Impaired memory

Class 5. Communication. Sending and receiving verbal and nonverbal information

Approved Diagnoses

00157	Readiness for enhanced communication
00051	Impaired verbal communication

Domain 6. Self-Perception

Awareness about the self

Class 1. Self-Concept. The perception(s) about the total self

Approved Diagnoses

00124	Hopelessness
00174	Risk for compromised human dignity
00054	Risk for loneliness
00121	Disturbed personal identity

00225	Risk for disturbed personal identity
00167	Readiness for enhanced self-concept

Class 2. Self-esteem. Assessment of one's own worth, capability, significance, and success

Approved Diagnoses

00119	Chronic low self-esteem
00224	Risk for chronic low self-esteem
00153	Risk for situational low self-esteem
00120	Situational low self-esteem

Class 3. Body Image. A mental image of one's own body

Approved Diagnoses

00118	Disturbed body image

Domain 7. Role Relationships

The positive and negative connections or associations between peoples or groups of people and the means by which those connections are demonstrated

Class 1. Caregiving Roles. Socially expected behavior patterns by people providing care who are not health care professionals

Approved Diagnoses

00104	Ineffective breastfeeding
00105	Interrupted breastfeeding
00106	Readiness for enhanced breastfeeding
00061	Caregiver role strain
00062	Risk for caregiver role strain
00056	Impaired parenting
00057	Readiness for impaired parenting
00164	Risk for enhanced parenting

Class 2. Family Relationships. Associations of people who are biologically related or related by choice

Approved Diagnoses

00058	Risk for impaired attachment
00063	Dysfunctional family processes
00060	Interrupted family processes
00157	Readiness for enhanced processes

Class 3. Role Performance. Quality of functioning in socially expected behavior patterns

Approved Diagnoses

00223	Ineffective relationship
00207	Readiness for enhanced relationship
00229	Risk for ineffective relationship
00064	Parental role conflict
00055	Ineffective role performance
00052	Impaired social interaction

Domain 8. Sexuality

Sexual identity, sexual function, and reproduction

Class 1. Sexual Identity. The state of being a specific person in regard to sexuality or gender

Class 2. Sexual Function. The capacity or ability to participate in sexual activities

Approved Diagnoses

00059	Sexual dysfunction
00065	Ineffective sexuality pattern

Class 3. Reproduction. Any process by which new individuals (people) are produced

00221	Ineffective childbearing process
00208	Readiness for enhanced childbearing process
00227	Risk for ineffective childbearing process
00209	Risk for disturbed maternal–fetal dyad

Domain 9. Coping/Stress Tolerance

Contending with life events and life processes

Class 1. Posttrauma Responses. Reactions occurring after physical or psychological trauma

Approved Diagnoses

00141	Posttrauma syndrome
00145	Risk for posttrauma syndrome
00142	Rape-trauma syndrome
00114	Relocation stress syndrome
00149	Risk for relocation stress syndrome

Class 2. Coping Responses. The process of managing environmental stress

Approved Diagnoses

00199	Ineffective activity planning
00226	Risk for ineffective activity planning
00146	Anxiety
00073	Compromised family coping
00071	Defensive coping
00073	Disabled family coping
00069	Ineffective coping
00077	Ineffective community coping
00158	Readiness for enhanced coping [individual]
00076	Readiness for enhanced community coping
00075	Readiness for enhanced family coping
00147	Death anxiety
00072	Ineffective denial
00101	Adult failure to thrive
00148	Fear
00136	Grieving
00135	Complicated grieving

00172	Risk for complicated grieving
00187	Readiness for enhanced power
00125	Powerlessness
00152	Risk for powerlessness
00210	Impaired individual resilience
00212	Readiness for enhanced resilience
00211	Risk for compromised resilience
00137	Chronic sorrow
00177	Stress overload

Class 3. Neurobehavioral Stress. Behavioral responses reflecting nerve and brain function

Approved diagnoses

00115	Risk for disorganized infant behavior
00009	Autonomic dysreflexia
00010	Risk for autonomic dysreflexia
00116	Disorganized infant behavior
00117	Readiness for enhanced organized infant behavior
00049	Decreased intracranial adaptive capacity

Domain 10. Life Principles

Principles underlying conduct, thought, and behavior about acts, customs, or institutions viewed as being true or having intrinsic worth

Class 1. Values. The identification and ranking of preferred modes of conduct or end states

Approved Diagnoses

00185	Readiness for enhanced hope

Class 2. Beliefs. Opinions, expectations, or judgments about acts, customs, or institutions viewed as being true or having intrinsic worth

Approved Diagnoses

00185	Readiness for enhanced hope
00068	Readiness for enhanced spiritual well-being

Class 3. Value/Belief/Action Congruence. The correspondence or balance achieved between values, beliefs, and actions

Approved Diagnoses

00184	Readiness for enhanced decision making
00083	Decisional conflict [specify]
00175	Moral distress
00079	Noncompliance
00169	Impaired religiosity
00171	Readiness for enhanced religiosity
00170	Risk for impaired religiosity
00066	Spiritual distress
00067	Risk for spiritual distress

Domain 11. Safety/Protection

Freedom from danger, physical injury, or immune system damage; preservation from loss; and protection of safety and security

Class 1. Infection. Host responses following pathogenic invasion

Approved Diagnoses

00004	Risk for infection

Class 2. Physical Injury. Bodily harm or hurt

Approved Diagnoses

00031	Ineffective airway clearance
00039	Risk for aspiration
00206	Risk for bleeding
00048	Impaired dentition
00219	Risk for dry eye
00155	Risk for falls
00035	Risk for injury
00045	Impaired oral mucous membrane
00087	Risk for perioperative positioning injury
00086	Risk for peripheral neurovascular dysfunction
00205	Risk for shock
00046	Impaired skin integrity
00047	Risk for impaired skin integrity
00156	Risk for sudden infant death syndrome
00036	Risk for suffocation
00100	Delayed surgical recovery
00220	Risk for thermal injury
00044	Impaired tissue integrity
00038	Risk for trauma
00213	Risk for vascular trauma

Class 3. Violence. The exertion of excessive force or power so as to cause injury or abuse

Approved Diagnoses

00138	Risk for other-directed violence
00140	Risk for self-directed violence
00151	Self-mutilation
00139	Risk for self-mutilation
00150	Risk for suicide

Class 4. Environmental Hazards. Sources of danger in the surroundings

Approved Diagnoses

00181	Contamination
00180	Risk for contamination
00037	Risk for poisoning

Class 5. Defensive Processes. The processes by which the self protects itself from the nonself

Approved Diagnoses

00218	Risk for adverse reaction to iodinated contrast media
00217	Risk for allergy response
00041	Latex allergy response
00042	Risk for latex allergy response

Class 6. Thermoregulation. The physiologic process of regulating heat and energy within the body for the purposes of protecting the organism

Approved Diagnoses

00005	Risk for imbalanced body temperature
00006	Hypothermia
00007	Hyperthermia
00008	Ineffective thermoregulation

Domain 12. Comfort

Sense of mental, physical, or social well-being or ease

Class 1. Physical Comfort. Sense of well-being or ease and/or freedom from pain

Approved Diagnoses

00214	Impaired comfort
00183	Readiness for enhanced comfort
00134	Nausea
00132	Acute pain
00133	Chronic pain

Class 2. Environmental Comfort. Sense of well-being or ease in or with one's environment

Approved Diagnoses

00214	Impaired comfort
00183	Readiness for enhanced comfort

Class 3. Social Comfort. Sense of well-being or ease with one's social situations

Approved Diagnoses

00214	Impaired comfort
00053	Social isolation

Domain 13. Growth/Development

Age-appropriate increases in physical dimensions, organ systems, and/or progression through the developmental milestones

Class 1. Growth. Increases in physical dimensions or maturity of organ systems

Approved Diagnoses

00113	Risk for disproportionate growth
00111	Delayed growth and development

Class 2. Development. Attainment, lack of attainment, or loss of recognized milestones in life

Approved Diagnoses

00112	Risk for delayed development
00111	Delayed growth and development

APPENDIX C

Selected NANDA International Axis Descriptors

Axis 1. The Diagnostic Focus—This describes the "human response or experience" that is the core of the diagnosis. Examples are activity tolerance, airway clearance, anxiety, and pain.

Axis 2. Subject of the Diagnosis—This is defined as the person(s) for whom a nursing diagnosis is determined. The values in Axis 2 are:

Individual	A single human being distinct from others, a person
Family	Two or more people having continuous or sustained relationships, perceiving reciprocal obligations, sensing common meaning, and sharing certain obligations toward others; related by blood or choice
Group	A number of people with shared characteristics
Community	A group of people living in the same locale under the same governance. Examples include neighborhoods and cities

Axis 3. Judgment—A descriptor or modifier that limits or specifies the meaning of the diagnostic focus (or concept). The values in Axis 3 are:

Descriptor	***Definition***
Complicated	Intricately involved, complex
Compromised	Damaged, made vulnerable
Decreased	Lessened (in size, amount, or degree)
Defensive	Used or intended to defend or protect
Deficient	Insufficient, inadequate
Delayed	Late, slow, or postponed
Disabled	Limited, handicapped
Disorganized	Not properly arranged or controlled
Disproportionate	Too large or too small in comparison with norm
Disturbed	Agitated; interrupted, interfered with
Dysfunctional	Not operating normally
Effective	Producing the intended or desired effect
Enhanced	Improved in quality, value, or extent
Excess	Greater than necessary or desirable
Failure	Cessation of proper functioning or performance
Imbalanced	Out of proportion or balance
Impaired	Damaged, weakened
Ineffective	Not producing the intended or desired effect
Insufficient	Quantity or quality that is not able to fulfill a need or requirement
Interrupted	Having its continuity broken
Low	Below the norm
Organized	Properly arranged or controlled
Perceived	Observed through the senses
Readiness for	In a suitable state for an activity or situation
Situational	Related to a particular circumstance

Axis 4. Location—The parts/regions of the body and/or their related functions. The values in Axis 4 are:

Auditory	Neurovascular
Bladder	Olfactory
Body	Oral
Bowel	Peripheral
Breast	Peripheral neurovascular
Cardiac	Peripheral vascular
Cardiopulmonary	Renal
Cerebral	Skin
Gastrointestinal	Tactile
Gustatory	Tissue
Intracranial	Vascular
Kinesthetic	Verbal
Liver	Visual
Mucous membranes	Urinary

Axis 5. Age—Refers to the age of the person who is the subject of the diagnosis. The values in Axis 5 are:

Fetus	School-age child
Neonate	Adolescent
Infant	Adult
Toddler	Older adult
Preschool child	

Axis 6. Time —The duration of the diagnostic concept (Axis 1). The values in Axis 6 are:

Acute	Lasting less than 6 months
Chronic	Lasting more than 6 months
Intermittent	Stopping or starting again at intervals, periodic, cyclic
Continuous	Uninterrupted, going on without stop

Axis 7. Status of the Diagnosis—Refers to the actuality or potentiality of the problem or to its categorization as a wellness/health promotion diagnosis. The values in Axis 7 are:

Actual	Existing in fact or reality, existing at the present time
Health Promotion	Behavior motivated by the desire to increase well-being and actualize human health potential (Pender, Murdaugh, & Parsons, 2006, cited in *NANDA-I Nursing Diagnoses: Definitions & Classification 2007–2008*)
Risk	Vulnerability, especially as a result of exposure to factors that increase the chance of injury or loss
Syndrome	Clinical judgment describing a specific cluster of nursing diagnoses that occur together, and are best addressed together and through similar interventions

Note: From *NANDA International Nursing Diagnoses: Definitions and Classification 2012–2014* by NANDA International, 2012. Ames, IA: Wiley-Blackwell.

APPENDIX D

Multidisciplinary (Collaborative) Problems Associated With Diseases and Other Physiologic Disorders

Cancer

***Potential Complications of Cancer:** Anemia, bowel obstruction, cachexia, clotting disorders, electrolyte imbalance, pathologic fractures, hemorrhage, obstructive uropathy, metastasis to vital organs (e.g., brain, lungs), pericardial effusions, tamponade, sepsis→septic shock, spinal cord compression, superior vena cava syndrome, tissue anoxia→necrosis

Potential Complications of Antineoplastic Medications: Specify for each drug (e.g., anemia, bone marrow depression, cardiac toxicity, CNS toxicity, congestive heart failure, electrolyte imbalance, enteritis, leukopenia, necrosis at IV site, pneumonitis, renal failure, thrombocytopenia)

Potential Complications of Narcotic Medications: Depressed respirations, consciousness, and BP; cardiovascular collapse, biliary spasm

Potential Complications of Radiation Therapy: Increased intracranial pressure, myelosuppression, inflammation, fluid and electrolyte imbalances

Cardiac Function Disorders

Potential Complications of Angina/Coronary Artery Disease: Myocardial infarction

Potential Complications of Congestive Heart Failure: Ascites, severe cardiac decompensation, cardiogenic shock, deep-vein thrombosis, gastrointestinal congestion→malabsorption, hepatic failure, acute pulmonary edema, renal failure

Potential Complications of Digitalis Administration: Toxicity

Potential Complications of Dysrhythmias: Decreased cardiac output→decreased myocardial perfusion→heart failure, severe atrioventricular conduction blocks, thromboemboli formation→stroke, ventricular fibrillation

Potential Complications of Myocardial Infarction: Cardiogenic shock, dysrhythmia, infarct extension or expansion, myocardial rupture, pulmonary edema, pulmonary embolism, pericarditis, thromboembolism, ventricular aneurysm

*Also see specific disorders, such as Gastrointestinal Function Disorders, for effects of cancer on those patterns.

Potential Complications of Pericarditis/Endocarditis: Cardiac tamponade, congestive heart failure, emboli (pulmonary, cerebral, renal, splenic, cardiac), valvular stenosis

Potential Complications of Rheumatic Fever/Rheumatic Heart Disease: Congestive heart failure, decreased ventricular function, endocarditis, pericardial effusion, valvular changes

Endocrine Function Disorders

Potential Complications of Adrenal Gland Disorders

Potential Complications of Addison Disease: Addisonian crisis (shock, coma), diabetes mellitus, thyroid disease

Potential Complications of Cushing Disease: Congestive heart failure, hyperglycemia, hypertension, pancreatic tumors, potassium and sodium imbalance, psychosis

Potential Complications of Diabetes Mellitus: Coma, coronary artery disease, hypoglycemia, infections, ketoacidosis, nephropathy, peripheral vascular disease, retinopathy

Potential Complications of Parathyroid Gland Disorders

Potential Complications of Hyperparathyroidism: Hypercalcemia→ cardiac dysrhythmias, hypertension, metabolic acidosis, pathologic fractures, peptic ulcers, psychosis, renal calculi, renal failure

Potential Complications of Hypoparathyroidism: Hypocalcemia→ cardiac dysrhythmias, convulsions, malabsorption, psychosis, tetany

Potential Complications of Pituitary Gland Disorders

Potential Complications of Anterior Pituitary Disorders: Acromegaly, congestive heart failure, seizures

Potential Complications of Posterior Pituitary Disorders: Loss of consciousness, hypernatremia, seizures

Potential Complications of Thyroid Gland Disorders

Potential Complications of Hyperthyroidism: Exophthalmos, heart disease, negative nitrogen balance, thyroid crisis

Potential Complications of Hypothyroidism: Adrenal insufficiency, cardiovascular disorders, myxedema coma, psychosis

Gastrointestinal (GI) Function Disorders

Potential Complications of Esophageal Disorders:

Potential Complications of Esophageal Diverticula: Obstruction, pulmonary aspiration of regurgitated food

Potential Complications of Esophageal Surgery: Reflux esophagitis, stricture formation

Potential Complications of Hiatal Hernia: Incarceration, necrosis→hemorrhage

Potential Complications of Gallbladder, Liver, and Pancreatic Disorders

Potential Complications of Cirrhosis: Ascites, anemia, diabetes mellitus, disseminated intravascular coagulation (DIC), esophageal varices, GI bleeding or hemorrhage, hepatic encephalopathy, hyperbilirubinemia, hypokalemia, splenomegaly, peritonitis, renal failure

Potential Complications of Cholelithiasis and Cholecystitis: Fistula, gallbladder perforation, intestinal ileus or obstruction, obstruction of common bile duct→liver damage, pancreatitis, peritonitis

Potential Complications of Hepatic Abscess: Fluid and electrolyte imbalance, hyperbilirubinemia

Potential Complications of Metronidazole or Iodoquinol Administration: Bone marrow suppression

Potential Complications of Hepatitis: Cirrhosis, hepatic encephalopathy, hepatic necrosis

Potential Complications of Pancreatitis: Ascites, cardiac failure, coma, delirium tremens, diabetes mellitus, hemorrhage, hypovolemic shock, hypocalcemia, hyperglycemia or hypoglycemia, pancreatic abscess, pancreatic pseudocyst, pleural effusion or respiratory failure, psychosis, renal failure, tetany

Potential Complications of GI Infections

Potential Complications of Appendicitis: Abscess, gangrenous appendicitis, perforated appendix, peritonitis, pylephlebitis

Potential Complications of Bacterial or Viral Infections (e.g., Food Poisoning): Bowel perforation, dehydration, hemolytic uremic syndrome, hypokalemia, hypovolemic shock, metabolic acidosis, metabolic alkalosis, peritonitis, respiratory muscle paralysis, thrombotic thrombocytopenic purpura

Potential Complications of Helminthic Infections: Anemia; bowel, biliary, or pancreatic duct obstruction; migration to liver or lungs

Potential Complications of Peritonitis: Hypovolemic shock, septicemia, septic shock

Potential Complications of GI Inflammatory Diseases (e.g., Diverticulitis, Gastritis, Peptic Ulcer, Ulcerative Colitis): Abscess, anal fissure, anemia, colorectal carcinoma, fistula, fluid and electrolyte imbalances, GI bleeding or hemorrhage, intestinal obstruction, intestinal perforation, peritonitis, pyloric obstruction, toxic megacolon

Potential Complications of Gastrectomy, Pyloroplasty: Dumping syndrome

Potential Complications of Structural and Obstructive GI Disorders

Potential Complications of Hemorrhoids and Anorectal Lesions: Anemia, infection, thrombosed hemorrhoid, sepsis

Potential Complications of Hernias: Bowel infarction, bowel perforation, hernia incarceration and strangulation, peritonitis

Potential Complications of Intestinal Obstruction: Bowel wall necrosis, gangrene, fluid and electrolyte imbalance, hypovolemic or septic shock, intestinal perforation, peritonitis

Potential Complications of Malabsorption Syndromes: Anemia, bleeding, delayed maturity, lack of growth, muscle wasting, rickets (and other nutrient deficiencies), tetany

Hematologic Disorders

Potential Complications of Aplastic Anemia: Congestive heart failure, hemorrhage, infections

Potential Complications of Coagulation Disorders: Hemorrhage (specific effects are determined by site of bleeding, for example, increased intracranial pressure in the brain, adult respiratory distress syndrome in the cardiovascular system), joint deformity or disability

Potential Complications of Leukemias: Anemia, bleeding difficulties or internal hemorrhage, bone infarctions, coma, hepatomegaly, infections, renal failure, seizures, splenomegaly, tachycardia

Potential Complications of Nutritional Anemias: Impaired neurologic function (e.g., problems with proprioception), impaired cardiac function

Potential Complications of Iron Therapy: Hypersensitivity, toxicity (cardiovascular collapse, liver necrosis, metabolic acidosis)

Potential Complications of Cyanocobalamin Therapy: Hypersensitivity, hypokalemia, peripheral vascular thrombosis, pulmonary edema

Potential Complications of Polycythemia: Bone marrow fibrosis, GI bleeding and ulcers, splenomegaly, thrombosis (various organs)

Potential Complications of Sickle Cell Anemia: Multisystem organ failure (e.g., congestive heart failure, hyperuricemia, hepatomegaly, hepatic abscesses and fibrosis, hyperbilirubinemia, gallstones, bone marrow aplasia, osteomyelitis, aseptic bone necrosis, skin ulcers, vitreous hemorrhage, retinal detachment), sickle cell crisis

Potential Complications of Sickle Cell Crisis: Aplastic crisis, CVA, hemosiderosis (from repeated transfusions), infections (e.g., pneumonia), seizures, splenic sequestration→circulatory collapse

Immune Function Disorders

Potential Complications of Altered Immune Function: Allergic reactions→anaphylaxis, autoimmune disorders (e.g., systemic lupus erythematosus), delayed wound healing, infections (e.g., nosocomial, opportunistic), sepsis→septicemia, acute or chronic tissue inflammation (e.g., granulomas), transplant or graft rejection

Potential Complications of Autoimmune Deficiency Syndrome (AIDS): HIV wasting syndrome; malignancies (cervical cancer, Kaposi sarcoma, lymphomas); neurologic (dementia complex, meningitis); opportunistic infections (e.g., candidiasis, cytomegalovirus infection, herpes infection, *Mycobacterium avium* infection, *Pneumocystis carinii* pneumonia, toxoplasmosis, tuberculosis)

Immobilized Patient

Potential Complications of Immobility: Contractures, decreased cardiac output, decubitus ulcers, embolus, hypostatic pneumonia, joint ankylosis, orthostatic hypotension, osteoporosis, renal calculi, thrombophlebitis

Musculoskeletal Disorders and Trauma

Potential Complications of Amputation: Contracture, delayed healing, edema of the stump, infection

Potential Complications of Fractures: Compartment syndrome, deep-vein thrombosis, delayed union, fat embolism, infection, necrosis, reflex sympathetic dystrophy, shock

Potential Complications of Gout: Nephropathy, uric acid stones→renal failure

Potential Complications of Osteoarthritis: Contractures, herniated disk

Potential Complications of Osteomyelitis: Cutaneous sinus tract formation, necrosis, soft tissue abscesses

Potential Complications of Osteoporosis, Osteomalacia: Fractures, neuropathies, posttraumatic arthritis

Potential Complications of Paget Disease: Bone tumors, cardiovascular complications (e.g., arteriosclerosis, hypertension, congestive heart failure), degenerative osteoarthritis, dementia, fractures, renal calculi

Potential Complications of Rheumatoid Arthritis: Anemia, bony or fibrous ankylosis, carpal tunnel syndrome, contractures, episcleritis or scleritis of the eye, Felty syndrome, muscle atrophy, neuropathy, pericarditis, pleural disease, vasculitis

Potential Complications of Corticosteroid Intra-Articular Injections: Intra-articular infection, joint degeneration

Potential Complications of Corticosteroid Systemic Administration: Atherosclerosis, cataract formation, congestive heart failure, Cushing syndrome, delayed wound healing, depressed immune response, edema, growth retardation (children), hyperglycemia, hypertension, hypokalemia, muscle wasting, osteoporosis, peptic ulcers, psychotic reactions, renal failure, thrombophlebitis

Potential Complications of Nonsteroidal Anti-Inflammatory Medications: Gastric ulcers or bleeding, nephropathy

Neurological Disorders

Potential Complications of Organic Brain Diseases (e.g., Alzheimer Disease): Aspiration pneumonia, dehydration, delusions, depression, falls, malnutrition, paranoid reactions, pneumonia

Potential Complications of Brain Injury and Intracranial Hemorrhage: Brain ischemia, herniation, increased intracranial pressure

Potential Complications of Brain Tumor: Hyperthermia, increased intracranial pressure, paralysis, sensorimotor changes

Potential Complications of Cerebrovascular Accident (CVA): Behavioral changes, brain stem failure, cardiac dysrhythmias, coma, elimination disorders, increased intracranial pressure, language disorders, motor deficits, respiratory infection, seizures, sensory-perceptual deficits (*NOTE:* The manifestations and complications of a CVA vary according to the area of the brain affected. Also, it is difficult to determine which effects are manifestations and symptoms and which are actually complications. Furthermore, many of the complications of CVA are due to the resulting immobility rather than to the pathophysiology of the CVA itself. Refer to *Immobilized patient.*)

Potential Complications of Increased Intracranial Pressure (e.g., Cerebral Edema, Hydrocephalus): CNS ischemic response (increased mean arterial pressure, increased pulse pressure, and bradycardia), coma, failure of autoregulation of cerebral blood flow, hyperthermia resulting from impaired hypothalamic function, motor impairment (decorticate or decerebrate posturing)

Potential Complications of Intracranial Aneurysm: Hydrocephalus, hypothalamic dysfunction, rebleeding, seizures, vasospasm

Potential Complications of Meningitis and Encephalitis: Arthritis, brain infarction, coma, cranial nerve damage, hydrocephalus, increased intracranial pressure, seizures

Potential Complications of Multiple Sclerosis: Pneumonia, dementia, sudden progression of neurologic symptoms (convulsions, coma), urinary tract infection

Potential Complications of Myasthenia Gravis: Aspiration, cholinergic crisis, dehydration, myasthenic crisis, pneumonia

Potential Complications of Parkinson Disease: Depression and social isolation, falls, infections related to immobility (e.g., pneumonia), malnutrition related to dysphagia and immobility, oculogyric crisis, paranoia and hallucinations, pressure ulcers

Potential Complications of Seizure Disorder: Accidental trauma (e.g., burns, falls), aspiration, head injury, status epilepticus→acidosis, hyperthermia, hypoglycemia, hypoxia

Potential Complications of Spinal Cord Injury: Autonomic dysreflexia, cardiac dysrhythmias, complications due to immobility (see Immobilized Patient), hypercalcemia, necrosis of spinal cord tissue, paralytic ileus, respiratory infection secondary to decreased cough reflex, spinal shock

Peripheral Vascular and Lymphatic Disorders

Potential Complications of Aortic Aneurysm: Dissection, hemiplegia and lower extremity paralysis (with dissection), rupture→ hypovolemic shock

Potential Complications of Femoral and Popliteal Aneurysms: Embolism, gangrene, rupture, thrombosis

Potential Complications of Hypertension: Aortic dissection, CVA, congestive heart failure, hypertensive crisis, malignant hypertension, myocardial ischemia, papilledema, renal insufficiency, retinal damage

Potential Complications of Lymphedema: Cellulitis, lymphangitis

Potential Complications of Peripheral Arterial Disease: Arterial thrombosis, cellulitis, CVA, hypertension, ischemic ulcers, tissue necrosis→gangrene

Potential Complications of Thrombophlebitis: Chronic leg edema, pulmonary embolism, stasis ulcers

Potential Complications of Varicose Veins: Cellulitis, hemorrhage, vascular rupture, venous stasis ulcers

Respiratory Function Disorders

Potential Complications of Asthma: Atelectasis, cor pulmonale, dehydration, pneumothorax, respiratory infection, status asthmaticus

Potential Complications of Corticosteroid Therapy: Hypertension, hypokalemia, hypoglycemia, immunosuppression, osteoporosis, ulcers

Potential Complications of Methylxanthine Therapy: Toxicity (seizures, circulatory failure, respiratory arrest)

Potential Complications of Chronic Obstructive Pulmonary Disease (COPD): Hypoxemia, respiratory acidosis, respiratory failure, respiratory infection, right-sided heart failure, spontaneous pneumothorax

Potential Complications of Pneumonia: Bacteremia→endocarditis, meningitis, peritonitis; lung abscess and empyema; lung tissue necrosis; pleuritis

Potential Complications of Pulmonary Edema: Cerebral hypoxia, multisystem organ failure, right-sided heart failure

Potential Complications of Pulmonary Embolism: Pulmonary infarction with necrosis, right ventricular heart failure, sudden death

Potential Complications of Tuberculosis: Bacteremia→extrapulmonary tuberculosis (e.g., genitourinary tuberculosis, meningitis, peritonitis, pericarditis), bronchopleural fistula, empyema

Potential Complications of Medications for Tuberculosis: Hepatotoxicity, hypersensitivity, nephrotoxicity, peripheral neuropathy (isoniazid), optic neuritis (ethambutol)

Sexually Transmitted Disease

Potential Complications of Chlamydial Infections:

Females: Abortion, infertility, pelvic abscesses, pelvic inflammatory disease, postpartum endometritis, spontaneous abortion, stillbirth

Males: Epididymitis, prostatitis, urethritis

Neonates: Ophthalmia neonatorum, pneumonia

Potential Complications of Genital Herpes:

All: Herpes keratitis

Females: Cervical cancer

Males: Ascending myelitis, lymphatic suppuration, meningitis, neuralgia, urethral strictures

Neonates: Potentially fatal infections; infections of eyes, skin, mucous membranes, and CNS

Potential Complications of Genital Warts:

All: Urinary obstruction and bleeding

Females: Increased risk of cancer of the cervix, vagina, vulva, and anus; obstruction of the birth canal during labor; transmission to neonate

Neonates: Respiratory papillomatosis

Potential Complications of Gonorrhea:

All: Secondary infection of lesions; fistulas; chronic ulcers; sterility

Females: Abdominal adhesions, ectopic pregnancy, pelvic inflammatory disease

Males: Epididymitis, nephritis, prostatitis, urethritis

Neonates: Ophthalmia neonatorum

Potential Complications of Syphilis: Blindness, paralysis, heart failure, liver failure, mental illness

Shock

Potential Complications of Shock: Cerebral hypoxia→coma, multiple organ system failure, paralytic ileus, pulmonary emboli, renal failure

Skin Integrity Disorders

Potential Complications of Burns: Airway obstruction (inhalation injury), Curling ulcer, hypothermia, hypovolemic shock, hypervolemia, infection secondary to suppression of immune system, negative nitrogen balance, paralytic ileus, renal failure, sepsis, stress ulcers

Potential Complications of Skin Lesions/Dermatitis/Acne: Cyst formation, malignancy, infection

Potential Complications of Herpes Zoster: Dissemination→visceral lesions, encephalitis, loss of vision

Potential Complications of Pressure Ulcer: Necrotic damage to muscle, bone, tendons, joint capsule; infection, sepsis

Urinary Elimination Disorders

Potential Complications of Cystitis: Bladder ulceration, bladder wall necrosis, renal infection

Potential Complications of Polycystic Kidney Disease: Renal calculi, urinary tract infection, renal failure

Potential Complications of Pyelonephritis: Bacteremia, chronic pyelonephritis, renal insufficiency, renal failure

Potential Complications of Acute Renal Failure: Electrolyte imbalance, fluid overload, metabolic acidosis, pericarditis, platelet dysfunction, secondary infections

Potential Complications of Chronic Renal Failure: Anemia, cardiac tamponade, pericarditis, congestive heart failure, fluid and electrolyte imbalance, GI bleeding, hyperparathyroidism, infections, medication toxicity, metabolic acidosis, pleural effusion, pulmonary edema, uremia

Potential Complications of Urolithiasis: Hydronephrosis, hydroureter, infection, pyelonephritis, renal insufficiency

APPENDIX E

Multidisciplinary (Collaborative) Problems Associated With Tests and Treatments

Test or Treatment	***Potential Complications (Collaborative Problems)***
Arteriogram	Allergic reaction, embolism, hemorrhage; hematoma, paresthesia, renal failure, thrombosis at site
Bone marrow studies	Bleeding, infection
Bronchoscopy	Airway obstruction or bronchoconstriction, hemorrhage
Cardiac catheterization	Cardiac dysrhythmias, infarction, perforation, embolism, thrombus formation, hypervolemia, hypovolemia, paresthesia, site hemorrhage or hematoma
Casts and traction	Bleeding, edema, impaired circulation, misalignment of bones, neurologic compromise
Chest tubes	Bleeding →hemothorax, blockage or displacement → pneumothorax, septicemia
Foley catheter	Bladder distention (tube not patent), urinary tract infection
Hemodialysis	Air embolism, bleeding, dialysis dementia, electrolyte imbalance, embolism, fluid shifts, hepatitis B, infection or septicemia, shunt clotting; fistulas, transfusion reactions
Intravenous therapy	Fluid overload, infiltration, phlebitis
Medications	Allergic reactions, side effects (specify), toxic effects or overdose (specify)
Nasogastric suction	Electrolyte imbalance, gastric ulceration hemorrhage
Radiation therapy	Fistulas, tissue necrosis, hemorrhage, radiation burns, radiation pneumonia
Tracheal suctioning	Bleeding, hypoxia
Ventilation, assisted	Acid–base imbalance, airway obstruction (tube plugged or displaced), ineffective O_2–CO_2 exchange, pneumothorax, respirator dependence, tracheal necrosis

Adapted from *Nursing Process & Critical Thinking* (4th ed., p. 165) by J. Wilkinson, 2001, Upper Saddle River, NJ: Prentice Hall .

APPENDIX F

Multidisciplinary (Collaborative) Problems Associated With Surgical Treatments

Format for problem statement:
"Potential Complication of [*column 1*]: [*column 2*],"

Example: Potential Complication of general surgery: *Atelectasis, bronchospasm, and so forth.*

Column 1 **Type of Surgery "Potential Complication of"**	***Column 2*** **Potential Complications (Multidisciplinary Problems)**
General surgery (complications that can occur regardless of type of surgery)	Atelectasis, bronchospasm or laryngospasm on extubation (with general anesthesia), electrolyte imbalance, excessive bleeding→ shock, fluid imbalance, headache from leakage of cerebrospinal fluid (with regional anesthesia), hypotension (with regional anesthesia), ileus, infection, stasis pneumonia, urinary retention→ bladder distention, venous thrombosis→ pulmonary embolism, wound dehiscence→ evisceration

Instructions: Choose complications from *General surgery* above; then choose those that apply to patient's particular type of surgery. Potential complications of various types of surgery follow; these complications are in addition to those of General surgery.

Abdominal surgery	Dehiscence, fistula formation, paralytic ileus, peritonitis, renal failure, surgical trauma (e.g., to ureter, bladder, or rectum)
Breast surgery	Cellulitis, hematoma, lymphedema, seroma
Chest surgery: coronary artery bypass graft	Cardiovascular insufficiency, renal insufficiency, respiratory insufficiency
Chest surgery: thoracotomy	Adult respiratory distress syndrome, bronchopleural fistula, cardiac dysrhythmias, empyema of the chest cavity, hemothorax, infection at chest tube sites, mediastinal shift, myocardial infarction, pneumothorax, pulmonary edema, subcutaneous emphysema

Craniotomy	Cardiac dysrhythmias, cerebral or cerebellar dysfunction, cerebrospinal fluid leaks, cranial nerve impairment, gastrointestinal bleeding, hematomas, hydrocephalus, hygromas, hyperthermia or hypothermia, hypoxemia, increased intracranial pressure, meningitis or encephalitis, residual neurologic defects, seizures
Eye surgery	Endophthalmos, hyphema, increased intraocular pressure, lens implant dislocation, macular edema, retinal detachment, secondary glaucoma
Musculoskeletal surgeries	Bone necrosis, fat embolus, flexion contractures, hematoma, joint dislocation or displacement of prosthesis, nerve damage, sepsis, synovial herniation
Neck surgeries	Airway obstruction, aspiration, cerebral infarction, cranial nerve damage, fistula formation (e.g., between hypopharynx and skin), flap rejection (in radical neck dissection), hypertension or hypotension, hypoparathyroidism (in thyroidectomy or parathyroidectomy), local nerve damage (e.g., to the laryngeal nerve), respiratory distress, tetany (in thyroidectomy), thyroid storm, tracheal stenosis, vocal cord paralysis
Rectal surgery	Fistula formation, stricture formation
Skin grafts	Edema, flap necrosis, graft rejection, hematoma
Spinal surgery	Displacement of bone graft (in laminectomy or spinal fusion), bladder or bowel dysfunction, cerebrospinal fistula, hematoma, nerve root injury, paralytic ileus, sensorineural impairments, spinal cord edema or injury
Urologic surgery	Bladder neck constriction, bladder perforation (intraoperative), epididymitis, paralytic ileus, retrograde ejaculation (in prostate resection or prostatectomy), stomal necrosis, stenosis, obstruction (in urostomy or nephrostomy), urethral stricture, urinary tract infection
Vascular surgery: Aortic aneurysm resection	Congestive heart failure, myocardial infarction, renal failure, rupture of the suture line→ hemorrhage, spinal cord ischemia
Vascular surgery: Other	Cardiac dysrhythmia, compartmental syndrome, failure of anastomosis, lymphocele, occlusion of graft

CREDITS

Permission from NANDA International (2012). *NANDA Nursing Diagnoses: Definitions and Classification 2012–2014*. Ames, IA: Wiley-Blackwell.

Labels, definitions, and activities for 100 NIC labels reprinted from *Nursing Intervention Classification*, 5th ed., Bulechek, Butcher, and Docterman (2008) with permission from Elsevier Science.

Labels, definitions, and activities for 60 NOC labels reprinted from *Nursing Outcomes Classification*, 4th ed., Moorhead, Johnson, Maas, and Swanson (2008) with permission from Elsevier Science.

INDEX

A

E

G

H

J

K

T

3

Wilkinson, Judith.

Pearson Nursing Diagnosis Handbook.